Integrative Healthcare Remedies for Everyday Life

Malinee Thambyayah, FRCP

Pediatric Neurologist
Pantai Hospital
Kuala Lumpur
Malaysia

ELSEVIER

Elsevier
3251 Riverport Lane
St. Louis, Missouri 63043

Notices

Practitioners and researchers must always rely on their own experience and knowledge in evaluating and using any information, methods, compounds, or experiments described herein. Because of rapid advances in the medical sciences, in particular, independent verification of diagnoses and drug dosages should be made. To the fullest extent of the law, no responsibility is assumed by Elsevier, authors, editors, or contributors for any injury and/or damage to persons or property as a matter of products liability, negligence or otherwise, or from any use or operation of any methods, products, instructions, or ideas contained in the material herein.

Director, Content Development: Laurie Gower
Senior Content Strategist: Lauren Boyle
Content Development Specialist: Denise Roslonski
Publishing Services Manager: Deepthi Unni
Senior Project Manager: Umarani Natarajan
Design Direction: Bridget Hoette

Printed in India

Last digit is the print number 9 8 7 6 5 4 3 2 1

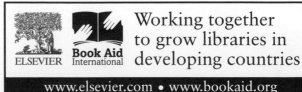

Foreword

In 2005, my colleagues and I produced for WHO the World Health Organization Global Atlas of Traditional, Complementary, and Alternative Medicine (TCAM), a two-volume public health atlas mapping the global trends in this sector. The most striking global trend was that the majority of the world's population was using some form of traditional or complementary medicine on a regular basis. And that, in most cases, was being paid for out of pocket. Something that is used regularly by the majority can't really be considered "alternative." And since then the terminology has changed. Now we are more likely to speak of Integrative Medicine, where both modern and complementary medicine combine in a holistic way to achieve safe and effective patient-centered care along with prevention of illness.

Asian healthcare traditions have globalized during this time. Chinese Medicine clinics are now found all over the world, offering herbal therapies, acupuncture, traditional forms of massage, and integrative exercise such as Tai Chi. At the same time, India's time-honored wellness pathways of yoga and meditation have become globally researched and applied as means for reducing stress and creating inner peace, while Ayurvedic medicine has taken its place on the world stage as a detox and integrative program for balanced living. Other traditions from Japan, Korea, Vietnam, Malaysia, and Indonesia, especially Bali, have emerged as features of wellness programs and destination resorts across Asia–Pacific and globally.

In her book *Integrative Healthcare Remedies for Everyday Life*, Dr. Malinee Thambyayah has combined her deep training as a pediatrician and child neurologist along with her lifelong experience, begun at her mother's knee, in the healthcare application of classical spices, foods, and herbal preparations from her family's Sri Lankan heritage. Dr. Malinee brings into focus simple ways to prevent and manage common health conditions. This is the kind of knowledge that generations of mothers across Asia have passed on for the homecare of their children based on the knowledge of how to live healthily simply. And now as a senior pediatrician, herself a mother of doctors, she puts this knowledge into clinical perspective guided by evidence, and offers a 21st century how-to or, as she describes it, "it is like a 'cookbook' for clinicians and parents interested in integrative medicine."

The Table of Contents is comprehensive and covers the following:

- Cardiovascular System
- Respiratory System
- Gastrointestinal System
- Renal System
- Endocrine and Metabolism
- Reproductive System
- Eyes
- Bones and Joints
- Skin, Hair, Nails, and Teeth
- Central Nervous System
- Mental Health
- Cancer
- Immune Boosters

This is a book built from a combination of generational heritage and a lifelong dedication to the highest standards of modern medicine. And it stems from a passionate and lifelong commitment to know more about how local health traditions of Asia and beyond can contribute to both home and clinical care, offering healthcare choices, early intervention, safety, and evidence-based pathways to integrative healthcare and well-being for families and individuals.

Integrative Healthcare Remedies for Everyday Life by Dr. Malinee Thambyayah will quickly become a standard household reference and will, in time, take its place as a classic in integrative healthcare practice in Asia and beyond.

Gerard Bodeker, PhD
Chair, Mental Wellness Initiative of the Global Wellness Institute & Department of Epidemiology
Columbia University
New York & Green Templeton College
University of Oxford

To dad and mum, *who brought us up on mostly natural medicine.*
To my children, *who also grew up on mostly natural remedies and some modern medicine.*
To my patients, family, and friends, *who also believe in natural medicine and urged me to write.*

About the Author

Dr. Malinee Thambyayah graduated from the All India Institute of Medical Sciences, New Delhi, in 1979, and did her pediatric neurology training under a British Council scholarship in the UK in 1988. She has been mentored by many well-known international neurologists. Of Sri Lankan Tamil roots, she was born and raised in Malaysia. She has worked 25 years in the national health system and then moved into private practice at two premier hospitals in Kuala Lumpur from 2004.

Her years of clinical excellence has earned her a reputation of diagnosing and treating difficult cases using Western diagnostics and healing with modern and complementary medicine. Her passion for natural medicine led her to earn a Siddha medicine qualification in 2014, and she embraces nutrition, naturotherapy, homoeopathy, Ayurveda, hyperbaric oxygen therapy, acupuncture, stem cells, and many other remedies to treat common and complex ailments.

Mission statement: *Many great views and ideas are really old and simple. Going back to basics and the roots are important. I am passionate about natural health, nutrition, and providing integrative pediatric medicine which integrates traditional, complementary, and alternative medicine and lifestyle with modern medicine. Start from young and lay the foundation for wellness and health.*

"The greatest medicine of all is to teach people how not to need it."

SUSHRUTA, INDIAN PHYSICIAN AND FATHER OF SURGERY (BORN AND DIED IN 600 BCE)

"The natural healing force within each one of us is the greatest force in getting well. Our food should be our medicine. Our medicine should be our food."

"Nature itself is the best physician."

"It is more important to know what sort of a person has a disease than to know what sort of disease a person has."

"A wise man ought to realise that health is his most valuable possession."

HIPPOCRATES, GREEK PHYSICIAN (460–377 BCE)

"The art of healing comes from nature and not from the physician. Therefore, the physician must start from nature with an open mind."

PARACELSUS, SWISS-GERMAN PHYSICIAN, CHEMIST, BOTANIST, ALCHEMIST ASTROLOGER, AND OCCULTIST (1493–1541)

"The art of medicine consists of amusing the patient while nature cures the disease."

"God gave us the gift of life. It is up to us to give ourselves the gift of living well."

"Doctors put drugs of which they know little into bodies of which they know less."

VOLTAIRE FRENCH, PHYSICIAN (1694–1778)

"Medicine is a collection of uncertain prescriptions, the results of which taken collectively, are more fatal than useful to mankind. Water, air, and cleanliness are the chief articles in my pharmacopeia."

NAPOLEON BONAPARTE, FRENCH STATESMAN (1769–1821)

"The doctor of the future will give no medicine but will interest his patients in the care of the human frame, in diet and in the cause and prevention of disease."

THOMAS EDISON, AMERICAN INVENTOR (1877–1930)

"The more you let Ayurveda and Yoga become the basis for your living, the easier living gets."

AYURVEDA

"Life (ayu) is the combination (samyoga) of body, senses, mind, and reincarnating soul."

"Ayurveda is the most sacred science, beneficial to humans in this world and the world beyond."

CHARAKA, INDIAN AYURVEDA PHYSICIAN (BORN AND DIED IN 300 BCE)

"The law of yin and yang is the natural order of the universe, the foundation of all things, mother of all changes, the root of life and death."

"A doctor who treats disease after it has happened is a mediocre doctor. A doctor who treats a disease before it happens is a superior doctor."

**CHINESE
THE YELLOW EMPEROR'S CLASSIC OF MEDICINE**

"There are no incurable diseases—only the lack of will. There are no worthless herbs—only the lack of knowledge."

AVICENNA, PERSIAN PHYSICIAN, ASTRONOMER, AND PHILOSOPHER (980–JUNE 1037)

Introduction on Integrative Medicine

Integrative medicine (IM) is a rapidly growing field and is highly credible. It combines modern mainstream medicine or treatments and the latest scientific advances together with the ancient healing systems (i.e., traditional, complementary, and alternative medicine [TCAM/CAM] or natural medicine).

According to the Stanford University School of Medicine website for the Pediatric Integrative Medicine Fellowship, IM can be defined as an approach to the practice of medicine that makes use of the best available evidence taking into account the whole person (body, mind, and spirit), including all aspects of lifestyle. IM is an emerging field that emphasizes the combination of both conventional and alternative approaches to address the biological, psychological, social, and spiritual aspects of health and illness. It emphasizes respect for the human capacity for healing, the importance of the relationship between the practitioner and the patient, a collaborative approach to patient care among practitioners, and the practice of conventional, complementary, and alternative healthcare that is evidence-based.

Treatment modalities included in this definition include but are not limited to: dietary supplements, botanicals, mind-body therapies, stress reduction, movement therapies, whole systems healing traditions such as Traditional Chinese Medicine (TCM) and Ayurveda, and diet counseling.

According to BMC Pediatrics 2012, the National Institutes of Health (NIH) defines complementary and alternative medicine (CAM) as a group of diverse medical and healthcare systems, practices, and products that are not generally considered part of conventional medicine. IM is defined as relationship-centered care that focuses on the whole person, is informed by evidence, and makes use of all appropriate therapeutic approaches, healthcare professionals, and disciplines to achieve optimal health and healing, and as such includes the best of evidence-based CAM therapies and evidence-based conventional therapies.

IM is similar to the biopsychosocial model of medicine in that it focuses on the whole person, but it also articulates a commitment to evidence-based practice using multiple therapeutic modalities including CAM therapies.

Rates of reported CAM usage among children vary between studies, but prevalence is notable across populations. Approximately 10% to 40% of healthy children and more than 50% of children with chronic, recurrent, or incurable conditions use CAM, most often in conjunction with conventional care. Although many families use CAM along with conventional care, only 20% to 65% discuss their CAM use with their physician; non-reporting usually occurs because they do not think it is relevant. Pediatric IM is emerging as a new subspecialty in the United States to better help address the 21st-century patient concerns.

According to many critics, complementary medicine (CM), CAM, integrative medicine or IM, and holistic medicine are among many rebrandings of the same phenomenon. Alternative therapies share in common that they reside outside medical science and rely on pseudoscience.

Mainstream of modern medicine is generally or definitely ideal for acute medical or surgical problems. It is standard and follows clinical practice guidelines in almost all countries. TCAM or natural medicine is better for chronic, longstanding medical problems. However, it varies from country to country. According to the World Health Organization (WHO), 80% of the world's population living in developing countries use herbal medicines as a primary treatment.

Nevertheless, some aspects of IM are evidence-based medicine and are truly holistic. It has the power to improve, transform, and heal one's physical, emotional, and spiritual health. In the WHO Global Report on Traditional and Complementary Medicine 2019, it states that "*more and more countries are recognizing the role of Traditional and Complementary Medicine in their national health systems amongst the 179 member countries. Countries aiming to integrate the best of Traditional and Complementary Medicine and conventional medicine would do well to look not only at the many differences between the two systems, but also at areas where both converge to help tackle the unique health challenges of the 21st century. In an ideal world, traditional medicine would be an option offered by a well-functioning, people-centered health system that balances curative services with preventive care. WHO is halfway through implementing the WHO Traditional Medicine Strategy 2014–2023.*"

As a practitioner of IM, it is my mission to share the knowledge and experience I have gained from my parents mostly and others too. I have tried to put together much information into a comprehensive guide. This compilation is a valuable resource book for you to also share with family and friends. It is a how-to guide combining kitchen or garden pharmacy with little or no modern drugs and various forms of safe TCAM practices to promote health and treat diseases. Caution needs to be exercised when combining certain foods with drugs as they can exacerbate certain symptoms. For example, taking vitamin K supplements for bone health or grapefruit juice together with anticoagulants can predispose to bleeding. It is important to inform your doctor if you are on natural medicines.

TCAM is generally not taught in medical schools. Hence, most doctors do not have a background in TCAM/CAM or feel comfortable to advise their patients.

TCAM may sound like folklore or based on testimonials and may not be backed up by robust clinical trials. Many TCAM studies also show a high level of bias. Often TCAM/CAM practitioners sound overenthusiastic about their treatments and even suggest stopping the mainstream/modern drugs. Even worse or unethical is when TCAM or herbal remedies are mixed with modern allopathic drugs (steroids, antiepileptic drugs, etc.) to achieve quick cures. Accurate assessment of risk-benefits of TCAM/CAM is difficult and also one must be very cautious about dangerous and unethical practices. However, many sage secrets or grandma's remedies have been backed up by scientific research now.

It is interesting to compare TCAM practices in each country, but this would be a colossal research project. Since Indian and Chinese civilizations are the longest, their ancient health systems, which are 4000 to 5000 years old, have been compared. Korean traditional medicine (Hanuihak) and Japanese traditional medicine (Kampo medicine) also share many Chinese practices. I am not an expert in these subjects and again you must refer to the masters or gurus in their fields. Western natural remedies also vary from country to country, but they have been grouped in this compilation. Aboriginal or tribal medicine also has rich roots in ethnobotany or phytomedicine, and I have no exposure to these TCAM sources, and these have not been compared.

For more details, readers are encouraged to refer to the original texts and references. For example, two medical treatises which are classical collections *(Samhita)* of ancient traditional Indian medicine on Ayurveda are called *Charaka Samhita* and *Sushruta Samhita*, which were written by the Ayurvedic scholars, Charaka (a physician) and Sushruta (a surgeon) around 300 BCE.

For more details on the comprehensive written work on TCM, reading of the treatise on *Yellow Emperor's Inner Classic* (*Huangdi Neijing* by Xuanyuan Huangdi) around 206 BCE to CE 25 and *Yellow Emperor's Classic of Internal Medicine* are recommended.

TCAM/CAM is here to stay. Many mainstream conventional doctors in the East also believe in the power of spiritual healing, and there is nothing wrong in seeking divine help. Our Eastern cultures and traditions are rich compared to the West, and it is impossible to subject the Eastern TCAM practices to rigorous clinical trials. Sometimes, a cure is achieved, and scientific explanations are not needed as to how this occurred. Many people are also not willing to pop pills these days.

Integrative medicine is like a happy marriage or relationship. Choose the right partner (or partners) in TCAM/TCM/CAM, and there will be a lifetime of happiness, health, and wealth.

It is important to establish the correct diagnosis at the onset of signs and symptoms. Diagnosis can be clinical, but laboratory tests are also necessary. Western diagnostic tests such as x-rays, blood or urine tests, etc. offer greater accuracy and must be encouraged.

Classification of Integrative Medicine

1. Traditional, Complementary, and Alternative Medicine (TCAM/CAM)
2. Modern/Mainstream Medicine

Classification of TCAM and Introduction

1. Herbal medicine/natural remedies/phytomedicine/phytobotanicals (Eastern and Western)
2. Traditional Indian medicine (Ayurveda, Siddha medicine, Unani)
3. Traditional Chinese medicine (acupuncture, acupressure, reflexology cupping, moxibustion, candling, tai chi, qigong, tuina)
4. Nutrition therapy/nutraceuticals/diet therapy
5. Energy medicine
   a. *Indian*: yoga, pranayama (breathing), Varmam/varma therapy, chakra healing, pranic healing, aura cleansing
   b. *Chinese*: acupuncture, cupping, moxibustion, candling, tai chi, qigong, tuina
   c. *Japanese*: reiki
   d. *Western/others*: theta healing and emotional freedom technique (EFT), thought field therapy (TFT), hypnosis, color therapy, quantum healing, crystal healing, magnet therapy, bio-resonance therapy, transcranial magnetic stimulation (TMS), transcranial direct current stimulation (tDCS), meditation, light therapy, spiritual healing, aura cleansing
6. Osteopathy, craniosacral therapy and chiropractic medicine, applied kinesiology (AK), Rolfing, Bowen therapy (Western CAM)
7. Massage therapy
8. Biofeedback
9. Homoeopathy (Western and Indian CAM)
10. Naturopathy
11. Others: hydrotherapy/aqua therapy, art therapy, pet therapy, aromatherapy, Bach flower therapy, ozone therapy, hyperbaric oxygen therapy (HBOT), stem cell therapy.

There is an overlap in the classification. For example, naturopathy can also include herbal medicine, nutritional therapy, use of nutraceuticals, osteopathy, or chiropractic medicine, etc. Massage therapy exists in both Eastern and Western practices.

Herbal Medicine/Plant Medicine/Phytomedicine/Natural Remedies: Eastern and Western

This will be discussed under each system (cardiovascular, respiratory, gastrointestinal, renal, endocrine and metabolism, reproductive, eyes, bones and joints, skin–hair–nails–teeth, central nervous system, mental health, and cancer). The mechanism of action and the health benefits of each herb or plant is described separately in the Glossary.

Medicinal plants contain several bioactive or phytochemical compounds, such as flavonoids, phenols, alkaloids, sterols, saponins, steroids, glycosides, tannins, terpenes (terpenoids and triterpenes), anthraquinones, hydrocarbons, and many others. These plant secondary metabolites have varying and specific or non-specific biological and pharmacological actions which include antioxidant, antimicrobial, anti-bacterial, anti-viral, anti-fungal, anti-parasitic, anti-helminthic, anti-inflammatory, analgesic, anti-allergy, antipyretic, anti-coagulant, anti-thrombotic, vasoactive, antidiabetic, anti-hypertensive, anti-hyperlipidemic, cardiotonic, expectorant, anti-catarrhal, carminative, antiemetic, laxative, anti-diarrheal, cholagogue, demulcent, astringent, hepatoprotective, diuretic, anti-lithogenic, wound healing, estrogenic or anti-estrogenic, aphrodisiac, neuroprotective, anti-convulsant, anti-aging, immune boosting, and anti-mutagenic (anticancer) effects in the human body.

Although plants or herbs are natural and generally regarded as safe (GRAS), it can be unsafe when used in prolonged or high doses or with some prescription items. It can also be unsafe during pregnancy or breast-feeding.

Traditional Indian Medicine

Ayurveda

Ayurveda means knowledge of life and longevity (*Ayur* = life/longevity, *veda* = knowledge).

Our body is made up of *five elements* (panchamahabhutas) and individual consciousness *(jivatman)*. These five elements are *earth* (the principle of inertia), *water* (the principle of cohesion), *fire* (the principle of radiance), *air/wind* (the principle of vibration), and *space/ether* (the principle of pervasiveness).

The combination of these elements gives rise to *three doshas*. Doshas are dynamic energy patterns that flow in our bodies to regulate our physical and mental well-being. A balance of the doshas results in health while an imbalance results in disease. There are three primary doshas: *vata, pitta, and kapha*. We are all born with all three of them but in unique and different proportions at various stages of life and which defines our temperament, physical, and mental characteristics. The doshas can change according to the food we eat, the seasons, and our thoughts and emotions. Under normal conditions, the ratio between vata, pitta, and kapha are 4:2:1, respectively. There is *prakruti* when the doshas are balanced and *vikruti* if there is a deviation from prakruti.

Doshas: Their Elements and Attributes

ELEMENTS OF THE THREE DOSHAS

Vata	Kapha	Pitta
Air + Ether	Earth + Water	Fire + Water

ATTRIBUTES OF THE THREE DOSHAS

Vata	Kapha	Pitta
Dry	Heavy	Oily
Light	Slow	Sharp (penetrating)
Cold	Cold	Hot
Rough	Oily	Light
Subtle	Slimy (smooth)	Mobile
Mobile	Dense	Liquid
Clear	Soft	Acidic
	Static (stable)	
	Cloudy (sticky)	

The *vata dosha type* (air + space) tends to be thin, fast-moving, and quick thinking. Vata locations are in the bones, joints, colon, skin, ears, brain, and the nerves. Vata disorders include arthritis, dry skin and hair, emphysema, pneumonia, flatulence, constipation, anxiety, nervousness, tics, twitches, and mental confusion and indecisiveness.

The *pitta dosha type* (fire + water) tends to have a fiery temperament with oily skin. Pitta locations are in the stomach, small intestine, liver, spleen, pancreas, eyes, blood, and sweat. Pitta disorders include gastritis, stomach ulcers, liver infections, and skin ailments (eczema, acne, skin inflammation).

The *kapha dosha type* (earth + water) tends to have a solid body frame with a calm personality. Kapha locations are in the throat, lungs, fat, tendons, and ligaments. Kapha disorders include cough, cold, flu (bronchitis, rhinitis, sinusitis), diabetes, obesity, and swellings.

General Characteristics of the Three Doshas

Characteristics	Vata	Kapha	Pitta
Location	Bones, joints, colon, skin, ears, brain, and nerves	Throat, lungs, fat, tendons, and ligaments	Stomach, small intestine, liver, spleen, pancreas, eyes, blood, and sweat
Somatotype (body structure)	Ectomorphic/thin	Endomorphic/broad	Mesomorphic/medium
Muscle	Poor growth	Well-developed	Moderate growth
Hair	Dry, brittle, and breaks easily	Strong, firm, and thick	Thin, oily, and premature graying
Skin	Dry and fissured	Smooth, clear, and firm	Soft, thin, and prone to acne and pigmentation (freckles, moles)
Memory	Fast to learn and grasp but poor retention	Slow to grasp but good retention	Moderate grasp and retention
Speech	Chatty and talkative	Less talk but speech is logical, organized, and methodical	Sharp, outspoken, and precise
Personality and emotions	Adventurous, energetic, flexible, and creative. Lively person and can take initiatives. Quick-tempered and quick to forgive	Affectionate, loving, strong, supportive, and shows excessive attachment. Also calm, patient, loyal, and thoughtful. Prefers routine	Practical, analytical, focused, ambitious, and intelligent
Movement	Fast/quick	Moderate	Slow/lethargic
Appetite	Frequent and irregular meals	Normal appetite with regular meals	High appetite for all foods and fluids with good digestion
Bowel habit	Irregular and variable bowels with constipation tendency and may have to strain. Stools are hard, dry, scanty, and pellet-like	Passes stools slowly and may feel incomplete. Stools are well-formed but sticky, slimy, or with mucus and difficult to clean	Frequent bowel movements, usually two to three times per day and passes stools quickly. Stools are hot, oily, semi-solid, or loose and tend to break apart
Weight gain	Difficulty to gain weight	Tendency to gain weight	Fluctuating weight
Metabolism of drugs and toxins	Moderate	Slow/poor	Fast/quick
Season preference	Cold intolerance	Tolerance to both cold and heat	Heat intolerance
Body immunity	Weak	Strong	Good
Related diseases	Arthritis, dry skin and hair, emphysema, pneumonia, flatulence, constipation, anxiety, nervousness, tics, twitches, and mental confusion, insomnia, and indecisiveness	Cough, cold, flu (bronchitis, rhinitis, sinusitis), diabetes, obesity, atherosclerosis, and swellings	Gastritis, stomach ulcers, liver infections, and skin ailments (eczema, acne, skin inflammation)
Ageing	Quick	Slow	Moderate

Sub-Doshas: There are five sub-doshas for each dosha with different locations and functions.

Vata Sub-Doshas

Prana Vata: Location—brain, head, heart, throat, and lungs—it governs the mind, perception through senses, and regulates breathing (heart–mind connection).

Udana Vata: Location—throat, lungs, and navel—it regulates speech, exhalation, vitality, strength, and enthusiasm.

Samana Vata: Location—stomach and small intestine—it governs peristalsis of the gut.

Vyana Vata: Location—heart—it controls heart rhythms, circulation, and movement.

Apana Vata: Location—pelvis from navel to anus—it controls all eliminations including urine, feces, menstrual blood, and semen.

Kapha Sub-Doshas

Kledaka Kapha: Location—upper stomach—it regulates the initial phase of digestion.

Avalambaka Kapha: Location—heart, chest, and lungs—it governs lubrication of the lungs and heart.

Bodhaka Kapha: Location—mouth, tongue, and throat—it governs taste and moistens food.

Tarpaka Kapha: Location—sinuses, head, and cerebrospinal fluid (CSF)—it regulates mood (happiness, stability, and calmness).

Shleshaka Kapha: Location—joints—it lubricates all the joints.

Pitta Sub-Doshas

Pachaka Pitta: Location—small intestine and stomach—it is the digestive fire. It regulates digestion and assimilation of food and separates waste and nutrients.

Ranjaka Pitta: Location—liver, gallbladder, and spleen—it is the fire for healthy blood and feces color. It controls the formation of red cells and imparts the color to blood and feces.

Sadhaka Pitta: Location—head and heart—it is the fire of the heart and mind. It governs memory, thought, intelligence, and contentment.

Alochaka Pitta: Location—eyes—it is the fire of sight and visual perception.

Bhrajaka Pitta: Location—skin—it is the fire for skin glow. It governs the pigmentation, complexion, and luster of skin.

Synchronization between sub-doshas maintains a disease-free state. For example, Pachaka Pitta, Samana Vata, and Kledaka Kapha work synchronously to ensure optimum digestion.

There are *seven basic tissues* (dhatu), which are plasma *(rasa)*, blood *(rakta)*, muscles *(māmsa)*, fat *(meda)*, bone *(asthi)*, marrow *(majja)*, and semen *(shukra)*. These seven tissues make up the structure of the body. *Shukra dhatu* means "pure and radiant" and refers to the female egg and male semen or the reproductive system. With aging, each dhatu will degenerate.

Malas are metabolic wastes that are eliminated or excreted regularly from the body. Urine, stool, and sweat are the main three *malas*.

Agni is the digestive fire for food digestion, metabolism, and assimilation so that there is overall good health. When *Agni* is weak, metabolic waste or *Ama* is generated. This *Ama* can penetrate in any of the seven *dhatus* causing disease.

In the Ayurveda concept, there are *20 gunas* (qualities or characteristics) which are considered to be inherent in all matters. These are arranged in 10 pairs: heavy/light, cold/hot, unctuous/dry, dull/sharp, stable/mobile, soft/hard, non-slimy/slimy, smooth/coarse, minute/gross, and viscous/liquid.

In Hindu philosophy, there are three main *gunas* which are *tamas* (dark, dull, and with inertia), *rajas* (active and moving), and *sattva* (harmonious and balanced). Each person possesses all three *gunas* in varying proportions.

It is believed eating Sattvic foods (most fresh fruits, vegetables, whole grains, nuts, and legumes are in this category) and cooked lightly with spices and ghee can give balance and harmony and increase the *Ojas* (vitality).

If anything exists in a state of incomplete transformation (example from improper or incomplete digestion), then *ama* exists (a Sanskrit word meaning *uncooked* or *undigested* toxic by-products). *Ama* formation and accumulation can lead to chronic disease. The *ama* must be lowered to obtain and remain in good health.

Ojas refers to the innate vitality and resides mainly in the heart. *Ojas* can be increased through proper diet, fasting, exercise, adequate sleep, stress reduction, and spirituality. A healthy and balanced kapha dosha promotes *Ojas* and prevents *Ojas* depletion.

Any vitiation (impairment or depletion) of the three doshas is called tridosha dushti. Any vitiation of agni or digestive fire is called agnimandya. Either of these vitiations can lead to *Ama* formation and *Ojas* depletion leading to chronic disease. A healthy *Agni* leads to healthy *Ojas*.

Based on the five senses, there are eight ways in which Ayurveda makes a diagnosis. They are *nadi* (pulse), *mootra* (urine), *mala* (stool), *jihva* (tongue), *shabda* (speech), *sparsha* (touch), *druk* (vision), and *aakruti* (appearance).

There are eight components of medicine according to Ayurveda. These are:
- *kāyachikitsā*: general medicine, medicine of the body
- *kaumāra-bhṛtya*: the treatment of children, pediatrics
- śalyatantra: surgical techniques and the removal of foreign objects
- *śhālākyatantra*: treatment of ailments affecting ears, eyes, nose, mouth, etc. ("ent")
- *bhūtavidyā*: appeasing of possessed spirits and the affected people whose minds are affected by such spirits
- agadatantra: toxicology
- *rasāyantantra*: revitalization and tonics for increasing longevity, intellect, and strength
- *vājīkaraṇatantra*: aphrodisiacs and therapies for increasing the quantity and quality of semen and sexual pleasure.

Treatment consists of two parts:

1. *Samshamana* or *Shamana* therapy or *Shamana Chikitsa*: This is a palliative and purification treatment to re-ignite the *agni* and balance the vitiated doshas through lifestyle changes (exercise, yoga, and meditation), diet (fasting once a week and mindful eating), and herbs (internal or external).

   Deepana or *dipana* herbs are taken just before or with meals to stimulate or kindle the *agni*. They are like appetizers. These include ginger, turmeric, coriander, cumin, fennel, cardamom, and pippali.

   Pachana herbs and spices are taken after meals to facilitate digestion of food and excretion of toxins. These include ginger, black pepper, cumin, coriander, cinnamon, chitrak, fennel, and trikatu.

2. *Samshodhana* or *Shodhana* therapy or *Shodhana Chikitsa*: This is a detoxification and cleansing treatment to prevent and treat disease via *Panchakarma* methods. The *Amas* (toxins or metabolic wastes) are expelled from the body.

   Panchakarma is a five-procedure therapy to balance the *doshas*, remove the *Ama* or toxins so as to purify the body and mind (detoxification and rejuvenation). These five procedures are:

   Vamana (Emesis): This is therapeutic vomiting. It is useful in kapha-related conditions like chronic asthma, sinusitis, diabetes, or lymphatic swelling.

   Virechana (Purgation): This is to remove blood toxins and cleanse the gastrointestinal system, kidneys, and sweat glands. Various oral purgatives such as triphala, castor oil, psyllium, senna, aloe vera, flaxseeds, dandelion root, bhumi amla, etc. are used.

   Basti (Enema): Medicated sesame oil and herbal enemas (*Niruha vasti and Anuvasana vasti*) are given to treat vata-related diseases (rheumatism, arthritis, slipped disc, constipation, bloating and gas, insomnia, etc.). Vata is present mainly in the colon and colon membrane is related to bone membrane.

   Nasya (Intranasal medications): There are five types of nasya:

   - *Cleansing (Virechana) nasya*: For kapha-related disorders, dry powder herbs (*brahmi, jatamansi, or vacha*) are sniffed into the nostrils.
   - *Nutritive (Bruhana) nasya*: For vata-related disorders, ghee-based herbs with *ashwagandha, shatavari*, etc. or medicated milk are instilled into the nose.
   - *Sedative (Shamana) nasya*: Based on the dosha type, medicated herbal oils, decoctions, or fresh herbal juices are given intranasally. Example: Brahmi ghee is used in pitta disorders.
   - *Navana nasya*: Specific fresh herbal juices are given into the nose. Example: *Vacha* (calamus) juice for vata diseases and *brahmi* juice for pitta disorders.
   - *Marsha nasya*: Few drops of coconut or sesame oil or ghee are rubbed into the nostrils with the finger and then sniffed daily to prevent nasal allergies or dryness.

   Rakta moshan (Blood detoxification): Blood is cleansed, purified, and toxins removed via venesection (bloodletting) especially for pitta disorders. Leeches can also be used (*Jalaukavacharana* or leech therapy/hirudotherapy).

   Pre-panchakarma (Purvakarma) procedures include *Snehana* (Oleation or oil massage) to lubricate and soften the whole body and *Swedana* (sweating via herbal steam bath) to eliminate the toxins. This is done usually for 3 days before *panchakarma*.

   Ayurvedic herbal formulations are available as:

   Kashayams/kashaya/kasayam/kwath. It is an herb-infused decoction/herbal brew/herbal tea used to treat common respiratory and gastrointestinal ailments.

   Lehyam/leham. It is a thick, jam-like, semi-solid, sweet and antioxidant-rich product made from polyherbs, honey, jaggery, ghee, and others with general tonic, immune- and energy-boosting, nervine, and aphrodisiac effects.

   Churnam/churna. It is a fine powder containing a mixture of dried herbs and/or minerals which have been pulverized and sieved. It is used to treat diabetes and liver and kidney disorders. Examples include ginger powder and trikatu.

   Arishtam. It is an alcohol-based tonic made by boiling herbs and then fermentation. It is used to treat intestinal disorders including piles, indigestion, and constipation.

   Ghrita. It is medicated ghee where fresh herbs or herbal decoctions are processed with ghee.

   Lepam. It is a topical herbal paste or cream applied on the affected skin to reduce inflammation.

   Bhasmam. It is a herbo-metal-mineral fine ash powder made from incineration of metals, minerals, and animal products (shells, horns, feathers) under very high temperatures and then calcined with various herbal extracts. It is regarded as nanomedicine to treat chronic diseases.

   Tailam/taila. It is medicated oil. Usually, sesame oil is used as the base oil and various herbs are added. It is used externally (as a massage) or internally (taken orally).

Chakras (means spinning wheel) are energy points that vibrate and channel the energy into the body and meridians. Meridian channels follow the same path that the autonomic nervous system does along the spine.

Chakra energy spins in a clockwise direction as it moves the energy of the body out into the field around us, and it spins counterclockwise to pull energy from our external world (and the people in it) into our body. It is the frequency state of the chakras that determines the direction our energy will flow as they either draw energy into our body or release it outward through the endocrine system and the nervous system.

Chakras are center points of energy, thoughts, feelings, and the physical body. It determines our experiences with emotions, desires or aversions, confidence or fear, and even physical symptoms.

There are seven chakras. Each chakra has a color. Visible light gives off electromagnetic waves, vibrating across the field through time and space. Red is a lower-frequency wave that looks like a slow roll. Purple is a high-frequency wave with sharp peaks and valleys. The chakra energies vibrate at their different frequencies and also have different colors.

Sahasrara: The *crown or thousand-petalled chakra* is located at the top of the head and is represented by violet. It is associated with the pineal gland, light sensitivity, sleep cycles, dreams, clarity, wisdom, and spirituality. It represents pure consciousness.

Ajna: The *command* or *third-eye chakra* is a meeting point between two important energy streams in the body. It is located between the eyebrows and under the frontal lobe of the brain. It corresponds to the colors violet, indigo, or deep blue. It relates to the pituitary gland, pineal gland and drives growth, development, and sleep. It is also related to decision-making, planning, orientation, self-esteem, clarity, wisdom, and intuition.

Vishuddha: The *throat/especially pure chakra* is represented by blue and is associated with the thyroid and metabolism. It relates to speech, hearing, and peaceful expression.

Anahata: The *heart/unstruck chakra* relates to green and pink colors. It is associated with the heart, lungs, and immune system. It relates to complex emotions, compassion, tenderness, unconditional love, equilibrium, rejection, and well-being. It emits tremendous electromagnetic energy.

Manipura: The *solar plexus/navel or jewel city chakra is* located between the navel and sternum and is represented by yellow. It is associated with the digestive system, pancreas, liver, and gallbladder. It relates to power, positivity (or fear, anxiety), developing opinions, and tendencies toward an introverted personality.

Svadhishthana: The *sacral (one's own base or pelvic)* chakra is located 2 or 3 inches below the navel. It is represented by orange and is associated with the reproductive organs, the genitourinary system, and the adrenal gland. It is associated with pleasure and is mind-body chakra.

Muladhara: The *root chakra or root support* is at the base of the spine in the coccygeal region and is represented by red. It contains natural urges relating to food, sleep, sex, and survival, fear, and avoidance. It is related to our grounding and connection with the Earth.

Each of the seven chakras is associated with one of the nine endocrine glands and a nerve plexus which correspond to specific functions.

The chakras represent the physical body and also parts of our consciousness.

Blocked energy in a chakra will trigger physical, mental, or emotional imbalances that will present with various symptoms such as anxiety, lethargy, or poor digestion. Yoga asanas can free energy and stimulate an imbalanced chakra.

Chakra	Root Muladhara	Spleen/Pelvic Svadhishthana	Plexus/Naval Manipura	Heart Anahata	Throat Vishuddha	3rd Eye/Brow Ajna	Crown Sahasrara
Location	Coccyx perineum	Lower abdomen	Solar plexus Stomach	Mid-chest	Throat	Forehead	Top of the head
Color	Red	Orange	Yellow	Green	Blue	Indigo	Violet
Psychological functions	Vitality	Emotions	Willpower	Love	Speech	Psychic abilities	Visionary
	Survival	Sensuality	Self-control	Peace, compassion, forgiveness, harmony	Expression	Intuition	Inspiration
	Support	Intimacy	Knowledge		Communication	Understanding	Awareness
	Stability	Procreation	Mind clarity			Self-realization	Wisdom
	Security	Movement	Awareness	Guilt	Creativity	Fearlessness	Mediation
	Grounding	Sociability	Curiosity	Relationships	Organization	Perception	High self
	Individuality	Freedom	Wit	Acceptance	Planning	Memory	Self-sacrificing
	Sexuality	Confidence	Humor	Renewal	Trust	Invention	
	Courage	Polarity	Laughter		Wisdom		Charisma
	Impulsiveness		Optimism		Caution		
Emotions	Passion	Emotions	Purpose	Balance	Expression	Imagination	Spirituality
		Desires	Sunshine	Love	Healing	Intuition	Bliss
Glands	Adrenals	Gonads	Pancreas	Thymus	Thyroid	Pituitary	Pineal
Associated body parts	Spine (chi, life force)	Ovaries	Stomach	Lung	Throat	Eyes	Cerebral
	Legs	Testes	Digestion	Heart thymus	Voice	Nose	Cortex
	Feet	Uterus	Liver	Gland	Mouth	Ears	Pituitary
	Bones	Kidney	Pancreas	Arms	Jaw	Sinuses	Hair growth
	Teeth	Urinary tract	Diaphragm	Hands	Parathyroid	Autonomic nervous system	
	Colon	Skin	Nervous system	Hypertension	Tongue		
	Prostate	Spleen	Metabolism	Muscles	Neck	Cerebellum	
	Bladder	Gallbladder	Small intestine		Shoulder	Pineal	
	Blood circulation	Recharges etheric body aura				Forebrain	
	Tailbone					Heals etheric body aura	

Chakra	Root Muladhara	Spleen/Pelvic Svadhishthana	Plexus/Naval Manipura	Heart Anahata	Throat Vishuddha	3rd Eye/Brow Ajna	Crown Sahasrara
Physical dysfunction	Anemia Fatigue Obesity Anus-rectum (hemorrhoids) Constipation Cold body Temperature Bladder infection Rebuild blood cells and hemoglobin Static Numbness Leukemia	Impotence Frigidity Ovaries and uterine problems Candida Eating disorders Drug use Depression Alcoholism Polarity Imbalance Gout allergies Asthma (oxygen deficiencies)	Ulcers Diabetes Hepatitis Hypoglycemia Blood sugar disorders Constipation Nervousness, timidity Addiction to stimulants Parasite and worms Toxicity Jaundice Poor memory	High blood pressure Passiveness Lethargy Asthma Immune system Breathing difficulties Pneumonia Emphysema Cell growth Muscle tension Heart problem Chest pain	Thyroid Flu Fever Blisters Infections—herpes Itching sores Tonsillitis Toothaches OCD Speech disorders Hyperactivity Melancholy Internal problem Swelling Hiccups PMS Mood swing	Blindness Vision Headaches Migraines Earaches Nightmare Sleep disorders Manic Depression Anxiety Schizophrenia Paranoia Equilibrium imbalances	Depression Alienation Neuralgia Confusion Senility Veins Blood vessels Lymphatic system Bacteria Warts Skin rashes Eczema

OCD, Obsessive compulsive disorder; *PMS,* premenstrual syndrome.

Siddha Medicine

Siddha means "established truth or perfection." Siddhars and Vaidyars are the teachers and practitioners of Siddha medicine in Tamil Nadu, South India. The principles of Siddha are similar to Ayurveda. It uses safe herbs and herbomineral (heavy metal) medicines for treatment together with lifestyle modifications and diet. (In Ayurveda, plant herbal medicines are used.)

Unani Medicine

Unani medicine (also called Unani tibb, Arabian medicine, or Islamic medicine) is a traditional healing system in the Indian subcontinent and Iran (previously called Persia).

Our bodies are made from four elements *(arkan arba)* (i.e., *nar* [fire], *maa* [water], *hawa* [air], and *arz* [earth]).

There are four humors *(akhlat* arba) (i.e., *dam* [blood], *balgham* [phlegm], *safra* [yellow bile], and *sauda* [black bile]). Based on age, there is more production of *safra* in young, *dam* in children, *sauda* in adults, and *balgham* in elderly persons.

These elements/humors are present in fluids and their balance leads to health. Each person has a unique mixture of these substances which determines the *mizaj* (temperament). Imbalance leads to illness due to failure of the *Quwwat-e-Mudabbira-e-Badan* or the body's ability to maintain its own balance and harmony.

Khilt is a liquid substance made up of *istehal awwal* (first metabolism) of food in the kabid (liver). The human body consists of four humors *(akhlat arba)*. *Khilt* is a liquid body which is enclosed in the vessels and cavity of the body to provide *badal ma tahallul* through conversion into *jauhar aza*. They provide nutrition to the *aza* which has the same *mizaj* as *akhlat*. Dam (blood) carries the *hararat gharizia* (inherent and intrinsic energy) from *qalb* (heart) to *aza* (organs). Harmony of *khilt* may be altered by specific *mizaj*, in different ages, seasons, residences, and different diets.

Abnormal humors may cause pathological changes in the tissues in the affected area to cause illness. A predominance of blood gives a sanguine temperament; a predominance of phlegm makes one phlegmatic. Yellow bile predominance makes one more bilious (or choleric) and black bile more melancholic.

Treatment follows a pattern (*Usool-e-ilaj*):
Izalae sabab (elimination of cause)
Tadeele akhlat (normalization of humors)
Tadeele aza (normalization of tissues/organs)

Treatment includes regimental therapy known as *Ilaj-Bil-Tadbeer*. These therapies include cupping, aromatherapy, bloodletting, bathing, exercise, and *dalak* (massaging the body). Medicines or surgery are also provided.

For more details, classical texts of Ayurveda like Sushrut Samhit should be referred to.

Traditional Chinese Medicine

In TCM, Qi (pronounced as Chi) is the universal life force or life energy. Qi is in a state of continuous flux. It changes and transforms endlessly from one aspect of Qi into another.

This Qi vibration alternates between Yin and Yang energies, producing all physical things.

Yin and Yang are continuously changing. They are opposite but are complementary and interdependent. It constantly adjusts, transforms endlessly one into the other and never separates. It is an eternal dance of becoming one. It is never created or destroyed. It merely changes in its manifestation.

Yin is derived from the earth and moves upward and includes manifestations of Qi that are relatively *material,* substantial, condensing, solid, heavy, descending, cold, moist, cooling, dark, passive, and quiescent. Yin is the female essence. It is negative, dark, black, feminine, and cooling. Yin helps to cool and moisten the body. The body will start to heat up if yin is deficient or out of balance. The main Yin organs are liver, spleen, heart, lungs, and kidneys. Blood is also Yin.

Yang includes aspects or manifestations of Qi that are *relatively immaterial,* amorphous, expanding, hollow, light, ascending, hot, dry, warming, bright, aggressive, and active. (It manifests as light, movement, heat, nerve impulses, thought, and emotion.) Yang is the male essence. Yang is positive, bright, masculine, white, and warming. The main Yang organs are stomach, small intestine, large intestine, gallbladder, urinary bladder, and the triple burner (this is a functional organ). Qi is also Yang.

Each Yin organ is paired with a Yang organ and this pair is associated with one of the five elements *(Refer to the Relationship table below).* For example, heart (Yin) and small intestine (Yang) are associated with the Fire element or phase. The five elements (or phases) of wood, fire, earth, metal, and water are connected with the five stages of life, i.e., birth, growth, development or maturation, death, and rebirth.

Everything that is Yin contains some element of Yang, and everything that is Yang contains some element of Yin. Nothing is pure Yin or pure Yang. All solid or material (Yin) substances will contain some vibratory energy (Yang). All kinetic or immaterial (Yang) substances will also contain some material component (Yin).

There are six types of Qi in nature that manifest in six different forms, i.e., wind, cold, heat, damp, dryness, and summer heat.

Good health is the result of a harmonious balance of Yin and Yang. Illness is said to be the consequence of an imbalance of Yin and Yang. Restoring balance helps with the body's immune system and resistance to pathogens, increase blood flow, and reduce pain.

There are *four types of basic Qi movements,* i.e., Ascending, Descending, Entering, and Exiting.

There are *four disharmonies of the Qi movement,* i.e., Qi Deficiency, Qi stagnation, Collapsed Qi, and Rebellious Qi.

Meridians are channels or energy highways that direct the flow of Qi through specific, closed pathways inside the body and not on the surface. Each side of the body is traversed by six meridians—three Yin and three Yang.

The 12 standard or principal meridians are divided into yin and yang groups.

The Yin meridians of the arm are lung, heart, and pericardium.

The Yang meridians of the arm are the large intestine, small intestine, and triple burner.

The Yin meridians of the leg are spleen, kidneys, and liver. The Yang meridians of the leg are stomach, bladder, and gallbladder.

Meridians are mapped throughout the body and exist in corresponding pairs. Each meridian has many acupuncture points along its path. There are 350 acupuncture points on the meridian system.

Some TCM Concepts

- *Zheng* means "pattern or syndrome." To make a diagnosis in TCM, TCM Zheng classification (eight principles of diagnosis) is combined with biomedical methods (four pillars of diagnosis).
- The eight principles of diagnosis are four pairs of opposites (i.e., two parameters in each pair). These four pairs are as follows: interior-exterior, heat-cold, excess-deficiency, and yin-yang.
  1. **Interior–Exterior**: Broadly, this refers to the location of the disease. Interior refers to the internal organs like brain, bone, and spine. Exterior refers to skin, joints, and muscles.

     The three common pathogens that can enter or invade the body from the exterior are Wind, Cold, and Heat.

     The common types of Exterior conditions are Wind Cold and Wind Heat invasions (rarely Wind Dryness). Painful Obstruction Syndrome occurs from blocked channels.

  2. **Heat–Cold**: Broadly, this refers to the temperature of the presenting symptom. For example, pallor and lethargy are due to cold. Hyperactivity or inflammation is related to heat. The different patterns are:

     Full heat pattern is due to excess Yang: The manifestations include constipation, dark scanty urine, red face, red eyes, red tongue with yellow coating, fever, thirst, and rapid full pulse.

     Empty heat is due to Yin deficiency: The manifestations include dry stools, dark scanty urine, dry mouth, dry throat, peeling tongue, feeling heat in the afternoon and in the soles, palms, and chest, night sweats, rapid floating pulse, and anxiety.

     Full cold is due to excess Yin: The manifestations include loose stools, copious clear urine, pale face, pale tongue with thick white coating, feeling cold with cold peripheries, preference for warm fluids, lack of thirst, abdominal pain worse with pressure, and full deep pulse.

     Empty cold is due to Yang deficiency: The manifestations include loose stools, copious clear urine, pale face, pale tongue with thin white coating, feeling cold with cold peripheries, lack of thirst, sweating, lethargy, and weak slow pulse.

  3. **Deficiency-Excess** (*also called Empty-Full*)
     - **Deficiency or Empty** is characterized by weak Qi and absence of a pathogenic factor.

There are four types of deficiency: Qi Deficiency (Empty Qi), Yang Deficiency (Empty Yang), Blood Deficiency (Empty Blood), and Yin Deficiency (Empty Yin).

Qi deficiency means low energy or weak Qi. This low energy can affect the whole body or specific organs and cause different symptoms. It is often associated with fatigue and chronic disease.

Types of Qi Deficiency include:

Spleen Qi deficiency: Manifestations include loss of appetite, acid reflux, gas or bloating, nausea, diarrhea, hemorrhoids, diabetes, eating disorders, varicose veins, difficulty waking in the morning, apathy, mental fatigue, and brain fog.

Kidney Qi deficiency: Manifestations include frequent urination, copious clear urine, incontinence, enuresis, spermatorrhea, miscarriage and infertility, cold limbs, hair loss, and asthma.

Lung Qi deficiency: This is a common pattern. Manifestations include shortness of breath with exertion, tendency to catch colds, recurrent mild cough, low-weak voice, daytime sweating, aversion to cold, pale tongue, and empty pulse.

Heart Qi deficiency: Manifestations include anxiety, palpitations, sweating, insomnia with restless sleep and nightmares, and mood changes.

Yang Deficiency. The manifestations include cold peripheries (including hands and feet) and facial pallor. There is also a dislike of the cold with preference for warm foods and drinks. The tongue is coated and there are tooth imprints on the tongue.

If Kidney Yang deficiency, there are cold limbs and cold and pain in the lumbar area.

Blood Deficiency. The digestion, assimilation, and transformation of food into blood occurs mostly in the Spleen. Blood is stored mainly in the Liver. The Blood carries the oxygen from the Lungs and the Heart pumps and circulates blood to all organs.

Blood deficiency occurs due to poor nutrition; mental stress and blood loss during menstruation, pregnancy, and childbirth; and internal or external bleeding.

Manifestations include gynecological problems (amenorrhea, scanty menses, miscarriage, and infertility) and general symptoms (pallor, cold peripheries, dry skin, hair loss, fatigue, anxiety, headache, insomnia, and poor wound healing).

There are three types of Blood Deficiency: Liver-Blood Deficiency, Heart-Blood Deficiency, Spleen-Blood Deficiency.

Yin deficiency. Dryness is the cardinal sign. Dry skin, dry hair, dry eyes, dry nails, cracks or red spots on the tongue with little or no tongue coating implies Yin deficiency or internal Heat imbalance or Empty Heat. Other common signs of Yin deficiency include dry stools, warmth in the periphery and chest, thirst in the afternoon, heat intolerance, night sweats, scanty periods, insomnia, hot flashes, nightmares, or vivid dreams.

These manifestations develop slowly over many years and are usually due to chronic stress from poor lifestyle (over-work, poor nutrition, and nourishment). The affected person cannot cool down, calm down, or develop harmony in the body.

There are many causes of Liver Yin deficiency especially in women (i.e., due to liver Blood deficiency from menorrhagia, childbirths, physical and emotional stress).

If a person has *Deficient Liver-Yin* with poor blood circulation to nourish the head, the manifestations include eye fatigue, dry eyes, eye floaters, blurring of vision, dizziness, and headache.

If the Liver-Yin is weak to nourish the tendons, there are stiff joints and weak knees.

If a person has *Deficient Kidney Yin* with poor nourishment to brain and ears, the manifestations include dizziness, tinnitus, deafness, and poor memory.

If deficient Kidney Yin with poor nourishment to the knees and lumbar regions, manifestations include weak knees and backache, constipation, spermatorrhea, and scanty dark urine, dry mouth, thirst, and night sweats.

In *Lung Yin Deficiency*, there is also dry unproductive cough with little sticky phlegm. It can be due to Lung Qi deficiency.

In *Stomach Yin Deficiency*, there is loss of hunger or appetite and epigastric discomfort. It is often due to bad eating habits like irregular or missing mealtimes.

In Yin-Deficiency-Heat (YDH) syndrome, when there has been prolonged Yin Deficiency, the Yang (warming) becomes excessive which then generates a lot of internal heat. In this YDH syndrome, there are symptoms of "Dryness" and "Heat."

To nourish and build Yin, it is important to eat whole and dark foods, healthy fats, and good quality protein, especially seafood and take the right herbal remedies. Avoid sugar, strong spices, alcohol, and caffeine. Lifestyle change is required.

- **Excess or Full** is characterized by intact Qi and the presence of a pathogenic factor.

  Manifestations include acute disease, scanty urine, constipation, red face, profuse sweating, restlessness, agitation, irritability, loud strong voice, strong breathing, pain aggravated by pressure, tinnitus, and full pulse type.

  4. **Yin–Yang**: Each Yin organ is paired with a Yang organ.

To assess the signs and symptoms and make a diagnosis, one parameter from each pair is used. The syndrome differentiation is made according to the above eight parameters, i.e., interior-exterior, heat-cold, excess-deficiency, and Yin–Yang.

Broadly and generally speaking, Yin symptoms tend to be interior, deficient, and cold and Yang symptoms tend to be exterior, excessive, and hot.

Blood stagnation or Blood stasis: This means that blood is not circulating or flowing properly to a focal area (in a fracture, bruise, or sprain) or it can be generalized poor circulation (with multisystem manifestations). Common manifestations of Blood Stasis include dark circles under the eyes, bruises, menstrual problems (irregular or painful periods or with blood clots), limb stiffness, or focal stabbing pain in the chest or abdomen which is aggravated with pressure.

Qi deficiency is the most common cause of Blood stasis.

Qi stagnation: This occurs when Qi stagnates or is blocked due to mainly emotional disturbances. Manifestations include physical symptoms (loss of appetite, abdominal pain, hiccups, lump in the throat, irregular or painful menses with premenstrual syndrome signs) or mental symptoms (labile moods, depression, or anger bouts). *Qi stagnation*: This can manifest as anxiety, depression, irritability, insomnia, sighing tendency, and being sentimental.

Types of Qi stagnation include:

Spleen Qi stagnation: The signs and symptoms include loss of appetite, nausea, acid reflux, abdominal distension, and pain.

Liver Qi stagnation: The signs and symptoms include low mood, irritability, right abdominal pain, and premenstrual or menstrual discomforts.

Lung Qi stagnation: The signs and symptoms include cough, shortness of breath, chest discomfort or pain, breathlessness or panting.

• **Phlegm-Dampness***:* Dampness is accumulation of too much moisture or water in the body due to impaired digestion. Phlegm is produced when the spleen is weak or challenged by a poor diet. Spleen is the main organ in the digestive system. The dampness will move to the lungs and cause cough and phlegm. The dampness will also move to the large intestines and cause loose stools with mucus and abdominal discomfort.

Characteristic features of Dampness include being heavy, sticky, going downward, lingering, delayed, recurring, and is difficult to eliminate. Specific characteristics depend on the affected organ (if skin, stomach, eyes, joints, etc.).

There are two types of Dampness:

Internal dampness is more common and combines heat or cold to cause damp-heat or damp-cold. Manifestations include edema, bloating, water retention, distended abdomen, weight gain, eczema, and sluggishness.

External dampness is due to humid conditions and manifests as joint pains and heaviness.

There is higher risk of hypercholesterolemia, allergies, chronic fatigue, and cancer.

Avoid dairy, cold, or greasy foods to prevent phlegm-dampness. Sauna, moxibustion, cupping, and acupuncture can also remove dampness.

Fire

Fire is an element which represents heat and summer. It is red in color and is associated with joy, love, passion, hate, and anger. It manifests in the heart and small intestine.

Manifestations of Deficient Fire include poor circulation, chills, poor digestion, hyposexuality, and emotional detachment. Excess Fire manifestations include hyperactivity, insomnia, and high libido. Other manifestations of Fire Imbalance include heart palpitations, excessive laughing, extreme love-hate emotions, and dependency on others.

Fire–Heat

Full Heat is caused by Excess of Yang, Qi stagnation which can lead to Heart Heat or Liver Heat. Consumption of heat-generating foods or spices and from Exterior conditions also contribute to Heat.

Common Full Heat symptoms include feeling of heat, red face, thirst, anxiety, dry stools, scanty-dark urine, tachycardia with full pulse, and a red tongue with yellow coating.

Types of Heat include:

Lung-Heat. Symptoms include feeling of heat, shortness of breath, cough, and mild-chest discomfort.

Heart-Heat. Symptoms include palpitations, insomnia, and agitation.

Stomach-Heat. Symptoms include nausea, vomiting, acid reflux, hunger pangs, and bad breath.

Liver-Heat. There are more mental symptoms with agitation, anger, dizziness, headache, and insomnia.

Spleen-Heat. Symptoms are similar to Stomach heat.

Damp Heat. Damp-Heat produces Phlegm and Phlegm-Heat. The Heat in Damp-Heat also becomes Phlegm. Characteristic features of Damp-Heat include nausea, vomiting, abdominal distension, sticky taste, loss of appetite, thirst but no desire to drink, loose foul stools, scant dark or turbid urine, difficulty passing urine, oily skin, eczema, sense of warmth, low-grade fever, night sweats, body aches, and lethargy.

Specific characteristics depend on the affected organ (stomach, spleen, small intestine, etc.).

Wind

Wind is a Yang excess and refers to movement. Manifestations of Wind include sudden fever, headache, sweating, nose block, sore throat, itching, and allergies. Wind diseases start and end suddenly and usually occur in the upper body. Examples include stroke, seizures, sinusitis, sore throat, skin rash, and eruptions.

External Wind is due to infectious pathogens or external factors which if untreated can stir Internal Wind and lodge in the deeper tissues.

There are different associations of Wind, i.e., Wind-Cold, Wind-Heat, Wind-Dryness, Wind-Humidity, and Wind-Phlegm which produce complex disease patterns and symptoms.

There are different types of Wind described. For example, Wind stirring, Great Feathery Wind, Scheming Wind, Breaking Wind, Ferocious Wind, Ominous Wind, Unpromising Wind, etc.

There are many wind-dispelling and wind-settling herbs and also specific wind acupuncture points to treat Wind disorder.

In summary, the common TCM syndrome types are: Blood Deficiency, Blood Stasis, Phlegm-Dampness, Fire-Heat, Qi Deficiency, Qi Stagnation, Yin Deficiency with and without Internal Heat, and Yang Deficiency.

The five elements consist of fire, earth, wood, water, and metal. It describes the interactions and relationships between things and correlates with different aspects of the natural world and the body.

Wood correlates with spring and wind in the natural world and to the eyes, liver, gallbladder, and tendons in the body.

Fire correlates with summer and heat in the natural world and to the heart, blood, and small intestines.

Earth correlates with late summer and dampness in the natural world, and to the mouth, stomach, muscles, and spleen.

Metal correlates with autumn and dryness in the natural world and to the nose, lungs, large intestines, and skin.

Water correlates with winter and cold in the natural world and to the kidney, bladder, bone, and ears.

Emotions also affect the organs:
- Love–heart
- Grief–lungs
- Anger–gallbladder and liver
- Fear–kidneys.

Example of someone who gets angry:
- Anger affects the liver.
- Liver gets hot.
- It leads to eye problems and stomach issues.

Someone living in grief:
- Grief injures the lungs.
- Grieve for a specific time.
- If it drags on too long, you will get sick.
- Do not be too sad or too happy.

Keep a happy balance in all things.

Relationship Between Five Elements, Nature, and the Body

	Wood	Fire	Earth	Metal	Water
Orientation	east	south	middle	west	north
Season	spring	summer	late summer	autumn	winter
Climate	wind	summer heat	dampness	dryness	cold
Cultivation	germinate	grow	transform	reap	store
Yin organ	liver	heart	spleen	lung	kidney
Yang organ	gallbladder	small intestine	stomach	large intestine	bladder
Orifice	eye	tongue	mouth	nose	ear
Tissues	tendon	vessels	muscles	skin and hair	bones
Emotion	anger	joy	pensiveness	grief	fear
Color	blue/green	red	yellow	white	black
Taste	sour	bitter	sweet	pungent	salty
Voice	shout	laugh	sing	cry	groan

Principles of Traditional Chinese Medicine

- TCM diagnosis embraces the four pillars. These are:
  - *Look.* This refers to inspection of tongue, face, skin color, movements, mental state, etc. Different parts of the tongue represent different organs. Tongue tip is heart, tongue center is spleen, and tongue back is intestines and kidneys.
  - *Listen, Smell, and Taste. Listen* refers to the Voice characteristics, i.e., shout, laugh, sing, weep, or groan. *Smell* refers to odor of breath, feces, or urine. *Taste* of urine is no longer done.
  - Each of the Voice characteristics correlates with one of the five elements. For example, Shout is Wood, Laugh is Fire, Sing is Earth, Weep is Metal, and Groan is Water. (Read more under Relationship Table below).
  - *Touch.* This involves Pulse analysis, Acupuncture points, presence of swellings, tenderness, etc.
  - *Ask.* This involves history taking about urine, stools, sweat, menses, taste, smell, sleep, etc.
- The term *Zheng* means "pattern, symptom, or syndrome." To make a diagnosis in TCM, TCM Zheng classification is combined with biomedical methods.

Treatment is symptom-based. Same, similar, or common symptoms can occur in different diseases. If there is stabbing pain in stable angina, dysmenorrhea, or stomachache, it can be treated with the same remedy.

However, if the stabbing pain in the angina is due to Blood stasis syndrome or Qi stagnation, then the remedy is different for each syndrome.

- TCM healing embraces *four pillars of holistic treatment* methods. These are:
  - Chinese herbs and diet
  - Acupuncture or acupressure
  - Exercise and movements (qigong or tai chi)
  - Massage and manipulation (tuina, cupping, and moxibustion)
  - They are used alone or in combination.
- Most Chinese herbal teas and brews are not often taken on their own. They are usually composed of many herbs and brewed together as an herbal decoction.
- They are best discussed with a reliable local sensei (trained TCM doctor) or grandma or any elderly person well versed in TCM.

Specially tailored recipes and dosages are often prescribed by the sensei and the patient's condition closely monitored (personalized medicine). These remedies are taken as directed, as different treatment methods vary depending on the type of energy deficiency causing the disease. Two persons may suffer from the same disease, but the treatment can be different for each person.

TCM herbal remedies are often available as commercial polyherbal preparations, or as pure herbs dried, ground powder, or as capsules.

- TCM remedies are often used as an adjunct to allopathic treatment and should be carefully monitored. If taking other allopathic medications, the medical professional should be informed about the concurrent TCM to ensure there are no negative interactions between the modern allopathic medications and the TCM.
- Infants, children below 12 years of age, and the elderly should take herbs only as directed by a sensei.

Most of these herbs should be used cautiously in children. An accurate diagnosis, treatment plan, and correct dosage information are important.

The author is not an expert in TCM treatments, and the appropriate TCM practitioners should be consulted for further information and clarification.

Nutritional Therapy

Nutritional therapy is an approach that is individualized and personalized to one's dietary needs and lifestyle. The goal is to maximize one's health in a holistic manner. Specific diets, meal plans, and recipes are recommended.

It can be used to benefit people with digestive issues, cardiovascular problems, hormonal imbalances, skin problems, autoimmune disorders, and mental health issues.

A detailed medical history, diet history, and lifestyle history are taken. Often natural, whole, and unprocessed foods are recommended. The nutritional therapist also advises nutritional supplements such as vitamins, minerals, and probiotics.

Nutraceutical is a substance that is considered a food or part of food which provides medical or health benefits to prevent disease. They are also called functional foods or medical foods. It is used by about 50% to 70% of the population in developed countries.

Diet therapy refers to the practical application of nutrition as a preventative or corrective treatment of disease. The existing diet and lifestyle are modified to promote optimum health. In some cases, a food elimination diet is necessary for overall well-being.

Energy Medicine

Indian Energy Medicine

Yoga

Yoga is a body–mind way of life with a 5000-year history of Indian philosophy. It combines physical postures, breathing techniques, and meditation or relaxation. It is a spiritual energy and uses breathing methods and mental focus. Now, it is a popular physical exercise based upon poses and postures that promote fitness, wellness, and mind–body control. One should choose a yoga type that is appropriate for one's fitness level.

Benefits of Yoga
- Improves mental focus.
- Reduces stress and improves mental well-being.
- Improves physical fitness and well-being (i.e., breathing, strength, flexibility).

Medical Evidence
- Decrease in stress hormone/cortisol.
- Increase in endorphins, enkephalins, and serotonin (feel-good neurotransmitters).
- Increase in alpha and theta waves in the brain.

Risks and Side Effects
Yoga is generally low impact and safe. Pregnancy and medical conditions such as high blood pressure, glaucoma, or sciatica are not absolute contraindications but certain poses or postures must be avoided or altered.

Serious injury due to yoga is not common. Beginners should avoid extreme poses (asanas) and difficult techniques such as headstand, lotus position, and forceful breathing.

Yoga is a good add-on therapy to the ongoing mainstream modern medicine.

The classification and terminology of yoga is rather complex and attempts are made to simplify based on different concepts and criteria.

The Eight Limbs of Yoga
Yama: Attitude toward our environment
Niyama: Attitude toward our self
Asana: Physical postures
Pranayama: Control of breathing (restraint or expansion)
Pratyahara: Withdrawal of the senses
Dharana: Concentration
Dhyana: Meditation
Samadhi: Complete integration

The Six Branches of Yoga
Raja yoga: This branch involves meditation. Its focus is to quiet the mind. It strictly adheres to the disciplinary steps known as the *eight limbs* of yoga (listed above).
Hatha yoga: This is the physical and mental branch to strengthen the body and mind.
Karma yoga: This is a path of service to others and to God. It aims to remove negativity and selfishness with focus on "be intent on action, not on the fruits of action."
Bhakti yoga: This is the path of devotion, a positive way to channel emotions and cultivate acceptance and tolerance. Devotional singing is a popular practice.
Jnana yoga: This branch of yoga is the yoga of knowledge. It is the wisdom and the path of the scholar to develop intellect through study.
Tantra yoga: This is the path of rituals, ceremonies, or consummation of a relationship.

The Styles and Types of Yoga
Hatha yoga: It refers to the generic term for any type of yoga that teaches physical postures. Asanas are the many physical postures in Hatha yoga. Hatha is a gentle introduction to the basic yoga postures.

Ashtanga yoga: This type of yoga applies six established sequences of postures that rapidly link every movement to breathing.

Iyengar yoga: This type focuses on finding the correct alignment in each pose using a range of props such as blocks, blankets, straps, chairs, and bolsters.

Bikram yoga: Bikram is done in artificially heated rooms at temperatures of nearly 105 degrees and 40% humidity. It consists of 26 poses and a sequence of two breathing exercises. It is also called *hot* yoga.

Jivamukti yoga: Jivamukti means liberation while living. It incorporates spiritual teachings and practices that focus on the fast-paced flow between poses rather than the poses themselves. This focus is called vinyasa. There is a theme in each class. This is explored through yoga scripture, chanting, meditation, asanas, pranayama, and music. Jivamukti yoga can be physically intense.

Kripalu yoga: Here practitioners learn to know, accept, and learn from the body. The practitioner or student finds his/her own level of practice by being introspective and looking inward. The classes usually begin with breathing exercises and gentle stretches, followed by a series of individual poses and final relaxation.

Kundalini yoga: Kundalini means coiled like a snake. Kundalini yoga is a system of meditation that aims to release pent-up energy. It begins with chanting and ends with singing. In between, it features asana, pranayama, and meditation customized to create a specific outcome.

Sudarshan kriya yoga (SKY): This is a guided meditation using breathing techniques. It is a purification process and uses the mind to control the breath. It improves mental and physical well-being. It is also recommended in stress, anxiety, and severe depression.

It involves initial slow-paced breathing (at 2 to 4 breaths/min and involves *Ujjayi breath*), then medium-paced and finally fast-paced breathing (at 30 breaths/min and involves *Bhastrika breath or Bellows breath*). This is done over 45 minutes and can be done at any time of the day but not after a meal.

Power yoga: This is a more active and athletic type of modern yoga based on the traditional ashtanga system.

Sivananda yoga: This system is a five-point philosophy which embraces proper breathing, relaxation, diet, exercise, and positive thinking together to form a healthy yogic lifestyle. Typically, it uses the same 12 basic asanas starting with sun salutations and ending with savasana (*corpse*) poses.

Viniyoga: Viniyoga can adjust and adapt to any person irrespective of physical ability. It requires in-depth training, and the Viniyoga teachers are experts on anatomy and yoga therapy.

Yin yoga: This is a quiet, meditative yoga practice. It is also called Taoist yoga. Yin yoga allows the release of tension in key joints, including the ankles, knees, hips, whole back, neck, and shoulders. Yin poses are passive, meaning that gravity shoulders most of the force and effort.

Pre/Peri/Post-natal yoga: Yoga uses postures in pregnancy, maintains health during pregnancy, and also helps in getting back into shape after pregnancy.

Restorative yoga: This is a restorative and relaxing method of yoga. Four or five simple poses with props like blankets and bolsters are used to get into deep relaxation without exerting any effort in holding the pose.

Yoga uses *asanas* (postures or poses), focused concentration on specific body parts, and *pranayama* (breathing techniques) to integrate the body, mind, and soul.

Yoga asanas (postures or poses) help condition the body. There are thousands of yoga poses, and these poses include *kriyas* (cleansing actions), *mudras* (seals), and *bandhas* (locks). A kriya focuses on the effort to move energy up and down the spine, yoga mudra is a gesture or movement to hold energy or concentrate awareness, and a bandha uses the technique of holding muscular contractions to focus awareness.

Pranayama

Pranayama is part of the eight limbs of yoga and is more of a spiritual practice. It has a set of exercises involving breath control. Pranayama is control of breath (*prana* means life force/breath and *ayama* to restrain or control the prana) via a set of breathing techniques.

The Eight Types of Pranayama

1. *Ujjayi Pranayama:* You have to inhale through your nostrils while making a sound from your throat. Hold the breath for a while and exhale from the left nostril. This is beneficial for thyroid problems and throat related issues.

2. *Bhramari Pranayama:* You have to close your ear with your thumb and eyes with the help of your fingers. Take a deep breath and while exhaling you have to chant, "Om" and try to focus on it while mumbling. This pranayama increases the concentration level in students and is beneficial for improving the memory.

3. *Suryabhedi Pranayama:* You have to inhale from the right nostril, hold the breath for a while and exhale from the left nostril. Maintain the breathing time ratio of 1:2:2 in the beginning. This can be increased later. This is beneficial in winters and maintains the heat in the body.

4. *Bhastrika Pranayama (Bellows Breath):* You have to inhale and exhale at a fast rate continuously, and after a few rounds, you have to hold your breath in the end. This is also beneficial in winters when your body needs to maintain the temperature.

5. *Sheetali Pranayama:* You have to roll your tongue and inhale through your mouth. Hold your breath and apply jalandhara bandha (chin lock position). After some time, exhale through your nostrils. This is beneficial for summers and reduces body temperature.

6. *Sheetkari Pranayama:* You have to inhale through your mouth with the sound of sheetkari which can be produced when you keep your tongue behind your teeth and inhale. Apply jalandhara bandha and hold your

breath. After a while, exhale from your nostrils. This is also beneficial in summers.

7. *Moorchha Pranayama:* You have to keep on exhaling again and again without inhaling. This will increase the concentration of carbon dioxide in your body, and after a while, you will be unconscious. Your body will regain your consciousness by automatically inhaling while you are asleep.

8. *Plavini Pranayama:* This pranayama is done in water. You have to work with your breath so that your body starts floating on the water surface. The moorchha and plavini pranayama are not meant for everybody and should be done by Siddha yogis only because they need a fair amount of practice.

The Five Types of Prana

Our life force, prana, divides itself into five vayus, each governing different functions.

Vayu	Area of Body	Function
Prana	Chest, head	Controls intake, inspiration, propulsion, forward momentum
Apana	Pelvis	Governs elimination, downward and outward movement
Samana	Navel	Governs assimilation, discernment, inner absorption, consolidation
Udana	Throat	Governs growth, speech, expression, ascension, upward movement
Vyana	Whole body	Controls whole circulation, expansiveness, pervasiveness

The Four Stages of Pranayama

1. *Arambha avastha*—this is the first stage which the practitioner enters when he has performed Nadi-shuddhi (purification of channels of energy in the body).

2. *Ghata avastha*—this is the second stage. This is achieved when the practitioner has learned to hold and stop his breath for long periods of time. By this time the yogi gains special powers including but not limited to levitation.

3. *Parichaya avastha*—this is the third and an advanced stage of spirituality.

4. *Nishpatti avastha*—the fourth stage where the practitioner reaches a state of perfect bliss. Now, he can do kevala kumbhaka where he can now go on for months without food and breathing.

The Four Stages of Breathing

1. Inhalation or puraka/*purak* (to inhale)
2. A pause or kumbhaka/*kumbhak* (to hold the breath)
3. Exhalation or rechaka/*rechak* (to exhale)
4. A *pause* before the cycle begins once again.

Four Kinds of Breathing

1. *High breathing* uses the upper part of the lungs with limited powers of absorbing oxygen.

2. *Low breathing* utilizes the lower part of the lungs and generally enables the breather with a rich supply of oxygen.

3. *Mid breathing* falls somewhere between these two.

4. *Complete breathing* is the deepest possible breath utilizing the lung capacity to its fullest.

Process of Breathing

1. *Inhalation:* During inhalation, air which contains 21% oxygen enters the lungs (from the nose to the alveoli). Oxygen then diffuses into the arterial blood and binds with hemoglobin. This oxyhemoglobin is transported to all organs in the body to ensure optimum functioning.

2. *Exhalation:* The venous blood then carries back the used deoxygenated blood containing carbon dioxide from the organs back to the lungs which then release the carbon dioxide via exhalation.

Patterns of Breathing

There are many kinds of breathing and a person goes through all these stages.

In *fast breathing or panting*, inhalation and exhalation alternate rapidly without the two pauses.

During *sleep*, there is automatic slow breathing where all these four stages are lengthened.

Varma Therapy

Varma Kalai is a traditional Tamil therapy in Siddha medicine. *Varmam* means body's pressure points and *Kalai* means knowledge. Specific varma points are stimulated using the fingers usually. There are 8000 varma points in the body, but only 108 varma points are used. These points are the reservoirs of subtle pranic energy which flow in the body through dasa nadis. When the flow of pranic energy is affected by injury, stress, abnormal physical activity, or eating habits, illness results. Manipulation of the correct varma points improves the flow of pranic energy resulting in the restoration of physiological and metabolic function of the organs. Varma points can be stimulated in 12 ways in which mathirai kanakku (depth) and pathi kanakku (pressure) are very important.

Varma therapy is targeted at the nerves, veins, tendons, soft tissues or ligaments, organs, and bone joints and is used commonly in several musculoskeletal conditions such as osteoarthritis of the knees, frozen shoulder, lumbar and cervical spondylosis with disc bulges, writer's cramp, foot drop, sciatica, etc. It is also used in autism management.

An example is illustrated for knee osteoarthritis.

Varma Points for the Treatment of Osteoarthritis (taken from Sivaranjani. *European Journal of Pharmaceutical and Medical Research*).

Varma Points	Location	Function
Kannady Kalam	Middle of upper 1/3 of nasal bridge	Strengthen the joint
Mootu Varmam	Middle of the popliteal fossa	Relieves knee pain
Veera Adangal	In the semitendinosus tendon	Relieves knee pain
Kudhirai Muga Varmam	Over the patellar tendon	Reduces pain
Chippi Munai Varmam	Medial border of the scapular region	Gives energy to the joint and enhances synovial fluid secretion
Adappa Kalam	Lateral wall of thorax	Gives energy to lower limbs
Vilangu Varmam	Depression below the middle of the clavicle	Gives mobility to the joint
Komberi Kalam	Middle of the leg along the medial border of tibia	Enhances energy to walk
Viruthi Kalam	At the level of distal end of first metatarsal bone	Strengthens leg and foot

Chakra Healing

The chakras can be open or closed, overactive or underactive, depending on the energy flow.

In a hurt relationship, one feels it in the heart. If we are anxious and nervous, our limbs tremble and the bladder becomes weak. If there is stress or tension in the consciousness, the chakra associated with that part of consciousness is detected by the nerve plexus associated with that chakra and communicated to the parts of the physical and energy body controlled by that plexus. Refer to the table below.

The opening and closing of our chakras work in unison. A negative experience with associated low-frequency energy will close the chakra so that the energy is blocked out. Any emotions that sit at the root chakra may result in a chakra energy constriction.

Chakra healing allows to open chakras and allow energy freely without obstruction.

Balance is essential in chakra healing. Even if one chakra is affected (closed or underactive), another chakra will be overactive. Hence, all seven chakras must be healed, balanced, open, and humming to allow energy to flow into and out of the body.

HOW YOU MAY FEEL OR ACT WHEN CHAKRAS ARE OVERACTIVE OR UNDERACTIVE

THE CHAKRAS AND ASSOCIATED GLANDS, ORGANS, AND SYMPTOMS

SIGNS AND SYMPTOMS

Chakra	Overactive	Underactive	Associated Endocrine Glands and Organs	Physical Symptoms of Unbalance
Root Sacral	Fearful, nervous, insecure, or ungrounded; materialistic or greedy; resistant to change	Lacking a sense of being at home or secure anywhere, co-dependent, unable to get into one's body, fearful of abandonment	Adrenal glands, spine, blood, and reproductive organs	Inability to sit still, restlessness, unhealthy weight (either obesity or eating disorder), constipation, cramps, fatigue or sluggishness
Sacral Chakra	Overemotional, very quick to attach and invest in others, attracted to drama, moody, lacking personal boundaries	Stiff, unemotional, closed off to others, lacking self-esteem or self-worth, possibly in an abusive relationship	Kidneys and reproductive organs: ovaries, testes, and uterus	Lower-back pain or stiffness, urinary issues, kidney pain or infection, infertility, impotence
Navel (Solar Plexus) Chakra	Domineering, aggressive, angry, perfectionistic, or overly critical of oneself or others	Passive, indecisive, timid, lacking self-control	Central nervous system, digestive system (stomach and intestines), liver, pancreas, metabolic system	Ulcers, gas, nausea, or other digestive problems, eating disorders, asthma or other respiratory ailments, nerve pain or fibromyalgia, infection in the liver or kidneys; other organ problems
Heart Chakra	Loving in a clingy, suffocating way; lacking a sense of self in a relationship; willing to say yes to everything; lacking boundaries, letting everyone in	Cold, distant, lonely, unable or unwilling to open up to others, full of grudge	Thymus gland and immune system, heart, lungs, breasts, arms, hands	Heart and circulatory problems (high blood pressure, heart palpitations, heart attack), poor circulation or numbness, asthma or other respiratory ailments, breast cancer, stiff joints, or joint problems in the hands

HOW YOU MAY FEEL OR ACT WHEN CHAKRAS ARE OVERACTIVE OR UNDERACTIVE — SIGNS AND SYMPTOMS

THE CHAKRAS AND ASSOCIATED GLANDS, ORGANS, AND SYMPTOMS

Chakra	Overactive	Underactive	Associated Endocrine Glands and Organs	Physical Symptoms of Unbalance
Throat Chakra	Overly talkative, unable to listen, highly critical, verbally abusive, condescending	Introverted, shy, having difficulty speaking the truth, unable to express needs	Thyroid, neck, throat, shoulders, ears, and mouth	Stiffness or soreness in the neck or shoulders, sore throat, hoarseness or laryngitis, earaches or infection, dental issues or TMJ, thyroid issues
Third-Eye Chakra	Out of touch with reality, lacking good judgment, unable to focus, prone to hallucinations	Rigid in thinking, closed off to new ideas, too reliant on authority, disconnected or distrustful of inner voice, anxious, clinging to the past and fearful of the future	Pituitary, eyes, brow, base of skull, biorhythms	Vision problems, headaches or migraines, insomnia or sleep disorders, seizures, nightmares (though this isn't a physical symptom per se, it is a common occurrence)
Crown Chakra	Addicted to spirituality, heedless of bodily needs, having difficulty controlling emotions	Not very open to spirituality, unable to set or maintain goals, lacking direction	Pituitary, pineal gland, brain, hypothalamus, cerebral cortex, central nervous system	Dizziness, confusion, mental fog, neurological disorders, nerve pain, schizophrenia or other mental disorders

TMJ, Temporomandibular joint.

Pranic Healing

The physical body can heal itself and by adding a catalyst, i.e., prana, this can accelerate the healing process. A pranic healer uses his hands to cleanse and energize a person's energy field and chakras with fresh prana to trigger the healing process. It is a no-touch technique.

Aura Cleansing

When there is stress or fatigue, there is an accumulation of positive ions around our energy field or in the home. This will then create more negative thoughts and emotions.

To recharge the body with more negative ions, salt or herbs can be used. This can be done by placing bowls with natural salt (sea salt or Himalayan salt) in the corners of a room or near the bed. This helps to remove negative energy and cleanse the home. Soaking in a salt bath (above salt or using Epsom salt) also helps to improve overall well-being. Salt also has purifying, disinfecting, and antibacterial properties.

Burning frankincense is common in many cultures. This is a plant aromatic resin from the Boswellia tree. Pieces of it are placed on a metal or ceramic vessel and then burned. The aroma from the smoke is cleansing, calming, and can reduce anxiety.

Sound Bath

This is a form of healing music where a particular soothing music or tune is played, usually from a percussion or wind instrument after a meditation session. These vibrations help to reduce stress, anxiety, depression, and insomnia. The Tibetan singing bowls meditation music is an example of healing sounds.

Chinese Energy Medicine

Acupuncture

The original traditional Chinese acupuncture involves inserting very thin needles at specific points on the skin at various depths. The qi flows through the meridians which can be tapped via 350 acupuncture points in the body.

Each acupoint relates to a specific organ in the body and hence can provide relief from certain symptoms. Acupuncture points are locations where nerves, muscles, and connective tissue are stimulated to increase blood flow. This then triggers the release of the body's natural painkillers (endorphins). Needles are inserted into these points with the right combinations and usually left for 15 to 30 minutes to restore the Qi energy flow balance. The benefits include pain relief and improved mood, energy, and body function. Acupuncture should never be attempted at home.

There are various sites, forms, and ethnic variations of acupuncture.

Body acupuncture. Needles are inserted at specific acupoints on the body to treat specific disorders.

Auricular (Ear) acupuncture. The ear represents all the different organs of the body. Needles or electrical currents are used to stimulate specific points. It is useful in pain and addiction management and infertility.

Scalp acupuncture. Needles are inserted on the scalp areolar layer. If inserted on the motor area, it is very helpful in stroke motor recovery. It is also useful in early-onset autism.

Tongue acupuncture. Needles are inserted on the tongue and it is useful in post-stroke dysphagia to improve swallow function.

Hand acupuncture & acupressure. The hand has many nerve endings and has a large cortical (brain) representation. The entire organs are mapped on each hand. Korean hand therapy includes hand acupuncture, hand acupressure, and hand reflexology.

Foot reflexology & Foot acupressure. The foot represents several reflex points which correspond to all the organs in the body. These reflex points are pressed or massaged by thumb-finger or a reflexology stick to target specific nerve points in foot reflexology. They are different from acupoints. Foot acupressure uses acupoints. Foot massage is non-specific and provides relaxation to a sore foot.

Needle acupuncture. Disposable fine stainless-steel needles are used to stimulate the acupuncture points.

- In *Japanese acupuncture,* fewer and shallower needles are used compared to Chinese acupuncture.
- In *Korean acupuncture,* more needles and usually copper needles are used.

Electroacupuncture. Minute electric currents are used to stimulate the needles at the body acupuncture points.

Laser acupuncture. Low energy laser beams stimulate the acupuncture points.

Acu-magnets. Magnets are taped over the acupuncture points. Auricular therapy using magnetic pearls can improve the quality and quantity of sleep among the elderly.

Herbal acupuncture. Purified herbal extract from a distilled herbal decoction is placed at the tip of the acupuncture needle which is then inserted at an acupoint.

Bee venom acupuncture. It is widely used in Korea. Diluted bee venom is placed at the tip of the acupuncture needle and this needle is inserted at the skin acupoint. It can treat musculoskeletal and neurological disorders such as osteoarthritis, rheumatoid arthritis, lumbar disc disease, lateral epicondylitis, adhesive capsulitis, stroke, and peripheral neuropathy.

Acupressure. Instead of needles, finger-thumb pressure is applied on the acupuncture points along the meridians. Needle acupuncture is more potent than acupressure. Acupressure is helpful in migraine headaches and morning sickness.

- *Zen shiatsu.* This is a Japanese form of hand acupuncture without needles.
- *Korean hand acupressure.* This is described above.

Teishin acupuncture. In this needle-free acupuncture, "blunt pressure needles" are tapped on the skin without skin penetration to stimulate the acupuncture points to relieve pain.

Approved indications by the WHO in 2003 (based on the effectiveness of acupuncture from evidence-based medicine) include the following conditions: headaches/migraine, stroke risk reduction, lower-back pain, neck pain, knee pain, osteoarthritis, high and low blood pressure, inducing labor, chemotherapy-induced nausea and vomiting, peptic ulcer, painful periods, dysentery, allergic rhinitis, facial pain, morning sickness, dental pain, rheumatoid arthritis, sciatica, sprains, and tennis elbow.

Approved indications by WHO (based on partial benefits) include the following conditions: tobacco and alcohol dependence, fibromyalgia, neuralgia, postoperative convalescence, spine pain, stiff neck, vascular dementia, whooping cough, Tourette syndrome, several infections including some urinary infections, and epidemic hemorrhagic fever.

Obstetric acupuncture can be used to treat various conditions during pregnancy and childbirth such as **morning sickness, lower-back and pelvic pain**, heartburn, swelling in the legs, constipation, carpal tunnel syndrome, sciatica, depression, headaches, sleep problems, breech correction, induction of labor, etc.

Acupuncture points such as LI4, BL32, and BL60 are used to treat back pain and heartburn in pregnancy between 12 and 36 gestational weeks.

Cupping

This involves placing cups on the skin or over main acupressure points to create suction to facilitate the flow of qi and blood and balance yin and yang or the negative and positive within the body.

There are two types of cupping:
- **Dry cupping** involves suction only.
- **Wet cupping** involves both suction and controlled medicinal bleeding.

Rounded ball-like glass cups which are open on one end are heated with fire using alcohol, herbs, or paper that are placed directly into the cup. Few heated cups are placed with the open side directly on the patient's skin for about five to ten minutes. This hot air inside the cup cools and creates a vacuum that draws the skin and muscle upward into the cup. The skin usually turns red.

In wet cupping, the cups are placed for a few minutes before they are removed, and small incisions are made to draw blood (bloodletting).

After the cups are removed, the cupped areas are covered with ointment and bandages to prevent infection. Bruises or other marks will resolve spontaneously after 7 to 10 days.

Cupping can be combined with acupuncture.

It is effective to treat muscle aches and pains, cervical spondylosis, and lumbar disc herniation. It may also help in digestive issues, cough, facial paralysis, etc.

Cupping is contraindicated in the elderly (mainly due to their fragile skin), children under four years, and in pregnancy or menstruation.

Adverse events may include light-headedness, dizziness, sweating, or nausea. Local events include transient circular marks, bruising, pain, infection, or skin scars.

Moxibustion

This involves burning moxa sticks which are placed on acupuncture points and certain locations of the body. The moxa sticks or cones are made from the dried leaves of the artemisia plant (mugwort).

It is believed to treat and prevent diseases and maintain health to help strengthen the organs and immune system. It warms the meridians and expels cold. It can be used to promote circulation over areas of chronic pain or muscle tension.

In pregnancy, women burn the moxa sticks close to their toes for about 15 to 20 minutes from anywhere to 1 to 10 times per day for up to 2 weeks. This treatment is usually started between 28 and 37 weeks of pregnancy specially to turn a breech baby. However, caution must be exercised.

Side effects of mugwort include allergies, sneezing and sinus-related symptoms, contact dermatitis, or rashes.

Candling

Ear candling is used to remove unwanted ear wax, impurities, and toxins from the ear for better physical and mental health. The person lies down in the lateral position with one ear facing up. A special cone-shaped wax candle with the pointed end is then placed inside the ear. The outer, wider candle end is lighted up.

The United States Food and Drug Administration (FDA) warns against the practice due to side effects including burns (from the dripping wax), perforated eardrums, ear canal blockages, and even hearing loss.

Tai Chi

Tai chi is a very effective exercise for the health of mind and body. There are many styles and forms of tai chi, the major ones being *Chen, Yang, Wu, Wu,* and *Sun.*

Essential principles include body–mind integration, control of movements and breathing, generating internal energy, mindfulness, *song* (loosening), and *jing* (serenity). *Qi* or life energy then flows well through the body, resulting in harmony. The flowing movements of tai chi contain much inner strength like water flowing in a river. Below the tranquil surface, powerful currents exist (i.e., the power for healing and wellness). With regular tai chi, the internal energy (*qi*) is converted to internal force (jing), and this will further produce more internal energy.

Tai chi improves muscle and joint strength, flexibility, fitness, and immunity, relieves pain, and improves quality of life. Flexibility exercises promote mobility, circulation, and healing.

Qigong

This is a holistic system of coordinated body posture and movement with coordinating slow flowing movement, deep rhythmic breathing and moving meditation, and calm meditative state of mind. It is used for the purposes of health, spirituality, and martial arts training. It cultivates and balances life energy/qi (chi).

It is used in medical conditions such as hypertension, pain, and cancer.

Tuina

With some background on Taoism and martial arts, the tuina practitioner will roll, knead, press, or knead the injured area in the patient using the knuckles, palms, and fingertips to eliminate the blockages along the meridians. It is a deep massage and is done on a fully dressed patient on a chair or couch. This will stimulate the qi and healing will be promoted. It is beneficial in soft tissue sports injuries.

Japanese: Reiki

Reiki is a simple form of spiritual healing. Rei means higher power and ki means life force energy. Hence, reiki is "spiritually guided life force energy." It involves "laying on hands" for stress reduction and relaxation, promoting healing, and improving quality of life. It is taught by a reiki master and the student taps into life force energy.

Western Energy Medicine

Theta Healing

Theta healing is a process of meditation which teaches people to develop natural intuition through changing their brain wave cycle to the more relaxed theta waves for emotional well-being.

In direct individual sessions, the therapist sits directly opposite the patient, listens, and questions the patient with empathy. It also can be done via telephone or internet. The therapist tunes into a person's energy to free the negative experiences and thought patterns via meditation.

It is believed that a person's conscious and unconscious mind impacts emotional well-being and hence on physical health. It is combined with mainstream medicine.

Emotional Freedom Technique

Emotional Freedom Technique (EFT) is a self-help method. It involves tapping near the end points of "energy meridian endpoints" present at various parts of the body (top of the head, eyebrows, under eyes, side of eyes, chin, collar bone, and under the arms). Eye movements are sometimes included. While tapping, specific phrases are recited to target an emotional component of a physical symptom. It is reported to be effective in reducing anxiety.

It combines acupuncture, neuro-linguistic programming, energy medicine, and TFT. With some reduction of cortisol levels and the body's stress response, relaxation occurs.

Thought Field Therapy

A variant form called TFT uses similar principles, but in TFT, different tapping sequences (known as algorithms) are used for each emotional problem (e.g., anger, guilt, anxiety, etc.).

Hypnosis and Hypnotherapy

Hypnosis is a state of concentration, focused attention, and inner absorption. Clinical hypnosis refers to an altered state of awareness, consciousness, or perception. It is used by licensed and trained doctors or therapists for treating a psychological or physical problem. Hypnotherapy is a therapy which is a psychological healing process that uses hypnosis to achieve a desired outcome. It promotes better communication between the conscious and the subconscious mind. It is a highly relaxed state.

Self-hypnosis can only work when one uses it to motivate oneself to work on reaching your goals and not when you try to use it to achieve your goals directly.

The American Psychological Association (APA) defines the practice as "a procedure during which a health professional or researcher suggests while treating someone, that he or she experiences changes in sensations, perceptions, thoughts, or behavior."

It teaches patients to use a deep relaxation state to address issues such as anxiety, phobias, substance abuse (e.g., smoking, alcoholism) weight control, chronic pain, or self-improvement.

There are different hypnotic inductions methods. These include suggestions for relaxation, calmness, and well-being. Hypnotic inductions include common instructions to imagine or think about pleasant or nice experiences.

It can be used in pain, depression, anxiety, stress, habit disorders, and many other psychological and medical problems. It has been shown to be particularly effective during anesthesia, surgery, painful medical procedures, childbirth, and in pediatric settings communication (e.g., dental extraction).

Hypnosis is generally a safe procedure. However, it may not be recommended for persons with depression or personality disorders, such as schizophrenic, borderline, or narcissistic disorders.

Color Therapy

Colors can change the way we feel and react to different situations. Color therapy (also called chromopathy, chromotherapy, or color healing) uses colors and their frequencies to heal, energize, and soothe one's physical and emotional problems. The light is delivered via color therapy equipment or enters into the body through the eyes.

Different colors produce different psychological effects on mood and emotion, so different colors are used for different mental conditions and mood problems.

Green enhances the emotions of love, joy, and inner peace. It brings hope, strength, and serenity. Green increases wisdom and facilitates change and independence. When one is feeling sad, hopeless, or depressed, green can improve your mood.

Blue is associated with wisdom, creativity, loyalty, and spirituality. It helps express one's feelings and inner truth. Light blue promotes serenity. It can also be used to help with insomnia. Blue is usually used for relaxation and meditation. Too much blue or blue that is too dark can lead to sadness, depression, and a feeling of emptiness.

Yellow brings out energy, action, happiness, and wisdom. Too much or too-bright yellows are associated with betrayal, cruelty, and deceit.

Orange signifies abundance, pleasure, well-being, and sexuality. It stimulates physical healing, increased mental energy, and feeling of connectedness between mind and body. However, it is not suitable for anxiety.

Red is more stimulating than orange. It influences emotional issues like financial independence and physical survival. It is mostly used for physical healing because its emotional effects can be extreme. Red is not indicated in severe mental conditions.

Purple is associated with beauty, spirituality, and bliss. It is used on the forehead and neck to initiate feelings of calm and relaxation.

Quantum Healing

Quantum healing is based on a mixture of quantum mechanics/electrodynamics, psychology, philosophy, and neurophysiology and is believed to govern health and well-being. Quantum ideas include wave-particle duality and virtual particles which are believed to relate to vibrational energy. It is generally regarded as pseudoscience.

Crystal Healing

Crystal healing uses semiprecious stones and crystals such as quartz, amethyst, bloodstone tourmaline, etc. Rose quartz is the master healing stone that can stimulate and align all seven chakras. Its properties include unconditional love, self-forgiveness, and acceptance. Tiger's eye brings good luck to the wearer and also gives better mental focus. Bloodstone improves blood circulation.

The crystals can be worn as a bracelet or necklace, placed in the underclothes, bedroom, or workplace, or used by the therapist. The selected stones/crystals are placed on different parts of the body corresponding to chakras, or they can be placed around the body to construct an energy grid so that healing energy surrounds the client.

The Tibetan Buddhists use 108 crystals as prayer beads (*malas*) during meditation or chanting mantras. The Catholics also use 108 rosary beads (made of quartz, amethyst, etc.) during prayers. Muslims use 99 prayer beads (*subha, misbaha, or tasbih*), made of precious stones, wood, or bone, mainly to proclaim Allah but also use it for meditation.

It is believed that stones or crystals have metaphysical or electromagnetic properties that give healing vibrations. Also, certain physical properties such as shape, color, and markings will determine the ailments that a stone can heal. Color selection and placement of stones are done according to concepts of grounding, energy grids, or chakras. Stone selection is also based on the individual's birthdate.

Magnet Therapy

Magnet therapy uses the weak, static magnetic fields of permanent magnets to the body for alleged health benefits. There are different effects assigned to different orientations of the magnet.

Our body emits weak electric or magnetic fields. Hemoglobin carries oxygen which is weakly diamagnetic (when oxygenated) or paramagnetic (when deoxygenated). However, the magnets used in magnetic therapy are too weak to have any measurable effect on blood flow.

Magnetic bracelets and jewelry, magnetic straps for wrists, ankles, knees, and back, shoe insoles, mattresses, magnetic blankets (blankets with magnets woven into the material), and *magnetized water* are worn or used by the patient.

Patients should be advised that magnet therapy has no proven benefits, and if any, its healing effect may be small.

Bio-Resonance Therapy

Electromagnetic waves can be used to diagnose and treat diseases. Electrical devices measure the skin resistance and stimulate a change of *bioresonance* in the cells, hence reversing the change caused by the disease. These transformed signals are believed to generate healing signals and effects. This therapy is controversial and there are reports of little or no benefit.

Transcranial Magnetic Stimulation

TMS is a non-invasive and painless procedure. Magnetic fields are used to stimulate the brain cells to improve symptoms of treatment-resistant depression when standard treatments have failed. When repetitive magnetic pulses are delivered, it is called repetitive TMS or rTMS.

During an rTMS session, an electromagnetic coil is placed against the scalp near the forehead. The electromagnet delivers a magnetic pulse that stimulates nerve cells in the area of the brain that controls mood and depression. It activates areas of the brain that have decreased activity in depression. The exact mechanism is not known.

rTMS does not require surgery or implantation of electrodes unlike vagus nerve stimulation or deep brain stimulation. Also rTMS does not require sedation or anesthesia unlike electroconvulsive therapy (ECT).

Generally, TMS is considered safe and well-tolerated. Some common side effects are headaches, light-headedness, scalp discomfort at the site of stimulation, tingling, and spasms or twitching of facial muscles. They are mild to moderate and are transient and will decrease over time with additional sessions. The level of stimulation can reduce these symptoms.

Uncommon side and rare side effects are seizures, mania especially in people with bipolar disorder, and hearing loss if there is inadequate ear protection during treatment.

In persons with any metal or implanted medical devices in the body *(aneurysm clips or coils, stents, vagus nerve or deep brain stimulators, pacemakers or medication pumps, electrodes for monitoring brain activity, cochlear implants for hearing, any magnetic implants, bullet fragments)*, rTMS is generally not recommended due to the strong magnetic field produced.

Other contraindications include personal or family history of epilepsy, mental health disorders such as substance misuse, bipolar disorder or psychosis, brain tumor, stroke, traumatic brain injury, frequent or severe headaches, and other serious medical conditions.

Transcranial Direct Current Stimulation

tDCS is also a non-invasive form of neuromodulation. A medical device is used to modulate cortical excitability. Weak, small direct electric currents are delivered via two scalp electrodes from a portable battery-powered stimulator. There are two types of stimulation. The anodal stimulation is usually excitatory. The cathodal stimulation is usually inhibitory. tDCS is used to treat chronic pain, depression, mood disorders, stroke, tinnitus, and schizophrenia. It can also decrease alcohol, nicotine, drug, or food cravings.

Side effects are mild and self-limiting and include local redness, tingling, burning sensation, and headaches.

Meditation

Meditation is a simple and cost-free strategy to promote better health and happiness through relaxation and better awareness of our stressful lives. It improves physical well-being and emotional health. It also can increase more connectivity between the neurons (brain cells) so as to boost memory, clarity, and sharpness.

There are many types of meditation created by various ethnic, spiritual, or religious groups to suit most people regardless of personality or lifestyle. There is no "right or perfect way" to meditate. One can explore and choose a type that works best for oneself. It is a skill that takes time and discipline to acquire and master. It is often frustrating and challenging to remain *present* and focus on the moment through a mantra without getting distracted. One must persist and accept thought intrusions as normal. Group meditation and a teacher's support may help one get started.

Prayer beads can be used during meditation or mantra chanting. *Rudraksha* beads (which are dried seeds from the *Elaeocarpus ganitrus* tree) are used mostly by Hindus. The Tibetans use 108 crystal beads to ward off negative energy and during mantra meditation. The Catholics also use 108 rosary beads (made of quartz, amethyst, etc.) during prayers. Muslims use 99 prayer beads *(subha, misbaha, or tasbih)* made of precious stones, wood, or bone for meditation.

Common and Popular Types of Meditation

Loving-Kindness Meditation

Loving-kindness meditation is also known as Metta meditation. It aims to cultivate and develop an attitude of love and kindness toward everything and everyone, including enemies and sources of stress. During deep breathing, practitioners open their minds to receive loving-kindness. They then send messages of loving-kindness to their loved ones, specific persons, and to the world. This act of messaging is done repeatedly. It promotes compassion and love for others and oneself. Positive emotions can increase and there may be reduced depression, anxiety, and post-traumatic stress disorder or PTSD. It can help those affected by anger, frustration, resentment, and interpersonal conflict.

Body Scan or Progressive Relaxation

In progressive relaxation or body scan meditation, the practitioner scans the body for areas of tension. The goal is to identify tension and to allow it to release. During this meditation session, the practitioner starts usually from the feet and upward to the head covering the whole body.

First, the muscles are made to tense and then relax. Another way is to visualize a wave, drifting over the body to release tension.

It promotes a sense of calm and relaxation slowly and steadily. It can help with chronic pain and sleep.

Mindfulness Meditation

Mindfulness is a form of meditation that urges practitioners to remain aware and be present in the moment. Awareness of the surroundings, mindfulness, and breath awareness are also important. The practitioner must be non-judgmental.

This kind of meditation can be done almost anywhere, whether standing in a queue in a mall or sitting in a crowded hall. Focus the attention to the areas of tension in the body while being aware of breathing. Mindfulness can reduce fixation on negative emotions, improve focus, improve memory, lessen impulsive and emotional reactions, and improve relationship satisfaction. Mindfulness can improve overall health, including blood pressure.

Breath-Awareness Meditation

This is a type of mindful meditation that encourages mindful breathing. The practitioner takes slow and deep breaths and counts the breaths. The aim is to focus on breathing only and to ignore other thoughts that enter the mind. The benefits of breath awareness are the same as in mindfulness, i.e., reduced anxiety, better concentration, and greater emotional flexibility.

Kundalini Yoga

Kundalini yoga is a physically active form of meditation that blends movements with deep breathing and mantras. The poses and mantras are usually taught by a teacher. It improves physical strength, reduces pain, and improves mental health by reducing anxiety and depression.

Zen Meditation

Zen meditation, sometimes called Zazen, is a form of meditation that is usually part of Buddhist practice. It involves specific steps and postures and is taught by a teacher. The aim is to focus on breathing and mindfully focus one's thoughts without judgment. It is similar to mindfulness meditation but requires more discipline and practice.

Transcendental Meditation

TCM, as it is usually called, is a spiritual form of meditation. One remains seated with the eyes closed, breathes slowly, and recites a mantra or a repeated word or series of words for 15 to 20 minutes twice a day. The aim is to transcend or rise above one's current state of being.

The teacher decides the mantra based on various factors, including the date of birth of the student practitioner and the year of the teacher's training. Practitioners of TCM report spiritual experiences and heightened mindfulness.

White Light Meditation (Visualization) or Jyoti Dhyana

Sit in a comfortable position (usually lotus position). Alternatively, one hand can be placed on the solar plexus chakra and the other hand on the sacral chakra. There can be some soothing music in the background if desired. Visualize an intense bright white light entering through the crown chakra at the top of the head. Let this light pass through every part of the body via the seven chakras and exit via the soles of the feet.

Breathe in slowly via the nose (inhale) and breathe out via the mouth (exhale).

This can reduce and release stress, tension, nervousness, and anxiety and promote self-healing.

Affirmation and Manifestation

An affirmation is a positive sentence or statement that one makes to indicate what you want to manifest. It can be said (self-talk), written as a daily nighttime ritual, or as visualization. The Universe can give you what you want through positive thoughts.

A written manifestation can be done in several ways.

The 55-5 rule is to write a sentence (your goal or dream), for example. "I will cure my cancer" or "I will be happy as I decide to be" (the affirmation) 55 times per day for 5 days.

The 3-6-9 rule is writing the affirmation three times in the morning, six times in the afternoon and nine times in the night.

Light Therapy

Light therapy (also called bright-light therapy or phototherapy) involves daily, scheduled exposure to intense doses of white light in order to regulate seasonal mood swings, improve sleeping patterns, and produce a general sense of well-being. The patient sits or works near a device called a light-therapy box. The box gives off artificial bright light that mimics natural outdoor light.

Light therapy is used as a treatment in seasonal affective disorder (SAD), non-seasonal mood disorders, jet lag, night shift, circadian sleep phase disorders, and dementia.

Lights may also be used in pregnant women to avoid pre- and postnatal blues with encouraging results.

It helps to reset the daily body clock (i.e., circadian rhythms) in people with SAD, which gets out of balance during the winter. It also increases the level of serotonin (a neurotransmitter that positively affects moods) which decreases in winter.

In light therapy, fluorescent light tubes are used with a recommended starting dose of 10,000 LUX for 30 minutes per day (LUX is the unit of measuring the illumination intensity of light) at a distance of 11 to 15 inches.

Response to bright-light therapy occurs quickly and significant improvement usually occurs within 1 week. Symptoms recur when bright-light therapy is stopped.

Incremental response to the bright-light therapy may still be seen after 2 to 4 weeks.

Side effects include headache, eye strain, agitation, insomnia, or difficulty getting to sleep which is usually due to *over-lighting*. They disappear when the light duration is reduced.

Relative contraindications to bright-light therapy include eye problems and photosensitizing medications.

Spiritual Healing

Spiritual healing is the laying on of hands coupled with prayer. There are different types.

Magnetic Healing: The healer will usually hold the patient's hands and tune in to the patient. This creates a blend of aura energies and the healer's energy is transferred to the patient.

Absent Healing: There is prayer and laying on of hands but without direct contact.

Distant Healing: Healing to a person is being given from a distance. The healer's hands are placed within 2 to 3 inches of the patient's body, but usually within the same room.

Near-to-the-Body Healing: Near-to-the-body healing is contact healing but with the hands removed a few centimeters from the body. Contact is not taking place. The healing energy is directed via the healer to the patient's aura and from there to the spirit.

Contact Healing: The healer's hands are placed upon the patient, and the healing energies are directed by the healer to the patient.

Trance Healing: The healer will enter a state of altered awareness to a degree whereby the healing energies are transmitted to the patient. This process is explained to the patient before the healing takes place.

Aura Cleansing

Various herbs such as sage can be used for aura cleansing to promote energy healing. Sage is a medicinal plant (herb) which has many benefits. It has antiseptic, anti-inflammatory, and antioxidant properties. Sage is burned in a ceramic vessel, and the smoke can transform the surrounding positive ions into beneficial negative ions to improve general well-being. Other herbs or plant essential oils used include frankincense, lemon, bergamot, rosemary, vetiver, geranium, patchouli, and many others.

Osteopathy/Craniosacral Therapy, Chiropractic Medicine, Applied Kinesiology, Rolfing, and Bowen Therapy

Cranial Osteopathy/Cranio-Sacral Therapy

Cranial osteopathy (also called cranial therapy or craniosacral therapy) is a form of osteopathic manipulative therapy.

The skeleton and connective tissues, especially the skull and sacrum, are manipulated. It is believed that there are subtle, rhythmic pulsations in the CSF which bathes the surface of the brain and the spinal cord. By gentle hand pressure, restrictions in the movement of cranial bones, and associated soft tissues are freed to stimulate the flow of CSF, blood, and lymph nodes to stimulate healing and also ensure alignment. Disturbances and distortions in the natural rhythms of the central nervous system may be due to birth trauma, childhood injuries, automobile accidents, and emotional trauma.

A full medical history is taken with details from birth to the present lifestyle. During treatment, patients are fully clothed and they lie down, face up.

During the physical exam, the limbs, head, spine, and ribs are felt and moved for any evidence of restricted motion. Treatment includes gentle hands-on manipulation of the cranial bones and the sacrum and other joints. A calming effect ensues and sometimes tingling sensation is felt during the treatment.

This therapy is used in pain management, migraine, disturbed sleep cycles, neck pain, temporomandibular joint (TMJ) syndrome, asthma, ENT problems including sinusitis, and Ménière disease.

It is also recommended in the treatment of colic in babies, infants with poor suckling, earaches, and hyperactivity in children.

Chiropractic Medicine

Chiropractic medicine covers the diagnosis and treatment of mechanical problems of the musculoskeletal system, especially the spine. Chiropractors use mainly hands-on spinal manipulation. Proper alignment of the spine mainly and the rest of the musculoskeletal system will enable the body to heal itself without surgery or medication. Manual therapy (i.e., manipulation) is used to restore mobility to joints and to relieve pain in joints and soft tissues.

It is commonly used in lower-back pain from various causes, including accidents, sports injuries, and muscle strains such as sitting without proper back support. Other uses are for pain in the neck, arms, and legs, headaches, and scoliosis.

Although evidence is lacking or conflicting, it is also used in non-musculoskeletal conditions, including attention deficit hyperactivity disorder (ADHD)/learning disabilities, dizziness, high blood pressure, vision conditions, asthma, infant colic, bedwetting, carpal tunnel syndrome, fibromyalgia, menstrual cramps, postmenopausal symptoms, insomnia, pelvic and back pain during pregnancy.

Chiropractic treatment is also used with mainstream medical treatment. The practitioners also use x-rays and CT scans.

The WHO regards chiropractic care as generally safe when utilized with skill.

Manipulation is regarded as relatively safe. However, complications and adverse effects can occur. Risks and contraindications include rheumatoid arthritis and conditions known to result in unstable joints.

Spinal manipulation is associated with frequent, mild, and temporary adverse effects, including new or worsening pain, stiffness or soreness in the affected region, mild headache, and briefly elevated pain fatigue. They occur in about 1/3 to 2/3 patients and frequently occur within an hour of treatment and disappear within 24 to 48 hours.

Serious complications include permanent disability or death in adults and children. Vertebrobasilar artery stroke (VAS) is statistically associated with cervical manipulative therapy in persons under 45 years of age.

Applied Kinesiology

Kinesiology or biomechanics is the study of body movement. AK is also referred to as muscle strength testing. It involves the diagnosis and treatment of various disorders. It is believed that various muscles are connected to particular organs and glands and that specific muscle weakness can indicate and signal distant internal problems such as nerve damage, reduced blood supply, chemical imbalances, or other organ problems. By correcting this muscle weakness, healing of the affected internal organ can take place.

It is used to diagnose and treat nervous system problems, nutritional deficiencies, or excesses and imbalances in the body's "energy pathways."

Detailed medical history is taken. Blood pressure is taken in the lying to sitting to standing positions to indicate any imbalances. Posture and gait are observed. Tests of skin sensitivity, reflexes, balance, and range of motion are also done.

Strength is tested against the pressure exerted by the practitioner. If the muscle strength is good and does not give way to resistance, it is regarded as *strong* or *locked*. The muscles that give way to resistance are considered *weak* or *unlocked*, and indicate a problem. Trigger points are also pressed to see if they will indicate muscle weakness.

When AK is used to determine whether a particular food or other substance weakens (or strengthens) a patient, the food is placed under the tongue or held in the hand as a muscle is tested. Emotional well-being by testing muscle strength can also be done while the patient imagines being in a troubling or tense situation or with a problematic person.

AK-related therapies also include deep massage, joint manipulation and realignment, craniosacral therapy, acupuncture, nutritional therapies, and dietary manipulation.

Rolfing

It is a mind–body system of soft tissue manipulation and movement education that organizes the whole body in gravity (it was created by Dr. Ida P. Rolf, an organic chemist of the United States).

Rolfing bodywork affects the body's posture and structure by manipulating the myofascial system (connective tissue). It is a deep-tissue approach involving all the layers of the body. It allows more efficient and economical muscle use, conserves energy, and refines patterns of movement. Rolfing speeds up recovery by reducing pain, stiffness, and muscle tension, improving movement and circulation around joints. It reduces chronic stress or muscle tension from previous physical and emotional traumas, reduces spinal lordosis, and enhances neurological functioning.

Professional athletes, dancers, and musicians use Rolfing to break up scar tissue, rehabilitate injuries, increase range of motion to improve comfortable performance, flexibility and avoid repetitive stress injuries. It is used by counsellors and therapists, and the practitioners are called Rolfers.

Rolfing is different from massage. Massage or deep-tissue massage often focuses on relaxation and relief of muscle discomfort. In Rolfing, there is soft tissue manipulation and movement education which then affect long-term body posture, structure, body alignment, and functioning.

Structural integration and alignment are usually carried out over a series of 10 sessions. There is loosening of superficial fascia and then deeper areas are worked starting with support in feet and legs and then higher structures.

Bowen Therapy

This is a gentle hands-on and non-manipulative technique that uses rolling movements to stimulate the soft tissues and release both physical and emotional pains associated in many conditions. It originated from Australia. Although popular, it is not evidence-based.

Massage Therapies

Massage is a technique to rub and knead different parts of the body using gentle or strong pressure to the muscles and joints using the hands.

Different types of massages are used in different countries with different names, but essentially the principles and techniques are similar. Depending on the type of massage, they can be done while fully clothed or naked. Some of the common and popular massages are listed here.

Indian Massage: Ayurvedic Massage

An Ayurvedic massage is a massage done using warm essential oils. It relieves pain, increases blood circulation, stimulates and strengthens the lymphatic system, and revitalizes and purifies the body.

The several types of Ayurvedic massages and their health benefits.

Abhyanga

This is a full-body massage with medicated warm herbal oils based on the dosha or the medical condition (dosha-specific abhyanga). For Vata dosha, do a warm oil massage in warm surroundings and avoid chills. For Pitta dosha, do room temperature oil massages. For Kapha dosha, little oil is used. Pressure is applied to the pressure points which stimulates different energy centers. This will eliminate the deep-seated toxins and improve the overall blood circulation. It should not be done during pregnancy or menstruation. Self-massage with dosha-specific oil should be done daily.

Benefits: It calms the nerves, strengthens muscles, joints, and bones, nourishes the entire body, increases circulation, eliminates impurities and toxins from the body, increases stamina, and improves sleep quality.

Pizhichil

This therapy combines two classical Ayurvedic treatments, Snehana (oleation/oil massage) and Swedana (sudation/heat treatment). The whole body is bathed in streams of lukewarm medicated oil with simultaneous soft massage using hands and special cotton cloths. Two to three therapists on either side attend to the client. More than 3 L of relaxing, medicated oil is used in this therapy. It is done daily for about 10 days.

It is indicated in rheumatic disorders, arthritis, neurological diseases, nerve weakness, paralysis, and sexual weakness.

Benefit: It improves overall blood circulation, strengthens the immune system, rejuvenates the whole body, improves muscle tone and development, and contributes to anti-aging.

Shirodhara

Shiro means head and *dhara* means flow. It involves gently pouring liquids over the forehead. The liquids used in shirodhara depend on the underlying dosha and disease but can include oil, milk, buttermilk, coconut water, or even plain water.

Different types of oils (*thailam*) are used for specific conditions. For example, *Narayana thailam* is useful in neuromuscular conditions, *Ksheerabala taila* is used to treat *Vata* conditions, etc.

The warm liquid is placed in a special pot called kindi. This pot is placed just above the mid-forehead, and it drips slowly onto the forehead. The type of medicated oil used is based on the dosha. The oil and the massage generate heat resulting in perspiration to maintain vata dosha stability.

Shirodhara usually starts with a full-body massage (i.e., Abhyangam). It is believed to calm the hypothalamus in the brain and normalize the functions of hormones that regulate sleep and emotions.

Benefits: It relieves headaches, improves clarity and focus, and diminishes mental fatigue. It is used in the treatment of eye diseases, sinusitis, allergic rhinitis, graying of hair, neurological disorders, memory loss, insomnia, hearing impairment, tinnitus, vertigo, Ménière disease, and psoriasis. It is also used at spas for relaxation. It helps in anxiety, mental stress, and improves sleep quality in those with sleep problems.

There are specialized forms of shirodhara called *ksheeradhara/dugadhadhara* (uses lukewarm medicated milk), *thakradhara* (uses buttermilk), tailadhara (uses warm medicated oil), and jaladhara (uses coconut water or plain water).

Udvartana

Udvartana is a deep-cleansing massage using dry herbal powder. It improves the skin, strengthens the muscles, and breaks down the fat.

Benefits: It exfoliates the skin, improves circulation, removes toxins, helps in weight loss, dries the Kapha dosha, which is heavy and moist, and improves muscle tone and joint mobility.

Gharshana

This massage does not involve oil or herbal powders. It does not require any lubricant. Raw silk gloves are used to massage and stimulate the body.

Benefits:
- It stimulates the lymphatic system which eliminates the toxins.
- It breaks down the fat cells in the body.
- It exfoliates the skin and makes it clean and glowing.

Njavarakizhi

This massage is customized to increase the sweating in the body. Medicated oil is applied and then pressurized massage is done as part of Njavarakizhi. The massage is done with the help of small cotton blouses that are filled with a special type of cooked rice called Njavara. These blouses are dipped in cow's milk, and herbal paste is applied to boost the production of sweat. This massage is beneficial for the skin, and it helps the senses to revitalize.

Ubtan and Elakizhi

Various herbal or animal-based products are used to nourish, treat, and rejuvenate the skin. The special massage technique helps to improve the skin quality and nourishes the body.

Nethra Tharpanam (Eye Oiling)

In this eye oil massage, a grain-based paste or cloth ring is placed around both eyes to retain the oil. The warm fluid medicinal ghee is poured over the closed eyes into this ring, and the patient is asked to blink. After about 30 minutes, the oil is dabbed off with some gauze, and the ring paste is removed. It has a cooling effect and helps to improve eyesight if done regularly.

Karna Pratisaranam/Purana (Ear Oiling)

Tilt the head sideways. Use a dropper and put 2 to 3 drops of warm sesame oil into the ear canal. Use the finger, press and rub the ear tragus to lubricate the ear canal or insert the little finger to rub it in. It can be done daily and helps to calm and ground a person. Alternatively, lie sideways and fill the ear canal with oil for 15 to 20 minutes. Drain it out and repeat in the other ear. This is done once a month. This procedure balances the three doshas apart from cleaning the ear wax. It is contraindicated in an ear infection or perforation.

Scalp Massage (Murdha Taila)

This massage is done with bhringraj oil or brahmi oil. It promotes hair growth, stimulates the senses, and is also anti-aging.

Face Massage

Use oil to massage the face at specific marma points to relieve tension and improve circulation and complexion.

Chinese Massage

Reflexology (also called zone therapy): It is used to complement standard medical treatments in various medical conditions (although there may be insufficient medical evidence). The reflexology chart indicates the areas of the feet which correspond with organs in the *zones* of the body. The therapist uses gentle to firm thumb/finger/hand pressure on different pressure points of the feet, hands, and ears of the patient and is done with the patient fully clothed.

Tuina: This is a pinch-and-pull technique where a trained traditional Chinese practitioner will brush, knead, roll, press, and rub his palms, fingertips, and knuckles to remove blockages along the meridians of the patient to stimulate qi and blood to promote healing. It is effective in tendon and bone-related injuries.

It is also helpful in children who suffer from cough, asthma, constipation, enuresis, autism, and other medical problems.

It is contraindicated in bone fractures, spinal cord injuries, open or bleeding wounds, cancers, and acute infections.

Balinese Massage

This is **a deep-tissue and whole-body therapy.** It combines acupressure, reflexology, gentle stretches, and aromatherapy. The combined therapies stimulate the flow of blood, oxygen, and *qi* (energy) in the body resulting in calmness and deep relaxation. Various techniques include skin rolling, kneading, and stroking, and pressure-point stimulation, combined with the aromas of essential oils.

It is carried out on a massage couch or on a floor mattress. Aromatherapy (i.e., scented massage) oils are used to soothe, relax, and facilitate fluid-like and friction-free massage strokes.

There are different types of Balinese massage including Javanese Lulur ritual (performed on brides in preparation to marriage), Balinese Boreh (a massage for rice farmers to ease pain using a paste of ground spices), Urat massage (nerve/tendon massage), Sasak massage, and Lombok massage.

Javanese Massage

This involves deep thumb pressure with stroking palm movements, kneading, and knuckling to loosen knotted muscles and stimulate lymphatic drainage. Scented massage oils such as lemongrass (*serai),* patchouli (*pokok nilam*), fennel, and sandalwood (*chandana*) are used.

It is believed that the body accumulates air or *winds* resulting in congestion, flu, or rheumatism. Since the wind is toxic, it is expelled via burps and farts with deep pressure and special strokes. It also reduces cellulite and improves blood and energy flow.

It benefits patients with chronic headaches/migraine, fibromyalgia, lower-back and neck pain, hypertension, sleep disorder, depression, and anxiety.

Compared to a Balinese massage, the Javanese massage is much rougher. One type of Javanese massage is using a coin to scrape the skin to let out air.

Balinese massage is more relaxing with techniques including Thai thumbing, Thai palming, reflexology, aromatherapy, fresh herbs, and body scrub. It is more suitable in a spa setting than the Javanese massage.

Thai Massage

This is a very active massage on the whole body using different movements to stretch and twist the body into various positions. Palms and fingers are used to apply firm pressure. It helps to improve flexibility and circulation. It is done on the floor.

Japanese Massage (Shiatsu)

This massage uses fingers, thumbs, feet, and palms, assisted stretching, and joint manipulation and mobilization. It is usually done on the floor.

Swedish Massage

This is a gentle type of full-body massage which is used for people with knotted muscles and who are sensitive to touch. It combines kneading, long flowing strokes in the direction of the heart, vibration, deep circular movements, tapping, and passive joint movements.

Others

Hot stone massage: Heated bricks or stones are placed on different areas around a specific area of muscle pain or tension or sometimes the whole body. It improves blood flow and reduces muscle tension.

Aromatherapy massage: This gentle massage uses diluted essential oils on the skin. It improves mood and reduces stress and anxiety as part of emotional healing.

Deep-tissue massage: This is a deep and strong massage. It uses slow strokes and deep finger pressure for chronic muscle pain and injury.

Trigger-point massage: This is a deep and gentle massage for chronic pain. It uses broad and flowing strokes with deep or strong pressure. Specific areas of tightness in the muscle or trigger points are massaged to relieve pain.

Sports massage: This can be used in repetitive use injury as prevention in injury-prone persons or in sportspersons to improve performance and flexibility. It can be used in targeted areas or the whole body.

Chair massage: This a quick massage using light to medium finger pressure on the neck, shoulder, and back while seated in a special chair.

Couple's massage: This is a massage done with another partner in the same room with a conversation going on if desired. Any of the above types of massages can be chosen and is carried out by two therapists.

Prenatal massage: Except during the first trimester, this massage is used during pregnancy especially on the lower back, hips, and legs to reduce body aches and muscle tension using mild pressure like the Swedish massage.

Post-natal massage: This is done for the mother after delivery usually for about one month. Techniques vary among various Asian cultures. Hot stones, steam, and herbs are used to improve circulation and cleanse and contract the uterus.

Infant massage: This can be done when the baby is a few days or weeks old during or after a bath or when the infant is awake and alert. Oil is usually used although dry massage can be done for the whole body or specific parts. Benefits include better sleep and prevention of fussiness, excessive crying, colic, and constipation.

Biofeedback Therapy

Biofeedback therapy is a non-invasive and non-drug treatment in which patients learn to control the autonomic and involuntary functions of the body such as blood pressure, heart rate, breathing, brain waves, muscle tension, skin conductance, and pain perception so that one can manipulate them at will.

In biofeedback, the patient is connected to electrical sensors to receive information (feedback) about the body which is then connected to a monitoring box.

The therapist views the measurements on the monitor, and via trial and error, identifies a range of mental activities and relaxation techniques that can help regulate the patient's bodily processes.

Changes to thoughts, emotions, and behavior can alter physiological changes and improve health and performance. Eventually, these changes may be maintained, and no equipment is required to biofeedback.

Biofeedback is recommended in the prevention or treatment of hypertension, migraine/headaches, chronic pain, insomnia, and incontinence. Neurofeedback biofeedback may help patients with ADHD, addiction, anxiety, seizures, and depression.

There are many types of biofeedback, but there are three common types of biofeedback therapy:

Thermal biofeedback measures skin temperature. A feedback thermometer detects skin temperature with a thermistor (a temperature-sensitive resistor) that is put on a finger or toe. Skin temperature mainly reflects arteriole diameter. Hand-warming involves arteriole vasodilation produced by a beta-2 adrenergic stimulation. Hand-cooling involves arteriole vasoconstriction due to the increased stimulation of sympathetic C-fibers.

Temperature biofeedback is used to treat chronic pain, headache (migraine and tension-type headache), stress and anxiety, essential hypertension, Raynaud disease, and edema.

Electromyography (EMG) measures muscle tension. An electromyograph (EMG) uses surface electrodes to detect muscle-action potentials from underlying skeletal muscles that initiate muscle contraction. Surface electromyogram (SEMG) is measured when one or more active electrodes are placed over a target muscle and reference electrodes are placed nearby.

EMG biofeedback is used to treat anxiety, chronic pain, headaches, lower-back pain, physical rehabilitation (cerebral palsy [CP], incomplete spinal cord lesions, and stroke), temporomandibular joint dysfunction (TMD), torticollis, and fecal incontinence, urinary incontinence, and pelvic pain.

Neurofeedback or EEG biofeedback focuses on electrical brain activity. There are different types of brain rhythms at different frequencies.

For example, beta rhythms consist of asynchronous waves and can be divided into low beta and high beta ranges (13 to 21 Hz and 20 to 32 Hz). Low beta is associated with attention and focused thoughts. High beta is associated with anxiety, hypervigilance, panic, and peak performance.

Neurofeedback is used to treat addiction, ADHD, learning disability, anxiety, obsessive-compulsive disorder, post-traumatic stress disorder, depression, migraine, and generalized seizures.

Homeopathy

Homeo means similar and *pathy* means science. It is based on the philosophy that "like cures like" and that the body can heal itself. It means that if a substance brings on symptoms in a healthy person, the same substance can in a very small dose treat an illness with similar symptoms. It uses tiny amounts of natural substances like plants and minerals to stimulate the healing process.

It was developed in the late 1700s in Germany and is common in many European countries.

Homoeopathy is based on the law of similars. Its treatment is based on the art of miasmatic prescribing by incorporating the miasmatic diagnosis into the plan of treatment. A miasm is a force within a person which causes a susceptibility or predisposition to certain kinds of illness. Miasmatic prescribing helps in eliminating the underlying cause of the disease and avoids increased susceptibility to future diseases.

Homoeopathy as a part of the integrative healthcare system can play a definitive role in the treatment of any disease with its personalized approach. It treats the child and adult holistically and can be integrated with other non-drug and even drug interventions.

Arnica, stinging nettle plant, Calcarea phosphorica, poison ivy, and crushed whole bees are some common homoeopathic remedies. This will trigger and stimulate the immune system to fight disease.

These ingredients are weakened by adding water or alcohol. The mixture is shaken as part of a process called *potentization*. It is believed this step transfers the healing essence. It is also believed that lower the dose, the stronger and more powerful the medicine will be. These remedies actually no longer contain any molecules of the original substance. They are available usually as sugar pellets or liquid drops and sometimes as creams, gels, and tablets.

It is useful in many chronic illnesses such as allergies, migraines, depression, chronic fatigue syndrome, rheumatoid arthritis, irritable bowel syndrome, premenstrual syndrome, etc. It can also be used for minor issues like bruises, scrapes, toothaches, headaches, nausea, coughs, and colds.

It is not recommended in life-threatening illnesses like acute asthmatic attack, cancer, and heart disease or in emergencies. It should not be a substitute for vaccines including some homoeopathic products called *nosodes* which are marketed as vaccine alternatives.

Caution must be exercised as some homoeopathic medicines can contain excessive heavy metals such as homoeopathic teething tablets and gels.

Naturopathy

Naturopathy is based on a belief that the body can heal itself through an internal, vital energy or force. Most naturopaths practice a holistic approach and avoid surgery and conventional medicines tending to reject evidence-based medicine.

A consultation begins with a long patient interview focusing on lifestyle, medical and psychological history, and physical exam. In some developed countries, naturopaths are primary care providers and can prescribe drugs, perform minor surgery, and integrate conventional medical approaches such as diet and lifestyle counselling with their naturopathic practice. Some naturopaths do not recommend vaccines and antibiotics.

Various treatments are provided by naturopaths. These include herbalism (botanical medicines), vitamins, minerals, homoeopathy, acupuncture, natural cures, physical therapies, AK, colonic enemas, chelation therapy, color therapy, cranial osteopathy, hair analysis, iridology, live-blood analysis, ozone therapy, reflexology, Rolfing, massage therapy, and TCM.

Natural cures include exposure to sunshine, fresh air, heat or cold, nutrition advice on fasting, vegetarian, whole food, sugar-free and alcohol-free meals, detoxification, and allergy treatments. Physical therapy includes bone or soft tissue manipulation, exercise, and hydrotherapy. Psychological counselling includes meditation, relaxation, lifestyle counselling, stress management.

Others: Hydrotherapy/Aquatic Therapy, Art Therapy, Pet Therapy, Ozone Therapy, Hyperbaric Oxygen Therapy, Stem Cell Therapy

Hydrotherapy

Hydrotherapy or aquatic therapy refers to exercises in warm water to treat various medical conditions. The temperature in the warm-water pool is normally between 33°C and 36°C, warmer than a typical swimming pool. Warm water improves movement of stiff or swollen joints, relaxes muscles, strengthens weak muscles, and reduces aches and pains in arthritis, rheumatism, or poor blood circulation. It also helps neurological conditions such as CP, muscular dystrophy, multiple sclerosis, and Parkinson disease.

It involves special exercises that are customized depending on the symptoms. The exercises consist of slow, controlled movements and include relaxing exercises, gentle stretching, strengthening exercises against the resistance of the water, flotation, and movement exercises.

Hydrotherapy treatment is usually available in the physiotherapy department of a hospital.

Initial assessment is carried out by the neuro physiotherapist or physiotherapist who is also a trained hydrotherapist to establish goals, physical ability and function, treatment plan, costume changing, access to the pool, and safety issues.

Hydrotherapy improves both fitness and general mobility. It also improves posture, reduces muscle tension or muscle spasm, and relieves pain in the limbs, supports aching muscles, and facilitates movement. It stimulates the release of endorphins which in turn promotes relaxation and pain relief. The slow movements and relaxing exercises can reduce stress and high blood pressure.

There is improved coordination and balance, increased metabolic rate and digestion activity, and decreased swelling/pain. Children and adults with CP who have difficulty in controlling their movements due to stiffness, unsteadiness, and unwanted involuntary movement on land do better in water. Spontaneous movements in water are more attainable than movements on land because of the buoyancy and weightlessness in the water. They are able to stand upright and walk by themselves in water.

Children and adults who are liable to lose strength, muscle bulk, and flexibility because of their inability to move independently benefit from hydrotherapy because they are supported in the water and are therefore able to move their limbs. The ability to swim is not a requirement for hydrotherapy.

Art Therapy

In art therapy, there is direct or indirect engagement, exchange, and interaction between the patient and therapist.

Art therapy involves and promotes humanism, self-awareness, personal growth, creativity, and emotional conflict resolution.

It can aid in many illnesses (cancer, heart disease, etc.). The patients can escape and hide the emotional pain of disease through art.

Some people cannot express the way they feel as it can be difficult to put into words. Hence, art can help people express their experiences. It is a coping mechanism.

Engaging women with cancers in different art programs such as drawing and painting or visual art (textiles, card making, collage, pottery, watercolor, acrylics) help them focus on positive life experiences, enhance their self-worth, maintain a social identity, and express their feelings in a symbolic manner. The creative art making itself is therapeutic.

It is used in various traumatic experiences during disasters or crisis intervention to help adults or children make art in response to their trauma. The symbolic expression can be interpreted by the therapist.

Art therapy is also used in autism, dementia, and schizophrenia.

Art therapy may provide an outlet for exploring strengths and emotions in children with eating disorders or any kind of child abuse because they may not know how to vocalize their emotions.

Pet Therapy

Pet therapy in general includes animal-assisted therapy and other animal-assisted activities.

Animal-assisted therapy uses dogs or other animals to help people recover or cope with various health problems such as heart disease, mental health disorders, or cancer.

Animal-assisted activities usually have a more general purpose such as providing comfort and joy for nursing home residents.

The assistance dog and its handler visit the patient in the hospital room. They stay for 10 or 15 minutes. The patient is invited to pet the dog and ask the handler questions.

Hippotherapy is a form of physical therapy using horseback riding as a therapeutic or rehabilitative treatment. It is widely used in CP, autism, and other special needs or disabilities. The benefits include better balance, posture, muscle strength, and coordination.

Dolphins are also used in the rehabilitation of CP children.

Animal-assisted therapy can significantly reduce pain, anxiety, depression, and fatigue in people with a range of chronic medical conditions including heart disease, cancer, dementia, and those in long-term care facilities.

Safety and sanitation are important issues in hospitals. The canines (dogs) must be clean, vaccinated, well-trained, and screened for appropriate behavior during the hospital visits.

Aromatherapy

Aromatherapy uses essential oils. These are aromatic, concentrated extracts from plants that are obtained through steam distillation, cold press, or resin tapping. The oils are usually diffused as a mist (via a diffuser) and inhaled through the nose or applied topically on the skin. It can be part of a bath, bath or cosmetic products, or used in spa treatments.

Essential oils are made from flower, herb, and tree parts like bark, roots, peels, and petals. A lot of plant product is needed to make pure and natural essential oils. More than 200 pounds of lavender flowers are used to make just 1 pound of lavender essential oil. Lemon, chamomile, lavender, cedarwood, frankincense, and bergamot are the commonly used essential oils.

The essential oil stimulates the smell receptors in the nose, and the electrical impulses are transmitted to the specific areas of the brain (i.e., limbic system) which affects the emotions and the brainstem area which produces serotonin neurotransmitters.

This therapy helps to calm, relax, and reduce stress, anxiety, and depression, improve sleep, give local pain relief, and reduce chemotherapy-associated nausea and vomiting.

Aromatherapy is generally safe. Occasional local irritation of the eyes, skin, or nose mucous membranes or mild allergic reactions may occur. Rarely essential oils are consumed, and there is a danger of liver or kidney damage or even seizures from inhalation.

Bach Flower Therapy

Bach flower remedies are used to treat emotional problems (anxiety, depression, stress) and pain. It uses small amounts of natural watered-down extracts from the flowers of wild plants preserved in grape-based brandy to restore mind–body balance and bring peace and happiness. There are 38 remedies with each remedy to treat a specific negative emotion.

There are seven broad categories of emotions, i.e., fear, uncertainty, lack of interest in present circumstances, loneliness, oversensitivity to influences and ideas, sadness or despair, care for others at the expense of self.

It is similar to homoeopathy, but fewer materials are used and only emotional issues are addressed. Physical problems are not treated.

Drops of Bach remedies (single or combined) are placed on the tongue or mixed into a glass of water and consumed. This can be taken two or three times per day.

Ozone Therapy

Ozone is a gas with three oxygen atoms whereas oxygen has two oxygen atoms. Ozone can also be toxic when inhaled.

Ozone activates the immune system to promote healing. It helps red blood cells to transport oxygen and improves circulation and general cell function. It has anti-inflammatory and anti-infective effects against bacteria, viruses, fungi, yeast, and protozoa. It is a powerful antioxidant and removes toxins.

There is an ozone layer in the Earth's stratosphere which protects the Earth from the sun's ultraviolet radiation, most of which it absorbs.

It is used as a gas for medical treatment, but it can damage the respiratory system.

It is used for treating infected wounds, eczema, circulatory disorders, macular degeneration, viral diseases, rheumatism and arthritis, cancer, SARS, and AIDS.

Ozone improves circulation by cleaning the arteries and veins, purifies blood and the lymph nodes, normalizes hormone and enzyme production, reduces pain and swelling, stops bleeding, prevents shock, limits stroke damage, reduces cardiac arrhythmia, reduces the risk of complications from diabetes, and improves brain function and memory.

Ozone can be administered to patients by bagging the gas over a skin infection or by blowing it into the ear, nose, mouth, and rectum. In major autohemotherapy, about 250 mL of blood is withdrawn into an intravenous bag which is then injected with ozone and then transfused back to the patient. Direct intravenous and vaginal routes are not recommended.

Ozone therapy is generally considered safe and serious adverse events are rare. Small amounts of ozone can irritate the lungs and throat, resulting in coughing, shortness of breath, burning of eyes, nausea or vomiting, or mild headaches.

Herxheimer reactions can also occur with flu-like symptoms. If ozone therapy is given, using insufflation via the rectum, there is mild discomfort, cramping, and passing wind. These side effects are temporary.

Serious adverse events include increased risk of stroke, damage to the eardrum via insufflation of the ear, bowel rupture because of insufflation of the rectum, and pulmonary embolism and death when given intravenously.

Positive side effects include longer and stronger nails and hair, healthier skin, better sleep, and more energy.

Hyperbaric Oxygen Therapy

HBOT is a medical treatment that uses pure 100% oxygen at pressures greater than normal atmospheric (sea level) pressure. It involves the systemic delivery of oxygen at levels two to three times greater than atmospheric pressure. It increases the oxygen transport capacity in the blood whereby the oxygen transport by plasma will be significantly increased under HBOT.

The patient breathes in 100% oxygen while placed in a comfortable hyperbaric chamber. These chambers come in many shapes and sizes but can broadly be classified into two main groups—monoplace, which is suitable for a single patient and multiplace, in which various numbers of patients can be treated depending upon the size of the chamber. Some multiplace chambers are also able to accept ventilated intensive care patients.

The monoplace delivers 100% oxygen directly to the patient without the need to use masks or hoods. It is significantly less costly to set up, occupies smaller space, and uses less manpower to operate, service, and maintain.

Oxygen therapy is an excellent type of therapy for all conditions where there is a loss of blood flow and thus a loss of oxygen, resulting in some cells dying. This may cause permanent damage. However, some cells will be dormant and not dead. It is these cells that the HBOT often salvages and restores to life (e.g., as in a difficult wound healing or in brain injury).

In the brain, it is the neurons that can be reawakened and restored. By giving the *sleeping cells/idling neurons* (dormant cells) pressurized oxygen, they will have the electrical spark needed to fire them electrically. The dormant cells need more oxygen so that they will have the ability to fully function. HBOT improves microcirculation. When these *idle, dormant cells or neurons* return to normal, through restored oxygen levels, brain functions such as cognitive, motor, visual, and auditory response are greatly improved in many patients. HBOT helps to speed and enhance the body's natural ability to heal.

The current approved indications by FDA and ANZHMG (Australia and NZ Hyperbaric Medical Group) include:
Acute ischemic conditions
Acute arterial insufficiency
Infective conditions
Radiation tissue damage
Non-healing wounds
Toxic gas poisoning and smoke inhalation
Ocular ischemia
Sudden deafness and tinnitus
Exceptional blood loss

The non-accepted conditions include sports, stroke, Bell palsy, multiple sclerosis, and CP.

Side effects or risks of HBOT are quite rare. The commonest is barotrauma to the ears, resulting in earache/pain (*crackling* in the ears). This can be prevented. Some patients may experience light-headedness for several minutes after treatment, but this would soon pass. On rare occasions, patients may develop temporary changes in eyesight, which will return to normal after the end of treatment.

Treatments are individualized to each patient. Some emergency cases require only one or two treatments. Wound healing cases and acute anoxic brain injury cases may require 20 to 30 duration of HBOT treatments for maximum benefit. The exact number of treatments will be determined by the patient's response to HBOT. For inpatients, treatments may be done twice a day. Outpatients are usually treated once a day for 5 or 6 days a week.

A HBOT treatment needs to be operated by certified hyperbaric technicians (CHTs).

Stem Cell Therapy

Cell therapy is a therapy where living whole and intact cells or cellular materials are administered to a patient for the treatment of a disease. It is also known as regenerative medicine and is an emerging branch in medical science. It promotes the repair of diseased, dysfunctional, or injured tissue using stem cells or their derivatives.

The cells can be derived from the same individual (autologous source) or from another individual (allogeneic source).

Stem cells can be obtained from various sources. These include embryo, amnion, fetus, placenta, cord blood, cord tissue (Wharton jelly), placenta, bone marrow, peripheral blood, adipose tissue, exosomes, and induced pluripotent stem cells (iPSCs, which are reprogrammed from skin fibroblasts).

Based on their differentiation potential, stem cells are classified into five groups: totipotent/omnipotent, pluripotent, multipotent, oligopotent, and unipotent.

Totipotent or *omnipotent* cells can differentiate into embryonic and extraembryonic tissues and generate a complete and viable organism. A fertilized egg (zygote) is an example of a totipotent cell.

Pluripotent cells can self-renew and differentiate into any of the three germ layers, ectoderm, endoderm, and mesoderm, from which all tissues and organs develop. Embryonic stem cells are the natural pluripotent stem cells.

Multipotent stem cells can self-renew and differentiate only in a closely related family of cells, for example: mesenchymal stem cells (MSC).

Oligopotent stem cells can self-renew and differentiate only into closely related cell types, for example hematopoietic stem cells that can differentiate into both myeloid and lymphoid lineages.

Unipotent stem cells can self-renew and differentiate into only one cell type, for example, muscle stem cells.

Based on their origin, stem cells can be grouped into five categories: embryonic, fetal, perinatal, adult, and iPS.

Embryonic and iPS cells are pluripotent.

Fetal and perinatal cells (amniotic, placenta, umbilical cord blood, and tissue) are generally multipotent.

Adult stem cells are usually oligo- or unipotent.

Embryonic stem cells are derived from embryos that are 3 to 5 days old. This embryo is called a blastocyst and has about 150 cells. They are pluripotent stem cells and can divide into more stem cells or can become any type of cell in the body.

A stem cell is the only type of cell out of the 220 cell types in the body that has the ability to continuously divide and differentiate into various other types of cells. The stem cell has the capacity to divide and self-renew for a long time. It also has the ability to differentiate.

A stem cell will undergo symmetric cell division to give rise to two identical cells with identical stemness characteristics for a long period of time. It has the potential to give rise to specialized cell types, for example, nerve cell, cardiac cells, blood cell, etc.

Two main types of stem cells are used hematopoietic stem cells (from bone marrow, peripheral blood, or cord blood) and MSC. They have their identification called cluster of differentiation (CD) markers.

The surface markers for hematopoietic stem cells are CD34+, CD38−, CD90+, and CD45−.

The surface markers for MSCs are CD29+, CD44+, CD105+, CD14−, CD31−, CD34−, CD45−, and CD133−.

The MSCs are like building blocks and are found in all the organs, tissues, blood, and immune system. They can regenerate into additional stem cells or differentiate into specialized cells. When they are transplanted into a patient's body, stem cells can repair or replace the patient's damaged or diseased cells.

The donor MSC is derived from the umbilical cord tissue (Wharton jelly), dental pulp of the tooth, bone marrow, or adipocyte (fat cell). MSCs can regulate immune responses, blood vessel growth, repair and regenerate tissues or home to the sites of inflammation, reduce scarring, and prevent premature cell death.

MSCs can proliferate extensively, differentiate into the desired cell type, and do not cause immune rejection. It has extensive potential medical therapeutic applications. There are also some reports that MSCs can also contribute to tumor pathogenesis. They has the potential to become any of the 220 types of different cells in the body. By enhancing and stimulating the stem cells, every organ can be revitalized and rejuvenated.

Amniotic cells contain epithelial and mesenchymal cells which have stem cell properties. The human amniotic epithelial cells are CD9, CD29, CD104, CD49, 49D, CD44 positive. They are effective to treat eye surface conditions, burns, and ulcers. They has immunomodulatory properties.

Exosomes are extracellular vesicles. They are substances that are released by most types of cells and have a role in cell-to-cell communication. They have different roles and targets and deliver efficiently many kinds of cargo to the target cells. They are frequently used to deliver therapeutic cargo for treatment. Exosomes may be natural or modified with other substances to increase the delivery ability.

Stem cells can be grown in the lab. They can be manipulated to specialize into specific types of cells, such as heart muscle cells, blood cells, or nerve cells. These specific and specialized cells can then be implanted. For example, in a patient with heart disease, the cells could be injected into the heart muscle or into the coronary artery. The healthy transplanted heart muscle cells help to repair the defective heart muscle.

All stem cells undergo stringent cell viability, sterility test, immunophenotyping, and karyotyping. The cells are stored in sterile cryovials, labelled, sealed prior to deep freezing in liquid nitrogen at −190°C.

Stem cells have been used in spinal cord injuries, type 1 diabetes, Parkinson disease, amyotrophic lateral sclerosis, Alzheimer disease, heart disease, stroke, burns, cancer, osteoarthritis, premature infants with bronchopulmonary dysplasia, and many more conditions.

References

8 Limbs Yoga Centers Staff. (n.d.). *About yoga*. https://8limbsyoga.com/about-yoga/. Accessed March 29, 2021.

ActionPotential Inc. (2011). *What is rolfing? How is it different from deep tissue massage?* http://www.rolfusa.com/rolfing.html.

Acupuncturetoday.com. (n.d.). *Ilex (mao dong qing)*. https://www.acupuncturetoday.com/herbcentral/ilex.php.

Ambardekar, N. (2018, January 11). *Aromatherapy & essential oils for stress relief*. WebMD. https://www.webmd.com/balance/stress-management/aromatherapy-overview#2.

American College of Hyperbaric Medicine. (n.d.). http://www.achm.org/amsimis/. Accessed July 12, 2020.

American Psychological Association. (n.d.). *APA dictionary of psychology*. APA. https://dictionary.apa.org/self-hypnosis.

American Society of Clinical Hypnosis. (2021). https://www.asch.net/aws/ASCH/pt/sp/home_page#Question1.

Anderson, S. (n.d.). *The 5 prana vayus chart*. Yoga International. https://yogainternational.com/article/view/the-5-prana-vayus-chart. Accessed March 29, 2021.

Bach, E. (n.d.). *The 38 bach flower remedies*. Information & Sales—The Original Bach Flower Remedies. http://www.bachflower.com/original-bach-flower-remedies/. Accessed July 12, 2021.

Barrett, S. (2015, March 28). *Reflexology: A close look*. Quackwatch. https://quackwatch.org/related/reflex/.

Berman, L. (2019, April 24). *Balancing your energy body: A complete guide to chakra healing*. Conscious Lifestyle Magazine. https://www.consciouslifestylemag.com/chakra-healing-energy-body-balancing/.

Bhat, V. (2015, June 6). *7 Types of ayurvedic massages you must know*. Onlymyhealth. https://www.onlymyhealth.com/health-slideshow/7-types-of-ayurvedic-massages-you-know-1433588565.html.

Bohonowych, J. (2017, April 12). *New evidence supports benefits of hippotherapy*. Foundation for Prader–Willi Research. https://www.fpwr.org/blog/new-evidence-supports-benefits-of-hippotherapy.

Bowen Therapy Professional Association. (n.d.). http://www.bowen-therapy.org. Accessed July 12, 2021.

Brazier, Y. (2017, December 21). *How does acupuncture work?* MedicalNewsToday. https://www.medicalnewstoday.com/articles/156488.

British Hyperbaric Association. (2021). https://www.ukhyperbaric.com/.

Cherniack, E. P., & Govorushko, S. (2018). To bee or not to bee: The potential efficacy and safety of bee venom acupuncture in humans. *Toxicon*, 154, 74–78. https://doi.org/10.1016/j.toxicon.2018.09.013.

Clogstoun-Willmott, J. (2021, April 21). *Liver Yin deficiency*. Acupuncture Points. https://www.acupuncture-points.org/liver-yin-deficiency.html.

Contemporary American Religion. (2021, June 17). *Quantum healing*. https://www.encyclopedia.com/religion/legal-and-political-magazines/quantum-healing.

D'Alberto, A. (n.d.). *The development of wind aetiology in traditional Chinese medicine—part two*. https://www.attiliodalberto.com/articles/the-development-of-wind-aetiology-in-chinese-medicine-part-two.php.

Davis, C. P. (2021, March 29). *Medical definition of siddha medicine*. https://www.medicinenet.com/siddha_medicine/definition.htm.

Dey, S., & Pahwa, P. (2014). Prakriti and its associations with metabolism, chronic diseases, and genotypes: Possibilities of new born screening and a lifetime of personalized prevention. *Journal of Ayurveda and Integrative Medicine*, 5(1), 15–24. https://doi.org/10.4103/0975-9476.128848.

Dhakal, A., & Sbar, E. (2021). *Jarisch herxheimer reaction* [E-book]. StatPearls Publishing.

Dharmananda, S. (2010, October). *Feng: The meaning of wind in Chinese medicine*. Institute of Traditional Medicine. http://www.itmonline.org/articles/feng/feng.htm.

Editors of Good Spa Guide. (2013, January 31). *What is balinese massage?* Good Spa Guide. https://goodspaguide.co.uk/features/balinese-massage-explained.

Editors of HappyMassage.com. (2013, November 7). *Indonesian javanese massage—massage wiki*. HappyMassage. http://www.happymassage.com/wiki/Indonesian_Javanese_Massage.

Editors of PhysioFunction. (2021, June 9). *Hydrotherapy (aquatic therapy)*. PhysioFunction. https://www.physiofunction.co.uk/neurological-services/hydrotherapy.

Ernst, E. (2009). Is reflexology an effective intervention? A systematic review of randomised controlled trials. *Medical Journal of Australia*, 191(5), 263–266. https://doi.org/10.5694/j.1326-5377.2009.tb02780.x.

Eu Yan Sang Editors. (n.d.). *Tuina: Ancient Chinese healing techniques*. Eu Yan Sang. https://www.euyansang.com.my/en_MY/tuina%3A-ancient-chinese-healing-techniques/eystcm8.html.

European Underwater and Baromedical Society. (2021). http://www.eubs.org.

Finegold, L., & Flamm, B. L. (2006). Magnet therapy. *BMJ, 332*(7532), 4. https://doi.org/10.1136/bmj.332.7532.4.

Fregni, F., Nitsche, M. A., Loo, C. K., Brunoni, A. R., Marangolo, P., Leite, J., et al. (2015). Regulatory considerations for the clinical and research use of transcranial direct current stimulation (tDCS): Review and recommendations from an expert panel. *Clinical Research and Regulatory Affairs*, 32(1), 22–35. https://doi.org/10.3109/10601333.2015.980944.

Galyen, W. (2020, December 20). *What is color therapy, what is it for, and is it right for me?* ReGain. https://www.regain.us/advice/therapist/what-is-color-therapy-what-is-it-for-and-is-it-right-for-me.

Hall, H. (2020, May 4). Applied kinesiology and other chiropractic delusions. *Skeptical Inquirer*, 44(3). https://skepticalinquirer.org/2020/05/applied-kinesiology-and-other-chiropractic-delusions/.

Hamilton-Parker, C. (2021, March 23). *Spirit healing: 6 types of spiritual healing explained*. Hamilton Parker Psychics. https://psychics.co.uk/blog/spirit-healing/.

Hear.com. (2021, February 2). *What is ear candling and why is it bad for you?* https://www.hear.com/useful-knowledge/ear-candling/.

Hurst, K. (2018, January 29). *A guide to healing crystals: 10 most effective healing stones*. The Law of Attraction. https://www.thelawofattraction.com/healing-crystal-guide/.

Hussein, R. A., & El-Anssary, A. A. (2019). Plants secondary metabolites: The key drivers of the pharmacological actions of medicinal plants. *Herbal Medicine, 1*(3). https://doi.org/10.5772/intechopen.76139.

Hyperbaric Health. (2013). *About hyperbarics and wound care*. http://www.hyperbarichealth.com/about.html.

iMedical Publishing Editors. (n.d.). Diet therapy. *Journal of Clinical Nutrition & Dietetics*. https://www.imedpub.com/scholarly/diet-therapy-journals-articles-ppts-list.php.

Ilic, D., & Polak, J. M. (2011). Stem cells in regenerative medicine: introduction. *British Medical Bulletin*, 98(1), 117–126. https://doi.org/10.1093/bmb/ldr012.

IMR—Pediatrics. (n.d.). The Andrew Weil Center for Integrative Medicine. https://integrativemedicine.arizona.edu/education/peds_imr.html. Accessed March 29, 2021.

Italian Society of Underwater and Hyperbaric Medicine. (2020). https://www.simsi.org/.

Jagtenberg, T., Evans, S., Grant, A., Howden, I., Lewis, M., & Singer, J. (2006). Evidence-based medicine and naturopathy. *The Journal of Alternative and Complementary Medicine*, 12(3), 323–328. https://doi.org/10.1089/acm.2006.12.323.

Lam, P. (2018). *What is Tai Chi?* Tai Chi for Health Institute. https://taichiforhealthinstitute.org/what-is-tai-chi/.

Lee, H.-Y., & Hong, I.-S. (2017). Double-edged sword of mesenchymal stem cells: Cancer-promoting versus therapeutic potential. *Cancer Science*, 108(10), 1939–1946. https://doi.org/10.1111/cas.13334.

Levy, J. C. (2019, October 13). *5 Emotional freedom technique or EFT tapping benefits for stress, pain & more*. Dr. Axe. https://draxe.com/health/emotional-freedom-technique-eft-tapping-therapy/.

Lüdtke, R., Kunz, B., Seeber, N., & Ring, J. (2001). Test-retest-reliability and validity of the kinesiology muscle test. *Complementary Therapies in Medicine*, 9(3), 141–145. https://doi.org/10.1054/ctim.2001.0455.

Ma, C. J., Li, X., & Chen, H. (2021). Research progress in the use of leeches for medical purposes. *Talent of Medical Research*, 6, 15. https://doi.org/10.12032/TMR20200207159.

Mahesh, S., Wele, A., Patgiri, B. J., & Porszasz, R. (2019). Review of pain: An ayurvedic approach. *International Research Journal of Pharmacy*, 10(9), 24–34. https://doi.org/10.7897/2230-8407.1009256.

Marcin, A. (2019, January 4). *What is cupping therapy?* Healthline. https://www.healthline.com/health/cupping-therapy#treatment.

Mayo Clinic Staff. (2017, February 8). *Light therapy*. MayoClinic. https://www.mayoclinic.org/tests-procedures/light-therapy/about/pac-20384604.

Mayo Clinic Staff. (2018, November 27). *Transcranial magnetic stimulation*. Mayo Clinic. https://www.mayoclinic.org/tests-procedures/transcranial-magnetic-stimulation/about/pac-20384625.

Mayo Clinic Staff. (2019, June 8). *Stem cells: What they are and what they do*. Mayo Clinic. https://www.mayoclinic.org/tests-procedures/bone-marrow-transplant/in-depth/stem-cells/art-20048117.

Mayo Clinic Staff. (2020, September 15). *Pet therapy: Animals as healers*. Mayo Clinic. https://www.mayoclinic.org/healthy-lifestyle/consumer-health/in-depth/pet-therapy/art-20046342?reDate=12072021.

Meditating Works. (2021, October 23). *White light meditation*. https://meditatingworks.com/white-light-meditation/.

MENAFN—Costa Rica News. (2020, February 4). *All you need to know about the "Yin Yang" philosophy*. Middle East North Africa Financial Network. https://menafn.com/1099957576/All-You-Need-To-Know-About-The-Yin-Yang-Philosophy.

Moen, R. D. (2017, March 2). *What is hydrotherapy?* Made for Movement. https://blog.madeformovement.com/what-is-hydrotherapy.

Mosher Optimal Health. (n.d.). *The five elements*. Accessed 2021. https://www.mosherhealth.com/mosher-health-system/chinese-medicine/yin-yang/five-elements.

Nair, V. P. (2017, May 3). *Types of ayurvedic massages and their health benefits*. Jeevana. https://www.jeevana.in/types-of-ayurvedic-massages-and-their-health-benefits/.

National Center for Complementary and Integrative Health. (2016, October). *Tai Chi and Qi Gong: In depth*. NCCIH. https://www.nccih.nih.gov/health/tai-chi-and-qi-gong-in-depth.

National Center for Complementary and Integrative Health. (2017, September). *Naturopathy*. NCCIH. https://www.nccih.nih.gov/health/naturopathy.

National Center for Complementary and Integrative Health. (2021, April). *Complementary, alternative, or integrative health: What's in a name?* NCCIH. https://www.nccih.nih.gov/health/complementary-alternative-or-integrative-health-whats-in-a-name.

Nature Health. (n.d.). *Understanding the five elements*. http://www.naturehealth.com.au/what-is-qi-gong/aspects-of-qi-gong/understanding-the-five-elements/. Accessed March 23, 2021.

Newman, T. (2017, September 6). *Everything you need to know about reiki*. MedicalNewsToday. https://www.medicalnewstoday.com/articles/308772.

Nichols, H. (2021, April 15). *How does yoga work?* MedicalNews Today. https://www.medicalnewstoday.com/articles/286745.

Nordqvist, J. (2018, August 8). *What is biofeedback therapy and who can benefit?* MedicalNewsToday. https://www.medicalnewstoday.com/articles/265802.

Nutritional Therapist of Ireland Editors. (2020, August 10). *What is nutritional therapy?* Nutritional Therapist of Ireland Ltd. https://www.ntoi.ie/what-is-nutritional-therapy/.

Oldham, P. (2019). *The mindful guide to the law of attraction: Meditations to manifest health, wealth, and love*. Rockridge Press.

Ratini, M. (2016a, December 12). *Naturopathic medicine: What you need to know*. WebMD. https://www.webmd.com/balance/guide/what-is-naturopathic-medicine#1.

Ratini, M. (2016b, December 13). Homeopathy: What it is, benefits, risks, and more. *WebMD*. https://www.webmd.com/balance/what-is-homeopathy#1.

Rekstis, E. (2022, January 21). *Healing crystals 101: Everything you need to know*. Healthline. https://www.healthline.com/health/mental-health/guide-to-healing-crystals#benefits.

ScienceDirect. (n.d.). Nutraceutical—an overview. *ScienceDirect Topics*. https://www.sciencedirect.com/topics/agricultural-and-biological-sciences/nutraceutical. Accessed March 29, 2021.

Seymour, T., & Biggers, A. (2020, May 11). *What is ozone therapy? Benefits and risks*. MedicalNewsToday. https://www.medicalnewstoday.com/articles/320759.

Shojai, P. (2019, January 6). What is Qi Gong? (And how you can start practicing today). *Yoga Journal*. https://www.yogajournal.com/yoga-101/what-is-qi-gong/.

Skarnulis, L. (2007, January 1). *Chiropractic care for back pain*. WebMD. https://www.webmd.com/pain-management/guide/chiropractic-pain-relief#1.

Soliday, E., & Hapke, P. (2013). Research on acupuncture in pregnancy and childbirth: The U.S. contribution. *Medical Acupuncture*, 25(4), 252–260. https://doi.org/10.1089/acu.2012.0950.

Staff of Massage Sense. (n.d.). *Javanese massage*. Massage Sense. https://massagesense.nl/massages/javanese-massage/. Accessed July 12, 2021.

Stanford Medicine. (n.d.). *Fellowship programs*. https://med.stanford.edu/pedsfellowships/programs.html. Accessed March 29, 2021.

Sussex Publishers. (2021). *Meditation*. Psychology Today. https://www.psychologytoday.com/us/basics/meditation.

The Ayurvedic Institute. (n.d.). *Doshas: Their elements and attributes*. https://www.ayurveda.com/resources/articles/doshas-their-lements-and-attributes.

The Editors of Encyclopaedia Britannica. (2017a, July 12). *Siddha medicine*. Encyclopedia Britannica. https://www.britannica.com/science/Siddha-medicine.

The Editors of Encyclopaedia Britannica. (2017b, July 21). *Unani medicine*. Encyclopedia Britannica. https://www.britannica.com/science/Unani-medicine.

The Foundation for Peripheral Neuropathy. (2017, November 20). *Biofeedback therapy*. https://www.foundationforpn.org/living-well/integrative-therapies/biofeedback-therapy/.

ThetaHealing Institute of Knowledge. (n.d.). *ThetaHealing: The process of meditation*. ThetaHealing. https://www.thetahealing.com/blog/thetahealing/. Accessed July 12, 2021.

Undersea & Hyperbaric Medical Society. (2021, May 3). Home. https://www.uhms.org/.

Villines, Z. (2017, December 22). *What is the best type of meditation?* MedicalNewsToday. https://www.medicalnewstoday.com/articles/320392.

Vohra, S. (2012, August 15). Pediatric integrative medicine: pediatrics' newest subspecialty? *BMC Pediatrics*, 12, 123. https://bmcpediatr.biomedcentral.com/articles/10.1186/1471-2431-12-123.

Watson, K. (2020, October 26). What is a sound bath? Everything you need to know. *Healthline*. https://www.healthline.com/health/sound-bath#vs-music-therapy.

Weil, A. (2018a, September 28). *Applied kinesiology*. DrWeil.Com. https://www.drweil.com/health-wellness/balanced-living/wellness-therapies/applied-kinesiology/.

Weil, A. (2018b, December 19). *Cranial osteopathy, craniosacral therapy*. DrWeil.Com. https://www.drweil.com/health-wellness/balanced-living/wellness-therapies/cranial-osteopathy/.

Wong, C. (2020, April 6). *What is acupuncture? What are the benefits?* Verywell Health. https://www.verywellhealth.com/acupuncture-health-uses-88407.

YJ Editors. (n.d.). *Yoga poses*. Yoga Journal. https://www.yogajournal.com/poses/.

Yoga Help 911 Staff. (n.d.). *Pranayama—Stages of breathing in yoga*. YogaHelp911. http://yogahelp911.com/stagesofbreathing.html.

Yoga Journal Editors. (n.d.). *Pranayama exercises & poses*. Yoga Journal. https://www.yogajournal.com/poses/types/pranayama/. Accessed March 12, 2021.

Yoga Logic Editor. (2020, December 29). *11 Types of pranayama breathing techniques with instructions*. Yogic Logic. https://yogic-logic.com/types-of-pranayama/.

Young Living Malaysia Sdn Bhd. (2021). *Young living products*. Young Living. https://www.youngliving.com/en_MY/products/c/home.

Yurchenko, I. (n.d.). *7 Types of ayurvedic massage you need to try ASAP*. Her Beauty. https://herbeauty.co/en/beauty/7-types-of-ayurvedic-massage-you-need-to-try-asap/. Accessed July 12, 2021.

Zope, S., & Zope, R. (2013). Sudarshan kriya yoga: Breathing for health. *International Journal of Yoga*, 6(1), 4–10. https://doi.org/10.4103/0973-6131.105935.

Acknowledgment

The author is grateful to Udyanee Jayaweera and Juanita Suhai for patiently and diligently typing the manuscript over countless nights and days. I am also thankful to family and friends who provided information on various ethnic traditional remedies. They have been a vast treasure trove.

Contributors

Danaraj Navaratnam, MBBS

Dr. Danaraj obtained his medical degree (MBBS) from Melaka Manipal Medical College. He is presently a medical officer at a public hospital in Malaysia. His travels to Sri Lanka and India have influenced his views on the importance of traditional and Eastern medicine. During the COVID-19 pandemic, his wellness was maintained via good nutrition, yoga, herbs, spices, and supplements. A severe knee football injury during his youth treated with surgery, stem cells, and supplements has made him believe that integrative healthcare is the future of medicine.

Devaraj Navaratnam, BMedSc (Hons), BMBS, MRCS

Dr. Devaraj holds an MBBS from the University of Southampton, UK, and an MRCS. He is doing his orthopedics training presently in the UK. His interest is in hip and knee problems especially in the elderly. He believes in preventive orthopedics and that bone and joint health must start from childhood, especially with good nutrition, exercise, sunshine, nutraceuticals, sports, and yoga. His spouse who is also a medical doctor believes in the power of holistic health through plant medicine, homemade vegetarian and vegan meals, fasting, and spiritual healing with meditation and mindfulness.

Sumitha Navaratnam, MBBS

Dr. Sumitha has a medical degree (MBBS) from Melaka Manipal Medical College, a joint program between India and Malaysia. Currently, she is interning in the UK. As part of her wellness strategy, she embraces Ayurveda, yoga, homoeopathy, reflexology, massages, meditation, nutrition, nutraceuticals, and sports. Having traveled widely across Asia, she strongly believes in the power of Eastern medicine, nutrition, and naturopathy as part of holistic healing. Her childhood coughs and colds were treated mostly with kitchen and garden remedies and some modern drugs. She is passionate about sharing her knowledge and practices on integrative medicine especially on TCAM.

Nicole Perrira, MBBS

Dr. Nicole graduated from Taylors University Medical College, Malaysia, with an MBBS. She is presently interning at a public hospital. Coming from a diverse cultural background, embracing Eastern and Western medicine was a natural progression and way of life. Growing up with two grandmothers of different ethnicity in a joint family, she was nourished with homemade herbal soups, rich broths, and mulligatawny (rasam) to fight infections and restore energy during childhood ailments. Their daily cuisine is also a natural antioxidant and anti-aging way of life.

Contents

1

Cardiovascular System

Introduction

Cardiovascular diseases are common in most adults. An estimated 17.9 million people die from heart-related problems each year, and it remains the leading cause of death in both men and women. The incidence of cardiovascular problems increases with age, as well as with several other risk factors, such as obesity, high blood pressure (BP), diabetes mellitus, and sedentary lifestyles.

The cardiovascular problems to be discussed include the following:
- Hypertension (high BP)
- Hyperlipidemia/hypercholesterolemia (high lipid/fat levels, including cholesterol in the blood)
- Ischemic heart disease (IHD)/coronary artery disease (CAD)
- Heart failure

Tests for Cardiovascular system (CVS) disorders include electrocardiogram (ECG), cardiac echocardiogram (ECHO) and stress ECHO, exercise stress test, 24-hour BP monitoring, computed tomography (CT) coronary angiogram, magnetic resonance imaging (MRI) of the heart, nuclear medicine perfusion testing, cardiac catheterization, angiogram (femoral or brachial), Doppler ultrasound, Holter monitoring, chest x-ray, and blood tests (lipids, High-sensitivity C-reactive protein (hs-CRP), B-type natriuretic peptide (BNP), glucose, troponin T, full blood count, kidney function tests, thyroid function tests, etc.). Wearable devices that use artificial intelligence (AI) are also evolving to identify life-threatening cardiac arrhythmias.

Hypertension (High Blood Pressure)

Hypertension refers to long-standing and persistent elevation of BP in the arteries. It can be primary or secondary, with lifestyle factors often contributing to both types. According to the American Heart Association, a normal value is less than 120/80 mm Hg. In hypertensive crises, there is sudden elevation of BP greater than 180/120 mm Hg. There are reference ranges for various age groups.

Causes

Risk factors include obesity, insulin resistance, high alcohol intake, high salt intake (in salt-sensitive patients), aging, sedentary lifestyle, stress, low potassium intake, and low calcium intake.

Hypertension can be primary or secondary. Most of the causes are due to primary or essential hypertension.

Essential/Primary/Idiopathic Hypertension: Causes
- Unknown cause in the majority
- Genetic variations or genes that are overexpressed or underexpressed and the intermediary phenotypes that they regulate can cause high BP.

Secondary Hypertension: Causes

Renal
  Parenchymal kidney disease
  Renovascular disease
Endocrine
  Pheochromocytoma
  Acromegaly
  Thyroid disease
  Parathyroid disease
  Primary aldosteronism
  Cushing syndrome
Vascular
  Coarctation of the aorta
  Takayasu arteritis
Drug induced/drug related
  Oral contraceptives, steroids, nonsteroidal antiinflammatory drugs, cyclooxygenase 2 inhibitors, and erythropoietin
Miscellaneous
  Sleep apnea

Tests include ambulatory 24-hour BP monitoring, ECG, ECHO, and basic blood biochemistry. Specific tests depend on the underlying cause.

Various natural remedies from the East and West are described as follows. A mix-and-match approach may be adopted for most of the oral recipes, depending on personal preference, because many of these recipes were sourced from the author's own personal experience and by word of mouth. Some of the remedies are universal and are used by many ethnic groups.

Indian Natural Remedies

There is no definite consensus in Ayurveda on the pathogenesis of hypertension. The vitiated Doshas occur from *Vyana*

Vata (in the mind), *Prana Vata* (in the head), *Sadhaka Pitta* (*pitta subdosha*, which is the fire of heart and mind), and *Avalambaka Kapha* (*kapha subdosha* in the chest around the pericardium and pleura), along with *Rakta* in their disturbed states. There is *Avarana* (obstruction) of *Vata Dosha* by *Pitta* and *Kapha*, which manifests in the *Rasa-Rakta Dhatu* (plasma and blood), which will then affect the functioning of the various *Srotas* (microchannels) of circulation.

Common Ingredients for Hypertension

Spices

Amla/Indian gooseberry (*Phyllanthus emblica*)
Black cumin (*Nigella sativa*)

Black pepper (*Piper nigrum*)
Cardamom (*Elettaria cardamomum*)
Cassia seeds (*Cassia obtusifolia L*)
(*Inula racemosa*)
Cinnamon (*Cinnamomum vera*)

Clove (*Syzygium aromaticum*)
Coriander (*Coriandrum sativum*)
Fenugreek (*Trigonella foenum-graecum*)
Garlic (*Allium sativum*)
Long pepper (*Piper longum*)
Onion (*Allium cepa*)

Saffron (*Crocus sativus*)
Turmeric (*Curcuma longa*)

Herbs/Leaves

Drumstick leaf (*Moringa oleifera*)
Indian snakeroot/Sarpagandha
(*Rauwolfia serpentina*)
Rose petals (*Rosa*)
Ashwagandha (*Withania somnifera*)
Pushkarmool

Punarnava (*Boerhavia diffusa*)

Chandana/sandalwood (*Santalum album*)
Bibhitaki/vibhitaki (*Terminalia bellirica*)
Haritaki (*Terminalia chebula*)
Arjuna (*Terminalia arjuna*)
Brahmi (*Bacopa monnieri*)
Jatamansi (*Nardostachys jatamansi*)

Gotu kola (*Centella asiatica*)
Gokshura (*Tribulus terrestris*)
Tulsi/holy basil

Miscellaneous

Lemon (*Citrus limon*)
Aloe vera (*Aloe barbadensis*)

Celery (*Apium graveolens*)
Honey

Moong dal
(Green gram dal)
Coconut water
Rudraksha (*Elaeocarpus ganitrus*)
Indian Coleus (*Coleus forskolii*)
Green tea (*Camellia sinensis*)
Beetroot (*Beta vulgaris*)
Fruits:
- Watermelon
(*Citrullus lanatus*)
- Pomegranate
(*Punica granatum*)
- Pineapple
(*Ananas comosus*)
Cucumber (*Cucumis sativus*)
Passion flower and leaf
(*Passiflora incarnata*)

Common Recipes

Oral

Teas/Brews/Juice/Others

Aloe vera juice. Wash and dry an aloe vera leaf. Slit the leaf in half, and remove the gel, discarding the greenish gel. Cut the remaining white gel into cubes, and store in a refrigerator. Add the gel to any fruit juice, and blend.

Amla juice. Lightly pound three to four amla fruits, and strain the juice. Take this juice on an empty stomach in the morning with a glass of warm water.

   Variation #1. *Amla paste.* Lightly pound three to four amla fruits, and mix with honey to make a paste. Take this paste every morning.

Ashwagandha brew. Mix 1 teaspoon of ashwagandha powder into a cup of warm milk. Add honey to taste.

Arjuna tea. Add a cup of water and a cup of milk. Warm gently. Add 1 teaspoon of arjuna powder, and mix well. Boil, and then simmer until the brew has been reduced to 1 cup. Strain, and add honey to taste.

Black cumin (nigella seeds) tea. Take 1 tablespoon of nigella seeds. Crush them. Add 1 cup of hot water. Steep for 10 minutes. Strain, and drink.

Black pepper tea. Take 1 teaspoon of black pepper powder, 1 teaspoon of tea leaves, and ½-inch ginger (chopped). Add 1 cup of water, and boil. Add ½ cup of milk. Strain, and add sugar to taste. Drink warm.

Beetroot juice. Peel and cut a fresh beetroot into small pieces. Add 1 cup water, and blend. Strain the mixture, and drink.

Brahmi juice. Take a handful of fresh brahmi leaves, and blend with little water until smooth. Drink 5 to 10 mL of the juice with 1 teaspoon of honey every day.

Cardamom powder. Finely grind cardamom seeds into a powder. Take ½ teaspoon of cardamom powder once a day.

Cassia seed tea. Place 15 to 20 g of cassia seeds into a pot with 1 cup of water. Boil, and simmer for 15 minutes before straining.

Celery juice. Cut two to three stalks of celery into smaller pieces, and blend with some water. Drink once a day.

Cinnamon paste. Mix ground cinnamon with honey to make a paste. Take 1 teaspoon of this mixture once a day.

Clove paste. Crush four to five cloves, and mix with honey to make a paste. Take this twice a week.

Coconut water. Consume fresh young coconut water.

Coriander and gokshura brew. Add one part of coriander powder and one part of gokshura to a pot of water. Boil gently for approximately 5 to 10 minutes. Allow to cool, and drink three times a day.

Cucumber juice. Cut one cucumber into smaller chunks. Blend until smooth, and drink.

Fenugreek tea. Take 2 teaspoons of fenugreek seeds. Lightly crush them. Add 1 cup of water. Boil, and then simmer for approximately 5 minutes till the water is pale yellow-brown. Strain, and consume the liquid. The seeds can be eaten at the same time. It can be taken once or twice a day.

Variation #1. Roast the fenugreek seeds lightly. Ground them, and store in an airtight bottle. Take 1 to 2 teaspoons of the powder, and add 1 cup of hot water. Allow to steep for 15 minutes, and consume.

Variation #2. Take a teaspoon of fenugreek. Add a glass of water, and soak overnight. Drink the water and eat the seeds on an empty stomach in the morning.

Garlic brew. Pound or blend two to three cloves of garlic. Add the garlic to a pot with a cup of milk. Gently heat the mixture for approximately 5 to 10 minutes. Consume.

Variation #1. *Fresh garlic cloves.* Consume one to four cloves of fresh garlic daily.

Gotu Kola tea. Steep a teaspoon of fresh or dried gotu kola leaves in a cup of hot water for approximately 10 to 15 minutes. Drink it warm.

Green tea. Steep 1 teaspoon of dried green tea leaves in a cup of hot water for approximately 10 to 15 minutes.

Gulkand (rose petal jam). Thoroughly wash a cup of fresh rose petals, and allow to dry. Chop the petals into thin slices, and mix with honey. Close the jar tightly, and allow it to sit in the sunlight for 7 to 10 days, mixing it with a clean spoon every other day. Take 1 to 2 teaspoons of Gulkand every day.

Indian coleus. Boil the roots of the coleus to make tea. It is also available as a supplement.

Indian snakeroot. The root powder or leaves are consumed as powder. It is also available as capsules.

Jatamansi brew. Add a pinch of jatamansi root powder to a cup of warm water, and take it twice a day.

Moringa leaf juice. Lightly pound some moringa leaves, and extract the juice. Mix with honey and take once a day. Dried leaf powder is also available.

Variation #1. *Moringa leaves.* Consume as a stir-fry.

Pineapple juice. Peel and cut a pineapple into small chunks. Blend with some water. Strain if required, and consume fresh.

Pomegranate juice. Blend the pomegranate until smooth. Strain if required. Consume fresh.

Punarnava tea. Add one part each of dried punarnava, one part of dried passion fruit flower, and two parts of dried hawthorn berries. Take approximately half a teaspoon of this mixture. Add 1 cup of hot water, and steep for approximately 10 minutes. Drink twice a day, after lunch and dinner.

Passion fruit and passion fruit leaf. The leaves are sliced finely and made into a sambal/sambola (mixed with sliced shallots, green chili, lime juice, and salt) and eaten as a salad in Sri Lankan cuisine.

Variation #1: To make tea, take 2 teaspoons of dried passion fruit leaves and/or flower. Add 1 cup of hot water. Steep for 5 to 10 minutes. Strain, and consume. Some fresh fruit pulp can also be added.

Variation #2: Cut two or three fruits. Scoop pulp with the seeds. Blend with some water and consume.

Pushkarmool. Take 1 to 3 g of the root powder with honey or with water twice a day.

Rudraksha. Place the Rudraksha in a copper jug or pot filled with 250 ml water. Leave it overnight. Consume this water first thing in the morning on an empty stomach.

For better efficacy, add 2 grams Rudraksha powder (churna) into 250 ml of water in a copper vessel. Leave overnight and consume the next morning. Alternatively, a decoction can be made by adding 5 grams Rudraksha churna into 400 ml water and boiling till the volume is reduced to 100 ml.

Copper may increase the antihypertensive property of Rudraksha.

Saffron tea. Add three to five strands of saffron to a cup of hot water, and cover. Steep for 5 to 10 minutes before straining. Drink warm.

Trikatu brew. Steep equal parts of black pepper, long pepper, and ginger in a cup of hot water. Steep for approximately 10 to 15 minutes. Drink it warm.

Triphala tea. Add half a teaspoon of triphala powder to 1 cup of hot water. Mix well, and drink it warm.

Tulsi tea. Place a handful of tulsi leaves into a pot of water. Bring to a boil, and reduce the heat. Allow the mixture to simmer for 5 to 10 minutes. Strain, and drink twice a day.

Turmeric paste. Mix 3 to 6 g of ground turmeric with honey or ghee to form a paste. Consume two to three times a day.

Turmeric tea. Take 2 teaspoons of turmeric powder into 3 to 4 cups of hot water. Stir, and steep for approximately 5 to 10 minutes. Strain. Add honey, fresh lemon juice, or milk to taste.

Watermelon juice. Blend the watermelon until smooth. Consume fresh.

Therapeutic Measures

Diet
Eat a healthy diet that is low in salt and fats and high in potassium and fiber. Consume plenty of whole grains, moong dal (green gram), and fruits and vegetables such as watermelon, lemon, celery, and cucumber. Add raw onion to meals to salads or as an appetizer. They can also be made into fresh juice.

Lifestyle
Keep fit and active with daily or regular exercises, yoga, or sports for at least 20 to 30 minutes per day for most days of the week to regulate BP.

Place a cold pack on the spine to reduce BP.

Limit or omit alcohol and cigarettes

Practice good sleep hygiene. Maintain adequate sleep of 7 to 8 hours.

Practice meditation or mindfulness.

Apply sandalwood essential oil on the temples or inhale.

Yoga Asanas
Aromatherapy with essential oils such as rose oil can help to manage stress

These include:

Surya Namaskar (sun salutation)

Shavasana (corpse pose)

Bhujangasana (cobra pose)

Balasana (child pose)

Setu Bandha Sarvangasana (bridge pose)

Sukhasana (easy pose)

Adho Mukha Svanasana (downward-facing dog pose)
Anulom Vilom Pranayam (alternate nostril breathing)

Purification (Detoxification)

Virechana (purgation): Virechana (therapeutic purgation) is part of the panchakarma treatments. Various Virechaka dravyas (oral purgatives) such as triphala, castor oil, trikatu, and dani are given by mouth.

Basti (enema): Medicated sesame oil and herbal enemas are used. *(Anuvasana Basti)*

Rakta mokshana (bloodletting). This is done via venesection.

Chinese Natural Remedies

In traditional Chinese medicine (TCM), hypertension is often attributed to four theories: yin deficiency–yang hyperactivity (YD), yin-yang deficiency (YY), liver-fire ascending syndrome (LF), and dampness-phlegm accumulation syndrome (DP).

Treatment is based on the principles to calm the liver, reinforce deficiency, and remove blood stasis. The herbs used will cover the liver, heart, and kidney meridians. Uncaria (cat's claw), *Scutellaria baicalensis* (skullcap), Achyranthes, and Poria are widely used together with other herbs as TCM polyherbal formula.

Common Ingredients for Hypertension

Spices	Herbs/Leaves/Flowers	Miscellaneous
Black cumin/xiao hui xiang (*Nigella sativa*)	Asian ginseng/ren shen (*Panax ginseng*)	Lemon/ning meng (*Citrus limon*)
	Chinese skullcap/huang qin (*Scutellaria baicalensis*)	Wolfberry fruit/gou qi zi (*Lycium barbarum*)
	Red sage/salvia/danshen (*Salvia miltiorrhiza*)	Hawthorn berry
	Moutan peony/mu dan pi (*Paeonia suffruticosa Andr.*)	Gastrodia rhizome/tian ma (*Gastrodia elata*)
	Chrysanthemum/ju hua	Gardenia fruit/zhi zi (*Fructus gardeniae*)
	Poria cocos/fu ling (*Wolfiporia extensa*)	Pearl shell powder
	Mulberry mistletoe/sang ji sheng (*Taxillus chinensis*)	Abalone shell/shi jue ming
	Anemarrhena rhizome/zhi mu (*Anemarrhena asphodeloides*)	Kudzu (*Pueraria montana*/*Pueraria lobata*)
	Gentian/qin jiao (*Gentiana scabra*)	
Ginger/sheng jiang (*Zingiber officinalis*)	Ox knee root/huai niu xi (*Achyranthes bidentata*)	
	Cat's claw/gou teng (*Uncaria tomentosa*)	Celery/qin cai (*Apium graveolens*)

Common Recipes

Oral

Teas/Brews/Juice

Cat's claw tea. Cat's claw is available as bark or in a powder form. To make the tea, boil some water and pour into a cup. Add one or two pieces of bark or 1 to 2 teaspoons of the powder to the water. Add a few drops of lemon juice, and mix well.

Celery juice. Wash and cut two stalks of celery. Add water, and blend till smooth. Strain, and drink the juice.

Celery leaf tea. Place a handful of celery leaves in a pot of boiling water. Boil, and then simmer for approximately 15 minutes. Strain the mixture, and drink.

Celery seed tea. Lightly crush ½ tablespoon of celery seeds. Steep in a cup of hot water for approximately 20 minutes. Strain the mixture, and drink.

Chrysanthemum tea. Take a handful of dried chrysanthemum flowers into a pot with 2 cups of water. Bring to a boil, and then remove from the heat. Strain, and drink throughout the day.

Gastrodia rhizome tea. Cut dry slices. Boil in hot water. Add honey to taste. Consume warm.

Ginger tea. Lightly pound approximately 1 to 2 inches of fresh ginger (if unavailable, use 1 to 2 teaspoons of ginger powder), and add to a cup of hot water. Allow to steep for 5 to 10 minutes. Strain, and drink while warm. Add honey to taste.

Ginseng brew. Add two to three slices of panax ginseng to a cup of hot water, and allow it to steep for 5 to 10 minutes. Drink it warm.

Hawthorn berry tea. Take approximately 1 teaspoon of dried hawthorn berries. Boil in hot water, and simmer for 10 to 15 minutes. Strain, and consume twice a day. Add honey if required.

Common Polyherbal Formula for Hypertension

Tian Ma Gou Teng Yin decoction (TGD). The commonly used 11 herbs include gou teng (cat's claw), tian ma (gastrodia rhizome), shi jue ming (abalone shell), huang qin (Chinese skullcap), fu ling (poria cocos), huai niu xi (ox knee root), du zhong (eucommia bark), sang ji sheng (mulberry mistletoe), zhi zi (gardenia), yi mu cao (Chinese motherwort), and he shou wu (fleeceflower root). It is also known as "Gastrodia and Uncaria granules."

Zhengan Xifeng decoction (ZGXFD). The commonly used 12 herbs include dai zhe shi (hematite), huai niu xi (ox knee), gui ban (turtle shell), long gu (dragon bone), mu li ke (oyster shell), chuan lian zi (Chinaberry), bai shao (peony), xuan shen (figwort root), tian men dong (Chinese asparagus tuber), gan cao (licorice), mai ya (barley sprouts), and yin chen (wormwood).

Ban Xia Bai Zhu Tian Ma Tang decoction. It contains tian ma (gastrodia rhizome), chen pi (tangerine peel), fu ling (poria cocos), bai zhu (atractylodes rhizomes), ban xia (crow-dipper rhizome), da zao (jujube dates), gan cao (liquorice), and sheng jiang (ginger).

Compound Danshen formula (CDF). The key ingredients include danshen (red sage), bing pian (borneol), and san qi (pseudoginseng).

Bushen Qinggan. The key ingredients include huang qin (skullcaps), gou teng (cat's claw), tian ma (gastrodia rhizome), du zhong (eucommia bark), and kuding cha (bitter butyl tea).

Songling Xuezhikang capsule. The key ingredients include powdered mu li (pearl oyster shell), ge gen (kudzuvine root), and song ye (pine needles).

Yiqi Huaju formula (huangqi, huanglian, pu huang, zexie, and yinchen). The key ingredients include Radix astragali (milk vetch root), Pollen typhae (cattail pollen), Artemisia capillaris (oriental wormwood), Rhizoma coptidis (Chinese gold thread), and Rhizoma alismatis (water plantain tuber).

Jiangya capsule. The key ingredients include Radix achyranthis (two formulations of achyranthes root used), Thallus sargassum pallidum (seaweed), Pheretima aspergillum (earthworm extract), Szechwan lovage rhizome (lovage root), and Rhizoma gastrodiae (orchid).

Pinggan Tishen Ditan Yin decoction. The key ingredients include Rhizoma gastrodiae (orchid), Alisma plantago-aquatica (mad-dog weed/common water-plantain), Radix achyranthis (achyranthes root), Uncaria rhynchophylla (gambir plant), Rhizoma atractylodis macrocephalae (bai zhu), Prunella vulgaris (common self-heal), and Pinellia ternata (crow-dipper), Thallus sargassum pallidum (seaweed), Cassia torae (sickle senna), Taxillus chinensis (loranthus), and Pheretima aspergillum (earthworm extract).

Calming Gan and suppressing hyperactive yang (CGSHY) decoction. The key ingredients include Rhizoma gastrodiae (orchid), Uncaria rhynchophylla (gambir plant), Radix achyranthis (achyranthes root) Concha haliotidis (abalone shell), and Concha ostreae (oyster shell).

Er Xian Tang. The key ingredients include yin yang huo (epimedium herbs), dang gui (dong quai), xian mao (curculigo rhizomes), ba ji tian (morinda roots), zhi mu (anemarrhena rhizomes), and huang bo (phellodendron bark).

Kudzu. Oral puerarin is available as a supplement.

Therapeutic Measures

Lifestyle
Tuina massage, tai chi, and qigong: These measures also help to lower BP. Refer under "TCM" pages 11 and 15.

Acupuncture
Refer to "TCM" page xxii and also below.

Acupressure
GB 20 (gallbladder 20) is an acupressure point also known as wind pool. It is located in the depression at the back of the neck on either side of the vertebra and at the base of the skull. With your fingers, firmly massage this area for up to 1 minute while breathing slowly and deeply. This point is believed to be able to stabilize BP and relieve headaches associated with hypertension.

GV 20 (governing vessel 20) is also known as hundred convergences. It is located at the top of the head, exactly halfway on an imaginary line drawn from ear to ear. Massage this point with your fingers for 1 to 2 minutes to relieve hypertension.

LI 11 (large intestine 11) is also called the crooked pond and is located on the outer edge of the elbow crease. Massage this area on both arms firmly for up to 1 minute to reduce BP and inflammation.

LI 4 (large intestine 4) is also known as the union valley and is found in the midpoint of the webbing between the index finger and thumb. Massage this area for up to 1 minute.

ST 36 (stomach 36) is also called the leg 3 miles and is found four finger widths below the lower edge of the kneecap and one finger width away from the shin bone on the outer edge of the leg. Massage this area firmly for approximately 1 minute.

PC 6 (pericardium 6) is known as the inner gate and is located on the midpoint approximately three finger widths below the wrist crease. Massage this area for approximately 1 to 2 minutes to aid circulation and hence reduce BP.

GB 34 (gallbladder 34) is also known as the yang hill spring and is found on the outer side of the lower leg in the hollow below the head of the fibula bone. This point should be stimulated by applying firm pressure for 1 to 2 minutes with an index finger.

LV 3 (liver 3) is also known as the "supreme rushing" or "great rushing" and is found on the top of the foot in the web between the big and second toe. This point should be massaged for approximately 1 minute to reduce BP. It calms irritability and anger.

HT 7 (heart 7) is also known as the spirit gate and is located on the wrist crease. Apply firm pressure with a thumb for approximately a minute.

KD 1 (kidney 1) is also called the "bubbling/gushing spring" and can be found on the sole of the foot between the second and third toes, approximately one-third of the way down the foot. This point should be firmly massaged for 1 to 2 minutes to reduce BP.

Western/Other Natural Remedies

Common Ingredients for Hypertension

Spices	Herbs/Leaves	Miscellaneous
Cardamom (*Elettaria cardamomum*)	Basil (*Ocimum basilicum*)	Beetroot (*Beta vulgaris*)
	Mint (*Mentha*)	Pomegranate (*Punica granatum*)
	Lavender (*Lavandula angustifolia*)	Dark chocolate
	Rooibos leaves (*Aspalathus linearis*)	Lemon (*Citrus limon*)

Spices	Herbs/Leaves	Miscellaneous
	Parsley (*Petroselinum crispum*)	Honey
	Watercress (*Nasturtium officinale*)	Cod liver oil or olive oil
	Buchu (*Agathosma betulina*)	Apple cider vinegar (*Malus pumila Mill.*)
	Guelder rose bark (*Viburnum opulus*)	Hibiscus (*Hibiscus rosa-sinensis*)
	Blackcurrant leaves (*Ribes nigrum*)	Olive leaf extract
	Cattail (*Typha angustifolia*)	Rose oil
Cayenne pepper (*Capsicum annuum*)	Rosemary (*Rosmarinus officinalis*)	Watermelon (*Citrullus lanatus*)
Cinnamon (*Cinnamomum vera*)	Marjoram (*Origanum majorana*)	Seeds: flax, pumpkin, sunflower
Ginger (*Zingiber officinalis*)	Oregano (*Origanum vulgare*)	Nuts: walnuts, peanuts, almond, pistachio, cashew

Common Recipes

Oral

Teas/Brews/Others

Apple cider vinegar. Add 5 to 10 drops of apple cider vinegar to a cup of hot water. Add honey to taste, and drink once a day in the morning.

Basil juice. Place a handful of fresh basil leaves into a pot of water. Boil, and then let cool. Allow the mixture to steep for approximately 5 to 10 minutes. Strain the mixture, and store it in a jar. Take 1 teaspoon twice a day.

Beetroot juice. Cut a fresh beetroot into smaller cubes. Place the beetroot cubes into a blender, and blend while gradually adding 1 cup of water to the blender. Strain the mixture, and drink.

Blackcurrant tea. Take 1 teaspoon of fresh chopped leaves (or 1 to 2 teaspoons of dried leaves), and add 1 cup of hot water. Steep for 5 to 10 minutes. Strain, and drink.

Buchu tea. Finely chop some fresh buchu leaves, and add approximately 1 teaspoon to an empty cup. Pour boiling water into the cup, and allow it to steep for approximately 10 minutes before straining and drinking the tea.

Cattail. The roots or young stems can be eaten raw, boiled or baked. The dried roots are also ground into powder and used as a thickener. The seeds, stem and pollen are also edible. The pollen is easily harvested, sieved and added to juices, shakes, or used as protein-rich flour.

Variation #1 Take 1 to 2 teaspoons of the dried root powder. Add 1 cup of water. Simmer for 5 minutes. Consume 4 to 6 cups a day.

Cayenne pepper. Add a pinch of cayenne pepper to a cup of soup.

Cinnamon tea. Add a stick of cinnamon to a pot of hot water, and allow it to steep for approximately 10 minutes. Add honey to taste, and drink.

Coconut water. Split a young coconut in half, and collect the juice in a cup. Drink once a day in the morning, preferably on an empty stomach.

Cod liver oil or olive oil. Consume 1 tablespoon of cod liver oil or olive oil once a day.

Dark chocolate. Consume one small square of dark chocolate every day to help lower BP.

Flaxseed. Blend 30 g of flaxseed, and add to salads or smoothies.

Ginger-cardamom tea. Lightly pound four to five slices of fresh ginger. Place into a pot of water, bring to a boil before lowering the heat, and simmer for 5 to 10 minutes. Add a teaspoon of cardamom powder to the mixture, and mix well.

Guelder rose bark (Cramp bark). Add 1 to 3 teaspoons of the broken-up cramp bark to a cup of hot water, and steep for 5 to 15 minutes. Alternatively, it can be simmered with 2 cups of water. Strain, and drink three times per day. Add honey to taste.

It is also available as a dietary supplement or tincture.

Hibiscus tea. Take three or four washed fresh hibiscus flowers. Remove the stamen and calyx. Add 1 cup hot water. Steep for approximately 5 to 10 minutes. Remove the decolorized petals. Consume warm or chilled. Add some lemon juice if desired (the tea will be more ruby-red) and/or some mint leaves.

Alternatively, use 1.5 teaspoons dried hibiscus flowers and steep longer.

Lavender leaves. Lavender can be added to baked goods, desserts, and marinades.

Lemon juice. Juice one lemon, and add the juice to a cup of water. Mix well, and drink once a day in the morning.

Marjoram tea. Add a few dried leaves into 1 cup of hot water. Steep for a few minutes. Drink warm.

Mint tea. Place a handful of mint leaves into a pot of water. Bring to a boil, and reduce the heat. Allow the mixture to simmer for 5 to 10 minutes. Strain, and drink twice a day.

Nuts. Consume 1 to 2 cups of nuts per week.

Olive leaf extract. Consume olive leaf extract capsules once a day.

Oregano tea. Add approximately 3 teaspoons of fresh oregano leaves to a cup of hot water, and steep for 5 to 10 minutes. Strain, and add honey to taste.

Parsley tea or juice. Cut a handful of fresh parsley into smaller pieces, and submerge fully in a pot of water. Boil for 3 to 4 minutes, and then cool completely. Strain, and drink three to four times a day.

Variation #1. Cut ¼ cup of parsley into smaller pieces, and place into a pot. Pour 1 cup of boiling water over the parsley, and allow it to steep for 5 to 10 minutes. The longer it steeps, the more bitter the drink becomes. Add honey to taste. Strain, and drink 1 to 2 cups every day.

Variation #2. To make fresh juice, place 3 cups of freshly cut parsley and little ginger (if desired) into a blender.

Blend until smooth, gradually adding up to 1 cup of water. Strain, and drink two to three times a week.

Pomegranate juice. Remove the pomegranate seeds, and place in a blender. Blend until smooth, and strain before drinking. Consume 150 mL of the juice daily.

Rooibos tea. Add 1 teaspoon of loose rooibos tea leaves into 1 cup of boiling water. Steep for approximately 5 to 10 minutes. Strain, and consume.

Rosemary tea. Add 1½ teaspoons of dry rosemary needles to a cup of hot water, and allow it to steep for 10 to 15 minutes. Drink it warm.

Watercress. Use as a garnish or add to salads, soups, smoothies, or sandwiches.

Watermelon juice. Refer to "Indian Natural Remedies" earlier.

Therapeutic Measures

Diet

Dietary approaches to stop hypertension (DASH diet): The DASH diet is an approach to healthy eating aimed at treating and preventing high BP. It encourages a reduction in sodium intake and to eat a variety of nutrient-rich foods that may help to lower BP (potassium, magnesium, calcium).

Inuit/Icelandic diet: The Icelandic people have diets rich in whale blubber fats, which are rich in omega-3 fatty acids. This has been found to be heart protective because it may help to decrease triglycerides, BP, and the risk of blood clotting.

Magnesium-rich foods: Nuts (cashew and almond) and seeds (pumpkin and sunflower).

Potassium-rich foods: Fruits (oranges and bananas), dried fruits (dates, raisins, prunes, and apricot), and vegetables (greens, tomatoes, and spinach).

High-fiber food: Consume whole grain foods such as whole wheat products and brown rice.

Lifestyle

Meditation is a way of life that has been found to be beneficial in reducing high BP.

New research has found a potential link between the number of push-ups and cardiovascular health. It has been found that individuals (regardless of gender) who are able to do more than 40 push-ups may have a lowered risk of developing cardiovascular disease.

Aromatherapy with essential oils such as rose oil can help to manage stress.

Modern Remedies

Antihypertensive Agents: Classification

No.	Category	Examples
1.	Calcium channel blockers	Verapamil, nifedipine, nimodipine, amlodipine, diltiazem, felodipine
2.	β-Blockers	Propranolol, metoprolol, atenolol, bisoprolol, labetalol
3.	Angiotensin-converting enzyme (ACE) inhibitors	Captopril, ramipril, enalapril, lisinopril
4.	Angiotensin II receptor blockers (ARBs)	Losartan, telmisartan, valsartan, olmesartan,
5.	Angiotensin receptor neprilysin inhibitor (ARNI)	Sacubitril/valsartan
6.	Diuretics	Chlorothiazide, hydrochlorothiazide, furosemide
7.	α-Blockers	Prazosin, terazosin, doxazosin
8.	Vasodilators	Diazoxide, sodium nitroprusside, hydralazine, minoxidil, nitroglycerin
9.	Centrally acting α_2 agonists	Clonidine, guanfacine, tizanidine, methyldopa (Aldomet)

Calcium Channel Blockers

Calcium channel blockers work by blocking calcium channels in vascular smooth muscles as well as in cardiac cells, hence reducing calcium entry into these areas. Because calcium is responsible for stimulating smooth muscle contraction and cardiac muscle contraction, a reduction in calcium leads to a reduction in stimulation of smooth muscle and cardiac muscle. This causes relaxation of the smooth muscle and cardiac muscle, decreased force of the heart pumping, and a decreased heart rate. It also dilates blood vessels in the body, reducing resistance to blood flow and reducing the burden on the heart, hence helping to reduce BP.

Examples: Verapamil, amlodipine, and nifedipine

β-Blockers

β-Blockers are a group of medication that binds to β receptors, which blocks the binding of epinephrine and norepinephrine. Epinephrine and norepinephrine are hormones that are released in response to stress and cause constriction of the blood vessels as well as an increased heart rate, leading to higher BP. By blocking the binding of these hormones, effects such as increased heart rate and vessel constriction are reduced. There are two types of β receptors: β_1 and β_2. Both these types of receptors are present in cardiac muscle, although β_1 receptors are the predominant receptors. β_2 Receptors are mostly present in vascular smooth muscle. There are three generations of β-blockers, depending on their individual binding sites in the body.

First-generation β-blockers are nonselective and block both β_1 and β_2 receptors in the body. Examples are propranolol and sotalol.

Second-generation β-blockers block only β_1 receptors located in the cardiac muscle. Examples are metoprolol, bisoprolol, and atenolol.

Third-generation β-blockers are medications that have vasodilator properties through the additional blocking of α receptors. Examples are carvedilol and nebivolol.

Angiotensin-Converting Enzyme Inhibitor

Angiotensin-converting enzyme (ACE) inhibitors cause vasodilation by inhibiting the formation of angiotensin II. Angiotensin II is a hormone that causes constriction of the blood vessels, as well as stimulating the hormone aldosterone, which causes retention of sodium and water in the kidneys, hence increasing blood volume. Its formation is inhibited by the blocking of the action of ACE, the enzyme responsible for the conversion of angiotensin I to angiotensin II. ACE inhibitors cause dilation of the blood vessels, hence reducing the workload of the heart. They also promote renal excretion of sodium and water, hence reducing blood volume and ultimately BP.

Examples: Enalapril, Lisinopril, and Captopril

Angiotensin II Receptor Blockers

Angiotensin II receptor blockers (ARBs) have a similar effect to ACE inhibitors but have a different mechanism of action. They function by competitively binding to angiotensin II receptors in the body, hence preventing angiotensin II from binding to the receptors and causing similar effects as ACE inhibitors. Ultimately, they reduce the workload of the heart, which thus reduces the BP.

Examples: Losartan, valsartan, and eprosartan

Angiotensin Receptor Neprilysin Inhibitor

Neprilysin is an enzyme that degrades atrial and brain natriuretic peptides, which are BP-lowering peptides and act by reducing the blood volume.

Example: *Sacubitril/valsartan* is a combination drug. *Sacubitril* is a prodrug that, when activated, becomes a neprilysin inhibitor. It is always combined with an ARB drug to block the excess angiotensin II. It is used in chronic heart failure.

Diuretics

Water retention often occurs if the kidneys are less effective at excreting fluid from the body and regulating fluid volume. This may lead to symptoms such as swelling in the ankles, feet, and hands. This can be controlled by reducing fluid and salt intake and through the use of medication called diuretics, which help the body to excrete more sodium and water. This means that the fluid volume in the body is reduced, relieving symptoms of water retention and lowering the BP. Diuretics are often taken once a day in the morning, and there are different types.

Thiazide diuretics: hydrochlorothiazide, metolazone, indapamide

Loop diuretics: furosemide, bumetanide

Potassium-sparing diuretics (mineralocorticoid receptor blockers): spironolactone, amiloride

Side effects of diuretics include electrolyte imbalance (low sodium, low or high potassium), headache, dizziness, increased glucose or uric acid, muscle cramps.

α-Blockers

These drugs bind to the α adrenergic (mostly α_1) receptors on the smooth muscle of blood vessels and dilate the arteries and veins. Side effects include nasal congestion, headache, dizziness, orthostatic hypotension, tachycardia, and fluid retention.

Vasodilators

They act directly on the blood vessel walls to cause vasodilatation, allowing more blood flow.

Centrally Acting α₂ Adrenergic Agonists

There is presynaptic inhibition of neurotransmitters (epinephrine and norepinephrine) in the brain stem, hence reducing sympathetic outflow. Side effects include dry nasal passage and mouth, constipation, bradycardia, and sedation.

Homeopathic Remedies

These include Crataegus oxycantha, Natrum muriaticum, Baryta carbonica, Rauwolfia serpentina, Adrenalinum, sulfur, Convallaria, Calcarea carbonica, Passiflora incarnata, Thuja occidentalis, Thyroidinum, Aurum metallicum, etc.

Hyperlipidemia/Hypercholesterolemia (High Lipid and Cholesterol Levels)

Cholesterol is a natural fatty substance in the blood. It is also a building block in vitamin D and steroid hormone synthesis in our body. It is important to keep blood cholesterol levels within the normal range. Excessive amounts can block arteries, leading to atherosclerosis and then heart disease or stroke.

There are three types of cholesterol (high-density lipoprotein [HDL], low-density lipoprotein [LDL], and very-low-density lipoprotein [VLDL]) and triglyceride. Normal total cholesterol level should be approximately 3 mmol/L (120 mg/dL).

Causes and contributing factors include poor lifestyle (high-fat diet, alcohol, and sedentary habits), family history, genetic factors (e.g., high homocysteine levels), or associated medical conditions (e.g., diabetes, liver disease).

A fasting lipid profile will identify the types and level of cholesterol.

Indian Natural Remedies

There is abnormal metabolism and accumulation of *meda* (fat) and *meda dhatu* (fat tissue) in the body from decreased *agni* and, initially, vitiated Kapha dosha, and then later Pitta and Vata dosha imbalance.

Common Ingredients for Hyperlipidemia

Spices	Herbs/Leaves	Miscellaneous
Black pepper (Piper nigrum)	Sweet broom (Scoparia dulcis) Pushkarmool (Inula racemosa)	Black gram/urad
Coriander seeds (Coriandrum sativum)	Guggulu (Commiphora wightii)	Grains: Unpolished rice, brown rice, millet, quinoa, oats
Cumin (Nigella sativa)	Coriander leaf (Coriandrum sativum)	Virgin coconut oil
Fennel (Foeniculum vulgare)	Trikatu	Salty lassi/ buttermilk

Spices	Herbs/Leaves	Miscellaneous
Fenugreek (*Trigonella foenum-graecum*)	Triphala	Curry leaf lassi/buttermilk
Garlic (*Allium sativum*)	Spinach (*Spinacia oleracea*)	Pulses/dried beans
Ground ginger (*Zingiber officinalis*)	Curry leaf (*Murraya koenigii*)	Lemon
Holy basil or tulsi (*Ocimum tenuiflorum*)	Alfalfa (*Medicago sativa*)	Yogurt
Turmeric (*Curcuma longa*)	Arjuna (*Terminalia arjuna*)	Sesame oil

Common Recipes

Oral

Teas/Brews/Others

Alfalfa juice. Place a handful of fresh alfalfa into a blender, and gradually add water. Blend till smooth. Drink on its own or mixed with other fruit or vegetable juice. Fresh alfalfa may also be added to salads.

Arjuna tea. Add a cup of water and a cup of milk to a pan and warm gently. Add 1 teaspoon of arjuna powder, and mix well. Boil, and then simmer until the brew has been reduced to 1 cup. Strain, and add honey to taste.

Coriander seed tea. Grind coriander seeds into a fine powder, and add 1 tablespoon of this to a pot of water. Bring to a boil, and reduce to heat to allow the mixture to simmer for 5 minutes. Drink once a day.

Coriander leaf tea. Place a handful of cut coriander leaves into a pot of water and bring to a boil. Reduce the heat, and simmer for 5 to 10 minutes. Strain, and drink twice a day.
Variation #1. Take 10 to 20 coriander leaves. Add water, and soak overnight. Strain, and consume in the morning on an empty stomach. Add fresh lemon juice if desired.

Curry leaf lassi/buttermilk. Grind or pound some curry leaves with a little water. Add 1 teaspoon of the curry leaf paste to a glass of buttermilk, and blend. Drink this on an empty stomach.

Curry leaves and turmeric. Add curry leaves and turmeric to cooked dishes to reduce cholesterol levels.

Garlic cloves. Consume one to four cloves of garlic (raw, grilled, or added to cooked dishes) daily.

Guggulu. Adults can take approximately 25 mg of guggulu supplements every day after a meal.

Lemon juice. Squeeze ½ a lemon into a glass of water. Drink on an empty stomach in the morning.

Pushkarmool. Take 1 to 3 g of the root powder with honey or with water twice a day.

Salty lassi/buttermilk. Place ¼ cup of yogurt, ¾ cup of water, a small piece of ginger (optional), cumin, black pepper, and salt in a blender. Blend together until smooth. Decorate with chopped fresh coriander if necessary. Add ice, and drink.
Variation #1. Take ¼ cup of yogurt, ¾ of cold water, and a pinch of salt into a blender. Blend briefly and discard the foam if necessary. Transfer the mixture to a cup. Add a little ground ginger, ¼ teaspoon of cumin powder, pepper, and ¼ teaspoon of ground coriander leaf.

Sesame oil. Use sesame oil in cooking because it is unrefined and unsaturated.

Spice mixture. Combine ground turmeric (three parts), ground cumin (six parts), ground coriander (six parts), ground fennel (six parts), ground fenugreek (two parts), ground ginger (one part), and ground black pepper (one part). Store the mixture in a jar, and use 1 teaspoon a day as seasoning in any cooked dish.

Sweet broom brew. Take seeds or a handful of leaves or whole plants. Add it into warm water. Leave overnight, and drink in the morning. Alternatively, the leaves can also be chewed.

Tiger nuts. It can be sprouted, roasted or dried and eaten.

Triphala tea. To be prepared as described under treatments for hypertension.

Trikatu tea. To be prepared as described under treatments for hypertension.

Tulsi tea. Place a handful of tulsi leaves into a pot of water. Bring to a boil, and reduce the heat. Allow the mixture to simmer for 5 to 10 minutes. Strain, and drink twice a day.

Polyherbs. Commercial formulations (e.g., Liposem) contain guggulu, Arjuna, Garcinia indica, Gokshura, and Saptaranga

Therapeutic Measures

Lifestyle
A healthy lifestyle should be adopted to reduce cholesterol levels. Quit smoking and drinking alcohol.

Regular exercise is also important. Yoga is also beneficial.

Diet
Avoid overly sweet, sour, or salty foods. Instead, opt for more bitter and astringent foods such as lentils (e.g., black gram), broccoli, cabbage, and cauliflower. Eat lots of greens such as spinach, kale, and mustard greens. Healthy grains such as oats, unpolished rice, brown rice, millet, and quinoa also boost fat metabolism in the body and hence help to reduce cholesterol levels.

Unrefined and unsaturated oils
Use healthy unsaturated and unrefined oils such as sesame oil, mustard oil, and extra virgin coconut oil in cooking. Avoid saturated fats and trans fats.

Chinese Natural Remedies

Certain herbs can strengthen specific organs, which in turn can help to reduce cholesterol levels. Symptoms of high cholesterol are believed to vary based on the specific organ causing high cholesterol. The organs that may cause high cholesterol are listed as follows.

Stomach. If the stomach receives too much food, it may produce symptoms such as excessive hunger and thirst, a craving for greasy food, dry stool, and yellow urine.

Spleen. A weak spleen means that nutrients are not absorbed effectively. A weak spleen may be caused by age, a weak constitution, chronic illnesses, high alcohol consumption, and excess consumption of oily food. Symptoms of high cholesterol caused by a weak spleen include shortness of breath, wet cough, palpitations, numb and heavy limbs, and a bloated stomach.

Kidneys. Weak kidneys may be caused by age, chronic illness, or a weak constitution. This leads to water retention and hence high cholesterol levels. Symptoms of kidney weakness induced by high cholesterol include water retention in the face and limbs, an aching back and knees, cold intolerance, and loose stool.

Liver. The liver may be weakened by age and is also believed to be weakened by negative emotions such as fear, anger, and depression. This may also cause high cholesterol with symptoms such as dizziness, insomnia, a dry mouth, and high BP.

Qi (energy levels). Qi circulation is another important aspect in TCM. It is believed that poor qi circulation can cause high cholesterol and several other health ailments.

- Most TCM herbs are taken as directed by a *sinseh* (sensei), and dosage is based on the patient's age, gender, general health, and other factors. For more information on dose, a local sensei should be consulted.
- TCM is not often used as a cure for high cholesterol levels. High cholesterol levels should be treated using Western medicine for immediate effect.
- TCM can be used in conjunction with Western medicine to help control cholesterol levels. A doctor should be consulted to ensure that there are no negative interactions between the medications.

Common Ingredients for Hyperlipidemia

Herbs	Fruit/Flower/Miscellaneous
Baikal skullcap/huang qin (Scutellaria baicalensis)	Gardenia fruit/zhi zi (Fructus gardeniae)
Cassia twig/gui zhi (Cinnamomum Cassia; Ramulus)	Orange/zhi shi (Citrus sinensis)
Chinese foxglove root/shu di huang (Rehmannia glutinosa)	Asiatic cornelian cherry fruit/shan yu rou (Cornus officinalis)
Female ginseng/dang gui (Angelica sinensis)	Jiaogulan
Magnolia bark/hou po (Magnolia officinalis)	Rhubarb/da huang (Rheum rhabarbarum)
Moutan peony bark/mu dan pi (Paeonia suffruticosa Andr.)	Hawthorn fruit/shan zha (Crataegus)
Peach seed/tao ren (Prunus persica)	Glossy privet berry/nu zhen zi (Ligustrum lucidum)
Pinellia tuber/ban xia (Pinellia ternata)	Figwort flower/xuan shen (Radix scrophulariae)
Red sage root/danshen (Salvia miltiorrhiza)	Natto
Tiger nuts (Cyperus esculentus)	Konjac root

Herbs	Fruit/Flower/Miscellaneous
White atractylodes rhizome/bai zhu (Atractylodes macrocephala)	Snake gourd/gua lou (Trichosanthes cucumerina)
White peony root/bai shao (Paeoniae radix lactiflora) and red peony root/chi shao (Radix paeoniae rubra)	Safflower/hong hua (Carthamus tinctorius)
Yam rhizome/shan yao (Rhizoma dioscoreae)	Wolfberry fruit/gou qi zi (Lycium barbarum)

Common Recipes

Oral

Blood Circulation. Safflower, hawthorn fruit, peach seed, red peony root, and red sage root are believed to aid blood circulation and hence lower cholesterol levels.

Kidneys. Cassia twigs, Asiatic cornelian cherry fruit, rehmannia root, and yam rhizome may be taken to strengthen the kidneys.

Liver. It is believed that tree peony bark, white peony root, female ginseng, jiaogulan, barbary wolfberry fruit, and glossy privet fruit may be of use in strengthening the liver.

Spleen. To strengthen the spleen, the following herbs and fruits may be used—orange fruit, snake gourd fruit, pinellia tuber, and bai zhu.

Animal fat, seafood, and sweet processed foods ought to be avoided because it is believed to lead to high cholesterol associated with *dampness*, such as in spleen weakness.

Stomach. For a weak stomach, the following herbs may be of use—rhubarb, magnolia bark, gardenia fruit, baikal skullcap root, and figwort flower.

Vegetables, fruits, and grains such as barley and oats should be consumed to aid digestion in the stomach.

Commercial Preparations

Hong Qu. Hong qu is commonly known as red yeast rice and is available as a supplement.

Jiao Gu Lan. This is also known as gynostemma and is believed to lower BP and cholesterol levels. It is also believed to inhibit platelet aggregation and blood clot formation.

Shan Zha. Shan zha is called the hawthorn fruit and is used in the treatment of high BP, angina, and high cholesterol. It is thought to cause dilation of the blood vessels.

Jue Ming Zi. Jue ming zi is known as cassia seed and is thought to be able to treat high cholesterol. It has a diuretic effect and hence is useful in lowering BP.

Ze Xie. This is known as the Oriental water plantain rhizome. It also has diuretic properties and is used for both high BP and cholesterol treatment.

Therapeutic Measures

Diet

Natto: This Japanese fermented soy product can reduce cholesterol, arterial calcification, and heart disease.

Konjac root: This Asian root vegetable can be boiled or processed into ground flour to make Japenese noodles (shirataki noodles) or snacks.

Lifestyle

Adopt a healthy lifestyle with regular exercise such as tai chi for 30 minutes a day, 5 days a week. This is thought to enhance qi circulation. Alcohol and smoking should be avoided.

It is also believed that negative emotions such as anger, fear, and depression cause heat in the body and may weaken the liver, leading to high cholesterol.

Spend time in a quiet environment with fresh circulating air. This is believed to enhance qi (energy) levels.

Western/Other Natural Remedies

Common Ingredients for Hyperlipidemia

Spices	Herbs/Leaves	Miscellaneous
Flaxseed (Linum usitatissimum)	Cattail (Typha angustifolia)	Walnuts (Juglans regia)
		Eggplant (Solanum melongena)
		Yogurt
		Evening primrose oil (Oenothera)
		β-Sitosterol
		Vitamin B complex (B6, B12, and folate)
Garlic (Allium sativum)	Alfalfa (Medicago satina)	Unrefined/ unsaturated oils
Onion (Allium cepa)	Artichoke (Cynara cardunculus var. scolymus)	Whole grains
Psyllium husk (Plantago ovata)	Olive leaf extract	Sunflower seed (Helianthus annuus)
Turmeric (Curcuma longa)	Green tea (Camellia sinensis)	Almonds (Prunus dulcis)

Common Recipes

Oral

Teas/Brews/Cholesterol-Lowering Foods

Alfalfa juice. Place a handful of fresh alfalfa into a blender, and gradually add water. Blend till smooth. Drink on its own or mixed with other fruit or vegetable juice. Fresh alfalfa may also be added to salads.

Almonds or walnuts. Snack on almonds or walnuts.

Artichokes. Incorporate artichokes in your diet.

β-Sitosterol. It can lower the total and LDL cholesterol. Foods high in β-sitosterol include avocado, pistachio, corn chips, and fava beans. It is also available as dietary supplement capsules.

Cattail. The roots or young stems can be eaten raw, boiled or baked. The dried roots are also ground into powder and used as a thickener. The seeds, stem and pollen are also edible. The pollen is easily harvested, sieved and added to juices, shakes, or used as protein-rich flour.

> Variation #1 Take 1 to 2 teaspoons of the dried root powder. Add 1 cup of water. Simmer for 5 minutes. Consume 4 to 6 cups a day.

Evening primrose. The seeds, flowers, and roots are edible. The seeds can be added to salads or smoothies. The seed oil is available as a dietary supplement.

> Variation #1. Take approximately 2 teaspoons of dried flowers. Add 1 cup of hot water, and steep for approximately 5 to 10 minutes. Drink twice a day.

Flaxseed, soybeans, and sunflower seeds. Incorporate these into the diet because these are high in unsaturated fats.

Garlic. Consume one to four cloves of garlic every day, preferably in the morning and on an empty stomach.

Green tea. Place 2 teaspoons of dried green tea leaves in a cup of hot water. Allow to steep for 10 to 15 minutes. Strain, and drink.

Olive leaf extract. Consume olive leaf extract capsules once a day.

Onion juice. Lightly pound some onion to extract approximately 1 tablespoon of juice. Add a few drops of honey, and mix well. Take it once a day for at least 2 weeks.

Psyllium husk. Take 2 to 3 teaspoons of psyllium husk with warm water, warm milk, or juice at night.

Turmeric-eggplant spread. Boil an eggplant until soft. Mash until smooth, and place 2 tablespoons of the mashed eggplant in a bowl. Add ¾ teaspoon of turmeric and 1½ teaspoons of hot water and little lemon juice to the mashed eggplant and mix well. This may be eaten as a spread on whole wheat bread.

Unrefined and unsaturated oils. Use unsaturated, unrefined oils such as sunflower oil or olive oil in cooking.

Vitamin B. B6, B9 (folate), and B12 can reduce homocysteine levels.

Whole grains. Eat whole grains such as wheat, oats, and barley because they contain fiber and β-glucan. These bind to cholesterol in the intestine and hence reduce cholesterol absorption and lower lipid levels. Eat approximately ½ cup of oatmeal every day.

Yogurt. Eat 1 cup of plain yogurt with active cultures every day.

Modern Remedies

Statins

Statins are a group of medications that inhibit cholesterol synthesis in the body and cause intracellular cholesterol to be taken up and used by the body. This leads to an increase in LDL (bad cholesterol) surface receptors and increases LDL use from the circulation. This in turn leads to a reduction in plasma LDL levels. They are often taken at night because LDL synthesis tends to spike in the early morning.

Examples: Atorvastatin, lovastatin, and pravastatin

Bile Acid Sequestrants

Bile acids are steroid acids synthesized by cholesterol in the liver. The reduction of bile acid causes more cholesterol to be converted to bile acids and hence used up. This causes an increased cholesterol uptake from circulation due to an increase in LDL receptors, which in turn leads to a decrease in plasma LDL levels. These drugs are often used as an adjunct to diet and lifestyle modifications.

Examples: Cholestyramine and colestipol

Nicotinic Acid

Nicotinic acid reduces lipid levels by inhibiting the enzyme lipase in adipose (fat) tissue. Lipase is responsible for lipolysis, which is the breakdown of fats and other lipids to release fatty acids. The reduction in fatty acid transport to the liver leads to a reduction in triglyceride synthesis. It also causes an increase in HDL cholesterol levels and a decrease in LDL levels.

Fibrates

Fibrates function by activating peroxisome proliferator-activated receptors (PPARs) in the body, a class of receptors that regulate carbohydrate and fat metabolism as well as fat tissue (adipose) differentiation. Activating PPARs leads to higher lipid metabolism, which helps to reduce plasma LDL levels.

Examples: Gemfibrozil, fenofibrate, and clofibrate

Ezetimibe

Ezetimibe is a selective cholesterol absorption inhibitor. It inhibits the absorption of cholesterol at the brush border of the small intestine mediated by the sterol transporter, Niemann-Pick C1-like-1 (NPC1L1) protein.

As monotherapy, it has been found to be able to reduce LDL levels by up to 15% and, when used in conjunction with statins, has been found to reduce LDL levels by up to 72%. Simvastatin-ezetimibe or atorvastatin combinations are available.

PCSK9 Inhibitors

There are monoclonal antibodies that are very effective in familial hypercholesterolemia.

Examples: Alirocumab and evolocumab

Lipid-Lowering Agents, Microsomal Triglyceride Transfer Protein Inhibitor

It decreases cholesterol via inhibition of the microsomal triglyceride transfer protein (MTP) pathway.

Example: Lopitamide

Messenger RNA Binders

The drug binds with apoB mRNA. It is an antisense oligonucleotide inhibitor of apoB100. It is used to treat homozygous familial hypercholesterolemia.

Example: mipomersen (weekly subcutaneous injection). It has been discontinued due to liver toxicity.

Liver Transplant

This may be a near-curative option in homozygous familial hypercholesterolemia.

Homeopathic Remedies

These include *alfalfa*, *Calcarea carb* (in obese person with boiled egg craving, excessive sweating, cold air sensitivity, and palpitations after food or night), *Strophnathus hispidus* (associated breathlessness and palpitations), *Curcuma*, *Allium sativum* (associated with meat craving and acid reflux), *Baryta muriaticum* (in elderly with hypertension, vertigo, and seizure), *Cardus marianus* (associated with fatty liver), *Chrysanthemum* (if overeating), *Berberis vulgaris* (overeating and sedentary life), *Avena sativum* (associated diabetes mellitus), *Crataegus oxyacantha* (associated with exertional dyspnea), *Nux vomica* (if excessive alcohol, fatty foods, constipation, and anger issues), and *Lycopodium* (it works well with person who are intelligent but physically weak, associated weak digestion and associated gas, bloating, and flatulence with cravings for hot drinks, and sweets).

Ischemic Heart Disease/Coronary Artery Disease

CAD refers to the build-up of plague in the walls of the coronary arteries. Hardening of the arteries is called arteriosclerosis. The commonest cause is atherosclerosis (fatty build-up). Risk factors include metabolic syndrome (diabetes, hyperlipidemia, and hypertension), obesity, and high homocysteine levels. Nonatheromatous arteriosclerosis is due to scarring or fibrosis in old age without any fatty plague.

Signs and symptoms include chest pain (angina), shortness of breath, fatigue, and light-headedness.

Test include blood biochemistry including lipid profile, hemoglobin, blood NT pro B-Type natriuretic peptide (BNP) and ECG, chest x-ray, cardiac ECHO, exercise stress ECG, cardiac catheterization via angiogram (femoral or brachial), CT angiogram, magnetic resonance (MR) angiogram and nuclear scans.

Indian Natural Remedies

Common Ingredients for Ischemic Heart Disease

Spices	Herbs/Leaves	Miscellaneous
Amla/Indian gooseberry (*Phyllanthus emblica*)	Jatamansi (*Nardostachys jatamansi*)	Snake gourd (*Trichosanthes cucumerina*)
Cardamom (*Elettaria cardamomum*)	Ashwagandha (*Withania somnifera*)	
Cinnamon (*Cinnamomum vera*)	Punarnava (*Boerhavia diffusa*)	
Fenugreek (*Trigonella foenum-graecum*)	Arjuna (*Terminalia arjuna*)	
Garlic (*Allium sativum*)	Guggulu (*Commiphora mukul*)	Jaggery
Ginger (*Zingiber officinale*)	Haritaki (*Terminalia chebula*)	

Spices	Herbs/Leaves	Miscellaneous
Gotu Kola (*Centella asiatica*)	Shankhpushpi (*Convolvulus pluricaulis*)	Lemon (*Citrus limon*)
Nutmeg (*Myristica fragrans*)	Tulsi/holy basil (*Ocimum tenuiflorum*)	Honey
Onion/Shallots (*Allium cepa*)	Brahmi (*Bacopa monnieri*)	
	Drumstick leaf (*Moringa oleifera*)	

Common Recipes

Oral

Teas/Brews/Others

Amla juice. Lightly pound three to four amla fruits, and strain the juice. Take this juice on an empty stomach in the morning with a glass of warm water.

Arjuna tea. To be prepared as described under treatments for hypertension.

Ashwagandha brew. To be prepared as described under treatments for hypertension.

Brahmi tea. Place approximately two to three stalks of fresh brahmi leaves into a cup. Pour boiling water over the leaves, and allow it to steep for approximately 10 to 15 minutes. Add honey to taste, and drink.

Cinnamon tea. Add a stick of cinnamon to a pot of hot water, and steep for approximately 10 minutes. Add honey to taste, and drink.

Drumstick (Moringa) leaves and snake gourd. Cook and consume these vegetables.

Fenugreek tea. Lightly crush fenugreek seeds. Pour the fenugreek seeds into a cup, and add a cup of boiling water. Allow to steep for approximately 10 to 20 minutes before straining the mixture. Add honey to taste, and drink.

Garlic brew. Lightly pound two to three cloves of garlic. Add the pounded garlic to a pot with a cup of milk. Gently heat the mixture for approximately 5 to 10 minutes. Strain, and consume this in the morning on an empty stomach.

Variation #1. Lightly crush four to five cloves of garlic. Place ½ a cup of water and ½ a cup of milk to a pot, and add the garlic to it. Simmer the mixture till it reduces to approximately ½ a cup. Consume this in the morning on an empty stomach.

Ginger-cardamom tea. Lightly pound approximately 3 to 4 cm of ginger and five to seven cardamom seeds. Add the ginger and seeds to a pot of water, and bring to a boil. Reduce the heat, and simmer for approximately 5 to 10 minutes. Strain, and add honey to taste.

Ginger-nutmeg tea. Lightly pound approximately ½ cm of fresh ginger. Place 1½ cup of water in a pot, and add the ginger. Bring the mixture to a boil. Reduce the heat, and simmer for approximately 15 to 20 minutes. Strain the mixture into a cup, and add a pinch of nutmeg. Mix well, and drink.

Ginger powder and jaggery. Consume approximately 5 g of ginger powder and 5 g of jaggery mixed.

Gotu kola tea. Steep a teaspoon of fresh or dried gotu kola leaves in a cup of hot water for approximately 10 to 15 minutes. Drink it warm.

Guggulu. It is available in the form of dietary supplements. Adults can take approximately 25 mg of guggulu supplements every day after a meal.

Variation #1. Take 1 cup of hot water. Add 1 tea bag of guggulu. Cover, and steep for 2 to 3 minutes. Drink it warm.

Jatamansi brew. Add a pinch of jatamansi root powder to a cup of warm water, and take it twice a day.

Lemon juice. Squeeze ½ a lemon into a glass of water. Drink on an empty stomach in the morning.

Pomegranate. Consume the fresh fruit or prepare juice.

Punarnava tea. Add one part each of dried punarnava, one part of dried passion fruit flower, and two parts of dried hawthorn berries. Steep approximately half a teaspoon of this in a cup of hot water for approximately 10 minutes. Drink twice a day, after lunch and dinner.

Many of the herbs listed previously are available as commercial preparations and may be taken as dietary supplements.

Shankhpushpi: Take five to six shankhpushpi (fresh blue pea) flowers. Add 1 cup of boiling water. Allow to steep for 5 to 10 minutes. Drink before bedtime.

Variation: Mix 1 teaspoon of ground shankhpushpi into 1 cup of warm milk. Drink warm twice a day.

Triphala tea. Add half a teaspoon of triphala powder to 1 cup of hot water. Mix well, and drink it warm. Triphala powder is made up of three ingredients: amla, haritaki, and bibhitaki.

Tulsi tea. Place five to seven fresh tulsi leaves in a pot with a cup of water. Boil for approximately 15 minutes, and then remove from the heat. Allow it to steep for approximately 5 minutes. Drink before bedtime every day.

Therapeutic Measures

Diet

Add fresh onions or shallots as part of the diet. Add them to curries, salads, and yogurt.

Lifestyle

The following yoga asanas and pranayama support a healthy heart:

Trikonasana (triangle pose)

Setu Bandhasana (bridge pose)

Virabhadrasana (warrior pose)

Bhujangasana (cobra pose)

Adho Mukha Svanasana (downward-facing dog pose)

Vrikshasana (tree pose)

Marjariasana (cat pose)

Bhramari pranayama (honey bee humming breath)

Chinese Natural Remedies

Qi (energy levels) qi circulation is an important aspect in TCM. It is believed that poor qi circulation can cause a number of ailments, including IHD.

Yang qi refers to heat energy. Yin qi refers to cold energy. These two energies should be in balance for an individual to maintain good health.

Heart yang deficiency with coldness can mean two things:

There is deficient qi, and hence the heart is unable to maintain sufficient blood circulation, leading to symptoms such as chest pain, palpitations, sweating, and shortness of breath. The patient is believed to have a pale tongue and face with a deep and weak pulse.

There is deficient yang, causing the body to be cold and hence constrict blood vessels. This causes symptoms such as a severe strangling chest pain that radiates to the back, cold extremities, a pale face, and purple lips or tongue.

Spleen-qi deficiency with phlegm is believed to be due to the spleen being unable to clear body fluids efficiently leading to phlegm production. This may be caused by an excessive intake of fat, greasy, sweet, or dairy-rich foods. It is also believed that emotional volatility may lead to spleen weakness.

Liver qi stagnation with blood stasis:

It is believed that the liver is the organ responsible for the smooth flow of qi in the body and can be affected by emotional volatility. This causes qi stagnation, which in turn causes blood stasis.

It is also thought that a deficiency in yin may cause blood stasis due to insufficient volume. The excess heat is believed to cause a reduction in the amount of blood, causing thickening and hence stasis.

Common Ingredients for Ischemic Heart Disease

Spices	Herbs/Leaves	Miscellaneous
Chinese cinnamon/ gui zhi (Cinnamomum Cassia; Ramulus)	Asian ginseng/ren shen (Panax ginseng)	Jujube/da zao (Ziziphus jujuba)
Ginger/sheng jiang (Zingiber officinale)	Wolfsbane/fu zi (Aconitum carmichaeli)	Chinese hawthorn/shan zha (Crataegus pinnatifida)
	White peony root/ bai shao (Paeoniae radix lactiflora)	Pinellia tuber/ban xia (Pinellia ternata)
	Pseudoginseng/ tian qi (Panax pseudoginseng)	Chinese cucumber/ gualou (Trichosanthes kirilowii)
	White atractylodes rhizome/bai zhu (Atractylodes macrocephala)	Red sage root/ danshen (Salvia miltiorrhiza)
	Pseudoginseng/ tian qi (P. pseudoginseng)	Peach seed/tao ren (Prunus persica)

Spices	Herbs/Leaves	Miscellaneous
	Kudzu (Pueraria montana/ Pueraria lobata)	Safflower/ hong hua (Carthamus tinctorius)
Liquorice/zhi gan cao (Glycyrrhiza glabra)	Astragalus root/ huang qi (Radix Astragali)	Tangerine peel/ chen pi (Citrus reticulata)

Common Recipes

Oral

Decoction for Heart Yang Deficiency With Coldness. Place 3 cups of water into a pot. Add 3 g of gui zhi (Chinese cinnamon), 3 g of bai shao (white peony root), 3 g of fresh sheng jiang (ginger), 2 g of zhi gan cao (liquorice), and three pieces of jujube (da zao) to the pot. Boil for approximately 30 minutes. Drink it warm (refer to the notes for more on this classification).

Other herbs used in this condition include ren shen (Asian ginseng), huang qi (astragalus), fu zi (wolfsbane root), and gua lou (Chinese cucumber).

Decoction for Spleen Qi Deficiency With Phlegm. Place 3 cups of water into a pot. Add 10 g of shan zha (Chinese hawthorn fruit) and 10 g of chen pi (tangerine peel) to the pot. Bring to a boil, and continue to boil gently for 30 minutes. Drink it warm.

Other herbs used to treat this condition are ren shen (Asian ginseng), bai zhu (white atractylodes), zhi gan cao (liquorice), and ban xia (pinellia tuber).

Decoction for Liver Qi Stagnation With Blood Stasis. Herbs used to treat this condition include *cooling* herbs such as danshen root (red sage root), tian qi (pseudoginseng), tao ren (peach seed), and hong hua (safflower).

Dosage and instructions on the use of these herbs should be obtained from a sensei.

Therapeutic Measures

Acupressure

Intravenous therapy. Intravenous puerarin is given in acute myocardial infarction.

Conception vessel 12 (CV 12), or middle cavity, is located on the midline of the abdomen, approximately 4 cm above the belly button.

Stomach 6 (ST 6), or the jaw bone, is located on the cheek approximately one finger width in front of and above the lower angle of the jawline. This point is most clearly felt at the muscle prominence with teeth clenched.

Stomach 40 (ST 40), or abundant bulge, is located on the lower leg approximately midway between the highest point of the outer ankle and the knee joint.

Treatment of liver qi stagnation with blood stasis includes acupressure at the following points:

Spleen 6 (SP 6) is also known as the three-yin intersection and is located on the inner side of the lower leg approximately 10 cm above the inner ankle.

Spleen 10 (SP 10), or sea of blood, is located (knee flexed) on the inner side of the thigh, approximately 6.5 cm above the top edge of the kneecap.

Urinary bladder 17 (UB 17), or diaphragm shu, is located on the back, approximately 5 cm to the side of the lower border of the 7th thoracic vertebra.

Lifestyle

Exercises to treat "spleen-qi deficiency with phlegm." Energy exercises such as the *self-tuina* massage may help to improve blood and qi circulation in the body. This exercise is performed by patting the arms, legs, and front and back of the body from the top down and patting the top of the head two to three times every day.

Western/Other Natural Remedies

Common Ingredients for Ischemic Heart Disease

Spices	Herbs/Leaves	Miscellaneous
Flaxseed (*Linum usitatissimum*)	Green tea (*Camellia sinensis*)	Pomegranate (*Punica granatum*)
	Cattail (*Typha angustifolia*)	Essential oils—lemon, lemongrass, frankincense, helichrysum, ginger
		Ozone
		Antioxidants: CoQ10, selenium, omega 3 oils
		Tomato extract (water soluble)
Garlic (*Allium sativum*)	Rosemary (*Rosmarinus officinalis*)	Honey
Ginger (*Zingiber officinale*)	Basil (*Ocimum basilicum*)	Apple cider vinegar (*Malus pumila Mill*)
Turmeric (*Curcuma longa*)	Thyme (*Thymus vulgaris*)	Lemon (*Citrus limon*)

Common Recipes

Oral

Teas/Brew/Others

Antioxidants. Coenzyme Q10 (CoQ10), selenium, and omega 3 oils supplements can lower heart disease.

Basil tea. Place approximately three to four fresh basil leaves into a pot of water. Bring to a boil before lowering the heat, and simmer for approximately 5 minutes. Strain, and add honey to taste. Drink it warm.

Cattail. The roots or young stems can be eaten raw, boiled or baked. The dried roots are also ground into powder and used as a thickener. The seeds, stem and pollen are also edible. The pollen is easily harvested, sieved and added to juices, shakes, or used as protein-rich flour.

Variation #1 Take 1 to 2 teaspoons of the dried root powder. Add 1 cup of water. Simmer for 5 minutes. Consume 4 to 6 cups a day.

Dark chocolate. Take a square of dark chocolate.

Flaxseed. It should be added to salads or smoothies.

Green tea. Steep 1 teaspoon of dried green tea leaves in a cup of hot water for approximately 10 to 15 minutes.

Heart Tonic. Place ½ cup of lemon juice and ¼ cup of apple cider vinegar in a pot. Lightly pound a piece of 2- to 3-cm-long ginger and three to four cloves of fresh garlic. Add the ginger and garlic to the pot. Bring the mixture to a boil, and boil gently until it thickens. Take off the heat, and allow it to cool. Add honey to taste. Store in the refrigerator, and take 1 teaspoon every morning on an empty stomach.

High fiber food. Eat a diet high in fiber such as vegetables and fruit, legumes, and beans. Healthy fats such as avocados, nuts, seeds, sunflower, and olive oil are also advisable to consume.

Pomegranate. Consume the fresh fruit, or prepare juice.

Rosemary tea. Add 1½ teaspoons of dry rosemary needles to a cup of hot water, and allow it to steep for 10 to 15 minutes. Drink it warm.

Thyme. It should be added as a spice to most cooked dishes.

Turmeric-ginger tea. Lightly pound a piece of 3- to 5-cm-long ginger, and add to a pot of water. Bring to a boil, and reduce the heat, allowing the mixture to simmer for approximately 10 to 15 minutes. Stir in 2 teaspoons of turmeric, and drink it warm.

Water-soluble tomato extract (from the gel around tomato seed). It contains several anti-platelet aggregation compounds such as polyphenols, flavonoids, and nucleosides.

Therapeutic Measures

Aromatherapy/Inhalation (Nasal)

Essential oils such as lemon, lemongrass, frankincense, helichrysum, and ginger have antiinflammatory properties, and their use may help to reduce the incidence of heart-related ailments. Dilute a few drops of the chosen essential oil with some water, and add the mixture to a humidifier/diffuser. If a humidifier is not available, sprinkle some of the essential oils on clothes or bed sheets.

Ozone Therapy

Ozone can be given intravenously.

Disclaimer: Most of these home remedies are meant to be for symptomatic relief, for prevention of heart ailments, or used as supplementation to other medication.

In the case of any acute chest pain, urgent medical attention is required to diagnose and treat the condition.

About 100 ml of blood is withdrawn, and ozone is then dissolved into the blood.

The blood and ozone mixture is then reinfused into the patient. This can improve circulation and help in detoxification.

Risks includes lung dysfunction and stroke.

Hematogenous Oxidation Therapy (HOT). About 50 ml of blood is withdrawn which is then exposed to high oxygen concentration and ultraviolet (UV) light. This improves cellular metabolism.

Modern Remedies

Nitrates

Nitrates are nitric oxide (NO) donors. NO is primarily produced by vascular endothelial cells in the body and has vasodilator properties, meaning that it dilates blood vessels in the body. It also inhibits platelet aggregation and has antiinflammatory properties. Nitrates are broken down in the body, releasing NO. This causes relaxation of blood vessels, hence reducing peripheral resistance, BP, and the workload on the heart. It also causes dilation of coronary vessels, improving blood flow to the heart and reperfusing the ischemic areas.

Examples: glyceryl trinitrate (GTN), isosorbide dinitrate (ISDN), and isosorbide mononitrate (ISMN).

Fibrinolytic Agents

Streptokinase

This is the most widely used agent. It is not fibrin specific, and it results in a lower patency rate of the occluded vessel at 60 minutes than fibrin-specific agents. Despite having a lower risk of intracranial hemorrhage, the reduction in mortality is less than with fibrin-specific agents.

Tenecteplase (TNK-tPA)

The benefit of using TNK-tPA is that it causes more rapid reperfusion of the occluded artery than streptokinase and is given as a single bolus dose.

Anticoagulants

These are blood thinners and are classified according to the route of administration.

Unfractionated Heparin (heparin)

It is administered intravenously. It requires regular blood tests and monitoring.

Low-Molecular-Weight Heparin (Enoxaparin, Dalteparin)

It is given subcutaneously. It does not require monitoring.

Non–Vitamin K Antagonist Oral Anticoagulant or Direct Oral Anticoagulants

Examples are *rivaroxaban, dabigatran,* and *apixaban.* Although expensive, they have a low risk of bleeding and do not require frequent blood monitoring.

Antiplatelet Therapy

Aspirin (Acetylsalicylic Acid)

Aspirin (acetylsalicylic acid) irreversibly inhibits prostaglandin H synthase (cyclooxygenase-1) in platelets and megakaryocytes and thereby blocks the formation of thromboxane A2.

Clopidogrel

It is an inhibitor of platelet activation and aggregation through the irreversible binding of its active metabolite to the $P2Y_{12}$ class of Adenosine diphosphate (ADP) receptors on platelets.

Clopidogrel, when given together with aspirin and fibrinolytic therapy in ST elevation myocardial infarction (STEMI), has been shown to reduce the odds of an occluded vessel, death, or reinfarction without increasing the risk of bleeding or cerebrovascular accidents.

Others. These include Ticagrelor and Prasugrel which are newer antiplatelet medications. They can be used in patients with normal or reduced renal function and they have less major bleeding risk.

Prevention

Polypill strategy. After a heart attack or an acute coronary syndrome, a single polypill consisting of aspirin, ramipril and atorvastatin is given to prevent recurrent cardiovascular events.

Percutaneous Coronary Intervention

Balloon Angioplasty

The catheter has a tiny folded balloon at the tip. Once the blocked or narrowed artery is reached, the balloon is inflated to open the artery. The balloon is then deflated and removed.

Angioplasty With Stent

In addition to balloon treatment, a stent is usually placed. This is a tiny mesh tube that is expanded and is left behind to keep the artery open. It has a coating that slowly releases special drugs which decreases scar tissue build-up. The newer dissolvable stent does not leave metal in the body permanently.

β-Blockers

Refer to "Hypertension."

Calcium Channel Blockers

Refer to "Hypertension."

Potassium Channel Activators

Nicorandil is a potassium channel activator that opens potassium channels in the vascular smooth muscle and causes dilation due to an efflux of potassium. It is a Nitric Oxide (NO) donor and hence causes dilation of blood vessels. The dilation of blood vessels means that the workload of the heart is reduced due to a reduced peripheral resistance. This allows the ischemic areas of the heart to receive the necessary blood flow and oxygen reperfusion.

Ranolazine

Ranolazine has antianginal and antiischemic effects. It blocks the late inward sodium currents and reduces calcium overload. This leads to improved coronary blood flow and is used in the treatment of chronic angina.

In an *acute myocardial infarction (heart attack) or acute coronary syndrome*, an aspirin may be taken and medical attention should be sought immediately. Acute treatment includes oxygen, sublingual and intravenous nitroglycerine (to improve blood flow), intravenous morphine (for pain relief), thrombolytics/fibrinolytics (streptokinase, recombinant tissue-type plasminogen activator, unfractionated heparin), antiplatelet agents (aspirin, clopidogrel, or prasugrel), and others (β-blockers, ACE inhibitor, angiotensin receptor blocker, statins).

Reperfusion or Revascularization Therapy

These include percutaneous intervention (PCI) (i.e., coronary angioplasty/stenting), coronary artery bypass graft (CABG), or cardiac stem cell therapy.

Homeopathic Remedies

These are generally not indicated for acute or severe life-threatening cardiac events such as acute myocardial infarction, although *Arnica montana, Calcarea phosphorica, cactus, Glonoine* (similar to GTN), and others have been tried in acute angina.

Baryta muriaticum and gold remedies (*Aurum mur, Aurum iod,* and *Aurum met*) are effective in arteriosclerosis.

Heart Failure

Heart failure means that the heart is not pumping well. A normal ejection fraction (EF) of the heart is between 55% and 70%. Less than 35% EF means severe pumping ability. There are two types of heart failure i.e.

Heart failure with reduced left ventricular function, and
Heart failure with preserved left ventricular function (HFpEF), also called diastolic heart failure

Causes and risk factors include coronary heart disease, hypertension, cardiomyopathy, congenital heart disease, diabetes, hyperlipidemia, anemia, and arrhythmias.

Signs and symptoms include breathlessness; cough or wheeze that is worse at night or on exertion; edema with swelling of feet, abdomen, or face; poor appetite; weight loss or weight gain; tachycardia; palpitations; dizziness; confusion; and fainting.

Investigations for heart failure: Refer to CAD subchapter.

Indian Natural Remedies

Common Ingredients for Heart Failure

Herbs/Leaves
Arjuna
(*Terminalia arjuna*)
Hibiscus flowers
(*Hibiscus rosa-sinensis*)
Indian coleus
(*Coleus forskohlii*)
Peepal leaf

Common Recipes

Oral
Teas/Brews
Arjuna tea. Take a cup of water and a cup of milk. Heat gently, and then add 1 teaspoon of arjuna powder. Boil, and then simmer until volume is reduced to 1 cup. Strain, and add honey to taste.
Arjuna supplement. It is available in the form of many commercial preparations and may be taken as a supplement. Take 500 mg of powdered arjuna bark three times a day

for up to 2 weeks. To relieve chest pain, 500 mg of powdered arjuna bark should be taken three times a day alongside other allopathic treatments for up to 3 months.
Hibiscus tea. Take ¼ cup of fresh or dried hibiscus petals. If fresh, macerate or bruise the petals first. Add hot water, and steep for 5 to 15 minutes. Other spices such as cinnamon, cloves, and ginger may be added. Strain, and drink. Add honey to taste.
Peepal tea. Take 2 g of Asvattha bark powder. Add 200 mL water. Boil, and reduce the volume till 50 mL. Add honey to taste. Consume twice a day.
Variation # 1. Boil some peepal leaves in 1 cup of water. Leave overnight. Strain, and drink in the morning.
Indian coleus. Boil the roots of the coleus to make tea. It is also available as a supplement.
Disclaimer. Natural remedies for heart failure should be used only as preventative measures or as an adjunct to conventional treatments. Consult a medical professional on the proper treatment of heart failure and the possible interactions between medications.

Chinese Natural Remedies

Common Ingredients for Heart Failure

Herbs/Leaves	**Miscellaneous**
Chinese hawthorn/shan zha (*Crataegus pinnatifida*)	Goldenseal (*Hydrastis canadensis*)
	Chinese goldthread/huang lian (*Rhizoma coptidis*)
	Oregon grape/gong lao mu (*Mahonia aquifolium* or *Berberis aquifolium*)
	Barberry/fu niu (*Berberis vulgaris*)
	Indian barberry (*Berberis aristata*)

Common Recipes

Oral
Berberine. It is a bitter-tasting yellow plant alkaloid found in many plants such as goldenseal, huang lian (goldenthread), gong lao mu (Oregon grape), fu niu (barberry), and Indian barberry. Berberine is available as a commercial preparation and can be taken orally in the form of a powder or capsule. It should not be used in infants or children younger than 12 years, due to a lack of safety information.
Hawthorn berry tea. Take approximately 1 teaspoon of dried hawthorn berries. Boil in hot water, and simmer for 10 to 15 minutes. Strain, and consume twice a day. Add honey if required.

Notes. It is important to remember that most of the studies involving the aforementioned natural remedies are lacking in long-term research and should not be used as a sole treatment for heart failure. Consult a medical professional for a safe diagnosis and treatment plan.

Western/Other Natural Remedies

Common Ingredients for Heart Failure

Miscellaneous

Banana
(*Musa*)

Salt substitutes/
  Potassium
  chloride

Fruits and vegetables high in
  potassium
Garlic
(*Allium sativum*)
Hawthorn berry
(*Crataegus*)

Co-Q10/ubiquinol

Nuts and legumes
Onion
(*Allium cepa*)

Common Recipes

Oral

Co-Q10/ubiquinol. Approximately 120 to 150 mg of Coq10 enzyme should be taken every day.

Garlic and onion. Take approximately three to five pips of garlic or one onion every day to improve heart health.

Hawthorn berry tea. Take approximately 1 teaspoon of dried hawthorn berries. Boil in hot water, and simmer for 10 to 15 minutes. Strain and consume twice a day. Add honey if required.

Nuts and legumes. They also contain large amounts of potassium, especially almonds and Brazil nuts, with about 800 mg of potassium in 4 ounces.

Salt and salt substitutes. Eliminate or reduce table salt (sodium chloride) intake. Salt substitutes, which contain potassium chloride, are available. It can be plain or mixed with regular salt (the latter is referred to as "lite" or low-sodium salt). One-quarter teaspoon per serving is recommended. Excessive potassium can be dangerous, and the intake of potassium chloride should be medically supervised.

Therapeutic Measures

Diet

Fruits and vegetables. Incorporate fruit and vegetables high in potassium into your daily diet. Potassium-rich fruits include banana, oranges, avocado, pomegranate, watermelon, honeydew melon, coconut water, dried apricots, prunes, and dates. Potassium-rich vegetables include beets, beans (white, black, edamame, kidney, soya, lentils), sweet potatoes, cooked spinach, cooked tomato or paste, broccoli, and leafy greens.

Lifestyle

A healthy lifestyle should be adopted. Quit smoking, and reduce alcohol intake. Exercise regularly to lose any excess weight.

Resistance training and exercise training are also very helpful in heart failure with preserved ejection fraction.

Enhanced External Counterpulsation

EECP is a noninvasive treatment used to lower the frequency and intensity of angina episodes. Three pairs of external inflatable cuffs are placed around the upper and lower legs and the buttocks. The cuffs continuously inflate and deflate depending on the heartbeat, increasing the amount of blood returning to the heart. This allows more oxygen to be transported to ischemic areas of the heart and reduces the incidence of chest pain as well as allowing the heart to function more effectively.

Notes. Most of the aforementioned natural remedies are to be used in combination with allopathic treatment, and for a proper treatment plan, a medical professional should be consulted.

Modern Remedies

Diuretics

Refer to "Hypertension."

Angiotensin-Converting Enzyme Inhibitor

Refer to "Hypertension."

Angiotensin II Receptor Blockers

Refer to "Hypertension."

Aldosterone Antagonist

Aldosterone antagonists work by blocking aldosterone receptors in the body. Aldosterone is a mineralocorticoid hormone in the body that plays a major role in sodium reabsorption and potassium excretion. This medication causes some excretion of sodium and functions as a low efficacy diuretic. This aids in reducing volume overload and hence decreases the workload on the heart. Examples of this drug are spironolactone and eplerenone. This medication has been found to reduce mortality in heart failure.

β-Blocker

Refer to "Hypertension."

SLGT-2 inhibitor

Sodium-glucose co-transporter inhibitors (eg. empagliflozin, dapagliflozin and canagliflozin) can improve heart failure with preserved ejection fraction.

Others

Some study trials have included calcium channel blockers and digoxin(digitalis)

Surgical Options

- Implantable cardioverter defibrillator (ICD) or cardiac resynchronization therapy (CRT). This is a treatment option if EF is below 35% and high arrhythmia risk.
- Stem cell treatment
- Heart transplant

Homeopathic Remedies

Although they are generally not recommended in the acute state, they can be useful in preventive and supportive heart care.

For example, *Crataegus oxycantha* is a hawthorn plant extract that removes calcareous deposits in the arteries and increases coronary blood flow. *Spigelia anthelmia* also improves circulation.

References

Hypertension

American Heart Association editorial staff. (2017, October 31). *Types of blood pressure medications*. Www.Heart.Org. Retrieved from https://www.heart.org/en/health-topics/high-blood-pressure/changes-you-can-make-to-manage-high-blood-pressure/types-of-blood-pressure-medications.

Ben-Yehuda, E. (2021a, June 2). *14 home remedies for high blood pressure*. RESPeRATE—Lower Pressure Blog. Retrieved from https://www.resperate.com/blog/hypertension/treatments/lifestyle/Home-Remedies-for-High-Blood-Pressure

Ben-Yehuda, E. (2021b, June 30). *18 herbs that naturally lower your blood pressure*. RESPeRATE blog. RESPeRATE. Retrieved from https://www.resperate.com/blog/hypertension/treatments/alternative-treatments/15-herbs-lower-high-blood-pressure.

Berry, J., & Carter, A. (2019, October 2). *What are the health benefits of cardamom?* Medical News Today. Retrieved from https://www.medicalnewstoday.com/articles/326532.

British Homeopathic Association. (n.d.). *Homeopathy UK*. Homeopathy UK. Retrieved from https://homeopathy-uk.org/.

Carretero, O. A., & Oparil, S. (2000). Essential hypertension. *Circulation, 101*(3), 329–335. Retrieved from https://doi.org/10.1161/01.cir.101.3.329.

Chauhan, V. (2021, March 24). *8 foods to eat daily for high blood pressure or hypertension*. Practo.Com. Retrieved from https://www.practo.com/healthfeed/top-9-ayurvedic-remedies-for-high-blood-pressure-or-hypertension-28097/post.

Chen, B., Wang, Y., He, Z., Wang, D., Yan, X., & Xie, P. (2018). Tianma Gouteng decoction for essential hypertension. *Medicine, 97*(8), e9972. Retrieved from https://doi.org/10.1097/md.0000000000009972.

Deesh, P. (2018, August 30). *10 wonderful benefits of Amla powder: A powerful superfood*. NDTV Food. Retrieved from https://food.ndtv.com/health/10-wonderful-benefits-of-amla-powder-a-powerful-superfood-1654043.

Gajendran, D. (2015, October 16). *10 useful acupressure points for controlling high blood pressure*. Modern Reflexology. Retrieved from https://www.modernreflexology.com/acupressure-for-high-blood-pressure/.

Gyanunlimited.com. (2020, November 17). *How to control high blood pressure naturally and quickly*. Gyanunlimited—A Hub of Alternative Medicine and Holistic Health. Retrieved from https://www.gyanunlimited.com/health/how-to-control-high-blood-pressure-naturally-and-quickly/9639/.

Harvard School of Public Health. (2021, July 6). *Dark chocolate*. The Nutrition Source. Retrieved from https://www.hsph.harvard.edu/nutritionsource/food-features/dark-chocolate/.

HealthCMi. (2020, June 20). *Acupuncture lowers hypertension finding*. HealthCMi. Retrieved from https://www.healthcmi.com/Acupuncture-Continuing-Education-News/1255-acupuncture-lowers-hypertension-new-finding.

Hebbar, J. V. (2020, July 2). *Triphala churna benefits, ingredients, dose, side effects, how to take*. AyurMedInfo. Retrieved from https://www.ayurmedinfo.com/2012/03/16/triphala-churna-benefits-ingredients-dose-side-effects-how-to-take/.

Huang, Y., Chen, Y., Cai, H., Chen, D., He, X., Li, Z., et al. (2019). Herbal medicine (Zhengan Xifeng Decoction) for essential hypertension protocol for a systematic review and meta-analysis. *Medicine, 98*(6), e14292. Retrieved from https://doi.org/10.1097/md.0000000000014292.

Klabunde, R. E. (2015, March 22). *Calcium-channel blockers (CCBs)*. Cardiovascular Pharmacology Concepts. Retrieved from https://cvpharmacology.com/vasodilator/CCB.

Klabunde, R. E. (2016, January 29). *Beta-adrenoceptor antagonists (beta-blockers)*. Cardiovascular Pharmacology Concepts. Retrieved from https://www.cvpharmacology.com/cardioinhibitory/beta-blockers.

Klabunde, R. E. (2017a, November 17). *Angiotensin converting enzyme (ACE) inhibitors*. Cardiovascular Pharmacology Concepts. Retrieved from https://cvpharmacology.com/vasodilator/ACE.

Klabunde, R. E. (2017b, November 17). *Angiotensin receptor blockers (ARBs)*. Cardiovascular Pharmacology Concepts. Retrieved from https://www.cvpharmacology.com/vasodilator/ARB.

Layne, K., & Ferro, A. (2016). Traditional Chinese medicines in the management of cardiovascular diseases: a comprehensive systematic review. *British Journal of Clinical Pharmacology, 83*(1), 20–32. Retrieved from https://doi.org/10.1111/bcp.13013.

Link, R., & Arnarson, A. (2020, March 12). *8 surprising health benefits of cloves*. Healthline. Retrieved from https://www.healthline.com/nutrition/benefits-of-cloves#_noHeaderPrefixedContent.

Magnifico, L. A. (2018, September 18). *7 home remedies for managing high blood pressure*. Healthline. Retrieved from https://www.healthline.com/health/high-blood-pressure-home-remedies.

Mayo Clinic Staff. (2021, June 25). *DASH diet: Healthy eating to lower your blood pressure*. Mayo Clinic. Retrieved from https://www.mayoclinic.org/healthy-lifestyle/nutrition-and-healthy-eating/in-depth/dash-diet/art-20048456.

Medicentres. (2019, June 3). *5 pressure points that will instantly lower your blood pressure!* Retrieved from https://medicentres.ae/2018/03/07/5-pressure-points-that-will-instantly-lower-your-blood-pressure/.

Menon, M., & Shukla, A. (2018). Understanding hypertension in the light of Ayurveda. *Journal of Ayurveda and Integrative Medicine, 9*(4), 302–307. Retrieved from https://doi.org/10.1016/j.jaim.2017.10.004.

Mercola, J. (2018, November 1). *Cat's claw potential health benefits*. Mercola.Com. Retrieved from https://articles.mercola.com/herbs-spices/cats-claw.aspx.

Ministry of Health. (2013). *Clinical practice guidelines: Management of hypertension* (4th ed.). Ministry of Health.

Morelli, J., & Ogbru, O. (2021, March 31). *High blood pressure (HBP) medications list, side effects, drug interactions & warning*. RxList. Retrieved from https://www.rxlist.com/high_blood_pressure_hypertension_medications/drugs-condition.htm.

Natura Magazine. (n.d.). *Alleviating hypertension naturally*. Eu Yan Sang. Retrieved from https://www.euyansang.com.sg/en/alleviating-hypertension-naturally/eyscardio13.html.

NDTV Food Desk. (2021, February 3). *Hypertension: 8 Ayurvedic remedies to manage high blood pressure*. NDTV.Com. Retrieved from https://www.ndtv.com/food/hypertension-8-ayurvedic-remedies-to-manage-high-blood-pressure-1943135.

NHS Website. (2020, March 18). *Treatment: High blood pressure (hypertension)*. Nhs.Uk. Retrieved from https://www.nhs.uk/conditions/high-blood-pressure-hypertension/treatment/.

Nicolas, D., Kerndt, C. C., & Reed, M. (2021). *Sacubitril/Valsartan*. StatPearls Publishing. Retrieved from https://www.ncbi.nlm.nih.gov/books/NBK507904/.

RxList (Ed.). (2021, June 11). *Black currant*. RxList. Retrieved from https://www.rxlist.com/black_currant/supplements.htm.

Sagon, B. C. (2011). *Harvard study: Dark chocolate can help lower your blood pressure*. AARP Bulletin. Retrieved from https://www.aarp.org/health/medical-research/info-03-2011/dark-chocolate-can-help-lower-your-blood-pressure.html.

Sheng-Nong Ktd. (Ed.). (2006). *High blood pressure and Chinese medicine*. Shen-Nong. Retrieved from http://www.shen-nong.com/eng/lifestyles/tcm_hypertension_high_blood_pressure_chinese_medicine.html.

Smith, A. A. (2020, December 15). *The 2020 practitioners guide to magnesium: Metabolics*. Metabolics High Quality Nutritional Supplements. Retrieved from https://www.metabolics.com/blog/the-definitive-guide-to-magnesium-and-magnesium-supplements.

Swasthi. (2019, July 14). *How to make aloe vera juice*. Swasthi's Recipes. Retrieved from https://www.indianhealthyrecipes.com/how-to-make-aloe-vera-juice/.

Tierra, L. (2018, May 15). *Hypertension II (Too!): A TCM look at types of high blood pressure*. East West School of Planetary Herbology. Retrieved from https://planetherbs.com/blogs/lesleys-blog/hypertension-ii-too-a-tcm-look-at-types-of-high-blood-pressure/.

Times Food (Ed.). (2018, May 17). *10 home remedies to reduce blood pressure naturally*. Times Food. Retrieved from https://recipes.timesofindia.com/articles/health/10-home-remedies-to-reduce-blood-pressure-naturally/photostory/64205222.cms.

Ware, M. (2017, November 2). *The health benefits of cabbage*. Medical News Today. Retrieved from https://www.medicalnewstoday.com/articles/284823#nutrition.

World Health Organization. (2019, June 11). *Cardiovascular diseases*. WHO. Retrieved from https://www.who.int/health-topics/cardiovascular-diseases/.

Zhang, D. Y., Cheng, Y. B., Guo, Q. H., Shan, X. L., Wei, F. F., Lu, F., et al. (2020). Treatment of masked hypertension with a Chinese herbal formula. *Circulation*, *142*(19), 1821–1830. Retrieved from https://doi.org/10.1161/circulationaha.120.046685.

Hyperlipidemia/Hypercholesterolemia

Busti, A. J. (2015, October). *The mechanism of action of Ezetimibe (Zetia) on the inhibition of cholesterol absorption*. Evidence-Based Medicine Consult. Retrieved from https://www.ebmconsult.com/articles/ezetimibe-mechanism-action-inhibit-cholesterol-absorption-intestine.

Chia, S. (2016, June 7). *Can TCM lower my cholesterol level?* AsiaOne. Retrieved from https://www.asiaone.com/health/can-tcm-lower-my-cholesterol-level.

Cooley, R. (2020, April 14). *Oregano oil may lower cholesterol naturally*. University Health News. Retrieved from https://universityhealthnews.com/daily/heart-health/herb-used-for-lowering-cholesterol-naturally/.

Datta, R. (2019, October 16). *6 most effective home remedies for cholesterol*. NDTV Food. Retrieved from https://food.ndtv.com/health/6-most-effective-home-remedies-for-cholesterol-1670512.

DrugBank Online Editorial Staff. (2005, June 13). *Atorvastatin: Uses, interactions, mechanism of action*. DrugBank. Retrieved from https://go.drugbank.com/drugs/DB01076.

Drugs.com (Ed.). (2021, June 30). *List of 48 high cholesterol medications compared*. Drugs.Com. Retrieved from https://www.drugs.com/condition/hyperlipidemia.html.

Harvard Health Editorial Staff. (2016, January 16). *Walnuts can lower cholesterol*. Harvard Health. Retrieved from https://www.health.harvard.edu/cholesterol/walnuts-can-lower-cholesterol.

Kalita, S., Khandelwal, S., Madan, J., Pandya, H., Sesikeran, B., & Krishnaswamy, K. (2018). Almonds and cardiovascular health: a review. *Nutrients*, *10*(4), 468. Retrieved from https://doi.org/10.3390/nu10040468.

Kumar, S. (2013). Chapter 39—Effect of *Terminalia arjuna* on cardiac hypertrophy [E-book]. In S. K. Maulik (Ed.), *Bioactive food as dietary interventions for cardiovascular disease* (1st ed., pp. 673–680). Academia Press. Retrieved from https://doi.org/10.1016/B978-0-12-396485-4.00036-0.

Kubala, J. (2017, November 4). *9 impressive health benefits of cabbage*. Healthline. Retrieved from https://www.healthline.com/nutrition/benefits-of-cabbage#TOC_TITLE_HDR_2.

Kubala, J., & Marengo, K. (2020, March 20). *9 benefits and uses of curry leaves*. Healthline. Retrieved from https://www.healthline.com/nutrition/curry-leaves-benefits.

Narsaria, R. (2021, January 28). *Homeopathic medicines, treatment and remedies for high cholesterol*. MyUpchar. Retrieved from https://www.myupchar.com/en/disease/high-cholesterol/homeopathy.

Nazario, B. (2004, December 8). *Which drugs lower my bad (LDL) cholesterol?* WebMD. Retrieved from https://www.webmd.com/cholesterol-management/guide/cholesterol-lowering-medication#1.

NHS Website. (2020, August 12). *Medicines for high cholesterol*. NHS.UK. Retrieved from https://www.nhs.uk/conditions/high-cholesterol/medicines-for-high-cholesterol/.

O'Brien, K. A. (2010). Alternative perspectives: how Chinese medicine understands hypercholesterolemia. *Cholesterol*, *2010*, 723289. Retrieved from https://doi.org/10.1155/2010/723289.

Ogbru, O. (2019, July 2). *Bile acid sequestrants: Drug facts, side effects and dosing*. MedicineNet. Retrieved from https://www.medicinenet.com/bile_acid_sequestrants/article.htm#what_are_bile_acid_sequestrants.

Park, R. (2018, August 14). *7 best remedies to lower high cholesterol levels naturally*. Remedies for Me. Retrieved from https://www.remediesforme.com/best-remedies-lower-high-cholesterol-naturally/.

Remedios, T. (2017, November 20). *Ayurveda tips to reduce high cholesterol*. The Times of India. Retrieved from https://timesofindia.indiatimes.com/life-style/health-fitness/health-news/ayurveda-tips-to-reduce-high-cholesterol/articleshow/19984193.cms.

Rosenfarb, A. (2007, August 1). The Yin and Yang of cholesterol hyperlipidemia. *Acupuncture Today*, *08*(08). Retrieved from https://www.acupuncturetoday.com/mpacms/at/article.php?id=31564.

Sitnikova, T. (2015, June 6). *12 best herbs to lower cholesterol and beat heart disease!* NaturalON—Natural Health News and Discoveries. Retrieved from https://naturalon.com/12-best-herbs-to-lower-cholesterol-and-beat-heart-disease/view-all/.

Staker, L. (2018, November 28). *Chinese herbs to lower cholesterol*. Healthfully. Retrieved from https://healthfully.com/chinese-herbs-to-lower-cholesterol-4771434.html.

StepIn2MyGreenWorld (Ed.). (2018, October 15). *6 essential herbs to lower your cholesterol naturally*. Step Into My Green World. Retrieved from http://www.stepin2mygreenworld.com/healthyliving/health/6-essential-herbs-for-cholesterol-health/.

WebMD (Ed.). (2011). *Amaranth*. WebMD. Retrieved from https://www.webmd.com/vitamins/ai/ingredientmono-869/amaranth.

Yoga U Editorial Staff. (2015, April 9). *Ayurvedic tips for lowering cholesterol naturally*. Yoga U Online. Retrieved from https://www.yogauonline.com/yoga-for-heart-disease/ayurvedic-tips-for-lowering-cholesterol-naturally.

Ischemic Heart Disease/Coronary Artery Disease

Bhargava, H. (2007, January 1). *Coronary artery disease*. WebMD. Retrieved from https://www.webmd.com/heart-disease/guide/heart-disease-coronary-artery-disease#1.

British Homeopathic Association. (n.d.). *Homeopathy UK*. Homeopathy UK. Retrieved from https://homeopathy-uk.org/.

Carey, E., & Whitworth, G. (2019, May 29). *The 6 best supplements and herbs for atherosclerosis*. Healthline. Retrieved from https://www.healthline.com/health/high-cholesterol/herbs-for-atherosclerosis#1.

Chauhan, M. (2019, April 30). *Ischemic heart disease*. Planet Ayurveda. Retrieved from https://www.planetayurveda.com/library/ischemic-heart-disease/.

Elvis, A., & Ekta, J. (2011). Ozone therapy: A clinical review. *Journal of Natural Science, Biology and Medicine, 2*(1), 66. Retrieved from https://doi.org/10.4103/0976-9668.82319.

Eu Yan Sang (Ed.). (n.d.). *Soothing a cough with TCM*. Eu Yan Sang. Retrieved from https://www.euyansang.com.sg/en/soothing-a-cough-with-tcm/eysihillnesses2.html.

Herbpathy (Ed.). (n.d.). *Atherosclerosis herbal treatment, prevention, symptoms, causes, cured by*. Herbpathy: Make Life Healthy. Retrieved from https://herbpathy.com/Herbal-Treatment-for-Atherosclerosis-Cid2449.

Jagalur, C. (2017, November 30). *Ayurvedic treatment for coronary artery blockage without surgery!* Lybrate. Retrieved from https://www.lybrate.com/topic/ayurvedic-treatment-for-coronary-artery-blockage-without-surgery/6bd2419e389c1e87c4cf72f3a164d16a.

Joy, A. (2017). *Coronary artery disease and its Ayurvedic treatment definition*. Ayurveda Treatment Methods. Retrieved from https://www.ayurveda-treatments.co.in/ayurvedatreatments/index.php/8-coronary-artery-disease-and-its-ayurvedic-treatment-defination-coronary-artery.

Khaliq, A. (2011, July 6). *Ayurvedic treatment for heart diseases*. Onlymyhealth. Retrieved from https://www.onlymyhealth.com/ayurvedic-treatment-for-heart-diseases-1298540356.

Kiefer, D., & Butler, N. (2017, September 2). *Herbs and supplements for heart disease*. Healthline. Retrieved from https://www.healthline.com/health/heart-disease/herbs-supplements.

Lade, H. (2014, July 23). *Acupuncture and Chinese herbs for coronary artery disease (CAD)*. The Acupuncture Clinic. Retrieved from https://www.theacupunctureclinic.co.nz/acupuncture-and-chinese-herbs-for-coronary-artery-disease-cad/.

Mayo Clinic Staff. (2020, June 5). *Coronary artery disease*. Mayo Clinic. Retrieved from https://www.mayoclinic.org/diseases-conditions/coronary-artery-disease/diagnosis-treatment/drc-20350619.

Stanford Health Care Editorial Staff. (2017, September 12). *Types of percutaneous coronary interventions*. Stanford Health Care. Retrieved from https://stanfordhealthcare.org/medical-treatments/p/percutaneous-coronary-revascularization/types.html.

Sweis, R., & Jivan, A. (2020, July). *Drug treatment of coronary artery disease*. MSD Manual Consumer Version. Retrieved from https://www.msdmanuals.com/home/heart-and-blood-vessel-disorders/coronary-artery-disease/drug-treatment-of-coronary-artery-disease.

WebMD (Ed.). (n.d.). *Ashwagandha*. WebMD. Retrieved from https://www.webmd.com/vitamins/ai/ingredientmono-953/ashwagandha.

Wong, C., & Fogoros, R. (2020, February 4). *Natural therapies for atherosclerosis*. Verywell Health. Retrieved from https://www.verywellhealth.com/can-alternative-medicine-fight-atherosclerosis-88836.

Wong, C. K. (2009, February). *The role of antiplatelet agents (No. 19)*. Bpac NZ. Retrieved from https://bpac.org.nz/BPJ/2009/february/docs/bpj19_antiplatelet_pages_32-37.pdf.

Xiumei Wu, M. (2017, September 6). *Traditional Chinese medicine for cardiovascular health*. Vitality Magazine. Retrieved from https://vitalitymagazine.com/article/traditional-chinese-medicine-for-cardiovascular-health/.

Heart Failure

Bharani, A., Ganguly, A., & Bhargava, K. (1995). Salutary effect of *Terminalia Arjuna* in patients with severe refractory heart failure. *International Journal of Cardiology, 49*(3), 191–199. Retrieved from https://doi.org/10.1016/0167-5273(95)02320-v.

Dwivedi, S., & Chopra, D. (2014). Revisiting *Terminalia arjuna*—An ancient cardiovascular drug. *Journal of Traditional and Complementary Medicine, 4*(4), 224–231. Retrieved from https://doi.org/10.4103/2225-4110.139103.

Flaws, B. (2002, January 1). Chinese medicine & congestive heart failure. *Acupuncture Today, 03*(02). Retrieved from https://www.acupuncturetoday.com/mpacms/at/article.php?id=27899.

Frankel Cardiovascular Center Staff. (n.d.). *EECP (Enhanced External Counter Pulsation) Treatment*. University of Michigan Cardiovascular Center. Retrieved from https://www.umcvc.org/conditions-treatments/eecp-enhanced-external-counter-pulsation-treatment.

Harvard Health. (2019, December 1). *Can a salt substitute cause high potassium levels?* Retrieved from https://www.health.harvard.edu/heart-health/can-a-salt-substitute-cause-high-potassium-levels.

Kaneka Ubiquinol (Ed.). (2021, January 28). *Ubiquinol for heart*. Kaneka Ubiquinol. Retrieved from https://www.kaneka-ubiquinol.com/health-benefits/heart-health/.

Kanne, H., Prasanna, V., Burte, N., & Gujjula, R. (2015). Extraction and elemental analysis of Coleus forskohlii extract. *Pharmacognosy Research, 7*(3), 237–241. Retrieved from https://doi.org/10.4103/0974-8490.157966.

Larrabee, B. (2019, March 1). *Medicines for congestive heart failure*. Kaiser Permanente. Retrieved from https://wa.kaiserpermanente.org/healthAndWellness/index.jhtml?itcm=%2Fcommon%2FhealthAndWellness%2Fconditions%2FheartDisease%2FchfMedications.html.

Maharishi AyurVeda Staff. (n.d.). *Ayurvedic heart health tips and recommendations*. Maharishi Ayurveda. Retrieved from https://mapi.com/blogs/articles/ayurvedic-heart-health-tips-and-recommendations.

Michigan Medicine Editorial Staff. (2021). *Health library*. The University of Michigan Health| Michigan Medicine. Retrieved from https://www.uofmhealth.org/health-library/hn-1193009.

Patel, K. (2018, June 15). *Terminalia arjuna*. Examine.Com. Retrieved from https://examine.com/supplements/terminalia-arjuna/.

PeaceHealth (Ed.). (2015, May 6). *Congestive heart failure (Holistic)*. PeaceHealth. Retrieved from https://www.peacehealth.org/medical-topics/id/hn-1193009.

Saul, A. W. (2019). *Congestive heart failure*. DoctorYourself.Com. Retrieved from http://www.doctoryourself.com/congestive.html.

Shoemaker, S. (2019, August 26). *9 impressive health benefits of Hawthorn Berry*. Healthline. Retrieved from https://www.healthline.com/nutrition/hawthorn-berry-benefits.

Sinatra, S. (2016, November 30). *Natural remedies for congestive heart failure*. Healthy Directions. Retrieved from https://www.healthydirections.com/articles/heart-health/natural-treatments-for-congestive-heart-failure.

Tang, W. H. W., & Nagarajan, V. (2019, January 20). *Aldosterone receptor antagonists*. The Cardiology Advisor. Retrieved from https://www.thecardiologyadvisor.com/home/decision-support-in-medicine/cardiology/aldosterone-receptor-antagonists/.

WebMD (Ed.). (n.d.). *Terminalia: Overview, uses, side effects, precautions, interactions, dosing and reviews*. WebMD. Retrieved from https://www.webmd.com/vitamins/ai/ingredientmono-811/terminalia.

WebMD (Ed.). (2017, February 13). *Potassium rich foods*. WebMD. Retrieved from https://www.webmd.com/diet/foods-rich-in-potassium#1.

Xia, L. M., & Luo, M. H. (2015). Study progress of berberine for treating cardiovascular disease. *Chronic Diseases and Translational Medicine, 1*(4), 231–235. Retrieved from https://doi.org/10.1016/j.cdtm.2015.11.006.

Zimney, E. (2008, February 7). *Hawthorn for heart failure—good news and bad news*. Everyday Health. Retrieved from https://www.everydayhealth.com/columns/zimney-health-and-medical-news-you-can-use/hawthorne-for-heart-failure-good-news-and-bad-news/.

2

Respiratory System
Cough, Cold, Flu, and Sore Throat

Cough, cold, and flu are common across all ages, especially in the very young and elderly. Natural remedies alone or together with judicious use of modern medicines are the best way to either beat these common ailments or provide temporary relief. Combining, complementing, and integrating traditional and modern medical practices is the basis of integrative medicine. Cold and flu symptoms are generally similar. Cold symptoms often come on gradually, whereas flu symptoms may occur suddenly. Signs and symptoms of flu include fever, headache, and extreme fatigue, whereas cold symptoms include stuffy nose, sneezing, congestion, and sore throat. Allergies may also be a factor.

Chronic cough is a cough that lasts 8 weeks or more. Common causes of chronic cough include asthma, Chronic obstructive pulmonary disease (COPD), pneumonia, bronchitis, acid reflux or Gastroesophageal reflux disease (GERD), post-nasal drip from rhinitis or rhinosinusitis, allergies, tonsillitis/adenoiditis/adeno-tonsillitis, tuberculosis, and drug-induced causes like Angiotensin - converting - enzyme (ACE) inhibitors. Uncommon causes include cystic fibrosis, heart failure, interstitial lung disease, lung tumors, bronchiectasis, sarcoidosis, and whooping cough. Chronic cough can lead to sleeplessness, chest pain, headaches, fatigue, and urinary incontinence. Other signs and symptoms include fever, night sweats, chills, hemoptysis (coughing blood), fast breathing, and weight loss.

Investigations include chest or paranasal sinus x-rays, CT thorax, bronchoscopy or biopsy to look at lower airways, rhinoscopy to look at the nasal passages, sputum for culture, throat and nose swabs for culture, spirometry or lung-function tests, fractional exhaled nitric oxide (FeNO), peak flow variability, blood counts and infection markers, allergy tests, skin prick tests, oximetry, arterial blood gas, and other disease-specific tests.

Asthma is characterized by airway inflammation causing cough, wheezing, shortness of breath, and—if severe—decreased activity, fatigue, and difficulty speaking. Causes and risk factors include allergens (commonly dust mite, pollen, dog or cat dander, mold, and cockroach droppings), food and food additives (commonly dairy, eggs, wheat, nuts, seafood, soy, and sulfite preservatives), medications (usually aspirin, NSAIDs, beta blockers), air pollution, smoking, weather changes, over-exercise, extreme emotions (excitement, laughter, stress), acid reflux, infections, rhinitis/rhinosinusitis, prematurity, and genetic predisposition. It can be life-threatening if there is a severe wheeze or anaphylaxis.

Rhinitis (hay fever or allergic rhinitis) is characterized by nasal passage inflammation with the presence of a blocked or runny nose with watery discharge, sneezing, and itchy, red, and watery eyes. It is often due to airborne allergens.

Sinusitis is inflammation of the lining inside the sinuses. It causes headaches and yellow or greenish nasal discharge. It is acute or chronic and is often associated with rhinitis and nasal polyps.

Pneumonia is inflammation of the lungs due to infection by a virus, bacteria, fungus, and parasite. Signs and symptoms include productive cough with yellow or greenish sputum and sometimes blood, fever with chills and rigors, fast breathing, and chest pain.

Chronic obstructive pulmonary disease (COPD): This is a progressive lung disease due largely to smoking and air pollution. There are two types: chronic bronchitis (a recurrent cough with mucus) and emphysema (which causes more lung damage).

Prevention and Long-Term Lung and Airway Health

Lung/airway health (respiratory) must start from a young age to build good, clean airways, strong bones, and muscles in the ribcage. Lifestyle practices such as adequate nutrition, sunlight exposure, exercise, and pollution-free environments are important.

Nutrition

Cod liver oil or emulsion and later capsules should be given daily from infancy through adulthood. It contains vitamin A and D, which are important for bone and respiratory mucosal health. In general, a well-balanced and antioxidant-rich diet ensures optimal health.

Exercise

Young children should be allowed to play in open fields, particularly in the morning sun. Rubbing some cod liver oil on the child's body and then sunning is an old practice to develop strong bones and lungs. All sports, regular exercises, and even dance should be encouraged as part of fitness.

Breathing

Yoga, especially pranayama breathing, must be taught from preschool to school and should become a way of life throughout adulthood. Do pranayama breathing daily. This includes Kapalbhati (skull-polishing breath), Bhastrika (bellows breath), Dirgha (three-part breath), and Ujjayi (ocean-sounding breath). Qigong can be practiced by everyone, especially the elderly.

Pollution and Allergen-Free Environments

Avoid smoking. Occupational health should also be addressed in workplaces. Safety measures such as masks should be provided to prevent inhalation of chemical pollutants. Age-old practices such as the sunning of bedding and regular washing of bed linens can eliminate dust mites and molds. Avoid airborne or ingested allergens.

Immune Boosters

These help ward off cold and flu and to strengthen the immune system. Before any travel, immune boosters such as vitamins A and C and herbal preparations like echinacea can be taken (read more under "Immune Boosters" chapter).

General Measures for Acute Respiratory Infections

Home-care measures are usually adequate. Most acute respiratory infections (ARIs) are self-limiting, as they are caused by viruses. Recovery is usually within 7 to 10 days. The following measures are advised.

Ensuring adequate rest and sleep.

Consuming plenty of warm fluids with honey, nourishing soups, herbal drinks, and soups and broths. Ice lollies can be given for painful sore throats.

Treating fever and pain with paracetamol or ibuprofen.

Maintaining a clean, cool, and humid environment free of smoke, other irritants, and pollutants.

Using saltwater/saline gargles and saline nasal sprays to clear, cleanse, and soothe the upper airways and throat.

Using over-the-counter remedies for colds and coughs.

Regular hand washing and using a face mask to prevent virus spread.

Diagnostic tests include blood counts, pulse oximetry, blood gas, sputum exams, allergy tests, chest x-ray, CT thorax, lung function tests (spirometry, body plethysmography and gas diffusion), ventilation-perfusion scan, bronchoscopy, thoracoscopy, pleural tap, lung biopsy, lymph node biopsy and specific tests (tuberculosis, antibodies, etc.).

Indian Natural Remedies

In Ayurveda, it is believed that allergy symptoms and phlegm are due to excessive Kapha dosha (water + earth elements).

Common Ingredients for Cough, Cold, Flu, and Sore Throat

Spices	Leaves/Herbs	Miscellaneous
Allspice	False black pepper (Embelia ribes)	
	Rudraksha (Elaeocarpus ganitrus)	
	Indian Coleus (Coleus forskolii)	
Bitter cumin (Centratherum anthelminticum)	Oregano (Origanum vulgare)	Axlewood/Ghatti gum (Anogeissus latifolia)
Black pepper (Piper nigrum)	Karpooravalli (Coleus amboinicus)	Rock sugar
Carom/ajwain (Trachyspermum ammi)	Lemongrass (Cymbopogon citratus)	Trikatu powder: long pepper (Piper longum), black pepper (Piper nigrum), ginger (Zingiber officinalis)
Cayenne pepper (Capsicum annuum)	Gum arabic/Babul (Vachellia nilotica)	
Cinnamon (Cinnamomum verum)	Kantakari (Solanum xanthocarpum)	
Coriander (Coriandrum sativum)	Liquorice (Glycyrrhiza glabra)	Palm sugar candy/ panam kalkandu
Cumin (Nigella sativa)	Tulsi/holy basil (Ocimum tenuiflorum)	Honey
Fenugreek (Trigonella foenum-graecum)	Nilavembu (Andrographis paniculata)	Apple cider vinegar
Garlic (Allium sativum)	Betel leaves (Piper betle)	Camphor (Cinnamomum camphora)
Ginger (Zingiber officinale)	Nirgundi/nochi (Vitex negundo)	Ghee
Green cardamom (Elettaria cardamomum)	Plantain weed/leaf (Plantago major)	
Red clover (Trifolium pratense)	Bala (Sida cordifolia)	
Tamarind (Tamarindus indica)	Giloy (Tinospora cordifolia)	Garden cress seeds
Turmeric (Curcuma longa)	Long peppers (Piper longum/ thippili)	Sea coconut (Lodoicea maldivica)

Common Recipes for Cough, Cold, Flu, and Sore Throat

Oral

Teas/Brews/Others (Respiratory Tonics and Immune Boosters)

Ajwain. Take 1 teaspoon of ajwain seeds (carom). Add 1 cup boiling water and 1 teaspoon of turmeric. Boil and reduce volume till ½ cup. Add some honey. Consume twice a day.

Axlewood. Chew the stem bark or swallow the sap.

Babul tree bark tea. Lightly pound dry babul tree bark and steep in a cup of hot water. Add honey to taste and drink warm.

Bala drink. Take ½ to 2 g of dried bala powder. Add warm or cold water.

Cayenne pepper tea. Mix a pinch of cayenne pepper and 1 tablespoon of apple cider vinegar or lime juice in a glass of hot water and consume.

To make a syrup version, mix ¼ teaspoon of cayenne pepper, ¼ teaspoon of dry ground ginger (powder), 1 tablespoon of honey, 1 tablespoon of apple cider vinegar, and 2 tablespoons of water. Consume 1 teaspoon of this mixture two or three times per day.

Clove oil-Garlic. Take 1 crushed garlic pip. Add 3 to 5 drops of clove oil and little honey. Suck slowly to soothe the throat.

Coriander brew. Take one to two handfuls of coriander seeds, 1 teaspoon of cumin, and some black peppercorn. Blend lightly and add to a pot of water and boil. Add rock sugar or panam kalkandu. Some karpooravalli or tulsi leaves can be added at last and cover the pot. Strain and drink a cupful several times a day.

Cumin (black). Take a pinch of black cumin, 3 to 5 peppercorn and little salt. Chew slowly.

Garden cress seeds. Soak the seeds in water and consume them.

Garlic-ginger brew. Flatten a piece of ginger and a few pips of garlic. Steep them in a glass of hot water. Drink twice a day with added honey if required.

Giloy. Take some giloy stems. Add 1 cup of water. Boil till ½ volume. Strain and consume daily.

Variation #1. Take some giloy stems. Add some ginger, amla powder, and black pepper. Blend and drink.

Variation #2. Alternatively, chew on the giloy stem.

Ginger-infused tea. Add boiling water to a slightly flattened piece of ginger. Drink when warm.

Hot coffee eggnog/hot toddy. For an older child, hot coffee eggnog/hot toddy may soothe the cough. To make this, whisk a raw egg with honey or palm sugar until well mixed. Add boiling coffee and milk to the egg mixture. Stir quickly or whisk, then add a teaspoon of whisky or brandy to it. Serve hot.

Hot Polyherbal Spice brew/tea. (also called decoction or kadha/kwath kashayam)

Each family has their own kadha recipe.

Various spices, herbs and leaves generate heat. These include ginger, pepper corn, tulsi (preferably black tulsi/basil), turmeric, honey, cumin, cloves, lemongrass, guava leaves, moringa leaves and jasmine leaves.

Cooling herbs, spices or foods include licorice, cardamom, coconut water, mint, rose water, oranges, and water melon

Basic recipe. Boil 2 cups of water in a saucepan. Add herbs and spices (quantity is usually by a pinch and handful measures).

These common herbs and spice ingredients include 1 inch peeled ginger, 5-6 peppercorn, 2 inches cinnamon stick, and 5 cloves. Crush them in a blender or pestle-mortar) Add to the boiling water and also 5-6 tulsi leaves. Simmer for about 15 to 20 minutes at low heat until the volume is reduced to half. Strain and add sweetener (honey, jaggery, rock sugar or palm sugar/panam kalkandu) and/or lemon juice if desired. Optional ingredients that can be added include licorice (mulethi)

Do not overboil when the herbs or spices are added to water. It can turn bitter and cause heartburn. Consume ½ cup per day for about 3 weeks and then stop for about 2 weeks Excessive or prolonged consumption can lead to " too much heat" in the body causing skin dryness, acne, urine infection, and constipation.

Variation #1. Ginger (1-2 inches lightly pounded), lemon slices, honey, and a pinch of salt may also be used.

Variation #2. Ginger (1-2 inches lightly pounded), tulsi leaves (10-20 leaves) and karpooravalli (10-12 leaves)

Variation #3. Cinnamon sticks (2-3 crushed sticks) pepper, coriander seeds, ginger fresh or dry, cumin, turmeric).

Variation #4. Coriander, cumin, and fenugreek brew. Put 3 tablespoons of coriander seeds + ½ tablespoon of cumin + ½ tablespoon of fenugreek in a pot of water. Boil and then simmer for about 30 minutes. Strain and add honey. Drink twice a day when unwell.

Variation #5. Add 1 teaspoon of crushed black peppercorn,1 teaspoon of crushed cumin, 1 piece of crushed ginger, 10 young neem leaves, 6 to 7 Kathpooravali leaves, 10 tulsi leaves, 1 betel leaf torn into smaller pieces. Bring to the boil and reduce till ½ volume. Add ¼ teaspoon turmeric and 2 teaspoons of palm sugar. Strain and drink ¼ cup three times per day for at least 7 to 10 days. Do not consume anything else for at least 1 hour after the brew.

Variation #6. Mix ground pepper (10%), ground fenugreek (10%), ground cumin (10%), karpooravalli – dried (50%), and tulsi – dried (20%). Add hot water. Steep for 5 to 10 minutes. Strain and drink.

Variation # 7. Boil 4 cups water in a saucepan. Take various ingredients (½ teaspoon crushed or grated ginger, 3-4 peppercorn, ½ teaspoon grated fresh turmeric and 2-3 cloves. Add to the boiling water and also 5-6 tulsi leaves. Simmer for about 15-20 minutes until the volume is reduced to half. Strain and add any desired sweetener

Variation # 8. Boil 1 litre of water in a saucepan. Take various ingredients (1 tablespoon crushed ginger, 2 teaspoons peppercorn, 2 inches cinnamon stick, 4-5 green cardamoms, and 2 teaspoon cloves. Crush them in a blender or pestle-mortar) Add these ingredients to the boiling water and also 1 handful each of washed, torn guava, tulsi, moringa and jasmine leaves. Simmer for about 15 to 20 minutes at low heat until the volume is reduced to half. Strain and add sweetener (honey, jaggery, rock sugar or palm sugar) if desired.

Kantakari. Take ½ teaspoon of kantakari powder. Add some water and honey. Consume twice a day.

Karpooravalli brew. Take three to five fresh leaves. Crush them and squeeze out the green juice with your hands.

> Variation #1. It can also be blended with little water. Squeeze out the juice and consume.
>
> Variation #2. The karpooravalli leaves can also be chewed slowly.

Lemongrass tea. Take five to six fresh leaves (1 teaspoon of dried leaves) or two bashed stalks of the lower stem. Boil in 1 cup of water and let it steep. Drink warm.

Liquorice tea. Take 1 teaspoon of dried ground root in 1 cup of water. Boil for 5 minutes. Drain and drink warm.

> Variation #1. Take a handful of liquorice sticks. Wash, pound, and flatten the sticks lightly in a mortar. Place in a saucepan of water and add a handful of raisins. Boil and simmer for about 15 to 20 minutes. Drink a cupful of this warm brew three to four times a day.
>
> Variation #2. Take 5 tablespoons of sliced liquorice roots (or some crushed sticks), 1 crushed cinnamon stick, and some fresh ginger slices. Add 5 cups of water. Boil and simmer for 15 to 20 minutes. Drink a cupful throughout the day.

Milk. Boil a glass of milk with two to three pips of blended/pounded garlic. Add a teaspoon of turmeric powder and honey. Consume twice a day.

> Variation #1. Add one teaspoon of turmeric, a pinch of cinnamon powder, some honey, or a pinch of pepper powder to a glass of hot milk. Drink this especially before bedtime.

Nilavembu tea. Take a handful of fresh nilavembu branches and pluck the leaves off. Break the stems into shorter segments and steep in water overnight. Discard the stems the next morning and drink the tea.

Plantain weed/leaf tea. Take a ¼ to ½ teaspoon of fresh leaves (or dried) and boil in 1 cup of water. Steep for 10 to 15 minutes. Cool and drink two to three times a day.

> Variation #1. Add 1 teaspoon of plantain leaves and 1 teaspoon of thyme into 100 mL of water. Boil the water. Add two drops of lime juice and honey to taste. Strain and drink.

Alternatively, for sore throat, gargle with plantain tea or apply the tincture under the tongue.

Rasam. Blend one handful coriander seeds, 1 tablespoon cumin and two to three pips of garlic. In a saucepan, heat up ghee (or oil), add in one to two dried chili, some mustard seeds, and some curry leaves. Add the blended mixture. Fry until aromatic. Pour about 3.5 cups of water into the saucepan, add tamarind and turmeric to the mixture. Add salt to taste and bring the mixture to a boil. Finally, add coriander leaves (optional) and turn off the heat.

Red clover tea. Take 2 teaspoons of red clover in 1 cup of water. Boil for 5 minutes. Allow it to steep. Drink warm.

Tulsi-infused tea. Add boiling water to 10 to 15 leaves of tulsi. Drink when warm.

Warm water. Drink a lot of warm water.

Pastes/Powders

Herb-spice paste. Place two cloves of garlic, half a small onion, one piece of turmeric, one piece of ginger, the juice of a lemon, a dash of cayenne pepper, and a teaspoon of raw honey into a blender. Blend until smooth and place in a clean, dry container. Store in a cool, dark place. Take 1 to 2 teaspoons when necessary.

Herbal-spice powder. Take methi/fenugreek (200 g), ajwain/carom seeds (100 g), kali jeeri/cumin (50 g). Roast together and keep the powder in a bottle. Take ¾ teaspoon daily to prevent coughs, colds, and flu.

Herbal-spice powder paste. Combine fenugreek (50 g), cumin (50 g), and black pepper (50 g). Roast lightly and pulverize. Mix ½ teaspoon with honey and consume two to three times a day.

Karpooravalli leaves. Chew karpooravalli leaves (five to six leaves) alone or with one to two black peppercorn or rock sugar to relieve sore throat and cough.

Liquorice paste. Mix ground liquorice with some honey. Consume the paste to treat coughs.

Onions (shallots). Pound or blend some onions (shallots) with a little turmeric. Add some honey. Consume 1 to 2 teaspoons to relieve sore throat and cough. Alternatively, eat raw onions (shallots) two to three times a day.

Rock sugar and black pepper. Make a paste of powdered rock sugar and black pepper powder with ghee. Consume it at night for sore throat.

> Variation #1. Mix rock sugar powder and black pepper powder with some warm water. Drink at night to clear a productive or wet cough with mucus.

Rudraksha paste. Mix some Rudraksha powder (churna), fresh tulsi leaf and honey and consume.

> Variation #1. Take ½ teaspoon Rudraksha churna and ½ teaspoon turmeric powder. Mix with 10 ml of honey. Place a few drops on the tongue and lick every 15 to 30 minutes in the acute stage and later 2 or 3 times per day if chronic.

Salt. Place some grains of salt on the tip of your tongue and push them to the back of the throat (to treat a sore throat).

Tamarind. Roll tamarind (pellet-sized) in a little salt and turmeric powder; suck on it to relieve sore throat.

Trikatu. Mix ¼ teaspoon of trikatu powder with little honey or crushed rock sugar and consume before meals at least twice a day. A pinch of turmeric may be added. Alternatively, the trikatu powder can be sprinkled over food or added into a glass of warm water and consumed.

Tulsi leaves. Chew tulsi leaves (5 to 10 leaves) alone or with 1 to 2 black peppercorns or some rock sugar to relieve sore throat and cough.

Therapeutic Measures

- **Induce vomiting.** (Infants/younger children tend to swallow their phlegm and they will feel and eat better if the phlegm is removed. The following herbs are used:

  Ginger. Pound ginger and squeeze the extract into a small container. Heat a knife over a flame till red hot and dip into the ginger juice extract. The bottom part will be the thick white sap/sediment. Discard this sediment. The upper part will be a translucent amber fluid. Mix this part with a little honey. Feed this mixture to the child.

Karpooravalli, tulsi, and betel leaf. Pound karpooravalli, tulsi, and betel leaf. Squeeze out the juice and feed the child to induce vomiting. (For the young infant use about 5 to 10 mL, and 10 to 15 mL for older children).

- **Nasal (Inhalational).**
  Use the following:
  - **Garlic vapor.** This is usually done for newborn babies. The garlic peel is placed in an incense pot and lit with some incense. A little frankincense can also be added. Keep the baby warm and let them inhale the garlic vapor.
  - **Steam inhalation.** The following items can be added to hot water in a pot or saucepan. Sit under a covered blanket or together if it is a child. Open the lid of the pot/pan in a controlled manner and according to tolerated steam level.
    Crushed camphor pieces (but beware of bronchospasm)
    Eucalyptus oil
    Menthol crystals
    Vicks
    Karpooravalli leaves. Place a few fresh karpooravalli leaves
    A combination mixture of crushed camphor, black peppercorn, and ajwain can be tied into a cloth and steeped into a pot of hot water and inhaled in the above manner.

  Also, a steamy bathroom can be created by running hot water from a tap. Sit in the bathroom for about 10 to 15 minutes with the infant on your lap.
  - **Nasal irrigation (saline sprays or neti pot).** Add 1 to 2 teaspoons of salt to a little hot water. Once salt is dissolved, add room temperature water till the salt solution is lukewarm and bearable to the touch. Pour some of the warm salt water into the cupped left hand. Close the right nostril with any right-hand finger and inhale the saline into the open left nostril from the cupped left palm. The salt solution can be felt at the back of the throat. Repeat three to five times. Do the same with the other nostril. Commercial saline nasal sprays are also available as single or multi-use. Alternatively, a *neti pot* may also be used. Do this daily. This cleanses the nasal passages and removes allergen particles or pollutants.
  - **Nasya.** Place some sesame oil into the nostril using the little finger, squirt bottle, or dropper. Other formulated or medicated nasya oils or ghee can also be used. A few drops of eucalyptus oil can be added into the sesame oil. Do this about 1 hour after the neti pot nasal saline irrigation.

  Ginger nasya can be done when the sinuses are clogged or congested. Add a pinch of ginger powder to a little warm sesame oil and water. Apply the ginger drops to each nostril and sniff deeply.
  - **Essential oil mist therapy.** Essential oils are extracts from various parts of the plants, such as roots, flowers, leaves, or stems. Various essential oils can be administered via a humidifier/diffuser. For cough, the following essential oils can be used—marjoram, lavender, cedar wood, or peppermint oil. For congestion, marjoram, lemon, lime, and lavender can be used. If a diffuser is not available, sprinkle a few drops of essential oil on the child's clothes or bed sheets.
  - **Camphor with peppercorn and caraway seeds.** One piece of camphor with little peppercorn and caraway seeds (ajwain) are ground and placed in a muslin cloth bag or handkerchief. This is pinned onto the pillow cover or to the child's clothing. The inhaled vapor will relieve nasal congestion.
  - **Nochi leaves.** Dried nochi leaves can be tied into a cloth knot and pinned onto the infant's shirt, especially at night.
  - **Breast milk.** A little breast milk may also be squirted into each of the baby's nostrils to relieve congestion.
- **Topical.**
  - **Vegetable oil.** Add 1 to 2 tablespoons of vegetable oil (coconut, mustard, or olive) to a pan and heat up. Chop one to two garlic pips, adding it to the hot oil. Brown the chopped garlic in oil over low heat until it emits an aroma. Pour this garlic oil into a small stainless-steel container. Instead of garlic, tulsi leaves with a pinch of camphor (non-edible) can also be added to the oil. To use, apply this warm oil with your two fingers onto the baby's face (i.e., the sides of the nose the cheeks, with a little on the forehead and throat. This will cover the nasal passages and sinuses). It can also be applied to the scalp to relieve nasal congestion.
  - **Vicks VapoRub (for infants).** Rub on the chest, neck, and soles of the feet before covering the feet with socks.
  - **Hot vegetable oil (coconut, mustard, or olive).** Massage on the chest and neck of the child.
  - **Rasna Choornam/Churna.** This is rubbed over the soft spot (vertex) of the head. A pinch of it can also be inhaled into the congested nostril. Refer to "Commercial Preparations."
  - **Mix spice.** Mix 1 g of cinnamon powder, 1 g of cardamom powder, and 125 mg of allspice. Add 1 teaspoon of honey. Lick three times a day for a few days for sore throat.
  - **False long pepper and ginger.** Crush some leaves of the false long pepper (vidanga) with ginger and use it as a mouthwash.
- **Diet.**
  Maintenance health brew. To maintain respiratory, gut, and overall health, make and take the following brews most days:
  Morning: Take a teaspoonful of ginger-honey mixture first thing in the morning on an empty stomach (thin slices, crushed or ground fresh ginger steeped in a bottle of honey).
  Midday: Take 1 teaspoon of dried ginger powder (chuku) mixed with a little ghee before lunch.

Evening: Take 1 teaspoon of kadukkai (Terminalia chebula/haritaki) powder before dinner.

Kapha-pacifying meals. Eat kapha-pacifying meals. Consume warm, fresh, and light foods cooked with a little ghee or olive oil. Avoid heavy or cold foods like meat, milk, wheat, iced drinks, and leftovers. This will spark and not dampen the digestive fire (agni).

Avoid foods that tend to produce phlegm such as yogurt, fried foods, sweets, and lentils.

Do not feed honey to children under 1 year of age due to risk of infantile botulism.

Water fast. Follow a 100% water fast for the first 2 to 3 days. Drink cool water. After the first 2 to 3 days, when the patient is able to swallow, they may be given coconut water and raw vegetable juices for another 2 to 3 days. Finally, some raw or steamed vegetables may be given. Many of the recipes appear similar, and there is no hard-and-fast rule. A mix-and-match style can be used.

- **Yoga**. Practice yoga, especially pranayama breathing daily, to maintain good lung health.
  Pranayama techniques include:
  Nadi shodhana pranayama (alternate nostril breathing)
  Kapalabhati pranayama (skull shining breath)
  Ujjayi pranayama (victorious breath)
  Yoga asanas include:
  Bhujangasana (cobra pose)
  Ardha chandrasana (half-moon pose)
  Dhanurasana (bow pose)
  Hasta Uttanasana (raised arm yoga pose)
  Chakrasana (wheel pose)
  Ustrasana (camel pose)
- **Others.**
  - Keep a cut onion in the bedroom. This may help prevent infection by absorbing the bacteria/virus. (It is difficult to say if this is folklore or fact.)
  - Suction out mucus from babies' nose and mouth (in young infants). A mucous extractor can be used. In the past, caregivers often performed mouth-to-face suction to clear the baby's congested nose and throat.
  - Keep the baby's head, hand, feet, and chest covered and warm with a cap, mitten, socks, and other warm clothing, especially in winter.
  - Bowel clearance using a mild enema is beneficial for clearing heat and toxins from the body.

Commercial Ayurvedic Preparations (Oral and Topical)

Commercial preparations with mixed herbs are also available, such as:

Oral

Pankajakasthuri. It is useful for chesty wet cough and contains the following ingredients: black pepper, long pepper, ginger, cardamom, cinnamon, Indian ginseng (*Withania somnifera*/ashwagandha), tamarind, cumin seeds, bael, arusa, mishri, haritaki (*Terminalia chebula*), vibhitaki, manjistha, and dusparsha.

Rasna choornam. Ribwort plantain (Rasna), Indian ginseng, Himalayan cedar (devadaru), Hellebore (katuka), white dammar (sarjarasa), costus (kottam), sweet flag (vayampu), Red ochre (gairika), turmeric, liquorice, country mallow (bala), nutgrass (mushta), black pepper, long pepper, ginger, Indian elm (puti), stinking gum, Vetiver (jala), khas grass (ushira), phenaka, sandalwood, aloes wood (aguru/agarwood), tamarind leaves.

Samahan. This is a polyherbal formulation containing 14 ingredients including vishnukranthi *(Evolvulus alsinoides)*, ginger, black pepper, cumin, coriander seeds, galangal, carom seeds *(Trachyspermum ammi)*, liquorice, long pepper, pathpadagam *(Hedyotis corymbosa)*, vasaka *(Justicia adhatoda)*, yellow vine *(Coscinium fenestratum)*, and Siritekku *(Premna herbacea)*. It can be taken orally after dissolving in hot water for cough or cold.

Sitopaladi churna. This is a five-herb powder that contains pippali *(Piper longum)*, vanshlochan *(Bamboo arundinaceu)*, cardamom *(Elettaria cardamom)*, cinnamon *(Cinnamonum zeylanicumm)*, and rock sugar candy/sitopala *(Saccharum officinarum)*. Take 1 teaspoon and mix with a little honey or ghee and consume three to four times per day after food.

Talisadi churna. This contains cinnamon, green cardamom, piper longum, peppercorn, ginger/zingiber officinale, tabashir, and sugar.

Topical

Himalaya cold relief balm. This contains eucalyptus, mint *(Mentha arvensis)*, camphor, nutmeg, and chir pine essential oils. It can be rubbed over the chest, back, throat, forehead, or nose two to three times per day to relieve nasal congestion. It should not be used for children under 2 years old.

Chinese Natural Remedies

In TCM, there are two main groups of coughs, and their causes are:

- The *acute cough* is usually due to external factors like pathogens and weather.
- The *chronic cough* is due to internal imbalances in the organ systems.
  The *acute cough* is due to:
- wind-cold (wet cough with usually clear or white phlegm and associated runny nose with clear nose drip, dry mouth, thirst and sweating, stiff neck, headache, and aversion to cold).
- wind-heat (wet coughing bouts with yellow sticky phlegm, sore throat, and associated runny nose with sticky nasal discharge, dry mouth, sweating, and aversion to heat).
- wind-dryness (non productive and dry coughing bouts) with itchy and dry throat and lips.
  The *chronic cough* lasts more than 3 weeks and is due to:
- damp cough (wet watery or foamy white phlegm with diarrhea, loss of appetite, and fatigue).

- damp-heat cough (wet cough with yellow sticky phlegm, rattly chest, fast breathing, and heat intolerance).
- liver-fire cough (lump-in-throat feeling, cough associated with emotional triggers, chest discomfort, dizziness).
- lung yin deficiency cough (dry and non productive cough or little phlegm, worse at 3 a.m. to 5 a.m.).

Similarly, the *common cold* is an exterior syndrome due to wind-cold type mainly, and wind-heat type and summer heat-dampness type.

Cold enters through the soles of the feet and upper thoracic spine. Wind enters via the nape of the neck. Risk factors include poor diet and lifestyle.

Common Ingredients for Cough, Cold, Flu, and Sore Throat

Spices	Herbs/Leaves	Miscellaneous	Fruit
Black pepper/hei hu jiao (Piper nigrum)	American ginseng (Panax quinquefolius)	Rock sugar	Chinese pear (Pyrus pyrifolia)
	Purple coneflower/echinacea (Echinacea purpurea)	Salt	Goji berries (Lycium barbarum)
	Astragalus (Radix Astragali)	Eucalyptus oil	Monk fruit/luo han guo (Siraitia grosvenorii)
	Liquorice/gan cao (Glycyrrhiza glabra)	Balloon flower root/jie geng (Platycodon grandiflorus; Radix)	Fritillary bulb/zhe bei mu (Fritillaria thunbergii bulb)
	Gentian	Ephedra/ma huang (Ephedra sinica)	Forsythia Fruit (Lian Qiao)
	Horny goat weed/Yin Yang Huo (Epimedium)	Lilyturf root/Mai Dong (Liriope muscari or Radix Ophiopogonis)	Rice/Glutinous rice
	Anemarrhena/zhi mu (Anemarrhena asphodeloides)	Wolfberry root bark/Di Gi Pi (Cortex lycii)	Eel
		Chinese wild ginger/xi xin (Asarum heterotropoides/ Asarum sieboldii)	
		Malva nuts (Pang Da Hai)	
		Honeysuckle flower (JinYin Hua)	
		Flos Magnoliae	
		Walnut (Juglans regia)	
		Snow fungus and black fungus	
Ginger/sheng jiang (Zingiber officinale)	Cordyceps (Ophiocordyceps sinensis)	Honey/Manuka Honey	Orange (Citrus sinensis)

Common Recipes for Wet Cough

Oral

Tea/Brews/Others

Astragalus tea. Take 1 tablespoon of sliced dried astragalus root. Boil in 2 cups of water for 20 to 30 minutes. Strain and drink warm.

Black sesame seed–ginger mix. Take 250 g black sesame and juice extract of 250 g ginger. Melt 200 g of rock sugar with some honey. Roast the sesame seeds and the fresh ginger juice until the mixture is dry. Add in the melted rock sugar syrup. Pour into an airtight container. Take one teaspoon of this mixture and add it into one glass of hot water. Consume twice a day.

Chive egg omelet. Take 100 g of Chinese chives. Wash and chop finely. Mix with two beaten eggs and fry as an omelet. Consume.

Di gu pi (wolfberry root bark). Wash and slice the roots. A water-based or alcohol-based decoction is prepared.

Hei hu jiao (black pepper) tea. Steep slightly pounded black pepper in hot water. Add honey to taste. Serve hot.

Inulin tea. Take ½ teaspoon of ground root. Add 1 cup of boiling water. Steep for 15 minutes. Strain and consume three to four times a day.

Jie geng tea. Take 5 g of jie geng (balloon flower root) and 5 g sliced gan cao (liquorice root). Steep in 1 cup of boiling water for about 5 minutes. Drink warm.

Radish ginger soup. Boil one radish in three bowls of water until soft. Add 15 g ginger and six sliced green onion bulbs. Simmer and reduce until one bowl remains. Take this concoction together with the softened ingredients. (For cough with copious phlegm.)

Rice gruel. Cook 60 g glutinous rice with 5 mL rice vinegar and some water until liquid. Add slices of five bulbs of green onion. Consume hot. (For wet cough, nose block and headache.)

Steamed salted orange. Cut the skin off the top of the orange like a lid and poke holes in it. Sprinkle ½ to

1 teaspoon of salt on the exposed orange flesh. Replace the lid of the orange and steam it for 15 to 20 minutes. Eat the flesh and drink the juice.

Tangerine peel brew. Take 2 g of tangerine and 2 g tea leaves. Add one cup of hot water and 30 g brown sugar. Allow it to steep. Strain and take one dose every day after lunch.

Zhe bei mu (fritillary bulb). Can be consumed as a decoction or a polyherbal mix.

For wind-cold cough:

- **Garlic.** Chew and suck slowly the juice of three garlic pips (when a cold starts).
- **Ginger decoction.** Take 10 g crushed ginger, 7 g tea leaves, and 15 g rock sugar or brown sugar. Add some water. Boil and simmer for 5 to 10 minutes. Consume after meals throughout the day.
- **Ginger spring onion soup.** Take three to five ginger slices, 1 tablespoon of Chinese apricot kernels, three stalks of spring onion white bulb with roots, and a dash of ground cinnamon. Add to a pot of water. Boil and then simmer for 10 to 15 minutes. Drink warm.

For wind-heat cough:

Chrysanthemum-mulberry leaf tea. Take 10 g chrysanthemum, 10 g mulberry leaf, and 5 g burdock seed. Add to a pot of water and boil. Simmer for 10 minutes and add 3 g peppermint. Strain and consume warm.

Polyherbals (which contain very cooling herbs such as honeysuckle, forsythia, and chrysanthemum)

- **Yin Chiao.** Contains licorice root, Angelica Dahurica, dried tangerine peel, Sichuan lovage root, forsythia root, honeysuckle flower, platycodon root, siler root, flos magnoliae, isatis root, and licorice root.
- **Gan Mao Ling.** Contains chrysanthemum flower, honeysuckle, evodia leaf, ilex root, isatis root, and vitex herb.

For damp-phlegm cough:

Polyherbal brew. Take equal amounts of 7 to 11 g of dried orange peel, poria cocos, pinellia ternata, radish seed, licorice root, perilla seed, and semen brassicae. A decoction is made.

Polyherbals

Ling Gan Wu Wei Jiang Xin Tang: It contains mainly five herbs: dried ginger, wild ginger, poria cocos mushrooms (fu ling), schisandra berries, and liquorice.

Da Qing Long Tang: The key ingredients are shi gao (gypsum), ma huang (ephedra), sheng jiang (fresh ginger), da zao (jujube), gui zhi (cinnamon), xing ren (apricot seeds), and gan cao (liquorice).

Xiao Qing Long Tang: Contains eight herbs including gui zhi (cinnamon), ma huang (ephedra), xi xin (wild ginger), wu wei zhi (five-flavor berry), gan jiang (dried ginger), ban xia (crow-dipper rhizome), gan cao (liquorice), and bai shao (white peony roots).

Hai Zao Yu Hu Tang: The key ingredients include 11 herbs compr hai zao, chuan xiong, kun bu, dang gui pian, jiang ban xia, qing pi, du huo, chen pi, lian qiao, zhe bei mu, and ye gan cao

Bei Mu Tang: The key ingredients are ma huang (ephedra), kuan dong hua (coltsfoot flower), zhe bei mu (fritillary bulb), gan cao, and xing ren (apricot seed).

Si Shun Tang: The key ingredients include zhe bei mu (fritillary bulb), zi wan (purple aster root), gan cao (licorice root), and jie geng (platycodon).

Er Mu San: The key ingredients are zhe bei mu (fritillary bulb) and zhi mu (anemarrhena rhizome).

Chuan Bei Pi Pa Gao: The key ingredients among the 15 herbs include fritillary bulb, *Eriobotrya japonica leaf, Typhonium flagelliforme rhizome, Fritillaria ussuriensis bulb, Platycodon grandiflorum root*

Common Recipes for Dry Cough

Oral

Tea/Brew/Others

Steamed Asian pear. Skin a pear and cut the top off to resemble a lid. Scoop the seeds out of the middle of the pear and fill with goji berries, water, and rock sugar. Steam for 15 to 20 minutes and serve. (Remove the goji berries for children under 2 years of age.)

Luo Han Guo (monk fruit) **brew.** Prepare it by cracking the fruit open and placing it in a pot of water and bringing it to a boil. Once it comes to a boil, lower the heat and allow it to simmer for about 50 to 60 minutes. Strain the mixture and drink it warm.

Egg stew. Take two eggs. Beat them in a little water. Add 50 mL vinegar and stew. Consume.

Sugar cane and water chestnut juice. Take 3 mL of sugarcane juice and add 15 mL of water chestnut extract. Add some warm water. Consume.

Peanut broth. Take 100 g of peanuts. Add some water and rock sugar. Boil and then simmer for 30 minutes. Drink this broth and consume the peanut.

Malva nut. Take one to two malva nuts (do not exceed three nuts). Add 1 cup of water. Steep for 30 minutes. Discard the skin and seed. Consume the liquid and pulp as a brew.

Variation #1. Take 100 g of malva nuts. Add 2 L of water and soak preferably overnight. Remove and discard the seed and thick outer skin the next morning. Strain the pulp (gel) via a coarse muslin cloth. Various spices or herbs can be added to the pulp.

Take 2 cups of water in a saucepan. Add pandanus (screwpine leaf) and brown sugar. Boil and simmer for 10 to 15 minutes. Add cinnamon stick, ginger slices, and licorice for additional flavors if desired. Strain. Add the malva nut pulp to the strained liquid and drink.

Variation #2. Other items such as red date, liquorice, chrysanthemum flower, jasmine tea, lilyturf root, haw and rock sugar can also be simmered together in water and then the malva nut pulp added.

Variation #3. Soaked basil seeds, sugar and ice can be added to the soaked malva nut pulp and drunk as a cooling drink.

Sesame seed brew. Take 15 g of unroasted sesame seeds. Add 1 cup hot water and some rock sugar. Steep for 15 to 30 minutes. Drink warm (for dry persistent night cough).

For *wind-dry cough,*

Snow fungus pear soup. Take one piece of snow fungus. Soak overnight or for 30 minutes and then break it into smaller pieces. Discard the hard stem. Take one Chinese pear and cut into small pieces and discard the seeds. Place these ingredients in a pot of water. Add 1 tablespoon Chinese apricot kernels and one piece honey date. Boil and then simmer for 30 minutes. Consume warm.

Black fungus. Consume black fungus as part of stir fries or soup.

Cold-Flu Remedies

Mung bean broth. Take 50 g mung beans (ground), 15 g rock sugar, and 5 g green tea. Add water. Boil and then simmer for 20 minutes. (For flu and sore throat.)

Garlic. Take three pips of garlic. Suck on it one at a time until the juice has gone out.

Rice congee mixture. Take 100 g of rice, cook it into a thin gruel. Add 30 g of raisins and some apple slices. Simmer for 5 minutes. Consume warm.

Glutinous rice congee. Take 100 g of glutinous rice and cook it into a thin gruel. Add slices of ginger and garlic (three pips) and add a handful of sliced bulbs of green spring onions. Sprinkle some white pepper if desired.
Variation #1. Parched rice 50 g can be used in place of glutinous rice.

Date-ginger brew. Take 30 g Chinese dates, 30 g brown sugar, and 15 g of sliced ginger. Add 3 cups of water, boil and then simmer for 10 to 15 minutes. Consume the brew warm, and eat the ingredients if desired.

Therapeutic Measures
Diet
- Consume more Lung qi strengthening foods. These are fresh natural foods that are generally white. For example: white vegetables (turnip, cauliflower, parsnip, rutabaga, potatoes, or daikon radish), white fruits (pear, apple), white grains (rice, oats), white herbs and spices (garlic, white peppercorn), and white seeds and nuts (sesame seeds, almonds).
- Avoid damp foods in chronic cough or wind-cold cough. These are dairy, cold fruits or juices (orange or tomato), sugars or fermented foods. Consume more hot or warm foods (ginger, garlic, onion, cayenne pepper, and cinnamon), and liquid such as soups.

Avoid heaty foods like chicken if there is a cough with yellow phlegm.
- Chicken soup with added shiitake mushrooms, astragalus, kombu or kelp are also warming and immune-boosting.

Nasal (Inhalation)
Steam inhalation. Add eucalyptus oil or Vicks to hot water in a saucepan or pot. (Refer to "Indian Natural Remedies" for cough above.)

Acupressure
Lie Que (Lung 07 or LU7): This acupoint is just above the styloid process of the radius, 1.5 cm above the transverse crease of the wrist. Massage the point slowly for 30 seconds to 1 minute (for sore throat or persistent coughing).

Lian Quan (CV 23): This acupoint is in the mid-neck in the depression between the clavicles just above the hyoid bone. Massage this point for 30 seconds. (For dry throat.)

LI20. This point is in the nasolabial groove. This can clear the nasal passages to relieve nasal congestion and itchy nose.
Guasha (Scraping or Stroking). To dispel wind-heat, use a coin or a spoon to stroke a few vertical lines from the shoulder blade down to the scapulae. Red lines will appear and then they become reddish purple bruises before they fade.
Moxibustion and Cupping. They can also remove dampness.

Prevention of Cough, Cold, Flu, and Sore Throat
This is to strengthen the immune system to promote lung health.

American ginseng. Consume the ginseng with water, juice, or tea. Take about ½ to 1 teaspoon of ginseng two to three times a day.

Cordyceps. Eat cordyceps supplements. Take about 5 to 10 g a day

Purple coneflower/Echinacea. Take echinacea supplements three times daily, 0.9 mL for 4 months and then increase to five times daily (the same dosage) at the first sign of a cold.

Eel. Cook the eel with millet and some wine and rice vinegar. Consume.
Note
- Ginseng should not be given to children.
- Echinacea supplements should not be given to children under 12 years due to potential severe allergic reaction

Western Natural Remedies/Others
Common Ingredients for Cough, Cold, Flu, and Sore Throat.

Spices	Herbs/Leaves/Fruit/Roots	Miscellaneous
Anise (Pimpinella anisum)	Marshmallow root (Althaea officinalis)	Salt
Black pepper (Piper nigrum)	Sage (Salvia officinalis)	Probiotics
Cinnamon (Cinnamomum vera)	Peppermint (Mentha piperita)	Apple cider vinegar
Clove (Syzygium aromaticum)	Slippery elm (Ulmus rubra)	Pineapple (Ananas comosus)
Ginger (Zingiber officinalis)	Thyme (Thymus vulgaris)	Honey/Manuka honey
Oregano	Common Mallow	Common couch (Elymus repens)
Turmeric (Curcuma longa)	Lobelia (Lobelia inflata)	Horseradish (Armoracia rusticana)
	Lemon (Citrus limon)	Essential oils (Cajeput, tea tree, thyme, oregano, eucalyptus, elemi and lavender)
	Elderberry (Sambucus canadensis)	White oak bark
	Ivy leaf (Hedera helix)	Muskmelon seeds

Spices	Herbs/Leaves/ Fruit/Roots	Miscellaneous
	Cyclamen (Cyclamen europaeum)	Shallots/Onions
	Mullein Leaf (Verbascum thapsus)	
	Horehound Leaf (Marrubium vulgare)	
	Wild Black Cherry (Prunus serontina)	
	Catnip (Nepeta cataria)	
	Cowslip (Primula veris)	
	Purple coneflower (Echinacea purpurea)	
	Hyssop (Hyssopus officinalis)	
	Rosemary (Rosmarinus officinalis)	
	Yarrow (Achillea millefolium)	
	Spearmint (Mentha spicata)	
	Chamomile (Matricaria chamomilla)	
	Marjoram (Origanum majorana)	
	Witch hazel leaf (Hamamelis virginiana)	
	Gentian root (Gentiana lutea)	
	Blackcurrant leaves	
	Rooibos (Aspalathus lincaris)	
	Lady's mantle	
	Meadowsweet (Filipendula ulmaria)	
	Goldenseal root	
	Geranium	
	Licorice (Glycyrrhiza glabra)	
	Curry plant (Helichrysum italicum)	
	Verbena (Verbena officinalis)	
	Aloe vera	
	Lamb's ear (Stachys byzantina)	
	Boneset (Eupatorium perfoliatum)	
	Passion fruit	

Common Recipes

Oral

Teas/Brews/Others

Aloe and onion cold syrup. Blend fresh aloe vera pulp (from 1 aloe leaf) and 1 red onion. Place in a glass bottle. Add the juice of 6 limes and enough honey to cover the mixture. Refrigerate and allow to steep for 3 to 4 days. Take 1 to 2 tablespoons of this mixture.

Anise tea. Add anise to boiling water and steep for about 15 minutes. Strain the mixture before adding honey to taste. Serve it hot.

Blackcurrant tea. Take 1 teaspoon of fresh chopped leaves (or 1 to 2 teaspoons of dried leaves) and add 1 cup of hot water. Steep for 5 to 10 minutes. Strain and drink.

Black pepper tea. Lightly crush and put 7 to 10 black peppercorns in a cup. Add boiling water and allow to steep for 10 minutes and then drink.

Boneset tea. Take ¼-½ teaspoon dried leaf and flowers. Add one cup of boiling water, allow to steep for 10-15 minutes. Consume when warm. Take maximum 3 cups per day.

Catnip tea. Place 2 teaspoons of dried catnip in a cup. Add hot water and allow to steep for 5 to 10 minutes. Add honey to taste and drink warm.

Chamomile tea. Add 3 to 4 tablespoons of fresh (or three to five dried) chamomile flowers into a cup. Pour 1 cup of boiling water over the flowers and allow to steep for 10 minutes. Strain and add honey to taste. Add mint if desired and drink warm.

Cinnamon tea. Mix one tablespoon of lukewarm honey with ¼ teaspoon of cinnamon powder to relieve the cough.

Common couch tea. Take 2 teaspoons of dried and sliced couch grass root in a cup of water. Boil and steep for 10 minutes. Consume three times a day. For sore throat, it also can be used as a mouth gargle.

Variation #1. **Common couch tincture.** Add 2 to 3 mL into a glass of water or fruit juice. Consume two to three times per day.

Cowslip tea. Take 1 teaspoon of cowslip flowers. Add 1 cup of water. Simmer for about 5 to 10 minutes and strain. Drink warm. Consume two to three times a day.

Elderberry cough syrup. Add dried elderberries, diced ginger, cinnamon powder, and clove powder to a small saucepan. Add water and bring it to a boil. Reduce the heat and simmer for about 30 minutes. Mash the mixture with a fork until pulpy. Allow to steep for about 10 minutes. Strain and stir in honey to taste. Store in the refrigerator. Take 1 tablespoon three to four times a day to prevent coughs, colds, and flu. Take about 2 tablespoons three to four times a day to treat.

Elderberry tea. Take 2 tablespoons of dried elderberry and 1 cinnamon stick. Add 2 cups of water. Boil and then simmer for 15 minutes. Strain and consume warm. Add honey if desired.

Some crushed ginger, turmeric or lemon slices may be added.

Gentian root tea. Take 1 to 2 teaspoons of gentian root. Boil in 1 cup of water for about 5 minutes. Strain and drink warm.

Geranium tea. Take 25 g of the flower buds or 50 g of the dried plant. Add 1 L of boiling water. Allow to steep for 20 minutes. Consume 3 to 4 cups per day.

Ginger tea. Lightly pound about 1 to 2 inches of fresh ginger (if unavailable, use 1 to 2 teaspoons of ginger powder) and add to a cup of hot water. Allow to steep for 5 to 10 minutes. Strain and drink while warm. Add honey to taste.

Goldenseal root. Take 1 teaspoon of goldenseal root or leaves. Add 2 or 3 cups of boiling water. Steep for 10 minutes. Strain and add honey or lemon to taste.

Variation #1. Consume 400 mg of goldenseal root powder.

Horehound leaf tea. Boil 1 cup of fresh horehound leaves (washed and chopped) in 2 cups of water. Steep for 10 minutes. Strain the brew and add 2 cups of water. Alternatively, ¼ cup of dried leaves can be used. Horehound leaves are also available as cough drops and lozenges.

Horseradish. Consume horseradish every day. It can be cooked (sauteed, grilled or boiled). The grated form is usually preserved in vinegar with salt and sugar.

Hot toddy. This is as discussed above, but if a non-stimulant is preferred at night, the coffee can be replaced with any other herbal brew and a dash of whisky.

Hyssop tea. Take 1 tablespoon of the dried leaves and 2 cups of water. Boil and steep for 10 minutes. Add honey to taste and drink warm.

Lady's mantle tea. Take 5 to 10 g lady's mantle. Add 1 L of boiling water and allow it to steep for 10 to 15 minutes.

Lemon balm tea. Take 2 tablespoons of dried leaves or five to six fresh leaves. Boil in 1 cup of water for 5 minutes. Strain and drink it warm.

Lamb's ear tea. Take 1 teaspoon of the dried leaves. Add 1 cup of boiling water. Steep for about 15 minutes. Consume three times a day.

Lemon tea. Squeeze half a lemon and add the juice to a glass of hot water. Add honey and drink it warm.

Liquorice tea. Take 1 teaspoon of dried ground root in 1 cup of water. Boil for 5 minutes. Drain and drink warm.

Variation #1. Take a handful of liquorice sticks. Wash, pound, and flatten the sticks lightly in a mortar. Put them in a saucepan of water, add a handful of raisins. Boil and simmer for about 15 to 20 minutes. Drink a cupful of this warm brew three to four times a day.

Variation #2. Take 5 tablespoons of sliced liquorice roots (or some crushed sticks), one crushed cinnamon stick and some fresh ginger slices. Add 5 cups of water. Boil and simmer for 15 to 20 minutes. Drink a cupful throughout the day.

Lobelia tea. Take 1 teaspoon of lobelia and ½ teaspoon of dried peppermint. Add 2 cups of boiling water. Steep for 30 minutes. Strain and add honey to taste. Drink 1 cup daily.

Mallow tea. Take some blue mallow flowers. Add 1 cup of boiling water. Allow to steep for 2 minutes and drink warm.

Manuka honey/Honey. Take one teaspoon of manuka honey/honey before each meal (to coat the throat).

Marjoram tea. Add a few dried leaves into one cup of hot water. Steep for a few minutes. Drink warm.

Marshmallow root tea. Add about 1 tablespoon of dried marshmallow root to 1.5 cups of water and bring to a boil in a pot or saucepan. Cover the pot and allow the mixture to simmer for about 20 minutes. Strain and add honey to taste. Serve hot.

Variation #1. Cold brew is preferred. Soak the roots in cold water for 30 minutes. Remove the skin. Cut the roots into smaller pieces. Place in a jug and fill with water. Leave overnight. Add some honey or rock sugar and some fresh orange juice. Consume.

Meadowsweet tea. Take 2 tablespoons of dried meadowsweet flowers or 4 teaspoons of fresh flowers. Add 1 cup of hot water. Steep for 10 minutes. Strain and consume it warm.

Mullein leaf tea. Add 1 to 2 teaspoons of dried mullein leaf (and/or flowers) to 1 cup of hot water. Allow to steep for 15 minutes. Strain and add honey to taste. This can be consumed three or four times per day.

Muskmelon seeds. Wash and dry the seeds. Eat the dried seeds or add them to foods. Alternatively, the fresh seeds can also be eaten.

Oat bark tea. Take 1 tea bag. Add 1 cup of boiling water. Steep. Strain, and drink.

Variation #1: Take 3 g of oat bark powder and add a few cups of water. Boil and then steep for 10 minutes. Strain and drink it.

Oregano tea. Take 2 teaspoons of dried oregano. Boil in 1 cup of water. Allow to steep and drink warm.

Passion fruit tea. Take two passion fruits. Clean them. Cut into half. Scoop out the pulp. Add the skin, pulp and seeds to a sauce pan. Fill with 1L of water. Boil and then simmer for 30 minutes. Add rock sugar to taste. Consume 1-2 cups per day for 1-3 days.

Variation #1. Boil 2 cut passion fruits and 1 small onion with 4 cups of water. Add sweetener as desired.

Pineapple slices. Eat pineapple slices. The pineapple can also be juiced and drunk warm.

Polyspice teas. Make one cup of brew with some chamomile, anise, licorice, fennel, caraway, black seed, saffron, and cardamom.

Variation #1. Make 1 cup of tea with 1 teaspoon lavender, 1 teaspoon elderberry, and 1 tablespoon of anise seeds.

Probiotics. They are important for good digestive health and immunity and hence may help with cold and flu prevention. Taking probiotics with at least 10 billion colony-forming units (CFU) dose during a cold/flu may reduce the symptoms.

Purple coneflower or echinacea tea. Place 1 tablespoon of dried echinacea (or 2 tablespoons of fresh leaves) in a cup. Simmer for about 10 minutes in 2 cups of water. Let it steep for another 10 minutes. Fresh flowers or leaves can also be used. Drain and drink.

Echinacea capsules (Blackmores Echinacea Forte or Nature's Way Echinacea Purpurea Herb) can be taken as immune boosters.

Rooibos tea. Add 1 teaspoon of loose rooibos tea leaves into 1 cup of boiling water. Steep for about 5 to 10 minutes. Strain and consume.

Rosemary tea. Add three to five sprigs of fresh rosemary (or 1½ teaspoons of dry rosemary leaf needles) to a cup of hot water and steep for 10 to 15 minutes. Drink warm.

Sage tea. Add three to five fresh sage leaves or (1 teaspoon of dried sage) into one cup of boiling water. Allow it to steep for 5 to 10 minutes. Strain and drink.

Shallots. Peel several shallots. Put the whole (or sliced or crushed) shallots in a glass jar . Steep with honey and refrigerate for few days. Consume one tablespoon of this mixture two to four times a day

Slippery elm lozenges or cough drops. Mix ¼ cup of slippery elm powder with 1 teaspoon of cinnamon powder, a pinch of salt, 2 to 3 tablespoons of honey, a few drops of vanilla (optional) and some cocoa powder (optional) in a bowl. Bind all the ingredients together to form a ball. Break small pieces to make little balls or pellets. Dry the balls at room temperature and store them in a container. Suck them as lozenges or cough drops many times a day.
Variation #1. The slippery elm powder can be mixed with honey and licorice root tea (1 teaspoon of licorice root, chopped, simmered in ½ cup of water and strained). It is then mixed and prepared as cough drops, as described above.

Slippery elm tea. Take 1 to 2 teaspoons of the powdered bark. Add 1 cup of boiling water. Add ginger or cinnamon as desired. Steep for a few minutes. Strain and add honey to taste.

Spearmint tea. Place six to eight spearmint leaves into a cup with boiling water. Cover and let sit for 5 to 10 minutes. Add lemon slices and drink it warm.

Thyme tea. Take three sprigs of fresh thyme (or two sprigs of dry thyme) and 1.5 cups of hot water. Keep for 5 minutes. Remove the sprigs and drink.

Thyme-Clove spice tea. Boil thyme and cloves together in water for about 10 minutes. Strain. Add honey to taste. Drink warm.

Turmeric tea. Add 1 to 2 teaspoons of ground turmeric to 1 cup of hot water. Mix well and add honey to taste. Drink one to two times a day. Alternatively, lightly pound 2 to 3 inches of fresh turmeric and add to a cup of boiling water. Allow to steep for 5 to 10 minutes and strain. Add honey to taste.

Valerian tea. Mix ½ teaspoon of dried valerian root (or 2 to 3 g teaspoon) in a cup of hot water. Cover and steep for 10 to 15 minutes. Consume 30 minutes to 2 hours before sleep.

Verbena tea. Take 1 tablespoon of fresh lemon verbena leaves or 1 teaspoon of dried leaves. Add 1 cup of boiling water. Steep or simmer for 15 minutes. Strain and consume warm with a desired sweetener.
To make a hot toddy, add some whiskey and spices (clove and cinnamon).

Wild black cherry tea. Take 2 tablespoons of black cherry bark. Add 2 cups of water and keep overnight. Heat and drink ½ cup two to three times a day. A decoction can also be made with 1 tablespoon of bark powder and 1 cup of hot water. Drink it warm.

Yarrow tea. Take 1 to 2 teaspoons of dried leaves and flowers or one twig of fresh yarrow. Boil in 1 cup of water. Mint or liquorice may also be added.
Variation #1. Boil 1 cup of water with ½ teaspoon of liquorice root. Add 1 to 2 teaspoons of dried yarrow leaves and flowers (one sprig of fresh yarrow) and several fresh mint (peppermint) or 1 teaspoon of dried leaves.

Therapeutic Measures

1. Gargles

    Saline gargle. Gargling saline is recommended if there is sore throat or cough. The saline can be made by adding 1 teaspoon of salt to ½ glass of warm water. Gargle a few times.
    Alternatively, place a pinch of salt on the tip of the tongue. Move the tongue tip and lick the throat a few times as if to paint the back of the throat.

    Witch hazel gargle. Take 1 teaspoon of witch hazel and add to 1 cup of water. Boil for 10 minutes. Wait till lukewarm and then gargle.

    Marshmallow gargle. Take some marshmallow flowers. Boil with some water, oil, honey and alum. When cool, use it as a gargle for sore throat.

    Geranium gargle: Make a decoction with rose geranium flowers and leaves. When cool, use it as a gargle for sore throat.

    Oat bark gargle. Make a decoction. Take 10 g of oak bark powder and add 2 cups of water. Simmer till reduced volume. When cool, use it as a gargle for sore throat.

    Licorice gargle. Take 1 teaspoon for licorice powder. Add half cup of warm water. Stir and use the solution to gargle.

2. Nasal Inhalation, Irrigation, and Sprays

    Steam inhalation. Add eucalyptus oil, Vicks or a few drops of Elemi essential oil to hot water in a saucepan or pot. (As above.) Mullein leaves may also be used.

    Saline sprays. As mentioned above in "Indian Natural Remedies."

    Essential oil mist therapy. As mentioned above in "Indian Natural Remedies."

    Carragelose/carrageenan containing nasal spray. This is a sulfated polysaccharide obtained from red seaweed. It binds directly to the virus and provides a physical barrier. It has a broad-spectrum antiviral effect and eliminates 99% of cold and flu viruses. It shortens the duration of the cold and flu symptoms by 2 days and reduces the severity of symptoms.

    Cyclamen europaeum nasal spray. This once a day nasal spray obtained from the extract of a flowering plant can reduce nasal congestion due to acute or chronic sinusitis.
    For nasal irrigation: Refer to "Indian Remedy."

    Ectoine nasal spray. Nasal spray with 2% Ectoine can reduce symptoms in mild to moderate allergic or non-allergic rhinitis/rhinosinusitis and sore throat.

    Betadine sore throat spray. This contains iodine and helps to relieve throat pain, discomfort, and hoarseness. It can be sprayed every 2 to 4 hours. It should not be used for children below 6 years of age if there is a history of thyroid problems or hypersensitivity to povidone.

3. **Juice fast.** A juice fast is advised for 2 to 3 days (raw vegetable juice or coconut water can be consumed).

4. **Talk less.** Rest the throat.

5. **Mild exercise.** Mild exercise is recommended, such as a walk. Avoid lying in bed all the time.

6. **Essential oils and aromatherapy.** Various essentials oils ie marjoram, curry plant (*Helichrysum italicum*) etc can be administered via humidifier/diffuser.

7. **Lozenges.** Lozenges can be sucked. They are hard, soft, or chewable. They are medicated or non-medicated and often with added flavors (mint, lemon, myrrh or blackcurrant) and sugar/honey. The active substances in the lozenge can provide anesthetic, analgesic, antitussive, or antiseptic effects. Benzocaine, betadine and menthol are common ingredients.

8. **Oral zinc.** This is available as lozenges and taken every few hours at the onset of the cold or flu.

9. **Vitamin C.** High doses of vitamin C usually 1 to 2 g are taken at the early cold/flu stage.

Commercial Preparations for Cough, Colds, and Sore Throat

Vicks/Baby Vicks ointment: This is applied to the baby's chest, neck, and soles of the feet.

Olbas oil: This is also applied as above. It contains various essential plant oils such as eucalyptus, cajuput (tea tree oil), clove, juniper berry, peppermint, levomenthol, and methylsalicylate (wintergreen) which can relieve nasal and bronchial congestion. Few drops can be sprinkled on the pillow cover, handkerchief, edge of the shirt or it can be inhaled via a diffuser.

(Vicks and Olbas may be prohibited in some countries and it should be used with caution only after the age of 3 months)

Herbal cough drops, lozenges, or candies (Herbal pharyngeal demulcents): They are commonly used for sore throat and cough.

   Fisherman's Friend lozenges. They contain different ingredients such as licorice, menthol, eucalyptus oil, capsicum tincture, tragacanth gum (dried sap from astragalus plant), mint, and aniseed.

   Ricola herbal candies. They contain various ingredients (i.e., peppermint, plantain, marshmallow, thyme, sage, elder, cowslip, lady's mantle, burnet, speedwell, yarrow, horehound, and menthol).

   Esberitox tablets: Echinacea purpurea, Echinacea pallida, Thuja occidentalis and Baptisia tinctoria.

   Strepsils. It contains amylmetacresol and 2,4-Dichlorobenzylalcohol as the main active ingredients which are antiseptic. Other ingredients include peppermint oil, star anise oil, and menthol.

Herbal cough syrups: There are various herbal cough syrups that can be used for sore throat and cough.

   Prospan cough syrup. This is an herbal remedy containing ivy leaf extract for a chesty cough. It liquefies and clears mucus from the airways.

Kaloba cough syrup. It is plant remedy containing *Pelargonium sidoides* extract for cough due to acute bronchitis and sinusitis.

Sinupret cough syrup or tablets. It contains cowslip flower, European elder flower, verbena, gentian root, and sorrel.

Others

Buteyko Breathing

It originated from Russia and is based on 3 core principles ie nasal breathing, reduced/controlled breathing, and relaxation

Modern Remedies

Bronchodilators

Bronchodilators are medications used to open the airways of the lungs. They do this by causing the bronchial (airway) muscles to relax. They are often used to treat conditions like asthma and allergic reactions as well as any other conditions that make breathing difficult. Bronchodilators are classified based on their mechanisms of action:

- Beta-adrenergic bronchodilators

  These bronchodilators are beta-2 agonists, which mean that they bind to beta-2 receptors in the bronchial muscles, causing them to relax and the airway to open. They are used as relievers or rescue medications during an acute wheeze.

  There are two main types of bronchodilators: short-acting and long-acting bronchodilators.

  - **Short-acting** bronchodilators i.e., short-acting beta2 agonists (*SABA*) have a quick onset of action within 5 minutes and last for about 2 to 4 hours. They are used to treat acute breathlessness and can be taken through a metered-dose inhaler or nebulizer. Oral forms (as tablets or syrups) are also available with the onset of action within 1 hour.

  Examples: salbutamol and terbutaline.

  - **Long-acting** bronchodilators (i.e., long-acting beta agonists (*LABA*)) have a slower onset of action and are used to reduce the incidence of breathlessness.

  Examples: salmeterol and formoterol.

- Muscarinic receptor antagonists ("Anticholinergic" bronchodilators)

  These bronchodilators prevent acetylcholine from binding to muscarinic receptors in the airway and nasal passages. This medication is also used to prevent and reduce the frequency of breathlessness attacks.

  Examples:

  Short-acting muscarinic antagonists (SAMA): *ipratropium bromide*

  Long-acting muscarinic antagonists (LAMA): *tiotropium; umeclidinium*

- Xanthine derivatives

  Xanthine derivatives function by blocking adenosine receptors. Adenosine binding to receptors causes stimulation of airway muscles and narrowing of the airway.

  Examples: *theophylline* (oral) and *aminophylline* (intravenous)

Steroids (Preventive)

In breathlessness, inflammation of the airway causes constriction and exacerbates breathing difficulties. Inhaled corticosteroids (ICS) are used to suppress airway inflammation and are often used in conjunction with other bronchodilators. They are used to prevent attacks of breathlessness and are often administered in the form of a metered-dose inhaler like other bronchodilator medications. They are often taken in the morning and evening. The most common steroids used are corticosteroids. Steroid nasal sprays are used in allergic rhinitis. Commonly used ICS for wheezing include *beclomethasone, budesonide, mometasone, and fluticasone. Oral prednisone or intravenous hydrocortisone* is given as a short sharp course for a few days during an acute attack.

Mast Cell Stabilizers

Mast cell stabilizers function by stabilizing mast cells, which are the cells in the body which release histamine. Mast cell stabilizers inhibit mast cell release of histamines due to exposure to allergens in the body. An example of a mast cell stabilizer is *sodium cromoglycate.*

Antihistamines

Antihistamines are a class of drug used to treat allergy symptoms and work by blocking the action of histamines. Histamines are a neurotransmitter in the brain responsible for allergic reactions and symptoms such as sneezing, watery eyes, and hives. Antihistamines come in various forms, such as tablets, capsules, liquid, injection, or nasal sprays. There are four histamine receptors in the body: H1, H2, H3, and H4. Antihistamines are classified by their antagonist action on various histamine receptors.

H1-antihistamines are antihistamines that selectively block the action of the H1 histamine receptors. These antihistamines can further be split into first- and second-generation antihistamines.

First-generation H1-antihistamines have relatively low selectivity for H1 receptors and may cause drowsiness. Examples include *diphenhydramine* (Benadryl), *promethazine* (Phenergan), *pheniramine* (Avil), and *chlorpheniramine* (Piriton). It is used in the treatment of acute allergies, coughs, flu, and hay fever.

Second-generation H1-antihistamines are far more selective for H1 receptors and do not cause drowsiness. Examples: *loratadine, desloratadine, cetirizine, levocetirizine, fexofenadine.*

Leukotrienes

Leukotriene receptor antagonists (LTRA) act by blocking the receptor LT1, which causes constriction of the airway. They reduce the number of white blood cells in mucus and reduce the incidence of airway inflammation and hypersensitivity due to allergies. Examples include *montelukast* and *zafirlukast.*

Expectorants and Mucolytics

Expectorants stimulate the glands in the airway, causing an increase in mucous production. This mucous secretion is much less viscous, making it easier to cough up.

Examples of expectorants: potassium citrate and ammonium chloride

Mucolytics are medications that break up the structure of the molecules forming mucus. They make mucus less viscous and thick and hence easier to cough up. This may also make it more difficult for bacteria to infect the mucous, causing an infection. Mucolytics are often given to patients with wet coughs who find it difficult to cough the mucus up.

Examples of mucolytics

Oral mucolytics: *bromhexine, ambroxol, carbocysteine, N-acetyl cysteine (fluimucil), guaifenesin (mucinex/robitussin)*

Inhaled mucolytics: *hypertonic saline, dornase alpha (Pulmozyme)*

Dornase alpha is a recombinant human DNA enzyme that cleaves long DNA strands in the white cells to thin the mucus in cystic fibrosis patients.

Cough Suppressants

Suppressants are also known as antitussives and work in the opposite way that expectorants do, by blocking the cough reflex. There are two types of suppressants: opioid suppressants and non-opioid suppressants. Opioid suppressants target the cough centre in the medulla of the brain but have high abuse potential. They can suppress the cough reflex for up to 6 hours. Non-opioid suppressants function in a similar way to opioid suppressants but do not have abuse potential. Suppressants should never be taken for wet coughs.

Examples:

Opioid suppressants: *codeine* and *noscapine.*

Non-opioid suppressants: *dextromethorphan.*

Nasal and Oral Decongestants

Nasal decongestants come in the form of nasal sprays as well as tablets and liquid medication. They function by narrowing the blood vessels in the nose and airways, effectively reducing swelling and inflammation. This allows air to pass through the airways more easily and allows mucous in the airways to drain. Decongestants should only be used to treat minor congestion. Nasal decongestants can be taken as topical medication, i.e., nasal spray (*oxymetazoline*) or oral medication (*pseudoephedrine*).

Antiseptic Throat lozenges (Pharyngeal Demulcents)

Difflam. It contains benzydamine (non-steroidal anti-inflammatory drug/NSAID), lignocaine (anesthetic), pholcodine (cough suppressant), and cetylpyridinium (antiseptic). It should not be used in children below 6 years old.

Anaesthetic lollipop. It contains lignocaine or tetracaine (more potent) and can soothe painful sore throat.

Antibiotics

Appropriate first-line antibiotics are usually given on the first visit whilst waiting for the culture's return. Oral penicillin for 10 days/amoxicillin with or without clavulanate or erythromycin is given for tonsillitis caused by group A

Streptococcus bacterium. Most are viral tonsillitis and do not require antibiotics. Macrolides like clarithromycin or azithromycin are used in sinusitis, pneumonia, or in mycoplasma infections. Fluoroquinolones (ciprofloxacin and levofloxacin) are also given. Hospital-acquired pneumonia will usually require specific and broad-spectrum intravenous antibiotics.

Antiviral Drugs

Most viral infections require supportive care only. Rarely, antiviral drugs are used for treatment or prophylaxis. Examples include:

Oseltamivir for influenza virus, *ribavirin* for respiratory syncytial virus (RSV), *acyclovir* for herpes simplex and *ganciclovir or Foscarnet* for cytomegalovirus

Allergen Immunotherapy

Sublingual immunotherapy (SLIT) and subcutaneous immunotherapy (SCIT) can benefit patients with severe allergic rhinitis and allergic asthma who are not controlled with regular spray or inhaled steroids, antihistamines, and bronchodilators.

Monoclonal Antibody (Biologics)

Mepolizumab can reduce the number of asthma exacerbations.

Mechanical or Assisted Ventilation

Machines are used to support or replace normal spontaneous breathing in disease states such as in severe pneumonia etc. This is done in intensive care units by specialized staff. Indications include fast, slow, or no breathing as in acute respiratory syndrome or acute lung injury.

Vaccines

Pneumococcal or flu vaccines are given to the older population or after recovery from pneumonia. Five doses of the DTaP vaccine and booster shots are given to infants and young children to protect from diphtheria, tetanus, and pertussis (whooping cough). 3D printed vaccine patches with microneedles provide much stronger immunity. They are painless and cheaper compared to conventional vaccines and may be the future for vaccine delivery. mRNA vaccines are also new.

EpiPen

It is a special auto-injector medical device that contains epinephrine (also called adrenaline). This is a life-saving drug and is used in serious allergic reactions or in an anaphylactic shock. It is self-administered or by a family member.

Therapeutic and Supportive Measures

These include chest physiotherapy, intravenous fluids, oxygen, antipyretics, nutrition, and rest.

Surgery

Adenoidectomy or tonsillectomy or adenotonsillectomy. They are done when indicated (usually more than seven infections per year, presence of obstructive sleep apnea, dysphagia, dyspnea, or peritonsillar abscess).

Functional endoscopic sinus surgery (FEES). This is a minimally invasive procedure done to restore sinus aeration and normal function in chronic sinusitis. Risks include bleeding, infection, recurrence of disease, and rare CSF leak or visual problems.

Balloon sinuplasty (sinus surgery). This is an office endoscopic procedure where a balloon catheter is inserted to inflate and drain the blocked sinus.

Polypectomy. The obstructive polyps in the nose or sinuses are removed via an endoscopic procedure.

Septoplasty. This is done for deviated nasal septum.

Turbinoplasty or turbinate reduction. This is done to reduce the swollen turbinate so that there is adequate sinus drainage and improve breathing.

Lung transplant. This may be an option in end-stage lung disease. One or both lungs are removed and replaced with lungs from a deceased donor. Only one lung lobe is removed if it is a living donor.

Homeopathic Remedies and Immunization

Homeopathic Remedies

Coughs that occur in pneumonia, croup, asthma, or other chest problems respond differently to different remedies such as *phytolacca, bryonia, pulsatilla, ferrum phos, kali mur, natrum mur, gelsemium, calcarea sulph, etc*. In chronic cases, *sulfur* and sometimes *silica* are administered.

Homeopathic Immunization

Homeopathic immunization may be an alternative to vaccinations (homeoprophylaxis). Read more on Dr Isaac Golden's *A Practical Handbook of Homeopathic Immunization*. Homeopathic flu shots taken in tablet form have been shown to be about 8% to 90% effective for prevention and during an acute flu episode.

References

Cough, Cold, Flu, and Sore Throat

American Academy of Allergy Asthma & Immunology. (2020, September 28). *Increasing rates of allergies and asthma*. Retrieved from https://www.aaaai.org/Tools-for-the-Public/Conditions-Library/Allergies/prevalence-of-allergies-and-asthma.

Amit, D. (2019, December 5). Pepper cumin rasam. *Dassana's Veg Recipes*. Retrieved from https://www.vegrecipesofindia.com/pepper-cumin-rasam-recipe/.

AromaWeb Editor. (n.d.). *Cardamom essential oil uses and benefits*. Aroma Web. https://www.aromaweb.com/essential-oils/cardamom-oil.asp.

Asgarpanah, J., & Kazemivash, N. (2012). Phytochemistry, pharmacology and medicinal properties of *Coriandrum sativum* L. *African Journal of Pharmacy and Pharmacology*, 6(31), 2340–2345. Retrieved from https://doi.org/10.5897/AJPP12.901.

Ashley, [Ashley's Conscious Life]. (2014, February 25). *How to use a neti pot* [Video]. YouTube. Retrieved from https://www.youtube.com/watch?v=EDSlUuAOnN0.

Berry, J. (2018, November 21). What are the benefits of licorice root? *Medical News Today*. Retrieved from https://www.medicalnewstoday.com/articles/323761.

Cronkleton, E., & Carter, A. (2019, August 8). *How to use camphor safely: Benefits and precautions*. Healthline. Retrieved from https://www.healthline.com/health/what-is-camphor.

Dada, G. (2017, August 23). *7 powerful home remedies for tonsillitis that work fast*. Fab How. Retrieved from https://www.fabhow.com/home-remedies-for-tonsillitis.html.

De, A. (2015, March 18). *Ayurvedic cure for tonsillitis*. Only My Health. Retrieved from https://www.onlymyhealth.com/ayurvedic-cure-for-tonsillitis-1311581517.

DerSarkissian, C. (2020, February 5). *What are "OTC" cough and cold medicines?* WebMD. Retrieved from https://www.webmd.com/cold-and-flu/otc-cold-medicines#1.

DerSarkissian, C. (2021, May 16). *A guide to cough medicine*. WebMD. Retrieved from https://www.webmd.com/cold-and-flu/cold-guide/cough-syrup-cough-medicine.

Dmello, S. (2017, August 14). *5 science-backed natural remedies for a sore throat*. AllAyurveda. Retrieved from https://allayurveda.com/blog/natural-remedies-with-these-ease-your-sore-throat/.

Doerr, S., Cunha, J. P., & Balentine, J. R. (2019, September 12). *Sore throat causes, remedies, symptoms, and medications*. MedicineNet. Retrieved from https://www.medicinenet.com/sore_throat_pharyngitis/article.htm.

Duda, K., & Menna, M. (2020, March 19). *Will a decongestant relieve your cold and flu symptoms?* Verywell Health. Retrieved from https://www.verywellhealth.com/what-are-decongestants-770588.

Dunkin, M. A., & Pathak, N. (2020, August 25). *Tonsillitis*. WebMD. Retrieved from https://www.webmd.com/oral-health/tonsillitis-symptoms-causes-and-treatments#1

Eu Yan Sang. (n.d.). *Soothing a cough with TCM*. Retrieved from https://www.euyansang.com.sg/en/soothing-a-cough-with-tcm/eysihillnesses2.html

Global Initiative for Asthma. (2021, June 17). GINA patient guide: You can control your asthma. *Global Initiative for Asthma—GINA*. Retrieved from https://ginasthma.org/gina-patient-guide-you-can-control-your-asthma/.

Go Health Editors. (2021, June 21). *20 at-home remedies for a sore throat*. GoHealth Urgent Care. Retrieved from https://www.gohealthuc.com/library/20-home-remedies-sore-throat.

Gotter, A., & Murrell, D. (2019, March 7). *Home remedies for tonsillitis*. Healthline. Retrieved from https://www.healthline.com/health/home-remedies-for-tonsilitis.

Hardie, A. (2015, May 4). *Behind the brew: Horehound*. The Daily Tea. Retrieved from https://thedailytea.com/taste/behind-brew-horehound/.

Health Benefits Times. (2018, May 21). *False daisy facts and health benefits*. Health Benefits. Retrieved from https://www.healthbenefitstimes.com/false-daisy/.

Healthy Matters. (2021, July 8). *Best Chinese medicine for coughs and colds at home*. Retrieved from https://www.healthymatters.com.hk/home-chinese-medicine-remedies-coughs-colds/.

Hebbar, J. V. (2013, February 21). *Rasnadi Choornam benefits, how to use, dosage, ingredients*. AyurMedInfo. Retrieved from https://www.ayurmedinfo.com/2012/05/11/rasnadi-choornam-benefits-how-to-use-dosage-ingredients/.

Herbal Academy. (2014, January 13). *8 herbal home remedies for colds and flu*. Retrieved from https://theherbalacademy.com/8-herbal-home-remedies-for-colds-and-flu/.

Huang, Y., Wu, T., Zeng, L., & Li, S. (2012). Chinese medicinal herbs for sore throat. *Cochrane Database of Systematic Reviews, 14*(3), CD004877. Retrieved from https://doi.org/10.1002/14651858.cd004877.pub3.

Indigo Herbs. (n.d.). *Bala benefits & information*. Retrieved from https://www.indigo-herbs.co.uk/natural-health-guide/benefits/bala.

Jirsa, A. (2020, November 30). *3 Herbs to soothe a stubborn cough*. Mind Body Green Health. Retrieved from https://www.mindbodygreen.com/0-7352/3-herbs-to-soothe-a-stubborn-cough.html.

Kerkar, P. (2017, May 26). *Herbal remedies to treat tonsillitis*. Pain Assist. Retrieved from https://www.epainassist.com/articles/herbal-remedies-to-treat-tonsillitis.

Khatri, M. (2019, September 25). *COPD (Chronic Obstructive Pulmonary Disease)*. WebMD. Retrieved from https://www.webmd.com/lung/copd/10-faqs-about-living-with-copd.

Kimberly. (2018, January 13). *Homemade elderberry syrup*. The Daring Gourmet. Retrieved from https://www.daringgourmet.com/homemade-elderberry-syrup-for-colds-coughs-and-flu/.

Knott, L., & Huins, H. (2018, November 27). *Mucolytics*. Patient. Retrieved from https://patient.info/chest-lungs/chronic-obstructive-pulmonary-disease-leaflet/mucolytics

Link Naturals Pvt Ltd. (2018). *Herbal health care products: Samahan*. Link Natural. Retrieved from http://linknaturalproducts.com/herbal-health-care-products/.

Marks, L., & Jasmer, R. (2015, November 25). *Antihistamine—Types, side effects & precautions*. Everyday Health.Com. Retrieved from https://www.everydayhealth.com/antihistamine/guide/.

Medtronic Editorial Staff. (n.d.). *Medical technology, services, and solutions global leader*. Medtronic. Retrieved from https://www.medtronic.com/us-en/index.html.

Meixner, M. (2019, March 21). *11 science-backed health benefits of black pepper*. Healthline. Retrieved from https://www.healthline.com/nutrition/black-pepper-benefits#1.-High-in-antioxidants-.

Morice, A. H., McGarvey, L., & Pavord, I. (2006). Recommendations for the management of cough in adults. *Thorax, 61*(Suppl. 1), i1–i24. Retrieved from https://doi.org/10.1136/thx.2006.065144.

Narayanan, S. (2018, May 30). *Ayurvedic treatment for cough and cold*. Speaking Tree. Retrieved from https://www.speakingtree.in/allslides/ayurvedic-treatment-for-cough-and-cold.

National Center for Homeopathy. (2021, May 13). *Homepage*. Retrieved from https://www.homeopathycenter.org/.

Natural Health Products Editor. (2017, February 28). *7 natural remedies with essential oils for cough or cold*. Young Living Canada Blog. Retrieved from https://www.youngliving.com/blog/canada/7-natural-remedies-for-cough-or-cold/.

National Institute for Health and Care Excellence. (2017, November 29). *Asthma: Diagnosis, monitoring and chronic asthma management*. NICE. Retrieved from https://www.nice.org.uk/guidance/ng80.

NDTV Food. (2018, August 22). *6 best home remedies for cough to give you instant relief*. Retrieved from https://food.ndtv.com/health/6-best-home-remedies-for-cough-to-give-you-instant-relief-1445513.

NDTV Food Desk. (2018, August 27). *Throat infection: 6 brilliant home remedies for throat infection*. NDTV Food. Retrieved from https://food.ndtv.com/health/6-brilliant-home-remedies-for-a-throat-infection-1678944.

NHS Website. (2020, January 15). *Steroid inhalers*. NHS.UK. Retrieved from https://www.nhs.uk/conditions/steroid-inhalers/.

NHS Website. (2021, February 10). *Tonsillitis*. NHS.UK. Retrieved from https://www.nhs.uk/conditions/tonsillitis/.

Nursing Times Contributor. (2019, August 3). *Echinacea allergy warning for children under 12*. Nursing Times. Retrieved from https://www.nursingtimes.net/archive/echinacea-allergy-warning-for-children-under-12-27-08-2012/.

Panesar, G. (2017, August 30). *8 incredible benefits of camphor: Pain killer, sleep inducer and more*. NDTV Food. Retrieved from https://food.ndtv.com/health/8-incredible-benefits-of-camphor-pain-killer-sleep-inducer-and-more-1648410.

Paydar, M., Moharam, B. A., Wong, Y. L., Looi, C. Y., Wong, W. F., Nyamathull, S., et al. (2013). *Centratherum anthelminticum* (L.) Kuntze a potential medicinal plant with pleiotropic pharmacological and biological activities. *International Journal of Pharmacology, 9*(3), 211–226. Retrieved from https://doi.org/10.3923/ijp.2013.211.226.

Proven Herbal Remedies. (2021, May 3). *Fritillaria (Chuan Bei Mu).* Chinese Herbs Healing. https://www.chineseherbshealing.com/proven-herbal-remedies/fritillaria.html.

Raina, K. (2019, April 30). *Benefits and side effects of betel leaf (Paan).* FirstCry Parenting. Retrieved from https://parenting.firstcry.com/articles/magazine-benefits-and-side-effects-of-betel-leafpaan/.

Robinson, J., & Liao, S. (2020, November 8). *How to get rid of a cough.* WebMD. Retrieved from https://www.webmd.com/cold-and-flu/cough-get-rid-home-hacks#1.

Rubin, B. (2007). Mucolytics, expectorants, and mucokinetic medications. *Respiratory Care, 52*(7), 859–865. Retrieved from https://www.researchgate.net/publication/6242212_Mucolytics_expectorants_and_mucokinetic_medications.

RxList (Eds.). (2021, June 11). *Basil.* RxList. Retrieved from https://www.rxlist.com/basil/supplements.htm.

Saha, A. (2018, August 30). *5 effective home remedies for tonsils.* NDTV Food. Retrieved from https://food.ndtv.com/health/5-effective-home-remedies-for-tonsils-1631116.

Shiel, W. C. (2019, October 9). *Chronic cough: Symptoms, signs, causes & treatment.* MedicineNet. Retrieved from https://www.medicinenet.com/cough/symptoms.htm.

Spritzler, F., & Arnarson, A. (2020, June 16). *15 natural remedies for a sore throat.* Medical News Today. Retrieved from https://www.medicalnewstoday.com/articles/318631.

Story, C. M., Gotter, A., & Wilson, D. R. (2017, March 29). *12 natural remedies for sore throat.* Healthline. Retrieved from https://www.healthline.com/health/cold-flu/sore-throat-natural-remedies.

Streit, L. (2020, November 3). *Gentian root: Uses, benefits, and side effects.* Healthline. Retrieved from https://www.healthline.com/nutrition/gentian-root#benefits.

The Crankshaft Publishing Staff. (n.d.). *Acute tonsillitis (common disorders of the sensory organs) (Chinese Medicine).* What-When-How. Com. Retrieved from http://what-when-how.com/chinese-medicine/acute-tonsillitis-common-disorders-of-the-sensory-organs-chinese-medicine/.

Times of India. (2018, December 6). *10 ways to get rid of a terrible sore throat.* The Times of India. Retrieved from https://timesofindia.indiatimes.com/life-style/health-fitness/home-remedies/10-ways-to-get-rid-of-terrible-sore-throat/articleshow/22091531.cms.

Times of India. (2020, September 2). *20 home remedies for common cold and cough.* The Times of India. Retrieved from https://timesofindia.indiatimes.com/life-style/health-fitness/health-news/15-home-remedies-for-common-cold-and-cough/articleshow/21952311.cms.

Top Sri Lankan Recipe [Top Srilankan Recipes]. (2018, March 10). *Simple rasam recipe without tomato and rasam powder (Healthy)* [Video]. YouTube. Retrieved from https://www.youtube.com/watch?v=a1m6WPe8F7s&t=16s.

U.S. National Library of Medicine. (2021, April 1). *Cold and cough medicines.* Medline Plus. Retrieved from https://medlineplus.gov/coldandcoughmedicines.html.

WebMD Editors. (n.d.-a). *ECHINACEA: Overview, uses, side effects, precautions, interactions, dosing and reviews.* WebMD. Retrieved from https://www.webmd.com/vitamins/ai/ingredientmono-981/echinacea.

WebMD Editors. (n.d.-b). *Soothe a sore throat.* WebMD. Retrieved from https://www.webmd.com/allergies/sinus-nose-tool/soothe-sore-throat.

White, L. B. (1998, September 1). *Best herbs for the common cold.* Mother Earth Living. Retrieved from https://content.motherearthliving.com/health-and-wellness/cold-busters/.

Yang, C., & Montgomery, M. (2021). Dornase alfa for cystic fibrosis. *Cochrane Database of Systematic Reviews, 3.* Retrieved from https://doi.org/10.1002/14651858.cd001127.pub5.

Zanni, G. R. (2014, November 10). *Treating sore throat.* Pharmacy Times. Retrieved from https://www.pharmacytimes.com/view/treating-sore-throat.

3

Gastrointestinal System

Introduction

Gastrointestinal disorders are common and affect people of all ages.

Signs and symptoms include:

1. Vomiting
2. Stomach ache/indigestion
3. Constipation
4. Diarrhea
5. Acid reflux
6. Gas/wind and bloating
7. Hemorrhoids (piles)
8. Irritable bowel syndrome (IBS)
9. Gallstones

Common causes of abdominal pain (based on organs) include the following:

GIT. Food poisoning, acute gastroenteritis, gastritis, indigestion, gas, gastroesophageal reflux disease (GERD), IBS, *Helicobacter pylori* gastritis, food allergy, appendicitis, gallstones, cholecystitis, diverticulitis, intestinal obstruction, pancreatitis, inflammatory bowel disease (Crohn's disease and ulcerative colitis), GIT tumors, abdominal aortic aneurysm, ischemic colitis, etc.

Gynecological. Menstrual cramps, endometriosis, ectopic pregnancy, ovarian [DMT1] cysts or cancer

Renal. Urinary tract infection (UTI), kidney stones

Psychogenic. Emotional factors can also contribute.

Infections such as viruses and bacteria are common causes in acute gastroenteritis or gastritis. Wrong foods or allergies can also contribute to some of these disorders.

There are overlaps in home remedies across different ethnic groups.

Diagnostic tests for the gastrointestinal (GI) system depend on the underlying disease. These include blood and stool tests for anemia, infection, presence of occult blood, and other specific tests. Procedures include upper GI endoscopy (OGDS), lower GI colonoscopy, capsule endoscopy, ERCP, CT abdomen with contrast, MRI abdomen, ultrasound abdomen, barium meal or barium enema, liver biopsy, plain x-ray abdomen, urea breath test, hydrogen breath test, esophageal pH monitoring, esophageal motility study, and rectal manometry.

Vomiting

Vomiting is throwing up food with associated sound. *Spitting up* is throwing up without sound. *Retching* is making sound without throwing up.

Indian Natural Remedies

Common Ingredients for Vomiting

Spices	Herbs/Leaves	Miscellaneous
Black cardamom (*Amomum subulatum*)		Baking soda (*Sodium bicarbonate*)
Carom seed/ajwain (*Trachyspermum ammi*)		
Cinnamon (*Cinnamomum vera*)		
Clove (*Syzygium aromaticum*)		
Cumin (*Nigella sativa*)		White rice (*Oryza sativa*)
Fennel (*Foeniculum vulgare*)		
Ginger (*Zingiber officinale*)	Mint/karpooravalli (*Coleus amboinicus/ Plectranthus amboinicus*)	Lime (*Citrus aurantiifolia*) or lemon (*Citrus limon*)
Green cardamom (*Elettaria cardamomum*)		Apple cider vinegar
Ground nutmeg (*Myristica fragrans*)	Chamomile (*Matricaria chamomilla*)	Essential oils
Onion (*Allium cepa*)		Honey

Common Recipes

Oral

Teas/Brews

Apple cider vinegar. Take 1 teaspoon of apple cider vinegar. Add 1 glass of warm water. Consume if there is nausea and before a meal.

Baking soda. Add ½ teaspoon of baking soda to ½ cup of warm water. Sip slowly if there is nausea.

Black cardamom tea. Lightly pound one to two black cardamom. Add 1 cup of hot water. Allow to steep for 5 to 10 minutes. Strain and drink warm.

Carom tea. Place a teaspoon of carom seeds into a pot of water and boil it. Strain the mixture and drink it warm.

Chamomile tea. Place some dried or fresh chamomile flowers into a cup. Pour boiling water over the flowers and allow to steep for 10 minutes. Strain and add honey to taste. Drink it hot. Drink two to three times a day.

Cinnamon tea. Add a stick of cinnamon to 1 cup of hot water and allow to steep for about 10 minutes. Add honey to taste and drink.

Clove tea. Lightly pound three to five cloves. Place into a cup of hot water and cover. Allow to steep for 5 to 10 minutes before straining. Drink warm.

Cumin brew. Lightly roast a teaspoon of cumin seeds and ground it into a fine powder. Add this powder to hot water. A dash of nutmeg powder may also be mixed into the brew. Honey may be added to taste. Drink it warm.

Fennel tea. Boil a teaspoon of fennel seeds (or fennel powder) in a pot of hot water. Strain the mixture. Drink three to four times a day.

Ginger-onion juice. Add about 1 teaspoon of ginger juice or pounded ginger to one teaspoon of onion juice.

Ginger tea. Lightly pound about 1 to 2 inches of fresh ginger (if unavailable, use 1 to 2 teaspoons of ginger powder) and add to a cup of hot water. Allow to steep for 5 to 10 minutes. Strain and drink while warm. Add honey to taste.

Honey lemon mix. Mix 1 teaspoon of lemon juice and mint juice with some lightly pounded ginger and some honey. Take this mixture two to three times a day to relieve nausea and vomiting.

Lime tea. Add about 10 drops of lime juice to a cup of water and stir in about ¼ teaspoon of baking soda. Add sugar to taste and drink.

Rice starch. Boil one cup of white rice in 2 cups of water. Strain the mixture and drink the excess water.

Spice tea. Steep a pinch of nutmeg and 1 teaspoon of cumin seeds in hot water. Drink it warm.

Chew/Suck

Cardamom seeds. Chew on one to two green cardamom seeds in order to prevent nausea.

Cloves. Chew on one to two cloves to provide relief from vomiting.

Ginger. Suck on a small piece of ginger.

Mint leaves. Chew on some mint leaves.

Therapeutic Measures

Aromatherapy (Inhalational)

Essential oil therapy. Lavender, peppermint, ginger, fennel seed, and lemon essential oils may be diluted with water and placed into a humidifier/diffuser. Keep the humidifier by the bedside. Alternatively, if a diffuser is not readily available, sprinkle some lavender oil on the child's bed sheets or on the clothes.

Topical

Apple cider vinegar. Warm ½ cup of apple cider vinegar. Place in a bowl. Soak a small towel in it. Place the towel gently on the abdomen.

Chinese Natural Remedies

Vomiting is due to the abnormal retrograde rise of stomach - qi resulting in the food in the stomach being expelled upward. The causes include:

Exterior conditions or exogenous evil (wind, cold, summer heat, dampness). These elements disrupt the harmonization and descent, forcing the stomach - qi to ascend. The stomach is located in the middle warmer (called Zhong Jiao). It receives and digests food and fluids and its qi must flow downward.

Dietary indulgence. Indigestion and food retention are often caused by overindulgence; overeating; or raw, cold, or greasy foods. This will then impair the functions of the spleen and stomach, leading to phlegm accumulation and then vomiting.

Internal injury due to strong emotions (anger, anxiety, mental health issues, etc.). These lead to the restriction of liver-qi movement. Disharmony between liver-qi and stomach-qi leads to indigestion of food and hence vomiting.

The following syndrome types will arise:

Liver-qi (Fire) attacking the stomach.

Deficiency of spleen and stomach-qi: This will lead to interior Cold.

Deficiency of stomach-Yin: This is often due to bad eating habits.

Common Ingredients for Vomiting

Spices	Herbs/Leaves	Miscellaneous
Cardamom (*Elettaria cardamomum*)	Red atractylodes/ cang zhu (*Rhizome*)	Tangerine peel/ Chen pi
Cinnamon bark (*Cinnamomum vera*)	White atractylodes rhizome/bai zhu (*Atractylodes macrocephala*)	Hawthorn berry/ shan zha (*Crataegus pinnatifida*)
Clove/Ding xiang (*Syzygium aromaticum*)	Pinellia tuber/ ban xia (*Pinellia ternata*)	Barley/Mai ya
Cumin	Aloeswood/chen xiang (*Lignum aquilariae resinatum*)	
	Poor man's ginseng/ dang shen (*Codonopsis pilosula*)	
	Eclipta/Han lian cao (*Herba eclipta prostrata*)	

Spices	Herbs/Leaves	Miscellaneous
	Ox knee/huai niu xi *(Radix achyranthes)*	
	Coptis/huang lian *(Rhizoma coptidis)*	
	Patchouli/huo xiang *(Herba agastaches)*	
	Phragmites/lu gen *(Rhizoma phragmitis)*	
	Loquat leaf/japonicae/ pi pa ye *(Folium eriobotryae)*	
	White mulberry leaf/ sang ye *(Folium mori albae)*	
	Bamboo shavings/ zhu ru *(Bambusae caulis)*	
	Perilla leaf/zi su ye *(Perillae folium)*	
	Sharp-leaf galangal/yi zhi ren	
Ginger *(Zingiber officinale)*	Chicken gizzard lining/ji nei jin	Rice/geng mi *(Oryza sativa)*
Sichuan Peppercorn	Thorowax root/ chai hu *(Radix Bupleuri)*	Honey

Common Recipes

Oral

Teas/Brews/Others

Bai zhu tea. Soak the bai zhu in warm water for approximately 10 minutes and rinse before use. Steep two to three pieces of bai zhu in hot water and drink it warm.

Black pepper tea. Lightly crush and put 7 to 10 black peppercorns in a cup. Add boiling water and allow it to steep for 10 minutes and then drink.

Chicken gizzard lining. It is often bought dry. It should be ground into powder. Six grams of chicken gizzard lining should be dissolved in hot water and consumed hot two times a day.

Cinnamon tea. Add a stick of cinnamon to a pot of hot water and allow to steep for about 10 minutes. Add honey to taste and drink.

Clove tea. Lightly pound three to five cloves. Place into a cup of hot water and cover. Allow to steep for 5 to 10 minutes before straining. Drink warm.

Cumin brew. Lightly roast a teaspoon of cumin seeds and ground it into a fine powder. Add this powder to hot water. A dash of nutmeg powder may also be mixed into the brew. Honey may be added to taste. Drink it warm.

Ginger tea. Lightly pound about 1 to 2 inches of fresh ginger (if unavailable, use 1 to 2 teaspoons of ginger powder) and add to a cup of hot water. Allow to steep for 5 to 10 minutes. Strain and drink while warm. Add honey to taste.

Hawthorn berry tea. Take about 1 teaspoon of dried hawthorn berries and steep in hot water. Add honey to taste and drink it warm.

Polyherbal teas. Many of the above listed herbs or leaves are available as mixed formulations.

Rice porridge. If unstrained, the rice water and soft rice is eaten as porridge.

Rice water. Boil a cup of rice in a pot of water, then simmer until the rice is soft. Strain the mixture and add some honey and lemon to the remaining rice water. Drink the rice water warm.

Sharp-leaf galangal polyherbal. It contains sharp-leaf galangal, dang shen (codonopsis roots), gan jiang (dried ginger), and bai shu (atractylodes rhizomes) (for nausea, vomiting, and abdominal pain).

Tangerine peel tea. Take three to five pieces of tangerine peel and steep in hot water. Drink it warm.

Therapeutic Measures

Acupressure (Topical)

- Pressure point P-6 (also known as neiguan) is on the inner arm, three finger widths below the wrist. Using your thumb, apply firm pressure on this point and massage it firmly for 2 to 3 minutes. This may relieve feelings of nausea and prevent vomiting.
- The outer gate acupressure point also helps to relieve nausea and vomiting. It is located on the back of the hand. It is located three finger widths below the wrist crease. Massage this area with your thumb for 2 to 3 minutes.
- Korean hand acupressure of the acupuncture point K-K9 can reduce postoperative vomiting in children after strabismus surgery. K-K9 point is located on the middle phalanx of the fourth finger on the lateral and palmar side.

Western/Other Natural Remedies

Common Ingredients for Vomiting

Spices	Herbs/Leaves	Miscellaneous
Allspice		Honey
Cinnamon		Essential oils—clove, lavender, chamomile, rose, peppermint
Clove		Ice cube
Cumin		Dry saltine crackers
Fennel	Chamomile	Lemon
Ginger	Mint	Ginger ale

Common Recipes

Oral

Teas/Brews/Others

Allspice tea. Take ½ teaspoon ground allspice. Add 1 cup of hot water. Steep for 10 minutes. Strain and consume it warm.

Chamomile tea. Place some dried or fresh chamomile flowers into a cup. Pour boiling water over the flowers and allow to steep for 10 minutes. Strain and add honey to taste. Drink it hot.

Cinnamon tea. Add a stick of cinnamon to a pot of hot water and allow to steep for about 10 minutes. Add honey to taste and drink.

Clove tea. Lightly pound three to five cloves. Place into a cup of hot water and cover. Allow to steep for 5 to 10 minutes before straining. Drink it warm.

Cumin brew. Lightly roast a teaspoon of cumin seeds and ground it into a fine powder. Add this powder to hot water. A dash of nutmeg powder may also be mixed into the brew. Honey may be added to taste. Drink it warm.

Fennel tea. Boil a teaspoon of fennel seeds (or fennel powder) in a pot of hot water. Strain the mixture. Drink three to four times a day.

Ginger ale. Drinking ginger ale may provide relief from nausea.

Ginger tea. Lightly pound about 1 to 2 inches of fresh ginger (if unavailable, use 1 to 2 teaspoons of ginger powder) and add to a cup of hot water. Allow to steep for 5 to 10 minutes. Strain and drink while warm. Add honey to taste.

Mint tea. Steep a few mint leaves in hot water and add honey to taste. Drink it warm.

Chew/Suck the following items:

Dry saltine crackers. Eat a *dry saltine cracker* to relieve nausea. It is believed that they help to absorb stomach acids.

Ginger. Suck on a small piece of *ginger.*

Ice cube. Sucking on an ice cube may provide relief from nausea.

Supplements. **Vitamin B-6.** The vitamin B-6 tablets may also be taken to relieve nausea and prevent vomiting.

Therapeutic Measures

Lifestyle

Opening windows to let fresh air in may also relieve feelings of nausea.

Deep, slow breathing may help to relieve nausea and prevent vomiting.

Nasal (Inhalational)

Lemon. Slice a lemon and inhale its scent.

Essential oil therapy. Dilute a few drops of essential oil (lavender, lemon, clove, peppermint, chamomile, or rose) in water. Place the mixture into a humidifier/diffuser. If a diffuser is not available, sprinkle a few drops of the essential oil onto clothes or bed sheets.

Modern Remedies

Antihistamines

Antihistamines work by inhibiting the effect of histamine at the H1 receptor in the body, hence limiting stimulation in the vomiting center. It is also thought that antihistamines work by dulling the inner ear's ability to sense motion and hence cause motion sickness and vomiting. Examples of antihistamines used as antiemetics include cyclizine and diphenhydramine as well as metoclopramide.

Anticholinergics

Anticholinergic drugs competitively bind to the acetylcholine receptors. Acetylcholine is a neurotransmitter that stimulates the vomiting center through the afferent reflexes. Blocking the effects of acetylcholine relieves feelings of nausea and vomiting. Examples of common anticholinergics are diphenhydramine and biperiden.

Serotonin (5-HT3) Antagonists

Serotonin (5-HT3) antagonists are used largely and are very effective in chemotherapy-induced nausea and vomiting and post-operative nausea and vomiting. They work by binding to serotonin receptors, hence blocking the effect of serotonin. Serotonin is a neurotransmitter that stimulates afferent neurons in the brainstem leading to vomiting. By blocking the effects of serotonin, this medication prevents feelings of nausea and vomiting.

Serotonin antagonists are divided into the first and second generation. Second-generation serotonin antagonists bind more tightly to serotonin receptors than first-generation serotonin antagonists. The effect of second-generation serotonin antagonists lasts for longer than the first generation. Examples of first-generation serotonin antagonists are dolasetron and ondansetron. Palonosetron is a common second-generation serotonin antagonist.

Steroids

The antiemetic action of steroids is not well understood as it is thought that they may work by antagonizing prostaglandins or release endorphins that improve one's mood and hence stimulate appetite. A common example of a steroid drug used to relieve nausea and vomiting is dexamethasone.

Dopamine Antagonists

Dopamine antagonists are bound to a dopamine receptor named D2 in the central nervous system and block the effects of dopamine. Dopamine stimulates the vomiting center, which leads to nausea and vomiting. Dopamine antagonists are often only given when vomiting is not controlled using other drugs. Sedation is a common side effect of dopamine antagonists, and serotonin antagonists are now more frequently indicated than dopamine antagonists. Dopamine antagonists are available in oral form and in rectal or parenteral forms.

Examples of dopamine antagonists include metoclopramide, domperidone, droperidol.

Metoclopramide has both antiemetic and prokinetic properties. It is often used in travel sickness and in GERD. Domperidone (also called Motilium) is both an antiemetic and an upper GIT prokinetic agent. It is a peripheral selective D2 receptor antagonist and does not enter the central nervous system, unlike metoclopramide. Side effects include dry mouth, nausea, diarrhea, and hyperprolactinemia.

Droperidol is also a dopamine antagonist but is considered outdated and not commonly used.

Homeopathic Remedies

These include *Ipecacuanha* or *Lacticum acidum* (for vomiting in pregnancy), *Arsenicum album* (especially in food poisoning), *Nux vomica* (vomiting with bloating and gas), *Carbo vegetalis* (in indigestion or reflux), *Ignatia* (in psychogenic vomiting), *Sepia officinalis* (in morning nausea before eating and vomit tendency after eating), and *Creosote* (in prolonged gastric stasis or cancers).

Stomach Ache and Indigestion

Abdominal pain, or stomach ache as it is usually referred to, is a very common symptom. It can be acute (starts within a few hours and lasts a few days), chronic (lasts a few days to weeks and is usually recurrent), or progressive (getting worse).

Indian Natural Remedies

In Ayurveda, *Shoola* means pain (usually colic). *Shoola roga* is described as a painful abdominal disorder associated with other clinical features but without any obvious localized swelling. The *Shoola* is due to vitiation of Vata Dosha from underlying *Srotas Awarodata* (microchannel obstructions) and *Dhatu Kshaya* (depletion of tissues/malnutrition).

An integrated and holistic approach in abdominal pain management is helpful (including addressing the emotional factors involved). The various Ayurvedic pain treatments include *Snehana* (external herbal oil massage), *Swedana* (sweating via herbal steam bath), *Basti* (medicated enemas), *Lepankarma* (topical herbal pastes), *Jalaukavacharan* (leech therapy), *Shaman chikitsa* (symptomatic pain relief), *yoga asanas, Satvavajaya chikitsa* (psychotherapy), and others.

Common Ingredients for Stomach Ache and Indigestion

Spices	Herbs/Leaves	Miscellaneous
Cardamom	Peepal leaf/Ashvattha	
Carom	Ceylon leadwort/chitrak (*Plumbago zeylanica*)	Molasses
Clove	Amla (*Phyllanthus emblica*)	Lime or Lemon
Coriander		
Fennel	Liquorice/yashtimadhu (*Glycyrrhiza glabra*)	Buttermilk
Garlic	Celery	Pomegranate
Ginger	Betel leaf	Nutmeg oil
Onion	Basil/tulsi	Honey
Peppercorn	Mint	Salt
Turmeric	Nagkesar	Ghee

Common Recipes

Oral

Teas/Brews/Juices/Others

Amla juice. Lightly pound a few pieces of amla and extract about 1 teaspoon of the juice. Drink this juice on an empty stomach every day to neutralize stomach acid.

Carom tea. Place a teaspoon of carom seeds into a pot of water and boil it. Strain the mixture and drink it warm.

Celery brew. Cut a stick of celery into shorter segments. Roast the celery sticks lightly and steep in hot water. Drink it warm.

Chitrak. Take 1 to 2 g of chitrak root powder. Mix with some honey and consume.

Clove tea. Take 8 to 10 cloves and steep in hot water. Drink it warm.

Coriander tea. Lightly crush 1 teaspoon of coriander seeds. Place the seeds in a cup and pour hot water over it. Let sit for 5 to 10 minutes before straining. Drink it warm.
  Variation #1. Coriander-Buttermilk. Take 4 to 5 teaspoons (or less) coriander powder. Add to a glass of fresh buttermilk. Drink before or after meals

Cumin-Buttermilk. Add 1 teaspoon of ground cumin seeds to a glass of fresh buttermilk. Consume it.

Fennel tea. Boil a teaspoon of fennel seeds (or fennel powder) in a pot of hot water. Strain the mixture. Drink three to four times a day.

Garlic mix. Pound one to two pips of garlic. Add 1 cup of hot water. Add some cumin seeds and peppercorns. Allow to steep for 10 minutes. Strain and drink.

Ginger paste. Lightly pound some fresh ginger to extract about 1 teaspoon of ginger juice. Mix this with ½ a teaspoon of ghee. Eat this paste to relieve abdominal pain.

Ginger tea. Blend lemon juice with ginger juice and drink. Alternatively, lightly pound some ginger and steep in hot water. Add a pinch of salt. Drink it warm.

Liquorice root tea. Add 1 to 2 teaspoons of ground liquorice root to a cup of boiling water. Allow it to steep for about 5 minutes. Add honey to taste and drink it warm.

Mint-lime-ginger juice. Pound mint and extract the juice. Mix this with lime juice. Add some ginger juice and a pinch of salt. Drink this mixture to relieve abdominal pain.

Mint tea. Lightly pound some mint leaves to extract about a teaspoon of mint juice. Mix this with water and add honey to taste.

Nagkesar. Take ¼ to ½ teaspoon of nagkesar powder. Mix with some honey or lukewarm water. Consume one to two times a day.

Onion. Consume onion as part of salad or cooked food.

Peepal tea. Take 2 g of Ashvattha bark powder. Add 200 mL water. Boil and reduce the volume till 50 mL. Add some jaggery and little salt. Consume twice a day.
  Variation #1. Take two to three peepal leaves and ground them. Add 50 g of jaggery. Make little pellets and chew on them three to four times a day.

Pomegranate-honey juice. Take a handful of pomegranate and blend. Mix the juice with a teaspoon of honey and consume to neutralize stomach acid.

Spice powder drink. Mix ½ a teaspoon of ginger powder and ½ a teaspoon of turmeric in a glass of warm water. Drink it warm.

Spice tea. Place a teaspoon of carom seeds into a pot of water and boil for about 5 minutes. Strain this mixture and add some salt.

Tulsi juice. Make some tulsi juice. Add a little cardamom powder and a pinch of chili powder. Consume this (if any stomach flu or infection).

Tulsi tea. Place a handful of tulsi leaves into a pot of water. Bring to a boil and reduce the heat. Allow the mixture to simmer for 5 to 10 minutes. Strain and drink twice a day.

Chew/Suck

Ginger. Slice fresh ginger and rub the slices in salt and lemon juice. Place it in the sun and dry thoroughly. Eat a piece after every meal to reduce bloating and hence relieve stomach aches.

Molasses. Consume molasses after every meal to aid digestion and prevent stomach aches.

Nutmeg oil-sugar paste. Mix some nutmeg oil with sugar and consume this paste to relieve stomach aches.

Topical

Betel leaf. Warm ½ teaspoon of castor oil. Apply gently on the abdomen around the navel. Place the betel leaf over the warm oil. Gently wrap with a cloth binder.

Ginger juice. Lightly pound some fresh *ginger* and extract the juice. Apply the juice on the bottom of the stomach and massage it gently to relieve stomach aches. This works as ginger has anti-inflammatory as well as analgesic (pain-relieving) properties.

Notes

Infants under the age of 2 years should not be given ginger.

Adults should take no more than 4 g of ginger a day, and pregnant women should not take more than 1 g of ginger a day.

Onion and garlic are high in insoluble fiber, fructans, and FODMAP. It may cause indigestion in some.

Chinese Natural Remedies

Common Ingredients for Stomach Ache and Indigestion

Spices	Herbs/Leaves	Miscellaneous
Ginger	Coptis/ Huang lian	Young tangerine peel/qing pi
Lilyturf root/ Mai Dong (*Liriope muscari* or *Radix Ophiopogonis*)	Mu-dan pi (*Paeonia suffruticosa*)	Honey
	Gardenia/zhizi	Rice
	Bai shao yao/ White Peony Root (*Radix Paeoniae Alba*)	
	Wu zhu yu/Evodia	

Spices	Herbs/Leaves	Miscellaneous
	Zhu ru (*Phyllostachys nigra*)	Tiger nuts (*Cyperus esculentus*)
	Phragmites/ lu gen	
	Glycyrrhiza/ gan cao	
	Bupleurum/ chai hu	
	Zhiqiao (*Poncirus trifoliata*)	
	Mint	

Common Recipes

Oral

Teas/Brews/Others

Ginger brew. Add six to eight slices of fresh ginger to a pot of water and boil it. Add honey to taste and steep a few mint leaves in the ginger tea. Drink it warm.

Herbal brew. Add huang lian (5 g), mu-dan pi (10 g), zhizi (10 g), bai shao yao (10 g), wu zhu yu (5 g), chuan lian zi (10 g), qing pi (10 g), zhu ru (10 g), lu gen (10 g), and gan cao (5 g) to a pot of water and boil. Drink it warm.

Polyherbal teas. Many of the above-listed herbs or leaves are available as mixed formulations.

Rice congee. Make congee by placing about ½ a cup of rice in a pot with water and bringing it to a boil. Once it begins to boil, bring the heat down and simmer for 40 to 50 minutes or until the rice is soft. Add ginger slices and simmer until the mixture becomes watery in texture.

Tiger nuts. It can be sprouted, roasted or dried and eaten.

Therapeutic Measures

Acupressure (Topical)

Zhong wan (CV 12) is located in the middle of the abdomen, halfway between the belly button and the base of your sternum. Place a finger on this point and apply firm pressure. Do not press for any more than 2 minutes at any time. This may also help to relieve abdominal pain.

The three-point mile (ST 36) is located four finger widths below the base of the knee cap. Massage this point for 2 to 3 minutes. This is also helpful in relieving abdominal pain.

Union valley (LI 4) is located on the flesh between the thumb and index finger. Massage this point with your thumb for about 2 to 3 minutes.

Western/Other Natural Remedies

Common Ingredients for Stomach Ache and Indigestion

Spices	Herbs/Leaves	Miscellaneous
Allspice	Yarrow leaf	Baking soda
	Basil	Figs
	Liquorice	Bread
	Cornflower	Essential oils
	Burning bush	Cranberry juice

Spices	Herbs/Leaves	Miscellaneous
		Coconut water
		Rose water
Fennel	Chamomile	Lemon
Ginger	Peppermint	Salt
Turmeric	Aloe vera	Apple cider vinegar

Common Recipes

Oral

Teas/Brews/Others

Allspice tea. Take ½ teaspoon ground allspice. Add 1 cup of hot water. Steep for 10 minutes. Strain and consume it warm.

Aloe vera juice. Wash one aloe vera leaf and pat dry. Slit it down the center and scoop out the white gel inside. Discard the greenish gel by rinsing it several times under running water. Add about 2 teaspoons of the white gel to a cup of warm water and place inside a blender. Blend until smooth and drink it warm.

Apple cider vinegar. Mix one tablespoon of apple cider vinegar with a cup of warm water. Add honey to taste and sip on it.

Baking soda. Mix 1 teaspoon of baking soda to a glass of warm water. Drink it warm.

Basil tea. Steep 3 to 5 fresh basil leaves in a cup of hot water. Drink it warm.

Burning bush tea. Take 2 to 3 teaspoons of dried burning bush leaves into a teapot with 2 cups of boiling water. Steep for 5 to 10 minutes and strain. Drink warm.

Chamomile tea. Add three to five dried or fresh chamomile flowers into a cup. Pour boiling water over the flowers and allow to steep for 10 minutes. Strain and add honey to taste. Drink hot.

Coconut water. Sip on up to 2 glasses of coconut water every 4 to 6 hours to relieve stomach pain.

Cornflower. Add 1 teaspoon of the dried cornflower in a cup of hot water. Allow to steep for 5 minutes then drink.

Cranberry juice: Drink about 2 cups of cranberry juice daily for 3 weeks (in *H. pylori* gastritis).

Fennel. Chew on two to three fennel seeds to relieve stomach ache. Alternatively, if raw fennel is available, slice a piece off and chew on it.

Figs. Soak two to four figs in water overnight. Consume them (both fruit and water) in the morning. Alternatively, they can be boiled and consumed.
Fig oil or syrup is also available.

Ginger-mint tea. Lightly crush some mint leaves and pound some ginger slices. Steep the pounded ingredients in a glass of warm water. Drink it warm.

Ginger mixture. Lightly pound some ginger slices and extract about 1 teaspoon of its juice. Do the same with some mint. Extract some lemon juice. Mix the juices and extracts and add a pinch of salt. Drink this mixture twice a day.

Liquorice root tea. Add 1 to 2 teaspoons of ground liquorice root to a cup of boiling water. Allow it to steep for about 5 minutes. Add honey to taste and drink it warm.

Mint. Chew on some mint leaves.

Rice water. Boil a cup of rice in a pot of water. Once the rice has come to a boil, bring the heat down and simmer until the rice is soft. Strain the mixture and add some honey and lemon to the remaining rice water. Drink it warm.

Rose water. Take 2 or 3 cups of fresh rose petals and place in saucepan. Add about 2 litres of distilled water or enough to cover the petals. Simmer in the saucepan for 30 to 45 minutes till the colour comes out from the petals. Cool, then strain and store in a clean bottle. Refrigerate and use for 1 month. Consume 1 glass daily.

Turmeric tea. Mix ½ teaspoon of turmeric in a cup of hot water. Drink it warm.

Yarrow tea. Add 1 to 2 teaspoons of ground yarrow leaves or flowers to a cup of hot water. Allow to steep for 10 to 15 minutes. Drink it warm.

Therapeutic Measures

Diet

BRAT diet: Consume low-fiber foods such as bananas, rice, applesauce, and toast. These foods are bland and do not contain any spices that may aggravate stomach pain.

Charred bread: Make some toast and char the bread. Charred bread is believed to be able to absorb toxins in the stomach, relieving any pain.

Sourdough bread. Consume sourdough bread to ease indigestion.

Lifestyle

Heating pad: Apply a heating pad to the abdomen to relax the muscles and reduce stomach cramps, relieving any stomach pain.

Nasal (Inhalational)

Essential oil therapy. Dilute *peppermint essential oils* with some water and add the mixture to a humidifier/diffuser. If a humidifier is not available, sprinkle some of the essential oils on clothes or bed sheets.

Modern Remedies

Antacids

Stomach ache may be caused by excess gastric acid (hydrochloric acid [HCL]) in the stomach. Antacids are medicines that contain alkaline ions. These ions neutralize the gastric acid in the stomach and hence relieve stomach ache. In the stomach, they react with HCL to form a salt compound and water, lowering the stomach's acidity levels.

Antacids

Examples	Composition
Alka-Seltzer	Aspirin, citric acid, sodium bicarbonate
Milk of Magnesia	Magnesium hydroxide
Gaviscon	Sodium alginate, sodium bicarbonate, calcium carbonate

Examples	Composition
Gelusil and Maalox plus	Aluminum hydroxide, magnesium hydroxide, simethicone
Mylanta	Aluminum hydroxide, magnesium hydroxide
Pepto-Bismol	Bismuth subsalicylate
Tums	Calcium carbonate
Alternagel	Aluminum hydroxide

Anti-Flatulence Agents

Anti-flatulence medication works by lowering the surface tension of gas in the stomach and intestines, which allows the gasses to break down more easily into bubbles. This allows the release of stomach gas as flatulence and prevents the build-up and formation of mucous-enclosed gas bubbles in the digestive tract, causing bloating and pain. A common example of anti-flatulence medication is simethicone.

Digestive Enzymes

Various enzymes will break down carbohydrates (amylase, lactate, invertase, cellulase), fats (lipase), and proteins (protease and bromelain).

Anti-Diarrhea Agents

Anti-diarrhea medication works by slowing down the movement of the gut and some have anti-inflammatory properties. It also inhibits the spread of some bacteria that cause diarrhea. Examples of anti-diarrhea medications are classified as below.

Antidiarrheal Agents

Anti-infective agents	ciprofloxacin, cotrimoxazole, erythromycin, doxycycline, metronidazole
Antimotility drugs (opiates/opioid agonists)	loperamide, diphenoxylate, difenoxin, codeine
Antisecretory agent (enkephalinase inhibitor) used in acute diarrhea to increase the availability of endogenous opioids (enkephalins)	racecadotril
Adsorbent drugs	pectin, kaolin, charcoal, bismuth subsalicylate, methylcellulose,
Antispasmodic/ Anticholinergic drugs	atropine, scopolamine, buscopan
Anti-inflammatory agents (for inflammatory bowel disease)	sulfasalazine, mesalazine
Somatostatin analogue (for chemotherapy-induced diarrhea or refractory diarrhea)	octreotide
Intestinal flora modifiers	probiotics

Laxatives

See under "Constipation."

Homeopathic Remedies

These remedies include *Natrum carbonicum* (associated dyspepsia and gas after fatty and starchy foods with the history of food, especially milk allergies in a sweet and gentle person). *Calcarea carbonica* (relieves chronic heartburn in obese persons and worse with milk), *N. vomica* (associated overindulgence, abdominal pain after food, always in a hurry, irritable, angry but less fearful), *Lycopodium* (prolonged heartburn up to the throat even after small snacks and with associated bloating), *Carbo vegetabilis* (associated gas and bloating), *Argentum nitricum* (associated gnawing upper abdominal pains, fear, always in a hurry, and diarrhea tendency), *Pulsatilla* (associated fatty foods and emotional upsets), *Anacardium* (associated recurrent upper abdominal pain when hungry and relieved by food briefly), *Phosphorus* (associated frequent vomiting tendency and cold-water craving). Others include *Bryonia, Mag phos, and Calcarea phosphorica.*

Constipation

Constipation is a common digestive problem and refers to infrequent or incomplete bowel movements (less than three times a week) or passing hard, dry stools. Causes and risk factors include low-fiber and fatty diet; lack of fluids; medications; pregnant, elderly, or bedridden persons; change in routine; IBS; and underlying medical conditions.

Further evaluation and tests such as abdominal x-ray, ultrasound, CT abdomen, Barium enema, colonoscopy, and blood tests are indicated if there is a change in bowel movements, weight loss, passage of blood, or signs of intestinal obstruction.

Indian Natural Remedies

Constipation is regarded as a *vata* disorder with cold and dry qualities. Hence the stools are dry and hard.

The following are simple Ayurveda home remedies.

Common Ingredients for Constipation

Spices	Herbs/Leaves	Miscellaneous
Ajwain (Carom seeds)	Giloy	Jaggery
Asafetida	Trivrit (*Operculina turpethum*)	China grass (agar-agar)
Cardamom	Figs (anjeer)	Ghee
Coriander seeds	Senna leaf	Bael fruit
Fennel	Dandelion root (*Taraxacum officinale*)	Flaxseed

Spices	Herbs/Leaves	Miscellaneous
Onions/Shallots	Bay leaf	Castor oil
	Chicory (Cichorium intybus)	Fruit juice, prune, pineapple, dates)
	Chirata	Amaltas (Cassia fistula)
		Guava fruit
		Malva nuts
Raw scallion	Liquorice root	Milk
Tamarind	Triphala	Psyllium

Common Recipes

Oral

Tea/Brews/Others

Amaltas brew. Take 1 to 2 teaspoons of the fruit pulp paste. Add 1 glass of warm water. Consume after dinner.

Asafoetida. Add asafetida as a spice to daily foods.

Bael fruit blend. Mix ½ cup bael fruit pulp with some tamarind water and one teaspoon of jaggery in the evening.

Variation #1. Take 1 cup of ripe bael fruit. Mix with some jaggery. Consume daily for 2 to 3 months.

Variation #2. Take ¼ to ½ teaspoon of bael powder. Add ½ to 1 cup of water. Drink twice a day after a meal.

Alternatively. To make bael juice, cut the bael fruit. Scoop out the pulp into a bowl and mash it and remove the seeds by hand. Blend the de-seeded pulp with some water. Add sugar to taste.

Bay leaf tea. Take 3 bay leaves and boil with 2 cups of water for about 10 minutes. Add a pinch of cinnamon. Honey or lemon juice to be added as desired.

Black cardamom tea. Lightly pound one to two black cardamom. Add 1 cup of hot water. Allow to steep for 5 to 10 minutes. Strain and drink warm.

Carom (ajwain) tea. Place a teaspoon of carom seeds into a pot of water and boil it. Strain the mixture and drink it warm.

Variation #1. Add ajwain seeds as a spice to daily foods.

Castor oil. Consume about 15 mL at bedtime (adult's dosage). It can be chilled in the fridge first or mixed with ½ teaspoon ginger powder to mask the taste.

Chicory. Drink 60 mL of chicory leaf juice regularly. Take five leaves. Blend with some water. Add any citrus fruit or beet.

Variation #1. Boil and consume chicory root as a vegetable. The young leaves can be added to salads or sautéed.

Variation #2. Make a hot brew. Take 2 tablespoons of ground chicory root. Add 1 cup of boiling water.

Variation #3. Take 10 to 12 g/day of chicory inulin supplement.

Variation #4. Take 30 g of fresh chicory leaves. Add in 1 L of water. Boil and consume 1 glass before each meal.

China grass. Cut some China grass into smaller segments and add to a cup of milk and some water. Place this mixture in a pot and lightly boil until the China grass has dissolved, and the mixture appears gelatinous. Remove from the heat and refrigerate until the mixture sets.

Chirata. Take the fresh chirata whole plant (or dry plant). Add 1 cup water. Boil until reduced to ¼ cup. Strain. Consume 3 to 4 teaspoons twice a day, after meals.

Coriander tea. Lightly crush 1 teaspoon of coriander seeds. Place the seeds in a cup and pour hot water over it. Let sit for 5 to 10 minutes before straining. Drink warm.

Variation #1. Roasted coriander seed powder can be added to curries.

Dandelion root tea. Boil 1 teaspoon of ground dandelion root in a pot of water. Drink three to four times a day. Dandelion root is also available in tablet form.

Figs. Soak figs in warm water and eat three to five figs every day.

Flaxseed tea. Take 1 tablespoon of flaxseed (whole or milled) every day with 1 to 2 cups of warm water.

Fruit juice. Consume a cup of fresh fruit juice (pineapple, prune, or dates) in the morning.

Giloy. Mix ½ g of giloy with some amla and jaggery (brown sugar) and consume at bedtime.

Guava fruit. Consume the guava fruit.

Ivy gourd. It can be cooked as a spicy stir-fry.

Variation #1. **Ivy gourd juice.** Place one to two cut ivy gourds into a blender and blend until smooth, gradually adding up to 1 cup of water. Strain and drink.

Liquorice root tea. Add 1 to 2 teaspoons of ground liquorice root to a cup of boiling water. Allow it to steep for about 5 minutes. Add honey or jaggery to taste and drink it warm. Liquorice is known to promote bowel activity.

Malva nut. Take 1 to 2 malva nuts (do not exceed 3 nuts). Add 1 cup of water. Steep for 30 minutes. Discard the skin and seed. Consume the liquid and pulp as a brew.

Variation #1. Take 100 g of malva nuts. Add 2 L of water and soak preferably overnight. Remove and discard the seed and thick outer skin the next morning. Strain the pulp (gel) via a coarse muslin cloth. Various spices or herbs can be added to the pulp

Take 2 cups of water in a saucepan. Add pandanus (screwpine leaf) and brown sugar. Boil and simmer for 10 to 15 minutes. Add cinnamon stick, ginger slices, and licorice for additional flavors if desired. Strain. Add the malva nut pulp to the strained liquid and drink.

Variation # 2. Other items such as red date, liquorice, chrysanthemum flower, jasmine tea, lilyturf root, haw, and rock sugar can also be simmered together in water and then the malva nut pulp added.

Variation #3. Soaked basil seeds, sugar, and ice can be added to the soaked malva nut pulp and drunk as a cooling drink.

Milk and ghee. Mix 1 to 2 teaspoons of ghee in a cup of hot milk and drink at bedtime.

Psyllium. Take 2 to 3 teaspoons of psyllium husk with warm water, warm milk, or juice at night.

Roasted fennel seeds. Lightly roast fennel seeds. Take 1 teaspoon of the seeds with a glass of warm water.

Scallion, shallots, and onions. Consume them raw as a part of salads.

Senna leaf and dried ginger powder. Take equal amounts (1 teaspoon) of both ingredients. Mix in warm water and consume at bedtime.

Tamarind brew. Boil about 80 g (5 to 6 tablespoons) of tamarind pulp and seed in a pot of water for about 10 minutes. Strain and drink throughout the day. Add some fresh calamansi or lemon juice and jaggery, if desired.

Triphala. It is available in paste, powder, or tablet form. The paste or powder may be dissolved in water or milk and taken at bedtime.

Trivrit and raisins. Make a fine powder of shweta (white) trivrit. Add 250 to 750 mg into a cup of warm milk or lukewarm water along with some raisins. Consume this.

Trivrit, triphala, ajwain, and rock salt. Take equal amounts of each ingredient and ground into fine powder. Add lukewarm water to 3 to 5 g of this powder and drink.

Commercial Preparations

Herbolax. It is a polyherbal tablet with prebiotic, prokinetic, and laxative actions. It contains trivrit (*Ipomoea turpethum*), senna (*Cassia acutifolia*), haritaki (*Terminalia chebula*), kasani (*Cichorium intybus*/blue daisy), *Zingiber officinale, Glycyrrhiza glabra* (liquorice/licorice), Kakamachi (*Solanum nigrum*/black nightshade), and vidanga/false black pepper (*Embelia ribes*).

Therapeutic Measures

Massage

- Take 1 cup of castor oil, 1 to 1 ½ inches long asafetida, three fresh garlic pips (crushed). Boil until they are melted. When cool, strain into a bottle. Apply on the umbilical and rub outward in a clockwise manner.
- Place a hot pack on the lower tummy. This can relax intestinal muscles, stimulate circulation and bowel activity, and relieve constipation.

Diet

Eat a vata dosha pacifying and balancing diet. Avoid cold and raw foods. Eat and drink warm and well-cooked foods.

A diet high in fiber of about 20 to 35 g/day is important to prevent constipation.

Avoid or limit oily foods, alcohol, and caffeinated beverages.

Lifestyle

Drink a glass of water (preferably warm) in the morning.

Make it a habit to open the bowels at a regular time. Avoid holding and answer nature's call.

Exercise regularly. This will improve circulation and stimulate bowel movements.

Yoga

The following asanas can help provide a "digestive massage" to relieve: Matsyasana (fish pose), Shavasana (corpse pose), Dhanurasana (bow pose), Suryanamaskar (sun salutation), Pawanmuktasana (wind relieving pose) Halasana (plough pose), Bhujangasana (cobra pose), and Supta Vajrasana (sleeping thunderbolt pose)

Practice mindfulness meditation.

Chinese Natural Remedies

Constipation is believed to be due to Qi deficiency mainly, and also Qi stagnation, blood deficiency, or blood stasis.

Common Ingredients for Constipation

Spices	Herbs/Leaves	Miscellaneous
Black sesame seed (hei zhi ma)	Trichosanthes	Rhubarb root
Cinnamon	Rehmannia	Dried tangerine peel/chen pi
Lilyturf root/ Mai Dong (*Liriope muscari* or *Radix Ophiopogonis*)	Chinese liquorice Konjac root	Honey
		Areca peel/da fu pi (*Areca catechu*) Tiger nuts (*Cyperus esculentus*)

Common Recipes

Oral

Teas/Brews

Black sesame seeds. Take 1 to 2 teaspoons of ground black sesame seeds with a cup of warm water. Alternatively, sprinkle black sesame seeds onto food.

Chinese liquorice tea. Place 2 to 3 teaspoons of ground Chinese liquorice and a stick of cinnamon into a pot of water and boil. Add honey to taste and drink it warm.

Glossy or slippery foods. Foods such as bananas and spinach are regarded as having lubricating effects on the intestines, hence relieving constipation.

Honey. Mix 1 teaspoon of *honey* in a cup of warm water. Drink before bedtime.

Konjac root. This Asian root vegetable can be boiled or processed into ground flour to make Japenese noodles (shirataki noodles) or snacks.

Lilyturf root. Slice the dried root. Make it into a decoction.

Rhubarb root tea. Place about 20 g of dried crushed rhubarb root into a pot and add about 1 L of water. Boil and then simmer gently for 10 to 15 minutes. Strain and drink one cup before two main meals of the day.

Sour food. Avoid *sour foods* like lime, *lemon, pickles, and vinegar.*

Tiger nuts. It can be sprouted , roasted or dried and eaten.

Commercial Preparations

- Many traditional Chinese medicines (TCMs) are sold as commercial preparations which contain herbs such as *trichosanthes* and *rehmannia* and are effective in treating constipation.

Some Chinese herbs have also been found to be able to relieve IBS-related constipation.

- **Daikenchuto extract powder.** This is a Japanese herbal medicine (part of Kampo medicine) containing Japanese pepper *(Zanthoxylum piperitum)*, ginseng, ginger, and maltose.
- **Daio Kanzo To.** This is a Japanese herbal medicine containing licorice root and rhubarb.
- **Keishikashakuyakuto.** This is a Japanese herbal medicine containing peony root, cinnamon bark, licorice root, jujube fruit, and ginger.

Therapeutic Measures

Acupressure (Topical)

Conception Vessel 6 (CV 6 or sea of qi) is located three finger widths below the belly button. Press it down with two fingers no more than 1 inch deep into the skin. Maintain firm pressure on the point for about 30 seconds while breathing normally and with your eyes closed.

Center of Power (CV 12) is in the midline of the abdomen, exactly between the base of the sternum and the belly button. Do not stimulate this point for more than 2 minutes at a time.

Three-mile Point (ST 36) is located four finger widths below the base of the knee cap.

Joining Valley Point (LI 4) is located on the webbing between the hub and the index finger. Stimulate this point gently but firmly for 2 to 3 minutes while taking long deep breaths.

Western/Other Natural Remedies

Common Ingredients for Constipation

Herbs/Leaves	Miscellaneous
Aloe	Coffee
Dandelion	Probiotics
Plantain weed/leaf *(Plantago major)*	Corn syrup
	Flaxseed
	Molasses
	Sodium bicarbonate
	Epsom salts
	Essential oils (peppermint, rosemary, lemon, ginger)
	Oils: Castor, Olive, Almond, Fig, Linseed
	Dates
Vegetable and fruit juices	Prunes

Common Recipes

Oral

Teas/Brews/Juice

Aloe vera juice. Wash and dry an aloe vera leaf. Slit the leaf down the center. Scrape out the white gel, discarding any of the yellow gel. Cut into smaller pieces and add to a blender. Blend until smooth. Add to a fruit/vegetable smoothie or warm water or drink alone. Take one to two times a day in the week.

Coffee. Drink a cup of coffee in the morning.

Corn syrup: Add 1 tablespoon of corn syrup to a glass of warm water and consume.

Dandelion tea. Steep three to five dried dandelion flowers in a glass of hot water. Drink it warm.

Dates. Consume five to six dates with some warm milk at bedtime, or soak a few dates overnight and eat them pre-meal.

Epsom salts. Mix 2 teaspoons of Epsom salts into a cup of water or fruit juice.

Figs. Soak two or four figs in water overnight. Consume them (both fruit and water) in the morning. Alternatively, they can be boiled and consumed.
Fig oil or syrup is also available.

Flaxseed. Consume 2 to 3 teaspoons of ground flaxseed with a glass of warm water.

Molasses. Consume 1 teaspoon of molasses on its own or mix it into a cup of warm water or tea.

Oils. Add 1 to 2 tablespoons of olive, almond, or castor oil to some warm milk. Consume at night.
Or consume 1 tablespoon of *castor oil* in the morning on an empty stomach.
Or take 1 teaspoon of linseed oil in ¼ cup of water before a meal.

Oil & Fruit juice: Mix ½ cup of olive oil (or 1 to 2 tablespoon of cold/chilled castor oil) and ½ cup orange juice. Consume at bedtime.

Plantain juice. Blend 2 cups of fresh plantain leaves and 3 cups of water. Drain and drink warm or with additives.
Variation #1. Take 2 teaspoons of plantain seeds (also called psyllium) and soak in 2 cups of water.

Probiotics. Consume foods with high probiotic content such as yogurt or sauerkraut.

Prunes. Soak two to three prunes in hot water overnight. Drink the water and consume the prunes in the morning. A few teaspoonfuls of prune juice can be given in infants under the age of 2. It should not be fed to babies under 4 weeks of age.

Sodium bicarbonate. Mix one teaspoon of sodium bicarbonate in a ¼ cup of warm water. Drink it warm.

Vegetable and Fruit juices: Fresh vegetable and/or fruit juices (preferably combined to suit one's needs and preference) can be made with spinach, carrot, apple, orange, figs, prunes, papaya, guava, aloe vera, etc. in the morning.
A mix of fig juice and prune juice or fresh lemon or lime juice in a glass or warm water (with honey if desired) are also effective remedies.

Therapeutic Measures

Nasal (Inhalational)

- **Essential oil therapy.** Ginger oil, peppermint oil, rosemary oil, or lemon oil may be used for constipation relief. It may be diluted with water and placed into a humidifier/diffuser. Keep the humidifier by the bedside. Alternatively, if a diffuser is not readily available, sprinkle some lavender oil on the child's bed sheets or on their clothes.

Abdominal Massages

- The above essential oils mixed with any carrier oil can be placed in the navel and the abdomen is then massaged in a clockwise manner.

Modern Remedies

Laxatives are medications given to relieve constipation. They are available in oral form (pills, powder, liquid) or as rectal suppository or enema. The onset of action varies from 5 to 10 minutes (usually enema and suppository) to 6 to 8 hours. They are classified in the following categories:

Laxatives

Category	Mechanism	Examples
Bulk-Forming Laxative	Bulk-forming laxatives are fiber supplements with either soluble fiber or insoluble fiber mainly. They are polysaccharides and cellulose from cereal grains, wheat bran, and psyllium husks. They mimic physiological gut activity more closely than other laxatives. They cause water retention in fecal matter, hence stimulating the bowel by the bulky stool mass. It also causes decreased intestinal transit time and increased defecation frequency. The soft, bulky stool is made easier to pass and there is relief from constipation.	**Predominantly soluble fiber laxative (more fermentable and gas-producing):** *calcium polycarbophil (FiberCon), wheat dextrin (Benefiber)* **Predominantly insoluble fiber laxative (less fermentable and less gas-producing:** *methylcellulose (Citrucel)* **Mixed soluble and insoluble fiber laxative:** *psyllium husk (Metamucil)*
Emollient Laxative	Emollient laxatives are stool softeners which contain docusate. Docusate is a surfactant which works to encourage bowel movements by increasing water and lipid (fat) absorption into the stool, preventing hard and dry stool. This helps to lubricate the passage of fecal material through the intestinal walls. It often takes a week or more before emollient laxatives become effective. Emollient laxatives are often indicated in patients with hemorrhoids as it helps to prevent straining and pain in passing stools.	Colace (Docusate sodium, DSS) and Surfak *(Docusate calcium)*.
Lubricant Laxative	Lubricant laxatives act on the colon and coat the stool with lipids, hence lubricating its passage through the intestinal passage. They also cause water retention in the fecal matter, promoting heavier and softer stool. It also decreases intestinal transit time. The onset of action is within 6–8 h.	*Mineral oils* (liquid paraffin oil or liquid petrolatum).
Hyperosmotic Laxative	Hyperosmotic laxatives work by creating an osmotic gradient and drawing water from the surrounding tissues into the bowels, hence increasing stool mass and softness **Hyperosmotic Saline laxative** Hyperosmotic saline laxatives, also known as salts, are used for rapid clearing of the bowels and lower intestine. They are enema preparations and are for short-term use only. **Hyperosmotic lactulose laxative** Lactulose is a synthetic sugar and is not digested in the intestine and is broken down in the colon by bacteria. This process draws water into the fecal matter, causing it to become bulky and soft. They are available as oral preparations. It acts more slowly than saline laxatives. **Hyperosmotic polymer laxative** This medication is a polyglycol, a large molecule that causes water retention in the stool. This causes the stool to become bulky and soft. It also increases the frequency of bowel movements. It is available as liquids, tablets, powder, and suppositories.	*Magnesium hydroxide (Milk of Magnesia), magnesium citrate, sodium biphosphate,* and *Sorbito Duphalac, Cholac, and Enulose.* MiraLax (polyethylene glycol).

Category	Mechanism	Examples
Stimulant Laxative	Stimulant laxatives work by speeding up muscle movement in the colon. Based on their mechanism of action, there are four main types of stimulant laxatives. Most of them are also lubricant laxatives.	**Bisacodyl (Dulcolax)** This medication stimulates the nerve endings in the colon, hence stimulating bowel movements. They are available in oral form and as a suppository. **Sodium Picosulfate** It is often used before intestinal surgery or other procedures like colonoscopy. It has a similar action to bisacodyl. **Anthraquinones** They stimulate the myenteric nerve plexus of the gastrointestinal system, hence causing bowel movements and relieving constipation. Examples of anthraquinones are senna leaf and pod, cascara, castor oil, buckthorn, aloe, or rhubarb root. **Glycerol** Glycerol is available as a suppository and has a mild irritant action on the rectum, hence stimulating bowel movements.
Target receptor stimulant (Selective stimulant)	Enzyme-targeted medication (Guanylate cyclase-C agonist) used in chronic idiopathic constipation in adults or constipation-predominant type of irritable bowel syndrome. Side effects include bloating, gas, and diarrhea. Selective type 2 chloride channel gut stimulant with increased chloride, sodium, and water secretion into the lumen so that stool is softened and motility is increased.	*Linaclotide (Linzess), Plecanatide (Trulance)* Lubiprostone

Note: Most laxatives are habit-forming and should not be used long term.

Others

Manual or digital evacuation of impacted stools may be required sometimes.

Homeopathic Remedies

These include *Bryonia alba* (for hard, dry, or lumpy stools that are hard to push), *N. vomica* (for scanty stools with ineffective bowel movement), *Natrum mur* (when stools are passed on alternate days), *Alumina* (when there is no desire or urge to defecate for days), *Silicea* (straining to pass soft stools but stools recede), *Podophyllum peltatum and Antimonium crudum* (for mixed IBS), *Lycopodium clavatum* (for associated bloating and flatulence), *Aesculus hippocastanum and Collinsonia canadensis* (for associated piles), *Ratanhia and Nitric acid* (for associated anal fissures), and *Opium and Chelidonium majus* (for hard, dry, and ball-like stools).

Diarrhea

Diarrhea is a sudden onset of loose, watery stools occurring three or more times per day. It can be acute (lasts usually for 1 to 2 days), persistent (lasts 2 to 4 weeks), or chronic (lasts more than 4 weeks and may be recurrent and intermittent). Associated mucus and blood can be present in the stools. Other signs and symptoms include abdominal pain, cramps, nausea or vomiting, fever with chills, and exhaustion. It can lead to dehydration and malabsorption.

Causes and contributing factors include infections (viral, bacterial, and parasitic), food allergies or intolerance (commonly dairy, wheat, soy, eggs, seafood), medicines (antibiotics or long-term drugs), intestinal surgery, and other digestive tract disorders (like IBS, celiac disease, ulcerative colitis, Crohn disease, and small intestine bacterial overgrowth).

Further evaluation and tests include a physical exam and stool tests (for microorganisms and reducing sugars). Blood tests, hydrogen breath tests, endoscopy (colonoscopy, sigmoidoscopy, or upper GI endoscopy), or ultrasound are usually indicated in persistent or chronic diarrhea.

Indian Natural Remedies

Diarrhea is called atisara in Ayurveda. When excess pitta or uncontrolled or vitiated vata occurs, this will decrease the agni (digestive-metabolic fire), resulting in more water drawn into the intestinal lumen and causing atisara. Also, there is slow absorption and assimilation of food resulting in more loss of undigested foods in the intestinal lumen.

Common Ingredients for Diarrhea

Spices	Herbs/Leaves	Miscellaneous
Ground cardamom	Amla (*Phyllanthus emblica*)	Yogurt
Ground cinnamon	Holy basil/tulsi (*Ocimum tenuiflorum*)	Whey
Ground ginger	Black nightshade (*Solanum nigrum*)	Mango seed
Nutmeg	*Terminalia arjuna*	Honey
Poppy seed	Bishop's weed (*Trachyspermum ammi*)	Wrightia antidysenterica/ kutaja
Saffron (Kumkum)	Gum arabic/ Babul (*Vachellia nilotica*)	Ghee
Sesame seed	Chamomile flower	Unripe banana
Tamarind pulp and seed	Mint	Pear
Turmeric	Haritaki/ Myrobalan (*Terminalia chebula*)	Buttermilk
	Mango	Bael fruit
	Guava leaf	Rice
	Indian sorrel	

Common Recipes

Oral

Teas/Brews/Others

Amla juice. Lightly pound three to four amla fruits and strain the juice. Take this juice on an empty stomach in the morning with a glass of warm water.

Babul tree bark tea. Lightly pound dry babul tree bark and steep in a cup of hot water. Drink it warm.

Bael fruit. Take unripe bael fruit pulp. Mix with some honey and consume.

Bishop's weed oil. Consume two to three drops of oil from bishop's weed seeds.

Black Nightshade leaf tea. Steep 5 to 10 black nightshade leaves in a cup of hot water. Drink it warm.

Chamomile tea. Steep 2 to 5 chamomile flowers and three to six mint leaves in a cup of boiling water. Strain the mixture and drink it about three times a day.

Ginger powder mixture. Mix ¼ teaspoon ginger powder, 1 teaspoon of ghee, and ¼ teaspoon of sugar. Take this paste two to three times a day for a few days.

Guava leaf. Take a handful of guava leaves. Add 100 mL of water. Boil until the volume is reduced to 25 mL. Consume twice a day.

   Variation #1. Take 4 to 6 washed guava leaves. Add 1 cup of boiling water. Steep for 10 to 15 minutes. Strain and consume.

Indian sorrel. Take 10 g of the Indian sorrel leaves and stem. Wash and dry them. Grind to make a powder. Add to a glass of buttermilk and consume twice a day (for bloody diarrhea).

Jamun, Mango, and Haritaki juice. Take the tender leaves of these three plants. Juice the leaves and add the extract to goat's milk and honey. This can treat bloody dysentery. The juice alone or mixed with little cardamom or cinnamon in goat's milk can also treat diarrhea in children.

Kutaja. Take ¼ to ½ teaspoon of dried seed powder and mix with water (or ghee). Consume after a light meal.

Lassi. Mix ½ a cup of plain yogurt with ½ a cup of water and some grated ginger.

Mango seed and yogurt. Lightly roast a mango seed and grind it into powder. Mix 1 teaspoon of ground mango seed and mix with ½ a cup of yogurt. Consume this mixture twice a day.

Mint tea. Make a tea by steeping four or five sprigs of fresh mint in 1 cup of boiling water for 5 minutes. Drink after meals.

Pomegranate-buttermilk. Finely grind dried pomegranate rind. Mix about 1 g of the pomegranate rind powder with buttermilk and drink. Take this twice a day.

Psyllium husk. Mix 1 teaspoon of psyllium husk with a cup of plain yogurt and take at bedtime.

Rice and yogurt. Add 1 tablespoon of ghee and ¼ cup of plain yogurt to 1 cup of cooked basmati rice. Mix it well and consume.

Saffron paste. Break a strand of saffron into smaller pieces and mix with 1 teaspoon of honey to make a paste. Take one to two times a day.

   Variation #1. To make tea add three to five strands of saffron to a cup of hot water and cover. Steep for 5 to 10 minutes before straining. Drink warm.

Sesame mixture. Finely grind 5 to 10 sesame seeds. Mix the seeds with warm water and add honey to taste. Drink it warm.

Spice powder. Mix ½ a teaspoon of fennel powder and ½ a teaspoon of ginger powder. Consume this mixture two to three times a day.

Spiced bananas: Chop one to two unripe bananas into small pieces. Add a teaspoon of warm ghee to the bananas as well as a pinch of cinnamon powder, cardamom powder, and nutmeg powder. Consume it.

Stewed apples. Peel and slice one to two apples. Place them in a saucepan with enough water to cover the apple slices. Add 1 teaspoon of ghee and a pinch of cinnamon powder, cardamom powder, nutmeg powder, saffron, and salt. Bring the mixture to a boil and then allow to simmer until the apples are mushy.

Tamarind brew. Boil about 80 g of tamarind pulp and seed in water for about 10 minutes. Drink throughout the day or until diarrhea is relieved.

Tulsi tea. Place five to seven fresh tulsi leaves in a pot with a cup of water. Boil for about 15 minutes and then remove from the heat. Allow it to steep for about 5 minutes. Drink before bedtime every day.

Turmeric-basil juice mixture. Mix the juice of 1 teaspoon of fresh turmeric and 1 teaspoon of holy basil and consume every 4 hours.

Udeechya (hrivera). Make a root decoction. Consume once daily in the morning for 3 to 4 days.

Whey. Consume whey protein instead of casein or lactose.

Therapeutic measures

Diet

Consume a pitta pacifying diet.

Eat cooling and nourishing foods and liquids like coconut water, coriander, and mint. Avoid salty, sour, sugary foods, and stimulants.

Chinese Natural Remedies

In TCM, chronic diarrhea is attributed to spleen deficiency.

Common Ingredients for Diarrhea

Spices	Herbs/Leaves	Miscellaneous
Cardamom	Liquorice root	
	Aconite	
	Indigo naturalis/ qing dai	
	Ku shen	
Cinnamon bark	Mint	White rice
Ginger	Atractylodes	
Nutmeg	Ginseng	

Common Recipes

Oral

Teas/Brews

Cinnamon tea. Steep a stick of cinnamon bark in hot water. Drink it warm.

Congee. Place ½ a cup of white rice in a pot with water and bring it to a boil. Once it begins to boil, bring the heat down and simmer for 40 to 50 minutes or until the rice is soft. Add ginger slices and simmer until the mixture becomes watery in texture then consume. The rice can be cooked faster in a pressure cooker.

Fu gui li zhong tang. Take aconite (30 g), ginseng (15 g), atractylodes (15 g), cinnamon bark (30 g), dry ginger (10 g), and liquorice (10 g). Place the herbs into a pot of boiling water. Bring to a boil and then reduce the heat and allow to simmer. Strain the mixture and drink it warm.

Ginger-cardamom tea. Lightly pound about 3 to 4 cm of ginger and five to seven cardamom seeds. Add the ginger and seeds to a pot of water and bring to a boil. Reduce the heat and simmer for about 5 to 10 minutes. Strain and add honey to taste.

Ginger tea. Lightly pound fresh ginger. Add into a pot of water and bring to a boil. Add honey to taste. Drink it warm.

Mint tea. Place a handful of mint leaves into a pot of water. Bring to a boil and reduce the heat. Allow the mixture to simmer for 5 to 10 minutes. Strain and drink twice a day.

Qing dai (Indigo naturalis). Oral qing dai powder is consumed twice a day for 4 months (in ulcerative colitis). It can also be administered as a rectal enema (Qing dai enema or polyherbal enema with added Ku Shen and Bai Tou Weng).

Therapeutic Measures

Acupressure (Topical)

Abdominal sorrow (SP 16) is located just below the rib cage boundary. Massage this point with an index finger for 2 to 3 minutes

Sea of energy (CV 6) is located two finger widths below the belly button. Massage this point with an index finger for 2 to 3 minutes.

Three-mile Point (ST 36) is located four finger widths below the base of the knee cap.

Grandfather-grandson Acupressure Point (SP 4) is located on the arch of the foot in the depression at the base of the first metatarsal bone.

Diet

Avoid foods such as spicy food, hot food, raw, cold, or greasy foods.

Avoid eating 2 to 3 hours before bedtime.

Eat small amounts of food frequently instead of large amounts infrequently.

Try to eat mostly whole, unprocessed foods.

Western/Other Natural Remedies

Common Ingredients for Diarrhea

Spices	Herbs/Leaves	Miscellaneous
Caraway	Chamomile flower	White rice
Cinnamon	Orange peel	Bananas
Nutmeg	Blackberry leaves	Applesauce
	Raspberry leaves	Toast
	Rooibos leaves	Probiotics
	Black haw (Viburnum prunifolium)	Honey
		Apple cider vinegar
		Essential oils

Common Recipes

Oral

Teas/Brews

Apple cider vinegar mixture. Mix 2 to 3 teaspoons of apple cider vinegar with a cup of water and drink.

Blackberry tea. Take 1 teaspoon of fresh crushed leaves (or 1 to 2 teaspoons of dried crushed fermented leaves) and add 1 cup of boiling water. Steep for about 5 to 10 minutes. Strain and drink warm.

To make the dried fermented leaves, wash the fresh leaves. Place them in a sterilized jar and allow them to ferment for 2 weeks or longer. Check intermittently for moldy growth. Then, remove and dry them. Crush the dried leaves to make tea.

Black haw tea. Add 1 teaspoon of black haw into 1 cup of boiling water. Steep for 5 minutes. Strain and drink three times a day.

BRAT diet. Consume a BRAT diet (bananas, rice, applesauce, and toast). These foods are bland and do not contain any spices or additives that may aggravate the symptoms further.

Buttermilk drink. Mix ½ teaspoon of ground, dried ginger into a cup of buttermilk. Drink three to four times a day.

Caraway tea. Steep a teaspoon of caraway seeds in hot water for about 15 minutes. Strain and drink it warm.

Chamomile tea. Steep three to five dried chamomile flowers in a cup of hot water. Strain and drink it warm.

Cinnamon tea. Take a pinch of cinnamon powder or steep a stick of cinnamon bark in a cup of hot water. Add a little lemon juice. Drink it warm.

Fresh orange peel tea. Peel a fresh orange. Steep the peel and a stick of cinnamon in a cup of hot water. Cover and allow it to steep until cool. Strain the mixture and add honey to taste.

Nutmeg -ghee. Take a spoonful of ghee and add a pinch of nutmeg powder. Consume.

Probiotics. Consume probiotics such as sauerkraut, kimchi, and yogurt to alleviate diarrhea.

Raspberry tea: Take 1 teaspoon of dried leaves. Add 1 cup of boiling water and steep for about 5 to 10 minutes. Strain and drink it warm.

Rooibos tea. Add 1 teaspoon of loose rooibos tea leaves into 1 cup of boiling water. Steep for about 5 to 10 minutes. Strain and consume.

White rice. Cook plain white rice and eat small quantities of it throughout the day.

Nasal (Inhalational)

Essential oil therapy. Dilute essential oils with some water and add the mixture to a humidifier/diffuser. If a humidifier is not available, sprinkle some of the essential oils on clothes or bed sheets. Some of the essential oils effective for diarrhea are peppermint, tea tree, lavender, ginger, chamomile, frankincense, and lemon.

Modern Remedies

General Management

Supportive hydration is the most important treatment in diarrhea. Oral rehydration salts should be given to maintain fluid and electrolyte balance.

Antidiarrheal agents

These can be given to relieve diarrhea and abdominal pain. Antimicrobial chemotherapy may be necessary in bacterial gastroenteritis such as Salmonella or Shigella dysentery, typhoid fever, cholera, clostridia, campylobacter infections.

Antidiarrheal Agents	
Anti-infective agents (Antibiotics)	ciprofloxacin, cotrimoxazole, erythromycin, doxycycline, metronidazole
Antimotility drugs(opiates) Mostly mu-opioid receptor agonists)	loperamide, diphenoxylate, difenoxin, codeine
eluxadoline	
Antisecretory agent (enkephalinase inhibitor) used in acute diarrhea to increase the availability of endogenous opioids (enkephalins)	racecadotril
Adsorbent drugs	pectin, kaolin, charcoal, bismuth subsalicylate, methylcellulose,
Antispasmodic/ Anticholinergic drugs	atropine, scopolamine (hyoscine), mebeverine, dicyclomine
Anti-inflammatory agents (for inflammatory bowel disease)	sulfasalazine, mesalazine
Somatostatin analogue (for chemotherapy induced diarrhea or refractory diarrhea)	octreotide
Intestinal flora modifiers	probiotics

Antibiotics. Usually acute gastroenteritis is self-limiting and is due to viral infection. Specific antibiotics are based on type of pathogen in bacterial gastroenteritis (whether cholera, salmonella, shigella, clostridia, etc.)

Antimotility agents. These medicines slow intestinal movements and hence reduce the frequency of diarrhea. They are classified into opioids and antimuscarinics:

Opioids increase the tone of the circular smooth muscles of the intestine while reducing longitudinal smooth muscle tone, hence reducing propulsion, and reducing diarrheal frequency. However, opioids have higher abuse potential compared to other antidiarrheal drugs.

Antimuscarinics drugs work by binding to the muscarinic acetylcholine receptor and hence block the effects of acetylcholine. Acetylcholine is a neurotransmitter that stimulates bowel movements. Antimuscarinics are rarely used on their own as they have many adverse effects such as urinary retention and blurred vision.

Antisecretory agents. They prevent fluid or electrolyte loss from the bowel as a result of acute diarrhea without affecting intestinal motility.

Adsorbent drugs. They adsorb intestinal luminal toxins and bacteria associated with some types of infectious diarrhea, and increase fecal elimination of the bacteria.

Antispasmodics. They are used to relieve abdominal cramps associated with diarrhea and are not used as a primary treatment for diarrhea. They cause relaxation of the smooth muscle in the intestines, hence reducing muscular spasms. This relieves abdominal pain due to muscle cramps. It is not advisable to use them in children.

Anti-inflammatory agents. See below.

Somatostatin analogue. It inhibits intestinal motility and secretions of the GI tract and pancreas. It is useful for the management of persistent diarrhea associated with neuroendocrine tumors, carcinoid tumors, and short bowel syndrome.

Probiotics. This is to restore the gut microbiome and reduce bacterial overgrowth. Consume probiotics such as sauerkraut, kimchi, and yogurt.

Colitis Management

For inflammatory bowel disease, i.e., ulcerative colitis and Crohn disease

5-aminosalicylic acid group of drugs (oral or rectal) are usually used as maintenance therapy (sulfasalazine, mesalamine, balsalazide, or olsalazine).

Steroids (oral or rectal) are used short-term for flare-ups.

Immunomodulator drugs are anti-inflammatory and immunosuppressive (azathioprine, mercaptopurine cyclosporine, or tofacitinib) and are used in moderate to severe disease.

Biologics class of drugs are derived from living organisms and block the immune system (examples: infliximab, adalimumab, golimumab, vedolizumab, ustekinumab). Tofacitinib is a Janus kinase (JAK) inhibitor drug that is used in the treatment of ulcerative colitis that is refractory to anti-integrin and anti-TNF therapies.

Supportive treatment includes antidiarrheals, analgesics, antibiotics, and nutritional supplements including iron, B12, calcium, vitamin D, probiotics, and prebiotics. Fish oil, aloe vera, turmeric, bromelain, and camel milk can also help to reduce inflammation. Nutrition therapy can include tube feeding or parenteral (intravenous) nutrition. A diet low in FODMAPs (fermentable oligosaccharides, disaccharides, monosaccharides, and polyols{sorbitol and mannitol} which are short-chain sugars) may also help.

Surgery is indicated to drain an abscess or close a fistula.

Homeopathic Remedies

These include *Arsenicum album* (in food poisoning or traveler's diarrhea with burning and watery loose stools, stomach cramps, thirst for sips of water, and feeling chilly), *Aloe socotrina* (with marked gurgling and gas with stool leak with slimy stools and is worse in the morning), *P. peltatum* (in explosive, watery, and copious stools and gas which are worse with food and fluids), *Phosphorus* (marked exhaustion and thirst and some relief with cold fluids or food and sleep), *Ipecacuanha* (associated vomiting and frequent frothy, greenish, and mucousy stools), *Sulfur* (hot smelly stools especially on waking with burning feeling in the rectum), *Cinchona officinalis* (associated marked bloating and indigestion and worse with hot weather and at night), and *Veratrum album* (in copious, painful diarrhea with marked exhaustion, vomiting, cold sweat, feeling chilly, and craving for cold fluids and foods).

Calcarea carb is preferred in infants (usually in chubby babies who are lethargic, pale with sweaty heads and have a sour body odor). *Chamomilla* is also given to fretful and irritable infants with smelly and greenish mucousy stools. Other remedies include *Agaricus* (with grass-green stools, perianal itching) and *Aconite* (with chopped spinach-like and watery stools).

In chronic diarrhea from colitis, *Asafoetida or Silicea* are helpful.

Irritable Bowel Syndrome (IBS)

IBS is a chronic and functional disorder that affects the bowels and causes abdominal pain, constipation, diarrhea, or both, bloating, gas, and mucus in the stools. Risk factors or triggers include stress, anxiety, food sensitivity, age below 50 years, associated diverticulitis, post-GI infection, and poor gut microbiota or bacterial overgrowth. The sub-types are IBS-diarrhea, IBS-constipation, and IBS-mixed.

General Principles

Non-Drug Approach: This should be the mainstay to relieve symptoms and include the following:

Lifestyle changes. Regular sleep, physical activity, and exercise are important.

Diet modification.

In constipation-predominant IBS, consume more fluids and high-soluble fiber foods.

In diarrhea-predominant IBS, avoid or eliminate gas-forming and fatty foods. Avoid known foods that may cause allergy or intolerance. Also limit or abstain from coffee and alcohol. Also avoid high FODMAP (fermentable oligosaccharides, disaccharides, monosaccharides, and polyols) foods (dairy, wheat, garlic, onions, leek, beans, legumes, fruits like apples, pears, mangoes, etc.) as they can increase gas, bloating, pain, and diarrhea.

Patient education. Many aspects of the non-drug approach have to be emphasized

Stress management. (Counseling, relaxation, massage, behavior therapy, meditation, mindfulness, hypnosis, hypnotherapy, biofeedback)

Indian Natural Remedies

The term *"Grahani"* in Sanskrit refers to IBS and has been described in the Ayurveda writings. The principles of Ayurvedic treatment include:

1. **Panchakarma.** This is a detoxification procedure which restores colon health. Vasti-herbal enemas are done for

constipation. Virechana is an herbal purgation to remove toxins. Shirodhara involves pouring medicated oil on the forehead (read more under Introduction on Ayurveda Page X).

2. **Rasayana.** This is a holistic therapy which incorporates all natural therapies including yoga and nutrition.

3. **Yoga Pranayama.** These are breathing techniques. Some of them include *Shitali* pranayama and *Sit Cari* (for acid reflux and constipation) and *Ujjayi* pranayama (gas bloating and diarrhea) and *Kapalabhati* pranayama (for chronic symptoms).

   Yoga Asanas for IBS, constipation. These include:

   Surya namaskar (sun salutation), Shavasana (corpse asana), Dhanurasana (bow pose), Matsyasana (fish pose), Ardha Matsyendrasana (half spinal twist pose), Halasana (plough pose), Pawanmuktasana (Wind-relieving pose), Bhujangasana (cobra pose), Mayurasana (peacock pose), Trikonasana (triangle pose), and Ustrasana (camel pose).

4. **Herbs.** These include triphala (helps with constipation), liquorice (reduces acidity and has mild laxative effect), bael fruit (immune booster), guduchi (antispasmodic), and ashwagandha (adaptogen).

   Others include ginger, fennel seeds, pepper, cumin, peppermint, and flaxseed.

5. Ayurvedic diet.

   Consume fresh buttermilk (takra), old rice, sorghum (jowar), amla, pudina (mint), asafoetida, cumin seeds, turmeric, coriander, moong dal (mung beans), coconut, pomegranate, pumpkin, bitter gourd, rock salt, ghee.

   Take frequent sips of hot water throughout the meal (preferably after meal). Avoid excessive coffee or tea.

   Avoid oily, spicy, salty, hot, heavy, and very cold foods.

   Avoid overeating.

6. Lifestyle
   - Avoid excess physical or mental stress and a negative attitude. Do meditation and have massages.
   - Avoid sedentary and irregular lifestyle
   - Avoid alcohol, smoking, etc.
   - Avoid excess drinking of water in morning especially
   - Avoid sleeping in the afternoon and staying awake till late night
   - Walk slowly for 15 to 20 minutes after every meal. It aids digestion of food.
   - Exercise for 30 minutes daily. Drink little lukewarm water after meals. It helps in proper digestion of food.

Common Ingredients for Irritable Bowel Syndrome

Herbs/Spices	Miscellaneous
Pudina	Millet (sorghum or jowar)
Spices: Cumin, coriander, turmeric, asafetida	Buttermilk
	Mung dal/mung bean
	Fruits: amla, Pomegranate, coconut
	Vegetables: pumpkin, bitter gourd
	Ghee

Note. Also avoid high FODMAP (fermentable oligosaccharides, disaccharides, monosaccharides, and polyols) foods (dairy, wheat, garlic, onions, leek, beans, legumes, fruits like apples, pears, mangoes, etc.) as they can increase gas, bloating, pain, and diarrhea.

Chinese Natural Remedies

The polyherbals used include the following:

Shun-Qi-Tong-Xie. The key ingredients include Xie Bai (Alli macrostemi Bulbus), Bai Shao (Paeonia Radix alba), Bai Zhu (Atractylodis macrocephalae Rhizoma), Fo Shou (Citri sarcodactylis Fructus), Che Qian Zi (Plantaginis Semen), and Bo He You (Oleum Mentha haplocalyx).

Tong Xie Yao Fang (TXYF). The key herbs are Rhizoma Atractylodis Macrocephalae, Citri Reticulatae Pericarpium, Paeoniae Radix Alba, and Saposhnikoviae Radix.

Western Natural Remedies

Refer to General Principles.

Therapeutic Measures

Hypnotherapy in IBS involves progressive relaxation, viewing of soothing imagery, and sensations focused on the individual's symptoms. This has been proven to improve overall well-being, quality of life, abdominal pain, constipation, and diarrhea.

Modern Remedies

Drugs: See table below

Pharmacological approach in Irritable Bowel Syndrome

Medication/Drug Group	Mechanism	Drug Examples
Laxatives	Refer "Laxatives"	Try OTC items—fiber supplements, emollients, or lubricants first. Then, the hyperosmolar agents or stimulants. In severe IBS-C, Lubiprostone or Linaclotide may be tried.
Antidiarrheal agents	Refer "Antidiarrheal agents" (Opioid receptor agonists)	Loperamide, diphenoxylate In severe IBS-D, Alosetron or Eluxadoline may be tried.
Antispasmodic agents	Anti-muscarinic receptor blocker Calcium channel blocker	Mebeverine, Trimebutine maleate Pinaverium bromide

Medication/Drug Group	Mechanism	Drug Examples
Probiotics	To restore gut microbiome and reduce bacterial overgrowth	Bifidobacterium, Lactobacillus
Prokinetic agents (Receptor stimulants)	5-HT4 agonists: non-selective and selective To increase bowel motility in IBS-C type	*Non-selective*: Domperidone, Metoclopramide, Cisapride, Tegaserod *Selective*: Prucalopride
Antibiotics	To inhibit bad-gut flora overgrowth and for gut decontamination	Metronidazole, Neomycin, Rifaximin
Psychiatry drugs	Anxiolytics, tranquilizers, Antidepressants	Tricyclic antidepressants, SSRI, Antidepressants

Fecal transplant/Fecal microbiota transplantation (FMT). Healthy donor gut bacteria are transplanted into the colon of the IBS patient.

Acid Reflux

Heartburn or acid reflux occurs when the lower esophageal sphincter (LES), a ring-shaped valve between the lower end of the esophagus and stomach, becomes lax and the HCL from the stomach enters to the esophagus. This reflux causes heartburn (chest pain behind the sternum), sour eructation or regurgitation, burping, hiccups, swallowing difficulty (dysphagia), or bloating. Dry cough, hoarse voice, or wheezing can even occur.

Many contributing factors lead to acid reflux. These include food factors (food allergies or intolerance, spicy foods, caffeine, alcohol, carbonated drinks, acidic foods like citrus or tomatoes, and eating large meals), obesity, drugs/medications (e.g., steroids, NSAID painkillers, osteoporosis medications like Fosamax, etc.), infections, and lying down or sleeping immediately after a meal. Pregnancy or smoking are also predisposing factors.

GERD is diagnosed if acid reflux occurs more than twice or thrice a week. It can be confirmed by upper endoscopy, esophageal pH test, esophageal manometry, or barium meal study.

Indian Natural Remedies

Common Ingredients for Acid Reflux

Spices	Herbs/Leaves	Miscellaneous
Arugampul/dhoob (*Cynodon dactylon*)		Ghee
Cinnamon (ground)		Honey
Cloves (ground)		Coconut water
Coriander seeds (ground)		Lemon juice with sugar
		Jaggery
		Yogurt
		Apple cider vinegar
		Buttermilk
Ginger	Basil leaf	Ripe banana

Common Recipes

Oral

Teas/Brews/Others

Apple cider vinegar mixture. Mix 2 to 3 teaspoons of apple cider vinegar with a cup of water and drink.

Arugampul juice. Take one to two handfuls of fresh washed arugampul (roots removed) and a few neem leaves. Add some water or coconut water and blend. Strain and drink fresh first thing in the morning on an empty stomach.

Banana. Consume bananas as part of the diet.

Basil leaves. Chew on some basil leaves.

Buttermilk drink. Mix ½ teaspoon of ground, dried ginger into a cup of buttermilk. Drink three to four times a day.

Cinnamon tea. Steep a stick of cinnamon bark in hot water. Drink it warm.

Clove tea. Lightly pound three to five cloves. Place into a cup of hot water and cover. Allow to steep for 5 to 10 minutes before straining. Drink warm.

Coconut water. Drink coconut water.

Coriander-Buttermilk. Take 4 to 5 teaspoons (or less) coriander powder. Add to a glass of fresh buttermilk. Drink before or after meals.

   Variation #1. Take ½ teaspoon coriander powder. Mix with little honey and consume it.

Ginger-ghee-sugar/honey paste. Mix 1 teaspoon of ghee with ¼ teaspoon of ginger powder and ¼ a teaspoon of sugar. Eat this paste two to three times a day for a few days.

Lemon juice. Drink lemon juice with water or some syrup.

Spice powder. Mix ½ a teaspoon of fennel powder and ½ a teaspoon of ginger powder. Consume this mixture two to three times a day.

Yogurt. Consume yogurt or make it into buttermilk.

Chinese Natural Remedies

Acid reflux is due to disharmony between the stomach and liver function.

Common Ingredients for Acid Reflux

Spices	Herbs/Leaves	Miscellaneous
Ginger	Liquorice root	Congee
	Pinelliae	Areca peel/da fu pi (*Areca catechu*)

Spices	Herbs/Leaves	Miscellaneous
	Chinese angelica	Chinese date
	Perillae	Poria (fu ling)
	White peony root	
	White atractylodes	
	Peppermint	
	Hare's Ear Root	

Common Recipes

Oral

Teas/Brews/Others

Cinnamon tea. Steep a stick of cinnamon bark in hot water. Drink it warm.

Congee. Refer under "Chinese remedies for diarrhea".

Ginger tea. Lightly pound about 1 to 2 inches of fresh ginger (if unavailable, use 1 to 2 teaspoons of ginger powder) and add to a cup of hot water. Allow to steep for 5 to 10 minutes. Strain and drink while warm. Add honey to taste.

Polyherbal formula combinations. Some of these include

- Zingiberis, Pinelliae, Perillae, Poriae.
- **Sini Powder (SNP) and the Zuojin Pill (ZJP).** The polyherbs include Paeoniae Radix Alba, Bupleuri Radix, Aurantii Fructus Immaturus, Paeonia lactiflora Pall, Glycyrrhizae Radix, Coptidis Rhizoma, and Evodiae Fructus.
- **Ban Xia Xie Xin Wan.** The key ingredients are Ban Xia, Huang Lian, Hou Po, Gan Jiang, Dang Shen, Shen Qu, Gan Cao, Huang Qin, and Wa Leng Zi
- **Xiao Yao. Wa.** The key ingredients are Bupleurum (chai hu), Poria (fu ling), Dong quai (dang gui), Peppermint (bo he), White peony root (bai shao), Licorice root (zhi gan cao), White atractylodes (bai zhu), and Quick fried ginger root (pao jian).

Therapeutic Measures

Diet

Avoid foods such as spicy food, hot food, raw, cold, or greasy foods.

Avoid eating 2 to 3 hours before bedtime.

Eat small amounts of food frequently instead of large amounts infrequently.

Try to eat mostly whole, unprocessed foods.

Acupressure (Topical)

"Inner Gate" (Neiguan P-6). Locate this point—three finger-widths above the wrist crease, between the two tendons on the inside of the left forearm. Exert firm pressure with the thumb and hold for 5 minutes. Repeat on the other arm.

"Middle Core"(CV-12). Locate this point- midway between the navel and the lower tip of your sternum. Apply mild pressure with 2 fingers using the index and middle fingers for 5 minutes. Then use the palm of hand, make and rub small circles at this point in a clockwise direction for 5 minutes (CV-12).

Western/Other Natural Remedies

Common Ingredients for Acid Reflux

Spices	Herbs/Leaves	Miscellaneous
Ginger	Aloe vera	Beet
	Chamomile flower	Apple cider vinegar
	Marshmallow root	Honey
	Liquorice root	Baking soda
	Slippery elm	Watermelon juice
	Blackberry leaves	Essential oils
	Raspberry leaves	Juniper berries
	Rooibos leaves	Mastic gum (Pistacia lentiscus)
	Meadowsweet	Apple juice

Common Recipes

Oral

Teas/Brews/Others

Aloe vera juice. Wash and dry an aloe vera leaf. Slit the leaf in half and remove the gel, discarding the greenish gel. Cut the remaining white gel into cubes and store in a refrigerator. Add the gel to any fruit juice and blend.

Apple cider vinegar mixture. Mix 2 to 3 teaspoons of apple cider vinegar with a cup of water and drink.

Baking soda water. Baking soda is known to have antacid properties and can relieve mild stomach pain. Mix one teaspoon of baking soda to a glass of warm water. Drink it warm.

Beet. Consume beet or make fresh juice.

Blackberry tea. Take 1 teaspoon of fresh crushed leaves and add 1 cup of boiling water. Steep for about 5 to 10 minutes. Strain and drink warm.

Variation #1. To make the dried fermented leaves, take the washed fresh leaves. Place them in a sterilized jar and allow them to ferment for 2 weeks or longer. Check intermittently for moldy growth. Then, remove and dry them. Crush the dried leaves to make tea.

BRAT diet. Consume a BRAT diet: bananas, rice, applesauce, and toast. These foods are bland and do not contain any spices or additives that may aggravate the symptoms further.

Caraway tea. Steep a teaspoon of caraway seeds in hot water for about 15 minutes. Strain and drink it warm.

Chamomile tea. Place some dried or fresh chamomile flowers into a cup. Pour boiling water over the flowers and allow it to steep for 10 minutes. Strain and add honey to taste. Drink it hot.

Ginger tea. Lightly pound 3 to 4 inches of fresh ginger and place into an empty cup. Pour boiling water into the cup and allow it to steep for about 10 minutes. Drink in the morning on an empty stomach.

Honey. Consume honey.

Juniper berry tea. Take 1 tablespoon of fresh berries and crush them. Add boiling water and steep for 10 minutes. Strain and drink. Add honey to taste.

Variation #1. Take 1 teaspoon of dried juniper berries. Crush it. Add 1 cup of boiling water. Steep for 20 minutes. Drink 1 cup twice a day.

Liquorice tea. Add 1 teaspoon of ground liquorice to a pot with 1 cup of boiling water. Allow it to simmer for 30 to 45 minutes before straining.

Marshmallow root tea. Place ¼ cup of dried marshmallow root into a cup and pour cold water over it. Allow to steep overnight and strain the next morning.

Mastic gum. Chew or suck on a piece of mastic gum.

Meadowsweet and apple juice. Take 2 cups of unsweetened fresh or pure apple juice and 2 tablespoons of apple cider vinegar. Bring to a boil. Add ½ teaspoon meadowsweet. Steep for 10 minutes. Strain and drink warm with 2 tablespoons of honey.

Probiotics. Consume probiotics such as sauerkraut, kimchi, and yogurt to alleviate diarrhea.

Raspberry tea. Take 1 teaspoon of dried leaves. Add 1 cup of boiling water and steep for about 5 to 10 minutes. Strain and drink it warm.

Rooibos tea. Add 1 teaspoon of loose rooibos tea leaves into 1 cup of boiling water. Steep for about 5 to 10 minutes. Strain and consume.

Slippery elm. Add 1 to 2 tablespoons of slippery elm to a glass of water and drink it after meals.

Watermelon juice. Drink watermelon juice.

White rice. Cook plain white rice and eat small quantities of it throughout the day.

Therapeutic Measures

Nasal (Inhalational). Various essential oils are used.

Essential oil therapy. Dilute essential oils with some water and add the mixture to a humidifier/diffuser. If a humidifier is not available, sprinkle some of the essential oils on clothes or bed sheets. Some of the essential oils effective for diarrhea are peppermint, tea tree, lavender, ginger, chamomile, frankincense, and lemon.

Modern Remedies

Antacids

Please refer to the list under "Stomach Ache."

H2 Receptor Antagonists

These drugs act on the histamine H2 receptors on the parietal cells in the stomach and decrease the amount of HCL produced. The onset of action is within 1 hour. They can also be used to treat peptic ulcer disease.

Examples: *Ranitidine, cimetidine, famotidine, and nizatidine.*

Proton Pump Inhibitors

These drugs block the proton pump on the parietal cells via enzyme inhibition in the stomach and decrease acid production. The onset of action is 1 to 4 days. Long-term side effects include headache, nausea, vomiting, diarrhea, risk of infections, fractures, B12 deficiency, kidney disease, dementia, and low magnesium.

Examples: *Omeprazole, esomeprazole, lansoprazole, and pantoprazole.*

Prokinetic drug

Itopride hydrochloride (Ganaton) can help with acid reflux, gas, and bloating. It has both anti-acetylcholinesterase and antidopaminergic and increases gut motility.

Others

Vonoprazan. This is a potassium-competitive acid blocker. It is used to treat acid reflux. It is also combined with antibiotics to treat *H. pylori* infection.

Therapeutic Measures

Diet

Eat more alkaline foods such as oats, green vegetables, apples, bananas, melons, and yogurt.

Coffee from dark roasted beans or espresso may be more tolerable as it has lower acid content.

In some people, some foods that heal acid reflux (e.g., banana, milk, mint, etc.) can paradoxically cause more heartburn.

Lifestyle

Maintain a healthy weight, avoid food triggers, set regular mealtimes, and eat small frequent meals. Eat and chew slowly (digestive enzymes are present in the mouth).

Wear clothes or belts that are loose-fitting.

Stop smoking.

Do not sleep or lie down flat after a meal. Wait 3 to 4 hours before bedtime.

Elevate the head of the bed at 15 degrees at least.

Acid Reflux: Surgery

When medications have failed, laparoscopic anti-reflux surgery (Nissen fundoplication) is done. This is a minimally invasive procedure.

Homeopathic Remedies

These include *Lycopodium* (there is prolonged burning up to throat and spine, relieved with belching and farting*)*, *C. vegetalis* (associated sour burps, bloating, and need for fresh air or fan, cold hands and feet), *N. vomica* (signs and symptoms of reflux in a highly stressed person who consumes various stimulants and gets angry easily, worse before breakfast), *Arsenicum album* (signs and symptoms of acid reflux, relieved with hot fluids and milk usually in an anxious person who fears to be alone and worse at night), *Pulsatilla* (associated sour burps after fatty foods, relief with fresh air in a mild-mannered and gentle person who fears to be alone), and *phosphorus* (burning is relieved with cold fluids and there is frequent vomiting of undigested foods). Other remedies include *Bryonia, Natrum carbonicum, Robinia,* and *Iris versicolor. Natrum phosphoricum* is often used for spitting infants with sour vomit.

Gas/Wind and Bloating

Excessive gas has different definitions and meanings for different individuals.

It can include:

- excessive belching or excessive burping (due to eating *wrong* foods or swallowed air).
- excessive passing of gas/flatulence/farts (*due to maldigestion or malabsorption of dietary sugars and polysaccharides that reach the colon undigested and become fermented. Smelly farts are often due to eating sulfur-rich foods or gas production by the colon bacteria*).
- fullness of the abdomen/bloating (due to excessive gas production by bacteria as in gut dysbiosis or bacterial overgrowth of the small intestine).
- distention of the abdomen (due to enlarged organs in the abdomen).

Other causes of bloating and gas include IBS, wheat and milk intolerance, acid reflux (GERD), or consumption of gas-producing foods.

Excessive gas or bloating can cause abdominal pain, discomfort, tightness, or cramps.

Passing gas about 14 to 23 times per day is considered normal.

Indian Natural Remedies

Common Ingredients for Gas/Wind and Bloating

Spices	Herbs/Leaves	Miscellaneous
Asafoetida (Hing)		
Carom seeds (ajwain)		
Coriander		
Cumin		
Fennel seed		
Ginger	Basil leaf	Vegetable pickles (achar)
Star anise	Chirata	Pumpkin seed
Turmeric		

Common Recipes

Oral

Ajwain tea. Place a teaspoon of ajwain seeds into a pot of water and boil it for 5 to 10 minutes. Strain the mixture and drink warm.

Basil tea. Place three to five fresh basil leaves in a pot of water. Allow it to boil for about 3 to 4 minutes. Add honey to taste and drink.

Chirata. Make a decoction from the plant and consume.

Fennel tea. Boil a teaspoon of fennel seeds (or fennel powder) in a pot of hot water. Strain the mixture. Drink three to four times a day.

Ginger tea. Lightly pound about 1 to 2 inches of fresh ginger (if unavailable, use 1 to 2 teaspoons of ginger powder) and add to a cup of hot water. Allow to steep for 5 to 10 minutes. Strain and drink while warm. Add honey to taste.

Herb-spice mix. For immediate relief from gas, mix 1 teaspoon dried ginger powder with a pinch of asafetida (hing) and a pinch of rock salt in 1 cup of warm water and drink.

Herbal powder. A mixture of roasted and blended carom seed, cumin, and anise powder is very beneficial for flatulence in the elderly. Take a small portion of this herbal powder three times a day.

Polyherbs. Ashta Choornam is a combination of eight herbs in equal amounts, i.e., long pepper *(Piper longum)*, black pepper *(Piper nigrum)* and ginger *(Zingiber officinalis)*, jeera or cumin *(Cuminum cyminum)*, krishna jeera/black cumin *(Carum bulbocastanum)* asafoetida *(Ferula assa-foetida)*, ajmoda *(Carum roxburghianum)*, rock salt and ghee

Pumpkin seed. Take a cup of pumpkin seeds. Consume them raw but preferably steamed, boiled, or roasted. Eat them daily.

Turmeric tea. Lightly pound about 2 to 4 inches of fresh turmeric. Place the turmeric into a pot with 2 cups of water. Bring to a boil and then allow to simmer for about half an hour. Add honey to taste and drink.

Therapeutic Measures

Diet

Eating one's *dosha* type can be helpful. *Vata dosha/air-ether elements* type of a person tends to experience the most amount of bloating.

Avoid ice-cold drinks or food as it slows the digestive fire *(agni)* and digestion.

For those with *vata (air and ether)* predisposition, cumin and fennel seeds are recommended.

For those with *pitta* (fire and water) predisposition, caraway and turmeric are recommended.

For those with *kapha* (earth and water) predisposition, ginger and cayenne pepper are recommended.

These spices can be consumed as tea once a day or used in cooking.

Chinese Natural Remedies

Common Ingredients for Gas/Wind and Bloating

Spices	Herbs/Leaves	Miscellaneous
Ginger	Liquorice root (Glycyrrhiza glabra Glycyrrhizae radix)	Orange/ tangerine peel/Chen pi (Citrus reticulata)
Star anise	Fu ling (poria cocos mushroom)	Barley/Maiya (Hordeum vulgare)

Spices	Herbs/Leaves	Miscellaneous
	Daikon radish seed	Hawthorn berry/
	Lai fu zi	Shan zha
	(Semen raphani sativi)	(Crataegus pinnatifida)
		Chicken gizzard/ Ji nei jin
		Geng me (Oryza sativa)
		Water caltrop/ Li Xi (Trapa bicornis)
		Tiger nuts (Cyperus esculentus)

In TCM, the liver, spleen, and stomach are important organs in digestion. The liver can also affect either the stomach or the spleen.

If the liver affects the spleen, there are symptoms such as irritability, abdominal distention, pain, poor sense of hunger and thirst, alternating constipation and diarrhea, and a lot of gas.

If the liver affects the stomach, there are more upper-digestive issues such as acid reflux, hiccups, belching, nausea and vomiting, food retention in the stomach, and upper abdomen distension.

Common Recipes

Oral

Chen pi (peel of an orange or tangerine). It regulates the whole digestive system and is good for spleen and stomach issues, including nausea, vomiting, belching, abdominal fullness, and distention or pain. It is also bitter and helps to drain dampness.

Chinese Four Herbs soup. This soup is prepared in a slow cooker for 4 hours with lotus seeds, gorgon fruit, Chinese yam, and poria. It is consumed once a week.

Geng mi/rice. It is cooked as congee as rice and is easily digestible.

Ginger tea. Lightly pound about 1 to 2 inches of fresh ginger (if unavailable, use 1 to 2 teaspoons of ginger powder) and add to a cup of hot water. Allow to steep for 5 to 10 minutes. Strain and drink while warm. Add honey to taste.

Alternatively, after meals, chew on fresh ginger slices soaked in lime juice to reduce gas production.

Ji nei jin (chicken inner golden/chicken gizzard). It promotes digestion, especially to move stagnant food. It is helpful for nausea, vomiting, diarrhea, moving undigested foods, and severe indigestion.

Lai fu zi (daikon radish seed). It has food moving properties and is high in digestive enzymes.

Mai ya (barley). It is good for food stagnation but facilitates the digestion of starches and carbohydrates well. Cooking with barley instead of rice or pasta can prevent or reduce bloating.

Mint tea. Make a tea by steeping four or five sprigs of fresh mint in 1 cup of boiling water for 5 minutes. Drink after meals.

Shan zha (hawthorn berry). Drink it as a tea after every meal. It is sweet and sour in taste. It promotes digestion and relieves food stagnation or food retention. It promotes digestion of meats and fats.

Shen qu (medicated leaven). It is also called *massa fermentata* and is a mixture of several herbs. It is combined with wheat flour, bran, flowering plants, artemisia, and apricot and then covered in hemp paper or mulberry leaves and left to ferment for about a week then cut into cubes and dried in the sun.

It relieves bloating, stomach pain, diarrhea, and chronic gastritis. The herb goes to the spleen and stomach meridians, strengthening the organs and improves digestion.

Tiger nuts. It can be sprouted, roasted or dried and eaten.

Water caltrop/chestnut. Add 15 to 20 water caltrop with ends trimmed and a piece of smashed sugar cane into a pot of water. Boil and simmer for about 30 minutes. Cool, strain, and drink (Pieces of water chestnut can be eaten). Alternatively, water chestnut can also be boiled with added sugar cane, 2 tablespoons of pearl barley, and rock sugar.

Therapeutic Measures

Acupressure for Flatulence

Locate the acupoint valley of harmony (LI-4 or Hegu), in the web between your thumb and index finger on your right hand. Use the left thumb and press this point for 2 minutes until sore. Repeat the same on the left hand.

Check the position for the acupoint upper great opening (ST-37 and ST-36-Zusanli). Place two hand-widths or eight finger widths below the outer indentation of the right knee next to the shinbone. Use the left thumb and apply steady and firm pressure. Hold for 2 minutes. Repeat on the left leg.

Qigong Exercise

Eight Treasures Called Raising the Hands to Adjust the Stomach and Spleen

1. Start by standing upright with the spine erect, feet close together and arms by the sides. Tilt the head slightly forward. Breathe in and out rhythmically.
2. Form a cup or plate with the right hand. Keep the palm facing the sky, breathe in (inhale), and make a large circular motion in front of you from the left to right while raising the arm above the head. As you complete this motion, move your left hand to your back with the palm facing the ground.
3. As the right hand reaches the highest point above the head, begin to stretch the body and stand on the ball of the feet. Exhale gently and at the same time push the left hand toward the ground. Ensure the push is in the opposite direction. For example, the right hand pushes to the sky and the left pushes to the ground.
4. Repeat this movement three times, inhaling as the arm goes up and exhaling during the stretch.

5. Change sides and repeat the exercise. Do this for 15 minutes twice daily.

The exercise helps to stretch the abdominal organs and stimulates the intestines, spleen, and stomach.

Western/Other Natural Remedies

Common Ingredients for Gas/Wind and Bloating

Spices	Herbs/Leaves	Miscellaneous
Allspice	Cilantro	Rose water
	Rosemary	
	Sage	
	Bay leaf (Laurus nobilis)	
	Basil	
	Coriander	
Anise	Peppermint	Green tea or herbal teas
Caraway	Oregano	Juniper berries
Cardamom	Chamomile	Apple cider vinegar
Fennel	Dandelion root	Manuka honey
Ginger	Mint tea	Baking soda
Turmeric	Dill	Essential oils

Common Recipes

Oral

Allspice tea. Take ½ teaspoon ground allspice. Add 1 cup of hot water. Steep for 10 minutes. Strain and consume warm.

Baking soda. To a glass of 4 ounces of warm water, add ½ teaspoon baking soda and drink.

Digestive aids. Herbal teas, honey, or apple cider vinegar can help reduce the burping or belching.

Elimination diet. This may help. Refer to "gas-forming/ gas-causing foods or *windy foods.*" Try removing one food at a time to see if the belching and flatulence or wind improves.

Essential oils. Oils derived from coriander seeds, star anise, or thyme. Consume not more than three to four drops.

Green tea. Add 1 teaspoon of green tea leaves to a pot with a cup of hot water. Boil and then simmer gently for 3 to 5 minutes and strain the mixture. Add honey to taste and drink three to four times a day.

Juniper berry tea. Take 1 tablespoon of fresh berries and crush them. Add boiling water and steep for 10 minutes. Strain and drink. Add honey to taste.

> Variation #1. Take 1 teaspoon of dried juniper berries. Crush it. Add 1 cup of boiling water. Steep for 20 minutes. Drink 1 cup twice a day.

Manuka honey. Take 1 teaspoon of manuka honey and add 1 cup of water. Some fresh lemon juice may also be added.

Rose water. Take 2 or 3 cups of fresh rose petals and place in saucepan. Add about 2 litres of distilled water or enough to cover the petals. Simmer in the saucepan for 30 to 45 minutes till the colour comes out from the petals. Cool, then strain and store in a clean bottle. Refrigerate and use for 1 month. Consume 1 glass daily.

Teas (to support liver and gallbladder function). Make tea by steeping 1 teaspoon (3 to 5 g) of any of the following herbs and spices in 1 cup of boiling water: dandelion root, dried dill, chamomile, oregano, cilantro, rosemary, sage, bay leaf, mint, cardamom, basil, coriander, ginger, anise, fennel, or turmeric. Drink this herbal tea infusion after each meal to prevent bloating and aid digestion.

Modern Remedies

Simethicone

Simethicone contains calcium phosphate tribasic and colloidal silicon dioxide. It changes the surface tension of gas bubbles in the gut so that they are broken and are easily eliminated.

Activated Charcoal

Take 2 charcoal tablets (500 mg) every hour until the symptoms subside.

Antacids

Aluminum and magnesium antacids work quickly to lower the stomach acidity

Probiotics

Probiotics with 3 to 5 million live CFU are recommended daily.

Digestive enzymes

Pancreatic enzymes (a mix of protease, lipase, and amylase) can help with digestion and improve absorption of essential nutrients. Take 3 to 4 g with each meal. Examples are Pancreatin, Creon.

Lactase enzyme (example: Dairy Ease or Lactaid) is specific for dairy products. Beano is useful when eating beans/legumes.

Therapeutic Measures

Diet

Eat small, frequent, and regular meals.

Take small bites and chew slowly.

Drink fluids and soups first.

Avoid flatulence or gas-producing foods (see the list below).

Avoid high-fiber foods.

Avoid excessive carbohydrate intake, carbonated beverages, beer, and chewing gum.

Consume fermented foods such as sauerkraut or pickled vegetables like radish, turnip, and carrot to aid digestion.

Take probiotics.

Flatulence-Producing Foods

Vegetables	Onions, radishes, broccoli, cabbage, cauliflower, mushroom, artichokes
Beans, legumes, and dhals	Most beans, peas, lentils(dhals), legumes
Whole grains with bran	Oats, wheat

Starchy foods	Potato, sweet potato
Dairy	Milk and other dairy products
Fruits:	Jackfruit, oranges
Others	Cashew nuts, yeast-containing products (most breads), beer, carbonated or sweetened drinks (with sorbitol)

Flatulence-Reducing Foods

Vegetables/herbs:	Carrots, pumpkin, coriander, parsley, cilantro, lemon, lime, chili
Spices:	Cumin, turmeric, caraway
Beans, legumes, and dhals:	It is advisable to soak these legumes overnight before cooking.
Grains:	Rice
Dairy:	Taking lactase enzymes may help if dairy is consumed.
Fruits:	Papaya
Others:	Seaweed

Lifestyle

Do not lie down or sleep soon after a meal. A slow walk is helpful.

Treat underlying problems such as acid reflux or food allergies.

Homeopathic Remedies

These are very effective for bloating and gas. They include graphite, carbo veg, abies can, magnesium phosphate, China, and raphanus.

Hemorrhoids (Piles)

Piles is a common painful condition.

Predisposing risk factors include obesity, pregnancy, diets which are more meat-based with little or no vegetables, low-fiber foods, over-spicy foods, excessive alcohol, constipation, old age, overindulgence in sex, sedentary lifestyle, and suppressing urges to defecate.

Hemorrhoids are swollen veins found in and around the anus and rectum. They can be either internal or external. There are two forms—dry or bleeding piles. Common symptoms include:

- intense itching around the anus
- painful or itchy swelling or lump near the anus
- painful bowel movements
- bleeding from the anorectal region during or after bowel movements
- irritation and pain around the anus
- leakage of stool

Classification of Piles

a. Based on the degree of protrusion or bulging
   First-degree pile: The pile is in the rectum.

Second-degree pile: The pile protrudes through the anus during defecation but reduces spontaneously.

Third-degree pile: The pile protrudes through the anus during defecation but is reduced manually with the finger.

Fourth-degree pile: The pile remains prolapsed outside the anus all the time.

b. Internal or external
c. Bleeding or non-bleeding

Indian Natural Remedies

There are three veins surrounding the anal region and rectum—visarajni, samvarni, and the pravahani. These veins get swollen and come out when there is excess pressure created inside the anal canal. The swollen veins in the anal canal will obstruct the normal process of passing stools. This will cause bleeding or painful prolapse, or produce discharge. This mainly occurs due to digestive disorders from the imbalances of the doshas inside the body.

When there are digestive disorders, the pitta dosha gets aggravated which causes accumulation of toxins in the digestive gut. These toxins are the vital causes of piles.

Types of Hemorrhoids According to Dosha

The dominant dosha determines the type of hemorrhoids experienced.

Vata type

The hemorrhoids are black with a rough, hard texture. They are extremely painful and give rise to constipation.

Pitta type

This pile is reddish, soft, inflamed, and bleeding. There is fever, thirst, and diarrhea.

Kapha type

Here the piles are large, soft, and slippery, light or whitish in color. There is very poor digestion.

There are four grades. Grade 1 and grade 2 are considered as initial stages while grade 3 and grade 4 are considered as the advanced stage. Ayurvedic treatment for these two stages are different:

Initial Stage: Grade 1 and 2
1. Personalized herbal medicine for dosha balancing
2. Diet and lifestyle modifications to improve digestion and have regular bowel movements
3. Strain-reducing yoga exercises. Example: Ashwini mudra in different seated or inverted postures

With these treatments, a complete cure is possible in grade 1 and 2 piles.

Advanced Stage: Grade 3 and 4
1. Advanced detoxification for cleansing
2. Customized medication and diet
3. Ksharsutra therapy (This is an herbal chemical cauterization and can also be used in other anal disorders such as anal fissure, anal fistula, and pilonidal sinus. A sterile

thread is coated 21 times in a special polyherbal solution and dried each time. This medicated thread is placed directly on the pile, fissure, or fistula.)

The piles usually bleed and prolapse. Treatment is a combination of advanced detoxification to cleanse ama and herbs to strengthen the excretory passage. Based on the individualized diagnosis, Kshar Sutra therapy may be recommended at this stage. It is safe with a minimal invasive surgery and reduces the risk of recurrence.

Common Ingredients for Hemorrhoids

Spices	Herbs/Leaves/Root	Miscellaneous
Black mustard seed (*Brassica nigra*)	Varun/Varuna/mavilinkam/three-leaf caper (*Crataeva nurvala*)	Ispaghula
	Trivrit/turpeth (*Operculina turpethum*)	Pomegranate
	Java plum/Jamun (*Eugenia jambolana*)	Buttermilk, Yogurt
	Ceylon leadwort/chitrak (*Plumbago zeylanica*)	White radish
	Bala (*Sida cordifolia*)	Banana
	Mimosa	
	Veld grape	
	Indian sorrel	
	White Dammar (*Vateria indica*)	
	Common rue	
Black pepper (*Piper nigrum*)	Vacha/vasambu/sweet flag (*Acorus calamus*)	Kollu
Ginger root/shunthi (*Zingiber officinale*)	Amla (*Phyllanthus emblica*)	Figs
Haridra/turmeric (*Curcuma longa*)	Pippali/pimpali/long pepper (*Piper longum*)	Amaltas (*Cassia fistula*)
Mustard seed (*Brassica juncea*)	Trikatu (blend of 3 peppers: black pepper + ginger + long pepper)	Bael leaves (*Aegle marmelos*)
	Korphad (*Aloe vera*)	Ashoka bark
	Suran/elephant foot yam (*Amorphophallus paeoniifolius*)	Malva nuts
Vidanga/false black pepper (*Embelia ribes*)	Haritaki (*Terminalia chebula*)	Kutaja
	Catechu	
	Acacia catechu	

Common Recipes

Oral

Tea/Brew/Others

Amaltas brew. Take 1 to 2 teaspoons of the fruit pulp paste. Add 1 glass of warm water. Consume after dinner.

Ashoka bark paste. Take ¼ to ½ teaspoon ashoka tree bark powder. Add little water or honey. Consume after meal.
Variation #1. Place 25 g of ashoka bark powder into a pot with 200 mL of water. Boil slowly until the water has reduced to about 50 mL. Add 50 mL of milk and continue to boil until only 50 mL of liquid is left. Strain and cool. Take 20 to 30 mL in the morning to reduce menstrual blood flow.
Variation #2. Take some ashoka tree bark and add about 200 mL of water. Boil and reduce to ¼ volume. Consume 40 to 50 mL twice a day.

Bael juice. Cut the bael fruit. Scoop out the pulp into a bowl and mash it and remove the seeds by hand. Blend the de-seeded pulp with some water. Add sugar to taste. Another variation. Take ¼ to ½ teaspoon of bael powder. Add ½ to 1 cup of water. Drink twice a day after a meal.

Bael leaves. Take a mixture of powdered dried bael leaf, carom seeds (ajwain), dried ginger, and black pepper. Add into a glass of buttermilk or lukewarm water and consume.

Bala drink. Take ½ to 2 g of dried bala leaf powder. Add warm or cold water. Cook and eat the leaves for bleeding piles.

Banana. Take one ripe banana. Blend or mash with one cup of milk. Consume this throughout the day.

Buttermilk mixture. Take a glass of buttermilk. Add in some ground black peppercorn, crushed ginger, and some Himalayan rock salt. Drink this twice a day, once in the morning and once in the evening.

Catechu. Apply catechu paste directly on the piles.

Chitrak root. Take 1 to 2 g of root powder and add it into buttermilk. Consume three times a day.

Common rue tea. Take 1 teaspoon of dried crushed rue leaves. Add ½ cup of boiling water. Steep for 15 minutes. Consume it.

Figs. Eat figs twice a day. Soak four figs in water overnight and eat them in the morning. Soak another four figs in the morning and eat them in the evening. Do not drink water before eating the figs. Repeat this every day for 4 weeks.

Goat milk yogurt. Take 250 mL of goat milk buttermilk (made from goat milk). Add in and blend 250 mL of carrot juice. Consume this mixture throughout the day.

Indian sorrel. Take 10 g of the Indian sorrel leaves and stem. Wash and dry them. Grind to make a powder. Add to a glass of buttermilk and consume twice a day (for bleeding piles).

Ispaghula. Take 2 teaspoons of Ispaghula and 2 teaspoons of palm sugar and mix with little water to make a paste. Place this paste on the middle of each leaf. Fold the leaf and consume it daily for 2 weeks.

Jamun. Eat the fruit with salt each morning. If bleeding piles, eat the fruit with honey.

Java plum (Jamun) juice. Take 10 to 15 washed black jamun fruits. Deseed and blend with 1 cup of water with added ¼ teaspoon of black salt and a small piece of ginger. Strain and drink. Add some honey and ice if desired.

Kollu. The grains are soaked and then cooked until soft. It is added to soups or mixed with rice or curries. Alternatively, soak 1 cup of seeds overnight. In the morning drain and consume on an empty stomach.

Kutaja. Take ¼- to ½ teaspoon of dried seed powder and mix with water (or ghee). Consume after a light meal.

Malva nut. Take one to two malva nuts (do not exceed three nuts). Add 1 cup of water. Steep for 30 minutes. Discard the skin and seed. Consume the liquid and pulp as a brew.

　Variation #1. Take 100 g of malva nuts. Add 2 L of water and soak preferably overnight. Remove and discard the seed and thick outer skin the next morning. Strain the pulp (gel) via a coarse muslin cloth. Various spices or herbs can be added to the pulp

　Take 2 cups of water in a saucepan. Add pandanus (screw-pine leaf) and brown sugar. Boil and simmer for 10 to 15 minutes. Add cinnamon stick, ginger slices, and licorice for additional flavors if desired. Strain. Add the malva nut pulp to the strained liquid and drink.

　Variation #2. Other items such as red date, liquorice, chrysanthemum flower, jasmine tea, lilyturf root, haw, and rock sugar can also be simmered together in water and then the malva nut pulp added.

　Variation #3. Soaked basil seeds, sugar, and ice can be added to the soaked malva nut pulp and drunk as a cooling drink.

Mimosa. Take 1 teaspoon of mimosa root and leaf powder. Add some milk. Consume two to three times a day.

Mustard seed. Take some ground black mustard seeds. Add to a bowl of yogurt. Consume this and then drink a glass of buttermilk.

Pomegranate peel. Take some pomegranate peel. Add 1 to 2 cups of water. Boil and simmer for 10 to 15 minutes. Cool and then strain. Consume twice a day.

Trikatu brew. Steep equal parts of black pepper, long pepper, and ginger in a cup of hot water. Steep for about 10 to 15 minutes. Drink it warm.

Vacha brew. Lightly pound some vacha root. Place 1 g of the root into a cup of boiling water and steep until completely cool. Mix some honey into the mixture and drink.

Varun. Take ½ to 1 teaspoon of varun powder and mix with honey. Consume after food.

Veld grape. Sauté some veld grape stems in a little ghee. Blend with a little water. Store in a bottle and refrigerate. Take ¼ teaspoon daily for 2 weeks.

Commercial Oral Preparations (for First-Degree Piles)

Herbolax. It is a polyherbal tablet with prebiotic, prokinetic, and laxative actions. It contains trivrit (*I. turpethum*), senna (*C. acutifolia*), haritaki (*T. chebula*), kasani (*C. intybus*/blue daisy), *Z. officinale*, *G. glabra* (liquorice), Kakamachi (*S. nigrum*/black nightshade), and vidanga/false black pepper (*E. ribes*).

Pilex tablets or ointment. They contain shilajit, *Azadirachta indica* (neem) seeds, *Commiphora wightii* (guggulu/shuddha), *Berberis aristata* (daruhaldi), Cassia fistula (amaltas), *T. chebula* (haritaki), *Phyllanthus emblica* (amla), *Terminalia bellirica* (vibhitaki), *Bauhinia variegata* (kanchanara), and *Mesua ferrea* (nagkesar). It also has a mild laxative function.

Pylowin tablets. They contain pepper longum, trivrit, nagkesar, aloe vera, sajjikhar—natural alkali, Berberis aristata, suran, guggulu, miri, and ginger.

Topical Treatment

Radish. Take some white radish juice. Mix with honey. Apply this mixture on the piles.

Rue oil. Take 1 tablespoon of crushed dry leaves. Add ½ cup of hot olive oil. Steep for 30 minutes or longer. Strain and store in a bottle. Apply this oil on the piles.

Sesame oil. Apply sesame oil on the external dry piles followed by warm fomentation (warm, moist compress or sitting in warm water). The easiest method is to sit in a tub with the buttocks submerged in warm water or warm saltwater.

Spice mix paste. Make a paste by mixing an equal amount of powdered long pepper and turmeric with milk (preferably cow's milk). Apply this paste on the external piles.

Herbal Application or Kshara/Kshara Karma

Kshara is a caustic, alkaline paste used to manage hemorrhoids. This paste is a mixture of herbs with chemical cauterizing properties mainly from *Achyranthes aspera* (apamarga) and *Euphorbia neriifolia* (snuhi) and an antiseptic (i.e., *Cucurma longa* [haridra]). The kshara is applied to the hemorrhoid which is open and bleeding using a device called a slit proctoscope. It is applied for 7 days and will cause the piles to shrink. This Kshara method is the best method for treating first- and second-degree hemorrhoids. There are no side effects or adverse reactions.

Depending on the dosha, specific medications are given to balance the body during recovery. Dietary or lifestyle adjustments must be continued.

Surgical Intervention or Sastra Chikitsa/Kshar Sutra

Kshar Sutra uses a special medicated alkaline thread to ligate at the base of the hemorrhoid. This cuts off the blood supply to the vein, allowing the hemorrhoid to shrink over the next 7 to 10 days. It will shrivel and detach on its own. This more invasive approach will be considered only when other treatments are not effective.

This is a quick and minimally invasive procedure. Patients can return to work the next day. Also, recovery is less painful than hemorrhoidectomy.

However, this procedure is contraindicated if there is infection, bleeding disorder, or blood-thinning medications.

Cauterization or Agnikarma

External hemorrhoids can be cauterized using infrared heat. There is increased pain or infection risk with cauterization. Five to six treatments over 5 to 6 weeks may be needed. Safer modern treatments may be better.

A combination of modern surgical intervention and Ayurvedic treatments are recommended.

Cauterization procedures and surgical procedures have a much higher risk with adverse effects such as tissue damage, bleeding, pain, infection, shock, leakage of stool, and recurrence of hemorrhoids.

It can be risky for a person experiencing hemorrhoids to choose the wrong treatment.

Therapeutic Measures

Diet

Eat more fruits such as papaya, oranges, and figs.

Drink plenty of fluids such as water, soups, juice, milk, buttermilk.

Avoid the intake of heavy, dry, cool, and stale foods.

Avoid refined foods like jams, pastries, packaged, and canned foods.

Also avoid tea, coffee, fizzy carbonated drinks, and alcohol.

Avoid nightshades including root vegetables, except radish and carrot.

Pickles should be avoided or eaten in moderation.

Lifestyle

- Avoid excessive fasting, overeating, eating during indigestion, and eating incompatible food.
- Use the squatting position during defecation.

Medication or Bhaishajya chikitsa. Based on the dosha type, the right remedies will be selected and any dietary or lifestyle changes are recommended to prevent a recurrence.

Chinese Natural Remedies

The Chinese have employed several remedies to heal piles. Traditional herbs will reduce the inflammation, and there will be less or no pain, swelling, irritation, and itching. Some of the Chinese medications for hemorrhoids are Formula H, Hemorrease, and Musk Hemorrhoids ointment.

There are five major patterns in Chinese medicine for hemorrhoid treatment. These are **intestinal wind, dry intestine, damp/heat, spleen deficiency, and blood stasis.**

Intestinal Wind

This condition is associated with fresh blood oozing out before or after passing bowels. There is blood on toilet paper or stool.

Dry Intestine

This is a condition of chronic constipation with dry stools. Straining to pass bowels may cause swelling of the tissues. Bleeding may occur before or after defecation. Chinese polyherbal medicines can relieve constipation and facilitate easy bowel movements.

Damp/Heat

This condition is associated with inflamed internal hemorrhoids. There is fresh blood oozing out before or after passing stools. The inflamed hemorrhoids are large and swollen and can cause burning pain, itching, and irritation.

Jing wan hong works like a topical ointment. It reduces the burning pain, itching, and irritation in the perianal region.

Other useful herbs are huang lian jie du wan and zhong guo zhi gen duan.

Spleen Deficiency:

Here the hemorrhoids are painful and protruding. The bleeding may be scanty or heavy.

Chinese remedies: Huang tu tang controls bleeding. Other useful herbs are fu zi li zhong wan, gui pi tang (wan), and bu zhong yi qi tang (wan).

Blood Stasis:

In chronic hemorrhoids, there is blood stasis which can cause continuous or severe pain and large dark fissures. Symptoms include bleeding, pain, irritation, and itching.

Chinese remedies: Tao he cheng qi tang helps to move the bowels better.

Jing wan hong is applied topically to relieve inflammation and dryness.

Other useful herbs are huo xue san yu tang, xue fu zhu yu tang, tong jing wan, and sheng tian qi pian.

Common Ingredients for Hemorrhoids

Atractylodes

Immature bitter orange

Konjac root

Qin jiao

Radix notoginseng (sanqi)

Rubia cordifolia (qian cao)

She Chuang Zi (Cnidium Monnieri Fruit)

Sophora tree flower

Water caltrop

White peony root

These are often Chinese proprietary medicines (available as tablets, capsules, or topical substances) or as polyherbal compounds.

Oral

Ba zhen tang (Eight Treasures). Mix 4.5 g of the herb powder in hot water and drink it as tea. Take two to three times daily.

Huai hua san. Grind together chao hua san, ce bai ye, jing jie sui, and fu chao zhi ke. Take 9-g dosages with 1 cup of hot water. Di yu may be added if the bleeding is heavy.

Konjac root. This Asian root vegetable can be boiled or processed into ground flour to make Japenese noodles (shirataki noodles) or snacks.

Qin jiao, bai zhu wan. Grind qin jiao *(Gentiana Macrophylla)* and bai zhu *(Atractylodes macrocephala)* to form 6 g pill balls and take it one to three times daily.

Sophora tree flower/huai hua mi. Take 1 tablespoon of dried flowers and buds. Make a hot tea decoction. Consume warm. Pills and capsules are also available.

Water caltrop juice. Drink the water caltrop juice together with sugarcane juice or eat the fruit to prevent hemorrhoids.

Commercial oral preparations for hemorrhoids

Fargelin is a specially formulated, widely used and very effective Chinese polyherbal herbal medicine for hemorrhoids. It is available in capsules.

Huai jiao wan. It is an oral polyherbal medication made from herbs Radix Sanguisorba Officinalis, Fructus Sophora Japonica, Flos Sophora Japonica, Radix et Rhizoma Rheum Palmatum, Radix Scutellaria Baicalensis, Radix Rehmannia Glutinosa, Radix Angelicae Sinensis, Radix Paeonia Lactiflora, Flos Carthamus Tinctorius, Radix Saposhnikoviae (Ledebouriella Divaricata), Spica Schizonepeta Tenuifolia, Fructus Citrus Aurantium. It is used to control bleeding and reduce the pain and irritation caused by hemorrhoids.

Ma zi ren wan. It is a polyherbal mixture with herbs including Semen cannabis sativae (huo ma ren or cannabis/hemp seed), Semen pruni armeniacae (xing ren or apricot seed), Fructus immaturus citri aurantii (zhi shi or immature bitter orange), Radix paeoniae alba (bai shao or white peony root), Cortex magnoliae officinalis (hou po or magnolia bark), and Radix et rhizoma rhei (dried root of da huang or Chinese rhubarb).

Run chang wan. This polyherbal formula works by moistening the bowels to alleviate the pain. It contains five herbs: Semen persicae (tao ren), Rhizoma seu Radix Notopterygii (qiang huo), Radix et Rhizoma Rhei (da huang), Radix angelicae sinensis (dang gui), and Semen cannabis (huo ma ren).

Yun nan bai yao. This polyherbal powder has Radix notoginseng (sanqi) as the main ingredient. Others include Rhizoma Dioscoreae, Rhizoma Dioscoreae Nipponicae, Ajuga Forrestii Diels, Dioscoreae Parviflora Ting, Herba Geranii, Herba Erodii Herba Inulae Cappae.

Zeng ye cheng qi tang. It is an herbal formulation made from xuan shen (Radix scrophulariae), mai men dong (Radix ophiopogonis), sheng di huang (Radix rehmanniae), da huang (Radix et Rz. Rhei), and mang xiao (Natrii sulfas). It works by moistening the bowels to alleviate the pain.

Zhong guo zhi gen duan. This polyherbal formula contains Panax notoginseng (sanqi), Rubia cordifolia (qian cao), Citrus aurantium (zhi ke), Styphnolobium japonicum, (huaimi), Sparganium eurycarpum (san leng), and magnesium.

Others. gu ben wan, liang xue di huang tang, and huai hua san.

Commercial Topical Preparations

Bai guo ye (Ginkgo biloba) is also known as Ginkgo or maidenhair. It is often used in the TCM treatment of hemorrhoids. It is available in many different forms including tea, extract, powder, and capsules.

Jing wan hong. This topical ointment can help get relief from itching and inflammation.

Ma ying long Musk Hemorrhoids ointment reduces inflammation, swelling, pain, bleeding, and itching. It is used externally as a topical ointment.

Therapeutic Measures

Acupuncture is also used to treat hemorrhoids.

Chinese Herbal Sitz Bath for hemorrhoids

Take 30 g of she chuang zi (Cnidium monnieri fruit). Add 2 L of warm water. Sit in the sitz bath for 10 to 15 minutes. Repeat two to three times per day for 1 week.

Western/Other Natural Remedies

Common Ingredients for Hemorrhoids

Spices	Herbs/Leaves	Miscellaneous
Ginger	Witch hazel leaf *(Hamamelis virginiana)*	Epsom salt
	Horse chestnut seed *(Aesculus hippocastanum)*	Vaseline or Petroleum jelly
	Tea tree oil	Granulated sugar
	Geranium (Cranesbill)	Vicks Vapor Rub
	Fleabane	White oak bark
	Oil of St John wort	White Dammar

Oral

Teas/Brews/Others

Butcher's broom. Take one teaspoon of chopped roots. Add one cup of boiling water. Steep for 10 minutes. Strain and consume it warm.

Fleabane tea. Make a decoction from the dried leaves and flowers. Consume for bleeding piles.

Variation #1. It can also be applied externally for bleeding piles.

Geranium tea. Take 1 to 2 teaspoons of the dried cranesbill root. Add 1 cup of water. Boil and simmer for 15 minutes. Strain and consume.

Variation #1. Take 2 to 3 tablespoons of the above and inject into the rectum as an enema after each passage of bloody stools.

Ginger tea. Lightly pound 3 to 4 inches of fresh ginger and place into an empty cup. Pour boiling water into the cup and allow it to steep for about 10 minutes. Drink in the morning on an empty stomach.

Horse Chestnuts. Take one teaspoon of horse chestnut bark or dried leaves. Add one cup of boiling water. Steep for 10 to 15 minutes. Strain and consume it warm.

Topical

Home Measures

- Sitz bath: If there are painful or inflamed piles, the patient is encouraged to sit in a bath of warm water with Epsom salt and glycerin at least three times a day for about 15 to 20 minutes.
- Apply or dab witch hazel, tea tree oil, Vicks Vapor Rub, or diluted apple cider vinegar on the external painful piles.
- Apply Vaseline or petroleum jelly on the piles for a soothing effect.
- Apply or put granulated sugar for prolapsed piles and leave for 15 to 20 minutes. Then attempt to reduce the prolapsed piles.
- Cold compresses or small ice packs can be placed on the piles for a few minutes.
- White oak bath. Take 5 g of ground oak bark. Add 4 cups of water. Boil. Add this mixture to bath water. Sit for 20 minutes,

  Fleabane. Use the fleabane decoction as a poultice for bleeding piles.

  Oil of St John wort. Apply on the piles to reduce pain and itching.

Commercial Preparation (Topical and Oral)

- *Healar* is an herbal product. It contains white lupin *(Lupinus albus)*, aloe vera, white dammar *(Vateria indica)*, and peppermint *(Mentha piperita)*. It is available as a cream, ointment, or suppository.
- *Preparation medicated H wipes*: These wipes contain witch hazel and sometimes also lignocaine.
- *Daflon;* This is an oral herbal remedy. It contains 90% diosmin and 10% hesperidin (both are flavones from citrus fruit peel). It takes a few days for painful and inflamed piles to shrink.
- *MemeThol Hemorrhoids Barrier Spray:* It is applied externally and once a day. It can be used for the 4 stages of piles. It relieves pain, itching, and complete cure of piles is also possible within 1 month. It contains a menthol derivative and propylene glycol (a solvent).

  Horse chestnut seed. The seed extract is available in the form of capsules.

Homeopathic Remedies

These include *Hamamelis virginiana*, *N. vomica*, *Collinsonia canadensis*, aloe vera, pulsatilla, graphites, *A. hippocastanum*, *Arnica montana*, thuja, sulfur, *Carbo vegetabilis*, phosphorus, *Paeonia officinalis*, and Calcarea fluorica.

Modern Remedies

Medications

a. Topical treatments

Various ointments, creams, suppositories, or pads are available which contain hydrocortisone or lignocaine. They can be used to relieve any inflammation, swelling, and discomfort.

Commercial Preparations

Anusol ointment, cream, or suppository contains zinc oxide (astringent), bismuth, and balsam peru. It reduces itching and has astringent properties. Anusol HC contains added hydrocortisone. Anusol plus has added pramoxine, a local anesthetic.

b. Painkillers

Common painkiller medications such as paracetamol can help relieve the pain of hemorrhoids.

Codeine painkillers should be avoided as they can cause constipation.

For painful hemorrhoids, local anesthetic injections can be given.

c. Laxatives

If there is constipation, stool softeners are given to move the bowels.

d. Antibiotics

If there is an infection after a surgical procedure, antibiotics may be necessary

Therapeutic Measures

Diet and Lifestyle (Non-drug)

- If constipation is the cause of hemorrhoids, bowel movements must be regular and without straining and with the passage of soft stools.
- Consume a fiber-rich diet such as fruits, legumes, whole grains, and vegetables.
- Drink plenty of water and avoid caffeine.
- Take probiotics.
- Use loose cotton clothes.

  Non-surgical treatments. If dietary changes and medications do not help, then non-surgical procedures such as banding and sclerotherapy are recommended for hemorrhoids in the upper anal canal.

a. Banding

Banding involves placing a very tight elastic band around the base of the hemorrhoids to cut off their blood supply. This will cause the hemorrhoids to fall off within a week after having the procedure.

Banding is done as an outpatient or day care procedure. Hence, most people return to their normal activities the next day.

b. Injections (sclerotherapy)

Sclerotherapy may be used as an alternative to banding. It involves injecting a chemical solution into the blood vessels in the anal canal. It relieves pain by numbing the nerve endings at the site of the injection.

It also forms a hard scar in the hemorrhoid. After about 4 to 6 weeks, the hemorrhoid should decrease in size or shrivel up and fall off.

c. Electrotherapy

Electrotherapy is another alternative to banding for people with small hemorrhoids. During the procedure, a device called a proctoscope is inserted into the anus to visualize the hemorrhoid. A small amount of electric current is then passed through a small metal probe placed at the base of the hemorrhoid. This will cauterize the pile at the base and thicken the blood in the blood vessels supplying the pile/hemorrhoid so that it will shrink.

Surgery. Most hemorrhoids can be treated using the methods described above, however, around 1 in every 10 people will require surgery.

Surgery is indicated for hemorrhoids that have developed below the dentate line.

Different types of surgery are available to treat hemorrhoids. They involve either removing the hemorrhoids or reducing their blood supply causing them to shrink.

a. Hemorrhoidectomy

A hemorrhoidectomy is an operation to remove hemorrhoids. It is done under general anesthesia. The procedure involves gently opening the anus so the hemorrhoids can be cut out.

b. Hemorrhoidal artery ligation

Hemorrhoidal artery ligation is an operation to reduce the blood flow to the hemorrhoids. It is done usually under general anesthesia. An ultrasound probe is inserted into the anus which produces high-frequency sound waves. This helps the surgeon to identify and locate the vessels supplying blood to the hemorrhoid.

Each blood vessel is sutured completely to block the blood supply to the hemorrhoid. This results in the shrinkage of the hemorrhoid over the next several days and weeks.

c. Stapling

Stapling is also known as stapled hemorrhoidopexy. It is used to treat a prolapsed hemorrhoid and is carried out under general anesthesia.

The anorectal region (lowermost part of the large intestine) is stapled. This reduces the risk of prolapse of the hemorrhoids. It also reduces the blood supply to the hemorrhoids with subsequent gradual shrinkage of the hemorrhoids.

This procedure is not routine as it carries more serious complications compared to other treatment modalities.

Gallstones

The gallbladder is a small pouch which is located under the liver. It stores and absorbs bile. Bile is a liquid which the liver produces to help digest fats. It passes through a series of channels (bile ducts) from the liver into the gallbladder. The bile is processed in the gallbladder and is more concentrated over time, which makes digestion of fat smoother.

Gallstones form within the gallbladder due to an imbalance in the chemical composition of bile. Raised levels of bile and excess cholesterol form into stones. They can be single or multiple stones of various sizes. Often, gallstones do not cause any symptoms. Biliary colic is caused by small stones trapped in biliary ducts. It can result in sudden intense abdominal pain, nausea, and vomiting.

Gallstones are classically more common in obese females over 40 years old and often there is a similar family history.

They are mostly cholesterol stones. Pigment gallstones are due to excessive bilirubin from some blood disorders and liver cirrhosis.

The diagnosis is confirmed by an ultrasound scan. The blood tests can show impaired liver function or signs of infection.

Cholecystitis refers to inflammation of gallbladder and cholangitis refers to inflammation of the bile ducts. This results in abdominal pain, fever, nausea, sweating, loss in appetite, yellowish discoloration (jaundice) in the skin and eyes.

Indian Natural Remedies

Common Ingredients for Gallstones

Spices	Herbs/Leaves	Miscellaneous
Black seed	Chicory (Cichorium intybus)	Psyllium husk
	Dandelion	
	Peppermint	
	Punarnavadi	
Turmeric	Gokshura (Tribulus terrestris)	Castor oil

Natural Ayurveda Remedies to treat gallstones

Black seed (Nigella sativa): Mix 250 g of black seeds (ground into powder) with 250 g of honey and 1 teaspoon of black seed oil. Add ½ cup of warm water and drink on an empty stomach.

Castor oil pack. Soak a thin towel or cloth in warm castor oil and place it on the abdomen. Place a hot pack on top of the oilcloth.

Chicory. Take 5 chicory leaves. Blend with some water. Add any citrus fruit or beet. Drink 60 mL of chicory leaf juice regularly.

Variation #1. Boil and consume chicory root as a vegetable. The young leaves can be added to salads or sautéed.

Variation #2. Make a hot brew. Take 2 tablespoons of ground chicory root. Add 1 cup of boiling water.

Variation #3. Take 10 to 12 g/day of chicory inulin supplement.

Variation #4. Take 30 g of fresh chicory leaves. Add in 1 L of water. Boil and consume 1 glass before each meal.

Dandelion. It can be consumed as a tea or its fresh leaves eaten as a salad or steamed.

Gokshura. Take ¼ to ½ teaspoon gokshura churna. Add little honey or milk. Consume twice a day after meals.

Variation #1. Capsules and tablets are also available.

Peppermint. It can be drunk as tea.

Psyllium husk. Mix 1 teaspoon of psyllium husk with a cup of plain yogurt and take at bedtime.

Punarnavadi (polyherbs of *Boerhaavia diffusa* mainly, turmeric, neem, ginger, *T. chebula, Cedrus deodara, Andrographis paniculata, Cyperus rotundus,* and *Luffa acutangula*). This is consumed as a decoction (*kashayam*).

Turmeric: Mix ½ teaspoon of turmeric powder in warm water every day.

Commercial Preparations to Treat Gallstones

- **Arogyavardhini vati.** It contains the following: *P. emblica*/amla, *T. bellirica*/Baheda, *T. chebula*/haritaki, Asphaltum/mineral wax)
- **Gokshuradi guggulu.** It consists of the following polyherbs: Dry ginger/sonth, *C. rotundus*/Nagarmotha, Piper longum/pippali, *P. emblica*/amla, *T. chebula*/haritaki, *T. bellirica*/Baheda, *P. nigrum*/black pepper, *C. wightii*/shuddha guggulu—purified
- **-Liverole.** It consists of the following polyherbs: *Terminalia arjuna, Picrorhiza kurroa*/Kutki, Navayas (iron-based polyherbal mix), Arogyavardhini ras/polymineral-polyherbal mix, *Aphanamixis rohituka, B. diffusa*/Punarnava, *P. nigrum*/black pepper, *Tinospora cordifolia*/giloy, *Eclipta alba*/bhringraj, *A. paniculata*, bhavna, and gum acacia

Therapeutic Measures to Prevent Gallstones

Diet
- Consume a low-fat diet and maintain an ideal weight.
- Eat fruits such as pineapple and papaya which contain digestive enzymes (bromelain and papain respectively) to improve liver and gallbladder metabolism.

Yoga
Yoga asanas can help improve liver and gallbladder metabolism.

These include the lotus pose (padmasana), cobra pose (bhujangasana), locust pose (shalabhasana), thunderbolt pose (vajrasana), back-stretching pose (paschimottanasana), bow pose (dhanurasana), and knee to chest (pawanmuktasana).

Chinese Natural Remedies

It is believed gallstone formation is due to the following: damp-heat in the liver and gallbladder, qi stagnation in the liver, liver yin deficiency, heat toxic stagnation, or blood stasis stagnation.

Various herb mixes (formula) are used for stone shrinking or stone dissolving and stone expulsion. Sometimes, animal bile is also added.

Herba lysimachia (gold coin grass). Consume 1 tablespoon once daily on an empty stomach, ½ hour before breakfast.

Commercial Formulation

Lysimachia GB formula: Herba lysimachia (gold coin grass), Radix bupleuri, Scutellaria, turmeric, dang shen (Codonopsis), capillaris (Herba artemisiae), gardenia fruit, bamboo shavings, melia fruit, white peony root, Chinese date, ginger, liquorice root.

Changgen/qian dan tong oral liquid: Herba lysimachia, Lysimachia christinae, Radix bupleuri, dandelion, oriental wormwood, Polygonum cuspidatum, root of red-rooted salvia Cyperus tuber, smoked plum, Semen cassiae torae.

Pai shi li dan granules. Lysimachia christinae, Radix bupleuri, Oriental wormwood, Radix gentianae, Radix paeoniae rubrathe (unpeeled), common peony root, Radix curcumae, Excrementum pteropi, Cattail pollen, glauber, Rheum officinale

Jin dan tablet. Lysimachia christinae, Radix gentianae, Polygonum cuspidatum, pig's bile

Therapeutic Measures

Acupuncture may help to relieve the pain (biliary spasm) associated with gallstones. The acupoints commonly used for the gallbladder, liver, and bladder meridians are riyue (GB24), danshu (BL19), and qiuxu (GB40).

Western/Other Natural Remedies

Common Ingredients for Gallstones

Spices	Herbs/Leaves	Miscellaneous
	Peppermint	Olive oil
	Dandelion	Sunflower oil
		Apple cider vinegar
		Apple juice
		Vegetable juice
		Pear juice
		Artichoke

Gallbladder Cleanse

There are various recipes and versions. Caution must be exercised in diabetic patients as there may be fasting in some methods.

Apple juice and apple cider vinegar cleanse. This is mixed together and is consumed on waking for 3 to 5 days. Some olive oil may be taken before this mixture.

Artichoke. It can be cooked in many ways. Extract is also available.

Dandelion. It can be consumed as a tea or its fresh leaves eaten as a salad or can be steamed.

Olive oil or sunflower oil flush. Drink 30 mL of olive oil or sunflower oil in the morning on waking. Then drink 120 mL of fresh lemon juice or grapefruit juice. This will stimulate the gallbladder to release and push the bile and the stones out. Some loose stools may be passed.

Pear juice. Mix ½ glass pear juice with ½ glass warm water and 2 tablespoons honey. Drink three times a day.

Peppermint tea. Place a handful of peppermint leaves into a pot of water. Bring to a boil and reduce the heat. Allow the mixture to simmer for 5 to 10 minutes. Strain and drink twice a day. Consume if there is acute pain during biliary colic.

Vegetable juice. Blend and mix equal parts of beet, carrot, and cucumber juice. Drink twice a day. This will help dissolve gallstones.

Modern Remedies

Medical Treatment

- For *biliary colic*, painkillers and anti-emetics are given. In acute cholecystitis, the patient is kept fasted, given intravenous fluids and intravenous antibiotics. A hot compress can be placed on the right side to relieve pain.
- *Bile acids,* i.e., ursodeoxycholic acid and chenodeoxycholic acid can be taken if the gallstones are small.

Surgical Treatment

Laparoscopic cholecystectomy is keyhole or minimally invasive surgery which is a gold standard. It is done to remove the gall bladder using a number of small incisions (about 1 to 2 cm) in the abdomen. The potential surgical risks are bile duct injury with bile leaks or bile duct stricture, biliary bleeding, bowel injury and rare recurring stones in the common bile duct, and postcholecystectomy syndrome.

In open cholecystectomy, the gallbladder is removed through a single large incision below the liver (about 10 to 15 cm).

The gallbladder is a useful organ but not essential. It can be removed safely without interfering with digestion as the liver can produce bile to digest food.

Homeopathic Remedies

Chelidonium (effective for the pain and obstructive jaundice), calcerea carb (in obese persons), lycopodium (especially if there is associated bloating and acidity), phosphorus (with associated sour belches and vomit after food), and carduus marianus (with associated pain and inflamed gall bladder).

References

Vomiting

Church, M., & Church, D. (2013). Pharmacology of antihistamines. *Indian Journal of Dermatology*, 58(3), 219–224. Retrieved from https://doi.org/10.4103/0019-5154.110832.

Cleveland Clinic Medical Professional. (2019, July 23). *Nausea & vomiting*. Cleveland Clinic. Retrieved from https://my.cleveland-clinic.org/health/symptoms/8106-nausea—vomiting.

DerSarkissian, C., & McMillen, M. (2019, October 28). *Tips for managing chemotherapy side effects*. WebMD. Retrieved from https://www.webmd.com/cancer/tips-for-managing-chemotherapy-side-effects.

Drugs.com (Eds.). (n.d.). *List of 64 nausea/vomiting medications compared*. Drugs.Com. Retrieved from https://www.drugs.com/condition/nausea-vomiting.html.

Familydoctor.org Editorial Staff. (2020, April 21). *Antiemetic medicines: OTC relief for nausea and vomiting*. Familydoctor.Org. Retrieved from https://familydoctor.org/antiemetic-medicines-otc-relief-for-nausea-and-vomiting/.

Flake, Z. A., Scalley, R. D., & Bailey, A. G. (2004). Practical selection of antiemetics. *American Family Physician*, 69(05), 1169–1174. Retrieved from https://www.aafp.org/afp/2004/0301/p1169.html.

Golembiewski, J., Chernin, E., & Chopra, T. (2005). Prevention and treatment of postoperative nausea and vomiting. *American Journal of Health-System Pharmacy*, 62(12), 1247–1260. Retrieved from https://doi.org/10.1093/ajhp/62.12.1247.

Health Engine (Ed.). (2011, May 30). *5-HT3 receptor antagonists (serotonin blockers) information | myVMC*. HealthEngine Blog. Retrieved from https://healthengine.com.au/info/5-ht3-receptor-antagonists-serotonin-blockers.

Hopkins Technology. (n.d.). *Vomiting*. Acupuncture.Com. Retrieved from http://www.acupuncture.com/Conditions/vomiting.htm.

Kandola, A., & Sethi, S. (2018, February 10). *What are the best ways to get rid of nausea?* Medical News Today. Retrieved from https://www.medicalnewstoday.com/articles/320877.

Kandola, A., & Wilson, D. R. (2018, June 5). *Which essential oils help with nausea?* Medical News Today. Retrieved from https://www.medicalnewstoday.com/articles/322032.

Kapoor, A. (2018, June 1). *6 effective home remedies to prevent vomiting*. NDTV Food. Retrieved from https://food.ndtv.com/health/6-effective-home-remedies-to-prevent-vomiting-1661727.

Khan, A. (2020, May 29). *13 effective home remedies for vomiting in children*. FirstCry Parenting. Retrieved from https://parenting.firstcry.com/articles/easy-home-remedies-for-vomiting-in-children/.

Kokalj, Z., & Unhawane, M. (2016, November 1). *Nausea remedies for quick relief the natural way*. All Ayurveda. Retrieved from https://allayurveda.com/blog/6-ways-to-get-rid-of-the-agony-of-nausea-fast/.

Kukreja, K., & Lytle, M. (2019, October 17). *13 effective home remedies to stop vomiting*. StyleCraze. Retrieved from https://www.stylecraze.com/articles/effective-home-remedies-to-stop-vomiting/#gref.

Moodie, T. (2013). *Anticholinergic medication*. DermNet New Zealand Trust. Retrieved from https://www.dermnetnz.org/topics/anticholinergic-medications/.

Schlager, A., Boehler, M., & Pühringer, F. (2000). Korean hand acupressure reduces postoperative vomiting in children after strabismus surgery. *British Journal of Anaesthesia*, 85(2), 267–270. Retrieved from https://doi.org/10.1093/bja/85.2.267.

Sengupta, S. (2018, June 1). *5 Ayurvedic home remedies for nausea and vomiting*. NDTV Food. Retrieved from https://food.ndtv.com/health/5-ayurvedic-home-remedies-for-nausea-and-vomiting-1802192.

The BabyCentre Editorial Team. (2012). *Can vitamin B6 relieve morning sickness?* BabyCenter. Retrieved from https://www.babycentre.co.uk/x2519/can-vitamin-b6-relieve-morning-sickness.

The Crankshaft Publishing. (n.d.). *Vomiting (common internal medicine disorders) (Chinese Medicine)*. What-When-How.Com. Retrieved from http://what-when-how.com/chinese-medicine/vomiting-common-internal-medicine-disorders-chinese-medicine/.

UCLA Center for East-West Medicine. (n.d.). *Acupressure point P6: Pericardium 6 or Nei Guan*. Explore Integrative Medicine. Retrieved from https://exploreim.ucla.edu/self-care/acupressure-point-p6/.

Stomach Ache and Indigestion

Brennan, D. (2020, September 2). *Health benefits of Ajwain*. WebMD. Retrieved from https://www.webmd.com/dicenet/health-benefits-ajwain#1.

British Homeopathic Association. (n.d.). *Homeopathy UK*. Homeopathy UK. Retrieved from https://homeopathy-uk.org/.

Chinese Herbs Info. (2021, March 31). *Gui Zhi (Cinnamon Twig, Ramulus Cinnamomi, Cassia Twig)*. Retrieved from https://www.chineseherbsinfo.com/the-benefits-and-side-effects-of-gui-zhi-cinnamon-twig.

Cummings, G. (2017, August 31). *10 common digestive herbs and how they benefit your health*. Evening Standard. Retrieved from https://www.standard.co.uk/reveller/foodanddrink/10-common-digestive-herbs-and-how-they-benefit-your-health-a3624266.html.

Dabcevic, M. (2020, December 28). *5 Chinese herbs to power up your digestion*. Mind Body Green Food. Retrieved from https://www.mindbodygreen.com/0-25201/5-chinese-herbs-to-power-up-your-digestion.html.

Dogra, T. (2021, February 9). *Upset stomach? Get relief from stomach pain with these effective home remedies.* Only My Health. Retrieved from https://www.onlymyhealth.com/home-remedies-for-stomach-pain-1352374107.

Drug Bank (Ed.). (n.d.). *Simethicone: Uses, interactions, mechanism of action | DrugBank Online.* DrugBank. Retrieved from https://go.drugbank.com/drugs/DB09512.

Drugs.com (Ed.). (n.d.). *Antacids.* Drugs.Com. Retrieved from https://www.drugs.com/monograph/antacids.html.

Gajendran, D. (2014, October 16). *9 best acupressure points to treat digestive problems.* Modern Reflexology. Retrieved from https://www.modernreflexology.com/acupressure-points-to-treat-digestive-problems/.

Ganesh, P., Kumar, R. S., & Saranraj, P. (2014). Phytochemical analysis and antibacterial activity of Pepper (*Piper nigrum* L.) against some human pathogens. *Central European Journal of Experimental Biology*, *03*(02), 36–41. Retrieved from https://www.scholarsresearchlibrary.com/articles/phytochemical-analysis-and-antibacterial-activity-of-pepper-piper-nigrum-l-against-some-human-pathogens.pdf.

Gupta, A., Kumar, R., Kumar, S., & Pandey, A. K. (Eds.). (2017). Pharmacological aspects of *Terminalia belerica*. In *Molecular Biology and Pharmacognosy of Beneficial Plants* (pp. 52–64). Delhi: Lenin Media Private Limited.

Health Benefits Times.com. (2017, July 17). *Allspice facts and health benefits.* Health Benefits | Health Benefits of Foods and Drinks. Retrieved from https://www.healthbenefitstimes.com/allspice/.

Health Benefits Times. (2019, July 28). *Health benefits of Doctorbush (Plumbago zeylanica).* Health Benefits. Retrieved from https://www.healthbenefitstimes.com/doctorbush-plumbago-zeylanica/.

Jessica, W. (2020, December 5). *5 common herbs and spices to relieve stomach pain naturally.* Off The Grid News. Retrieved from https://www.offthegridnews.com/alternative-health/5-common-herbs-and-spices-to-relieve-stomach-pain-naturally/.

Link, R. (2018, October 15). *7 health benefits and uses of anise seed.* Healthline. Retrieved from https://www.healthline.com/nutrition/anise#TOC_TITLE_HDR_10.

Lobo, J., & Olsen, N. (2019, March 8). *5 homemade ayurvedic tonics that help calm your stomach ASAP.* Healthline. Retrieved from https://www.healthline.com/health/food-nutrition/ayurvedic-tonics-stomach-disorder.

Monica, B. (n.d.). *3 Ayurvedic remedies for tummy troubles.* HeyMonicaB. Retrieved from https://www.heymonicab.com/blog/3-ayurvedic-remedies-for-tummy-troubles.

Practo. (2017). *Stomach/abdominal pain: Causes, diagnosis, & treatment.* Retrieved from https://www.practo.com/health-wiki/stomach-abdominal-pain-causes-diagnosis-treatment/175/article.

RxList (Ed.). (2021, June 11). *Basil.* RxList. Retrieved from https://www.rxlist.com/basil/supplements.htm.

Srinivasamurthy, N. (2017, March 28). *Stomach pain—Know its Ayurvedic remedies!* Lybrate. Retrieved from https://www.lybrate.com/topic/stomach-pain-know-its-ayurvedic-remedies/e55c-77c56b0b6ad53d81e2b3d05773ac.

The Crankshaft Publishing. (n.d.). *Stomachache (Common Internal Medicine Disorders) (Chinese Medicine).* What-When-How.Com. Retrieved from http://what-when-how.com/chinese-medicine/stomachache-common-internal-medicine-disorders-chinese-medicine/.

Trust Herb. (2021, February 1). *5 health benefits of Amaltas.* Trust The Herb. Retrieved from https://trustherb.com/health-benefits-of-amaltas/.

WebMD (Ed.). (2009). *Bismuth subsalicylate oral: Uses, side effects, interactions, pictures, warnings & dosing—WebMD.* WebMD. Retrieved from https://www.webmd.com/drugs/2/drug-3596/bismuth-subsalicylate-oral/details.

WebMD (Ed.). (2017, May 25). *How to treat stomach pain in adults.* WebMD. Retrieved from https://www.webmd.com/first-aid/abdominal-pain-in-adults-treatment.

Yarlagadda, K. (2021, September 1). How to Make Your Own Rose Water for Beauty, Wellness, and Relaxation. Healthline. https://www.healthline.com/health/beauty-skin-care/how-to-make-rose-water

Constipation

Banyan Botanicals. (2021, February 2). *An Ayurvedic approach to constipation relief.* Retrieved from https://www.banyanbotanicals.com/info/ayurvedic-living/living-ayurveda/cleansing/an-ayurvedic-guide-to-healthy-elimination/an-ayurvedic-approach-to-constipation-relief/.

Basu, S. (2021, March 19). *Amaltas: Benefits, uses, formulations, ingredients, method, dosage and side effects.* Netmeds. Retrieved from https://www.netmeds.com/health-library/post/amaltas-benefits-uses-formulations-ingredients-method-dosage-and-side-effects.

Bolen, B., & Rufo, P. A. (2019, November 20). *How to use stimulant laxatives for constipation.* Verywell Health. Retrieved from https://www.verywellhealth.com/stimulant-laxatives-for-constipation-1944782.

Boyle, C. (2020, May 29). *Smooth moves: Yoga poses for constipation.* Healthline. Retrieved from https://www.healthline.com/health/fitness-exercise/yoga-for-constipation.

Brinckmann, J., & Smith, T. (n.d.). *Senna.* Herbalgram.Org. Retrieved from https://www.herbalgram.org/resources/herbalgram/issues/120/table-of-contents/hg120-herbpro-senna/.

Bruce, D. B. (2007, June 25). *How to safely use laxatives for constipation.* WebMD. Retrieved from https://www.webmd.com/digestive-disorders/laxatives-for-constipation-using-them-safely#1.

Cadman, B., & Wilson, D. R. (2020, January 2). *What makes moringa good for you?* Medical News Today. Retrieved from https://www.medicalnewstoday.com/articles/319916#_noHeaderPrefixedContent.

Cirino, E., & Luo, E. K. (2019, March 7). *How to make yourself poop.* Healthline. Retrieved from https://www.healthline.com/health/digestive-health/how-to-make-yourself-poop.

Cunha, J. P., & Marks, J. W. (2019, July 18). *Laxative types for constipation relief, weight loss & side effects.* MedicineNet. Retrieved from https://www.medicinenet.com/laxatives_for_constipation/article.htm.

Demers, C. (2020). *Ayurvedic tips for constipation.* Yoga International. Retrieved from https://yogainternational.com/article/view/ayurvedic-tips-for-constipation.

Drass, J. (2021, March 12). *The pros and cons of probiotics for kids.* Geisinger Health. Retrieved from https://www.geisinger.org/health-and-wellness/wellness-articles/2018/02/09/13/53/the-pros-and-cons-of-probiotics-for-kids.

Gajendran, D. (2015, August 28). *6 important acupressure points for treating constipation.* Modern Reflexology. Retrieved from https://www.modernreflexology.com/acupressure-points-for-constipation/.

Hirata, J. (2019, November 17). *How to relieve constipation naturally.* Vibrant Wellness Journal. Retrieved from https://vibrantwellnessjournal.com/2013/10/17/relieve-constipation-naturally/.

Johnson, J., & Wilson, D. R. (2018, July 30). *Nine herbal teas for constipation.* Medical News Today. Retrieved from https://www.medicalnewstoday.com/articles/322624.

Watson, S. (2019, March 8). *How to use castor oil to relieve constipation.* Healthline. Retrieved from https://www.healthline.com/health/digestive-health/castor-oil-for-constipation.

McDermott, A., & Choi, N. (2018, September 30). *What are bulk-forming laxatives?* Healthline. Retrieved from https://www.healthline.com/health/digestive-health/bulk-forming-laxatives.

Nogrady, B. (2015, October 9). *Chinese herbs bring relief from IBS constipation.* Family Practice News. Retrieved from https://www.mdedge.com/familymedicine/article/103449/gastroenterology/chinese-herbs-bring-relief-ibs-constipation.

Panoff, L., & Bjarnadottir, A. (2019, September 17). *8 surprising health benefits of coriander.* Healthline. Retrieved from https://www.healthline.com/nutrition/coriander-benefits.

Rana, S. (2018a, July 11). *8 effective remedies for constipation suggested by Ayurveda.* NDTV Food. Retrieved from https://food.ndtv.com/health/8-effective-remedies-for-constipation-suggested-by-ayurveda-1837216.

Rana, S. (2018b, September 8). *Triphala for constipation: How to use this Ayurveda wonder to manage digestive issues.* NDTV. Retrieved from https://www.ndtv.com/food/triphala-for-constipation-how-to-use-this-ayurveda-wonder-to-manage-digestive-issues-1912465.

Rodriguez, A. (2019, March 7). *Stool softeners vs. laxatives.* Healthline. Retrieved from https://www.healthline.com/health/constipation/stool-softeners-laxatives#types.

Schofield, K., & Wilson, D. R. (2017, November 19). *6 natural constipation remedies.* Healthline. Retrieved from https://www.healthline.com/health/6-natural-remedies-constipation.

Sharma, V. (2019, February 18). *10 best homeopathic medicines for constipation.* DrHomeo.Com: All About Homeopathy. Retrieved from https://www.drhomeo.com/constipation/homeopathic-medicine-constipation/.

Shefi, E., & Schoenbart, B. (2007, August 14). *How to treat constipation with traditional Chinese medicine.* HowStuffWorks. Retrieved from https://health.howstuffworks.com/wellness/natural-medicine/chinese/how-to-treat-constipation-with-traditional-chinese-medicine.htm.

Shukla, L. (2018, September 14). *Bottle gourd juice benefits, uses and side effects.* MyUpchar. Retrieved from https://www.myupchar.com/en/tips/lauki-juice-benefits-and-side-effects-in-hindi.

Streit, L. (2019, November 14). *5 emerging benefits and uses of chicory root fiber.* Healthline. Retrieved from https://www.healthline.com/nutrition/chicory-root-fiber.

WebMD (Ed.). (2014). *Bael.* WebMD. Retrieved from https://www.webmd.com/vitamins/ai/ingredientmono-164/bael.

WebMD (Ed.). (2013). *Mineral oil laxative oral: Uses, side effects, interactions, pictures, warnings & dosing—WebMD.* WebMD. Retrieved from https://www.webmd.com/drugs/2/drug-153865/mineral-oil-laxative-oral/details.

WebMD (Ed.). (2015). *Adult probiotic oral: Uses, side effects, interactions, pictures, warnings & dosing.* WebMD. Retrieved from https://www.webmd.com/drugs/2/drug-163888/adult-probiotic-oral/details.

West, H., & Sethi, S. (2020, July 15). *13 home remedies for constipation.* Medical News Today. Retrieved from https://www.medicalnewstoday.com/articles/318694.

Diarrhea

Alter, T. (n.d.). *Herbal and Ayurvedic treatment for diarrhea.* Street Directory. Retrieved from https://www.streetdirectory.com/travel_guide/110901/alternative_medicine/herbal_and_ayurvedic_treatment_for_diarrhea.html.

Ambardekar, N. (2019, August 6). *Understanding diarrhea treatment.* WebMD. Retrieved from https://www.webmd.com/digestive-disorders/understanding-diarrhea-treatment#1.

Atanu, F. O., Ebiloma, U. G., & Ajayi, E. I. (2011). A review of the pharmacological aspects of *Solanum nigrum* Linn. *Biotechnology and Molecular Biology Review, 06*(01), 01–07. Retrieved from https://academicjournals.org/journal/BMBR/article-full-text-pdf/0E4825611574.

Banyan Botanicals. (2020, September 24). *An Ayurvedic approach to diarrhea relief.* Retrieved from https://www.banyanbotanicals.com/info/ayurvedic-living/living-ayurveda/cleansing/an-ayurvedic-guide-to-healthy-elimination/an-ayurvedic-approach-to-diarrhea-relief/.

Charoensiddhi, S., & Anprung, P. (2008). Bioactive compounds and volatile compounds of Thai bael fruit (*Aegle marmelos* (L.) Correa) as a valuable source for functional food ingredients. *International Food Research Journal, 15*(03), 287–295. Retrieved from http://ifrj.upm.edu.my/15%20(3)%202008/06.%20Suvimol%20C.pdf.

Dharmananda, S. (2010, July). *Treatment of chronic diarrhea with Chinese herbs and oriental diet therapy.* Institute of Traditional Medicine. Retrieved from http://www.itmonline.org/articles/diarrhea/diarrhea.htm.

Ecklund, L. L. (2020, December 11). *Treating children with traditional Chinese medicine.* Pacific College. Retrieved from https://www.pacificcollege.edu/news/blog/2014/06/27/treating-children-with-traditional-chinese-medicine.

Freedom Chinese Medicine. (2018, January 10). *Medicinal foods for loose stools or diarrhea.* Retrieved from https://freedomchinesemedicine.com/medicinal-foods-loose-stools-diarrhea/.

Gajendran, D. (2016, June 23). *Best acupressure points to treat diarrhea for immediate relief.* Modern Reflexology. Retrieved from https://www.modernreflexology.com/acupressure-points-for-diarrhea/.

Guandalini, S., Frye, R. E., & Tamer, M. A. (2021, January 31). *Diarrhea treatment & management: Medical care, consultations, diet.* Medspace. Retrieved from https://emedicine.medscape.com/article/928598-treatment.

Healthcare Medicine Institute. (2020, June 20). *Chinese herb & acupuncture clear ulcerative colitis research.* HealthCMi. Retrieved from https://www.healthcmi.com/Acupuncture-Continuing-Education-News/814-ulcerativecolitis67.

Madormo, C. (2021, March 30). *9 home remedies for diarrhea.* The Healthy. Retrieved from https://www.thehealthy.com/digestive-health/diarrhea/home-remedies-diarrhea/.

Mayo Clinic Staff. (2020, June 16). *Diarrhea—Symptoms and causes.* Mayo Clinic. Retrieved from https://www.mayoclinic.org/diseases-conditions/diarrhea/symptoms-causes/syc-20352241.

National Institute for Health and Care Excellence. (2021). *Diarrhoea and vomiting.* NICE. Retrieved from https://www.nice.org.uk/guidance/conditions-and-diseases/digestive-tract-conditions/diarrhoea-and-vomiting.

Negi. (2020, August 26). *10 amazing health benefits of buttermilk (Chaas).* Amritsr: The Maharaja of Indian Cuisine. Retrieved from https://amritsruae.com/blog/health-benefits-of-buttermilk/.

Ogbru, O., & Marks, J. W. (2019, December 12). *Anticholinergic, antispasmodic drug names, uses, side effects.* MedicineNet. Retrieved from https://www.medicinenet.com/anticholinergics-antispasmodics-oral/article.htm.

Spritzler, F. (2018, September 6). *8 science-based health benefits of coconut water.* Healthline. Retrieved from https://www.healthline.com/nutrition/8-coconut-water-benefits.

Sturluson, T. (2019, July 31). *Medicinal herbs for diarrhea treatment and relief.* The Herbal Resource. Retrieved from https://www.herbal-supplement-resource.com/diarrhea-natural-herbs.html.

Sugimoto, S., Naganuma, M., Kiyohara, H., Arai, M., Ono, K., Mori, K., et al. (2016). Clinical efficacy and safety of oral Qing-Dai in patients with ulcerative colitis: A single-center open-label prospective study. *Digestion, 93*(3), 193–201. Retrieved from https://doi.org/10.1159/000444217.

Taste for Life (Ed.). (n.d.). *Natural home remedies for diarrhea.* Taste for Life. Retrieved from https://tasteforlife.com/conditions-wellness/digestion/diarrhea-natural-remedies.

The Miracle of Essential Oils Editorial Staff. (2018, September 28). *7 best essential oils for diarrhea & how to use.* The Miracle of Essential Oils. Retrieved from https://www.themiracleofessentialoils.com/essential-oils-for-diarrhea/.

Times of India. (2019, August 21). *Home remedies for diarrhea.* The Times of India. Retrieved from https://timesofindia.indiatimes.com/life-style/health-fitness/home-remedies/home-remedies-for-diarrhea/articleshow/33073000.cms.

Ullman, D. (1992). Homeopathic medicines for diarrhea. In *Homeopathic medicine for children and infants* (pp. 15–32). TarcherPerigee. Retrieved from https://homeopathic.com/homeopathic-medicines-for-diarrhea/.

Walt, R., & Campbell, E. (2011). Antimotility and antisecretory drugs. In A. Evers, M. Maze, & E. Kharasch (Eds.), *Anesthetic pharmacology: Basic principles and clinical practice* (pp. 842–854). Cambridge: Cambridge University Press. doi:10.1017/CBO9780511781933.054.

Wang, X., & Wu, H. (2010). How do you treat constipation and diarrhea in your practice? *Medical Acupuncture, 22*(01), 5–10. Retrieved from https://doi.org/10.1089/acu.2009.2008.

Weil, A. A. (2020). Approach to the patient with diarrhea. In J. B. Harris & R. C. LaRocque (Eds.), *Hunter's tropical medicine and emerging infectious diseases* (10th ed., pp. 172–177). Philadelphia: Elsevier. Retrieved from https://doi.org/10.1016/B978-0-323-55512-8.00022-3.

Wong, C., & Syn, M. (2020, September 29). *Bael fruit nutrition facts and health benefits.* Verywell Fit. Retrieved from https://www.verywellfit.com/the-health-benefits-of-bael-fruit-89602.

World Health Organization. (‚Äé2005)‚Äé. *The treatment of diarrhoea: A manual for physicians and other senior health workers, 4th rev.* World Health Organization. Retrieved from https://apps.who.int/iris/handle/10665/43209.

Irritable Bowel Syndrome (IBS)

5 Ways to Treat Symptoms of IBS. (2020, August 7). Ayurherbs clinic Melbourne. Retrieved from https://www.ayurherbs.com.au/5-ways-to-treat-symptoms-of-ibs/.

Ambulkar, P. (2016, September 5). *Prikkelbaar darm syndroom (PDS).* Het Ayurveda Institute. Retrieved from https://www.ayurvedainstituut.com/en/prikkelbaar-darm-syndroom-pds-ayurveda.

Bhargava, H. D. (2020, June 16). *Irritable bowel syndrome.* WebMD. Retrieved from https://www.webmd.com/ibs/guide/digestive-diseases-irritable-bowel-syndrome#1.

California College of Ayurveda Students. (2014, June 16). *Irritable bowel syndrome: The Ayurvedic approach by Branislava Petric.* California College of Ayurveda. Retrieved from https://www.ayurvedacollege.com/blog/ibs/.

Christen, M. (1990). Action of pinaverium bromide, a calcium-antagonist, on gastrointestinal motility disorders. *General Pharmacology: The Vascular System, 21*(6), 821–825. Retrieved from https://doi.org/10.1016/0306-3623(90)90439-s.

Colino, S. (2011, January 4). *5 stomach-soothing herbs and spices.* Live Right Live Well/Health24. Retrieved from https://www.news24.com/health24/Natural/Natural-living/5-stomach-soothing-herbs-and-spices-20120721.

DrugBank Online. (2015, September 15). *Trimebutine: Uses, interactions, mechanism of action.* Retrieved from https://go.drugbank.com/drugs/DB09089.

Gastrointestinal Society. (2020, April 14). *Chinese medicine alleviates irritable bowel syndrome (IBS).* Retrieved from https://badgut.org/information-centre/a-z-digestive-topics/chinese-medicine-alleviates-ibs/.

Herndon, J. (2019, March 8). *Everything you want to know about IBS.* Healthline. Retrieved from https://www.healthline.com/health/irritable-bowel-syndrome#ibs-diet.

Khandelwal, P. (2016, March 29). *What Ayurveda says about irritable bowel syndrome (IBS)?* Practo. Retrieved from https://www.practo.com/healthfeed/what-ayurveda-says-about-irritable-bowel-syndrome-ibs-10392/post.

Khatri, M. (2019, August 30). *Alternative treatments for irritable bowel syndrome (IBS).* WebMD. Retrieved from https://www.webmd.com/ibs/alternative-therapies#1.

Lacy, B. E., Weiser, K., & de Lee, R. (2009). Review: The treatment of irritable bowel syndrome. *Therapeutic Advances in Gastroenterology, 2*(4), 221–238. Retrieved from https://doi.org/10.1177/1756283x09104794.

Mayo Clinic Staff. (2020, October 15). *Irritable bowel syndrome.* Mayo Clinic. Retrieved from https://www.mayoclinic.org/diseases-conditions/irritable-bowel-syndrome/diagnosis-treatment/drc-20360064.

Monash University. (n.d.). *High and low FODMAP foods.* Retrieved from https://www.monashfodmap.com/about-fodmap-and-ibs/high-and-low-fodmap-foods/.

Rajan, S. (2018, April 11). *7 herbal remedies for IBS.* Z Living. Retrieved from https://www.zliving.com/health/complementary-alternative-medicine/ibs-7-herbal-remedies-for-ibs-98471/.

Rawls, B. (2018, July 9). *Irritable bowel syndrome natural remedies that work.* RawlsMD. Retrieved from https://rawlsmd.com/health-articles/irritable-bowel-syndrome-natural-remedies-that-work.

Sanger, G. J., & Quigley, E. M. (2010). Constipation, IBs and the 5-HT4 receptor: What role for prucalopride? *Clinical Medicine. Gastroenterology, 3,* CGast.S4136. Retrieved from https://doi.org/10.4137/cgast.s4136.

Scottish Government National Health Service. (2020, February 14). *Irritable bowel syndrome (IBS).* NHS Inform. Retrieved from https://www.nhsinform.scot/illnesses-and-conditions/stomach-liver-and-gastrointestinal-tract/irritable-bowel-syndrome-ibs.

Shen, Y. A., & Nahas, R. (2009). Complementary and alternative medicine for treatment of irritable bowel syndrome. *Canadian Family Physician, 55*(02), 143–148. Retrieved from https://www.ncbi.nlm.nih.gov/pmc/articles/PMC2642499/.

Wheat, C. (2018, June 22). *My 5 top herbs for IBS (that don't include ginger or mint!).* Health Union. Retrieved from https://irritablebowelsyndrome.net/living/top-herbs.

Acid Reflux

Arnarson, A. (2017, January 22). *14 ways to prevent heartburn and acid reflux.* Healthline. Retrieved from https://www.healthline.com/nutrition/heartburn-acid-reflux-remedies.

Bhargava, H. D. (2000, November 2). *Get the facts about gastroesophageal reflux disease (GERD).* WebMD. Retrieved from https://www.webmd.com/heartburn-gerd/guide/reflux-disease-gerd-1.

Cleveland Clinic Medical Professional. (2020, January 22). *Heartburn: Causes, symptoms & treatment.* Cleveland Clinic. Retrieved from https://my.clevelandclinic.org/health/diseases/9617-heartburn-overview.

Dharmananda, S. (2010, July). *Treatment of chronic diarrhea with Chinese herbs and oriental diet therapy.* Institute for Traditional Medicine. Retrieved from http://www.itmonline.org/articles/diarrhea/diarrhea.htm.

Diamond, L. (2021, June 28). *8 home remedies for GERD and heartburn your stomach will thank you for.* The Healthy. Retrieved from https://www.thehealthy.com/digestive-health/heartburn-gerd/gerd-home-remedies/.

Fanous, S. (2020, August 28). *7 amazing uses for aloe vera*. Healthline. Retrieved from https://www.healthline.com/health/7-amazing-uses-aloe-vera.

Gao, X., Wang, W., Wei, S., & Li, W. (2009). Review of pharmacological effects of Glycyrrhiza radix and its bioactive compounds. *Zhongguo Zhong yao za zhi = Zhongguo zhongyao zazhi = China Journal of Chinese Materia Medica*, 34(21), 2695–2700.

Grant, A. (2020, November 16). *Red raspberry herbal use—How to harvest raspberry leaf for tea*. Gardeningknowhow.com. Retrieved from https://www.gardeningknowhow.com/edible/fruits/raspberry/harvest-raspberry-leaf-for-tea.htm.

Haider, P. (2015, January 13). *10 health benefits of Bermuda grass juice*. Linkedin. Retrieved from https://www.linkedin.com/pulse/10-health-benefits-bermuda-grass-juice-dr-paul-haider/.

Hamilton, A. (n.d.). *Fermented blackberry leaf tea*. The Other Andy Milton. Retrieved from https://www.theotherandyhamilton.com/fermented-blackberry-leaf-tea/.

Health Benefits Times. (2018, August 9). *Bermuda Grass facts and health benefits*. Health Benefits. Retrieved from https://www.healthbenefitstimes.com/bermuda-grass/.

Holland, K. (2018, November 2). *Can essential oils relieve the symptoms of heartburn?* Healthline. Retrieved from https://www.healthline.com/health/digestive-health/essential-oils-for-heartburn.

Mayo Clinic Staff. (2020a, April 17). *Heartburn—Diagnosis and treatment*. Mayo Clinic. Retrieved from https://www.mayoclinic.org/diseases-conditions/heartburn/diagnosis-treatment/drc-20373229.

Mayo Clinic Staff. (2020b, May 22). *Gastroesophageal reflux disease (GERD)—Diagnosis and treatment*. Mayo Clinic. Retrieved from https://www.mayoclinic.org/diseases-conditions/gerd/diagnosis-treatment/drc-20361959.

McGrane, K. (2020, June 12). *What are Licorice root's benefits and downsides?* Healthline. Retrieved from https://www.healthline.com/nutrition/licorice-root#uses.

NDTV Food. (2020, November 24). *12 amazing home remedies for acidity: Easy tips to reduce the pain*. Retrieved from https://food.ndtv.com/health/12-amazing-home-remedies-for-acidity-1449021.

Sweet, J. (2020, January 17). *Essential oils for heartburn and acid reflux to relieve chest pain*. Woman's World. Retrieved from https://www.womansworld.com/posts/health/essential-oils-for-heartburn-158786.

The Healthline Editorial Team. (2019, March 22). *Everything you need to know about acid reflux and GERD*. Healthline. Retrieved from https://www.healthline.com/health/gerd.

Ullman, D. (2017, January 23). *Homeopathic medicines for indigestion, gas, and heartburn: Natural remedies you can stomach*. Homeopathic. Com. Retrieved from https://homeopathic.com/homeopathic-medicines-for-indigestion-gas-and-heartburn-natural-remedies-you-can-stomach/.

Gas/Wind and Bloating

Dabcevic, M. (2020, December 28). *5 Chinese herbs to power up your digestion*. Mind Body Green. Retrieved from https://www.mindbodygreen.com/0-25201/5-chinese-herbs-to-power-up-your-digestion.html.

Great Secret of Life. (n.d.). *Water chestnut barley drink—Barley water chestnut drink*. Great Secret of Life—Tasty Recipes. Retrieved from https://www.great-secret-of-life.com/2013/07/water-chestnut-barley-drink-barley.html.

Jaret, P. (2010, March 23). *Bloating 101: Why you feel bloated*. WebMD. Retrieved from https://www.webmd.com/digestive-disorders/features/bloated-bloating.

Jiva Ayurveda. (2019, June 3). *Excessive belching embarrassing you? Try these home remedies for relief*. Retrieved from https://store.jiva.com/excessive-belching-embarrassing-you-try-these-home-remedies-for-relief/.

Keshavarz, A., Minaiyan, M., Ghannadi, A., & Mahzouni, P. (2013). Effects of *Carum carvi* L. (Caraway) extract and essential oil on TNBS-induced colitis in rats. *Research in Pharmaceutical Sciences*, 8(1), 1–8. Retrieved from https://www.ncbi.nlm.nih.gov/pmc/articles/PMC3895295/#__ffn_sectitle.

Landon, R. [Rommel Landon]. (2013, April 11). *8 treasures Qigong Part I* [Video]. YouTube. Retrieved from https://www.youtube.com/watch?v=madK_R7C78c.

Lockett, E. (2020, November 9). *5 acupressure points for gas and bloating*. Healthline. Retrieved from https://www.healthline.com/health/acupressure-points-for-gas.

Marcene, B. (2020, July 4). *30 essential oil benefits and uses*. Natural Food Series. Retrieved from https://www.naturalfoodseries.com/30-essential-oil-benefits-uses/.

Marks, J. W., & Shiel, W. C. (2019, September 11). *How to get rid of intestinal gas pain: Causes, symptoms & treatment*. MedicineNet. Retrieved from https://www.medicinenet.com/intestinal_gas_belching_bloating_flatulence/article.htm.

McGrane, K., & Hatanaka, M. (2020, February 4). *All you need to know about dill*. Healthline. Retrieved from https://www.healthline.com/nutrition/dill.

Me & Qi. (2021a). *Poria-cocos mushrooms (Fu Ling)*. Retrieved from https://www.meandqi.com/herb-database/poria-cocos-mushroom.

Me & Qi. (2021b). *Radish seeds (Lai Fu Zi)*. Retrieved from https://www.meandqi.com/herb-database/radish-seeds.

Nagdeve, M. (2021, July 21). *7 surprising benefits of pickles*. Organic Facts. Retrieved from https://www.organicfacts.net/health-benefits/other/health-benefits-of-pickles.html.

Ni, M. S. (2016). *Gas & flatulence relief: Diet, herbs, self-acupressure*. Natural-Treatments-For.Com. Retrieved from http://www.natural-treatments-for.com/natural-treatments-for-flatulence.html.

Shiel, W. C. (2019, October 9). *Intestinal gas: Symptoms, signs, causes & treatment*. MedicineNet. Retrieved from https://www.medicinenet.com/gas/symptoms.htm.

Souter, K. (2021). *Digestive problems*. Homeopathy UK. Retrieved from https://homeopathy-uk.org/homeopathy/how-homeopathy-helps/conditions/digestive-problems.

WebMD (Ed.). (2016). *Bay leaf*. WebMD. Retrieved from https://www.webmd.com/vitamins/ai/ingredientmono-685/bay-leaf.

Women's Weekly Diet & Nutrition. (2020, January 29). *10 herbal teas to beat the festive bloat*. Women's Weekly. Retrieved from https://www.womensweekly.com.sg/gallery/beauty-and-health/diet-and-nutrition/10-herbal-teas-beat-festive-bloat-chinese-new-year/.

Hemorrhoids (Piles)

Ayurdhamah, A. (2018, March 23). *Ways to treat piles with herbal remedies and naturals solutions*. Medium. Retrieved from https://medium.com/

Digestive Health Team. (2020, October 16). *5 simple ways you can prevent hemorrhoids*. Health Essentials from Cleveland Clinic. Retrieved from https://health.clevelandclinic.org/5-simple-ways-you-can-prevent-hemorrhoids/.

Gotter, A. (2017, April 19). *8 home remedies for hemorrhoids*. Healthline. Retrieved from https://www.healthline.com/health/home-remedies-for-hemorrhoids.

Gotter, A. (2019, March 27). *Ayurvedic treatment for piles (Hemorrhoids)*. Healthline. Retrieved from https://www.healthline.com/health/ayurvedic-treatment-for-piles.

Health Benefits Times (Ed.). (2019, August 19). *Elephant Yam facts and health benefits*. Health Benefits. Retrieved from https://www.healthbenefitstimes.com/elephant-yam/.

Jiva Ayurveda (Ed.). (2021). *Best Ayurvedic treatment for piles: Fistula, Fissure & Ano Medicines*. Jiva Ayurveda. Retrieved from https://www.jiva.com/diseases/digestive/ano-rectal.

Kahn, A. (2018, February 26). *Bleeding disorders*. Healthline. Retrieved from https://www.healthline.com/health/bleeding-disorders.

Kahn, A., & Jewell, T. (2021, January 5). *Hemorrhoids*. Healthline. Retrieved from https://www.healthline.com/health/hemorrhoids.

Kivi, R. (2019, December 24). *What you need to know about fecal incontinence*. Healthline. Retrieved from https://www.healthline.com/health/bowel-incontinence.

Kshar Sutra Therapy. (2021). *Kshar Sutra therapy: Best treatment for piles, fissure, fistula & pilonidal sinus*. Retrieved from https://www.ksharsutratherapy.com/.

Nall, R. (2019, July 11). *Everything you need to know about anal itching*. Healthline. Retrieved from https://www.healthline.com/health/itchy-anus.

NHS website. (2018a, August 9). *Local anaesthesia*. NHS.UK. Retrieved from https://www.nhs.uk/conditions/local-anaesthesia/.

NHS website. (2018b, August 22). *How to get more fibre into your diet*. NHS.UK. Retrieved from https://www.nhs.uk/live-well/eat-well/how-to-get-more-fibre-into-your-diet/.

NHS website. (2018c, December 17). *Ultrasound scan*. NHS.UK. Retrieved from https://www.nhs.uk/conditions/ultrasound-scan/.

NHS website. (2019, August 14). *Water, drinks and your health*. NHS.UK. Retrieved from https://www.nhs.uk/live-well/eat-well/water-drinks-nutrition/.

NHS website. (2021a, February 17). *Paracetamol for adults*. NHS.UK. Retrieved from https://www.nhs.uk/medicines/paracetamol-for-adults/.

NHS website. (2021b, April 13). *Constipation*. NHS.UK. Retrieved from https://www.nhs.uk/conditions/constipation/.

NHS website. (2021c, July 2). *General anaesthesia*. NHS.UK. Retrieved from https://www.nhs.uk/conditions/general-anaesthesia/.

Progressive Health. (2018, November 22). *Best ointment for hemorrhoids*. ProgressiveHealth.Com. Retrieved from https://www.progressivehealth.com/hemorrhoid-ointment.htm.

Progressive Health. (2020a, March 6). *Oat straw effective for hemorrhoids*. ProgressiveHealth.Com. Retrieved from https://www.progressivehealth.com/oat-straw-and-hemorrhoids.htm.

Progressive Health. (2020b, August 8). *Chinese medicine for hemorrhoids*. ProgressiveHealth.Com. Retrieved from https://www.progressivehealth.com/hemorrhoids-chinese-medicine.htm.

Progressive Health Editorial Staff. (2020c, August 8). *Traditional Chinese medicine for anal itching*. ProgressiveHealth.Com. Retrieved from https://www.progressivehealth.com/hemorrhoids-chinese-medicine.htm.

Roth, E. (2019, June 10). *Blood thinners for heart disease*. Healthline. Retrieved from https://www.healthline.com/health/heart-disease/blood-thinners.

Sanchez, C., & Chinn, B. (2011). Hemorrhoids. *Clinics in Colon and Rectal Surgery, 24*(01), 005–013. Retrieved from https://doi.org/10.1055/s-0031-1272818.

Stang, D. (2019, March 8). *Hemorrhoid surgery*. Healthline. Retrieved from https://www.healthline.com/health/hemorrhoid-surgery.

TCM Simple (Ed.). (n.d.). *Chinese medicine treatment for hemorrhoids (piles)*. Tcmsimple.Com. Retrieved from https://www.tcmsimple.com/hemorrhoids.php.

Villalba, H., & Abbas, M. (2007). Hemorrhoids: modern remedies for an ancient disease. *The Permanente Journal, 11*(02), 74–76. Retrieved from https://doi.org/10.7812/tpp/06-156.

WebMD (Ed.). (n.d.). Black Nightshade: Overview, uses, side effects, precautions, interactions, dosing and reviews. *WebMD*. Retrieved from https://www.webmd.com/vitamins/ai/ingredientmono-821/black-nightshade.

Gallstones

All Ayurveda (Ed.). (2018). *Gallstones*. All Ayurveda. Retrieved from https://allayurveda.com/kb/gallstones/.

Chen, Q., Zhang, Y., Li, S., Chen, S., Lin, X., Li, C., & Asakawa, T. (2019). Mechanisms underlying the prevention and treatment of cholelithiasis using traditional Chinese medicine. *Evidence-Based Complementary and Alternative Medicine, 2019*, 1–9. Retrieved from https://doi.org/10.1155/2019/2536452.

Dharmananda, S. (2001, August). *Treatment of gallstones with Chinese herbs and acupuncture*. Institute for Traditional Medicine. Retrieved from http://www.itmonline.org/arts/gallstones.htm.

Gogia, V. (2018, March 9). *Bid goodbye to gallstones with these 3 simple yoga poses*. Only My Health. Retrieved from https://www.onlymyhealth.com/bid-good-bye-to-gallstones-three-simple-yoga-poses-1273558322.

Khatri, M. (2021, April 22). *Prevention of gallstones*. WebMD. Retrieved from https://www.webmd.com/digestive-disorders/understanding-gallstones-prevention.

Macon, B. L., & Rogers, G. (2019, March 22). *Understanding gallstones: Types, pain, and more*. Healthline. Retrieved from https://www.healthline.com/health/gallstones.

NHS website. (2019, August 15). *Acute cholecystitis*. NHS.UK. Retrieved from https://www.nhs.uk/conditions/acute-cholecystitis/.

NHS website. (2020, November 16). *Gallstones*. NHS.UK. Retrieved from https://www.nhs.uk/conditions/gallstones/.

Taylor, T. (2020, August 2). *Gallbladder*. Innerbody Research. Retrieved from https://www.innerbody.com/image_digeov/dige04-new.html#continued.

WebMD (Ed.). (2010). *Chicory*. WebMD. Retrieved from https://www.webmd.com/vitamins/ai/ingredientmono-92/chicory.

Yan, C. (2013). *Chinese medicine preparation for treating gall-stone (CN102178889A)*. China. Retrieved from https://patents.google.com/patent/CN102178889A/en.

4

Renal System

Introduction

Kidney problems are usually secondary to other underlying primary diseases such as cardiovascular diseases, hypertension, diabetes, autoimmune disorders (e.g., SLE/lupus), or chronic infections. Other factors such as genetics, diet, and environment may also contribute.

Some of the kidney problems discussed include:
1. Kidney stones
2. Urinary tract infection (UTI)
3. Chronic kidney failure (CKF)
4. Urinary incontinence

Kidney Stones

Kidney stones (also called renal calculi or urolithiasis) are more common in males. They usually present with pain during urination (dysuria), blood in urine (hematuria), back or abdominal pain, nausea or vomiting or fever with chills (if associated urine infection). Small stones may be asymptomatic or found incidentally during imaging. They can be found in the kidneys, ureters, or bladder.

Risk factors include obesity, inadequate fluid intake, dehydration, family or personal history of stones, high protein, salt or oxalate diet, previous intestinal bypass surgery, history of polycystic kidney disease, metabolic disorders (like renal tubular acidosis, hyperuricemia), hyperparathyroidism states, medication use (thiazide diuretics, calcium or vitamin D supplements, and antiepileptic drugs like topiramate or levetiracetam). Geographical and regional variability of kidney stones are also prevalent in various countries.

Kidney stones are classified based on the type of crystals of which they are made: .
- **Calcium stones.** They are the most common and they occur as calcium phosphate or calcium oxalate stones.
- **Uric acid stones.** They occur usually in hyperuricemia (genetic or from a high-protein diet, malabsorption, chronic diarrhea, and gout). Uric acid stones form when urine is too acidic due to high amounts of uric acid in the urine.
- **Struvite stones.** They often form due to an infection such as UTIs or kidney infections. They are large stones that are made of calcium, phosphate, magnesium, and ammonium.
- **Cystine stones.** They are rare and occur in cystinuria, a genetic disorder that often affects the transport of cystine in the body, resulting in excess cystine in the urine and the formation of cystine stones.

Tests include abdominal ultrasound, urine exam, blood tests, plain abdominal x-ray, and sometimes CT abdomen with contrast or stone analysis.

Indian Natural Remedies

Kidney stones or renal calculi (*Mutrashmari*, in Sanskrit) occur due to an imbalance of Vata and Kapha dosha. This imbalance causes obstruction (*Sanga*) in the urinary tract (*Mutravaha Srotas*) and leads to urination problems. There are many herbs that have diuretic (*Mutral*) and Vata-Kapha balancing effects.

Common Ingredients for Kidney Stones

Spices	Herbs/Leaves	Miscellaneous
Anise (*Pimpinella anisum*)	Shilapushpa (*Didymocarpus pedicellata*)	Fig
Arugampul/dhoob (*Cynodon dactylon*)	Punarnava (*Boerhavia diffusa*)	Salt
Black peppercorn (*Piper nigrum*)	Pashanabheda/Pakhanbed ka Beeda (*Bergenia ligulata*)	Tomato (*Solanum lycopersicum*)
Cardamom	Prajmoda/parsley	Honey
Cinnamon	Ashwagandha/winter cherry (*Withania somnifera*)	Banana stem
Coriander seeds	Picrorhiza (*Picrorhiza kurroa*)	Dates
Fenugreek	Boerhavia (*Boerhavia diffusa*)	Pineapple

Spices	Herbs/Leaves	Miscellaneous
Gokshura/bindii (*Tribulus terrestris*)	Varuna (*Crataeva nurvala*)	Coconut water
Kalonji (*Nigella sativa*)	Keelanelli/Gale of the wind (*Phyllanthus niruri*)	Bottle gourd (*soraka/sorakkai*)
Kollu/Horse gram (*Macrotyloma uniflorum*)	Tulsi/holy basil	Lemon
Manjistha (*Rubia cordifolia*)	Patharchatta/Katti Pottal (*Bryophyllum Pinnatum*)	Turnip
	Sweet broom	Bakul
	Ashoka (*Saraca asoca*)	Jasmine (*Jasminum auriculatum*)
	Guduchi	
	Basil	
	Moringa oleifera	
	Kantakari (*Solanum xanthocarpum*)	
	Aerva lanata	
	Bakul (*Mimusops elengi*)	
	Hairy rupturewort (*Herniaria hirsuta*)	
	Khella (*Ammi visnaga*)	
	Keelanelli	
Nutmeg	Gokshura/Small caltrops	Kidney beans (*Phaseolus vulgaris*)
Onion	Bearberry/uva ursi (*Arctostaphylos uva-ursi*)	Pomegranate
Radish seed	Shatavari (*Asparagus racemosus*)	Lady's finger/okra (*Abelmoschus esculentus*)

Common Recipes

Oral

Teas/Brews

Aerva lanata. Take a large handful of fresh sprigs with the flowers and leaves. Wash and air dry for a few days. Store them. Take a few dried sprigs. Add 1 to 2 cups of water and simmer for 10 to 15 minutes. Strain and consume 1 cup daily.
Tea bags with the dried leaves are also available.

Anise tea. Add anise to boiling water and steep for about 15 minutes. Strain the mixture before adding honey to taste. Serve it hot.

Amla juice. Lightly pound three to four amla fruits. Strain and add a pinch of turmeric. Mix well and drink 20 mL of juice in the morning on an empty stomach.

Arugampul juice. Take one to two handfuls of fresh-washed arugampul (roots removed) and a few neem leaves. Add some water or coconut water and blend. Strain and drink fresh first thing in the morning on an empty stomach.

Ashoka bark. Take 1 to 2 teaspoons of the bark powder and drink with a glass of water daily.

Bakul. Take 1 to 2 g of dried flowers and add 50 to 60 mL water. Make a cold decoction. Consume 40 to 50 mL daily.

Banana stem juice. Cut the stem of the banana plant and soak in water for an hour to soften. Cut the soaked stem into smaller pieces and place into a blender. Blend until smooth. Strain the mixture and mix in 1 teaspoon of cardamom powder. Add honey to taste. Drink twice a day on an empty stomach or 10 minutes before food.

Basil paste. Take five to seven basil leaves and wash them. Cut into smaller pieces and lightly pound to extract the juice. Mix about 1 tablespoon of the juice with some honey to make a paste. Take it once a day in the morning for 6 months. Alternatively, fresh basil leaves can also be chewed.

Basil juice. Consume water infused with basil juice.

Cardamom tea. Lightly pound black to two black cardamom. Add 1 cup of hot water. Allow to steep for 5 to 10 minutes. Strain and drink warm.

Cinnamon tea. Add one cinnamon stick to a cup and pour boiling water over it. Allow it to steep for about 10 minutes. Add honey to taste. Drink in the morning on an empty stomach.

Coconut water. Drink a cup of coconut water from a young, raw green coconut once a day.

Coriander water. Soak some coriander seeds overnight in a glass of water. Consume early in the morning or twice a day.
Variation #1. Take ½ to 1 teaspoon of coriander powder. Add a glass of water. Consume early in the morning or twice a day.
Variation #2. Take ½ teaspoon of coriander powder with water.

Dates. Soak a few dates in water overnight. Consume the dates and water in the morning.

Fenugreek brew. Lightly roast some fenugreek seeds and grind into a fine powder. Mix one teaspoon of the powder in 1 cup of warm water. Drink in the morning on an empty stomach. Alternatively, soak some seeds in water overnight. Drink the water the next morning and chew on the seeds.

Fig brew. Place two figs into a pot of water. Bring to a boil and allow to simmer over low heat for about 10 minutes. Drink the liquid in the morning on an empty stomach once a day.

Gokshura. Take 3 to 6 g of gokshura powder. Mix with 1 teaspoon of honey. Consume daily. Capsules are also available.

Guduchi juice. Place a handful of fresh guduchi leaves in a blender and blend until smooth. Strain and add honey to taste. Drink this daily in the morning on an empty stomach.

Herb mix. Take about 10 g of powdered varun/varuna, 10 g of powdered Bermuda grass, and 10 g of powdered horse gram. Mix this with water and drink three to four times a day.

Jasmine. Make a decoction from the root or flowers of the jasmine. Consume 50 to 60 mL.

Kalonji. It can be eaten raw or mixed with water. Take ¼ to ½ teaspoon of kalongi's seeds. Then add 1 glass of water. Soak overnight. Strain and drink the kalonji water in the morning.

> Variation #1. Swallow a few kalonji seeds with warm water.

> Variation #2. It can be lightly roasted and then used whole or ground and added to bread dough curry or cereal.

Kantakari. Take ½ teaspoon of kantakari powder. Add some water and honey. Consume twice a day.

Keelanelli juice. Blend the leaves and make fresh juice. Drink 15 to 20 mL (2 to 4 teaspoons) daily on an empty stomach with a glass of water before breakfast. Powders and capsules are also available.

Khella tea. Take 1 teaspoon powdered khella fruit (or crushed seeds). Add 1 cup of boiling water. Steep for 10 to 15 minutes. If crushed seeds are used, infuse longer.

Kidney bean brew. Soak the kidney beans overnight. Boil or cook the soaked red kidney beans in a pressure cooker until soft. Strain and drink the broth of the cooked kidney beans. Consume the broth several times a day. The cooked beans and the broth with added spices can also be eaten with rice as a dhal or a lentil dish.

Kollu. The grains are soaked and then cooked until soft. It is added to soups or mixed with rice or curries.

Kollu (Horse gram) soup. Add 1 cup of horse gram to half a liter of water in a pot. Boil until the water is reduced to ⅓ of the original volume. Strain and cool the mixture completely. Drink this mixture every day.

Kushmanda juice. Cut a slice of the fruit and remove the peel. Cut into small pieces and blend. Blend until smooth, gradually adding up to 1 cup of water. Strain and drink.

Lady's finger juice. Cut three to four fresh lady's fingers into smaller pieces. Soak in water overnight. Squeeze out the pulp of the lady's fingers and mix into a cup of water. Drink three times a day. It can also be included in the diet.

Lemon-olive oil. Extract about ¼ cup of fresh lemon juice and mix this with ¼ cup of olive oil. Add 240 mL of water and mix well. Drink two to three times a day. It is believed that the citric acid in lemon juice helps to break down kidney stones while the olive oil helps to ease the passage of the stones.

Manjistha tea. Take ¼ teaspoon of manjistha powder. Add 1 cup of hot water. Allow it to steep for about 5 minutes.

Moringa leaf brew. Add ½ cup of fresh moringa leaves to a pot with 1 ½ cup of water. Bring to a boil and then remove from the heat. Drink when cool. Alternatively, ground dried moringa leaves may be used to make tea. Stir 1 teaspoon of the ground moringa into a cup of hot water.

Onion brew. Take about two to three small red onions and roughly chop them. Place in a pot with one cup of water and bring to a boil. Allow it to continue boiling for about 15 minutes. Strain the mixture and add honey to taste. Drink three times a day.

Pomegranate juice. Blend pomegranate until smooth and strain to separate the liquid from the sediment. Drink throughout the day. It can also be drunken neat without straining.

Prajmoda (Parsley) tea or juice. Cut a handful of fresh parsley into smaller pieces and submerge fully in a pot of water. Boil for 3 to 4 minutes and then cool completely. Strain and drink three to four times a day.

> Variation #1. Cut ¼ cup of parsley into smaller pieces and place into a pot. Pour 1 cup of boiling water over the parsley and allow it to steep for 5 to 10 minutes. The longer it steeps, the more bitter the drink becomes. Add honey to taste. Strain and drink 1 to 2 cups every day.

> Variation #2. To make fresh juice, place 3 cups of freshly cut parsley and little ginger (if desired) into a blender. Blend until smooth, gradually adding up to 1 cup of water. Strain and drink two to three times a week.

Pashanabheda/Pakhanbed ka Beeda. Take 1 to 3 g of the pashanabheda root powder. Make a paste or consume with some water after a meal once or twice a day.

> Variation #1. Take three washed leaves. Trim the stem. Take 2 teaspoons of Ispaghula and 2 teaspoons of palm sugar and mix with little water to make a paste. Place this paste on the middle of each leaf. Fold the leaf and consume it daily for 2 weeks.

Patharchatta (Katti Pottal). Take four to five leaves. Wash them. Fold and chew the leaves or consume them with a glass of water in the morning on an empty stomach for about 2 months.

Pineapple spice juice. Place fresh pineapple slices into a blender and blend until smooth. Strain and mix in a pinch of ground cinnamon and nutmeg. Drink once in the morning and once before bedtime.

Radish juice. Cut radish into cubes and soak in water overnight. Strain the mixture and drink twice a day.

Radish leaf juice. Place the radish leaves in a blender and blend until smooth. Strain the mixture and drink throughout the day.

Radish seed brew. Place 2 teaspoons of radish seeds into a pot with one cup of water. Bring to a boil, and boil until the mixture has reduced to half a cup in volume. Strain and drink ½ cup twice a day.

Shatavari brew. Slightly warm 120 mL of milk in a pot. Meanwhile, add 1 teaspoon of ground shatavari to a pot along with ⅛ teaspoon of cinnamon powder and a pinch of ginger powder. Pour a little milk over the powder and mix to form a paste. Slowly add the remaining milk, stirring well until no lumps remain. Add honey to taste and drink.

Shilapushpa. Take some flowers and blend. Add 2 cups of water. Boil for 15 minutes. Reduce to ¼ volume. Strain and drink 10 to 15 mL twice a day.

Sorakkai soup/rasam. Cook as part of soup or rasam.

Sweet broom. Take seeds or a handful of leaves or whole plants. Add it into warm water. Leave overnight and drink in the morning.

Variation #1. The leaves can also be chewed.

Variation #2. Take the whole plant. Blend with little water to extract the juice. Mix with ½ glass of milk. Consume daily 3 to 4 days.

Tomato juice. Take three very ripe tomatoes and roughly chop them. Blend until smooth. Add a pinch of salt and ground black peppercorn. This helps to dissolve the mineral salt deposits in the kidney. This remedy should not be used in oxalate stones.

Tulsi tea. Place five to seven fresh tulsi leaves in a pot with a cup of water. Boil for about 15 minutes and then remove from the heat. Allow it to steep for about 5 minutes. Drink before bedtime every day.

Turnip juice. Blend two turnips with some water and make fresh juice. Consume daily on an empty stomach. Some lime juice or water cress may be added.

Uva ursi. Take 3 g of dried leaves and soak in 150 mL of water for 12 hours. Drain and drink three to four times a day. This is drunken as a cold infusion.

Variation #1. To make a warm brew, take 1 tablespoon of the dried leaves and add 2 cups of hot water. Steep for 40 minutes. Strain and add honey or lemon to taste. Drink ½ cup twice a day for 5 days.

Variation #2. Take 1 teaspoon of tincture form and add 1 cup of water. Consume.

It is also available as tablets or capsules.

Varun. Take ½ to 1 teaspoon of varun powder and mix with honey. Consume after food.

Commercial Oral Preparations. Many commercial preparations are available for the treatment of kidney stones.

- *Himalaya Cystone tablets:* It has three main ingredients: Shilapushpa (*Didymocarpus pedicellata*), pashanabheda (*Bergenia ligulata*), and small caltrops (gokshura).
- *Organic India LKC.* The vegetarian capsules contain gale of the wind (*Phyllanthus niruri*), boerhavia (*Boerhavia diffusa*), and picrorhiza (*Picrorhiza kurroa*). It heals and protects the liver and kidney.
- *Gokshura churna:* It contains seven herbs in equal amounts: gokshura (*Tribulus terrestris*), punarnava (*B. diffusa*), dry ginger or shunthi (*Zingiber officinalis*), wet ginger or adrak (*Z. officinalis*), garlic (*Allium sativum*), haritaki (*Terminalia chebula*) and devdaru (*Cedrus deodara*)

Add 1 tablespoon of Gokshura churna and 1 tablespoon of *honey* to a cup of warm milk.

Consume this once a day before meals for 1 week.

- StonAid. It contains pashanabheda (*B. ligulata*), punarnava (*B. diffusa*), varuna (Crataeva nurvala), shilapushpa (*D. pedicellata*) and gokshura (*T. terrestris*).

Therapeutic Measures

- Diet

  Consume a sattvic diet with mostly vegetables and fruit. Abstain or minimize meat intake.

  Maintain adequate hydration. Consume 12 glasses of fluids per day. Drink water ½ hour before meals and 1 hour after meals.

  Pre-breakfast: warm water or herbal tea. Lunch: buttermilk. Dinner: soup

  For those with oxalate stones, eat low-oxalate foods. Avoid okra, spinach, beets, brinjal,

  Almonds, nut butter, and potato chips.

- Hot compresses, baths, and back massages may relieve pain induced by kidney stones.
- **Yoga asanas:** They can help maintain kidney health.

  Camel pose (Ustra asana), raised leg pose (Uttanpadasana), cobra pose (Bhujangasana), Pawanmuktasana: (wind relieving pose), bow pose (Dhanur Asana), half spinal twist (Ardha Matsyendrasana)

Chinese Natural Remedies

Common Ingredients for Kidney Stones

Spices	Herbs/Leaves	Miscellaneous
Cinnamon	Dandelion (pu gong ying)	Parsley
Ginger	Phellodendron/ huang bo (*Phellodendri cortex*)	Chicken gizzard lining (ji nei jin)
	Ox knee root/huai niu xi (*Achyranthes bidentata*)	Oriental water plantain rhizome/ ze xie (*Alisma Plantain d'Eau*)
	Gold coin grass/jin qian cao (*Herba Lysimachiae/ Lysimachia christinae*)	Polyporus/zhu ling (*Polyporus umbellatus*)
	Japanese climbing fern (*Lygodium japonicum*)	Poria/fu ling (*Wolfiporia extensa*)
		White atractylodes rhizome/bai zhu (*Atractylodes macrocephala*)

Common Recipes

Oral

Teas/Brews

Dandelion juice. Place 3 cups of dandelion greens into a blender along with two to three pieces of fresh ginger. Blend until smooth, gradually adding up to 1 cup of water. Strain and drink. Dandelion stimulates the production of bile, which aids in toxin elimination.

Huang bo tea. Take about 3 to 12 g of the powder once a day. Place the powder into a cup of hot water and mix well. Huang bo is also available as sliced, dried pieces of bark.

Jin qian cao tea. Place 2 to 3 teaspoons of dried jin qian rao into a cup of hot water and allow it to steep for 40 minutes. Drink 2 to 3 cups a day.

Parsley-ginger juice. Place 3 cups of freshly cut parsley and two to three pieces of fresh ginger into a blender. Blend until smooth, gradually adding up to 1 cup of water. Strain and drink two to three times a week.

Parsley tea. Cut a handful of fresh parsley into smaller pieces and submerge fully in a pot of water. Boil for 3 to 4 minutes and then cool completely. Strain and drink three to four times a day.

> Variation #1. Cut ¼ cup of parsley into smaller pieces and place into a pot. Pour 1 cup of boiling water over the parsley and allow it to steep for 5 to 10 minutes. The longer it steeps, the more bitter the drink becomes. Add honey to taste. Strain and drink 1 to 2 cups every day.

Water plantain root tea: Place 2 teaspoons of the dried root into about 300 mL of hot water and allow it to steep for 30 minutes. Drink three times a day.

Polyherbal formulas

Lygodium japonicum. It is added to other polyherbal formulas.

Polyporus Mix. This includes polyporus, corn silk, red atractylodes, poria, and alisma.

Wu ling san mixture. This mixture is made up of water plantain root, *Polyporus umbellatus, Atractylodes macrocephala, Wolfiporia cocos,* and cinnamon bark. It can be purchased as a ready-mixed powder from Chinese herbal shops. In the form of a powder, it should be taken twice a day, 6 to 9 g each time. Alternatively, 4 to 5 tablets should be taken twice a day.

Western/Other Natural Remedies

Common Ingredients for Kidney Stones

Herbs/Leaves	Miscellaneous
Basil	Lemon
Birch leaf	
Celery	Apple cider vinegar (ACV)
Celery seed	Rose hip (Rosa canina L.)
Cleavers	Bladderwrack (Fucus vesiculosus)
Common couch (Elymus repens)	Berberis vulgaris (barberry root bark)
Goldenrod (Solidago spp.)	Evening primrose seed oil
Green tea (Camellia sinensis)	Lily of the valley
Horsetail (Equisetum arvense)	Tribulus terrestris fruit
Joe Pye weed (Eutrochium purpureum)	Hibiscus flower (Hibiscus rosa-sinensis)
Parsley (Petroselinum crispum)	
Raspberry leaf (Rubus idaeus)	Oregano
Stinging Nettle	Juniper berries
Verbena (Verbena officinalis)	
Wheatgrass (Triticum aestivum)	Kidney bean

Common Recipes

Oral

Teas/Brews/Others

Apple cider vinegar. Add 2 tablespoons of ACV to about 250 mL of water. Drink throughout the day.

Basil juice. Place about 5 to 10 fresh basil leaves into a blender and blend until smooth. Drink 1 teaspoon a day.

Birch leaf tea. Take 3 fresh birch leaves or 2 teaspoons of dried leaves and a few young twigs (preferably roasted and ground). Add 1 cup of hot water. Steep for 10 minutes. Strain and consume.

Bladderwrack tea. Add 1 to 2 teaspoons of dried bladderwrack to a cup of hot water. Allow it to steep for 5 to 10 minutes. Strain and add honey to taste. Drink two to three times a day.

Celery juice. Cut about three stalks of celery into smaller pieces. Blend until smooth and drink throughout the day.

Celery seeds. Eat the seeds as a spice or as an addition to salads.

Celery tea. Cut two celery stalks into smaller pieces and place in a pot of water. Boil for 3 to 4 minutes. Cool and drink throughout the day.

Cleavers. There are various recipes to use cleavers.

> Variation #1. Take 3 tablespoons of dried or fresh leaves. Add 2 cups of boiling water. Steep for 10 minutes. Strain and drink tea.

> Variation #2. Take 1 teaspoon of freshly chopped cleavers into a clean jar. Add 250 mL of filtered water. Cover and keep for 8 to 12 hours. Strain and add honey to taste. Drink as a cold infusion.

> Variation #3. To make a smoothie, take 1 cup of fresh leaves and blend with other fruits or vegetables (such as pineapple, cucumber, ginger, celery, green apple, and green tea).

Common couch. Take 2 teaspoons of dried and sliced couch grass root in a cup of water. Boil and steep for 10 minutes. Consume the tea three times a day.

Evening primrose tea. Place about 2 teaspoons of dried leaves into about 300 mL of hot water and steep for at least 45 minutes. Drink twice a day.

Goldenrod. Chop some goldenrod flowers. Place in a jar. Cover it with apple cider vinegar. Allow to steep for 6 weeks. Consume 1 teaspoon daily. This can also be mixed with olive oil to make a salad dressing.

Variation #1. Take 2 tablespoons of dried goldenrod flowers (or stem or leaves). Add 1 cup of hot water. Steep for 15 minutes. Strain and consume. Add honey to taste. Consume 3 to 5 cups a day.

Green tea. Add 1 teaspoon of green tea leaves to a pot with a cup of hot water. Boil and then simmer gently for 3 to 5 minutes and strain the mixture. Add honey to taste and drink three to four times a day.

Hibiscus. Place 2 teaspoons of dried hibiscus petals into 300 mL of hot water and steep for 20 minutes. Drink the tea two to three times a day.

Horsetail. Place a handful of dried, chopped horsetail into 2 to 3 cups of hot water. Allow it to steep for at least 15 minutes. Drink the tea throughout the day.

Joe Pye Weed. There are many variations of the tea recipe.

Variation #1. To make the root tea, take 1 ounce of dried crushed root. Add ½ L of water. Boil for 30 minutes and drink ½ a cup every 2 hours.

Variation #2. To make flower tea, take 1 teaspoon of the dried flowers. Add 1 cup of boiling water. Steep for 10 minutes.

Juniper berry tea. Take 1 tablespoon of fresh berries and crush them. Add boiling water and steep for 10 minutes. Strain and drink. Add honey to taste.

Variation #1. Take 1 teaspoon of dried juniper berries. Crush it. Add 1 cup of boiling water. Steep for 20 minutes. Drink 1 cup twice a day.

Kidney bean broth. Soak the kidney beans overnight. Boil for several hours or cook the soaked red kidney beans in a pressure cooker. Strain and drink the broth of the cooked kidney beans. Consume the broth several times a day.

Lemon juice. Juice one lemon and mix into a cup of warm water. Add honey to taste and drink.

Alternatively, drink 8 oz of freshly squeezed lemon juice (from 10 to 15 lemons) with added honey or stevia. Then drink diluted lemon juice every 1 hour several times (i.e., 1 oz lemon juice mixed in 1 glass of water with the above sweetener).

Take also high-dose magnesium around 1000 mg to relax the ureters to facilitate stone passage.

Lily of the valley tincture. Take fresh flowers and half-fill a jar. Add alcohol or vodka until full. Steep for 2 weeks. Strain. Take 10 to 15 drops and add some water to consume.

Oregano tea. Add 3 teaspoons of fresh oregano leaves or 1 teaspoon of dried leaves to 1 cup of boiling water. Steep for 5 to 10 minutes before straining.

Parsley. Refer to "Indian Natural Remedies" for kidney stones.

Raspberry tea. Take 1 teaspoon of dried leaves. Add 1 cup of boiling water and steep for about 5 to 10 minutes. Strain and drink it warm.

Rose hip tea. Place four to eight dried rose hips in 1 cup of water. Steep for 10 to 15 minutes. Drain and drink. Drink three times a day.

Stinging nettle tea. Boil 1 cup of fresh leaves in 2 to 4 cups of water. Steep for 5 to 10 minutes. Strain and drink the cooked leaves, which can also be added to food.

St. John's wort tea. Place 2 tablespoons of St. John's wort in a teapot with about 6 cups of hot water. Cover and let steep for 3 to 10 minutes before straining. Add a little honey to taste. Drink warm.

Tribulus terrestris. It is available as powder or pill form. Take ½ to 1 teaspoon of the powder two times a day for 1 week.

Verbena tea. Take 1 tablespoon of fresh lemon verbena leaves or 1 teaspoon of dried leaves. Add 1 cup of boiling water. Steep or simmer for 15 minutes. Strain and consume warm with a desired sweetener.

Wheatgrass. Take about 30 g of fresh wheatgrass in a blender and blend until smooth. This juice may be drunken on its own or blended into other fruit juices. Alternatively, wheatgrass supplements can also be bought and consumed.

Therapeutic Measures
Diet

- Drink adequate amounts of water to ensure that the body is able to flush out minerals and toxins that may be responsible for the formation of kidney stones.
- Reduce salt content in food.
- Avoid sugary drinks such as sodas and energy drinks as they dehydrate the body and predispose to kidney stones.
- Avoid cola or carbonated drinks as they are high in phosphates.
- Maintain a low uric acid diet: For uric acid stones, reduce or omit red meat, offal (pancreas, liver, intestines) fish, eggs, and poultry.
- Go on a low-oxalate diet: For oxalate stones, avoid oxalate-rich foods such as spinach, beets, bran, nuts, rhubarb, French fries, and chocolate.
- Magnesium-rich foods: Consume foods high in magnesium content such as bananas, avocados, and leafy green vegetables. Magnesium prevents the binding of calcium to oxalate and hence prevents the formation of stones.

Modern Remedies

Painkillers
Smaller kidney stones often do not require medication and often pass out of the body on their own with adequate hydration. However, they may cause discomfort, which may be treated with painkillers. Painkillers such as ibuprofen or acetaminophen may be prescribed.

Thiazide Diuretic
Thiazide diuretics may be helpful in the treatment of calcium kidney stones as they lower the amount of calcium in urine by stimulating the sodium/calcium pump in the body and causing it to reabsorb a higher amount of calcium into the blood, hence lowering the amount of calcium to be excreted in the urine.

Examples: Chlorothiazide, metolazone, and indapamide

α-Blockers

α-Blockers have been found to help relax the ureter, which allows the kidney stone to pass with less difficulty and pain. This medication works by blocking the α-adrenergic receptors, which are present along the length of the human ureter. Stimulation of these receptors increases the force of ureteral contraction and peristalsis, causing pain as the stone attempts to pass through. Hence, by taking α-blockers, the α-adrenergic receptors are not stimulated, allowing the ureter to relax and the stone to pass through more easily.

Examples: Tamsulosin, terazosin, and doxazosin

Surgical

If a kidney stone is too big to pass naturally (6 to 7 mm), various procedures are done to remove them.

ESWL (extracorporeal shockwave lithotripsy). It uses ultrasound waves to break the stone into smaller pieces so that it can be passed in the urine. It is very effective (99%) for stones up to 20 mm in size.

Ureteroscopy. This procedure can be done if a kidney stone is stuck in the ureter. It involves passing a long thin telescope through the urethra into the bladder. It is then passed into the ureter where the stone is stuck. For stones up to 15 mm, this procedure is done.

PCNL (percutaneous nephrolithotomy). It is done for large stones. It involves using a thin telescopic instrument called a nephroscope. A small incision is made in the back, and a nephroscope is passed into the kidney to remove the stone.

Open surgery. This is rarely done nowadays but it is used for very large stones or in a person with abnormal anatomy.

Homeopathic Remedies

These include Berberis vulgaris and Cantharis.

Urinary Tract Infection

UTIs are common and recurrent in adult women, especially during pregnancy, post-menopause, associated vaginal infections, and diabetes mellitus. It can occur in any part of the urinary tract, but cystitis (infection of the bladder) is common and is usually due to gut bacteria (*Escherichia coli*). In noninfective cystitis, urine culture is negative. Tight and noncotton underwear or trousers, bubble baths, chemical fragrances can also predispose to UTI. In children, constipation and threadworms are predisposing factors. Symptoms and signs include painful or burning urination, which may be frequent and scanty, bladder discomfort, passage of cloudy or blood-stained urine, and fever.

Investigations include urine exams for microscopy and culture, renal ultrasound, blood tests and sometimes micturating cystogram (MCU) or radio-isotope scans (DMSA and DTPA).

General Therapeutic Measures

Perineal hygiene. Wiping from back to front can cause bacteria from the rectum to enter the urethra. Wiping the bottom from front to back can eliminate this.

Bowels. Avoid constipation.

Probiotics. They promote a healthy gut microbiome and can prevent UTIs.

Underclothing. Wear cotton underwear and loose clothing to ensure that the genital areas are adequately dry and clean.

Chemicals. Avoid scented products when cleaning genital areas. They can cause irritation and lead to UTIs.

Habits. Do not hold in urine as it causes bacteria to multiply in the bladder and cause a UTI. Double or triple voiding empties the bladder and prevents urine reflux. Practice also good menstrual hygiene with regular sanitary pad or tampon changes. Pads are preferred during UTI.

Pre and post-intercourse. Pass urine and wash the groin and genital area before and after sex if possible.

There are mixed views on using spermicidal creams with antibiotics or antiseptic creams with povidone iodine, which may help prevent UT1. Water-based lubricants and estrogen-based creams for post-menopausal women are preferable.

Diet. Consuming functional foods or medicinal plants regularly can reduce the risk of recurrent UTIs. Avoid bladder-irritant foods like strong spices, excessive alcohol, or caffeine.

Indian Natural Remedies

In Ayurveda, UTI is called *Mutrakricchra*. This is due to a combination of vitiated tridoshas and *mandagni* (from reduced agni and undigested foods). This affects the *mutra vaha srotas* (urinary tract) and leads to UTI.

Common Ingredients for Urinary Tract Infection

Spices	Herbs/Leaves	Miscellaneous
Ajwain	Basil/tulsi (*Ocimum sanctum*)	Horseradish
Anise (*Pimpinella anisum*)	Couch grass (*Elymus repens*)	Raisin
	Shilapushpa (*Didymocarpus pedicellata*)	Lady's finger
	Uva ursi	Cucumber (*Cucumis sativus*)
	Guava leaf	Blue pea flower (*Clitoria ternatea*)
	Drumstick/ Moringa leaves	Pineapple (*Ananas comosus*)
	Haritaki (*Terminalia chebula*) or Triphala	Black gram /Urad
	Java plum/ Jamun	Pomegranate (*Punica granatum*)
	Keelanelli	

Spices	Herbs/Leaves	Miscellaneous
	Chicory leaf	
	Black-jack (Bidens pilosa)	
	Neem (Azadirachta indica)	
	Nilavembu (Andrographis paniculata)	
	Babul (Acacia nilotica)	
	Indian abutilon/ Indian mallow	
	Common barberry	
Black mustard seeds (Brassica nigra)	Green tea leaf	Honey
Chandan (Santalum Album)	Varun/varuna	Bottle gourd/ Lauki (Lagenaria siceraria)
Cinnamon	Tinospora cordifolia (guduchi)	Hibiscus
Coriander	Boerhavia diffusa (punarnava)	Aloe vera
Garlic	Tribulus terrestris (gokshura)	Coconut water
Ginger	Coriander	Essential oils (lemongrass, lemon, cinnamon leaf, clove, cajeput, sandalwood)
Turmeric	Spinach	Carrot

Common Recipes

Oral

Teas/Brews/Others

Ajwain tea. Place a teaspoon of ajwain seeds into a pot of water and boil it for 5 to 10 minutes. Strain the mixture and drink warm.

Aloe vera juice. Wash and dry an aloe vera leaf. Slit the leaf down the center. Retain the white gel and discard any of the greenish-yellow gel. Place the white gel in a blender. Blend until smooth. Strain the mixture. This may be taken on its own or blended into any other fruit juice.

Anise. Add anise to boiling water and steep for about 15 minutes. Strain, add honey, and drink warm.

Babul tree bark tea. Lightly pound dry babul tree bark and steep in a cup of hot water. Add honey and drink warm.

Variation #1. Take ¼ to ½ teaspoon Babul churna. Mix with some water or honey and consume.

Barberry. It is available as a commercial preparation and can be taken orally as a powder or capsule. Dried roots of barberry can be used in tea.

Basil juice. Place about 5 to 10 fresh basil leaves into a blender. Blend until smooth. Drink 1 teaspoon a day.

Variation #1. Basil tea. Place three to five fresh basil leaves in a pot of water. Allow it to boil for about 3 to 4 minutes. Add honey to taste and drink.

Bidens tea. Take the young bidens shoot and brew as tea.

Variation #1. Take 45 to 90 drops of bidens tincture and add to a glass of water. Consume three to four times a day.

Variation #2. Add the fresh leaves to salads or add to stews or soups. The flowers are also edible and can be added to rice.

Black mustard seeds. Add the mustard seeds with other spices during sauteing or tempering.

Blue pea flower tea. Take five to six fresh blue pea flowers. Remove the green calyx. Add 1 cup of boiling water. Allow to steep for 5 to 10 minutes. Strain or discard the flowers. Add some lemon juice if desired and consume warm or chilled.

Bottle gourd juice. Blend the peeled bottle gourd with little water and mix with some lime juice. Consume it.

Carrot and spinach broth. Place a handful of fresh spinach greens in a pot with some cut carrots. Add ½ a L of water and simmer for about 30 to 40 minutes. Remove from the heat and mash until it forms a thick soup. Drink twice a day.

Cinnamon tea. Add 2 tablespoons of cinnamon powder and 1 teaspoon of honey in a glass of warm water and drink.

Coconut water. Consume coconut water every day to hydrate the body and to flush out bacteria.

Coriander and gokshura brew. Add one part of coriander powder and one part of gokshura to a pot of water. Boil gently for about 5 to 10 minutes. Allow to cool and drink three times a day.

Couch grass plus. Take 2 teaspoons of couch grass, cornsilk, and buchu. Add 1 cup of water. Boil and simmer for 5 minutes. Strain and consume two to three times a day.

Cucumber. Take the cucumber seeds. Mix with some rock salt and consume.

Variation #1: Blend the cucumber with some water. Consume.

Drumstick (Moringa) leaf. Cook and consume the leaves.

Garlic. Consume two to five fresh garlic pips every day.

Green tea. Place 2 teaspoons of dried green tea leaves in a cup of hot water. Allow it to steep for 15 to 20 minutes. Add honey to taste and drink.

Guava leaf. Take a handful of guava leaves. Add 100 mL of water. Boil until the volume is reduced to 25 mL. Consume twice a day.

Variation #1. Take four to six washed guava leaves. Add 1 cup of boiling water. Steep for 10 to 15 minutes. Strain and consume.

Guduchi juice. Place a handful of fresh guduchi leaves in a blender and blend until smooth. Strain and add honey to taste. Drink this daily in the morning on an empty stomach.

Haritaki tea. Take ¼ to ½ teaspoon of haritaki powder. Add 1 cup of warm water. Consume once or twice a day.

Hibiscus tea. Take three to four fresh washed hibiscus flowers. Remove the stamen and calyx. Add 1 cup of hot water. Steep for 5 to 10 minutes. Strain and drink. Add some fresh lemon juice if desired.

> Variation #1. Place 2 teaspoons of dried hibiscus petals into 300 mL of hot water and steep for 20 minutes. Drink two to three times a day.

Horseradish. Consume horseradish every day. It can be cooked (sauteed, grilled or boiled). The grated form is usually preserved in vinegar with salt and sugar.

Indian abutilon. Take some Indian Mallow (Tuturu Benda) leaves. Add some water and soak for a few hours. Add some rock candy and consume regularly.

> Variation # 1. Take some Indian Mallow leaves. Add some cumin seeds. Blend them together. Add some water. Strain and consume regularly until burning urine ceases.

Java plum (Jamun) juice. Take 10 to 15 washed black jamun fruits. Deseed and blend with 1 cup of water with added ¼ teaspoon black salt and a small piece of ginger. Strain and drink. Add some honey and ice if desired.

Keelanelli juice. Blend the leaves and make fresh juice. Drink 15 to 20 mL (2 to 4 teaspoons) daily on an empty stomach with a glass of water before breakfast. Powders and capsules are also available.

Neem tea. Crush four to five neem leaves and add to a cup of hot water. Allow to steep for about 10 minutes. Strain and drink.

> Variation #1. Chew four to five neem leaves or take 1 teaspoon of neem extract.

Nilavembu tea. Take a handful of fresh nilavembu branches and pluck off the leaves. Break the stems into shorter segments and steep in water overnight. Discard the stems the next morning and drink the tea.

Pineapple. Blend some pineapple slices with some water. Consume.

Pomegranate juice. Blend the pomegranate until smooth. Strain if required. Consume fresh.

Punarnava tea. Add one part each of dried punarnava, one part of dried passion fruit flower, and two parts of dried hawthorn berries. Steep about a ½ teaspoon of this in a cup of hot water for about 10 minutes. Drink twice a day after lunch and dinner.

Raisins. Eat about 15 to 20 of each daily (to prevent constipation).

Shilapushpa. Take some flowers and blend. Add 2 cups of water. Boil for 15 minutes. Reduce to ¼ volume. Strain and drink 10 to 15 mL twice a day.

Spade flower. A decoction can be made by boiling the whole plant. Capsules are also available.

Turmeric-ginger tea. Add three to five slices of lightly pounded ginger to a pot of water and bring to a boil. Reduce the heat and add 1 to 2 teaspoons of turmeric. Mix well. Allow it to simmer for about 5 to 10 minutes. Add honey to taste and drink.

Uva ursi. Take 3 g of dried leaves and soak in 150 mL of water for 12 hours. Drain and drink three to four times a day. This is drunken as a cold infusion.

> Variation #1. To make a warm brew, take 1 tablespoon of the dried leaves and add 2 cups of hot water. Steep for 40 minutes. Strain and add honey or lemon to taste. Drink ½ cup twice a day for 5 days.

> Variation #2. Take 1 teaspoon of tincture form and add 1 cup of water. Consume.

Varun. Take ½ to 1 teaspoon of varun powder and mix with honey. Consume after food.

Polyherbal brews. Some of these include:

> *Punarnavadi kashayam.* It contains neem, punarnava, guduchi, haritaki, kiratatikta, ginger, Devadaru, Patola, and Haridra.

> *Gokshuradi tablet.* It contains amla, haritaki, bibhitaki, long pepper, gokshuradi, mushta, black pepper, ginger, guggulu.

> *Varanadi kashayam.* It contains varuna, shatavari, saireyaka, bilwa, chitrak, murva, haritaki, brihati, kitamari-*Aristolochia bracteolata*, karanja-*Millettia pinnata/Pongamia pinnata*, putikaranja, kantakari, moringa, bhallataka (marking nut), agnimantha, and darbha grass

Topical

Essential oils. They do not cure UTI but may help prevent recurrent infections. They should never be applied directly into the urethra or vagina. The essential oil (5 drops) can be mixed with a carrier oil (30 mL of coconut oil or olive oil) and then massaged over the skin over the pubic area, inner thighs, and lower back at the tailbone to kill surface bacteria. Alternatively, it can be inhaled via a humidifier/diffuser or sprinkled on the child's bed sheets or on their clothes.

Therapeutic Measures

Diet. Consume more functional foods and eat a pitta-pacifying diet. Consume chicory leaves, moringa leaves, buttermilk, and coconut water. Avoid meat.

Lifestyle. Essential oil inhalation therapy. As above via a diffuser.

Yoga. These include *Surya namaskara* (sun salutation), *Savasana* (Corpse pose), *Setu Bandha Sarvangasana* (Bridge pose), *Utkatasana* (Chair Pose) and *Malasana* (Wall Squat Pose), *Bhujangasana* (Cobra pose), and *Dhanurasana* (Bow pose).

Pranayama. These include *Moola bandha* (Root lock), *Nadi Shodhana* (Alternate nostril breathing), *Bhastrika pranayama* (Bellow breathing), *Jalandhara bandha* (throat/chin lock), and *Sheetali* (cooling breath)

Chinese Natural Remedies

It is believed that UTIs or problems are due to dampness, damp-heat, or qi stagnation.

Common Ingredients for Urinary Tract Infection

Herbs

Anemarrhena/zhi mu (*Anemarrhena asphodeloides*)
Asiatic cornelian cherry fruit/shan zhu yu (*Cornus officinalis*)
Baikal/huang qin (*Scutellaria baicalensis*)
Chinese foxglove root/shu di huang (*Rehmannia glutinosa*)
Chinese thorowax root/chai hu (*Radix bupleuri*)
Cortex radicis moutan (mu dan pi)
Gentian root/long dan cao (*Gentiana scabra*)
Honeysuckle
Oriental water plantain (ze xie)
Phellodendron/Huang bo (*Phellodendri cortex*)
Poria/fu ling (*Wolfiporia extensa*)
Rice paper pith
Yam rhizome/shan yao (*Rhizoma dioscoreae*)

Common Recipes

Oral

Huang bo tea. Take about 3 to 12 g of the powder once a day. Place the powder into a cup of hot water and mix well. Huang bo is also available as sliced, dried pieces of bark.

Rehmannia six formula (liu wei di huang wan). Rehmannia six formula is one of the most widely used Chinese herbal formulas and is made up of *Rehmannia glutinosa,* cornus, oriental water plantain, cortex radicis moutan, *Poria sclerotium,* and *Dioscorea opposita.* Rehmannia and Oriental water plantain are believed to normalize kidney function and clear it of any *coldness.* Cornus and cortex radicis moutan help to improve liver function and *moisten* the kidneys. Finally, dioscorea and Poria sclerotic are believed to improve spleen function.

This herbal mixture is readily available as a commercial preparation or pure powder. For powder preparations, 24 g of Rehmannia should be taken, 12 g of cornus, 12 g of dioscorea, 9 g of Oriental water plantain, 9 g of moutan, and 9 g of *P. sclerotium.*

Rice paper pith. A decoction is made with water, and other herbs are usually added.

Skullcap tea. Place 1 cup of hot water into a pot and bring to a low boil. Turn off the heat. Add 2 teaspoons of dried skullcap to the pot and cover with a lid. Allow it to sit for 5 to 10 minutes. Strain and drink.

Commercial Preparation. Wenglitong capsule. It contains many herbs, including yi yi ren (coix barley seed), zhe bei mu (fritillary bulb), gou ya hua (cape jasmine), xuan fu hua (Japanese inula flower), jin yin hua (Japanese honeysuckle flower bud), zhi gan cao (liquorice root), huang qi (astragalus root), etc. It can be combined with tolterodine for better OAB relief.

Therapeutic Measures

Acupressure

Ren 3 (middle summit) is located on the midline of the lower abdomen, about 13 cm below the belly button. Massage this point with an index finger for about 1 to 2 minutes to relieve pain caused by UTI.

Spleen 9 (yin-mound spring) is located under the medial condyle of the tibia in the depression behind and below the inner side of the tibia. Place a finger on this point and massage for 1 to 2 minutes firmly.

Notes. The acupressure points cannot cure a UTI but are commonly used to strengthen the organs and to relieve pain and discomfort caused by the UTI.

Most traditional Chinese medicine (TCM) formulas should be taken as directed by a sensei.

Western/Other Natural Remedies

Common Ingredients for Urinary Tract Infection

Spices	Herbs/Leaves	Miscellaneous
Corn silk (*Zea mays*)	Stinging nettle/ common nettle	Yogurt
Garlic	Cleavers (*Galium aparine*)	Cranberry (*Vaccinium oxycoccos*)
Rosemary	Horsetail (*Equisetum arvense*)	Lemon
Sage (*Salvia officinalis*)	Marshmallow root (*Althea officinalis*)	Apple cider vinegar (ACV)
	Common mallow (*Malva sylvestris*)	Pomegranate
	Goldenseal	Probiotics
	Dandelion leaf	Prune
	Buchu (*Agathosma betulina*)	Couch grass/ Common couch
	Oregon grape	Essential oils (oregano, thyme, lavender, tea tree, eucalyptus)
	Juniper	African cherry (*Prunus africana*)
	Burdock root	Peacock flower (*Caesalpinia nuga*)
	Celery (*Apium graveolens*) and celery seeds	
	Peppermint	
	Meadowsweet	
	Birch leaf	
	Saw palmetto (*Serenoa repens*)	
	Verbena (*Verbena officinalis*)	

Common Recipes

Oral

Teas/Brews/Juices

African cherry. Blend the African cherry until smooth. Strain if required. Consume it fresh.

Pyegeum extract is available as capsules.

Apple cider vinegar. Add 1 tablespoon of apple cider vinegar to 3 tablespoons of water and drink once a day.

Birch leaf tea. Take 3 fresh birch leaves or 2 teaspoons of dried leaves. Add 1 cup of hot water. Steep for 10 minutes. Strain and consume it.

Buchu tea. Finely chop some fresh buchu leaves and add about 1 teaspoon to an empty cup. Pour boiling water into the cup and allow it to steep for about 10 minutes before straining and drinking the tea.

Burdock root tea. Roughly chop fresh or dried burdock root into smaller chunks. Add 2 tablespoons of the chopped root to a pot with water. Allow to simmer gently for about 10 minutes before turning off the heat. Strain and drink warm.

Variation #1. Take 1 teaspoon of dried burdock root. Add 1 cup of hot water. Steep for 10 to 15 minutes. Strain and consume three times a day.

Variation #2. Consume 10 to 25 drops of burdock root tincture three times a day.

Celery juice. Wash and cut 2 stalks of celery. Blend with water until smooth. Strain and drink the juice.

Variation #1. Consume 1 cup of fresh chopped celery stick or sauté with other vegetables.

Variation #2. Celery seed tea. Lightly crush ½ tablespoon of celery seeds. Steep in a cup of hot water for about 20 minutes. Strain the mixture and drink it.

Cleavers. Take 3 tablespoons of dried or fresh leaves. Add 2 cups of boiling water. Steep for 10 minutes. Strain and drink tea.

Variation #1. Take 1 teaspoon of freshly chopped cleavers into a clean jar. Add 250 mL of filtered water. Cover and keep for 8 to 12 hours. Strain and add honey to taste. Drink as a cold infusion.

Variation #2. To make a smoothie, take 1 cup of fresh leaves and blend with other fruits or vegetables (such as pineapple, cucumber, ginger, celery, green apple, and green tea).

Couch grass plus. It can also be combined with buchu, yarrow, and uva ursi to make a brew.

Couch grass tea. Take 2 teaspoons of dried and sliced couch grass root and 1 cup of water. Boil and steep for 10 minutes. Consume three times a day.

Couch grass tincture. Add 2 to 3 mL of tincture into a glass of water or fruit juice. Consume two to three times per day.

Corn silk. Take 2 tablespoons of dried corn silk. Add 2 cups of water. Boil and simmer for 10 minutes. Steep for another 30 minutes. Strain and consume. Add honey to taste.

Cranberry juice. Cranberry juice is available as a commercial preparation.

Dandelion tea. Place dandelion roots or leaves into a pot with 1½ cups of water. Bring to a boil and allow to simmer for about 15 minutes. Strain and drink three times a day.

Garlic extract. Peel three to five cloves of garlic. Place the garlic in a food processor and pulse until the oil starts to separate from the garlic pieces. Strain the garlic. The liquid from the garlic is called extract. Consume a tablespoon of this every day. Alternatively, roasted three to four garlic pips can be consumed.

Goldenseal root. Take 1 teaspoon of goldenseal root or leaves. Add 2 or 3 cups of boiling water. Steep for 10 minutes. Strain and add honey or lemon to taste.

Variation #1. Consume 400 mg of goldenseal root powder every day.

Homemade juice. Put about 450 g of fresh or frozen cranberries into a pot with 4 cups of water. Boil, simmer until the berries burst, and then cool. Strain through a piece of muslin cloth. Add honey to taste and cool completely. Drink this juice throughout the day.

Horsetail tea. Place a handful of dried, chopped horsetail into 2 to 3 cups of hot water. Allow it to steep for at least 15 minutes. Drink throughout the day.

Juniper berry tea. Take 1 tablespoon of fresh berries and crush them. Add boiling water and steep for 10 minutes. Strain and drink. Add honey to taste.

Lemon juice. Juice a lemon and mix with one cup of warm water. Add honey to taste.

Mallow root tea. It is prepared as marshmallow root tea.

Variation #1. Prepared as above in marshmallow leaves and flowers.

Variation #2. The young leaves or flowers can be added to salads and eaten raw or cooked. The seeds are also edible.

Marshmallow root tea. Place ¼ cup of dried marshmallow root into a cup and pour cold water over it. Allow to steep overnight and strain the next morning.

Variation #1. Take the flowers and leaves (whole plant without root). Place in a jug. Add boiling water. Steep for 3 hours. Consume 250 mL daily for 4 days. Stop for a few days. Then repeat.

Variation #2. The young leaves can be added to salads and eaten raw. They can also be sautéed or added to soups.

Meadowsweet tea. Take 2 tablespoons of dried meadowsweet flowers or 4 teaspoons of fresh flowers. Add 1 cup of hot water. Steep for 10 minutes. Strain and consume it warm.

Oregon grape root tea. Take 2 teaspoons of dried root into a pot with 1 cup of boiling water. Bring to a boil before reducing the heat and simmer for 15 minutes. Strain and drink it warm.

Peacock flower. All parts of the plant, i.e., leaves, roots and bark are boiled together to make tea.

Peppermint tea. Place a handful of peppermint leaves into a pot of water. Bring to a boil and reduce the heat. Allow the mixture to simmer for 5 to 10 minutes. Strain and drink twice a day.

Pomegranate juice. Blend the pomegranate until smooth. Strain if required. Consume it fresh.

Probiotics. Consume probiotics with Lactobacillus or yogurt to maintain gut health.

Prune juice. Take 8 ounces of prune juice a day. It is available as a commercial preparation.

Variation #1. Take 1 cup of dried pitted prunes and add 5 cups of boiling water. Allow the prunes to soak overnight or 12 to 24 hours. Add the prunes and the water to a blender and blend until smooth. Strain and discard any solid pieces. Dilute with boiled water until there is about a liter of prune juice. Add honey to taste.

Rosemary tea. Add two to three sprigs of fresh rosemary (or 1⅓ of dried leaf needles) into a pot with 2 cups of water. Allow it to boil for about 1 minute. Remove from the heat and strain.

Sage. Take 1 tablespoon of washed fresh salvia leaves. Chop them and add to 2 cups of boiling water. Simmer for 5 to 15 minutes. Add honey or milk. Drink it warm.

Saw palmetto. Take ¼ cup of fresh saw palmetto berries. Add 2 cups of boiling water. Add 1 tablespoon of honey and ¼ teaspoon of vanilla or almond extract. Strain and consume it warm. It is also available in supplement form.

Stinging nettle tea. Boil 1 cup of fresh leaves in 2 to 4 cups of water. Steep for 5 to 10 minutes. Strain and drink the cooked leaves, which can be added to food.

Verbena tea. Take 1 tablespoon of fresh lemon verbena leaves or 1 teaspoon of dried leaves. Add 1 cup of boiling water. Steep or simmer for 15 minutes. Strain and consume warm with a desired sweetener.

Topical

Essential oils. As above under *Indian Herbs for UTI.*

Therapeutic Measures

Essential oil inhalation therapy. As above via a diffuser under *Indian Herbs for UTI.*

Apply a heating pad, hot water bottle or a towel soaked in hot water over the lower abdomen or lower back if there is cramping pain. Keep it for 15 to 20 minutes.

Modern Remedies

Mild cases, especially in women, will often get better by themselves within a few days. However, women who have recurrent infections, women who are pregnant or immunocompromised, men, and children usually will require antibiotic treatment. *E. coli* is the most common bacteria.

Antibiotics. Different antibiotics act differently via any of the five mechanisms (listed below), all of which cause bacterial cell death. (These are called bactericidal drugs.)

- Inhibiting enzymes in the bacteria responsible for cell wall synthesis, protein synthesis, or nucleic acid synthesis
- Interfering with bacterial cell membrane permeability
- Interfering with bacterial cell wall synthesis
- Interfering with bacterial DNA synthesis
- Interfering with bacterial protein synthesis

However, due to increasing rates in *E. coli* antibiotic resistance, minor, uncomplicated UTIs are not treated with antibiotics. Cephalosporins are a group of antibiotics that are divided into four generations with each later generation having greater antimicrobial effectiveness than the last. They function by disrupting the synthesis of peptidoglycan, a structural molecule in the bacterial cell wall, resulting in bacterial cell death. As human cells do not have peptidoglycan, the antibiotics are able to specifically target bacteria cells.

Examples: Amoxicillin, clavulanate, and cephalosporins such as *cefpodoxime* or *cefaclor*

Homeopathic Remedies

These include *Nux vomica* (UTI symptoms in a highly stressed individual and with chills), *Cantharis* (severe burning throughout urination with some blood and increased sexual desire), *Pulsatilla* (in young girls or women who are shy and emotional or leak after sneezing, coughing, or laughing), *Sepia* (in recurrent UTI with frequent antibiotic use and painful sex), *Arnica montana* (in UTI following childbirth with associated perineal injuries), *Staphysagria* (in UTI after sex or pelvic procedures or history of repressed anger, sadness, or sexual abuse in a person who is meek and mild-mannered), Aconite (UTI after cold exposure and there is marked fear), and *Sarsparilla* (in UTI with pain after voiding and relieved with standing when voiding). Others include *Mercurius, Berberis, and Apis mellifica.*

Chronic Kidney Failure

Chronic kidney failure (CKF) or chronic kidney disease (CKD) refers to damage to the kidneys with the inability to filter waste products, excess fluids, and toxins.

Main causes include diabetes and hypertension. Others are glomerulonephritis, kidney infections, hypercholesterolemia, obstructive uropathy from stones or enlarged prostate, polycystic kidney disease, and medications (such as NSAIDs and lithium).

Although herbs, herbs and nutritional supplements are natural and can maintain optimum health, if they are taken in megadoses, they can cause kidney injury or failure. Examples include

Vitamin C and oxalate stones;

Turmeric and oxalate stones;

Creatine (body-building supplement) and rhabdomyolysis;

Lysine (antiviral agent for cold sores) and tubulointerstitial nephritis; and

Chromium (for weight loss or diabetes) and kidney enlargement and inflammation, proteinuria, and acute tubular necrosis.

Medicinal teas and heavy metal contamination with nephrotoxicity risk.

Signs and symptoms of CKF include anorexia, nausea, anemia, edema of feet or face, hematuria, proteinuria, oliguria, nocturia, fatigue, muscle cramps, itching, shortness of breath, or erectile dysfunction. Often, it is asymptomatic in the early stage.

Tests include urinalysis, kidney ultrasound, and routine blood biochemistry, including renal functions.

Indian Natural Remedies

Common Ingredients for Chronic Kidney Failure

Spices	Herbs/Leaves	Miscellaneous
Black peppercorn *(Piper nigrum)*	Radish leaf	Watermelon
	Holy basil (Tulsi)	Beetroot
		Fig
		Coconut water
		Carrot
		Bottle gourd (lauki)
		Honey
		Tomato *(Solanum lycopersicum)*
		Salt

Common Ingredients for Kidney Failure

Herbs/Leaves	Miscellaneous
Horny goat weed/Yin Yang Huo *(Epimedium)*	Dodder seeds/tu si zi *(Cuscuta chinensis Lam)*
Milkvetch/huang qi *(Fabaceae astragalus)*	Asiatic cornelian cherry fruit/ shan yu rou *(Cornus officinalis)*
	Yam rhizome/ shan yao *(Rhizoma dioscoreae)*
	Poria
	Oriental water plantain/ ze xie *(Alisma Plantain d'Eau)*
Rehmannia glutinosa (sheng di huang/ Chinese foxglove)	Goji berry

Common Recipes

Oral

Teas/Brews

Basil-honey paste. Pound three to five fresh basil leaves. Squeeze the basil juice out of the pounded basil. Take 1 tablespoon of the juice and mix it with some honey to make a paste. Take this every morning on an empty stomach for 5 to 6 months.

Beetroot juice. Place 2 cups of freshly cubed beetroot in a pot with enough water to submerge the beetroot. Allow it to boil until the beetroot becomes soft. Mash beetroot and strain through a piece of muslin. Drink 2 to 3 cups of this juice every day.

Bottle gourd juice. Place 1 cup of peeled and chopped bottle gourd into a blender and add one cup of water. Blend until smooth and drink.

Carrot juice. Place 1 cup of peeled and cubed carrot into a blender. Add one cup of water and blend until smooth. Strain and drink it.

Coconut water. Consume coconut water every day to cleanse the kidneys.

Fig brew. Place two figs into a pot with one cup of water. Bring to a boil. Allow it to simmer under low heat for 15 to 20 minutes. Drink every morning on an empty stomach for a month.

Radish leaf juice. Place a handful of radish juice in a blender. Blend until smooth. Strain and drink twice a day.

Tomato juice. Take about three very ripe tomatoes and roughly chop them. Add to a blender and blend until smooth. Add a pinch of salt and ground black peppercorn. This helps to dissolve the mineral salt deposits in the kidney.

Watermelon juice. Place 2 cups of fresh cubed watermelon into a blender. Blend until smooth. Alternatively, eat watermelon slices every day.

Chinese Natural Remedies

Various Chinese herbs, if taken correctly, can improve (and not injure) symptoms in end-stage kidney disease.

Common Recipes

Oral

There are several different energy deficiencies that may cause CKD. Qi (energy levels) circulation is an important aspect of TCM. It is believed that poor qi circulation can cause several health ailments. Yang qi refers to heat energy. Yin qi refers to cold energy. These two energies should be in balance for an individual to maintain good health.

- *Qi deficiency of spleen and kidneys.* This refers to an energy deficiency that leads to weakness of the spleen and kidneys, producing symptoms such as a pale complexion, physical weakness, difficulty breathing, loose stools, bloating, poor appetite, a sore lower back or knees, and a pale tongue. There are many forms of commercial preparations for treating this condition such as bu zhong yi qi tang (tonify the middle and augment the qi decoction) and rao yuan tang (preserve the basal decoction).

- *Yang deficiency of liver and kidneys.* A yang deficiency means that there is coldness in the body, leading to weakness of the liver and kidneys. Symptoms of yang deficiency are an ashen complexion, mental and physical fatigue, poor appetite, loose stools, cold intolerance, and a pale tongue. Remedies include zhen wu tang (true warrior decoction), shi pi yin (bolster the spleen decoction).

- *Yin deficiency of liver and kidneys.* This energy imbalance means there is excess heat in the body leading to weakness in the liver and kidneys. Symptoms of this energy deficiency are a sallow complexion, a dry mouth with an unpleasant taste, a preference for cold drinks, dry eyes, constipation, and hot palms and soles of the feet, dizziness, tinnitus, and an overly pink or red tongue. Remedies include qi lu di huang tang, which is made up of lycium fruit, chrysanthemum, and rehmannia.

Dodder seeds. They are available as supplements (including powder, tablets, or capsules) and can be taken alongside food and other vitamins.

Horny goat weed tea. Take 5 g of dried leaves or powder. Simmer in 250 mL of water. Strain and drink warm.

Western/Other Natural Remedies

Common Ingredients for Chronic Kidney Failure

Spices	Herbs/Leaves	Miscellaneous
	Hydrangea (Hydrangea paniculata)	Seaweed
		Grape
		Cranberry
		Rice

Common Recipes

Oral

Teas/Brews/Others

Cranberry juice. Cranberry juice is available as a commercial preparation but may also be prepared at home. Put about 450 g of fresh or frozen cranberries into a pot with 4 cups of water. Boil, then simmer on low heat until the berries burst. Remove from heat. Strain through a piece of muslin cloth. Add honey to taste and cool. Drink this juice throughout the day.

Grapes. Consume grapes every day (unless there is hyperkalemia).

Hydrangea root tea. Hydrangea root herbs are available for purchase as dried herbs. Place about 3 teaspoons of this herb into a cup of hot water and steep for 10 to 15 minutes before drinking.

Seaweed. Consume seaweed as a part of the diet.

Modern Remedies

There is no cure for CKD, but treatment can help relieve the symptoms and prevent progression of the disease. Treatment will depend on the stage of CKD.

Medication. This is given to treat *high blood pressure*, diabetes, and *high cholesterol*.

Dialysis. This treatment is indicated in advanced (stage 5) chronic kidney disease (CKD) to maintain kidney functions.

Kidney transplant. This may be needed in advanced CKD (stage 5).

Therapeutic Measures

Lifestyle

1. Lifestyle changes are recommended for people with kidney disease to remain as healthy as possible. These include:
   - no smoking;
   - eating a healthy, balanced diet;
   - reducing the salt intake to less than 6 g (0.2 oz) a day;
   - keeping a safe limit of not more than 14 alcohol units a week;
   - doing regular exercise; 150 minutes a week is recommended;
   - losing weight if overweight or obese; and
   - not abusing NSAID painkiller medications, such as ibuprofen, unless indicated. These medicines can cause more kidney damage.
2. Medications/treatment of underlying conditions predisposing to CKD

Symptoms/Disease	Treatment	Notes
i. High blood pressure	**Calcium Channel Blockers** Examples: Verapamil, amlodipine, and nifedipine **β-Blockers** First-generation β-blockers are nonselective and block both β-1 and β-2 receptors in the body. Examples: Propranolol and sotalol Second-generation β-blockers only block B1 receptors located in the cardiac muscle. Examples: Metoprolol, bisoprolol, and atenolol Third-generation β-blockers are medications that have vasodilator properties through the additional blocking of α-receptors. Examples: Carvedilol and nebivolol. **Angiotensin-Converting Enzyme Inhibitor (ACE Inhibitor) and Angiotensin II Receptor Blockers (ARBs)** Examples: Enalapril, lisinopril, and captopril Examples of ARBs are losartan, valsartan, and eprosartan. **Diuretics** Hydrochlorothiazide, metolazone, and indapamide	

Symptoms/Disease	Treatment	Notes
ii. High cholesterol	Statins Examples: Atorvastatin, lovastatin, and pravastatin	Chronic kidney disease is a risk factor for developing strokes and heart attacks. The incidence of this can be decreased through careful control of lipid levels in the blood, including cholesterol. Lipid levels may be controlled through several ways, most commonly through the use of statins. ***Statins*** Statins are a group of medications that inhibits cholesterol synthesis in the body. This in turn leads to a reduction in plasma LDL levels. They are often taken at night, as LDL synthesis tends to spike in the early morning.
iii. Anemia	• Iron supplements • Erythropoietin injections	Many people with later-stage kidney disease develop *anemia*, which is a lack of red blood cells. Symptoms of anemia include: tiredness lack of energy *shortness of breath* a pounding, fluttering, or irregular heartbeat *(palpitations)* Erythropoietin is a hormone medication that will produce more red blood cells from the bone marrow. Iron supplements are also given if there is iron deficiency.
iv. Bone problems	To decrease high levels of calcium in blood—calcium acetate and calcium carbonate Low in vitamin D—cholecalciferol or ergocalciferol	Calcium and phosphate in the right amount maintain healthy bones in a healthy person. In kidney failure, there is increased phosphate and low calcium, which can lead to osteoporosis (bone thinning). It is advised to limit the amount of high-phosphate foods in the diet such as red meat, dairy products, eggs, and fish. Phosphate binders are given if diet measures do not work. Low calcium is treated with calcium supplements like calcium acetate and calcium carbonate. Low levels of *vitamin D* are treated with cholecalciferol or ergocalciferol to increase vitamin D levels.
v. Glomerulonephritis	Steroids or immunosuppressants cyclophosphamide	Kidney disease can be caused by kidney inflammation such as *glomerulonephritis* due to autoimmune diseases. A kidney biopsy is done to determine the cause, *steroid medication*, or immunosuppressants (e.g., cyclophosphamide is necessary for immune-mediated diseases).

Treatment of Severe Chronic Kidney Disease. If the disease worsens, the kidneys will stop working, hence the next stage of treatment is more aggressive. There are two options: dialysis or kidney transplant. This depends on multiple factors, and it is usually decided by the specialist to enable the patient to have a comfortable life.

Dialysis. This is a procedure to remove extra water, waste, and impurities from the blood. There are two main types of dialysis:

Hemodialysis: This involves diverting blood into an external machine (artificial kidney), where it is filtered before being returned to the body. Hemodialysis is done about three times a week, either at the hospital or at home. Each session takes about 4 hours. A fistula or graft must be created in the arm for hemodialysis.

Peritoneal dialysis (PD): This involves pumping dialysis fluid into the space inside the abdomen to draw out waste products from the blood passing through vessels lining the inside the abdomen. Peritoneal dialysis is usually home-based and is carried out several times a day or overnight. There are two main types of PD.

In continuous ambulatory peritoneal dialysis (CAPD), there is no machine, and the patient can do this about four or five times a day at home and/or at work.

In automated peritoneal dialysis (APD), there is a cycler machine that determines the number of cycles or exchanges to be done. Each cycle usually lasts 1 to ½ hours, and the exchanges take place during sleep time.

Although the average life expectancy on dialysis is about 5 to 10 years, many survive well on dialysis for 20 to 30 years.

Kidney Transplant. An alternative to dialysis for people with severely reduced kidney function is a kidney transplant. This can be a *living donor transplant* (can last 15 to 20 years), *deceased donor transplant* (can last 10 to 15 years), *paired kidney exchange* transplant, and *incompatible kidney transplant.*

This is often the most effective treatment for advanced kidney disease, but it involves major surgery and taking life-long medications to stop rejection (i.e., the body attacking the donor organ [immunosuppressants]).

Dialysis must be continued while waiting for a transplant.

Nowadays, overall survival rates for kidney transplants are very good. About 90% of transplants still function after 5 years, and many return to work for 10 years or more.

Homeopathic Remedies

These may be used as supportive care and include *Ammonium carbonicum, Aurum metallicum, A. mellifica, Arsenic album, Chelidonium majus,* phosphorus, arsenicum, etc.

Urinary Incontinence

Urinary incontinence refers to the lack of voluntary control over urination.

Causes and risk factors include postmenopausal age, pregnancy, childbirth, obesity (BMI >30), post-hysterectomy, previous pelvic surgery or trauma, excessive alcohol or caffeine, associated medical conditions (diabetes mellitus, chronic cough, connective tissue disease, etc.), UTI, medications (diuretics, β-blockers, ACE inhibitors, sedatives, psychotropics, benzodiazepines), family history of urinary incontinence, and local factors (overactive bladder [OAB], enlarged prostate of BPH, incompetent urethral sphincter, and bladder outlet obstruction).

Tests include urine analysis, blood tests, kidney and pelvis ultrasound, urodynamics, cystoscopy, cystogram, fluid charts, and bladder diary.

Types of urinary incontinence

Stress incontinence (SUI)

There is poor bladder closure. Urine leak occurs due to pressure on the bladder from raised intra-abdominal pressure during a bout of cough, sneeze, laugh, or exercise.

Urge incontinence (UUI)

There is OAB from detrusor muscle overactivity due to a higher density of the M2 and M3 (muscarinic) receptors, absent urothelium or over-expression of suburothelial TRPV1 (transient receptor potential vanilloid-1) receptors. A strong urge to urinate followed by an involuntary loss of urine occurs. Underlying UTI, constipation, neurologic disorder, diabetes, and excessive caffeine or alcohol can lead to frequency, urgency, and nocturia.

Overflow incontinence (OUI)

There is constant or frequent urine leak due to incomplete emptying of the bladder from a bladder obstruction due to enlarged prostate, constipation, or bladder stones.

Mixed incontinence (MUI)

There is a urine leak due to urgency and increased abdominal pressure.

Functional incontinence

A physical or mental disorder that prevents one from holding urine in the bladder and reaching the toilet on time.

Indian Natural Remedies

Common Ingredients for Urinary Incontinence

Spices	Herbs/Leaves	Miscellaneous
Cinnamon powder	Amla (Indian gooseberry)	Chili pepper
Cumini/dry jamun seed powder *(Syzygium jambolanum)*		Dhanwantharam oil
		Honey
Fennel seeds		Turnip *(Brassica rapa subsp. rapa)*

Common Recipes

Oral

Juices/Brews/Others

Amla (Indian gooseberry). Take two or three amla. Cut the pulp into small pieces and discard the seed. Add a pinch of turmeric and 1 teaspoon of honey. Consume this daily in the morning for 4 weeks. This strengthens the prostate.

Chili peppers. This contains capsaicin, which can desensitize pain receptors.

Cinnamon powder. A teaspoon of ground cinnamon with some honey is added in a glass of warm water. Drink it warm. It has antiseptic properties. However, it can also be a bladder irritant in some.

Dhanwantharam oil. This polyherbal sesame oil is consumed in the prescribed dose to pacify the apana vata and improve bladder incontinence. A cotton cloth or gauze soaked in the oil can also be placed on the lower abdomen for 30 minutes.

Fennel seeds. Steep or boil some fennel seeds in hot water. Strain and drink this as an herbal tea. Alternatively, 1 teaspoon of fennel and 1 teaspoon of honey can be added to a glass of warm milk and consumed.

Honey. Take 2 teaspoons before bedtime.

Syzygium jambolanum/cumini (dry jamun seed powder). Take 1 teaspoon twice a day.

Turnip juice. Drink 30 mL of fresh turnip juice twice a day. This is for the prostate's health.

Therapeutic Measures

Yoga asanas. The squat pose (malasana), chair pose (utkatasana), triangular pose (trikonasana), and legs-up-the-wall pose (viparita karani) help to reduce SUI by about 70% by strengthening the pelvic floor muscles.

Chinese Natural Remedies

Common Ingredients for Urinary Incontinence

Herbs	Miscellaneous
Ginseng	Reishi mushroom/lingzhi *(Ganoderma lucidum)*
Sharp-leaf galangal/Yi zhi ren	Walnut

Common Recipes

Oral

Ginseng tea. Add about two to four slices of ginseng to a cup. Pour boiling water over the ginseng and allow it to steep for about 10 to 15 minutes.

Reishi mushroom. It is often cooked as food (stewed or sauteed) or added to soups. It is also added as a food supplement in various formulations.

Walnut. Boil oats and walnuts with some water for a few minutes. Add goji berries. Consume.

Polyherbal Mixtures.

Ba-wei-di-huang-wan (BWDHW): It contains Rehmanniae radix, Dioscoreae rhizoma, Cornus officinalis, Poria cocos, Alismatis rhizoma, Cinnamomi cortex, Moutan radicis cortex, and Aconiti radix. It is reported to have anti-M2 (muscarinic) receptor activity and warms the kidney yang, especially in diabetes-related incontinence.

Ji-sheng-shen-qi-wan (JSSQW)/gosha-jinki-gan (GJG in Japanese): In addition to the above herbs in BWDHW, it also contains Plantaginis semen and Achyranthis radix. It is effective in reducing incontinence in men with BPH and in women with OAB. Side effects include nausea.

Suo-quan-wan (SQW): It contains Alpinia oxyphylla Miq, *D. opposita* thunb and Lindera radix. It regulates the TRPV1 receptors and improves bladder outlet obstruction.

Sang-piao-xiao-san (SPXS): There are many formulas with Mantidis ootheca as the key herb component.

Wenglitong capsule: It contains many herbs, including yi yi ren (coix barley seed), zhe bei mu (fritillary bulb), gou ya hua (cape jasmine), xuan fu hua (Japanese inula flower), jin yin hua (Japanese honeysuckle flower bud), zhi gan cao (liquorice root), huang qi (astragalus root), etc. It can be combined with tolterodine for better OAB relief.

Suo Quan Wan: It contains yi zhi ren (sharp-leaf galangal), Lindera root (Wuyao), and Dioscorea/yam (Shan yao).

Therapeutic Measures

Diet

Maintain normal fluid intake but limit 2 to 3 hours before bedtime.

Restrict or avoid alcohol, caffeine, and carbonated drinks. Follow the "Bladder Diet" and avoid bladder irritants.

Lifestyle

Lose weight if BMI >30.

Stop smoking.

Avoid or treat constipation.

Plan travel time and avoid embarrassing situations.

Use absorbent products like protective pads, panty liners, and diapers, especially for the elderly.

Bladder Retraining (Behavioral Treatment)

Empty the bladder at a strict time schedule (hourly).

Delay urination time if urge is present. This is to increase the holding time.

Do double or triple voiding, and bend forward to empty the bladder.

Practice distraction techniques or do something that requires concentration.

Sit on a hard seat or across a tightly rolled towel.

Pelvic Floor Muscle Exercises/Squeezes/Kegels Exercises. Do regular voluntary contractions and relaxations of the pelvic floor muscles. This will improve urethral resistance and pelvic visceral support by increasing the strength of the voluntary pelvic floor muscle contraction. Improvements can take up to 6 months with a success rate around 65% to 75%. It is not successful in women who cannot locate and properly contract their pelvic floor muscles.

Acupuncture. It can help with bladder incontinence. Acupuncture points SP6, CV4, and K13 in the lower legs are stimulated with needle electrodes. Treatment is usually weekly.

Foot and Hand Reflexology. This may reduce the bladder spasms although the data is not strong.

Western Natural Remedies

Common Ingredients for Urinary Incontinence

Herbs/Leaves	Miscellaneous
Bearberry/uva ursi *(Arctostaphylos uva-ursi)*	
Chamomile	Beta-sitosterol
Horsetail *(Equisetum arvense)*	Pumpkin seeds

Herbs/Leaves
Nettle (*Urtica dioica*)
Peppermint
Sharp-leaf galangal
Valerian (*Valeriana officinalis*)

Miscellaneous
Saw palmetto
Apple cider vinegar

Magnesium

Common Recipes

Oral

Tea/Brews

Apple cider vinegar. Mix one tablespoon of apple cider vinegar into one cup of warm water. Drink in the morning on an empty stomach.

Baking soda. Mix 1 teaspoon of baking soda to a glass of warm water. Drink it warm.

Beta-sitosterol. It is a plant sterol. Consume nuts, beans and avocado. It is also available as oral supplements. It can increase urinary flow in benign prostatic hyperplasia (BPH).

Chamomile tea. Place some dried or fresh chamomile flowers into a cup. Pour boiling water over the flowers and allow it to steep for 10 minutes. Strain and add honey to taste. Drink it hot.

Goldenseal root. Take 1 teaspoon of goldenseal root or leaves. Add 2 or 3 cups of boiling water. Steep for 10 minutes. Strain and add honey or lemon to taste.
Variation #1. Consume 400 mg of goldenseal root powder every day.

Herbal infusion teas. Many herbs are available. Take 1 tablespoon of the herb. Pour hot water. Steep for 10 to 15 minutes. Strain and drink. These herbs include:

Horsetail tea. Place a handful of dried, chopped horsetail into 2 to 3 cups of hot water. Allow it to steep for at least 15 minutes. Drink throughout the day.

Magnesium. Take magnesium supplements and consume magnesium-rich foods, which include bananas, corn, potatoes, and pumpkin seeds.

Peppermint tea. Place a handful of peppermint leaves into a pot of water. Bring to a boil and reduce the heat. Allow the mixture to simmer for 5 to 10 minutes. Strain and drink twice a day.

Pumpkin seeds. Consume pumpkin seeds.

Saw palmetto. Take ¼ cup of fresh saw palmetto berries. Add 2 cups of boiling water. Add one tablespoon of honey and ¼ teaspoon of vanilla or almond extract. Strain and consume warm. It is available as a supplement.

Sharp-leaf galangal. It can be consumed as food.

Stinging nettle tea. Boil 1 cup of fresh leaves in 2 to 4 cups of water. Steep for 5 to 10 minutes. Strain and drink the cooked leaves, which can also be added to food.

Uva ursi. Take 3 g of dried leaves and soak in 150 mL of water for 12 hours. Drain and drink three to four times a day. This is drunken as a cold infusion.
Variation #1. To make a warm brew, take 1 tablespoon of the dried leaves and add 2 cups of hot water. Steep for 40 minutes. Strain and add honey or lemon to taste. Drink ½ cup twice a day for 5 days.

Variation #2. Take 1 teaspoon of tincture form and add 1 cup of water. Consume.
It is also available as herbal tea, tablets, or capsules.

Valerian tea. Mix ½ teaspoon of dried valerian root (or 2 to 3 g teaspoon) in a cup of hot water. Cover and steep for 10 to 15 minutes. Consume 30 minutes to 2 hours before sleep.

Modern Remedies

1. Drugs for Urge Urinary Incontinence (UUI)
   a. Anticholinergic drugs/Antimuscarinic drugs for OAB
   These medications relax the bladder muscles and increase the volume of urine held in the ladder. These include an oxybutynin tablet or a patch (sold under different brand names such as Lyrinel XL tablet, Ditropan tablet, and patch and Kentera patch), Darifenacin (Emselex), Solifenacin (Vesicare), Tolterodine (Detrusitol), Trospium (Regurin), Propiverine (Detrunorm), and Fesoterodine (Toviaz).
   The oxybutynin transdermal patch is available as an OTC item. It is applied on the skin twice every week (every 3 to 4 days). About 50% women will have up to 50% improvement.
   Side effects include dry mouth, nausea, constipation, dry eyes and dizziness, heart rate changes, and cognitive issues.
   b. β-3 adrenergic agonist
   Mirabegron (Myrbetriq) relaxes the bladder muscles. Although it has a delayed onset of action, it is effective in about 50% cases and is well-tolerated. Side effects include high blood pressure, backache, headache, joint pain, dizziness, and flu symptoms. It can be combined with Solifenacin.
2. Drugs for Stress Urinary Incontinence (SUI)
   a. Selective serotonin and noradrenaline reuptake inhibitor (SSNRI)
   Duloxetine is used in moderate to severe SUI. It increases the urethral closure pressure and electrical activity of the sphincter. Side effects include gastrointestinal disturbances, dry mouth, headache, and suicidal ideation.
   b. α-adrenergic agonists
   These include pseudoephedrine and phenylephrine.
3. Drugs for Urge or Overflow Incontinence
   a. α-blockers (α-adrenergic antagonists)
   It relaxes the muscle fibers in the prostate and the bladder neck muscles and hence decreases the overflow incontinence. Examples include tamsulosin, silodosin, alfuzosin, doxazosin, and terazosin.
4. Topical Estrogen Creams
   The vaginal estrogen cream can improve muscle tone and strength and improve coordination at the urethra and vagina.
5. Miscellaneous
   a. Vaginal cones
   The weighted cones are inserted vaginally for short periods to strengthen the pelvic floor muscles. Change

daily with increasing weights and retain the cone for 10 to 20 minutes each time. The cure/improvement rate is about 60% (mild to moderate).

b. Vaginal pessary

It is used to support the vaginal wall, urethra, uterus, and bladder and helps to control incontinence.

c. Urethral insert

It is a small disposable device inserted into the urethra by women with stress incontinence before any activity or sport to prevent a leak. It is removed when passing urine.

6. Surgery for Stress Incontinence

Anterior Colporrhaphy (Anterior Vaginal Surgery)

This vaginal surgery treats moderate or severe SUI and the anterior vaginal wall prolapse. The bladder neck is elevated with deep sutures on either side. Stitches are also inserted to para-urethral tissue and anterior portion of pubococcygeus. The continence rate at 5 years is about 50% to 70%.

Burch Colposuspension: Laparoscopic or Open Abdominal Retropubic Suspension

The bladder neck and base are elevated by suturing the upper lateral vaginal walls to the iliopectineal ligaments. It is highly effective for SUI with a continence rate at 5 years around 85%. The complications include genitourinary prolapse, voiding disorders, and detrusor overactivity.

Sling surgery (Bladder Suspension Surgery/Bladder Sling)

Slings can be autologous or of synthetic mesh materials. Slings can be sub-urethral, mid-urethral, or pubovaginal in position. It causes urethral closure when the sling is stretched.

Autologous sling: Here, strips of rectus fascia are placed in a sling under the bladder neck. There is about 70% improvement of SUI after 5 years.

Tension-free vaginal tape (Transvaginal tape, TVT)

A tape made of synthetic polypropylene mesh is inserted vaginally to provide mid-urethral support for SUI. The 5-year cure rate is around 88%. It is a simple procedure. Rare complications include vascular and bladder injuries, UTI, voiding difficulties, OAB, and tape erosion.

Trans-obturator tape (TOT) sling

The permanent tape mesh is suspended under urethra through the obturator and puborectalis muscles. It avoids blind entry into the retropubic space hence reduces the risk of damage to internal organs. The 5-year cure rate is around 88%. Complications include OAB and voiding difficulties. Pelvic mesh complications include vaginal mesh extrusion and mesh/tape erosion into the urethra/bladder.

TVT or TOT may be combined with a prolapse repair.

Urethral Bulking

Collagen material (bovine origin), Calcium hydroxyapatite *(Coaptite)* or usually a plastic hydrogel *(Bulkamid* is polyacrylamide hydrogel) is injected around the urethra into the submucosal space at the bladder neck to reduce its width. The success rate in SUI is about 50%, and the effect lasts about 3 to 9 months. Adverse reactions include UTI, immune reaction, or extrusion of the bulking agent.

Surgical Procedures for Urge Incontinence Done by a Urologist (Only after Failed Medical Treatment)

- **Sacral neuromodulation, SNM (sacral nerve root stimulation):** An electrode is implanted to the 3rd or 4th sacral nerve, which delivers an electrical stimulus. The 5-year cure rate for UUI is about 67% to 80%. The battery lasts about 7 years. Adverse reactions include implant site pain, lead migration, electric shocks, and infection.
- **Botulinum toxin A injections:** The injections are given at about 30 sites into the bladder muscle, except the trigone area via a cystoscopy every 6 to 12 months. The success rate is 65% to 100% and the effect lasts about 3 to 9 months.
- **Artificial sphincter:** An artificial valve or sphincter is inserted to regulate and control the flow of urine from bladder to urethra.
- **Partial detrusor myomectomy (bladder auto augmentation):** The success rate is about 60% and is a simple procedure for refractory OAB.
- **Laparoscopic or robotic augmentation cystoplasty (bladder augmentation):** It is usually done for the neurogenic bladder in children and refractory OAB.
- **Cell therapy:** Autologous muscle cells are taken from the thigh and expanded in vitro and then implanted at the bladder neck.
- **Intravesical instillation of vanilloids (i.e., capsaicin or resiniferatoxin):** It is effective in neurogenic detrusor overactivity in spinal cord injuries. *Capsaicin* is derived from the *capsicum* plants (chili peppers). *Resiniferatoxin* is a C-nerve fiber neurotoxin, a natural chemical derived from *Euphorbia resinifera (cactus family)* and is 1000 times more potent than capsaicin. Either of the compounds in the alcohol solution is instilled into the bladder for 30 minutes. It desensitizes the bladder's sensory nerves.

Miscellaneous

- **Percutaneous posterior tibial nerve stimulation:** The posterior tibial nerve at the ankle is stimulated to treat OAB as it also affects sacral nerve root function. This is a neuromodulation technique or like electro-acupuncture. It is done for 30 minutes once a week for 12 weeks with subsequent boosters. The benefits are short-term.
- **Specific surgery for BPH** include transurethral resection of prostate (TURP), transurethral microwave therapy (TUMT), transcatheter prostate artery embolism, prostatic urethral lift with implants (Urolift), Holmium laser enucleation of prostate (HoLEP), Photoselective Vaporization of Prostate (PVP) (i.e., Greenlight laser vaporization with 180 W, 532 nm wavelength laser), convective radiofrequency transurethral water vapor thermal therapy (Rezum), and conductive radiofrequency thermal therapy (Prostiva).

Homeopathic Remedies

These remedies include *Ferrum phosphoricum* (if daytime wetting especially when standing), *belladonna* (if leaking more when chilled or cold and associated wild dreams), *kreosotum* (more for functional incontinence), *Arnica* (for post-op dribbling), *causticum* (wetting more in winter and fear of sleeping in the dark), *cantharis* (if strong urge and burning pain when urinating), etc.

References

World Health Organization. (2020, December 9). *The top 10 causes of death*. WHO. Retrieved from https://www.who.int/news-room/fact-sheets/detail/the-top-10-causes-of-death.

Kidney Stones
Acharya, D., & Shrivastava, A. (2016, May 17). *7 Wonder herbs to cure kidney stones*. Medium. Retrieved from https://medium.com/

Acupuncture Today. (2021). *Phellodendron (huang bai)*. Acupuncture Today. Retrieved from https://www.acupuncturetoday.com/herb-central/phellodendron.php.

Bazilian, W. (2014, August 12). *Spice up your diet: 7 kidney-friendly seasonings*. National Kidney Foundation. Retrieved from https://www.kidney.org/news/ekidney/august13/Spice_Up_Your_Diet_with_7_Kidney-Friendly_Seasonings.

Cleveland Clinic medical professional. (2015, February 17). *Oxalate-controlled diet for kidney stones: Benefits*. Cleveland Clinic. Retrieved from https://my.clevelandclinic.org/health/articles/11066-kidney-stones-oxalate-controlled-diet.

de Arriba, S. G., Naser, B., & Nolte, K. U. (2013). Risk assessment of free hydroquinone derived from *Arctostaphylos Uva-ursi folium* herbal preparations. *International Journal of Toxicology*, 32(6), 442–453. Retrieved from https://doi.org/10.1177/1091581813507721.

Doctor NDTV. (2018, July 18). *Kidney stones: 5 best ayurvedic cures to get rid of stones*. Doctor.NDTV.com. Retrieved from https://doctor.ndtv.com/living-healthy/kidney-stones-5-best-ayurvedic-cures-1878975.

Gopalakrishnan, L., Doriya, K., & Kumar, D. S. (2016). Moringa oleifera: A review on nutritive importance and its medicinal application. *Food Science and Human Wellness*, 05(02), 49–56. Retrieved from https://doi.org/10.1016/j.fshw.2016.04.001.

Govindasamy, K. [Krishnan Govindasamy]. (2018, February 19). *Sorakkai (bottle gourd) soup for uric acid* [Video]. YouTube. Retrieved from https://www.youtube.com/watch?v=5RTW_0H7yz8.

Group, E. (2017, March 14). *10 Natural remedies for kidney stones*. Global Healing. Retrieved from https://explore.globalhealing.com/remedies-for-kidney-stones/.

Healthcare Medicine Institute. (2017, December 5). *Acupuncture and herbs force expulsion of kidney stones*. HealthCMi. Retrieved from https://www.healthcmi.com/Acupuncture-Continuing-Education-News/1807-acupuncture-and-herbs-force-expulsion-of-kidney-stones.

Khatri, M. (2019, September 15). *Kidney stone treatment: What should I expect?* WebMD. Retrieved from https://www.webmd.com/kidney-stones/understanding-kidney-stones-treatment#1.

Khatri, M., & Brown, S. (2019, September 17). *High oxalate foods that can cause kidney stones*. WebMD. Retrieved from https://www.webmd.com/kidney-stones/kidney-stones-food-causes.

Lipkin, M., & Shah, O. (2006). The use of alpha-blockers for the treatment of nephrolithiasis. *Reviews in Urology*, 08(04), S35–S42. Retrieved from https://www.ncbi.nlm.nih.gov/pmc/articles/PMC1765041/.

Mattison, L. D. (2021, June 25). *Your guide to all the different types of basil*. Taste of Home. Retrieved from https://www.tasteofhome.com/collection/types-of-basil/.

Mayo Clinic Staff. (2020, May 5). *Kidney stones*. Mayo Clinic. Retrieved from https://www.mayoclinic.org/diseases-conditions/kidney-stones/symptoms-causes/syc-20355755.

National Institute of Diabetes and Digestive and Kidney Diseases. (2017, May). *Treatment for kidney stones*. Retrieved from https://www.niddk.nih.gov/health-information/urologic-diseases/kidney-stones/treatment.

National Kidney Foundation. (2019, June). *Kidney stones Diet plan and prevention*. Retrieved from https://www.kidney.org/atoz/content/diet.

Neelima. (2017, July 25). *Sorakaya soup/bottle gourd soup for weight loss in Telugu with English subtitles* [Video]. YouTube. Retrieved from https://www.youtube.com/watch?v=HBmsr5aT5_U.

NHS website. (2019, May 9). *Treatment: Kidney stones*. NHS.UK. Retrieved from https://www.nhs.uk/conditions/kidney-stones/treatment/.

Pacific College of Health Science. (2019, January 8). *Oriental medicine offers natural remedies for kidney stones*. Pacific College. Retrieved from https://www.pacificcollege.edu/news/press-releases/2015/05/14/oriental-medicine-offers-natural-remedies-for-kidney-stones.

Palsdottir, H. (2019, October 16). *8 Natural remedies to fight kidney stones at home*. Healthline. Retrieved from https://www.healthline.com/nutrition/kidney-stone-remedies.

Reller, P. L. (2017, August 3). *Kidney and urinary stone prevention and cure*. Acupuncture Integrated. Retrieved from http://www.acupunctureintegrated.com/articles/kidney-stone-prevention.

Russell, S. (2017, October 2). *Easy herbal remedies for kidney and gall bladder stones*. Dimmak Herbs. Retrieved from https://www.dimmakherbs.com/2009/02/16/easy-herbal-remedies-for-kidney-and-gall-bladder-stones/.

Saleem, M. (2018, January 13). *Ayurveda home remedies for effective relief from kidney stones*. Ayurveda. Retrieved from https://www.practo.com/healthfeed/ayurveda-home-remedies-for-effective-relief-from-kidney-stones-31266/post.

Shehab, A., Bhagavathula, A. S., Mahmoud Al-Khatib, A. J., Elnour, A. A., & AlKalbani, N. M. S. (2015). Ammi Visnaga in treatment of urolithiasis and hypertriglyceridemia. *Pharmacognosy Research*, 7(4), 397–400. Retrieved from https://doi.org/10.4103/0974-8490.167894.

Swasthi, S. (2021, February 28). *Wheatgrass juice recipe*. Swasthi's Recipes. Retrieved from https://www.indianhealthyrecipes.com/wheatgrass-juice-recipe/.

The Indian Med. (2020, July 17). *Amazing Arugampul benefits that will interest you!* The Indian Med. Retrieved from https://theindianmed.com/amazing-arugampul-benefits-that-will-interest-you/.

The Yoga Institute. (2017, September 11). *Yoga healing for kidney stones*. Retrieved from https://theyogainstitute.org/yoga-healing-for-kidney-stones/.

Tulane University School of Medicine. (2019, October 31). *Thiazide diuretics*. TMedWeb. Retrieved from https://tmedweb.tulane.edu/pharmwiki/doku.php/thiazides.

Watson, B. (2020). *Home remedies for kidney stones and prevention*. MyMed. Retrieved from https://www.mymed.com/diseases-conditions/kidney-stones-renal-lithiasis-nephrolithiasis/home-remedies-for-kidney-stones-and-prevention.

Winston, D. (2011). Herbal and nutritional treatment of kidney stones. *Journal of the American Herbalists Guild*, 10(02), 61–71. Retrieved from https://www.americanherbalistsguild.com/files/journal/vol%2010%20no%202/Kidney%20Stones%20V10N2.pdf.

Wong, C., & Bull, M. (2021, February 1). *Health benefits of Bishop's weed*. Verywell Health. Retrieved from https://www.verywellhealth.com/the-benefits-of-bishops-weed-88612.

Zanni, G. R. (2013, September 13). *Kidney stones*. Pharmacy Times. Retrieved from https://www.pharmacytimes.com/view/kidney-stones.

Zelman, K. (2010, September 23). *The truth about coconut water.* WebMD. Retrieved from https://www.webmd.com/food-recipes/features/truth-about-coconut-water.

Urinary Tract Infection

All Ayurveda. (2018). *Urinary disorders.* Retrieved from https://allayurveda.com/kb/urinary-disorders/.

Aviva Romm. (2021, March 5). *Natural remedies for bladder infections and UTIs.* Aviva Romm MD. Retrieved from https://avivaromm.com/treating-bladder-infections-naturally/.

Bandukwala, N. Q. (2019, October 31). *Antibiotics for UTIs: What to know.* WebMD. Retrieved from https://www.webmd.com/a-to-z-guides/what-are-antibiotics-for-uti#1.

British Homeopathic Association. (2021). *Urinary tract infections.* Homeopathy UK. Retrieved from https://homeopathy-uk.org/homeopathy/how-homeopathy-helps/conditions/urinary-tract-infections.

Danahy, A. (2021, March 9). *Does Uva Ursi work for urinary tract infections?* Healthline. Retrieved from https://www.healthline.com/nutrition/uva-ursi#side-effects-and-safety.

Dharmananda, S. (n.d.). *Rehmannia six formula.* Institute for Traditional Medicine. Retrieved from http://www.itmonline.org/arts/rehm6.htm.

Doctor NDTV. (2018, April 9). *5 super effective home remedies for urinary infection.* Doctor.NDTV.Com. Retrieved from https://doctor.ndtv.com/living-healthy/5-wonderful-home-remedies-for-urinary-problems-1776705.

Flower, A., Lewith, G., Liu, J. P., & Li, Q. (2013). Chinese herbal medicine for treating recurrent urinary tract infections in women. *Cochrane Database of Systematic Reviews.* https://doi.org/10.1002/14651858.cd010446

Julius, M. (2017, August 16). *Urinary tract infections (UTI) and TCM.* Acupuncture Remedies™ NYC. Retrieved from https://aprpc.com/urinary-tract-infections-uti-tcm-new-york-ny/.

Koullouros, A. (2016, February 23). *7 herbal remedies for urinary tract infections.* Stuff: Life & Styles. Retrieved from https://www.stuff.co.nz/life-style/well-good/teach-me/77170050/7-herbal-remedies-for-urinary-tract-infections.

Link, R. (2018, April 23). *6 home remedies for urinary tract infections.* Healthline. Retrieved from https://www.healthline.com/nutrition/uti-home-remedies.

Mayo Clinic Staff. (2021, April 23). *Urinary tract infection (UTI).* Mayo Clinic. Retrieved from https://www.mayoclinic.org/diseases-conditions/urinary-tract-infection/diagnosis-treatment/drc-20353453.

Mooney, S. (2011, March 6). *Ayurvedic support for urinary tract infections.* Banyan Botanicals. Retrieved from https://www.banyanbotanicals.com/info/blog-the-banyan-insight/details/ayurvedic-support-for-urinary-tract-infections/.

Olmstead, C. B. (2019, February 2). *Skullcap: Why this hooded herb deserves your attention.* Mercola: Take control of your health. Retrieved from https://articles.mercola.com/herbs-spices/skullcap.aspx.

Sheng Foong. (2013, June 21). *Liu Wei Di Huang Wan (Rehmannia Six Formula/Six Flavor Rehmannia Pill).* Amazon.Com. Retrieved from https://www.amazon.com/Huang-Rehmannia-Formula-Flavor-Pill/dp/B00DJ7GE5G.

Stevens, M. (2020, December 11). *5 herbs for UTI relief within hours!* Eat Beautiful. Retrieved from https://eatbeautiful.net/5-herbs-that-heal-utis-within-hours/.

Villines, Z., & Wilson, D. R. (2018, April 23). *Can essential oils treat a UTI?* Medical News Today. Retrieved from https://www.medicalnewstoday.com/articles/321582.

Wong, C., & Menna, M. (2021, July 7). *How a urinary tract infection is treated.* Verywell Health. Retrieved from https://www.verywellhealth.com/urinary-tract-infections-treatments-89319.

Chronic Kidney Failure

Arora, P. (2021, February 21). *Chronic Kidney Disease (CKD) Treatment & Management: Approach considerations, delaying or halting progression of chronic kidney disease, treating pathologic manifestations of chronic kidney disease.* MedScape. Retrieved from https://emedicine.medscape.com/article/238798-treatment.

Fields, C. (2016, August 17). *World-famous celebrity chef shares top 10 herbs & spices for CKD & dialysis patients.* KidneyBuzz. Retrieved from https://www.kidneybuzz.com/world-famous-celebrity-chef-shares-top-10-herbs-spices-for-ckd-dialysis-patients/2016/8/17/world-famous-celebrity-chef-shares-top-10-herbs-spices-for-ckd-dialysis-patients.

Kubala, J., & Arnarson, A. (2019, November 18). *The 20 best foods for people with kidney disease.* Healthline. Retrieved from https://www.healthline.com/nutrition/best-foods-for-kidneys#3.-Sea-bass.

Motshakeri, M., Ebrahimi, M., Goh, Y. M., Othman, H. H., Hair-Bejo, M., & Mohamed, S. (2014). Effects of brown seaweed (*Sargassum polycystum*) extracts on kidney, liver, and pancreas of type 2 diabetic rat model. *Evidence-Based Complementary and Alternative Medicine, 2014,* 1–11. Retrieved from https://doi.org/10.1155/2014/379407.

Myhre, J., Sifris, D., & Wosnitzer, M. (2021, July 1). *How chronic kidney disease is treated.* Verywell Health. Retrieved from https://www.verywellhealth.com/kidney-disease-treatments-4170060.

NHS website. (2018, October 30). *10 self-help tips to stop smoking.* NHS.UK. Retrieved from https://www.nhs.uk/live-well/quit-smoking/10-self-help-tips-to-stop-smoking/.

NHS website. (2020a, January 9). *Get fit for free.* NHS.UK. Retrieved from https://www.nhs.uk/live-well/exercise/free-fitness-ideas/.

NHS website. (2020b, February 21). *High cholesterol.* NHS.UK. Retrieved from https://www.nhs.uk/conditions/high-cholesterol/.

NHS website. (2020c, April 22). *Dialysis.* NHS.UK. Retrieved from https://www.nhs.uk/conditions/dialysis/.

NHS website. (2020d, June 25). *Eat well.* NHS.UK. Retrieved from https://www.nhs.uk/live-well/eat-well/.

NHS website. (2020e, July 20). *Kidney transplant.* NHS.UK. Retrieved from https://www.nhs.uk/conditions/kidney-transplant/.

NHS website. (2020f, December 1). *Start the NHS weight loss plan.* NHS.UK. Retrieved from https://www.nhs.uk/live-well/healthy-weight/start-the-nhs-weight-loss-plan/.

NHS website. (2021a, March 2). *Ibuprofen for adults (including Nurofen).* NHS.UK. Retrieved from https://www.nhs.uk/medicines/ibuprofen-for-adults/.

NHS website. (2021b, June 23). *Tips on cutting down.* NHS.UK. Retrieved from https://www.nhs.uk/live-well/alcohol-support/tips-on-cutting-down-alcohol/.

NHS website. (2021c, June 25). *High blood pressure (hypertension).* NHS.UK. Retrieved from https://www.nhs.uk/conditions/high-blood-pressure-hypertension/.

Nohr, M. (2021, May 19). *Healthy kidneys: Best foods and natural remedies.* DrJockers.Com. Retrieved from https://drjockers.com/kidneys-health-natural-remedies/.

Ranjan, R., & Kumar, H. (2021, January 5). *Chronic kidney disease in Ayurveda.* Himveda. Retrieved from https://himveda.com/chronic-kidney-disease-ayurveda/.

The Council on Renal Nutrition. (2019, April). *Herbal supplements and kidney disease.* National Kidney Foundation. Retrieved from https://www.kidney.org/atoz/content/herbalsupp.

The Healthline Editorial Team. (2019, October 3). *How to prevent kidney failure*. Healthline. Retrieved from https://www.healthline.com/health/kidney-health/how-to-prevent-kidney-failure#11-tips.

Urinary Incontinence

Carewatch. (2018, October 10). *6 natural remedies for incontinence*. Carewatch. Retrieved from https://www.carewatch.co.uk/6-natural-remedies-for-incontinence/.

Cherney, K., & Wilson, D. R. (2019, March 7). *What home remedies work for an overactive bladder?* Healthline. Retrieved from https://www.healthline.com/health/overactive-bladder/home-remedies.

Drugs.com. (2021, March 22). *Uva Ursi*. Drugs.com. Retrieved from https://www.drugs.com/npp/uva-ursi.html.

Feng, T., & Anger, J. T. (2013). Surgical management of stress urinary incontinence: Trends in older women. *Aging Health*, *09*(05), 515–518. Retrieved from https://doi.org/10.2217/ahe.13.57.

Johns Hopkins Medicine. (2021). *Urinary incontinence*. Health. Retrieved from https://www.hopkinsmedicine.org/health/conditions-and-diseases/urinary-incontinence.

Kelleher, C., Hakimi, Z., Zur, R., Siddiqui, E., Maman, K., Aballéa, S., et al. (2018). Efficacy and tolerability of mirabegron compared with antimuscarinic monotherapy or combination therapies for overactive bladder: a systematic review and network meta-analysis. *European Urology*, *74*(03), 324–333. Retrieved from https://doi.org/10.1016/j.eururo.2018.03.020.

Lalwani, H. (2018, April 6). *Home remedies and ayurvedic treatment for urinary incontinence*. Nirogam. Retrieved from https://nirogam.com/blogs/news/home-remedies-and-ayurvedic-treatment-for-urinary-incontinence.

Lee, W. C., & Liu, Y. L. (2018). Traditional Chinese medicine and herbal supplements for treating overactive bladder. *Urological Science*, *29*(05), 216–222. Retrieved from https://doi.org/10.4103/uros.uros_8_18.

Magowan, B. A., Owen, P., & Thomson, A. (2018). *Clinical obstetrics and gynaecology* (4th ed.) [E-book]. Elsevier.

Mamut, A., & Carlson, K. V. (2017). Periurethral bulking agents for female stress urinary incontinence in Canada. *Canadian Urological Association Journal*, *11*(6S2), 152. Retrieved from https://doi.org/10.5489/cuaj.4612.

Mayo Clinic Staff. (2021, March 9). *Urinary incontinence*. Mayo Clinic. Retrieved from https://www.mayoclinic.org/diseases-conditions/urinary-incontinence/diagnosis-treatment/drc-20352814.

McIntosh, C. (n.d.). *Bladder problems*. Homeopathy UK. Retrieved from https://homeopathy-uk.org/homeopathy/how-homeopathy-helps/conditions/bladder-problems.

Monga, A., & Dobbs, S. (2011). *Gynaecology by ten teachers* (19th ed.). Boca Raton, FL: CRC Press.

Paik, S. H., Han, S. R., Kwon, O. J., Ahn, Y. M., Lee, B. C., & Ahn, S. Y. (2013). Acupuncture for the treatment of urinary incontinence: a review of randomized controlled trials. *Experimental and Therapeutic Medicine*, *06*(03), 773–780. Retrieved from https://doi.org/10.3892/etm.2013.1210.

Shaw, G., & Nazario, B. (2011, July 22). *New treatments for OAB*. WebMD. Retrieved from https://www.webmd.com/urinary-incontinence-oab/features/treatment-advances.

Watanabe, T., Yokoyama, T., Sasaki, K., Nozaki, K., Ozawa, H., & Kumon, H. (2004). Intravesical resiniferatoxin for patients with neurogenic detrusor overactivity. *International Journal of Urology*, *11*(04), 200–205. Retrieved from https://doi.org/10.1111/j.1442-2042.2003.00782.x.

5

Endocrine and Metabolic System

Introduction

Some of the topics discussed under the endocrine and metabolic system are:

1. Obesity
2. Diabetes mellitus
3. Hypothyroidism
4. Hyperthyroidism
5. Poor appetite

Obesity

Obesity is defined by the WHO as "abnormal or excessive fat accumulation that presents a risk to health." It is estimated that 39% of adults aged 18 and above are overweight with 13% of this population who are obese. Obesity is caused by larger amounts of calories consumed than calories used due to either an increased energy-dense, high-fat food intake or a sedentary lifestyle. Underlying medical, endocrine, genetic causes, and medications can also lead to obesity.

There are many hormones that are involved in food satiation (i.e., glucagon-like peptide-1 [GLP1], cholecystokinin [CCK] and peptide YY [PYY]).

The hormones that regulate appetite and hunger include ghrelin, leptin, and adiponectin.

Ghrelin is produced in the gastrointestinal tract, induces hunger, and increases appetite. It is a hunger pang-signaling hormone.

Leptin and adiponectin are cytokines (collectively called adipokines) produced by fat cells in the white adipose tissue.

Leptin inhibits hunger and decreases appetite. It is an appetite suppressant. Leptin is increased in obesity and heart disease.

Adiponectin is both proinflammatory and anti-inflammatory. It induces hunger. It is reduced in obesity, atherosclerosis, and diabetes.

The enzyme, AMP-activated protein kinase (AMPK), is present in the hypothalamus. When the enzyme is activated, it stimulates hunger. When the enzyme is inhibited, hunger is inhibited.

- *Body mass index (BMI)*. The formula is (weight in kg)/(height in m)^2.
  BMI of 25 to 29.9: Overweight

BMI greater than 30: Obese
- *Hip to waist ratio*. Abdominal obesity is defined as:
  waist-hip ratio greater than 0.90 (male)
  waist-hip ratio greater than 0.85 (female)
- Waist circumference
  Normal waist circumference for males: 94 to 102 cm
    greater than 102 cm: Obese
  Normal waist circumference for females: 80 to 88 cm
    greater than 88 cm: Obese

Obesity is considered a major risk factor for developing other health problems such as diabetes, heart-related ailments, and cancer. Diabesity refers to a combination of diabetes and obesity.

General Therapeutic Measures

Diet

High protein diets. They can boost metabolism and aid with weight loss.

Low-carbohydrate and **low-fat foods** are recommended to provide a low-calorie diet.

- Avoid processed foods, refined oils, trans fats, starchy vegetables, sugary and fatty foods, and baked goods.
- Snack on healthy foods such as fruits, nuts, and yogurt.
- Drink lemon water first thing in the morning. Then warm water (or lemon water or green tea) throughout the day. Drinking water before meals leads to a decreased calorie intake.
- Chew foods slowly when eating to facilitate digestion. Mindful eating and being thankful can also reduce stress and overeating.
- Avoid big meals before bedtime. The main or biggest meal should be during the day.
- Avoid fad diets.
- Avoid snacking.

Short-term fasting. Intermittent short-term fasting done regularly can induce ketosis and promote weight loss.

Nutrigenomics and nutrigenetics look at how food affects gene expression and how the genes can affect nutrition, respectively. This genetic information can predict a person's health status and risk for cancer or chronic diseases. The test uses salivary DNA to identify molecular markers.

Lifestyle

Lifestyle changes. Make healthy lifestyle changes such as eating at regular times. Dinner should be the lightest meal and before 7 p.m.

- Regular exercise or sports should be a daily routine. These can include 20- to 30-minute walks, yoga, pilates, tai chi, or qigong, etc.
- Adequate sleep also aids with weight loss.
- Reduce stress factors.

Indian Natural Remedies

In Ayurveda, obesity is termed as *Atisthaulya*. This is due to excessive *Meda* (fat) and *Mamsa* (muscle) accumulation from underlying *Santarpanottha Vikaras* (excessive calories and nutrition). The excessive fat tissue will obstruct the Strotas (microchannels), hence blocking *Vata* (air), and increasing Agni (digestive fire), and causing repetitive hunger urges. A weakened or decreased Agni can also lead to fat accumulation.

Medo Dushti refers to fat metabolism disorders. There are many *Medohara and Lekhaniya* (anti-obesity and hypolipidemic) herbs or drugs with specific properties that help with weight loss. The following herbs contain these properties:

- bitter taste *(Tikta Rasa)* e.g., neem, giloy
- astringent *(Kashaya)* e.g., bibhitaki, haritaki,
- pungent *(Katu Vipaka)* e.g., pippali
- hot potency *(Ushna Veerya)* e.g., ashwagandha
- light and dry *(Laghu and Ruksha Guna)* e.g., green gram, pomegranate
- anti-phlegmatic *(Vata Kapha hara)* e.g., ginger

It is not uncommon for herbs to have multiple properties (e.g., neem is both bitter and pungent.)

Herbal remedies listed below should be used only as an adjunct to proper lifestyle and diet changes.

Common Ingredients for Obesity

Spices	Herbs/Leaves	Miscellaneous
Black peppercorn (*Piper nigrum*)	Guggulu (*Commiphora mukul*)	Buttermilk
Cardamom	Coriander	Hibiscus tea
Chili	*Centella asiatica*	
	Neem leaf	Chickpea
	Triphala (amla, haritaki, and bibhitaki)	Black gram/Urad
	Ceylon leadwort/chitrak (*Plumbago zeylanica*)	Indian gooseberry/Amla
	Guava leaf	Kallimudayan (*Caralluma Fimbriata/Caralluma adscendens*)
	Barberry (*Ber beris aristata*)	Green gram (moong/mung bean)
	Moringa leaves	
	False black pepper/Vidanga (*Embelia ribes*)	
	Agnimantha (*Premna integrifolia*)	
	Jalkumbhi/Water hyacinth (*Pontederia crassipes*)	
	Guduchi/Giloy (*Tinospora cordifolia*)	
	Nutgrass/Mustaka (*Cyperus rotundus*)	
	Vacha (*Acorus calamus*)	
Cinnamon	Punarnava *Boerhavia diffusa*	Lemon
Coriander	Kutki (*Picrorhiza kurroa*)	Jaggery
Cumin seed	Mint	Hawthorn berries
Fennel	Gurmar (*Gymnema sylvestre*)	Kollu
	Gotu kola	Banana flower

Spices	Herbs/Leaves	Miscellaneous
Fenugreek (methi)	Vijaysar Malabar kino (*Pterocarpus marsupium*)	Passion fruit flower
Garlic	Brahmi (*Bacopa monnieri*)	Aloe vera
Ginger/Shunthi	Haritaki/myrobalan (*Terminalia chebula*)	Honey
Kalonji (Nigella seeds)	Indian coleus (*Coleus forskohlii*)	Trikatu (black pepper + long pepper + ginger)
Long pepper (*Piper longum*)	Arugampul/dhoob (*Cynodon dactylon*)	Vrikshamla (*Garcinia cambogia*) or HCA or HCA-containing *Garcinia* extract
Turmeric	Bibhitaki (*Terminalia bellirica*)	Barberry/Daruharidra (*Berberis vulgaris*)

Common Recipes

Oral

Teas/Brews

Agnimantha. Pound the agnimantha leaves and extract 20 mL juice. Consume this twice a day for 3 months.
   Variation # 1. To make a decoction, take 25 g of the Agnimantha root powder. Add 400 mL water. Boil and reduce the volume to 100 mL. Consume this daily.

Aloe vera juice. Wash and dry an aloe vera leaf. Slit the leaf in half and discard the greenish gel. Cut the remaining white gel into cubes and store in a refrigerator. Add the gel to any fruit juice and blend.

Arugampul juice. Take one to two handfuls of fresh washed arugampul (roots removed) and a few neem leaves. Add some water or coconut water and blend. Strain and drink fresh first thing in the morning on an empty stomach. Alternatively, take 3 teaspoons of the dried arugampul powder.

Amla juice. Lightly pound three to four amla fruits and strain the juice. Take this juice on an empty stomach in the morning with a glass of warm water.

Banana flower. It can be chopped finely and sauteed with various spices (usually onion, garlic, cumin, and curry leaves).
   Variation #1. To make banana flower dosai or adai, take 1 cup of rice, ¼ cup of toor dhal (yellow split pea), 2 tablespoons of black dal (urad), 1 tablespoon of chickpeas (chana dal) and 1 tablespoon of green/mung bean (moong dal). Soak overnight. Blend with some grated coconut, two red chilis, 1 teaspoon of cumin seeds, a little asafoetida and 1 cup chopped boiled banana flower. Take two scoops and make the pancake on a skillet.

Barberry tea. Take 1 to 2 teaspoons of crushed berries or 1 to 2 teaspoons of dried barberry root. Add 1 cup of hot water. Steep for 10 minutes. Strain and consume three times a day.

Black gram. Consume black gram on most days as a part of the daily diet.

Brahmi tea. Place about two to three stalks of fresh brahmi leaves into a cup. Pour boiling water over the leaves and allow it to steep for about 10 to 15 minutes. Add honey to taste and drink.

Cardamom powder. Finely grind cardamom seeds into a powder. Take ½ a teaspoon of cardamom powder once a day.

Chickpea. Consume chickpeas on most days and as a part of daily diet.

Chitrak. Take 1 to 2 g of chitrak root powder. Mix with some honey and consume.

Cinnamon paste. Mix some cinnamon with honey to make a paste. Take this three times a day.

Cinnamon tea. Add one cinnamon stick to a cup and pour boiling water over it. Allow to steep for about 10 minutes. Add honey to taste. Drink in the morning on an empty stomach.

Coleus forskohlii. Coleus forskohlii is available as pickle or as an extract of 10% forskohlin. The recommended dose in adults is 250 mg of coleus (10% forskolin) twice a day.

Coriander tea. Grind coriander seeds into a fine powder and add to a cup of hot water. Allow to steep for 10 minutes and drink.

False black pepper/Vidanga. Consume fresh juice made from the fruits and leaves. The leaves can also be cooked, or the raw fruits eaten.

Fennel tea. Grind fennel seeds into a fine powder and add to a cup of hot water. Allow to steep for 10 minutes and drink.

Fenugreek. Brew lightly, roast some fenugreek seeds, and grind into a fine powder. Mix 1 teaspoon of the powder in 1 cup of warm water. Drink in the morning on an empty stomach. Alternatively, soak some seeds in water overnight. Drink the water the next morning and chew on the seeds.

Garcinia cambogia/HCA or HCA-containing *Garcinia* extract. This herb is available as a commercial preparation as a capsule.

Garlic paste. Take one clove of garlic a day. Pound one clove of garlic until smooth and add to a cup of water. Mix well and drink.

Giloy juice. Place a handful of giloy leaves into a blender and blend until smooth. Strain and drink. Alternatively, chew on fresh giloy leaves or consume as a powder.

Gotu kola tea. Steep a teaspoon of fresh or dried gotu kola leaves in a cup of hot water for about 10 to 15 minutes. Drink it warm.

Guava leaf. Take a handful of guava leaves. Add 100 mL of water. Boil until the volume is reduced to 25 mL. Consume twice a day.

> Variation #1. Take four to six washed guava leaves. Add 1 cup of boiling water. Steep for 10 to 15 minutes. Strain and consume.

Guggulu. It is available in the form of dietary supplements. Adults can take about 25 mg of guggulu supplements every day after a meal. Alternatively, 1 teaspoon of ground guggulu can be mixed with some ground ginger and honey to make a paste. Take this paste three times a day.

Gurmar brew. Gurmar is available as a powder or in the form of dried leaves. Alternatively, make gurmar brew by mixing 1 teaspoon of gurmar powder (or 1 to 2 g of dry leaves) in 1 cup of warm water. Add honey to taste and drink. Consume ½ hour after lunch and dinner.

> Variation #1. Gurmar juice. Take some fresh washed leaves. Blend with a little water and make fresh juice. Consume 20 to 30 mL once or twice a day.
>
> Variation #2. Gurmar leaves. Chew on one or two fresh gurmar leaves every day.

Hawthorn berry tea. Take about 1 teaspoon of dried hawthorn berries and steep in hot water. Add honey to taste and drink it warm.

Herb mixture. Mix equal parts of chitrak, trikatu, and kukti. Consume half a teaspoon of this mixture with water. Take this mixture one to two times a day.

Hibiscus tea. Place a handful of dried or fresh hibiscus petals into a teapot with a cup of boiling water. Steep for 10 to 15 minutes and strain. Add a pinch of cinnamon and honey to taste. Alternatively, fry two hibiscus flowers in ghee and consume with a cup of warm milk once a day.

> Variation #1. Add 2 teaspoons of dried hibiscus flower petals to a teapot. Pour 2 cups of boiling water over the petals. Allow it to steep for about 10 minutes. Strain and add honey to taste.
>
> Variation #2. Take about 1 cup of fresh hibiscus petals. Wash and dry them. Steep them in some honey in a bottle and expose it to the sun for about 7 days. Consume 1 spoon daily.

Jaggery and lemon juice. Mix 1 teaspoon of fresh lemon juice into 1 cup of warm water. Add a piece of jaggery to the lemon water. Mix well and drink in the morning on an empty stomach. This is believed to be able to boost metabolism and help with weight loss.

Jalkumbhi juice. Place a handful of fresh jalkumbhi leaves in a blender and gradually add up to 1 cup of water. Blend until smooth. Pour into a cup and drink.

Kalonji seeds. Eat four to five seeds with some water after lunch and dinner.

Kollu. The grains are soaked and then cooked until soft. It is added to soups or mixed with rice or curries.

Kutki. Take ½ teaspoon of kutki powder. Add 1 tablespoon of aloe vera juice and 1 teaspoon honey. Consume three times a day after meals.

Mint tea. Place a handful of mint leaves into a pot of water. Bring to a boil and reduce the heat. Allow the mixture to simmer for 5 to 10 minutes. Strain and drink twice a day.

> Variation #1. Fresh mint leaves can also be eaten as food.

Neem tea. Chew four to five neem leaves or take 1 teaspoon of neem extract. Alternatively, lightly crush four to five neem leaves and add to a cup of hot water. Allow to steep for about 10 minutes. Strain and drink.

Nutgrass/Mustaka tea. Take 1 tablespoon of the nutgrass root powder. Add 1 cup of water. Boil until volume is reduced to 50 to 75 mL. Strain and consume warm.

Punarnava tea. Add one part each of dried punarnava, one part of dried passion fruit flower, and two parts of dried hawthorn berries. Steep about half a teaspoon of this in a cup of hot water for about 10 minutes. Drink twice a day after lunch and dinner. The passion fruit leaf is often chopped up and eaten in a salad in Sri Lankan cuisine.

Spice buttermilk. Add some grated ginger, ground cumin seeds, and chopped coriander leaves to a cup of fresh buttermilk. Mix well and sprinkle with some salt.

Spices. The spices in the above list can be mixed or rotated every day as tea or as food seasoning. Do not exceed more than 1 tablespoon per day.

Trikatu brew. Steep equal parts of black pepper, long pepper, and ginger in a cup of hot water. Steep for about 10 to 15 minutes. Drink it warm.

Triphala tea. Add half a teaspoon of Triphala powder to one cup of hot water. Mix well and drink it warm.

Turmeric tea. Lightly pound about 2 to 4 inches of fresh turmeric. Place the turmeric into a pot with 2 cups of water. Bring to a boil and then allow to simmer for about half an hour. Add honey to taste and drink.

Vacha brew. Lightly pound some vacha root. Place 1 g of the root into a cup of boiling water and steep until completely cool. Mix some honey into the mixture and drink.

Vijaysar. Vijaysar is available as a commercial preparation, in the form of a powder to be taken with water.

Polyherbal Compound Formulations

Some of these include:

Navayasa lauha. It contains amla, haritaki, vibhitaki, pippali, vidanga, chitraka, mustaka, ginger, and lauha bhasma (processed iron).

Trikatu. It contains pippali, black pepper, and ginger.

Vidangadi churna. It contains amla, vidanga, ginger, barley, processed iron, and carbonate of potash.

Navaka Guggulu. It contains amla, haritaki, vibhitaki, pippali, vidanga, chitraka, mustaka, ginger, and guggulu.

Takrarishta. It contains buttermilk, amla, haritaki, black pepper, ajwain, sea salt, black salt, and efflorescence salt.

Trimad. It contains mustaka, vidanga, and chitraka.

Herbal polyherbal formula, HFO-O2. It contains triphala, trimad, guggul, and vrikshamla/Garcinia.

Garcinia Plus. It contains vrikshamla/Garcinia, Citrus auranti, Atractylodes, and chromium.

Therapeutic Measures

Diet and Lifestyle

- Eat foods according to the dosha type. For example, the *Vata*-dominant person tends to be "dry and cold" and hence needs more fats and warmer foods. Also, the meals should be small and frequent. Avoid astringent foods and fruits and consume sweet, juicy fruits.
- Eat freshly cooked and warm meals.
- Consume *sattvic foods*, which are fresh seasonal fruits, vegetables, whole grains, nuts, legumes, and dairy.
- Eat meals with all six tastes (i.e., sweet, sour, salty, bitter, astringent, and pungent).
- Include digestives like dried ginger, cumin, cinnamon, fenugreek, garcinia, tamarind, or triphala to facilitate fat digestion.
- Vegetarian or vegan meals can help with weight loss.
- Do not eat until the stomach is full. The general rule is: Fill the stomach with ½ solid foods, ¼ liquid foods, and ¼ left empty.
- There is no true intermittent fasting in Ayurveda. The 4 to 6 hours' interval between 4 to 6 meals per day allows for complete digestion. Hence, do not snack between meals.
- Sip hot fluids or hot water between meals. This also aids digestion.
- Regular fasting *(Upavasa)* is done as part of Shamana (palliative) treatment, usually once a week or once a month, to restore good physical, mental, and spiritual health. It is a detoxification and spiritual ritual.

  There is complete abstinence of foods, fluids, and all other pleasures. Fasting improves Sattvic behaviors (purity in thoughts and deeds). Fasting should not be done at extreme ages (pediatric and geriatric), during pregnancy, and in debilitating or some medical conditions.

  A post-fasting meal is usually a warm, light, and freshly cooked rice porridge with digestive spices and herbs or fruits. It should not be a mindless feast.
- Overall, an Indian diet is largely lacto-vegetarian. It consists of vegetables, fruits, whole grains, legumes (dal), spices, dairy, and healthy fats. Grain portions and sugars must be reduced.
- Refer also to the above for the general therapeutic measures.

  Panchakarma procedures can help to purify the body and help in weight loss.

Upavasa or Langhana fasting. Complete fasting or liquid fasting can increase digestive fire *(Agni)*, remove toxins, and improve health.

Ruksha Udvartana. This is a deep-cleansing massage using dry herbal powder. It improves the skin, strengthens the muscles, and breaks down the fat.

Kizhi. This one's a hot fermentation therapy with the help of medicated pouches.

Vamana (therapeutic vomiting). Various herbal decoctions are used for emetic therapy.

Virechana (therapeutic purgation). This is to remove blood toxins and cleanse the gastrointestinal system, kidneys, and sweat glands. Various oral purgatives such as triphala, castor oil, psyllium, senna, aloe vera, flaxseeds, dandelion root, bhumi amla, etc., are used.

Basti (enema). Medicated sesame oil and herbal enemas are used. *Lekhana basti*, a form of medicated enema, is used to treat Sthaulya disorders.

Pre-panchakarma (Purvakarma) procedures include *Snehana* (oleation or oil massage) to lubricate and soften the whole body and *Swedana* (sweating via herbal steam bath) to eliminate the toxins. This is done usually for 3 days before panchakarma.

Yoga asanas for weight loss include the following:

Chaturanga Dandasana (plank pose), Dhanurasana (bow pose), Adho Mukha Svanasana (downward dog pose), Trikonasana (triangle pose), Setu Bandha Sarvangasana (bridge pose), Virabhadrasana (warrior pose), Parivrtta Utkatasana (twisted chair pose), Surya Namaskar (sun salutation), and Sarvangasana (shoulder stand).

Chinese Natural Remedies

Common Ingredients for Obesity

Spices	Herbs/Leaves	Miscellaneous
Black pepper (Piper nigrum)	Pu-erh tea leaf	Hawthorn berry/shan zha
	Codonopsis root/ dang shen	Rangoon creeper fruit/ shi jun zi (Combretum indicum)
	Licorice root/ gan cao	Radish seed/(lai fu zi
	Chinese yam/ huai shan	Peach seed/tao ren
	Coix seed/Yi Yi Ren (Coix lacryma-jobi)	Biota seed/bai zi ren (Platycladus orientalis)
	Poria (fu ling)	Rhubarb/da huang
	Inula flower (xuan fu hua)	Black sesame/hei zhi ma (Sesamum indicum)
	Senna leaf/fan xie ye (Cassia acutifolia/Cassia angustifolia)	Red bean/hong dou (Vigna angularis)
	White atractylodes/ bai zhu	Plantain seed/che qian zi (Plantago asiatica/Plantago depressa)
	Pinellia tuber/ ban xia (Pinellia ternata)	Fructus hordes germinates/mai ya
	Jiaogulan	Ginseng
	Fructus forsythiae suspensae (lian qiao)	Areca peel/da fu pi (Areca catechu)
	Semen raphani sativi (lai fu zi)	Atractylodes
	Berberine	
	Konjac root	

Spices	Herbs/Leaves	Miscellaneous
Cinnamon	Oolong tea leaf	Dried tangerine peel/ (chen pi)
Ginger	Green tea leaf	Unripe orange/ zhi shi

Common Recipes

Oral

- **Remedies for strengthening the spleen:** Codonopsis root, licorice root, Chinese yam, coix seed, and poria. In TCM, it is believed that spleen weakness causes body fluid and toxin accumulation.
- **Remedies to boost digestion and metabolism:** Unripe orange, hawthorn berry, Rangoon creeper fruit, radish seed, and dried tangerine peel. These herbs are believed to stimulate the secretion of digestive fluid, hence boosting digestion and metabolism.
- **Remedies to promote bowel movements:** Black sesame, radish seed, peach seed, biota seed, and rhubarb. These remedies are used to promote waste excretion and toxin buildup in the body, which is thought to cause weight gain.
- **Remedies to prevent fluid retention:** Coix barley, red bean, inula flower, plantain seed, senna leaf, cinnamon and ginger, and white atractylodes. These remedies are thought to have a diuretic effect on the body, promoting fluid excretion from the body. These herbs are thought to be *warming* herbs and can resolve cold dampness in the body, which is thought to cause weight gain.

  Jiaogulan tea. This is consumed twice a day 30 minutes before meals.

  Barberry tea. Take 1 to 2 teaspoons of crushed berries or 1 to 2 teaspoons of dried barberry root. Add 1 cup of hot water. Steep for 10 minutes. Strain and consume three times a day.

  Cinnamon tea. Add one cinnamon stick to a cup and pour boiling water over it. Allow it to steep for about 10 minutes. Add honey to taste. Drink in the morning on an empty stomach.

  Konjac root. This Asian root vegetable can be boiled or processed into ground flour to make Japanese noodles (shirataki noodles) or snacks.

  Ginger tea. Lightly pound 3 to 4 inches of fresh ginger and place into an empty cup. Pour boiling water into the cup and allow it to steep for about 10 minutes. Drink in the morning on an empty stomach.

- **Oolong/green/Pu-erh tea.** Oolong, green tea, and Pu-erh are available in the form of dried leaves or tea bags. Place the tea leaves or tea bag into a cup and pour boiling water over it. Allow it to steep for about 10 minutes. Ginger may also be added to the cup.
- **Black pepper tea.** Lightly crush and put 7 to 10 black peppercorns in a cup. Add boiling water and allow it to steep for 10 minutes and then drink.
- **Ginseng tea.** Add about 2 to 4 slices of ginseng to a cup. Pour boiling water over the ginseng and allow it to steep for about 10 to 15 minutes.

  Coix seed. It can be cooked as a porridge or drunken as a brew. Boil the seeds for 30 minutes and drink the liquid.

  Rangoon creeper. Take 1 tablespoon and consume as a decoction.

  Red beans. It can be cooked and consumed as a soup or puree for dessert.

Commercial Oral Preparation

- **Bao he wan.** This is used for the treatment of bloating as well as to boost digestion and metabolism. It is made up of hawthorn berry, zhi ban xia, fu ling, dried tangerine peel, lian qiao, lai fu zi, and mai ya. Adults should take five to eight pills after meals two to three times a day. This herbal preparation should not be taken by those with liver, heart, or kidney diseases.
- **Berberine.** This is available as a commercial preparation. The active ingredient berberine is derived from the barberry plant. The recommended dose of berberine is 250–300 mg daily.

Western/Other Natural Remedies

Common Ingredients for Obesity

Spices	Herbs/Leaves/Fruit/Flower	Miscellaneous
Black peppercorn	Rosemary	Grain of Paradise (*Aframomum melegueta*)
Cayenne pepper	Green tea leaf	Probiotics
Cinnamon	Yerba mate (*Ilex paraguariensis*)	Yogurt
Ginger	Parsley	Apple cider vinegar
Oregano	Peppermint leaf	Honey
	Celery	Chitosan
	Sage	• Vitamins and vitamin-like compounds
		• B (B3, B5, and B7, choline and inositol)
		• A, D, E, K
		• Alpha lipoic acid
	Plantain weed/leaf	*Minerals* (chromium, selenium, zinc, magnesium, and calcium)

Spices	Herbs/Leaves/Fruit/Flower	Miscellaneous
	Rose hip	*Amino acids and Derivatives*
	(*Rosa canina L.*)	Conjugated linoleic acid
		Choline
		Acetyl-L-carnitine
		Asparagine
		Glutamine
		Cysteine
	Damiana	Almond
	(*Turnera diffusa*)	
	Artichoke	*Gynostemma pentaphyllum*
	Watercress	Kelp/Brown algae seaweed (fucoxanthin)
	Aloe vera	Eggs
	Lemon	African mango seed powder (*Irvingia gabonensis*)
	Grapefruit	Caffeine
		• Green coffee bean extract
		• Green tea
		• Cocoa
		• Guarana
	Rose petal	White kidney bean (Cannellini) extract
	Dandelion	*Griffonia simplicifolia* seeds (5-HTP extract)
	Hibiscus	Glucomannan
	Cranberry	Hordenine
	Forskolin	Yohimbine
		Protein powder supplements
		Soluble fiber
		(*From psyllium husk, glucomannan, guar gum, or beta glucans*)
		Raspberry ketone
		Adiponectin
		7- Keto DHEA
		Naringenin

Common Recipes

Oral

Teas/Brews/Others

Acetyl L-carnitine. It is available in the form of supplements.

Adiponectin. This dietary supplement can help with weight loss. Consume omega-3 fish oil or other monounsaturated fats (olive oil, avocados, nuts) or herbs (ginger, fennel, sage marjoram) to increase adiponectin levels.

African mango seed powder. Consume as a part of a regular diet. It is also available as commercial preparations.

Almonds. Consume five to six almonds daily.

Aloe vera juice. Wash and dry an aloe vera leaf. Slit the leaf in half and discard the greenish gel. Cut the remaining white gel into cubes and store in a refrigerator. Add the gel to any fruit juice and blend.

AMPK activators. AMPK is an enzyme found in all cells, which stops fat storage. Botanical extracts like *Gynostemma pentaphyllum* and *Hesperidin* can activate AMPK activity. Reduced AMPK activity is found in fat tissue and with older age.

Apple cider vinegar. Mix 1 tablespoon of apple cider vinegar into 1 cup of warm water. Drink in the morning on an empty stomach.

Artichoke. Consume artichoke as part of food.

Beta-hydroxybutyrate. This is an exogenous ketone supplement that reduces appetite, acts as a fuel source, and reduces fat mass. Side effects include abdominal pain, diarrhea, and constipation. It is available as ketone salts or ketone esters.

Cayenne pepper. Add cayenne pepper to cooked dishes. Alternatively, add a pinch of cayenne pepper to a cup of water and mix well. Add honey to taste and drink.

Celery juice. Wash and cut two stalks of celery. Blend with water until smooth. Strain and drink the juice.

Variation #1. Celery leaf tea. Place a handful of celery leaves in a pot of boiling water. Bring the mixture to a boil then reduce the heat and allow it to simmer for about 15 minutes. Strain the mixture and drink.

Chitosan. This is available as a dietary supplement and is taken just before meals.

Cinnamon tea. Lightly crush one stick of cinnamon bark and place in a cup. Pour boiling water into the cup and steep for about 5 minutes. Add honey to taste and drink.

Conjugated linoleic acid. This is an omega-6 fatty acid or natural trans fat in the body. It is also available as a supplement and may reduce body fat.

Cranberry juice. Place a cup of frozen or fresh cranberries in a pot and add about 2 cups of water. Cook until the berries burst and strain through a piece of muslin. Add honey to taste.

Damiana polyherbal. It contains damiana, guarana, yerba mate, and an inulin-based soluble fiber.

Damiana tea. Take 1 teaspoon of the dried leaves and add 1 cup of boiling water. Steep for 10 minutes. Strain and drink warm.

Dandelion-peppermint tea. Place equal parts of dried dandelion and peppermint leaves into a cup. Pour 1 cup of boiling water over the leaves and allow it to steep for 5 to 10 minutes. Drink twice a day.

Eggs. Consume an egg daily for breakfast.

Glucomannan. It is taken with water three times a day at least 1 hour before meals.

Green tea and ginger. Lightly pound 2 to 4 inches of fresh ginger. Place 2 teaspoons of dried green tea leaves and the ginger into a teapot. Pour 1 cup of boiling water into the teapot and allow it to steep for 5 to 10 minutes. Strain and drink.

Hibiscus tea. Add 2 teaspoons of dried hibiscus flower petals' to a teapot. Pour 2 cups of boiling water over the petals. Allow it to steep for about 10 minutes. Strain and add honey to taste. Hibiscus has been found to have diuretic properties and stimulate bowel movements.

Lemon tea. Squeeze half a lemon and add the juice to a glass of hot water. Add honey and drink it warm.

Lemon and black pepper tea. Mix about 2 tablespoons of lemon juice to a cup of warm water and mix well. Lightly pound 5 to 10 black peppercorns and add to the cup of lemon water. Steep for about 5 to 10 minutes. Strain and drink.

Naringenin. This is available as a dietary supplement or combined with other ingredients.

Parsley tea. Chop two to three stalks of fresh parsley into smaller pieces. Place the parsley into a cup and pour hot water into the cup. Allow it to steep for 5 to 10 minutes.

Plantain weed/leaf. Consume 3 g of plantain leaf in 250 mL of water. Take three times a day ½ hour before each meal. Young leaves can be eaten as a salad green.

Probiotics. Consume high-dose probiotics with at least 30 CFU.

Rose hip tea. Place four to eight dried rose hips in 1 cup of water. Steep for 10 to 15 minutes. Drain and drink. Rose hip supplements are also available.

Rose petal tea. Place a handful of organic fresh or dried rose petals into a pot with 2 cups of water. Allow it to simmer until the petals have lost their color. Strain and drink.

Rosemary-lemon tea. Put about 1 tablespoon of chopped fresh rosemary in a pot and add 2 cups of water. Boil for about 1 minute. Cool and then add the juice of one lemon. Mix well and strain. Add honey to taste.

7-Keto DHEA. This supplement is taken to increase thermogenesis and metabolism and promote weight loss.

Raspberry ketones. This dietary supplement combined with vitamin C may help with weight loss.

Sage tea. Place three to five sage leaves in a cup of boiling water. Cover and let steep for 5 to 10 minutes. Drink warm.

Soluble fiber. It absorbs water and becomes gel-like to fill the stomach and gives a sense of fullness. This can be from psyllium husk, glucomannan, guar gum, and beta glucans.

Xanthigen. This is a nutraceutical supplement containing brown marine algae fucoxanthin and pomegranate seed oil (PSO), which can facilitate weight loss.

Yerba mate brew. Add 1 tablespoon of dried yerba mate to a teapot and pour 2 cups of boiling water over the herbs. Allow it to steep for about 5 minutes. Strain and drink.

Yogurt. Consume yogurt or buttermilk.

Yohimbine. This is available as a dietary supplement.

Vitamins and Vitamin-like Compounds

- **Vitamin B**: *B3 (niacin)* increases the adiponectin level. *B5(pantothenic acid)* activates the lipoprotein lipase enzyme. *B7 (biotin)* decreases insulin level so that less fat cells are formed.

  Choline can reduce body weight quickly.

  Inositol can increase adiponectin levels.

  Alpha lipoic acid can help with weight loss.

- **Vitamin A** promotes gene expression for the formation and size of fat cells.

- **Vitamin D** regulates carbohydrate metabolism and fat storage.

- **Vitamin E** prevents the immature fat cells from becoming mature fat storage cells.

- **Vitamin K** regulates sugar and fat metabolism.

Minerals

Calcium can prevent the synthesis of fat cells and helps with the fat oxidation.

Chromium increases the sensitivity of insulin, decreases body fat, and increases muscle.

Selenium regulates the thyroid hormones and hence decreases body fat.

Magnesium also increases insulin sensitivity and decreases fat absorption.

Zinc increases leptin levels. In obesity, there are low zinc and high leptin levels.

Amino Acids and Derivatives

Asparagine. It increases insulin sensitivity. The glucose is stored in the muscle instead of being changed to fat.

Glutamine. It increases glucose uptake into the muscle.

Cysteine. It is an antioxidant that reduces body fat storage.

Carnitine. It carries fatty acids into the cell so they can be burned for fuel; helps reduce visceral adiposity (belly fat).

Lipoic acid. It enhances glucose uptake into cells.

Commercial Preparations

There are many types of weight loss or diet pills available. They contain various herbs such as *G. cambogia* extract/ HCA, Green coffee bean extract, *Caralluma*, white kidney bean extracts, *Griffonia simplicifolia* extracts, Grain of Paradise, cinnamon, and vitamins and minerals. They are appetite suppressants that modulate the hunger (decrease ghrelin) and satiety hormones, or can inhibit the starch digestive enzymes, or are thermogenic fat burners, or are keto diet pills.

For example,

LeanBean contains glucomannan, caffeine (green coffee bean), Garcinia cambogia, black pepper, turmeric, acai berry, chromium picolinate, choline, vitamins B6 and B12, zinc, and potassium.

Java Burn is a beverage (usually coffee) additive, which contains green tea extract (EGCG catechin and caffeine), green coffee bean extract from Coffea arabica (chlorogenic acid and caffeine), chromium chloride, carnitine, theanine, and vitamins B6, B12, and D3.

Therapeutic Measures

Meal replacement shakes/protein shakes/protein bars/ protein powders/smoothies. Some store-bought shakes are wholesome (low sugar or additives) and contain adequate vitamins, minerals, protein (whey, pea, soy, egg, casein, chia, or hemp) and fiber with various flavors such as chocolate, coffee, or vanilla.

Multigrain such as barley, millet, brown rice, green pea, red beans, or oats are present in the powder formulations.

Homemade smoothies can be made with fresh yogurt, protein powder, nuts, or seeds and with a variety of fruits or greens blended with crushed ice. Various recipes are available. Consume about 30 g of protein, 10 g of fat, 5 g of fiber per meal to provide about 300 to 400 calories.

Diets. Many weight-loss diets are available. Calorie restriction is the main goal, and the diets generally follow the 1200 calorie per day rule. None are guaranteed and each diet type may work for one person and not another. Many are described as fad diets and not FDA-approved.

- *Paleo diet.* It consists of lean meat, fish, vegetables, fruits, and dairy-free, whole grain-free, and legume-free.
- *Keto or Ketogenic diet.* It consists of 75% fats, 10% to 30% protein, and 5% carbohydrates per day. Ketones instead of glucose are used as the main fuel in this diet. Carbohydrates are restricted to 20 g/day to induce ketosis. It is usually done in a hospital setting with medical supervision.
- *Modified Atkins diet.* It is less restrictive than the ketogenic diet. There is no calorie, protein, or fluid restriction. The protein intake is about 35%. Foods are not weighed. There is no fasting or hospitalization.
- *Vegan diet.* It is completely plant-based with no animal or animal-derived products. It is dairy-free and egg-free. There is risk of vitamins (D, B12), minerals (calcium, iron, iodine, zinc), and omega-3 deficiencies.
- *Mediterranean diet.* It comprises plenty of vegetables, fruits, whole grains, nuts, seeds, legumes, fish or seafood, and extra virgin olive oil. Dairy, eggs, and poultry are consumed in moderation. Red meat is restricted.
- *DASH diet* (Dietary Approaches to Stop Hypertension). It includes plenty of vegetables, fruits, whole grains, and lean meats with low salt, low sugar, and low-fat intake. Red meat is restricted. Based on the caloric intake, the number of servings allowed is proportioned. An average meal plan will have seven servings of whole-grain carbohydrates, five servings of vegetables, five servings of fruit, two servings of fish or lean meat, and two servings of low-fat dairy. Nuts and seeds are allowed two or three times per week.

- *Zone diet.* It is a low glycemic index (GI) diet, which consists of low GI carbohydrates with fruits, vegetables (⅓ to ⅔), and proteins (⅓), and a little monounsaturated fat. Small, frequent meals are eaten with the first meal or snack consumed 1 hour after waking.
- *Ornish diet.* This is largely a vegetarian or vegan diet that is low in fats, low in calories, and high in complex carbohydrates and fiber (fruits and vegetables).
- *hCG diet.* This is a low 500 calorie per day diet for 8 weeks while getting hCG (human chorionic gonadotropin) hormone injections or homeopathic oral hCG.
- *Dukan diet.* This consists of an initial unrestricted high-protein diet and oat bran only for a few weeks followed by nonstarchy vegetables, and then low-carb and low-fat foods.
- *Ultra-low-fat diet.* The fat consumed per day is 10% from the total calories per day from a largely plant-based diet.
- *Lectin-free diet.* This diet avoids beans, legumes, bell peppers, and nightshades, which are rich in lectins. However, they are safe when cooked properly or eaten in moderation.
- *Military diet.* Eat low-calorie foods from the strict preset menu for breakfast, lunch, and dinner and without snacks for 3 days. Then for the next 4 "off" days, eat normal calorie foods.
- *Alkaline diet.* This is a largely plant-based diet with plenty of vegetables, fruits, seeds, nuts, legumes, whole grains, dairy, and occasional meat.
- *Pegan diet.* It is a mix of a vegan and paleo diet. It consists of unprocessed, whole foods, which are organic or responsibly produced. They are mainly fruits and vegetables (making up 75%). Meat, fish, legumes, seeds, and nuts are eaten in moderation. Small amounts of gluten-free grains, healthy fat, and sugar are allowed (making up 25%).
- *Intuitive eating.* This is not a true weight-loss diet plan. Here, one eats when hungry and stops when satiated. A variety of healthy, sensible, and favorite foods can be eaten within limits, without binging or craving and most of all, to feel happy.
- *Functional foods* are often recommended, usually based on nutrigenomic testing. Functional foods have inherent anti-inflammatory, antioxidant, antimicrobial, and anticancer properties. They also have fat-burning, cholesterol lowering, or diuretic effects. They are natural foods that are rich with bioactive compounds such as lycopene, beta-carotene, flavonoids, resveratrol, and more. Nutraceuticals are usually dietary supplements.

Intermittent fasting. There are many variations with pros and cons with each diet type.

- **Complete fasting 2 days a week/weekly 24-hour fast (eat-stop-eat method).** Eat for 5 or 6 days. Fast for 1 or

2 nonconsecutive days. No food is eaten. Only zero-calorie fluids are consumed. There is a risk of lethargy, headaches, or irritability.

- **Partial fasting 2 days a week (5:2 diet/fast diet).** Eat normal calorie foods for 5 days. Eat low-calorie foods, 500 to 600 calories per day on the 2 fasting days.
- **Alternate day fasting.** No food or low-calorie foods on fasting days. Eat normal calorie foods the next day.
- **Fasting 12 h/day.** Fast for 12 hours. Eat normal calorie foods for 12 hours.
- **Fasting 16 h/day/16:8 diet/Leangains diet.** Fast for 16 hours, including skipping breakfast. Eat 2 meals (usually lunch and dinner with normal calorie foods over 8 hours).
- **Warrior diet.** Fast 20 hours and eat 1 meal (usually dinner with normal calorie foods over 4 hours) Another variation is to eat some low-calorie fruits and vegetables during the day and one big meal at night.
- **OMAD** (One Meal a Day) Diet. Fast for 22 or 23 hours. Eat 1 meal a day, usually dinner over 1 to 2 hours.

Vibration machines. These are shaking platforms or shaking machines that produce whole-body vibrations, which make the body muscles undergo reflex contraction with subsequent weight loss and muscle gain. Various exercises like squats can be done while standing on the vibrating machine.

Exercises:

- *Resistance training,* such as weightlifting and cardio workouts, are also excellent. Spin cycling is also another form of cardio training that helps with more weight loss compared to exercise bike cycling.
- *H.I.I.T (high-intensity interval training).* Here, there is a cycle of warm up (for about 3 minutes), then vigorous and intensive anaerobic exercise (e.g., cycling, sprinting uphill walking, stair climbing or rowing) for 20 to 60 seconds, followed by medium-intensity exercises (walking or slow jog) then rest or a cool down for 10 seconds. Repeat for 8 to 12 cycles. It can help young obese females.

Modern Remedies

Beta-Methyl-Phenylethylamine (Fastin)

This medication is a central nervous system stimulant that has been found to increase the metabolism of fat in the body.

Orlistat (Xenical)

Orlistat functions by inhibiting gastric and pancreatic lipases. Lipases are enzymes that break down triglycerides in the intestine. When the action of these enzymes is blocked, triglycerides are not broken down into free fatty acids and absorbed. Instead, they are excreted from the body unchanged. The prevention of absorption of fatty acids in the body reduces caloric intake and aids in weight loss. Orlistat is available as capsules.

Phentermine

Phentermine is a norepinephrine reuptake inhibitor. Its mechanism of action is not particularly well understood now. It is thought to treat obesity by suppressing appetite.

Sibutramine

Sibutramine is a centrally acting stimulant, which functions as an appetite suppressant. It reduces the reuptake of nor-epinephrine, serotonin, and dopamine. This leads to an increase in the levels of these substances in the synaptic clefts, which leads to feelings of satiety and suppresses appetite. Sibutramine has been removed from several global markets due to association with increased risk of cardiovascular events such as heart attacks and strokes.

Glucagon-like Peptide-1 (GLP-1) Agonists

Liraglutide (Saxenda), Semaglutide (Ozempic)

Prescription Combination Formula

- Phentermine-Topiramate (Qsymia)
- Bupropion-naltrexone (Contrave)

Intensive Behavioral Therapy

This mind-body intervention is done to change one's lifestyle to improve eating and exercise habits.

Family Therapy

This intervention is helpful in childhood obesity. Standardized Obesity Family Therapy (SOFT) is a systemic and solution-focused program for family interactions.

Weight Loss Surgery

It is also called bariatric surgery. It is sometimes used to treat people who are severely obese and have serious health conditions such as type 2 diabetes or hypertension.

There are several types of weight loss surgery. The most common types are:

Gastric band: A band is placed around the stomach, so less food is consumed.

Gastric bypass: The top part of the stomach is joined to the small intestine so that a feeling of fullness occurs sooner, and there is less calorie absorption from food.

Sleeve gastrectomy: Part of the stomach is removed so that less food is consumed, and the feeling of fullness occurs sooner.

Aesthetic and Plastic Surgery

These include liposuction and tummy tuck procedures, which are done by a trained plastic surgeon.

Liposuction (lipoplasty or body contouring) is a surgical procedure done to remove fat from specific areas of the body (usually abdomen, hip, thigh, buttocks, etc.) that have failed to respond to diet and exercise. Ultrasound, laser, and power-assisted liposuction are available. The most common type is tumescent liposuction is where saline and lignocaine are injected into the area of treatment.

Complications include swelling, infection, fluid overload, fat embolism, numbness, and lignocaine toxicity.

Tummy tuck (abdominoplasty) is a surgical procedure that involves removal of excessive skin and fat and tightening of the underlying fascia (connective tissue) with sutures.

Homeopathic Remedies

These may include:

Calcarea carbonica (pot belly, sweating over forehead, anxiety, fear of night, shortness of breath, and hunger after eating, slow metabolism, associated thyroid problem);

Graphites (associated fatigue, flatulence, irregular periods, melancholy);

Natrum muriaticum (with more fat over thighs and buttocks, heat intolerance, salt craving, associated stress, and depression);

Lycopodium (fat over buttocks and thighs mostly, associated hypothyroidism, gastric or liver problems, constipation, flatulence, cravings for sweet and hot drinks, quick temper);

Ammonium mur (obese trunk, buttocks with thin legs, heel pain, inability to cry);

Nux vomica (in sedentary lifestyle, associated cold intolerance, constipation, overeating, and craving for spicy and fried foods and quick temper);

Ammonium carb (associated nasal congestion, nervous tendency, cardiac problems, not contented);

Phytolacca (associated dry throat with difficulty swallowing, tongue blisters, pallor, body aches, and sciatic pain); and

Fucus vesiculosus (associated thyroid problems, indigestion, and flatulence).

Others include *Pulsatilla nigrans* and *ignatia*.

Diabetes Mellitus

Diabetes is a chronic metabolic and multisystem disease that is characterized by high blood sugar levels (hyperglycemia), either due to impaired insulin production by the pancreas or inefficient insulin use in the body. Insulin is a hormone that controls the blood sugar levels in the body. Over time, high blood sugar can cause several adverse effects in the body, such as damage to the eyes, nerves, brain (with increased Alzheimer's disease risk), kidneys, and blood vessels. Diabetes is classified into type 1 and type 2.

Type 1 Diabetes (also called insulin-dependent diabetes, IDDM)

Type 1 diabetes is caused by insufficient insulin production by the pancreas due to autoimmune disease. It is controlled through daily administration of insulin. Symptoms of type 1 diabetes include thirst, frequent excessive urination, constant hunger, weight loss, and fatigue. The onset is usually in childhood or in neonates (neonatal diabetes mellitus).

Type 2 Diabetes (also called non-insulin-dependent diabetes, NIDDM/maturity-onset diabetes mellitus of the young, MODY)

Type 2 diabetes is due to inefficient use of the body's insulin. Type 2 diabetes is caused by excess body weight and a lack of physical activity. Symptoms are similar to that of type 1 diabetes but are less evident, which means that type 2 diabetes may be diagnosed only several years after onset.

General Management Principles

Relevant tests include regular fasting blood sugar, glucose tolerance test (GTT), glycosylated hemoglobin (HbA1c), lipid profile, renal profile, urinalysis, ECG, and fundus exam.

Treatments include lifestyle optimization, prevention of obesity, maintenance of normoglycemia with optimum HbA1C of less than 6.5% with self-monitoring of glucose daily or continuously, avoidance of hypoglycemia risk, use of appropriate diabetic drug and management of comorbidities.

Indian Natural Remedies

In Ayurveda, diabetes mellitus *(Madhumeha)* is classified as a *Prameha* (urological disorder). It is attributed to tridosha imbalance from increased *medo dhatu*(fat) and *dhatu kshaya* (depletion of tissues). There is also overeating (excessive sweet, salty, oily, sour, or heavy foods), *asya sukha* (sedentary lifestyle), *vyayama* (lack of exercise), *atinidra* (excess sleep), and lack of *samshodhana* (detoxification) therapy.

Ayurvedic herbs have inherent *prameha ghana* (antidiabetic), *medohara* (antihyperlipidemic), and *rasayana* (antioxidant) properties, which ensure good glycemic control along with diet and lifestyle measures.

There are many medicinal herbs with anti-diabetic or antihyperglycemic actions. The various plant parts contain many and specific bioactive or phytoactive chemical constituents (flavonoids, alkaloids, tannins, and phenolic compounds) with single and/or multiple mechanisms of action. Tannins can stimulate insulin secretion. Quercetin is a polyphenol antioxidant.

For example:

Momordica charantia (Bitter gourd/bitter melon). It can regenerate and repair the β-cells of islets of Langerhan in the pancreas, stimulate the secretion of GLP-1 via the Gβγ-signaling pathway, and lower HbA1c levels.

Abelmoschus esculentus (Okra). It is an α-glucosidase and α-amylase inhibitor and hence lowers blood glucose.

Emblica officinalis (Amla), *Terminalia chebula* (Haritaki), *Terminalia bellirica* (Bibhitaki).

It promotes insulin secretion from the pancreas, inhibits glucose absorption in the intestines, and inhibits formation of advanced glycosylation end products (AGEs).

In Ayurgenomics, personalized treatment is based on the individual's *prakriti* status. For example, in kapha imbalance, a combination of kapha-modifying anti-diabetic plant herbs is used (i.e., *Anogeissus latifolia* [axlewood], *Berberis aristata* [common barberry], *Embelia ribes* [vidanga], and *Acacia catechu* [catechu]). In pitta imbalance, pitta-modifying antidiabetic herbal combinations are used (i.e., *Azadirachta indica* [neem], *Phyllanthus emblica* [amla], *Tinospora cordifolia* [guduchi], and *Trichosanthes dioica* [pointed gourd]).

Often, the polyherbal formulations are proven anti-diabetic herbs and combined with other herbal plants with antihyperlipidemic, hepatoprotective, adaptogenic, and immunomodulating actions.

Common Ingredients for Diabetes Mellitus

Spices	Herbs/Leaves	Miscellaneous
Allium cepa (onion)	Banyan tree bark (Ficus benghalensis)	Ivy gourd/Kovai (Coccinia indica)
Asafetida (Ferula assa-foetida)	Bibhitaki (Terminalia bellirica)	Milk
Bay leaf (Laurus nobilis)	Neem (Azadirachta indica)	Banana flower and pseudostem
Black cumin (Nigella sativa)	Berberis vulgaris root (barberry)	Bitter melon
Caraway (Carum carvi)	Moringa/drumstick (Moringa oleifera)	Wood apple (Limonia acidissima)
	Banaba/Queen's flower (Lagerstroemia speciosa)	Black gram/Urad
	Mango leaf	Amla (Phyllanthus emblica)
	South Africa leaf/African Bitter Leaf (Veronia amygdalina)	Hemp seed (Cannabis sativa)
	Sadabahar/Periwinkle/Madagascar periwinkle (Lochnera rosea/Catharanthus roseus)	Sweet potato/Sakkargand (Ipomoea batatas)
	Arugampul/Dhoob (Cynodon dactylon)	Hibiscus (Hibiscus rosa-sinensis)
	Guava leaf and fruit (Psidium guajava)	Garlic
	Triphala	Onion
	Mulberry (Morus indica)	Aegle marmelos (Indian bael)
	Anantmool/Indian sarsaparilla (Hemidesmus indicus)	Mango/Mango leaf and seed (Mangifera indica)
	Saptaranga (Salacia chinensis)	Gray nicker Caesalpinia bonducella
	Indrayan (Citrullus colocynthis)	Custard apple (Annona squamosa)
	Mustaka/Nagarmotha (Cyperus rotundus)	Green tea (Camellia sinensis)
	Gorakhmundi (Sphaeranthus indicus)	Cashew nut (Anacardium occidentale)
	Water lily (Nymphaea stellata)	Chicory (Cichorium intybus)
	Gambhari (Gmelina arborea)	Coconut oil (Cocos nucifera)
	Sweet broom (Scoparia dulcis)	Foxtail millet (Setaria italica)
	Babul (Acacia arabica)	Wood apple (Limonia acidissima)
	Keelanelli (Phyllanthus amarus)	Ponnanganni leaves/Matsyakshi (Alternanthera sessilis)
	Jute leaf (Corchorus olitorius)	Aloe vera
	Lodhra (Symplocos cochinchinensis)	Chundakkai/Turkey berry/Terung pipit (Solanum torvum)
	Indian abutilon/Indian mallow (Abutilon indicum)	Senna/Avarampoo (Cassia angustifolia/Cassia auriculata)
	Bhringraj (Eclipta alba)	Bilimbi (Averrhoa bilimbi)

Spices	Herbs/Leaves	Miscellaneous
	Spiral banner/Insulin plant (*Costus igneus*)	
	Nirgundi (*Vitex negundo*)	
	King of bitters/Nilavembu (*Andrographis paniculata*)	
	Jalkumbhi/Water hyacinth (*Pontederia crassipes*)	
Cinnamon (*Cinnamomum zeylanicum*)	Haritaki (*Terminalia chebula*)	Honey
Coriander (*Coriandrum sativum*)	Ivy gourd (*Coccinia indica*)	Lady's finger/Okra (*Abelmoschus esculentus*)
Cumin (*Cuminum cyminum*)	Holy basil/Tulsi	Noni (*Morinda citrifolia*)
Ginger	Vijaysar churna (*Pterocarpus marsupium*)	Java plum/Jamun (*Eugenia jambolana/Syzygium cumini*)
Mustard (*Brassica nigra, Brassica juncea*)	Gurmar (*Gymnema sylvestre*)	Punica granatum (pomegranate)
Piper nigrum (black peppercorn)	Giloy (*Tinospora cordifolia*)	Snake gourd (*Trichosanthes cucumerina*)
Trigonella foenum (fenugreek seed/methi dana)	Kutki (*Picrorhiza kurroa*)	Pointed gourd (*Trichosanthes dioica*)
Turmeric	Punarnava (*Boerhavia diffusa*)	Bitter gourd/bitter melon (*Momordica charantia*)

Other less well-known plants with anti-diabetic effects include:

Achyranthes aspera (chaff-flower), *Acosmium panamense* (chakte), *Alangium lamarckii* (ankolam or ankola), *Afzelia africana* (African mahogany), *Albizia odoratissima* (Mimosa), *Argyreia nervosa* (elephant creeper), *Artemisia pallens* (Davana), *Artocarpus lacucha* (monkey fruit/monkey jack fruit), *Artocarpus heterophyllus* (jackfruit), *Averrhoa bilimbi* (bilimbi), *Axonopus compressus* (tropical carpet grass);

Barleria prionitis (porcupine flower/koranti), *Biophytum sensitivum* (life plant/Mukkutti), *Bombax ceiba* (red cotton tree), *Borassus flabellifer* (palmyra palm), *Bryonia alba* (white bryony), *Butea monosperma* (flame of the forest);

Caesalpinia bonducella (gray nicker/putikaranja), *Cajanus cajan* (pigeon pea), *Capparis decidua* (karira), *Capparis spinosa* (capers and caperberries), *Chaenomeles sinensis* (Chinese quince), *Centaurium erythraea* (common centaury), *Chloroxylon swietenia* (Ceylon satinwood/East Indian satinwood), *Chenopodium album* (bathua), *Costus speciosus* (crepe ginger), *Cyclocarya paliurus* (wheel wingnut);

Dillenia indica (elephant apple or chalta), *Diospyros peregrina* (tinduka), *Dorema aucheri* (bilhar);

Eugenia uniflora (Pitanga), *Enicostema littorale* (Mamejava); *Ficus racemosa* (cluster figs), *Fraxinus excelsior* (common ash); *Gossypium herbaceum* (Levant cotton);

Helicteres species (*H. angustifolia* [Avartani]) and *H. isora* (Indian screw pine), *Hybanthus enneaspermus* (blue spade flower), *Hypoxis hemerocallidea* (African potato/African star grass);

Lippia nodiflora (creeping frog fruit), *Lithocarpus polystachyus* (stone oak), *Ophiopogon japonicus (dwarf lily-turf)*;

Marrubium vulgare (White horehound), *Marsdenia tenacissima* (murva), *Myrica bella* (sweet gale or bayberry);

Portulaca oleracea (purslane), *Prangos ferulacea* (jashir); *Rhus coriaria* (sumac);

Securinega virosa (white berry bush), *Semecarpus anacardium* (bhallataka/marking nut), *Solanum torvum (chundakkai/turkey berry), Solanum xanthocarpum* (kantakari);

Tetraena alba/Zygophyllum album;

Uvaria chamae (finger root/Bush banana);

Vaccinium arctostaphylos (Caucasian whortleberry), *Viscum schimperi*;

And many others.

Common Recipes

Oral

Teas/Brews/Others

African Bitter Leaf. Take three to five of fresh leaves, wash and add 2 cups of water. Let it simmer for ½ hour till about 1 cup. Strain, allow to cool, and then drink. Drink daily or twice a day.

The leaves can be dried and brewed as tea. The fresh leaves can also be added into stews or soups.

Amla juice. Lightly pound three to four amla fruits. Strain and add a pinch of turmeric. Mix well and drink 20 mL of juice in the morning on an empty stomach.

Arugampul juice. Take one to two handfuls of fresh washed arugampul (roots removed) and a few neem leaves. Add some water or coconut water and blend. Strain and drink fresh first thing in the morning on an empty stomach.

Asafetida. This spice can be added to Indian cooking.

Avarampoo. Make a tea decoction of the dried flowers and consume.

Babul gum powder. Take ½ teaspoon of babul gum powder. Add 1 cup of hot water. Steep for 5 to 10 minutes. Consume once a day.

Bael leaf juice. Soak 10 bael leaves in warm water overnight. Lightly pound the leaves and strain through a piece of muslin cloth. Mix the bael leaf extract with some ground black pepper and consume once a day. Alternatively, mix the bael leaf extract with 5 g of honey and consume three times a day.

Banaba (Queen's flower). Take banaba fruits and leaves. Dry for 2 weeks. Cut the leaves into smaller pieces. Take 1 cup of the fruits and leaves. Add 1 cup of boiling water. Steep for 30 minutes. Strain and consume several times a day.

Banyan brew. Place 20 g of dried Banyan tree bark or tender leaves into a pot with 4 cups of water. Bring the mixture to a boil and allow to cook until the water has been reduced to about 1 cup in volume. Allow to cool completely before drinking.

Take ½ tablespoon of banyan powder with a glass of milk.

Barberry tea. Take 1 to 2 teaspoons of crushed berries or 1 to 2 teaspoons of dried barberry root. Add 1 cup of hot water. Steep for 10 minutes. Strain and consume three times a day.

Bay leaf, turmeric, and aloe vera paste. Grind bay leaves into a fine powder. Mix ½ a tablespoon of ground bay leaf with ½ a tablespoon of turmeric. Slit an aloe vera leaf down the center and remove the white gel, discarding any yellow gel. Add 1 tablespoon of aloe vera gel to the turmeric and bay leaf powder. Mix well to form a paste and consume twice a day, preferably before lunch and dinner.

Bhringraj. Make a decoction of the leaves and consume. It is usually part of a polyherbal formula.

Bitter gourd dish. It can sauteed with onions and spices and eaten as a vegetable. It can also be blended, strained, and consumed as a fresh juice. The fresh grated form can be mixed with yogurt, some grated green mango, onion, pepper, and eaten as a salad.

Bitter gourd juice. Remove the seeds from a fresh bitter gourd and cut into smaller chunks. Place in a blender and blend until smooth, gradually adding up to about ¼ cup of water. Strain the mixture and drink 30 mL in the morning on an empty stomach.

Chicory. The chicory root powder is a popular coffee substitute. The young leaves are also edible as a salad.

Cinnamon tea. Add 3 to 4 tablespoons of cinnamon powder to about 1 L of water in a pot. Allow to simmer gently for about 20 minutes. Strain the mixture and let it cool completely. Drink once a day.

Cumin. This spice is widely used in Indian cuisine. It can also be consumed as tea.

Fenugreek (sprouted). Take ½ cup of fenugreek seeds. Soak them in 1 to 1½ cups of water overnight. Strain them through a muslin cloth. Discard (or consume) the water. Tie the muslin cloth containing the seeds and lay it in a bowl or tray. Place the bowl/tray in a warm and dark environment for about 12 to 24 hours until they sprout.

Fenugreek brew. Soak 4 tablespoons of fenugreek seeds in about 300 mL of warm water overnight. In the morning, place the soaked seeds into a blender and blend until smooth. Strain the mixture and drink once a day for at least 3 months.

Fenugreek microgreens. Put some fenugreek seeds in a pot with potting soil. It will germinate within 3 days to produce edible microgreens.

Fenugreek seeds. Soak 4 tablespoons of fenugreek seeds in warm water overnight. Chew on the soaked seeds in the morning.

Fenugreek-turmeric milk. Grind 100 g of fenugreek seeds into a fine powder and mix with 25 g of ground turmeric. Stir this mixture into a glass of warm milk and drink twice a day.

Fruits. These include custard apple, guava, jackfruit, belimbi, wood apple, mango, and amla.

Garlic. Garlic should be consumed due to the presence of allicin, a compound that reduces sugar levels in the body.

Giloy. Take some giloy stems. Add 1 cup of water. Boil until ½ volume. Strain and consume daily.

Variation #1. Take some giloy stems. Add some ginger, amla powder, and black pepper. Blend and drink.

Variation #2. Alternatively, chew on the giloy stem.

Guava leaf. Take a handful of guava leaves. Add 100 mL of water. Boil until the volume is reduced to 25 mL. Consume twice a day.

Variation #1. Take four to six washed guava leaves. Add 1 cup of boiling water. Steep for 10 to 15 minutes. Strain and consume.

Variation #2. Consume guava fruit regularly.

Gurmar brew. Gurmar is available as a powder or in the form of dried leaves. Alternatively, make gurmar brew by mixing 1 teaspoon of gurmar powder (or 1 to 2 g of dry leaves) in 1 cup of warm water. Add honey to taste and drink. Consume ½ hour after lunch and dinner.

Gurmar juice. Take some fresh washed leaves. Blend with a little water and make fresh juice. Consume 20 to 30 mL once or twice a day.

Gurmar leaves. Chew on one to two of fresh gurmar leaves every day.

Hemp seed oil. Consume 1 to 2 teaspoons of hemp seed oil daily.

Hibiscus tea. Take three to four washed fresh hibiscus flowers. Remove the stamen and calyx. Add 1 cup hot water. Steep for about 5 to 10 minutes. Remove the decolorized petals. Consume warm or chilled. Add some lemon juice if desired (the tea will be more ruby-red) and/or some mint leaves.

Indian Mallow. Take some Indian Mallow leaves. Add some cumin seeds. Blend them together. Add some water. Strain and consume regularly.

Variation #1. Take ½ teaspoon of the powder. Mix with some warm water. Consume twice a day after meals.

Ivy gourd. It can be cooked as a spicy stir-fry.

Variation #1. Ivy gourd juice. Place one to two cut ivy gourds into a blender and blend until smooth, gradually adding up to 1 cup of water. Strain and drink.

Variation #2. The leaves can be cooked and eaten.

Jalkumbhi juice. Place a handful of fresh jalkumbhi leaves in a blender and gradually add up to 1 cup of water. Blend until smooth. Pour into a cup and drink.

Jamun leaf/*Eugenia jambolana*. Chew on jamun leaves. It is also available as a seed extract in the form of capsule, tablets, or powder.

Jamun seed drink. Grind jamun seeds into a fine powder. Mix 1 teaspoon of the seed powder into 1 cup of warm water. Drink before each meal.

Java plum (Jamun) juice. Take 10 to 15 washed black jamun fruits. Deseed and blend with 1 cup of water with ¼ teaspoon of black salt and a small piece of ginger. Strain and drink. Add some honey and ice if desired.

Jute leaf. This can be eaten as a curry, soup, stew, stir-fry, or made into a tea.

Mango and Mango seed powder. Ripe and unripe mango fruit can be eaten. The unripe green mango seed or its dried mango seed powder is used in Indian cuisine.

Mango leaf tea. Place 10 to 15 fresh young tender mango leaves into a pot and cover with water. Boil gently for 15 to 20 minutes. Leave to steep overnight. Drink this strained liquid in the morning on an empty stomach.

Moringa leaf brew. Add a ½ cup of fresh moringa leaves to a pot with 1½ cup of water. Bring to a boil and then remove from the heat. Allow it to cool completely before drinking. Alternatively, ground dried moringa leaves may be used to make tea. Stir 1 teaspoon of the ground moringa into a cup of hot water.

Mulberry leaf tea. Place a handful of fresh mulberry leaves into pot with 4 cups of water. Simmer over low heat for 10 to 15 minutes and then remove from the heat. Add honey to taste and drink.

Mustard. The seeds are widely used as a tempering spice. The mustard leaves are cooked and eaten.

Neem tea. Place a handful of neem leaves into a cup and pour boiling water over the leaves. Allow to steep for 5 to 10 minutes. Add honey to taste and drink.

Neem-tulsi-bael extract. Soak 10 fresh neem leaves, 10 fresh tulsi leaves, and 10 fresh bael leaves in warm water overnight. The next morning, lightly pound the leaves and strain through a piece of muslin cloth. Drink this strained liquid in the morning on an empty stomach.

Nilavembu tea. Take a handful of fresh nilavembu branches and pluck off the leaves. Break the stems into shorter segments and steep in water overnight. Discard the stems the next morning and drink the tea.

Nirgundi. Place 5 to 10 nirgundi leaves into a pot with water. Allow to boil gently for about 5 to 10 minutes before straining. Drink warm.

Noni juice. To make the fresh quick juice, wash, dry, and peel the fruit. Cut into pieces and blend. Strain the puree and discard the fruit flesh. Drink the juice.

Variation # 1. To make the slow fermented noni juice, wash the fruit, and then sun dry it for a few hours. Pack the fruits into a sterilized mason jar or glass bottle. Allow to ferment for 6 to 8 weeks. Then, strain the juice and discard the fruit.

Variation #2. The unripe fruit can also be cooked as a stir-fry with curry spices and coconut milk.

Okra. Take five okras. Wash them, top and tail off the ends, then split lengthwise. Soak and squeeze them in 3 cups of water. Leave it overnight. Strain and drink the okra water in the morning on an empty stomach. The fresh okra vegetable also has a low glycemic index and is rich in soluble and insoluble fiber when cooked. Dried powdered okra is also available.

Onion. It is widely used in Indian cooking

Polyherbal brew. Take one teaspoon of licorice powder, one teaspoon of crushed coriander seeds, three pods of crushed cardamom and a piece of cinnamon bark. Add 1 cup of boiling water. Allow to steep for 5 to 10 minutes. Strain. Add 1 teaspoon of honey. Drink warm first thing in the morning.

Pomegranate juice and seeds. It is polyphenol antioxidant-rich, and the juice can regulate blood sugar and lipid levels.

Sadabahar (Periwinkle). Chew three or four washed fresh leaves before a meal. If taking the dried leaf powder, add 1 teaspoon to a cup of water or fresh fruit juice. To make a brew, take the pink flowers and boil them in 1 cup of water. Strain and consume it every morning on an empty stomach.

Saptaranga tea. Take 1 to 2 g of the Saptaranga root powder. Make a decoction and consume.

Snake gourd decoction. Place equal amounts of snake gourd, neem leaves, pounded amla fruit, and giloy stems in a pot with ½ cup of water. Bring to a boil and reduce the heat, allowing to simmer for 10 minutes. Cool completely and take three times a day.

Spices. The items listed under the Spices column are used in daily Indian cooking.

Spiral banner. Chew two leaves of *Costus igneus* morning and evening. The powder form is also available.

Sweet potato. The tuber can be boiled and eaten.

Triphala tea. Add a ½ teaspoon of triphala powder to 1 cup of hot water. Mix it well and drink it warm.

Vijaysar brew. Place one cube of vijaysar into a cup of water and allow it to steep overnight. Consume this in the morning on an empty stomach. Alternatively, mix ground vijaysar bark in warm water and drink twice a day before meals. The leaves can also be chewed or brewed as tea.

Wood apple juice. Cut the wood apple fruit. Scoop out the pulp into a strainer to remove the seeds and fiber. Add coconut milk (or any milk) and blend with jaggery. A pinch of cardamom powder or rock salt can be added.

Commercial Oral Preparations

Many simple and compound polyherbal and herbo-mineral formulations have various ingredients. These are mostly herbal plants and/or some calcined metals or minerals or gemstones. Some of them include:

Nishamalaki churna. This mixture contains two herbs in equal amounts (i.e., amla *[E. officinalis]* and turmeric *[Curcuma longa]*).

Madhumehantak churna. This is a polyherbal mixture of vijaysar, *B. aristata,* neem, *Gymnema sylvestre, Salacia chinensis,* bitter gourd seeds, fenugreek, tulsi leaves, *Aegle marmelos,* jamun seeds, *Acacia arabica* and *Lochnera rosea.* It is consumed with some warm milk or water.

Sapatarangyadi ghanavati. This is a polyherbal mixture of Saptarangi *(S. chinensis),* Fenugreek *(Trigonella foenumgraecum),* Karvellaka *(M. charantia),* Triphala and Guduchi *(T. cordifolia).*

Mustadi kwatha ghanavati. This is a polyherbal mixture of triphala, indrayan, turmeric *(C. longa),* murva *(M. tenacissima),* lodhra *(Symplocos racemosa),* nutgrass *(Cyperus rotundus),* and cedarwood *(Cedrus deodara).*

Diabecon. This is a polyherbal formula containing Amla, *Asparagus racemosus, Abutilon indicum, Aloe vera, B. aristata, Boerhavia diffusa, Commiphora wightii, Casearia esculenta, C. longa, E. jambolana, Glycyrrhiza glabra, Gmelina arborea, G. herbaceum, G. sylvestre, M. charantia, Ocimum sanctum, Piper nigrum, Phyllanthus amarus, Pterocarpus marsupium, Rumex maritimus, Shilajeet, Sphaeranthus indicus, Syzygium cumini, Swertia chirata, T. cordifolia, Tribulus terrestris,* and *Triphala.*

Glucocare. This is a polyherbal formula containing *G. sylvestre* (Mesasringi), *M. charantia* (Karavallaka), *C. wightii* (Guggulu), *P. marsupium* (Asana), *C. esculenta,* (Cilhaka bheda), *S. cumini* (Jambu), *A. racemosus* (Shatavari), *Boerhaavia diffusa* (Punarnava), *T. cordifolia* (Guduchi), *T. terrestris* (Gokshura), *P. amarus* (Keelnellikai), *Aloe vera,* Triphala, *P. nigrum* (Marica), *O. sanctum* (Tulsi).

Syndrex. This is germinated fenugreek seed extract.

Others include Glyoherb, Diasulin, Diabeta, Dia-Care

Therapeutic Measures

Diet

Various Ayurvedic diets are available. A wholesome, high fiber, vegetarian, and non-dairy diet *(Pathya Ahara)* is recommended, i.e.,

- low-glycemic grain cereals: millet, red rice, amaranth, quinoa, barley, whole wheat, and oats.
- pulses: green gram, chickpea, horse gram and toor dal/pigeon peas.
- bitter and astringent vegetables: moringa, bitter gourd, ivy and pointed gourd, unripe green banana, banana flower and stem, chundakkai, amaranth, fenugreek leaves/methi, bathua, ponnanganni leaves/Matsyakshi
- spices: fenugreek, garlic, ginger, garlic, turmeric, black pepper, asafetida, rock salt, black salt, mango seed powder
- fruits: amla, pomegranate, jamun (Java plum), monkey fruit, monk fruit, wood apple, palmyra
- seeds: lotus seeds
- oils: mustard oil, coconut oil, flaxseed oil
- sweeteners: pure honey, stevia

Copper vessel. Drink water from a copper vessel. Store the water in a copper jug overnight.

Yoga

Practice the following Yoga asanas to stimulate the pancreas:

Suryanamaskar (sun salutation), *Paschimottan asana* (seated forward bend), *Adomukhi svanasana* (downward dog pose), *Balasana* (child's pose), *Dhanurasana* (bow pose), *Vakrasana* (twisted pose), and *Manduka asana* (frog pose). Practice the following pranayamas:

Bhramari pranayama, Agnisar pranayama, and Kapalbhati kriya.

Panchakarma

Samshodhana chikitsa (Detoxification). Vamana, virechana, and vasti are carried out if obese.

Chinese Natural Remedies

Common Ingredients for Diabetes Mellitus

Herbs/Leaves	Miscellaneous
Achryanthes bidentata (huai niu xi)	Abalone shell (*Haliotis diversicolor*)
Alisma plantar (ze xie)	Forsythia fruit (*Forsythia suspensa*)
American ginseng/xi yang shen (*Panax quinquefolius*)	*Momordica charantia* (bitter melon/balsam pear)
Anemarrhena/zhi mu (*Anemarrhena asphodeloides*)	Paeonia suffruticosa (mu dan pi)
Cornus officinales/shan yu rou	Kelp
Dendrobium nobile (shi hu)	Senna leaf
Dioscorea batata (shan yao)	*Coptis chinensis*
Guava/fan shi liu (*Psidium guajava*)	*Lagenaria siceraria* (bottle gourd)
Gypsum fibrosum (shi gao)	Rice (jing mi)
Konjac root	
Lilyturf root/mai dong *Radix Ophiopogonis/Ophiopogon japonicus*	Chrysanthemum morifolium flowers (ju hua)
Poria (fu ling)	Oyster mushroom (*Pleurotus ostreatus*)
Radix ginseng (ren sheng)	Aloe vera (lu hui)
Rehmannia glutinosa (shu di huang)	Wolfberry fruit/gou qi zi (*Lycium barbarum*)
Spinach	
Tribulus terrestris (bai ji li)	Tiger nuts (*Cyperus esculentus*)
Trichosanthes kirilowii root (tian hua fen)	Cordyceps (*Ophiocordyceps sinensis*)

Common Recipes

Oral

- Treatment for "Upper warmer diabetes involving the lungs and stomach":
  - Symptoms of this condition are thirst, dry mouth and tongue, and frequent, large volumes of urine, and a red tongue.
  - The most common herbal decoction is bai hu ten shen tang: Ren shen (10 to 15 g), shi gao (20 to 30 g), zhi mu (9 to 12 g), and jing mi (15 to 20 g).
- Treatment for "Middle warmer diabetes involving the stomach heat and stomach yin deficiency":
  - Yu nu jian herbal decoction: Shi gao (10 to 15 g), shu di huang (10 to 15 g), mai men dong (3 to 6 g), and huai niu xi (3 to 6 g).
- Treatment for "Lower warmer diabetes involving the kidneys":
  - Liu wei di huang herbal decoction: Shan yu rou (10 to 15 g), shan yao (9 to 12 g), ze xie (6 to 9 g), fu ling (9 to 12 g), and mu dan pi (6 to 9 g).
- Treatment for diabetes complications:
  - For visual problems (glaucoma, cataracts), an herbal decoction called ming mu di huang is used, consisting of gou qi zi (6 to 9 g), ju hua (6 to 9 g), bai ji li (6 to 9 g), and abalone shell (20 to 30 g).
  - **Spinach tea.** Place a handful of spinach leaves into a pot with 2 cups of water. Bring to a boil and then reduce the heat, allowing the mixture to simmer for 10 minutes. Drink 1 cup three times a day.

Western/Other Natural Remedies

Common Ingredients for Diabetes Mellitus

Spices	Herbs/Leaves	Miscellaneous
Caraway	Green tea leaf	Cumin seed oil (*Nigella sativa*)
Carum carvi fruit		
	Rosemary	Oatmeal
	Oregano	Aloe vera
	Sage	Black plum
	White mulberry leaf	Alpha-lipoic acid
	Bitterwood/Jamaican Quassia	Chromium
	(*Picrasma excelsa*)	Vanadium
	Artichoke leaf	Vitamin D
	Watercress	Avocado
	(*Nasturtium officinale*)	(*Persea americana*)
	Geranium/Cranesbill	Oyster mushroom/ping gu (*Pleurotus ostreatus*)
	Fleabane	Prickly pear cactus (*Opuntia*)
	Stinging/Common nettle	Calendula
	(*Urtica dioica*)	
	Chamomile	Olive leaf extract
	Chamaemelum nobile	
	Halim seeds	Resveratrol
	(*Lepidium sativum*)	Glucomannan
		Adiponectin supplements
Cinnamon	*Althea officinalis* (marshmallow root)	Chondrus crispus (Irish moss)
Flaxseed	Basil leaf	Coffee
Garlic	*Polygonatum officinale* (Solomon's seal root)	Essential oil (cilantro, myrrh)
Ginger	*Ulmus fulva* (slippery elm bark)	Iceland moss
Oregano	Milk thistle	Bitter gourd
(*Origanum vulgare*)	(*Silybum marianum*)	

Konjac root. This Asian root vegetable can be boiled or processed into ground flour to make Japanese noodles (shirataki noodles) or snacks.

Tiger nuts. It can be sprouted, roasted or dried and eaten.

Therapeutic Measure

Diet

In TCM, diabetes is believed to be a yin deficiency and due to excess heat in the body. Hence, *cooling* foods such as spinach, soybeans, pumpkin, celery, and turnips. Fruits should be taken sparingly, but recommended fruits include mulberries, guava, strawberries, and crab apples. Small, frequent meals should be eaten at regular intervals throughout the day.

Kelp. There are several types of powdered kelp available.

Lifestyle

Qi gong: This is a form of exercise thought to strengthen the connection between mind and body. It is recommended as an adjunct to lifestyle modifications and medication to control diabetes.

Tui na: Tui na is a form of Chinese massage that stimulates specific acupressure points and can be used to treat symptoms of diabetes. It is often used in place of acupuncture, especially in pediatric patients.

Note. Most of the TCM remedies should be used as an adjunct to lifestyle and diet changes as well as other medication to control diabetes.

Common Recipes

Oral

Teas/Brews

Adiponectin supplement. Consume this dietary supplement to regulate blood glucose.

Aloe vera juice. Slit one aloe vera leaf down the center. Remove the white gel, discarding any yellow gel. Cut the white gel into smaller chunks and add to a blender. Blend until smooth and drink.

Alpha-lipoic acid. It has antioxidant and anti-inflammatory actions. A dose of 300 to 600 mg/day can decrease insulin resistance, improve blood glucose levels, and improve diabetic neuropathy. Higher doses have also been tried.

Artichoke. Consume boiled artichoke during a meal.

Avocado. Consume avocado as a snack or combine with other foods as a part of the diet.

Basil tea. Add three to five basil leaves to a pot with 1 cup of water. Bring to a boil and then lower the heat, allowing it to simmer for 3 to 5 minutes. Remove from the heat and strain.

Bitter gourd juice. Remove the seeds from a fresh bitter gourd and cut into smaller chunks. Place in a blender and blend until smooth, gradually adding up to about ¼ cup of water. Strain the mixture and drink 30 mL in the morning on an empty stomach.

Bitterwood. Take 30 g of bitterwood and boil in 4 L of water for 15 minutes. Then, let it sit for 1 hour. Strain, pour into bottles and refrigerate. Consume 1 cup daily in the morning or twice a day. It is also available as tablets.

Black plum. Black plum is thought to have antioxidant qualities and may be beneficial for those with type 1 or 2 diabetes.

Calendula tea. Add 1 tablespoon of fresh flowers (2 teaspoons of dried flower) into 1 cup of boiling water. Steep for 10 to 15 minutes. Drink it warm.

Chamomile tea. Place some dried or fresh chamomile flowers into a cup. Pour boiling water over the flowers and allow to steep for 10 minutes. Strain and add honey to taste. Drink hot.

Chromium picolinate. It is an antioxidant and can reduce insulin resistance in obese type 2 diabetes. A dose of 200 to 1,000 μg in two or three divided doses is taken for 3 to 4 months. Side effects include stomach irritation, dizziness, headaches, liver, and kidney damage.

Cinnamon tea. Add one cinnamon stick to a cup and pour boiling water over it. Allow it to steep for about 10 minutes. Add honey to taste. Drink in the morning on an empty stomach.

Flaxseed brew. Grind flaxseed until it forms a fine powder. Add 1 teaspoon of the flaxseed powder to 1 cup of boiling water and mix well. Allow it to steep for 10 to 15 minutes. Strain and add honey to taste.

Fleabane tea. Make a decoction from the dried leaves and flowers. Consume 2 to 4 ounces up to four times a day.

Garlic. Add garlic to cooked dishes or chew on one to two cloves of garlic every day.

Geranium tea. Take 25 g of the flower buds or 50 g of the dried plant. Add 1 L of boiling water. Allow to steep for 20 minutes. Consume 3 to 4 cups per day.
> Variation #1. Take 1 to 2 teaspoons of the dried cranesbill root. Add 1 cup of water. Boil and simmer for 15 minutes. Strain and consume.

Ginger tea. Add 2 to 4 inches of ginger to a cup and pour boiling water over the ginger. Steep for 5 to 10 minutes and drink.

Glucomannan. It is taken with water three times a day at least 1 hour before meals.

Green tea. Place 1 to 2 teaspoons of dried green tea leaves into a cup and pour boiling water over the leaves. Allow it to steep for 5 to 10 minutes and drink.

Halim seeds. Soak 1 tablespoon of halim seeds overnight. Consume them first thing in the morning with some added lemon juice. It can also be added to stews and soups.

Marshmallow root tea. Place ¼ cup of dried marshmallow root into a cup and pour cold water over it. Allow to steep overnight and strain the next morning.

Oatmeal. Consume oatmeal regularly as it is known to help to control blood sugar levels in the body.

Olive leaf extract. Consume olive leaf extract capsules once a day.

Oregano tea. Add 3 teaspoons of fresh oregano leaves or 1 teaspoon of dried leaves to 1 cup of boiling water. Steep for 5 to 10 minutes before straining.

Oyster mushrooms. Consume oyster mushrooms as a part of the diet.

Prickly pear cactus (opuntia or nopal). Remove the spines from the young prickly pear pads. Trim the edges and the base. Dice into small pieces. Blanch in boiling water for about 5 minutes until tender. Rinse and drain. It can be added to salad and consumed.

Rosemary tea. Add 2 to 3 sprigs of fresh rosemary (or 1⅓ of dried leaf needles) into a pot with 2 cups of water. Allow it to boil for about 1 minute. Remove from the heat and strain.

Sage tea. Add three to five fresh sage leaves or (1 teaspoon of dried sage) into one cup of boiling water. Allow it to steep for 5 to 10 minutes. Strain and drink.

Slippery elm tea. Slippery elm bark is often sold as a powdered herb, which can be used to make tea. Add 1 teaspoon of slippery elm powder to a cup and pour boiling water into the cup. Mix well and allow it to steep for 3 to 5 minutes before drinking.
> The seed and leaf extracts are available as powder, a tablet, tea, or tincture. Steep a tea bag in a cup of hot water for 5 minutes and consume.

Stinging nettle tea. Place 1 cup of fresh stinging nettle leaves in a cup. Boil 2 to 3 cups of hot water and pour over the stinging nettle leaves. Steep for 10 to 15 minutes and drink. Alternatively, dried stinging nettle may also be purchased to make tea.

Vanadium. It can lower blood glucose and improve insulin sensitivity. A dose of vanadyl sulfate 10 mg (containing

2 mg elemental vanadium) is recommended. Side effects include hypoglycemia and kidney damage.

Vitamin D. It is also believed to improve insulin sensitivity.

Watercress. Use as a garnish or add to salads, soups, smoothies, or sandwiches.

White mulberry leaf. The dried leaf is available as tablets or powder form and is consumed three times a day. The young leaves also can be cooked and eaten.

Therapeutic Measures

- **Essential oil therapy:** Add 2 to 3 drops of myrrh or cilantro oil to a diffuser and dilute with water. It is believed that cilantro oil may promote the secretion of insulin. Myrrh oil is thought to have antioxidant properties that may lessen the effects of diabetes on the body.
- **Lifestyle and diet:** Exercise regularly to lose any excess weight as being overweight may decrease insulin sensitivity, which means that the cells are less able to use the sugar in the blood. Control the amount of carbohydrates such as rice and pasta. Increase fiber intake as it reduces sugar absorption and carbohydrate digestion, hence causing a more gradual sugar level increase. Drink enough water throughout the day as it may help to control blood sugar levels.

  Notes
- The remedies stated above should be used as adjunctive therapy to other forms of diabetes medication, as well as the implementation of proper lifestyle and dietary changes.
- Consult a medical professional on the safety of the above herbs when used in conjunction with allopathic medication to avoid any adverse interactions between medications.

Modern Remedies

Injectable Insulin

Insulin is a hormone that controls blood sugar levels in the body. It does this by regulating how the body uses and stores glucose and fat. Insulin signals the liver, muscle, and fat cells to use glucose in the bloodstream in the form of energy. Any excess glucose is stored by the liver as glycogen.

In type 1 diabetes, insulin must be injected every day to control blood sugar levels in the body due to the pancreas's inability to produce sufficient insulin. It is used in type 2 diabetes as an add-on to oral hypoglycemic agents. The human insulin is of recombinant DNA origin. There are different types of injectable insulin available:

- **Rapid-acting insulin:** Rapid-acting insulin is usually taken immediately before a meal to prevent a blood glucose spike from the food intake. It is usually taken in conjunction with a longer-acting insulin. Its onset is between 4 and 15 minutes, and its effects peak from between 1.5 to 3 hours. Its effects last for 3 to 5 hours. Examples: insulin aspart (NovoRapid), insulin lispro (Humalog), insulin glulisine (Apidra), faster-acting insulin aspart (Fiasp)
- **Short-acting (or bolus) insulin:** Short-acting insulin is usually taken about 30 minutes before a meal to prevent a blood glucose spike. It is usually taken in conjunction with a longer-acting insulin. Its onset is between 15 and 30 minutes with effects that peak at about 2 to 5 hours. Its effects last for up to 12 hours. Examples: insulin regular (Humulin R, Entuzity)
- **Intermediate-acting insulin:** This type of insulin often functions by preventing blood glucose spikes when the effects of shorter-acting insulins has run out and is taken twice a day. Its effects start at about 1.5 to 3 hours, and peaks at about 5 to 8 hours. Its effects last for up to 18 hours. Examples: insulin NPH (Humulin N)

Premixed insulins are mixtures of fixed-dose insulins:
Examples:
Intermediate- and short-acting insulin: Humulin 70/30, Humulin 50/50, Novolin 70/30
Intermediate- and rapid-acting insulin: Humalog Mix 75/25, Humalog Mix 70/30

- **Long-acting insulin:** Long-acting insulin is often used conjunctively with a shorter-acting insulin. It lowers blood glucose levels when the effects of shorter-acting insulin run out and is taken one to two times a day. It has a more gradual effect that starts in about 1.5 hours and lasts for up to 24 hours. Examples: insulin glargine (Lantus), insulin glargine biosimilar (Basaglar), and insulin detemir (Levemir)
- **Basal insulin analogs** (or background insulin) can last 24 to 36 hours, and it regulates blood glucose between meals, during fasting, and when asleep. Examples include insulin glargine (Lantus and Toujeo) and insulin degludec (Tresiba). Side effects include hypoglycemia, weight gain, and respiratory infections.

Basal-bolus regimes are preferred over premixed insulins as there is better dose flexibility and less hypoglycemia risk.

The insulin can be delivered via a needle, pen, or an insulin pump implant.

Biguanides

Usually given in type 2 diabetes, metformin lowers the glucose production in the liver and increases the peripheral utilization of glucose by increasing sensitivity of insulin receptors to insulin in the body. It should not be used in kidney or heart failure.

Example: Metformin (Glucophage) or its extended-release formulation

Side effects include diarrhea, nausea, B12 deficiency, lactic acidosis, and hepatotoxicity

Sulfonylurea

Sulfonylureas stimulate the beta cells in the pancreas to produce insulin.

Examples:

First-generation sulfonylureas: Chlorpropamide, Tolbutamide

Second-generation sulfonylureas: Glimepiride (Amaryl), Glibenclamide (Daonil), Glipizide (Glucotrol), Glyburide, Gliclazide (Diamicron)

Side effects include weight gain, hunger, skin rash, nausea, and dark urine.

Meglitinides/Glinides

Meglitinides function in a similar way like sulfonylureas. It stimulates the beta cells of the pancreas to produce more insulin. It targets the postprandial blood glucose. They are faster acting than sulfonylureas and the effect in the body lasts for a shorter duration.

Examples: Repaglinide (Prandin), Nateglinide (Starlix)

Side effects include hypoglycemia and weight gain.

Thiazolidinediones (Insulin Sensitizers)

This type of medication works by increasing the body's tissue sensitivity to insulin in type 2 diabetes. They stimulate the production of new fat cells in the body, which are more sensitive to insulin hence can use them more effectively. It is an agonist for the peroxisome proliferator-activated receptor-gamma (PPARy).

Examples: Rosiglitazone (Avandia), Pioglitazone, Troglitazone. There is restricted use in some countries.

Side effects include weight gain, edema, heart failure, bone fracture, stroke risk, and macular edema.

Sodium-Glucose Co-transporter 2 (SGLT2) Inhibitors

It works by decreasing the renal threshold for glucose excretion. Sodium-glucose co-transporter 2 (SGLT2) proteins are expressed in the proximal convoluted tubule of the kidneys, and they reabsorb the filtered glucose.

Examples: Empagliflozin, Dapagliflozin, Canagliflozin

Side effects include yeast and urinary tract infections and diabetic ketoacidosis.

Combination drugs: dapagliflozin/metformin (Xigduo), empagliflozin/linagliptin (Glyxambi)

GLP-1 Receptor Agonists/GLP-1 RA (Incretin mimetics): Hormone Therapy

GLP-1 is an incretin (a gut hormone), which increases the insulin from the pancreas after a meal and decreases the glucagon from the liver during digestion. It lasts for only a few minutes only. The GLP1 receptor agonist mimics the action of the natural GLP1 and lasts for hours to days. It targets fasting and postprandial blood glucose levels. It promotes weight loss. It is an injection given subcutaneously in type 2 diabetes. Semaglutide is the first oral form (Rybelsus) of GLP-1 RA (daily dose). It is also available as an injection (Ozempic) given weekly.

Examples: exenatide, liraglutide, dulaglutide, lixisenatide, semaglutide, albiglutide

These drugs are biologics. Side effects include diarrhea, constipation, nausea, vomiting, dizziness, hypotension, tachycardia, headaches, weakness, acute pancreatitis, thyroid cancer, gall bladder problems, kidney problems, and suicidal thoughts.

Combination drugs: Basal insulin + GLP-1RA as fixed ratio combination is available. It is given as a single daily or weekly injection.

Dipeptidyl Peptidase (DPP4) Inhibitor/Gliptins

DPP-4 is an enzyme that destroys the hormone incretin. The DPP4-inhibitor blocks the action of this enzyme and hence increases incretin (GLP-1). It targets mostly the postprandial blood glucose. It reduces appetite and weight gain.

Examples: Sitagliptin (Januvia), Vildagliptin (Galvus), Saxagliptin (Onglyza), Alogliptin, Linagliptin (Tradjenta)

Combination drugs: Sitagliptin + Metformin (Janumet), Vildagliptin + Metformin (Eucreas)

Side effects include diarrhea, nausea, pancreatitis, skin rash, and flu symptoms

Alpha Glucosidase Inhibitors

Glucosidase is an enzyme that breaks down carbohydrates in the small intestine to simple sugars (i.e., glucose which is then absorbed into the blood). The alpha glucosidase inhibitors (AGIs) delays the absorption of glucose from the small intestine and targets the postprandial blood glucose and insulin levels.

Examples: Acarbose, Voglibose, Miglitol

Side effects include gas, bloating, abdominal pain, and diarrhea.

Amylin Analogs (Hormone Therapy)

Amylin is a hormone secreted by the beta cells of the pancreas. It delays gastric emptying, decreases appetite, increases satiety, and targets mostly postprandial blood glucose. The synthetic analog is injected subcutaneously along with mealtime insulin and is used in type 1 and type 2 diabetes. It is not widely used due to cost and limited efficacy.

Example: Pramlintide

Insulin-Secretagogues

These stimulate the beta cells in the pancreas to secrete insulin.

Examples: Sulfonylureas, Glinides

Other Emerging Therapies (in type 1 diabetes)

- Beta cell replacement therapy
  Pancreas or islet cell transplantation has been tried with insulin independence rate of about 50% and 10% at 1 and 5 years, respectively.
  The donor islet cells are injected into the portal vein. Long-term immunosuppressive drugs are required.
- Immunotherapy
  These include cyclosporine, azathioprine, methotrexate, etc., but are limited due to serious side effects.
- Cell therapy
  Mesenchymal stem cells, cord blood transfusion, and dendritic cells have been trialed
- Inhaled insulin
  This is a rapid-acting insulin and is given before meals together with a long-acting insulin. Side effects include cough, throat irritation, and bronchospasm.
- Immunomodulators
  Tumor necrosis factor (TNF)-alpha inhibitors and granulocyte colony stimulating factor are being tried
- Monoclonal antibody
  Tepilizumab, an anti-CD3 monoclonal antibody has shown some success.

Homeopathic Remedies

These include *Syzygium jambolanum* (to treat the polyuria, thirst, and burning urine), *Uranium nitricum* (to treat the polyuria, burning urine, nausea, and swelling), *Conium* (relieves the numbness in the feet and hands from diabetic neuropathy), *Plumbum* (for peripheral neuropathy and tinnitus), phosphoric acid (for impaired memory, hair loss, night urination, and poor erection), *Calendula* (treats infected ulcers), and *Candida* (for yeast infections). Others include *Helonias/False unicorn root, Iodum,* and *Bryonia alba.* However, these remedies are not substitutes for insulin.

Hypothyroidism

Hypothyroidism is defined as a lack of thyroid hormones in the bloodstream due to an underactive thyroid gland. The thyroid gland is a butterfly-shaped organ and located in the front of the neck. It converts iodine into thyroid hormones triiodothyronine (T3) and thyroxine (T4). The thyroid hormones have a number of effects on the body, such as to regulate the body's metabolism and to keep warm.

Common causes of hypothyroidism include Hashimoto's thyroiditis, which is an autoimmune disease in which the thyroid gland becomes inflamed due to an attack by the body's own antibodies. Another cause is thyroid removal or congenital thyroid agenesis (congenital lack of a thyroid). A tumor in the pituitary gland (in the brain) may affect the production of thyroid-stimulating hormone (TSH), which stimulates the production and secretion of thyroid hormones.

Indian Natural Remedies

Common Ingredients for Hypothyroidism

Spices	Herbs/Leaves	Miscellaneous
Black peppercorn (Piper nigrum)	Commiphora Mukul (guggulu)	Cucumber
Ginger	Centella asiatica (gotu kola)	Milk
Long pepper (Piper longum)	*Tribulus terrestris* (gokshura)	Pulses (moong dal, bengal gram)
	Bacopa monnieri (brahmi)	Coconut oil
	Nardostachys (jatamansi)	Honey
	Boerhavia diffusa (punarnava)	Mineral pitch/ shilajit
	Withania somnifera (Indian ginseng/ ashwagandha)	Hawthorn berry
	Ceylon leadwort/ chitrak (*Plumbago zeylanica*)	Passion fruit flower
	Moringa oleifera (moringa)	Indian gooseberry (amla)
Coleus forskohlii (Indian coleus)		Flaxseed
Trikatu		Shilajit

Common Recipes
Oral
Teas/Brews

- **Amla paste.** Crush amla to form a paste and mix with honey. Take in the morning on an empty stomach.
- **Ashwagandha.** Add 2 tablespoons of ashwagandha to a glass of hot milk. Stir in 1 teaspoon of ghee. Drink twice a day.
- **Brahmi juice.** Remove and discard the brahmi stems from the plant. Place a handful of the fresh brahmi leaves into a blender and add up to 1 cup of water. Blend until smooth. Add honey to taste and drink.
- **Brahmi tea.** Place about two to three stalks of fresh brahmi leaves into a cup. Pour boiling water over the leaves and allow it to steep for about 10 to 15 minutes. Add honey to taste and drink.
- **Coleus forskohlii.** Coleus forskohlii is available in the form of a powder or capsule. Adults can take 50 to 100 mg of Coleus forskohlii every day.
- **Cucumber juice.** Cut one cucumber into smaller chunks and place into a blender. Blend until smooth and drink.
- **Flaxseed brew.** Grind flaxseed until it forms a fine powder. Add 1 teaspoon of the flaxseed powder to 1 cup of boiling water and mix well. Allow it to steep for 10 to 15 minutes. Strain and add honey to taste.
- **Gotu Kola tea.** Steep a teaspoon of fresh or dried gotu kola leaves in a cup of hot water for about 10 to 15 minutes. Drink it warm.
- **Guggulu.** Guggulu is the sap produced by the Indian bdellium tree and is believed to have cholesterol-reducing properties. It is available in the form of dietary supplements. Adults can take about 25 mg of guggul supplements every day after a meal. Alternatively, 1 teaspoon of ground guggulu can be mixed with some ground ginger and honey to make a paste. Take this paste three times a day.
- **Jatamansi brew.** Add a pinch of jatamansi root powder to a cup of warm water and take twice a day.
- **Moringa brew.** Add a ½ cup of fresh moringa leaves to a pot with 1½ cup of water. Bring to a boil and then remove from the heat. Allow it to cool completely before drinking. Alternatively, ground dried moringa leaves may be used to make tea. Stir 1 teaspoon of the ground moringa into a cup of hot water.
- **Punarnava tea.** Add one part each of dried punarnava, one part of dried passion fruit flower, and two parts of dried hawthorn berries. Steep about half a teaspoon of this in a cup of hot water for about 10 minutes. Drink twice a day after lunch and dinner. The passion fruit leaf is often chopped up and eaten in a salad in Sri Lankan cuisine.

- **Shilajit.** Mix a pea-sized portion of shilajit in a cup of hot milk or tea and drink. Alternatively, put the shilajit under the tongue until it dissolves or swallow a piece with water. Consume three times a day.
- **Trikatu tea.** Steep equal parts of black pepper, long pepper, and ginger in a cup of hot water. Steep for about 10 to 15 minutes. Drink it warm.

Chinese Natural Remedies

Common Ingredients for Hypothyroidism

Spices	Herbs/Leaves	Miscellaneous
Cinnamon (rou gui)	Aconite (fu zi)	Fructus corni officinalis/ shan yu rou
	Rehmannia glutinosa (shu di huang)	Poria mushroom (fu ling)
	Rhizoma dioscoreae oppositae (shan yao)	Colla cornus cervi (deer antler gel/lu jiao jiao)
	Cortex moutan (mu dan pi)	Turtle shell gel/gui ban jiao (Chinemys reevesii)
	Water plantain rhizome (ze xie)	Fructus lycii chinensis (goji berry/gou qi zi)
	Radix rehmanniae (sheng di huan)	Dodder seeds/tu si zi (Cuscuta chinensis Lam)
	American ginseng/xi yang shen (Panax quinquefolius)	Radix Achyranthis Bidentatae (niu xi)
	Acanthopanax root/wu jia pi (Acanthopanax senticosus/ Eleutherococcus senticosus)	
	Chinese ginseng (ren shen)	
	Licorice (gan cao)	
	Codonopsis pilosula (bastard ginseng/ dang shen)	
	Five-flavor berry/wu wei zi (Schisandra chinensis)	

Common Recipes

Oral

Teas/Brews

- **American ginseng brew.** Place two to four slices of American ginseng into a teacup and pour boiling water over it. Cover and steep for 5 to 10 minutes. Drink one to three times a day.
- **Bastard ginseng tea.** Place three to five slices of bastard ginseng into a cup and fill with boiling water. Allow it to steep for 5 to 10 minutes before drinking. Alternatively, consume this herb by simmering two to four sticks of bastard ginseng in a soup.

- **Chinese ginseng tea.** Chinese ginseng tea should be taken as a strong formula. Place 10 to 30 g of Chinese ginseng into a special ginseng cooker. Drink 118 to 236 mL of this tea one to two times a day.
- **Licorice tea.** Licorice may be taken in the form of a tincture, powder, or tea. Place about ¼ cup of dried licorice into a teapot and add about 2 cups of boiling water. Allow to steep for 5 to 10 minutes and drink one to three times a day. Alternatively, mix 1 to 4 g of licorice powder into 1 cup of warm water. Drink once a day.
- **Magnolia vine tea.** Steep 10 g of dried magnolia vine in 1 L of cold water overnight. Strain in the morning and add honey to the liquid. Drink one to four times a day. Alternatively, this may be used as a jam.
- **Rehmannia tea.** Rehmannia is available in the form of capsules, powder, or dried herbs. To make tea, place a 3-inch-long piece of rehmannia in a pot with about 1 L of water. Boil and then simmer for about half an hour. Drink one to four times a day.
- **Siberian ginseng root tincture.** Siberian ginseng may be taken in the form of a tincture, extract, capsule, or decoction. Take 10 to 60 drops of Siberian ginseng root tincture mixed into water one to two times a day.

Commercial Preparations

Jin gui shen qi wan. This herbal preparation is available in the form of capsules and ingredients, including shu di huang, shan yao, shan yu rou, fu ling, mu dan pi, ze xie, fu zi, and rou gui. Adults should take two to three capsules, two to three times a day.

Zuo gui wan. This herbal preparation may be taken in the form of tablets, and adults should take 5 tablets, two to three times a day. Ingredients include shu di huang, shan yao, sia zhu yu, lu jiao jiao, goji berry, tu is zi, and niu xi.

Gui Lu Erxian Jiao. The key ingredients include lu jiao, gui ban (tortoise shell), ginseng and lycium (goji berry).

Dodder seeds. They are available in the form of supplements (including powder, tablets, or capsules) and can be taken alongside food and other vitamins.

Western/Other Natural Remedies

Common Ingredients for Hypothyroidism

Spices	Herbs/Leaves	Miscellaneous
Flaxseed	Bladderwrack (Fucus vesiculosus)	Essential oil (rosemary, frankincense)
Ginger	Stinging nettle leaf	Coconut oil
	Rhodiola (Rhodiola rosea)	Kelp
		Honey
		Black walnut

Common Recipes

Oral

Teas/Brews

- **Black walnut tincture.** Black walnut is available fresh, or as a powder and capsules. To make black walnut tincture, place about 10 to 12 under-ripe, halved black walnut hulls into a jar. Add about 3 to 4 cups of 40% or higher-proof vodka. Close the cap tightly and place it in a cool dark area for 6 weeks. Shake the jar once a day. After 6 weeks, strain the mixture and store the liquid in a dark bottle. Mix 15 drops in a ½ cup of water and drink three times a day. Black walnut hulls are high in iodine and can increase thyroid hormone levels in the body.
- **Bladderwrack tea.** Add 1 to 2 teaspoons of dried bladderwrack to a cup of hot water. Allow it to steep for 5 to 10 minutes. Strain and add honey to taste. Drink two to three times a day.
- **Flaxseed drink.** Grind flaxseed into a fine powder and mix into a glass of milk. Take it once a day.
- **Ginger tea.** Add about 1 inch of ginger to a cup of hot water. Allow it to steep for 5 to 10 minutes. Add honey to taste. Alternatively, chew on small pieces of ginger.
- **Kelp supplements.** Kelp is a type of seaweed that is rich in iodine. Consume 150 to 175 mg of kelp supplements every day.
- **Rhodiola tea.** Add 2 tablespoons of dried rhodiola root to 1 cup of hot water. Allow it to steep for 10 to 15 minutes. Add honey to taste; strain and drink.
- **Stinging nettle leaf tincture.** Stinging nettle may be taken in the form of tea or a tincture. They are also available as capsules. To make a tincture, place about 110 g of fresh-cut nettle leaves into a 500 mL jar and add enough glycerin to fill the jar. Cover the jar tightly and leave in a cool dark place for 2 to 3 weeks, shaking the jar daily. Afterward, strain the mixture and store the tincture into a dark bottle. Mix 1 to 3 drops of the tincture into about half a cup of water and drink.
  - Variation #1. Stinging nettle tea. Boil 1 cup of fresh leaves in 2 to 4 cups of water. Steep for 5 to 10 minutes. Strain and drink the cooked leaves, which can also be added to food.

Therapeutic Measures

- Essential oil therapy: Add 3 to 4 drops of rosemary or frankincense oil to your bath and soak in it for 15 to 20 minutes. Rosemary is thought to regulate the secretion of thyroid hormones in the body.
- Diet: Consume large amounts of eggs, meat, fish (omega-3 oil), vegetables, gluten-free grains like rice, quinoa, chia seeds, and flaxseeds. Avoid cruciferous vegetables such as broccoli, spinach, and cabbage—they contain goitrogens that suppress thyroid hormone production in the body. Fruits such as peaches, pears, and strawberries also have goitrogens.

Modern Remedies

Synthetic Thyroid Hormone (Levothyroxine)

The thyroid produces a hormone called triiodothyronine (T3) and thyroxine (T4). These hormones regulate the body's temperature, heart, weight, and metabolism. A lack of thyroid hormone (hypothyroidism) in the body causes symptoms such as cold intolerance, weight gain, decreased appetite, and a low heart rate. Hypothyroidism is caused by the body not producing enough thyroid hormone. In this case, synthetic thyroid hormones like levothyroxine (an exogenous source of T4) can be taken to increase thyroid hormone levels in the body. Levothyroxine is de-iodinated in the body to form T3 to supplement the body's lack of T3 production.

Hyperthyroidism

Hyperthyroidism is a condition characterized by an excess of thyroid hormones in the bloodstream due to an overactive thyroid gland. The excess of thyroid hormones (T3 and T4) in the body causes an increase in the body's metabolism, breathing, heart rate, and body temperature, leading to symptoms such as heat intolerance, tremors, rapid heartbeat, and feelings of anxiety.

Common causes of hyperthyroidism include an inherited autoimmune disorder known as Graves's disease, in which the body produces an antibody called thyroid-stimulating immunoglobulin (TSI), which stimulates the thyroid gland and causes an overproduction of thyroid hormones. Hyperthyroidism may also be caused by a goiter, lumps in the thyroid gland that stimulate overproduction of thyroid hormones. Inflammation of the thyroid gland (thyroiditis) due to a virus may also cause hyperthyroidism. A diet high in iodine may also stimulate overactivity of the thyroid gland.

Indian Natural Remedies

Common Ingredients for Hyperthyroidism

Spices	Herbs/Leaves	Miscellaneous
Coriander seed	Indian ginseng (Withania somnifera/ ashwagandha)	Ghee
Ginger	Kale	Moringa drumstick (Moringa oleifera)
	Spinach	(Indian gooseberry/ amla) (Phyllanthus emblica)
	Commiphora Mukul (guggulu)	
	Terminalia bellirica (bibhitaki)	
	Terminalia chebula (haritaki)	

Spices	Herbs/Leaves	Miscellaneous
	Giloy (*Tinospora cordifolia*)	
	Gokshura (*Tribulus terrestris*)	
	Convolvulus pluricaulis (shankhpushpi)	
	Nardostachys jatamansi (jatamansi)	
	Bacopa monnieri (brahmi)	
	Triphala	
	Trikatu	
Piper longum (long pepper)	Cabbage (*Brassica oleracea*)	Radish
Piper nigrum (black peppercorn)	Mustard greens	Essential oils— lemon and sandalwood

Common Recipes

Oral

Teas/Brews

- **Amla juice.** Lightly pound three to four amla fruits and strain the juice. Take this juice on an empty stomach in the morning with a glass of warm water.
- **Ashwagandha.** Add 2 tablespoons of ashwagandha to a glass of hot milk. Stir in 1 teaspoon of ghee. Drink twice a day.
- **Brahmi tea.** Place about two to three stalks of fresh Brahmi leaves into a cup. Pour boiling water over the leaves and allow it to steep for about 10 to 15 minutes. Add honey to taste and drink.
- **Coriander seed brew.** Place 10 g of coriander seeds into a pot with 1 cup of water. Boil and then cool. Strain and drink twice a day.
- **Giloy juice.** Place a handful of giloy leaves into a blender and blend until smooth. Strain and drink. Alternatively, chew on fresh giloy leaves or consume in the form of powder.
- **Gokshura tea.** Place dried gokshura herbs into a teapot and pour boiling water over it. Allow it to steep for 10 minutes. Strain and drink.
- **Guggulu.** Guggulu is the sap produced by the Indian bdellium tree and is believed to have cholesterol-reducing properties. It is available in the form of dietary supplements. Adults can take about 25 mg of guggulu supplements every day after a meal. Alternatively, 1 teaspoon of ground guggulu can be mixed with some ground ginger and honey to make a paste. Take this paste three times a day.
- **Jatamansi brew.** Add a pinch of jatamansi root powder to a cup of warm water and take twice a day.

- **Trikatu brew.** Steep equal parts of black pepper, long pepper, and ginger in a cup of hot water. Steep for about 10 to 15 minutes. Drink it warm.
- **Triphala tea.** Add half a teaspoon of triphala powder to 1 cup of hot water. Mix well and drink it warm. Triphala powder is made up of three ingredients: amla, haritaki, and bibhitaki.
- **Vegetable juice.** Place cabbage, mustard greens, kale, spinach, and radish into a blender. Blend until smooth and drink twice a day.

Commercial Preparations

Many Ayurvedic commercial preparations are available as pastes or powders and may be used in the symptomatic treatment of hyperthyroidism.

- Relieving excessive sweating
  - Kamdudha ras: Mukta pishti (pearl calcium), praval pishti (coral calcium), shukti pishti (pearl oyster shell calcium), kapardak bhasma (cowries), shankh bhasma (conch shell powder), shuddha sonageru (haematite), giloy satva (*T. cordifolia*).
  - Praval-Panchamrut: Mukta pishti (pearl calcium), praval pishti (coral calcium), shukti pishti (pearl oyster shell calcium), kapardak bhasma (cowries), shankh bhasma (conch shell powder).
  - Chandrakala-Ras: Cardamom, camphor, amla, nutmeg, Bombax malabaricum, purified and processed mercury, tin calcium, iron calcium, giloy satva, honey.
  - Sutshekhar-Ras: Purified and processed mercury, gold calcium, borax, purified Aconitum ferox, ginger, black pepper, long pepper, datura metel, purified and processed sulfur, copper calcium, cardamom, cinnamon, *Cinnamomum tamala*, *Mesua ferrea*, shankh bhasma (conch shell powder), bael fruit, *Curcuma zedoaria*.
- Relieving tremors, nervousness, and agitation
  - Brahmi-*Bacopa monnieri*
  - Jatamansi-Nardostachys jatamansi
  - Shankhpushpi-Convolvulus pluricaulis
  - Sarpagandha: Indian snakeroot/Rauwolfia serpentina
  - Saraswatarishta: brahmi, *A. racemosus*, *Pueraria tuberosa*, Vetiveria zizanioides, *Foeniculum vulgare*, honey, sugar candy, ashwagandha, giloy satva, cardamom, cinnamon, *Terminalia bellirica*, cloves.
  - Dashmoolarishta: Bilva root, agnimantha root, shyonaka root, patala root, kashmari root, brihati root, kantakari root, shalaparni root, prishniparni root, gokshura root, water, honey, jaggery, giloy, amla, haritaki, licorice.

Miscellaneous

- Dip a piece of cloth in water containing a paste of moringa bark. Allow to dry and tie loosely around the neck at night. This is thought to reduce enlargement of the thyroid gland. It should only be used for a maximum of 15 days, as long-term use may cause emaciation of the neck muscles.

Chinese Natural Remedies

Common Ingredients for Hyperthyroidism

Herbs/Leaves

Anemarrhena/zhi mu (*Anemarrhena asphodeloides*)	Oyster shell/mu li	
Burdock root/niu bang zi (*Arctium lappa*)	Radix glycyrrhizae preparata (zhi gan cao)	Jie geng
Chinese thorowax root/chai hu (*Radix bupleuri*)	Fructus lycii (gou qi zi)	Radix ginseng (ren sheng)
Cortex moutan (mu dan pi)	Radix ophiopogonis (mai dong)	Folium perillae (zi su ye)
Fructus corni/shan yu rou	Heal-all spike/xia ku cao (*Spica prunellae*)	Radix astragali (huang qi)
Fructus gardeniae (zhi zi)	Radix glehniae seu adenophorae (sha shen)	Cortex magnoliae officinalis (hou po)
Poria (fu ling)	Rhizoma cyperi (xiang fu)	Radix scrophulariae (xuan shen)
Radicis angelicae sinensis (dang gui shen)	Fructus toosendan (chuan lian zi)	Chinese senega roots/yuan zhi (*Polygala tenuifolia*)
Radix glycyrrhizae (gan cao)	Rhizoma pinelliae (ban xia)	Radix asparagi (tian men dong)
Radix paeoniae alba (bai shao)	Pericarpium citri reticulatae (chen pi)	Fructus schisandrae chinensis (wu wei zi)
Radix rehmanniae (sheng di huan)	Rhizoma zingiberis recens (sheng jiang)	Radix salviae miltiorrhizae (dan shen)
Rhizoma alismatis (ze xie)	Szechuan ox knee/chuan niu xi (*Cyathula officinalis; Radix*)	
Rhizoma dioscoreae (shan yao)	Carapax trionycis (bie jia)	Radix saposhnikoviae (fang feng)
Rhizoma ligustici chuanxiong (chuan xiong)	Radix paeoniae alba (zhi qiao)	Biota seeds/bai zi ren (*Platycladus orientalis*)
Semen ziziphi spinosae (suan zao ren)	Phellodendron/huang bo (*Phellodendri cortex*)	Fritillary bulb/zhe bei mu (*Fritillaria thunbergii bulb*)

Common Recipes

Oral

- **Treatment for liver fire:** An excess of liver fire in the body manifests as irritability, increased appetite, palpitations, a red tongue, and a rapid, wiry pulse. Zhi zi qing gan tang is an herbal concoction used to treat this condition, made up of Fructus gardeniae, Cortex moutan, Radix bupleuri, Radicis angelicae sinensis, Radix paeoniae alba, poria, Rhizoma ligustici chuanxiong, Fructus arctii, and Radix glycyrrhizae.

- **Treatment for qi and yin deficiency:** Symptoms include fatigue, shortness of breath, dry eyes, palpitations, excessive sweating, dry mouth and thirst, a red tongue, and a rapid, thready pulse. The most common herbal preparation is "yi guan jian," consisting of the following ingredients: Radix rehmanniae (30 g), Radix glehniae seu adenophorae (15 g), Radix ophiopogonis (15 g), Fructus lycii (15 g), Fructus toosendan (8 g), Radix angelicae sinensis (15 g).

- **Treatment for qi and phlegm stagnation:** Symptoms are irritability, a feeling of pressure on the chest, enlarged thyroid gland, a red tongue, and a slippery, wiry pulse. Two herbal remedies are used for this diagnosis.
  - **Chai hu shu gan tang:** Radix bupleuri (19 g), Pericarpium citri reticulatae (19 g), Rhizoma ligustici chuanxiong (14 g), Rhizoma cyperi (14 g), Radix paeoniae alba (14 g), Radix glycyrrhizae preparata (5 g).
  - **Ban xia hou po tang:** Rhizoma pinelliae (28 g), Rhizoma zingiberis recens (26 g), poria (21 g), Cortex magnoliae officinalis (16 g), Folium perillae (10 g).

- **Treatment for liver, kidney, and heart yin deficiency:** Symptoms are irritability, insomnia, anorexia, dry mouth with red tongue, and a rapid, thready pulse. There are two herbal decoctions available:
  - **Tian wang bu xin dan:** Radix Rehmannia (31 g), Radix ginseng (4 g), Poria (4 g), Radix polygalae (4 g), Fructus schisandrae chinensis (8 g), Radix scrophulariae (4 g), Platycladus orientalis (8 g), Radix platycodonis (4 g), Radix asparagi (8 g), Radix salviae miltiorrhizae (4 g), Semen ziziphi spinosae (8 g), Radicis angelicae sinensis (8 g), and Radix ophiopogonis (8 g).
  - **Zhi bai di huang wan:** Radix rehmanniae preparata (28 g), Fructus corni (14 g), Rhizoma dioscoreae (14 g), Cortex moutan (10 g), Rhizoma alismatis (10 g), Poria (10 g), Radix anemarrhenae (7 g), Cortex phellodendri (7 g).

- **Treatment for liver fire with phlegm and qi and yin deficiency:** Symptoms are low-grade fever, high heart rate, hand tremors, enlarged thyroid gland, swollen and bulging eyes, palpitations, excessive sweating, irritability, increased appetite, and high blood pressure. The remedy for this condition is called the "empirical formula for hyperthyroidism," and includes Radix scrophulariae, Radix anemarrhenae, Spica prunellae, Carapax trionycis, Radix cyathulae, Concha ostreae, Fritillaria thunbergii bulb, Radix polygalae, Radix astragali, Radix saposhnikoviae, and Radix glycyrrhizae.

  Notes
- In traditional Chinese medicine (TCM), hyperthyroidism is caused by several imbalances: Qi and yin deficiencies,

liver fire excess, and phlegm stagnation. The qi and yin deficiencies are thought to represent weakness and fatigue while liver fire is thought to mean excitation of the body due to the high thyroid hormone levels in the body. Phlegm stagnation is thought to refer to the enlargement of the thyroid gland.

- Qi (energy levels)—qi circulation is another important aspect in TCM. It is believed that poor qi circulation can cause high cholesterol and several other health ailments. Yang qi refers to heat energy. Yin qi refers to cold energy. These two energies should be in balance for an individual to maintain good health.

- It is believed that three organs are involved in regulating thyroid hormone levels in the body: the heart, the liver, and the kidneys. Treatments are often symptom-specific and are aimed at the organ that is thought to be causing the hyperthyroidism.

- Dosages are tailored to the patient's age, gender, health status, and other factors. Please consult a sensei for an accurate diagnosis and treatment plan.

Western/Other Natural Remedies

Common Ingredients for Hyperthyroidism

Herbs/Leaves	Miscellaneous
Bugleweed	Honey
Irish moss *(Chondrus crispus)*	
Lemon balm	
Motherwort *(Leonurus cardiaca)*	
Mullein leaf	
Stinging nettle	

Common Recipes

Oral

Teas/Brews

- **Bugleweed tea.** Bugleweed is available in the form of a dried herb or as capsules or pills. To make bugleweed tea, place some dried bugleweed into a teapot and pour boiling hot water into it. Steep for 5 to 10 minutes and drink.
- **Irish moss tea.** Irish moss is a seaweed available in the form of a gel, powder, or dried seaweed. To make Irish moss tea, place 3 tablespoons of Irish moss gel into a cup and add in 1 L of warm water. Mix well and drink. Alternatively, mix 1 tablespoon of powder into 1 cup of hot water and drink.
- **Motherwort tea.** Motherwort is available fresh as a dried herb, extract, or as a capsule. Place 1 tablespoon of dried motherwort herb into a cup and add 1 cup of boiling water over the herbs. Cover and steep for 15 to 20 minutes. Strain and drink.
- **Motherwort tincture.** Take 10 to 30 drops of motherwort extract and mix into a small amount of water. Drink twice a day.
- **Mullein leaf tea.** Place about 2 teaspoons of dried Mullein leaves into a cup and pour 1 cup of boiling water over the leaves. Allow it to steep for 10 to 15 minutes and strain before drinking.
- **Lemon balm tea.** Lemon balm is available fresh, dried, or as capsules. Place ¼ of freshly chopped lemon balm leaves into a cup and add 1 cup of boiling water. Steep for 10 minutes. Add honey to taste and drink it warm.
- **Nettle tincture.** Stinging nettle may be taken in the form of tea or a tincture. They are also available as capsules. To make a tincture, place about 110 g of freshly cut nettle leaves into a 500 mL jar and add enough glycerin to fill the jar. Cover the jar tightly and leave in a cool dark place for 2 to 3 weeks, shaking the jar daily. Afterward, strain the mixture and store the tincture into a dark bottle. Mix 1 to 3 drops of the tincture into about a ½ cup of water and drink.

Therapeutic Measures

Diet

Eat a healthy, balanced diet consisting of fresh vegetables, fruits, legumes, and whole grains.

Freshwater fish and flaxseeds are good sources of omega-3.

Lentils are high in protein and fiber.

Consume cruciferous vegetables such as broccoli, kale, and cabbage. They contain goitrogens, which block thyroid hormone production.

Calcium-rich foods such as almonds, parsley, and fresh turnip should also be eaten regularly.

Avoid too much seaweed due to the high iodine content, which can stimulate the thyroid gland and worsen hyperthyroidism.

Lifestyle

- Exercise regularly and lose weight if overweight.
    Notes
- Consult a medical professional before taking any of the natural remedies. Some may be used as adjuncts to modern treatments, but some may also have adverse interactions with allopathic medication and should be taken with care.
- Patients who are pregnant or have cardiovascular illnesses should consult a medical professional on the safety of the above natural remedies.

Modern Remedies

1. Antithyroid Agents
    Antithyroid agents are often used to treat hyperthyroidism, especially conditions such as Graves disease or goiter.
    - **Methimazole:** Methimazole has a similar function to PTU but does not block peripheral conversion of T4 to T3. Its effects are also far more potent than that of PTU.
    - **Propylthiouracil (PTU):** This medication functions by preventing thyroid hormone synthesis. It does this by inhibiting the thyroid peroxidase-catalyzed reactions and blocking the incorporation of iodine into

thyroglobulins (organification of iodine). It also blocks the peripheral conversion of T4 into T3.

- **Potassium iodide:** Iodide inhibits thyroid hormone release from the thyroid gland and inhibits the synthesis of thyroid hormones by inhibiting the enzyme thyroidal peroxidase in the thyroid gland. This form of therapy is often only given for a few weeks as the thyroid gland sometimes *escapes* from the iodide block. It is often used in conjunction with other anti-thyroid medication.

2. Iodine-131 (radioactive iodine)

Radioactive iodine is rapidly absorbed and concentrated in the thyroid and incorporated into storage follicles in the thyroid gland. It emits beta rays, which destroy parenchymal cells in the thyroid with little damage to other tissues in the body. After treatment with radioactive iodine, however, hypothyroidism may occur, which may be treated using thyroid hormone replacement medication.

3. Beta Blockers

Beta blockers such as propranolol or atenolol are helpful to ease the symptoms if there are palpitations, hand tremors, or hyperactivity.

4. Surgery

Partial or total thyroidectomy (removal of part or all the thyroid gland) is usually the treatment of choice for younger patients with large goiters and for those with severe disease.

Homeopathic Remedies

These may be used as supportive care and include Natrum muriaticum, phosphorus, Lachesis, and conium.

Poor Appetite

Poor appetite refers to a loss of desire to eat and a lack of interest in food, leading to weight loss and fatigue. It may be caused by several problems, such as digestive disorders (Crohn disease, irritable bowel syndrome), diabetes, chronic kidney or liver diseases, HIV and AIDS, or hypothyroidism. It may also refer to a general small appetite without any pathological reason. These remedies are intended to boost appetite but should be taken as an adjunct to lifestyle and diet changes and allopathic medication where necessary.

Indian Natural Remedies

Common Ingredients for Poor Appetite

Spices	Herbs/Leaves	Miscellaneous
Black peppercorn (Piper nigrum)		Nuts (almonds, walnuts)
Cardamom		Honey
Cinnamon	Ashwagandha (Indian ginseng)	Custard apple (Anonna squamosa)
Clove		Yashtimadhu (licorice)
Fenugreek seed		Milk
		Fruits (Mango, Banana, Custard apple, Fig)
		Gur (sugarcane jaggery)
		Palm date
		Beans
Garlic	Shatavari (Asparagus racemosus)	Chyawanprash
Ginger	Peepal fruit	Raisins (Vitis vinifera)
Saffron		Ghee

Common Recipes

Oral

Teas/Brews

- **Almond milk.** Mix 1 tablespoon of crushed almonds with 1 cup of hot milk. Drink once a day.
- **Ashwagandha.** Add 2 tablespoons of ashwagandha to a glass of hot milk. Stir in 1 teaspoon of ghee. Drink twice a day.
- **Banana milkshake.** Blend 1 banana and add gradually 250 mL of milk. Pour into a cup and sprinkle with cinnamon if desired.
- **Chyawanprash.** Mix 1 teaspoon of chyawanprash powder into a glass of milk. Drink twice a day. Chyawanprash is believed to increase appetite.
- **Custard apple.** Eat two custard apples a day for their high calorie and iron content.
- **Fenugreek paste.** Fry 5 g of fenugreek seeds in a teaspoon of ghee. Grind to a paste and mix with a ½ teaspoon of honey. Eat this paste once a day.
- **Fig, almond, and palm date milk.** Place two figs, two pieces of date palm, and three to five almonds into a pot with 1 cup of milk. Bring to a boil before reducing the heat. Allow it to simmer for 10 minutes. Strain the mixture. Drink once a day.
- **Mango and milk.** Eat mangoes with 250 mL of milk. Mango is a carbohydrate-rich fruit.
- **Nut and dry fruit mix.** Take 50 g each of figs, almonds, palm dates, and raisins. Add 100 g of gur to this mixture. Sautee this in ghee until it reaches a jelly-like consistency. Consume this twice a day after meals.
- **Peepal fruit.** Consume ripe peepal fruit.
  - Consume beans regularly as they have high protein and fiber content.
  - Snack on nuts such as almonds and walnuts throughout the day as they are calorie-dense foods.
- **Raisins and figs.** Place 5 to 8 dried figs and 10 to 12 raisins in a bowl of water. Leave to soak overnight and eat in two doses the next day.
- **Saffron milk.** Mix one strand of saffron into a cup of warm milk. Drink once a day.
- **Shatavari.** Add 2 to 5 g of shatavari powder to a glass of milk. Drink twice a day.
- **Spices** such as cinnamon, garlic, ginger, cardamom, black peppercorn, and cloves are believed to increase appetite. Take a pinch of these spices every day.

Chinese Natural Remedies

Common Ingredients for Poor Appetite

Spices	Herbs/Leaves	Miscellaneous
Ginger	Gentian (long dan cao)	Licorice
	Dandelion root	Chen pi
	Skullcap	Bird's nest

Common Recipes

Oral

Teas/Brews

Bird's nest. Consume bird's nest drink or soup.

Chen pi-ginger tea. Add about ½ an orange worth of chen pi and about 2 to 3 inches of freshly pounded ginger to an empty cup. Boil about 2 cups of water and pour into the cup over the chen pi and ginger. Let the tea sit for about 2 minutes and drink.

Dandelion root tea. Break fresh dandelion roots into smaller chunks and place in a pot with some water. Bring to a gentle simmer and allow to simmer for about 15 minutes. Allow the mixture to settle for about 5 minutes, then strain and drink.

Gentian tea. Gentian tea is available in the form of tea bags, capsules, powder, or as dried roots and stems. Place about 2 to 2.5 g of dried gentian or gentian powder and place into a pot with water. Boil for about 5 minutes then remove from the heat and allow to cool completely before drinking.

> The standard recommended dose for different preparations of gentian are as follows: capsule: 500 mg, taken two to three times a day (with meals); powdered gentian root, 1 to 4 g a day; dried gentian, 2 to 2.5 g a day; gentian extract, 5 to 30 drops (0.3 to 2 mL).

Ginger tea. Steep lightly pounded ginger in a cup of hot water and sip.

Licorice root tea. Add 1 to 2 teaspoons of ground licorice root to a cup of boiling water. Allow it to steep for about 5 minutes. Add honey to taste and drink it warm.

Western/Other Natural Remedies

Common Ingredients for Poor Appetite

Miscellaneous

Fruits (avocado, banana, and figs)	
Milk (cow's milk and almond milk)	
Nuts (walnuts, almonds, sunflower seeds, flaxseeds)	Royal jelly
Peanut butter	Eggs
Potatoes	Chamomile

Common Recipes

Oral

- **Figs** contain polyunsaturated fats, which aid with weight gain.
- **Eggs.** Include eggs into the daily diet.
- **Almond milk.** Soak about 200 g of almonds in water overnight. Peel the skins off the next morning. Add about 4 cups of water and blend until smooth. Strain through a piece of muslin and drink.
- **Chamomile tea.** Place some dried or fresh chamomile flowers into a cup. Pour boiling water over the flowers and allow to steep for 10 minutes. Strain and add honey to taste. Drink hot.
- **Royal jelly.** Give 5 to 10 mL daily to children above 3 years old after breakfast.
- **Nut mix.** Snack on nuts such as sunflower seeds, almonds, walnuts, and flaxseeds throughout the day.
- **Dense, high-calorie fruits.** Snack on bananas or avocados. Milkshakes can be made by blending one banana or two deseeded avocados with 1 cup of milk.
- **High-carbohydrate/high-fat diet** is recommended to gain weight. Suggested high caloric foods:

Food	kcal/100 g
Walnut	654
Almond	622.5
Sunflower seed	585.3
Banana	89
Fig	74.09
Avocado	160
Boiled egg	155
Smooth peanut butter	588

Homeopathic Remedies

These include *alfalfa* (ideal for any loss of appetite and anorexia nervosa), *psorinum* (especially after recovery from an illness), *China* (associated fullness, bloating, food aversion), *ignatia* (associated with depression), *colchicum* (associated nausea at the smell or thought of food), and *Antimonium crudum* (post-illness). In children, depending on the symptoms, *Carica papaya, chelidonium, Ferrum metallicum,* and *pulsatilla* are used.

References

Obesity

Abidov, M., Ramazanov, Z., Seifulla, R., & Grachev, S. (2010). The effects of Xanthigen in the weight management of obese premenopausal women with non-alcoholic fatty liver disease and normal liver fat. *Diabetes, Obesity and Metabolism, 12*(1), 72–81. Retrieved from https://doi.org/10.1111/j.1463-1326.2009.01132.x.

Altneu, K. (2017, December 18). *Solutions for obesity & weight loss in Chinese medicine.* The Point, Acupuncture & Chinese Medicine in Denver. Retrieved from https://thepointdenver.com/blog/chinese-medicine-solutions-obesity-weight-loss/.

Brabaw, K. (2016, January 6). *13 herbs and spices scientifically proven to help you lose weight.* Prevention. Retrieved from https://www.prevention.com/weight-loss/a20493821/herbs-and-spices-for-weight-loss/.

Brazier, Y., & Bubnis, D. (2018, November 14). *What are the treatments for obesity?* Medical News Today. Retrieved from https://www.medicalnewstoday.com/articles/323691.

Brody, B. (2013, December 20). *Dean Ornish's spectrum diet*. WebMD. Retrieved from https://www.webmd.com/diet/a-z/ornish-diet-spectrum-what-it-is.

Chertoff, J., & Wilson, D. R. (2019, May 21). *Can homeopathic medicine help with weight loss?* Healthline. Retrieved from https://www.healthline.com/health/homeopathic-medicine-for-weight-loss.

Drug Bank. (2003, June 13). *Phentermine: Uses, interactions, mechanism of action*. DrugBank Online. Retrieved from https://go.drugbank.com/drugs/DB00191.

Drug Bank. (2005, June 13). *Orlistat: Uses, interactions, mechanism of action*. DrugBank Online. Retrieved from https://go.drugbank.com/drugs/DB01083.

Elliott, B. (2018, May 7). *8 great reasons to include chickpeas in your diet*. Healthline. Retrieved from https://www.healthline.com/nutrition/chickpeas-nutrition-benefits.

Fei-Li, H. (2011). *Cosmetology in Chinese medicine (DVD included) (International Standard Library of Chinese Medicine)* (1st ed.). Shelton, CT: People's Medical Publishing House.

Finer, N. (2002). Sibutramine: Its mode of action and efficacy. *International Journal of Obesity, 26*(S4), S29–S33. Retrieved from https://doi.org/10.1038/sj.ijo.0802216.

Gaikwad, S. T., Gaikwad, P., & Saxena, V. (2017). Principles of fasting in Ayurveda. *International Journal of Science, Environment and Technology, 6*(1), 787–792. Retrieved from https://www.researchgate.net/publication/313250061_Principles_of_Fasting_in_Ayurveda.

Group, E. (2018, October 4). *The top 12 herbs for weight loss*. Dr. Group's Healthy Living Articles. Retrieved from https://explore.globalhealing.com/top-herbs-for-weight-loss/.

Gupte, P., Harke, S., Deo, V., Bhushan Shrikhande, B., Mahajan, M., & Bhalerao, S. (2020). A clinical study to evaluate the efficacy of Herbal Formulation for Obesity (HFO-02) in overweight individuals. *Journal of Ayurveda and Integrative Medicine, 11*(2), 159–162. Retrieved from https://doi.org/10.1016/j.jaim.2019.05.003.

Haider, P. (2015, January 13). *10 health benefits of bermuda grass juice*. Linkedin. Retrieved from https://www.linkedin.com/pulse/10-health-benefits-bermuda-grass-juice-dr-paul-haider/.

Hamdy, O. (2021, June 9). *Obesity treatment & management: Approach considerations, patient screening, assessment, and expectations, weight-loss goals*. Medscape. Retrieved from https://emedicine.medscape.com/article/123702-treatment.

Health Benefits Times (Ed.). (2018, July 20). *Black cardamom health benefits*. Health Benefits. Retrieved from https://www.healthbenefitstimes.com/black-cardamom/.

Hebbar, J. V. (2013). *Triphala Churna benefits, ingredients, dose, side effects, how to take*. Ayur Med Info. Retrieved from https://www.ayurmedinfo.com/2012/03/16/triphala-churna-benefits-ingredients-dose-side-effects-how-to-take/.

Karchmer, E. (2021, February 25). *5 ways to use bao he wan to support the digestive system*. DAO Labs. Retrieved from https://mydaolabs.com/blogs/the-way/5-ways-to-use-bao-he-wan-to-support-the-digestive-system.

Leonard, J. (2020, April 16). *Seven ways to do intermittent fasting*. Medical News Today. Retrieved from https://www.medicalnewstoday.com/articles/322293#tips-for-maintaining-intermittent-fasting.

Link, R. (2018a, January 6). *Amaranth: An ancient grain with impressive health benefits*. Healthline. Retrieved from https://www.healthline.com/nutrition/amaranth-health-benefits.

Link, R. (2018b, July 23). *13 herbs that can help you lose weight*. Healthline. Retrieved from https://www.healthline.com/nutrition/weight-loss-herbs.

Magee, E. (2005, February 18). *Your "hunger hormones."* WebMD. Retrieved from https://www.webmd.com/diet/features/your-hunger-hormones.

Mayo Clinic Staff. (2019, July 20). *Tummy tuck*. Mayo Clinic. Retrieved from https://www.mayoclinic.org/tests-procedures/tummy-tuck/about/pac-20384892.

Mayo Clinic Staff. (2020, August 25). *Paleo diet: What is it and why is it so popular?* Mayo Clinic. Retrieved from https://www.mayoclinic.org/healthy-lifestyle/nutrition-and-healthy-eating/in-depth/paleo-diet/art-20111182.

Mayo Clinic Staff. (2021, April 23). *Liposuction*. Mayo Clinic. Retrieved from https://www.mayoclinic.org/tests-procedures/liposuction/about/pac-20384586.

McPherson, G. (2021, June 22). *What is African Mango and its extract? Weight loss and more*. Healthline. Retrieved from https://www.healthline.com/nutrition/african-mango.

Mercola, J. (2012, November 26). *10 herbs and spices for proper weight management*. Mercola.Com. Retrieved from https://articles.mercola.com/sites/articles/archive/2012/11/26/herbs-and-spices.aspx.

Midland, N. (2021, March 9). *Chinese herbs for weight loss: A holistic approach to shake up your metabolism*. BetterMe Blog. Retrieved from https://betterme.world/articles/chinese-herbs-for-weight-loss/.

NDTV Food. (2018, March 28). *7 incredible benefits of drinking bottle gourd (Lauki) juice*. Retrieved from https://food.ndtv.com/food-drinks/7-incredible-benefits-of-drinking-of-bottle-gourd-lauki-juice-1452828.

Nicolai, J. P., Lupiani, J. H., & Wolf, A. J. (2018). Chapter 37—An integrative approach to obesity. In *Integrative medicine* (4th ed., pp. 382–394). Amsterdam: Elsevier Inc. Retrieved from https://doi.org/10.1016/B978-0-323-35868-2.00037-2.

Rana, S. (2020, January 30). *Weight loss: 10 Ayurvedic remedies to lose weight*. NDTV Food. Retrieved from https://food.ndtv.com/weight-loss/weight-loss-6-ayurvedic-remedies-to-cut-belly-fat-1888165.

Schreck, J. (2019, January 22). *Chinese herbs for obesity, diet and weight loss*. Shen Clinic.Com. Retrieved from https://shenclinic.com/blogs/herbs-for-ailments/chinese-herbs-for-diet-and-weight-loss.

Sengupta, S. (2019, June 19). *8 amazing health benefits of carrots: From weight-loss to healthy eyesight*. NDTV Food. Retrieved from https://food.ndtv.com/food-drinks/8-amazing-health-benefits-of-carrots-from-weight-loss-to-healthy-eyesight-1767963.

Smith, M. W. (2002, April 12). *Prescription weight loss drugs*. WebMD. Retrieved from https://www.webmd.com/diet/obesity/weight-loss-prescription-weight-loss-medicine.

Stanborough, R. J. (2019, July 22). *Can Ayurvedic medicine be used for weight loss?* Healthline. Retrieved from https://www.healthline.com/health/ayurvedic-medicine-for-weight-loss#dosha-eating.

Staughton, J. (2020, July 29). *18 best health benefits of carom seeds (Ajwain)*. Organic Facts. Retrieved from https://www.organicfacts.net/carom-seeds.html.

Swasthi, S. (2019, July 14). *How to make aloe vera juice*. Swasthi's Recipes. Retrieved from https://www.indianhealthyrecipes.com/how-to-make-aloe-vera-juice/.

The Indian Spot. (n.d.). *5 effective ayurvedic herbs for weight loss*. The Indian Spot. Retrieved from https://theindianspot.com/5-effective-ayurvedic-herbs-for-weight-loss/.

Times of India. (2015, September 28). *Top 20 herbs for weight loss*. The Times of India. Retrieved from https://timesofindia.indiatimes.com/life-style/health-fitness/diet/top-20-herbs-for-weight-loss/articleshow/19574894.cms.

World Health Organization. (2020, February 21). *Obesity*. Retrieved from https://www.who.int/health-topics/obesity.

Yin Yang House. (n.d.). *Chinese herbal and acupuncture treatment protocols for obesity (weight loss)—Formulas, protocols, TCM diagnoses*. Retrieved from https://theory.yinyanghouse.com/conditions-treated/alternative-natural-options-for-obesity.

Diabetes Mellitus

Aduloju, I. E., Omachi, A. B., & Olagunju, I. (2019). Nutritive and phytochemical analysis of bay leaf (*Laurus nobilis*), Nutmeg seed (*Myristica fragrans*) and Shepherd's purse seed (Capsella Bursa-Pastoris). *International Journal of Current Research, 11*(12), 9068–9071. Retrieved from https://doi.org/10.24941/ijcr.36832.12.2019.

American Association of Clinical Endocrinology. (2020). *Comprehensive type 2 diabetes management algorithm (2020)—Executive summary*. Retrieved from https://pro.aace.com/disease-state-resources/diabetes/clinical-practice-guidelines-treatment-algorithms/comprehensive.

American Diabetes Association. (n.d.). *Treatment & care*. Retrieved from https://www.diabetes.org/diabetes/treatment-care.

Behl, M. S. (2019, September 28). *14 amazing herbs that lower blood sugar*. Sepalika. Retrieved from https://www.sepalika.com/type-2-diabetes/14-amazing-herbs-that-lower-blood-sugar/.

Biswas, A. (2021, November 15). *7 best natural medicines for diabetes*. Practo. Retrieved from https://www.practo.com/healthfeed/7-best-natural-medicines-for-diabetes-25482/post.

BMJ Publishing Group. (2021). *Type 1 diabetes mellitus—Emerging treatments*. Retrieved from https://bestpractice.bmj.com/topics/en-us/25/emergingtxs.

Cafasso, J., & Wilson, D. R. (2018, June 16). *Homeopathy for diabetes*. Healthline. Retrieved from https://www.healthline.com/health/homeopathy-diabetes.

Choudhury, H., Pandey, M., Hua, C. K., Mun, C. S., Jing, J. K., Kong, L., et al. (2018). An update on natural compounds in the remedy of diabetes mellitus: A systematic review. *Journal of Traditional and Complementary Medicine, 8*(3), 361–376. Retrieved from https://doi.org/10.1016/j.jtcme.2017.08.012.

Diabetes Digital Media Ltd. (2020, January 27). *Diabetes community, support, education, recipes & resources*. Diabetes.co.uk. Retrieved from https://www.diabetes.co.uk/.

Diabetes UK. (n.d.). *Type 2 diabetes*. Retrieved from https://www.diabetes.org.uk/type-2-diabetes.

Dineshwori, L. (2020, September 4). *Ayurvedic diet chart for diabetes to keep your blood sugar under control | TheHealthSite.com*. The Health Site. Retrieved from https://www.thehealthsite.com/ayurveda/heres-what-a-typical-ayurvedic-diet-chart-for-diabetics-looks-like-766461/.

Dolson, L., & Kausel, A. M. (2020, May 31). *Steps to reducing your risk of diabetes*. Verywell Health. Retrieved from https://www.verywellhealth.com/diabetes-prevention-2242259.

Gope, A. (2020, February 14). *Health benefits of Cassia fistula | Sarakondrai*. The Indian Med. Retrieved from https://theindianmed.com/health-benefits-of-cassia-fistula-sarakondrai/.

Greenough, K. (2020, December 22). *TCM for diabetes mellitus*. Pacific College. Retrieved from https://www.pacificcollege.edu/news/blog/2017/03/28/tcm-for-diabetes-mellitus.

Haider, P. (2015, January 13). *10 health benefits of Bermuda grass juice*. Linkedin. Retrieved from https://www.linkedin.com/pulse/10-health-benefits-bermuda-grass-juice-dr-paul-haider/.

Hebbar, J. V. (2020, July 2). *Triphala Churna benefits, ingredients, dose, side effects, how to take*. AyurMedInfo. Retrieved from https://www.ayurmedinfo.com/2012/03/16/triphala-churna-benefits-ingredients-dose-side-effects-how-to-take/.

Hsia, D. S., Grove, O., & Cefalu, W. T. (2017). An update on SGLT2 inhibitors for the treatment of diabetes mellitus. *Current Opinion in Endocrinology, Diabetes, and Obesity, 24*(01), 73–79. Retrieved from https://www.ncbi.nlm.nih.gov/pmc/articles/PMC6028052/.

Iliades, C., & Marcellin, L. (2012, November 5). *Botanicals and herbs for type 2 diabetes*. Everyday Health. Retrieved from https://www.everydayhealth.com/alternative-health/botanicals-and-herbs-for-type-2-diabetes.aspx.

Jana, K., Bera, T. K., & Ghosh, D. (2015). Antidiabetic effects of *Eugenia jambolana* in the streptozotocin-induced diabetic male albino rat. *Biomarkers and Genomic Medicine, 7*(3), 116–124. Retrieved from https://doi.org/10.1016/j.bgm.2015.08.001.

Joseph, B., & Jini, D. (2013). Antidiabetic effects of *Momordica charantia* (bitter melon) and its medicinal potency. *Asian Pacific Journal of Tropical Disease, 3*(2), 93–102. Retrieved from https://doi.org/10.1016/s2222-1808(13)60052-3.

Joslin Diabetes Center. (n.d.). Education programs and classes. Retrieved from https://www.joslin.org/patient-care/education-programs-and-classes.

Kelly, E., & Kubala, J. (2020, September 21). *The 16 best foods to control diabetes*. Healthline. Retrieved from https://www.healthline.com/nutrition/16-best-foods-for-diabetics.

Khan, F. (2018). A newer approach in the management of diabetes and reduction of HbA1c level by the use of natural remedies over synthetic drugs. *Pharmacy & Pharmacology International Journal, 6*(5), 357–361. Retrieved from https://doi.org/10.15406/ppij.2018.06.00201.

Leontis, L. M., & Hess-Fischl Ms, A. (2014, July 14). *Thiazolidinediones (TZDs or Glitazones) for type 2 diabetes*. EndocrineWeb. Retrieved from https://www.endocrineweb.com/conditions/type-2-diabetes/thiazolidinediones-tzds-or-glitazones-type-2-diabetes.

Marino, M. (2009, October 9). *Meglitinides*. Diabetes Self-Management. Retrieved from https://www.diabetesselfmanagement.com/blog/meglitinides/.

Marks, L., & Sinha, S., (2015, December 1). *Sulfonylureas—Side effects & precautions*. Everyday Health. Retrieved from https://www.everydayhealth.com/sulfonylureas/guide/.

Mathur, M., Soni, D., & Kanodia, L. (2019, August 30). *Bael*. 1mg. Retrieved from https://www.1mg.com/ayurveda/bael-96.

Medical Health Guide (Ed.). (2011). *Cinnamon herbal medicine, health benefits, side effects*. Medical Health Guide. Retrieved from http://www.medicalhealthguide.com/herb/cinnamon.htm.

Modak, M., Dixit, P., Londhe, J., Ghaskadbi, S., & Devasagayam, T. P. A. (2007). Indian herbs and herbal drugs used for the treatment of diabetes. *Journal of Clinical Biochemistry and Nutrition, 40*(3), 163–173. Retrieved from https://doi.org/10.3164/jcbn.40.163.

Nazario, B. (2019, November 7). *Understanding diagnosis and treatment of diabetes*. WebMD. Retrieved from https://www.webmd.com/diabetes/guide/understanding-diabetes-detection-treatment#1.

Panoff, L. (2019, October 28). *Is buttermilk good for you? Benefits, risks, and substitutes*. Healthline. Retrieved from https://www.healthline.com/nutrition/buttermilk.

Raman, R. (2018, February 22). *Cilantro vs coriander: What's the difference?* Healthline. Retrieved from https://www.healthline.com/nutrition/cilantro-vs-coriander.

Rana, S. (2018, October 29). *Diabetes: 4 Ayurvedic herbal remedies to manage blood sugar levels naturally*. NDTV. Retrieved from https://www.ndtv.com/food/diabetes-4-ayurvedic-herbal-remedies-to-manage-blood-sugar-levels-naturally-1938040.

Rose, S., & Kumar-Singh, A. (2021, March 12). *The uses, benefits & side effects of 9 Ayurvedic herbs & spices*. Mindbodygreen. Retrieved from https://www.mindbodygreen.com/articles/ayurvedic-herbs-and-spices.

Shoemaker, M. S. (2020, October 15). *Indian Gooseberry: Benefits, uses, and side effects*. Healthline. Retrieved from https://www.healthline.com/nutrition/indian-gooseberry.

Singh, K., Ashok, B., Kaur, M., Ravishankar, B., & Chandola, H. (2014). Hypoglycemic and antihyperglycemic activity of Saptarangyadi Ghanavati: An Ayurvedic compound formulation. *AYU (An International Quarterly Journal of Research in Ayurveda), 35*(2), 187. Retrieved from https://doi.org/10.4103/0974-8520.146248.

Sinha, R. (2018, May 6). *Top 6 herbs and spices for diabetes.* Cultural Health Solutions. Retrieved from https://www.culturalhealthsolutions.com/herbs-spices-diabetes/.

Spritzler, F., & Bella, A. M. (2017, January 29). *13 ways to prevent type 2 diabetes.* Healthline. Retrieved from https://www.healthline.com/nutrition/prevent-diabetes.

Tinsley, G. (2018, March 23). *Chromium picolinate: What are the benefits?* Healthline. Retrieved from https://www.healthline.com/nutrition/chromium-picolinate#supplements.

Tierra, M. (2018, May 13). *Diabetes mellitus the TCM approach to treatment.* East West School of Planetary Herbology. Retrieved from https://planetherbs.com/research-center/therapies-articles/diabetes-mellitus/.

Watson, S., & Basina, M. (2020, February 27). *Everything you need to know about diabetes.* Healthline. Retrieved from https://www.healthline.com/health/diabetes.

WebMD (Ed.). (2010). *Ivy Gourd: Overview, uses, side effects, precautions, interactions, dosing and reviews.* WebMD. Retrieved from https://www.webmd.com/vitamins/ai/ingredientmono-1104/ivy-gourd#:%7E:text=Diabetes%3A%20Ivy%20gourd%20might%20lower,control%20during%20and%20after%20surgery.

WebMD (Ed.). (n.d.). *Metformin oral: Uses, side effects, interactions, pictures, warnings & dosing.* WebMD. Retrieved from https://www.webmd.com/drugs/2/drug-11285-7061/metformin-oral/mctformin-oral/details.

WebMD (Ed.). (n.d.). *Uva Ursi.* WebMD. Retrieved from https://www.webmd.com/vitamins/ai/ingredientmono-350/uva-ursi.

World Health Organization. (2019, May 13). *Diabetes.* WHO. Retrieved from https://www.who.int/health-topics/diabetes#tab=tab_1.

Xie, W., Zhao, Y., & Zhang, Y. (2011). Traditional Chinese medicines in treatment of patients with type 2 diabetes mellitus. *Evidence-Based Complementary and Alternative Medicine, 2011*, 1–13. Retrieved from https://doi.org/10.1155/2011/726723.

Hypothyroidism

Ayurvedacharya, M. (2016, November 23). *Ayurvedic herbs that help you in relieving thyroid—By Dr. Malik Ayurvedacharya.* Lybrate. Retrieved from https://www.lybrate.com/topic/ayurvedic-herbs-that-help-you-in-relieving-thyroid/b8ab29db7ab8faf404dc50fd55309cd0.

Berber, E., & Sargis, R. M. (2014, February 6). *Causes of hypothyroidism.* EndocrineWeb. Retrieved from https://www.endocrineweb.com/conditions/hypothyroidism/causes-hypothyroidism.

Borten, P. (2013, May 23). *Lu Rong—Velvet deer antler.* Chinese Herbal Medicine. Retrieved from https://chineseherbinfo.com/lu-rong-young-velvet-deer-antler/.

California College of Ayurveda Students. (2017, August 12). *The Ayurvedic Management of Hypothyroidism by Cassandra McDonough.* California College of Ayurveda. Retrieved from https://www.ayurvedacollege.com/blog/management-of-hypothyroidism/.

DrugBank Online. (2005, June 13). *Levothyroxine: Uses, interactions, mechanism of action.* DrugBank Online. Retrieved from https://go.drugbank.com/drugs/DB00451.

Hu, H. (2012, December 5). *TCM views and treatment of hypothyroidism.* Yang-Sheng.Com. Retrieved from http://yang-sheng.com/?p=8717.

Joybilee Farm. (2020, June 29). *Don't compost those black walnut hulls! Make a black walnut tincture instead.* Retrieved from https://joybileefarm.com/black-walnut-tincture/.

Knapp, J. (2017, January 6). *12 natural herbs for hypothyroidism treatment.* Hypothyroidism Natural Treatments. Retrieved from https://hypothyroidismnaturaltreatments.com/12-natural-herbs-for-hypothyroidism-treatment.

Orlander, P. R. (2021, June 26). *Hypothyroidism treatment & management.* MedScape. Retrieved from https://emedicine.medscape.com/article/122393-treatment.

Osansky, E. (2016, March 31). *7 spices most thyroid sufferers should consume.* Natural Endocrine Solutions. Retrieved from https://www.naturalendocrinesolutions.com/7-spices-most-thyroid-sufferers-should-consume/.

Pacific College of Health and Science. (2019, February 22). *Traditional Chinese medicine and thyroid disease.* Pacific College. Retrieved from https://www.pacificcollege.edu/news/press-releases/2015/05/14/traditional-chinese-medicine-and-thyroid-disease.

Purdue, P., & Kroner, A. (2020, June 17). *Treating thyroid disease with traditional Chinese medicine.* Verywell Health. Retrieved from https://www.verywellhealth.com/chinese-medicine-for-thyroid-disease-3231507.

Remedy Health Media. (2019, March 20). *Hypothyroidism: Overview, causes, and symptoms.* EndocrineWeb. Retrieved from https://www.endocrineweb.com/conditions/thyroid/hypothyroidism-too-little-thyroid-hormone-0.

Russo, A. T. (2018, May 3). *8 simple natural remedies for hypothyroidism.* Nutrition Key with Angela T Russo. Retrieved from https://nutritionkey.com/simple-natural-remedies-hypothyroidism/.

Shen Clinic. (n.d.). *Zuo Gui Wan | Extra Strength.* Shenclinic.Com. Retrieved from https://shenclinic.com/products/zuo-gui-pian-wan-active-herb-200-pills.

Wszelaki, M. (2020, October 5). *8 herbs for your thyroid (weight gain, fatigue, hair loss, dry skin).* Hormones & Balance. Retrieved from https://hormonesbalance.com/articles/8-herbs-thyroid-weight-gain-fatigue-hair-loss-dry-skin/.

Hyperthyroidism

Allayurveda. (2017, May 3). *Natural hyperthyroidism diet and treatments that work.* Retrieved from https://allayurveda.com/blog/natural-hyperthyroidism-diet-and-treatments-that-work/.

Chen, J. (2010a, January). *Treatment of hyperthyroidism: Western medicine vs. traditional Chinese medicine.* Elotus Update| Lotus Institute of Integrative Medicine. Retrieved from https://www.elotus.org/article/treatment-hyperthyroidism-western-medicine-vs-traditional-chinese-medicine.

Chen, J. (2010b, November 1). Treatment of hyperthyroidism. *Acupuncture Today, 11*(11). Retrieved from https://www.acupuncturetoday.com/mpacms/at/article.php?id=32299.

CureJoy Editorial. (2016, October 13). *8 Ayurvedic remedies for thyroid problems you should try.* CureJoy. Retrieved from https://curejoy.com/content/treat-thyroid-with-ayurvedic-therapy/.

Douillard, J. (2019, August 31). *Two Ayurvedic herbs for your thyroid: Ashwagandha + Guggul.* John Douillard's LifeSpa | Ayurveda and Natural Health. Retrieved from https://lifespa.com/two-ayurvedic-herbs-thyroid/.

Ferguson, S., & Wilson, D. R. (2019, June 10). *How to control hyperthyroidism naturally.* Healthline. Retrieved from https://www.healthline.com/health/hyperthyroidism-natural-treatment.

Health Benefits Times. (2019, July 3). *Agnimantha facts and health benefits.* Health Benefits. Retrieved from https://www.healthbenefitstimes.com/premna-integrifolia/.

Hebbar, J. V. (2011a, June 18). *Dasamoolarishtam uses, ingredients, dose, side effects, research.* AyurMedInfo. Retrieved from https://www.ayurmedinfo.com/2011/06/18/dasamoolarishtam-ingredients-uses-dose-and-side-effects/.

Hebbar, J. V. (2011b, August 31). *Saraswatarishta uses, dose, side effects and ingredients*. AyurMedInfo. Retrieved from https://www.ayurmedinfo.com/2011/08/31/saraswatarishta-uses-dose-side-effects-and-ingredients/.

Hebbar, J. V. (2012a, March 16). *Triphala Churna benefits, ingredients, dose, side effects, how to take*. AyurMedInfo. Retrieved from https://www.ayurmedinfo.com/2012/03/16/triphala-churna-benefits-ingredients-dose-side-effects-how-to-take/.

Hebbar, J. V. (2012b, May 14). *Chandrakala Ras benefits, dosage, side effects, ingredients*. AyurMedInfo. Retrieved from https://www.ayurmedinfo.com/2012/05/14/chandrakala-vati-benefits-dosage-side-effects-ingredients/.

Hebbar, J. V. (2012c, July 27). *Praval Panchamrit Ras—Benefits, dosage, ingredients, side effects*. AyurMedInfo. Retrieved from https://www.ayurmedinfo.com/2012/07/27/praval-panchamrit-ras-benefits-dosage-ingredients-side-effects/.

Jiva Ayurveda. (n.d.). *Ayurvedic medicine for thyroid*. Retrieved from https://www.jiva.com/diseases/endocrine/thyroid.

Milas, K. (2020, February 5). *Radioactive iodine for hyperthyroidism*. EndocrineWeb. Retrieved from https://www.endocrineweb.com/conditions/hyperthyroidism/radioactive-iodine-hyperthyroidism.

Nazario, B. (2021, January 18). *What are the treatments for hyperthyroidism?* WebMD. Retrieved from https://www.webmd.com/a-to-z-guides/treatments-hyperthyroidism.

Norman, J. (2021a, June 24). *Hyperthyroidism: Overactivity of the thyroid gland*. EndocrineWeb. Retrieved from https://www.endocrineweb.com/conditions/hyperthyroidism/hyperthyroidism-overactivity-thyroid-gland.

Norman, J. (2021b, June 24). *Hyperthyroidism: Overactivity of the thyroid gland*. EndocrineWeb. Retrieved from https://www.endocrineweb.com/conditions/hyperthyroidism/hyperthyroidism-overactivity-thyroid-gland.

Sharma, H. (2015, May 27). *Treat hyperthyroidism with Ayurveda*. Onlymyhealth. Retrieved from https://www.onlymyhealth.com/hyperthyroidism-treatment-in-ayurveda-1346757789.

Sharma, V. (2019, March 7). *Top homeopathic remedies for hyperthyroidism, and goitre*. Homeopathy at DrHomeo.Com. Retrieved from https://www.drhomeo.com/thyroid/homeopathic-remedies-for-hyperthyroidism-goitre-and-graves-disease/.

Sha Wellness Clinic. (2015, March 25). Dietary recommendations to hypothyroidism and hyperthyroidism. Retrieved from https://shawellnessclinic.com/en/shamagazine/dietary-recommendations-to-hypothyroidism-and-hyperthyroidism/.

Sheng-Nong Limited. (2006). *Hyperthyroidism: Causes*. Retrieved from http://www.shen-nong.com/eng/health/hyperthyroidism_causes.html.

Singh, J. (2015, December 14). *Kamdudha Ras*. Ayur Times. Retrieved from https://www.ayurtimes.com/kamdudha-ras/.

Surjushe, A., Vasani, R., & Saple, D. (2008). Aloe vera: A short review. *Indian Journal of Dermatology, 53*(4), 163–166. Retrieved from https://doi.org/10.4103/0019-5154.44785.

Tulane University School of Medicine. (2013, August 30). *Antithyroid drugs*. Tmedweb.Tulane. Retrieved from https://tmedweb.tulane.edu/pharmwiki/doku.php/antithyroid_drugs.

Walfish, B. (2021, July 12). *What is hyperthyroidism?* EndocrineWeb. Retrieved from https://www.endocrineweb.com/conditions/hyperthyroidism/hyperthyroidism-overview-overactive-thyroid.

Poor Appetite

Bhat, V. (2015, February 16). *7 Miraculous herbs for faster weight gain*. Onlymyhealth. Retrieved from https://www.onlymyhealth.com/health-slideshow/7-miraculous-herbs-for-faster-weight-gain-1424082030.html.

Boldsky Admin. (2016, June 20). *5 Ayurvedic remedies to increase appetite*. Boldsky. Retrieved from https://www.boldsky.com/health/wellness/2016/five-ayurvedic-remedies-tp-increase-appetite-102594.html.

Clossen, A. (2015, April 2). *Acupuncture and herbs for weight management*. Vitality Magazine. Retrieved from https://vitalitymagazine.com/article/acupuncture-and-herbs-for-weight-management/.

Contursi, J. (n.d.). *Herbs that increase appetite*. LiveStrong.com. Retrieved from https://www.livestrong.com/article/388436-herbs-that-increase-appetite/.

Dix, M., & Falck, S. (2018, September 29). *Supplements, medications, and lifestyle changes to help stimulate appetite*. Healthline. Retrieved from https://www.healthline.com/health/appetite-stimulant.

Foster, S. (1997, October 1). *Herbs for health: Bitter herbs for appetite and indigestion*. Motherearthliving.Com. Retrieved from https://content.motherearthliving.com/health-and-wellness/herbs-for-health-an-appetite-for-herbs/.

Karkala, P., & Kramer, A. (2021, January 29). *Natural appetite stimulant: Home remedies, exercises, and medicines*. Style Craze. Retrieved from https://www.stylecraze.com/articles/simple-home-remedies-to-improve-appetite/#gref.

Morrow, A., & Lacy, J. (2020, October 11). *8 ways to treat a loved one's loss of appetite*. Verywell Health. Retrieved from https://www.verywellhealth.com/how-to-whet-an-appetite-1132085.

Semeco, A. (2017, September 18). *16 ways to increase your appetite*. Healthline. Retrieved from https://www.healthline.com/nutrition/16-ways-to-increase-appetite.

Sharma, V. (2019, February 28). *Homeopathic treatment for loss of appetite*. Homeopathy at DrHomeo.com. Retrieved from https://www.drhomeo.com/homeopathic-treatment/homeopathic-treatment-loss-appetite/.

Sissons, B., & Biggers, A. (2018, December 17). *What causes a loss of appetite?* Medical News Today. Retrieved from https://www.medicalnewstoday.com/articles/324011.

Streit, L. (2021, April 7). *8 surprising benefits of Cherimoya (custard apple)*. Healthline. Retrieved from https://www.healthline.com/nutrition/cherimoya#TOC_TITLE_HDR_8.

6
Reproductive System

Introduction

Some of the reproductive problems discussed are:
1. Heavy periods (menorrhagia)
2. Period cramps (dysmenorrhea)
3. Irregular periods
4. Endometriosis
5. Polycystic ovarian syndrome (PCOS)
6. Fibroids
7. Vaginal discharge
8. Infertility

Heavy Periods (Menorrhagia)

Heavy periods can be caused by a variety of disorders such as structural abnormalities in the reproductive tract, bleeding disorders, or hormonal imbalances. Heavy periods are defined as excessive uterine bleeding (i.e., a total menstrual flow of >80 mL per cycle or soaking through a normal pad or tampon every 2 hours or less or uterine bleeding lasting longer than 7 days).

It is often the loss or reduction of normal daily activities that is more debilitating to women than the actual volume of blood loss. It can be caused by uterine fibroids, endometriosis, hormonal imbalance with high or low estrogen, medications, uterine cancer, and medical conditions like hypothyroidism, and kidney and liver disorders.

Menorrhagia (heavy periods) are often associated with dysmenorrhea (painful periods) and there is an overlap in the traditional remedies described below.

General principles

- Use a period tracker app to monitor onset, duration and frequency of periods, amount of menstrual flow and pain level.
- A menstrual cup is preferred to a pad or a tampon.
- Eat more iron-rich foods and take iron supplements or health tonics. Consume more fluids to stay normovolemic.
- Carry a kit with extra pads, underwear, disposable bags, and some painkillers in case of unexpected heavy or painful flow.
- Heavy flow beyond 7 days should be assessed.

Indian Natural Remedies

"Asrigdara" means excessive blood flow (menorrhagia) in Sanskrit.

The specific signs and symptoms of asrigdara (menorrhagia) is classified into four groups:

Pittaja asrigdara: reddish-black and warm bleeding

Vataja asrigdara: frothy and painful bleeding

Kaphaja asrigdara: thick, slimy, and pale bleeding

Sannipataja asrigdara: mixed signs and symptoms with associated fever and fainting

Specific and different treatments are available for each type of asrigdara.

In a *pitta-prakriti* female, there are heavy periods and swollen breasts.

In a *kapha-prakriti* female, there are heavy periods with clots.

Common Recipes

Oral

Teas/Brews/Others

Aloe vera. Consume aloe vera juice.

Amla juice. Lightly pound three to four amla fruits and strain the juice. Take this juice on an empty stomach in the morning with a glass of warm water.

Asafetida. Fry a pinch of asafetida with some ghee. Add some goat milk and honey. Consume daily for 1 month.

Ashoka bark paste. Take 25 g of ashoka bark powder and add 200 mL of water. Boil slowly until the water has reduced to about 50 mL. Add 50 mL of milk and continue to boil until only 50 mL of liquid is left. Strain and cool. Consume 20 to 30 mL in the morning.

Variation #1. Take some ashoka tree bark and add about 200 mL of water. Boil and reduce to ¼ volume. Consume 40 to 50 mL twice a day.

Banana flower-curd. Take ¼ to ½ cup chopped banana flower. Add little water, salt, and turmeric. Boil until soft. When cooled, add ½ teaspoon roasted cumin seed powder, some chopped green chili, and 1 to 2 tablespoons grated coconut. Add ½ to 1 cup thick yogurt. Mix well. Consume in the morning or with rice.

Variation #1. Banana flowers can be stir-fried with some turmeric powder, cumin seeds, salt, and peppercorn.

TABLE 6.1 Common Ingredients for Heavy Periods

Spices	Herbs/Leaves	Miscellaneous
Asafetida	Arugumpul/Durva (Cynodon dactylon)	Banana flower
	Pavonia odorata (udeechya)	Curd
	Indian sarsaparilla/ sariva (Hemidesmus indicus)	Mango bark
	Holy basil (thulasi/ tulsi)	Niranjan Phal (Sterculia lychnophora)
	Licorice	Guava flower
		Aloe vera
		Radish
Cinnamon	Tribulus terrestris (gokshura)	Raisins (Vitis Vinifera)
Coriander	Nelumbo nucifera (lotus stamen)	Saraca asoca (ashoka tree bark)
Crocus sativus (saffron)	Woodfordia fruticosa (dhataki)	Wrightia antidysenterica/kutaja
Fennel seed	Asparagus racemosus (shatavari)	Honey
Ginger	Bala (Sida cordifolia)	Sugar candy
Mustard seed	Mesua ferrea (nagakesara)	Rice water
Phyllanthus emblica (amla)	Vetiveria zizanioides (ushira)	Salmalia malabarica (mocharasa/gum of the silk cotton tree)
Tamarind	Mimosa pudica (lajjalu/shameplant)	Santalum album (Sandalwood)
Turmeric	Lodhra (Symplocos racemosa)	Bitter gourd

Variation #2. To make banana flower dosai or adai, take 1 cup of rice, ¼ cup of toor dhal (yellow split pea), 2 tablespoons of black dal (urad), 1 tablespoon of chickpeas (chana dal) and 1 tablespoon of green/mung bean (moong dal). Soak overnight. Blend with some grated coconut, 2 red chili, 1 teaspoon of cumin seeds, a little asafetida and 1 cup chopped boiled banana flower. Take 2 scoops and make the pancake on a skillet.

Bitter gourd juice. Remove the seeds from a fresh bitter gourd and cut into smaller chunks. Place in a blender and blend until smooth, gradually adding up to ¼ cup of water. Strain and drink. Bitter gourd is thought to aid with blood clotting, hence reducing heavy menstruation.

Cinnamon tea. Add 1 teaspoon of ground cinnamon to a cup of hot water and mix well. Add honey and drink one to two times a day.

Variation #1. Lightly pound one cinnamon stick and add to a cup. Pour boiling water over the cinnamon and steep for 15 minutes. Add honey to taste.

Coriander paste. Grind 2 teaspoons of coriander seeds into a fine powder. Mix with ¼ cup yogurt and consume twice a day.

Variation #1. Take 1 teaspoon of coriander seeds. Boil in 1 cup of water. Add ½ teaspoon of cinnamon. Reduce to half volume. Add 1 strand of saffron and 1 teaspoon of honey. Consume.

Variation #2. Take 2 tablespoons of coriander seeds. Add 200 mL or 1 cup water. Boil until reduced to half volume. Consume three to four times per day.

Variation #3. Take 2 tablespoons of coriander seeds and one stick of cinnamon. Add 200 mL or 1 cup water. Boil until reduced to half volume. Strain, add some honey, and consume the brew twice a day.

Dhataki brew. Take 1 teaspoon of dried flowers. Mix with some water. Consume twice a day after meals.

Fennel seed drink. Place a handful of fennel seeds in half a cup of warm water. Allow to soak overnight. Drink the water and the seeds in the morning on an empty stomach.

Variation #1. Take 1 teaspoon of ground fennel seed powder. Add 1 cup of boiling water. Steep for 10 minutes. Consume warm.

Guava flower. Take 1 g of the dried flower powder. Mix with some honey and consume three times a day.

Variation #1. To make the tea, take a handful of guava leaves. Add 100 mL of water. Boil until the volume is reduced to 25 mL. Consume twice a day.

Indian sarsaparilla (Sariva) tea. Add ½ to 1 teaspoons of the root powder into a cup of hot water. Cover and steep for 5 to 10 minutes. Strain and drink twice a day.

Kutaja. Take ¼ to ½ teaspoon of dried seed powder and mix with water (or ghee). Consume after a light meal.

Lajjalu paste. Crush the whole lajjalu plant to make a paste. Mix with rice water and drink.

Variation #1. Crush the whole lajjalu plant to make a paste. Mix with fresh juice of durva.

Licorice. Take one licorice root (or 1 tablespoon of licorice root slices or 1 teaspoon of dried powder). Add 1 cup boiling water. Steep for 5 to 10 minutes. Strain and consume three times per day for 5 days.

Lodhra brew. Place 3 g of lodhra bark powder into 100 mL of hot water and mix well. Drink once a day.

Lotus stamen paste. Pound three to six white lotus stamen and mix with rice water and sugar candy to make a paste. Consume one to two times a day.

Mango bark brew. Mix 10 mL of mango bark extract into a cup of hot water. Take 1 tablespoon of this mixture every hour for 3 to 4 days.

Mocharasa. Consume mocharasa as a part of the polyherbal formula i.e., pushyanug churna.

Mustard paste. Crush 2 teaspoons of mustard seeds into a fine powder. Mix with ¼ cup of yogurt and take twice a day.

Variation #1. Take ½ teaspoon of ground mustard powder and add to 1 cup of warm milk (or water). Consume twice a day.

Nagkesar. Take ¼ to ½ teaspoon of nagkesar powder. Mix with some honey or lukewarm water. Consume one to two times a day.

Niranjan phal. Soak the fruits overnight in a cup of water until it swells. Crush and squeeze the pulp into the water. Consume on an empty stomach in the morning. Add honey or sugar if desired.

Variation #1. Take 1 to 2 nuts. Add 1 cup of boiling water. Allow to steep and consume.

Radish. Take 1 small fresh radish. Blend with little water. Add 1 cup of yogurt. Consume daily.

Saffron paste. Break a strand of saffron into smaller pieces and mix with 1 teaspoon of honey to make a paste. Take one to two times a day.

Shatavari brew. Slightly warm 120 mL of milk in a pot. Meanwhile, add 1 teaspoon of ground shatavari to a pot along with ⅛ teaspoon of cinnamon powder and a pinch of ginger powder. Pour a little milk over the powder and mix to form a paste. Slowly add the remaining milk, stirring well until no lumps remain. Add honey to taste and drink.

Tamarind brew. Place two to three seedless tamarind into a pot with a cup of water. Boil for 15 minutes. Drink warm or cool with added honey.

Variation #1. Take about 10 pieces of tamarind and 5 dried plums. Add 500 mL water. Soak overnight. Blend in the morning. Add 2 to 3 tablespoons of honey. Refrigerate and consume daily for 5 days.

Tulsi tea. Place five to seven fresh tulsi leaves in a pot with a cup of water. Boil for about 15 minutes and then remove from the heat. Allow it to steep for about 5 minutes. Drink before bedtime every day.

Turmeric tea. Add 1 to 2 teaspoons of ground turmeric to 1 cup of hot water. Mix well and add honey to taste. Drink one to two times a day. Alternatively, lightly pound 2 to 3 inches of fresh turmeric and add to a cup of boiling water. Allow it to steep for 5 to 10 minutes and strain. Add honey to taste.

Udeechya (hrivera). Add hrivera together with sandalwood and rock sugar. Consume it with rice water.

Therapeutic Measures

Diet

Eat pitta, kapha-, and vata-pacifying foods.

Consume amla, ghee, honey, wheat products, dates, and pomegranate.

Avoid sour and salty foods, as well as fish, alcohol, spicy foods, horse gram, garlic, and black gram.

Include vegetables such as ash gourd, snake gourd, and bitter gourd.

Bitter gourd dish: Cut the bitter gourd into small, thin slices. Add a small amount of oil and salt to a frying pan. Place the bitter gourd in the pan and add onions. Fry for 10 to 15 minutes and eat.

Lifestyle

Yoga asanas, which can help reduce heavy periods and cramps, include:

Baddha konasana (Butterfly pose), *Kumbhakasana* (plank pose), *Paschimottanasana* (seated forward bend), *Uttanasana* (standing forward bend), and *Ardha Chandrasana* (half moon pose).

Chinese Natural Remedies

TABLE 6.2 Common Ingredients for Heavy Periods

Herbs/Leaves	Miscellaneous
Baikal skullcap/Huang Qin (*Scutellaria baicalensis*)	Cattail pollen/Pu Huang (*Typha angustifolia*)
Bamboo leaf tea	
Bugbane rhizome	
Caulis sargentodoxae (da xue tang)	
Charred garden burnet root	
Charred India madder rhizome	Semen coicis (yi ren)
Chinese motherwort (*Leonurus japonicus*)	Glossy privet fruit
Colla corii asini (e jiao)	Os draconis (long gu)
Concha ostreae (mu li)	Fructus lycii (gou qi chi)
Cortex moutan (mu dan pi)	Sesame seed
Eucommia bark/du zhong (*Eucommia ulmoides*)	
Folium artemisia argyi (ai ye)	

Continued

TABLE 6.2	Common Ingredients for Heavy Periods—cont'd	
Herbs/Leaves	**Miscellaneous**
Heal-all spike/xia ku cao *(Spica prunellae)*	
Herba agrimoniae (xian he cao)	
Herba ciresi japonici (da ji)	
Herba cirsii (xiao ji)	
Herba epimedii (epimedium/xian ling pi)	
Nelumbo nucifera (lotus stamen	
Nodus nelumbinis rhizomatis (ou jie)	Rhizoma dioscoreae (chinese yam/shan yao)
Patriniae herba (bai jiang cao)	
Petiolus trachycarpa (zong lu tan)	Fructus corni (shan yu rou))
Phellodendron/huang bo *(Cortex phellodendri)*	
Radix angelicae sinensis (dang gui)	Colla cornus cervi (Lu Jiao Jiao)
Radix astragali (Astragalus roo/huang qi)	
Radix astragali (huang qi)	
Radix codonopsis pilosulae (dang shen)	
Radix glycyrrhizae (gan cao)	Dodder seeds/tu si zi *(Cuscuta chinensis Lam)*
Radix morindae officinalis (morinda root/ba ji tian)	
Radix notoginseng (san chi)	Plastrum testudinis (zhi gui jia)
Radix rehmanniae (rehmannia root)	Carbonized hair
Radix salvia miltiorrhizae (dan shen)	Licorice
Radix sanguisorbae (di yu)	Os sepiae (hai piao xiao)
Resina commiphora myrrha (mo yao)	Jujube leaf and fruit
Rhizoma atractylodis (cang zhu)	
Rhizoma atractylodis macrocephalae (bai shu)	
Rhizoma cyperi (xiang fu)	
Rhizoma ligustici chuanxiong (chuan xiong)	Fructus gardeniae (zhi zi)
Rhizoma rehmanniae preparata (shu di)	
Rhizoma zingiberis preparata (pao jiang)	
Wolfberry root bark/Di Gu Pi *(Lycii cortex)*	Feces trogopterori (wu ling zhi)/ Flying squirrel feces

Common Recipes

Oral (Polyherbs)

- Decoction for "Heat in the Uterus"
  - Modified "Clear Heat and Consolidate Menstruation Decoction": Cattail pollen, carbonized hair, motherwort herb, huang qin, zhi zi, sheng di, di gu pi, di yu, e jiao, ou jie, zong lu tan, zhi gui jia, mu li, gan cao.
- Decoction for "Stasis in the Uterus"
  - Modified "Revolve Stasis and Stop Menorrhagia Decoction": Cattail pollen, charred Indian madder rhizome, dang gui, chuan xiong, san chi, mo yao, wu ling zhi, mu dan pi, dan shen, ai ye, e jiao, hai piao xiao, long gu, mu li.
- Decoction for "Damp-Heat in the Uterus"
  - Modified "Three Wonders Sargent glory Vine-Stem Decoction": Huang bo, cant zhu, yi yi ren, da xue tang, bai jiang cao, da ji, xiao ji, xian he cao, motherwort herb, xia ku cao, xiang fu.
- Decoction for "Qi Deficiency Failing to Retain Blood"
  - Modified "Consolidation and Stop Menorrhagia Decoction": Chinese yam, bugbane rhizome, charred

Indian madder rhizome, shu di, bai shu, dang shen, dang gui, huang qi, pao jiang.
- Decoction for "Kidney Yin Deficiency"
  - Modified "Restore the Left Kidney Decoction": Glossy privet fruit, charred garden burnet root, shu di, shan yao, shan yu rou, gou qi chi, tu si zi, lu jiao jiao, gui jia.
- Decoction for "Kidney Yang Deficiency"
  - Modified "Restore the Right Kidney Decoction": Astragalus root, morinda root, epimedium, shu di, shan yao, shan yu rou, gou qi chi, lu jiao jiao, tu is zi, du zhong, dang gui.

Bamboo leaf tea. Take 1 to 2 teaspoons of dried bamboo leaves (or 1 to 2 tea bags). Add 1 cup of boiling water. Allow to steep for 5 to 10 minutes. Strain, add honey to taste, and consume twice a day. (To make the dried leaves, collect some fresh green bamboo leaves from the stem. Air-dry them in a cool dry place for 5 to 7 days, then crush and store them in an airtight container).
  Variation #1. A cold infusion can be made by soaking the leaves overnight.

Dodder seeds. They are available in the form of supplements (including powder, tablets, or capsules) and can be taken alongside food and other vitamins.

Eucommia bark decoction. Take 10 to 15 g of eucommia bark. Add water and boil.

Jujube tea. Add 15 g of fresh jujube leaves and a spoonful of red dates to a cup of boiling water. Steep for 10 to 15 minutes before straining. Drink daily during the menses or 8 to 10 times a month, particularly during the menstrual cycle.

Licorice brew. Peel some licorice root and grind into a fine powder. Add 4 g of the powder to a cup of hot water and mix well. Drink once a day for 5 days.

Sesame seed brew. Grind 3 teaspoons of white sesame seeds into a fine powder and mix into one cup of hot water. Drink twice a day.

Lotus tea. Take 2 teaspoons of dried lotus flowers (petals and stamen) with 2 cups of hot water. Steep for 5 minutes. Add ½ teaspoon of fresh lotus seeds if desired. Drink thrice a day.

Notes
- **Heat in the Uterus**
  - This condition presents as sudden heavy vaginal bleeding (or persistent spotting). The blood is dark red and thick. Symptoms include a dry mouth, flushed face, dizziness, irritability, and scanty urine. The pulse will be taut and rapid.
  - The principles of the remedy used are to clear the body heat, cool the blood, consolidate the thoroughfare vessel, and stop the menstrual bleeding.
- **Stasis in the Uterus**
  - This condition presents as irregular periods, persistent spotting, or missed periods followed by sudden exaggerated menstruation. The blood is often dark purplish and has clots. The lower abdomen usually feels tender until the blood clots have been passed.

- The principles of the remedy used are to activate the blood, resolve stasis, consolidate the thoroughfare vessel, and stop or reduce menstrual bleeding.
- **Damp-Heat in the Uterus**
  - This condition presents as irregular periods, persistent spotting, or sudden profuse vaginal bleeding. The blood is often dark red or purplish red and is thick and sticky. Foul, excessive vaginal discharge may also be present, as well as abdominal pain and distension. There may be a feeling of general tiredness and fever.
  - The principles of the remedy are to clear the body's heat, resolve dampness, and reduce or stop the vaginal bleeding.
- **Qi Deficiency Failing to Retain Blood**
  - This condition presents as irregular periods that start off heavily then reduces to persistent spotting. The blood may be light in color and thin. The patient may be pale, fatigued, weak, short of breath, and have palpitations.
  - The principles of the remedy used are to replenish the body's qi, invigorate the spleen, and nourish the blood.
- **Kidney Yin Deficiency**
  - This condition presents as irregular periods, excessive vaginal bleeding, and persistent spotting. The blood is bright red and thick. Other symptoms include general weakness, fatigue, dizziness, sweaty palms and soles of the feet, irritability, weakness, and insomnia.
  - The principles of the remedy used are to nourish the kidney yin, consolidate the thoroughfare vessel, and reduce or stop menstrual bleeding.
- **Kidney Yang Deficiency**
  - This condition presents as irregular periods, excessive vaginal bleeding, and persistent spotting. The blood is thin. Other symptoms include limb coldness, frequent and excessive urination, and loose bowels.
  - The remedy aims to warm and invigorate the kidney yang.
- In general, treatment should be given continuously for three to four menstrual cycles to regulate the menstrual cycle.
- The sensei will evaluate each patient individually, often depending on a range of factors such as age group (adolescent girls, childbearing-aged women, and premenopausal women). The prescriptions and dosages of each medication will be modified accordingly.

Western/Other Natural Remedies

Common Recipes
Oral
Teas/Brews
Aloe vera juice. Slit an aloe vera leaf down the center. Scrape out the white gel, discarding any of the yellow gel. Cut into smaller pieces and blend until smooth. Add three teaspoons of the blended gel into a cup of hot water and mix well. Add honey to taste and drink twice a day in the morning and before bed.

TABLE 6.3	Common Ingredients for Heavy Periods	
Spices	**Herbs/Leaves**	**Miscellaneous**
Cayenne pepper	Raspberry leaf	Apple cider vinegar
	Sage	Black haw (*Viburnum prunifolium*
	Symphytum (comfrey leaf)	Blackstrap molasses
	Achillea millefolium (yarrow leaf)	Honey
	Thyme leaf	Hawthorn flower
	Rose hip (*Rosa canina L.*)	Marigold flower
	Jojoba leaf	Aloe vera
	Wood apple leaf (*Limonia acidissima*)	Flaxseed
	False unicorn (*Chamaelirium luteum*)	
	Geranium/Cranesbill	
	Fleabane	
	Chamomile	
Cinnamon	Capsella bursa-pastoris (shepherd's purse leaf)	Black cohosh (*Cimicifuga racemosa*)
Ginger	Alchemilla (lady's mantle leaf)	Chasteberry or chaste tree (*Vitex agnus-castus*)

Apple cider vinegar. Mix 1 tablespoon of apple cider vinegar in 1 cup of water. Drink once a day throughout menstruation.

Black cohosh. Add ½ to 1 teaspoon of dried black cohosh root to a pot with 1 cup of water. Boil and then simmer for about 15 minutes. Remove from the heat and steep for about 5 minutes. Strain and drink twice a day.

Black haw. Add 1 teaspoon of black haw into 1 cup of boiling water. Steep for 5 minutes. Strain and drink three times a day.

Blackstrap molasses. Add 1 to 2 teaspoons of blackstrap molasses to a cup of hot water. Mix well and drink once a day.

Cayenne pepper tea. Add a pinch of cayenne pepper to a cup of hot water and mix well. Add honey to taste. Drink twice a day during menstruation.

Chamomile. Take a few fresh chamomile leaves. Add 1 cup of boiling water.

Chasteberry tea. Take 1 teaspoon of dried chasteberry or three to six crushed berries. Steep in hot water for about 10 minutes. Consume one to two times daily for a few weeks. Capsules or tinctures are also available.

Cinnamon tea. Add 1 to 2 teaspoons of ground cinnamon to a pot with 1 cup of water. Boil for about 20 minutes. Add honey to taste. Drink before bedtime.

Comfrey leaf tea. Add a handful of comfrey leaves to a pot with a cup of water and bring to a boil. Steep for 5 to 10 minutes, strain, and consume.

Feverfew tea. Place 1 tablespoon of fresh or dried feverfew leaves in a cup. Pour 1 cup of boiling water over the herbs and let steep for 30 to 60 minutes. Strain and drink warm.

Fleabane tea. Make a decoction from the dried leaves and flowers. Consume 2 to 4 ounces up to four times a day.

Variation #1. Take 10 to 30 drops of the fresh whole plant extract. Add other herbs (½ teaspoon calendula flower, ½ teaspoon yerba mansa, and 1 teaspoon marshmallow root). Add 1 cup of boiling water. Steep, strain, and drink.

Geranium tea. Take 25 g of the flower buds or 50 g of the dried plant. Add 1 L of boiling water. Allow to steep for 20 minutes. Consume 3 to 4 cups per day.

Variation #1. Take 1 to 2 teaspoons of the dried cranesbill root. Add 1 cup of water. Boil and simmer for 15 minutes. Strain and consume.

Ginger tea. Add 1 to 2 teaspoons of ginger powder to a pot with a cup of hot water. Allow it to simmer for 5 minutes. Drink twice a day after meals.

Jojoba tea. Place a handful of jojoba leaves into a pot with a cup of hot water and simmer for about 15 to 20 minutes. Strain and drink once a day.

Lady's mantle tea. Take 5 to 10 g lady's mantle and add into 1 L of boiling water. Allow it to steep for 10 to 15 minutes. Drink 1 cup every day a week before menstruation.

Marigold tea. Add four to six marigold flowers to a pot with 1 cup of hot water. Simmer gently for about 30 minutes. Strain and drink 120 mL in the 3 days before menstruation and during the first 2 days of menstruation.

Raspberry leaf tea. Place 1 teaspoon of dried raspberry leaves into a cup of boiling water. Steep for 5 to 10 minutes and strain. Add honey and drink one to two times a day.

Rose hip tea. Place four to eight dried rose hips in 1 cup of water. Steep for 10 to 15 minutes. Drain and drink. Take 3 cups of rose hip tea every day.

Sage tea. Place 2 tablespoons of fresh sage leaves in a cup of boiling water. Allow it to steep for 5 to 10 minutes and strain. Drink twice a day.

Shepherd's purse tea. Take 3 to 4 teaspoons of dried shepherd's purse into boiling water and allow it to steep for 10 minutes. Strain and add honey to taste. Drink 1 to 3 cups a day.

Thyme tea. Add 3 teaspoons of dried thyme or 2 tablespoons of fresh thyme leaves to a cup of boiling water. Steep for 5 to 10 minutes, strain, and consume.

Wood apple leaf tea. Take fresh wood apple leaves into a cup of boiling water and steep for 15 minutes. Drink two times a day. Alternatively, consume wood apple fruit to reduce menstrual blood flow.

Yarrow tea. Place some yarrow leaves into a cup of boiling water. Steep until the water changes color. Add honey to taste and drink 1 cup every day. Yarrow is thought to work by constricting the blood vessels.

Therapeutic Measures

Lifestyle

- **Cold compress:** Wrap some ice cubes in a clean cloth and place on the lower abdomen for 20 minutes. Refrigerated cold packs can also be used. Repeat every 2 hours. The cold causes vessel constriction hence reducing blood flow.
- **Diet:** Eat more omega-3-rich foods (like cold oily fish, flaxseeds, walnuts, almonds, and olive oil).

Modern Remedies

Choice of management would depend on the patient's reproductive wishes and contraceptive needs. Hence the following medical management is divided as follows:

Contraceptive Effect

Combined oral contraceptive pills—The combined oral contraceptive (COCP) consists of estrogen and progestogen and is generally given for 3 weeks. This is followed by a pill-free week in which the woman experiences a hormone withdrawal bleeding. With this COCP, there is about a 50% reduction in blood loss, and there is the additional benefit of regulation of bleeding. The COCP can be *tri-cycled*—three packets can be taken consecutively without the pill-free weeks. The menstrual frequency and blood loss volume are reduced. Hence it is a preferred option for many women.

Levonorgestrel (Mirena)—This popular intrauterine system (IUS) contains an androgenic progestogen, levonorgestrel (LNG). LNG is slowly released from the IUS to act on the local endometrial environment, preventing proliferation and inducing an atrophic endometrium.

Oral Progesterone—Oral progesterone (such as norethisterone, a man-made progestin) functions as an anti-estrogen by minimizing the effects of estrogen on the target cells. This causes the endometrium of the uterus to remain thin and reduce blood flow during menstruation.

Injectable Progesterone—Medroxyprogesterone injection is given every 12 weeks.

No Contraceptive Effect

Non-Steroidal Anti-Inflammatory Drugs (NSAIDs)—NSAIDs exert their anti-inflammatory effect through inhibition of cyclooxygenase, which is the enzyme that catalyzes the transformation of arachidonic acid to prostaglandins and thromboxane. Hence, this will reduce tissue damage during menstruation and stop the prolonged menstrual bleeding.
Example: Mefenamic acid

Tranexamic Acid—Tranexamic acid treats menorrhagia by inhibiting the activation of plasminogen to plasmin. This reduces blood clotting. It prevents fibrinolysis and blood-clot breakdown by inhibiting the endometrial plasminogen activator. It also stops the small blood vessels in the uterus lining from bleeding.

Surgical Techniques

- Hysteroscopic endometrial ablation
  - Rollerball ablation
  - Transcervical endometrial resection
  - Laser diathermy
- Non-hysteroscopic endometrial ablation
  - Cryoablation therapy
  - Radiofrequency probe
  - Bipolar electrodes (Novasure system)
  - Thermal balloon therapy (Thermachoice)
- Myomectomy. This is done to remove some fibroids.
- Uterine artery embolization. This is a minimally invasive procedure done to reduce blood flow to the fibroid for about 6 months.
- Hysterectomy

Homeopathic Remedies

These include *Crocus sativus, Ferrum metallicum, belladonna, phosphorus, cyclamen, millefolium, Crotalus horridus, erigeron, Calcarea carbonica, lycopodium, Lachesis, Natrum muriaticum,* and others.

Period Cramps (Dysmenorrhea)

Period cramps are defined as pain in the lower abdomen immediately before or during menstruation. The pain may range from mild to severe. During menstruation, prostaglandins involved in pain and inflammation trigger uterine muscle contractions, leading to period cramps. Hence, higher prostaglandin levels cause more severe period cramps. Period cramps may also be caused by many problems such as endometriosis or fibroids, both of which will also be discussed.

TABLE 6.4	Common Ingredients for Period Cramps	
Spices	**Herbs/Leaves**	**Miscellaneous**
Cardamom		Unripe papaya
Cinnamon	Punarnava	Sesame oil
Cumin seed		Honey
Fenugreek	Aloe vera	Hot compress
Garlic		Ghee
Ginger	*Asparagus racemosus* (shatavari)	Lemon
Nutmeg		Ashok tree bark
Piper nigrum (black peppercorn)	Lady's mantle	Milk
Saffron		Hibiscus petal
Turmeric		Rose petal

Indian Natural Remedies

Common Recipes

Oral

Teas/Brews

Aloe vera. Consume as fresh juice (see below under Western natural remedies).

Ashoka bark paste. Place 25 g of ashoka bark powder into a pot with 200 mL of water. Boil slowly until the water has reduced to about 50 mL. Add 50 mL of milk and continue to boil until only 50 mL of liquid is left. Strain and cool. Take 20 to 30 mL in the morning to reduce menstrual blood flow.

> Variation #1. Take some ashoka tree bark and add about 200 mL of water. Boil and reduce to ¼ volume. Consume 40 to 50 mL twice a day.

Cumin tea. Grind cumin seeds into a fine powder and add 2 to 3 tablespoons of the crushed seeds to a cup of boiling water. Allow it to steep for 10 to 15 minutes and drink.

Fenugreek brew. Soak a handful of fenugreek seeds in warm water overnight. Drink and consume the amber water with the swelled seeds in the morning on an empty stomach.

Garlic-turmeric milk. Lightly crush three cloves of garlic and place in a pot with 1 cup of milk. Bring to a boil and then add ¼ teaspoon of turmeric powder. Constantly stirring the milk, continue to boil until the garlic softens. Remove from the heat. Add a pinch of black pepper powder and honey to taste. Drink and eat the garlic cloves.

Ginger and black pepper tea. Lightly pound 2 to 3 inches of fresh ginger and place into a teapot. Add 5 to 10 pieces of black peppercorn and pour boiling water into the teapot. Steep for 10 to 15 minutes and strain. Drink one to two times a day.

Hibiscus tea. Place a handful of dried or fresh hibiscus petals into a teapot with a cup of boiling water. Steep for 10 to 15 minutes and strain. Add a pinch of cinnamon and honey to taste.

Lady's mantle tea. Take 5 to 10 g of lady's mantle and add into 1 L of boiling water. Allow it to steep for 10 to 15 minutes.

Lemon water. Mix the juice of half a lemon into a cup of water. Drink in the morning on an empty stomach.

Punarnava paste. Grind punarnarva into a fine powder and mix with 1 teaspoon of honey to make a paste.

Rose petals. Place a handful of dried or fresh rose petals into a teapot with a cup of boiling water. Steep for 10 to 15 minutes and strain. Add a pinch of cinnamon and honey to taste.

> Variation #1. **Rose petal jam**. Take 2 cups of fresh, clean rose petals. Place in a pot with 1 cup of water and simmer for 10 minutes. Add a cup of cane sugar, ½ cup of lemon juice, and some grated lemon rind. Stir until it forms a gel-like consistency.

Shatavari kalpa. Roast about 28 g of shatavari with 1 to 2 tablespoons of ghee until light brown. Add two strands of saffron and a pinch of cardamom powder. Eat it.

Spice milk. Turmeric has anti-inflammatory properties while nutmeg has been found to be an antispasmodic. Add a teaspoon of each spice to a cup of warm milk. Mix well and drink at bedtime.

Unripe papaya. This can be consumed as a salad.

Therapeutic Measures

Ginger-soda bath. Add ⅓ cup of ground dried ginger and ⅓ cup of baking soda to a bathtub filled with hot water. Soak in the bathtub and get out when you begin to sweat. Sit in a warm bathroom until you begin to cool down before drying off and getting dressed.

Hot compress. Place a hot water bottle or hot pack on the lower abdomen. Heat relaxes the uterine muscles and reduces period cramps.

Chinese Natural Remedies

Common Recipes

Oral

Teas/Brews

Cinnamon tea. Lightly crush one stick of cinnamon and add to a cup. Pour 1 cup of boiling water over the cinnamon and allow it to steep for 10 to 15 minutes. Drink it warm.

Dang Gui tea. Add 1 to 2 teaspoons of dried dang gai to a cup of hot water. Steep for 5 to 10 minutes and strain. Drink hot. Dang gai is thought to *harmonize* the blood and have antispasmodic properties. It has also been found to contain coumarin, a chemical that dilates blood vessels and relaxes the uterine muscles, relieving menstrual cramping.

Fennel tea. Place 1 teaspoon of dried fennel seeds into a cup. Pour boiling water over the seeds and allow it to

TABLE 6.5	Common Ingredients for Period Cramps	
Spices	**Herbs/Leaves**	**Miscellaneous**
Cinnamon	Red peony root	Longan (Dimocarpus longan)
	Angelica sinensis (Chinese angelica root/dang gui)	Fennel fruit
	Fennel	Peach seed
	Chinese motherwort/yi mu cao (Leonurus japonicus)	Safflower
	Millettia/ji xue teng (Spatholobus suberectus)	Brown sugar
	Szechuan lovage roots/chuan xiong (Ligusticum chuanxiong)	Corydalis/yan hu suo (Corydalis yanhusuo)
Ginger	Licorice root	Red date

steep for about 10 minutes. Drink hot one to two times a day in the week prior to and during your period.

Ge Xia Zhu Yu Tang. It is a 12-polyherb formula containing yan hu suo (corydalis), chuan xiong (Szechuan lovage roots), tao ren (peach seeds), hong hua (safflowers), wu ling zhi (flying squirrel feces), chi shao (red peony roots), dang gui (female ginseng), zhi ke (bitter oranges), wu yao (lindera roots), xiang fu (coco-grass rhizome), gan cao (licorice), and mu dan pi (moutan peony bark).

Ginger, red date, and longan tea. Add two to three slices of ginger, three red dates, and two dried longan fruits to a pot with 1 cup of hot water. Bring to a boil and then reduce the heat, allowing the mixture to simmer for 5 to 10 minutes. Add brown sugar to taste and drink hot. Drink one to two times a day in the week before your period and whenever you experience period cramps.

Ginger tea. Place three to five slices of ginger into a pot with 1 cup of water. Boil and then simmer for 5 to 10 minutes. Add 1 tablespoon of brown sugar. Stir until it dissolves. Strain and drink it warm one to two times a day in the week before your period and whenever you experience period cramps. Ginger is believed to be *warming* and can reduce uterine cramps due to coldness in the body.

Licorice root tea. Add 1 to 2 teaspoons of ground licorice root to a cup of boiling water. Allow it to steep for about 5 minutes. Add honey to taste and drink it warm.

Millettia stem. Prepare a decoction using ½ to 1 tablespoon of the dried powder. Alternatively, millettia stem is also available in the form of tablets.

Peach seed tea. Peach seed is available as a powder and may be added to a cup of hot water and taken in the form of a tea.

Safflower tea. Safflower is thought to invigorate blood, which aids in the passing of blood out of the body and reduces period cramps. Add 2 teaspoons of dried safflower petals to a cup of boiling water. Allow it to steep for 5 to 10 minutes before straining. Drink it hot.

Shao Fu Zhu Yu Tang. It is a polyherbal formula containing 10 herbs, including xiao hui xiang (fennel seeds), chuan xiong (Szechuan lovage roots), rou gui (cinnamon bark), gan jiang (dried ginger), wu ling zhi (flying squirrel feces), dan gui (female ginseng), chi shao (red peony roots), yan hu suo (corydalis), pu huang (cattail pollen), and mo yao (myrrh).

Therapeutic Measures

- **Hot compress.** Place a hot pack or hot water bottle over the lower abdomen. Heat is believed to relieve menstrual cramping due to excessive coldness in the body and uterus.
- **Acupuncture.** Acupuncture is thought to reduce menstrual cramps by increasing blood flow to the uterus and nourishing it. Acupuncture should only be used while not menstruating.

Notes

- Traditional Chinese medicine practitioners believe that menstrual cramping may be caused by several reasons:
  - Qi stagnation in the body, due to liver dysfunction (due to fluctuating negative emotions such as anger, sadness, or stress)
  - Blood stagnation in the body due to excessive *coldness* in the uterus (drinking/eating raw, cold foods or a cold environment)
  - Blood deficiency in which the blood does not provide sufficient nutrition to the organs

Western/Other Natural Remedies

Common Recipes

Oral

Teas/Brews/Others

Aloe vera juice. Wash and dry an aloe vera leaf. Slit the leaf down the center. Scrape out the white gel, discarding any of the yellow gel. Cut into smaller pieces and add to a blender. Blend until smooth. Add to a fruit/vegetable smoothie or warm water or drink alone. Take one to two times a day in the week leading up to the start of menstruation.

Black cohosh tea. Add 1 teaspoon of black cohosh to a pot with 1 cup of water. Bring to a boil and then allow to simmer for about 20 minutes. Remove from the heat and steep for about 5 minutes. Strain and drink twice a day.

Black haw tea. As above under "Menorrhagia."

Blackstrap molasses. Add 1 to 2 teaspoons of blackstrap molasses to a cup of hot water. Mix well and drink once a day.

Blue cohosh tea. Prepare a decoction with some chopped roots. Strain and consume.

Chamomile tea. Place some dried or fresh chamomile flowers into a cup. Pour boiling water over the flowers and allow it to steep for 10 minutes. Strain and add honey to taste. Drink it hot.

TABLE 6.6 Common Ingredients for Period Cramps

Spices	Herbs/Leaves	Miscellaneous
Cinnamon	Actaea racemosa (black cohosh)	Hot compress
Fenugreek	Scutellariae (skullcap)	Peppermint oil
Ginger	Green tea leaf	Chamomile flower
White turmeric/ Zedoary (Curcuma zedoaria)	Dioscorea villosa (wild yam)	Pickle
	Blackstrap molasses	Aloe vera
	Cramp bark (Viburnum opulus)	Lemon
	Motherwort (Leonurus cardiaca)	Essential oil— frankincense, myrrh
	Salix alba (white willow bark)	Black cohosh
	Black haw (Viburnum prunifolium)	Blue cohosh
	Verbena (Verbena officinalis)	

Cinnamon tea. Lightly crush one stick of cinnamon and add to a cup of boiling water. Allow it to steep for 5 to 10 minutes and strain. Add honey to taste and drink. Alternatively, mix 1 to 2 teaspoons of cinnamon powder into a cup of boiling water and drink it warm. Cinnamon may also be added to food such as oatmeal or added to smoothies.

Cramp bark and ginger tea. Add ¼ cup of dried ginger and ¼ cup of dried cramp bark to a pot with 2 cups of water. Bring to a boil and then reduce the heat, allowing it to simmer for 10 to 15 minutes. Remove from the heat and steep for another 10 minutes. Strain and drink hot.

Fenugreek tea. Lightly crush 2 to 3 teaspoons of fenugreek seeds and place in a cup. Add boiling water to the cup and cover, allowing the mixture to steep for 3 to 5 minutes. Strain and add honey to taste. Drink it warm.

Ginger tea. Place 2 to 3 inches of fresh ginger into a cup of boiling water. Allow it to steep for 5 to 10 minutes and drink it warm. Drink one to two times a day, especially in the week leading up to your period. Alternatively, add 2 to 3 inches of fresh ginger to fruit or vegetable juices and smoothies.

Green tea. Add 1 teaspoon of green tea leaves to a pot with a cup of hot water. Boil and then simmer gently for 3 to 5 minutes and strain the mixture. Add honey to taste and drink three to four times a day. Green tea is thought to have anti-inflammatory and pain-relieving properties.

Lemon water. Juice ½ a lemon and mix the juice into a cup of warm water. Add honey to taste. Drink in the morning on an empty stomach.

Motherwort tea. Motherwort has been found to reduce period cramps by lessening uterine muscle spasms.

Motherwort is available as a tincture but may also be taken as a tea. Pour 1 cup of boiling water over 1 tablespoon of dried motherwort. Steep for 15 to 20 minutes and strain. Add honey to taste and drink.

Pickle juice. Drink ½ a cup of pickle juice when you begin to feel the menstrual cramps.

Skullcap tea. Place 1 tablespoon of dried skullcap in a teapot with 2 cups of boiling water. Cover and steep for 10 minutes. Add honey to taste and strain. Drink it hot.

Verbena tea. Take 1 tablespoon of fresh lemon verbena leaves or 1 teaspoon of dried leaves. Add 1 cup of boiling water. Steep or simmer for 15 minutes. Strain and consume warm with a desired sweetener.

White turmeric tea. White turmeric is available in the form of a powder and can be mixed into hot water to make a tea. Drink it warm.

White willow bark tea. Take 2 teaspoons of dried willow bark into a pot with 2 cups of water. Allow to gently simmer for 10 to 15 minutes before removing it from the heat. Continue to steep for half an hour before straining. Drink it hot. Variation #1. It is available as a tincture.

Wild yam tea. Add 1 teaspoon of wild yam powder to a cup of hot water. Mix well and strain. Drink it hot. Consume whenever you experience menstrual cramps.

It is available as a dietary supplement and can reduce menstrual cramps.

Therapeutic Measures

- **Essential oil therapy:** Frankincense or myrrh essential oils may be diluted with water and placed into a humidifier/diffuser. Keep the humidifier by the bedside. Alternatively, if a diffuser is not readily available, sprinkle some essential oil onto clothes or bed sheets.

- **Hot compress:** Place a hot water bottle or hot pack on the lower abdomen. Heat relaxes the uterine muscles and reduces period cramps.

Modern Remedies

Non-Steroidal Anti-Inflammatory Drugs

NSAIDs exert their anti-inflammatory effect through inhibition of cyclooxygenase, which is the enzyme that catalyzes the transformation of arachidonic acid to prostaglandins and thromboxane. Hence, this will reduce tissue damage at the time of menstruation and stop the prolonged menstrual bleeding.

Example: Mefenamic acid

Combined Oral Contraceptive Pills (COCP)

COCP consists of estrogen and progestogen and is generally given for 3 weeks. This is followed by a pill-free week in which the woman experiences a hormone withdrawal bleeding. With this COCP, there is about a reduction in blood loss of 50%, and there is the additional benefit of regulating bleeding. The COCP can be *tri-cycled*—three packets can be taken consecutively without the pill-free weeks. The menstrual frequency and blood loss volume are reduced. Hence, it is a preferred option for many women.

Surgical Treatment

Surgical options may also be considered for severe menstrual cramps that negatively impact the individual's daily activities and quality of life. Surgery is often indicated for some causes of menstrual cramps such as endometriosis, fibroids, or ovarian cysts. A number of surgical options exist, such as:
- Endometrial ablation
- Hysterectomy
- Laparoscopy

Homeopathic Remedies

These include belladonna, pulsatilla, Magnesium phosphoricum, Cimicifuga, Cocculus, Chamomilla, Colocynthis, Caulophyllum, Nux vomica, calcarea carb, and others.

Irregular Periods

A normal menstrual cycle lasts about 28 days. Periods are considered irregular if they occur more frequently than every 21 days, or last for longer than 8 days. They are often caused by several reasons such as polycystic ovarian syndrome (PCOS), stress or thyroid disorders. However, irregular periods may also be present without any underlying disease. This section aims to provide natural remedies from different cultures that may aid in regulating menstruation.

Indian Natural Remedies

Common Recipes

Oral

Teas/Brews

Asafetida. Fry a pinch of asafetida with some ghee. Add some goat milk and honey. Consume daily for 1 month.
Variation #1. Add a pinch of asafetida to buttermilk or to the diet.

Ashoka bark decoction. Take 10 g of ashoka bark. Add 2 cups of water. Boil and reduce volume to 1 cup. Add jaggery or honey and consume.

Bael leaf paste. Grind some bael leaves into a fine paste and take with 1 teaspoon of warm water.

Cinnamon milk. Mix a teaspoon of cinnamon powder into a cup of warm milk and drink once a day. Cinnamon is a warming herb and is believed to aid menstrual cycle regulation.

Coriander seed tea. Place 1 teaspoon of coriander seeds into a pot with 2 cups of water and boil until it reduces to one cup in volume. Add rock candy to taste and drink it warm. Drink two to three times a day.

Cumin tea. Place 2 teaspoons of cumin seeds in a cup of warm water overnight. Drink once daily in the morning on an empty stomach.

Garlic. Eat two to three cloves of raw garlic after each meal every day in the week leading up to menstruation.

Ginger tea. Lightly pound 2 to 3 inches of fresh ginger and add to a pot with 1 cup of water. Bring to a boil and then reduce the heat, simmering gently for 10 to 15 minutes. Add honey to taste and drink. Drink three times a day after meals.

Hibiscus tea. Place a handful of dried or fresh hibiscus petals into a teapot with a cup of boiling water. Steep for 10 to 15 minutes and strain. Add a pinch of cinnamon and honey to taste.
Variation #1. Fry two hibiscus flowers in ghee and consume with a cup of warm milk once a day.

Licorice and rice water tea. Mix 5 g of powdered licorice with 20 g of rice water. Add some jaggery or rock sugar to taste. Consume two times a day for about 2 to 3 months.
Variation #1. Add 1 to 2 teaspoons of ground licorice root to a cup of boiling water. Allow it to steep for about 5 to 10 minutes. Add honey or rock sugar to taste and drink it warm.

Lodhra brew. Place 3 g of lodhra bark powder into 100 mL of hot water and mix well. Drink once a day. Lodhra is believed to relax the uterine tissues, hence reducing blood flow.

Mint paste. Grind 1 teaspoon of dried mint leaves into a fine powder and mix with 1 teaspoon of honey to make a paste. Take this paste three times a day.

Niranjan phal. Soak the fruits overnight in a cup of water until it swells. Crush and squeeze the pulp into the water. Consume on an empty stomach in the morning. Add honey if desired.
Variation #1. Take one to two nuts. Add 1 cup of boiling water. Allow to steep and consume.

Saffron tea. Add 1 teaspoon of saffron to a pot with half a cup of water and boil the mixture until it reduces to

TABLE 6.7	Common Ingredients for Irregular Periods		
Spices	**Herbs/Leaves**	**Miscellaneous**
Asafetida		Rice water
Cinnamon	*Symplocos racemosa* (lodhra)	Rock sugar (mishri)
Coriander seed	Shilajit (black asphalt)	Ghee
Cumin	*Saraca indica* (ashoka tree bark)	Honey
Garlic	*Glycyrrhiza glabra* (licorice)	*Rosa sinensis* (hibiscus)
Ginger	Bael leaf	Castor oil
Saffron	Ferula foetida (asafetida)	Jaggery
Santalum album (chandan/ sandalwood)		Niranjan phal
Turmeric	Mint (pudina)	Unripe papaya

1 tablespoon in volume. Divide the mixture into three portions. Dilute the portion with ½ a cup of water and drink three times a day after meals. Repeat this for a few days.

Sandalwood brew. Add dried sandalwood roots or leaves to a cup of cow's milk and place in a pot. Boil and simmer for 10 minutes and strain. Drink it warm.

Shilajit. Dose is as recommended depending on the formulation.

Turmeric milk. Add ¼ teaspoon of turmeric to a cup of warm milk. Mix well and add honey or jaggery to taste. Take it once a day until the menstruation cycles regulate.

Unripe papaya. Cut an unripe papaya into small chunks and place into a blender. Blend until smooth and drink. Consume unripe papaya juice for a few months but never while menstruating. It can also be eaten as a salad.

Therapeutic Measures

Castor oil pack. Coat one side of a cotton cloth in warm castor oil. Cover the lower abdomen with the oiled side of the cotton cloth. Leave the cotton cloth for 30 to 60 minutes. Remove the cloth at the end of the 30 to 60 minutes and wipe with a damp cloth.

Chinese Natural Remedies

Common Recipes

Oral

- Decoction for "Heat in the Blood"
  - Modified "Qingjing San/Powder": Mu dan pi, di gu pi, bai shao, sheng di huang, huang bai, qing hao, yi mu cao, sheng di yu.
  - Soak the herbs in water for 2 hours or more. Then place the herbs and water in a pot and simmer for 25 to 30 minutes. Strain the mixture and drink half of it

TABLE 6.8	Common Ingredients for Irregular Periods	
Spices	**Herbs/Leaves**	**Miscellaneous**
Ramulus cinnamomi (gui zhi)	Cortex moutan radicis (mu dan pi)	Longan (*Dimocarpus longan*)
	Cortex lycii (di gu pi)	Flos carthami (hong hua/safflower)
	Radix paeoniae alba (bai shao)	Semen persicae (tao ren/peach kernel)
	Radix rehmanniae (sheng di huang)	Fructus evodiae (wu zhu yu)
	Herba artemisiae (qing hao)	
	Herba leonuri (yi mu cao)	
	Radix sanguisorbae (sheng di yu)	
	Rhizoma atractylodis macrocephalae (bai zhu)	
	Proa cum radix pini (fu shen)	
	Radix astragali (huang qi)	
	Semen ziziphi spinosae (suan zao ren)	
	Radix ginseng (ren shen)	
	Radix Aucklandiae (mu xiang)	
	Radix glycyrrhizae praeparata (zhi gan cao)	
	Radix angelicae sinensis (dang gui)	
	Chinese senega roots/yuan zhi (*Polygala tenuifolia*)	
	Folium artemisia argyi (ai ye tan)	
	Rhizoma zingiberis preparata (pao jiang)	
	Radix paeoniae rubra (chi shao)	
	Rhizoma chuanxiong (chuan xiong)	
	Rhizoma zingiberis recens (sheng jiang)	
	Radix glycyrrhizae (gan cao)	
	Poria (fu ling)	
	Radix bupleuri (chai hu)	
	Herba menthae (bo he)	

in the morning and the remaining mixture in the evening.

- Decoction for "Deficiency of Qi"
  o "Gui Pi Tang": Bai zhu, fu shen, huang qi, suan zao ren, ren shen, mu xiang, zhi gan cao, dang gui, yuan zhi, ai ye tan, pao jiang.
  o Soak the herbs in water for 2 hours or more. Then place the herbs and water in a pot and simmer for 25 to 30 minutes. Strain the mixture and drink half of it in the morning and the remaining mixture in the evening.
- Decoction for "Blood Stasis"
  - "Tao Hong Siwu Tang": Shu di huang, dang gui, shi shao, chuan xiong, tao ren, hong hua.
  - Soak the herbs in water for 2 hours or more. Then place the herbs and water in a pot and simmer for 25 to 30 minutes. Strain the mixture and drink half of it in the morning and the remaining mixture in the evening.
- Decoction for "Coldness in the Blood":
  - Modified "Wen Jing Tang": Wu zhu yu, dang gui, bai shao, chuan xiong, ren shen, gui zhi, mu dan pi, sheng jiang, gan cao.
  - Soak the herbs in water for 2 hours or more. Then place the herbs and water in a pot and simmer for 25 to 30 minutes. Strain the mixture and drink half of it in the morning, and the remaining mixture in the evening.
- Decoction for "Stagnation of Qi":
  - "Xiaoyao San": Zhi gan cao, dang gui, fu ling, bai shao, bai zhu, chai hu, bo he.
  - Soak the herbs (except bo he) in water for 2 hours or more. Then place the herbs and water in a pot, including the bo he. Simmer for 25 to 30 minutes. Strain the mixture and drink half of it in the morning and the remaining mixture in the evening.

Notes

- Heat in the Blood
  - Symptoms of this cause of irregular menstrual cycle are early menstruation, profuse bleeding of thick, sticky dark-red or bright-red, menstrual blood. Other symptoms include flushing, restlessness, a dry mouth, and a rapid pulse.
  - The principles of the remedy are to clear the excess heat from the body and regulate menstruation.
- Deficiency of Qi
  - Symptoms of this cause of irregular menstrual cycle are early menstruation, profuse bleeding of light-colored and thin-textured blood. There may also be a loss of appetite, loose stools, fatigue, and a weak pulse.
  - The principles of the remedy are to strengthen the spleen to maintain blood flow to the blood vessels and to regulate menstruation.
- Blood Stasis
  - Symptoms of this cause of irregular menstrual cycle are delayed menstruation, scanty menstruation with

dark-colored, clot-filled blood. There may also be a tender lower abdomen that is relieved by passage of the blood clots.
  - The principles of the remedy are to promote blood circulation and prevent blood stasis, hence regulating menstruation.
- Coldness in the Blood
  - Symptoms of this cause of irregular menstrual cycle are delayed menstruation, scanty, clot-filled menses, and abdominal pain relieved by warmth.
  - The principles of the remedy are to warm the body and dispel the excess coldness, hence regulating periods.
- Stagnation of Qi
  - Symptoms of this cause of irregular menstrual cycle are irregular menstruation, scanty or profuse bleeding of purplish or hesitant blood flow, irritability, and breast distension.
  - The principles of the remedy are to regulate the qi in the liver and to nourish the blood to regulate menstruation.

Western/Other Natural Remedies

Common Recipes

Oral

Teas/Brews

Alfalfa juice. Place a handful of fresh alfalfa into a blender and blend until smooth. Drink it by itself or with other fruit or vegetable juices.

Black cohosh. Add 1 teaspoon of black cohosh to a pot with 1 cup of water. Bring to a boil and then allow to simmer for about 20 minutes. Remove from the heat and steep for about 5 minutes. Strain and drink twice a day.

TABLE 6.9 Common Ingredients for Irregular Periods

Spices	Herbs/Leaves	Miscellaneous
Flaxseed	Alfalfa	
	Trifolium pratense (red clover)	
	Tribulus terrestris (tribulus)	
	Lepidium meyenii (maca)	
	Serenoa repens (saw palmetto)	
	Actaea racemosa (black cohosh)	
	Motherwort *(Leonurus cardiaca)*	
Saffron	Bladderwrack *(Fucus vesiculosus)*	Honey
Turmeric	Blue cohosh	*Vitex agnus-castus* (chasteberry)

Bladderwrack tea. Add 1 to 2 teaspoons of dried bladderwrack to a cup of hot water. Allow it to steep for 5 to 10 minutes. Strain and add honey to taste. Drink two to three times a day.

Chasteberry tea. Refer to "Western/Other Natural Remedies" under "Heavy Periods."

Flaxseed tea. Add 2 to 3 teaspoons of flaxseed to a cup of boiling water. Steep for 10 to 15 minutes and strain. Drink hot. Flaxseeds are rich in essential fatty acids. Essential fatty acids are important in regulating hormone production in the body.

Motherwort tea. Motherwort is available as a tincture but may also be taken as a tea. Pour 1 cup of boiling water over 1 tablespoon of dried motherwort. Steep for 15 to 20 minutes and strain. Add honey to taste and drink.

Saffron tea. Add saffron strands to a pot with 1 cup of water. Boil for 3 to 4 minutes and reduce the heat, allowing it to simmer for another 7 to 8 minutes. Strain and add honey to taste. Drink it warm.

Turmeric tea. Add 1 to 2 teaspoons of ground turmeric to 1 cup of hot water. Mix well and add honey to taste. Drink one to two times a day. Alternatively, lightly pound 2 to 3 inches of fresh turmeric and add to a cup of boiling water. Allow it to steep for 5 to 10 minutes and strain. Add honey to taste.

Modern Remedies

Irregular periods are not common conditions that need treatment unless they are caused by underlying problems such as PCOS or a thyroid problem. However, a number of options exist that may help to regulate periods:

Hormone Therapy

As irregular menstrual cycles are often due to hormonal imbalances, oral contraceptive pills may be prescribed. They contain estrogen and progesterone, which help to regulate periods.

Homeopathic Remedies

These include pulsatilla, *Cimicifuga racemosa*, Caulophyllum, Lycopodium, Lachesis, Sepia, and others.

Endometriosis

Endometriosis is thought to affect 3% to 10% of reproductive-aged women. It is a condition that occurs when uterine lining tissue grows on other organs in the body, usually in the lower abdomen or pelvis. Women with endometriosis often experience symptoms such as pelvic or lower abdominal pain, menstrual pain, and pain during intercourse. The pain is often at its worst right before or during menstruation. There are many theories as to the cause of endometriosis, such as retrograde menstruation. This theory proposes that during menstruation, some blood and uterine tissue travel into the abdominal cavity through the fallopian tubes.

TABLE 6.10	Common Ingredients for Endometriosis	
Spices	**Herbs/Leaves**	**Miscellaneous**
Flaxseed	Fennel	
	Asparagus racemosus (shatavari)	
Ginger	*Commiphora wightii* (guggulu)	
Turmeric	*Tinospora cordifolia* (giloy)	Castor oil

Another theory proposes that cells outside of the uterus may change into uterine lining cells. Endometriosis should be diagnosed by a medical professional, and these natural remedies are to be used as adjunctive treatment to allopathic medication or to help cope with the negative effects of endometriosis.

Indian Natural Remedies

Common Recipes

Oral

Teas/Brews

Fennel tea. Place 1 teaspoon of fennel seeds into a cup and pour hot water over the seeds. Cover and steep for 10 minutes before drinking. Drink it warm one to three times a day.

Flaxseed brew. Add 2 to 3 teaspoons of flaxseed to a cup of warm water. Steep overnight. In the morning, drink the water and consume the flaxseeds.

Giloy juice. Place a handful of giloy leaves into a blender and blend until smooth. Strain and drink. Alternatively, chew on fresh giloy leaves or consume in the form of powder.

Giloy tea. Add dried giloy leaves or powdered giloy to a cup of boiling water and mix well. Drink it warm.

Ginger tea. Add 1 to 2 teaspoons of ginger powder to a pot with a cup of hot water. Allow it to simmer for 5 minutes. Drink twice a day after meals.

Guggulu supplements. Guggulu is the sap produced by the Indian bdellium tree and is available in the form of dietary supplements. Adults can take about 25 mg of guggulu supplements every day after a meal.

Shatavari brew. As above.

Turmeric tea. Add 1 to 2 teaspoons of ground turmeric to 1 cup of hot water. Mix well and add honey to taste. Drink one to two times a day. Alternatively, lightly pound 2 to 3 inches of fresh turmeric and add to a cup of boiling water. Allow it to steep for 5 to 10 minutes and strain. Add honey to taste.

Therapeutic Measures

- **Enemas (Basti):** Basti involves the introduction of medicated liquids through the anal or vaginal route for detoxification and is believed to remove obstruction in the passages and reduce pain during sexual intercourse, hence improving fertility.

- **Ayurvedic oil massages:** Oil massages are believed to help improve hormonal balance in the body, promote fertility, and remove toxins from the body. They are also thought to block pain signals to the brain, hence reducing endometriosis pain.

Commercial Preparations

- **Pradrantak churna:** *Symplocos racemosa, Saraca indica, Ficus glomerata, Terminalia arjuna*
- **Shatavari capsules:** *Asparagus racemosus*
- **Boswellia-Curcumin:** Boswellia extract, serratiopeptidase, turmeric extract, piperine

Chinese Natural Remedies

Common Recipes

Oral

Traditional Chinese medication used to treat endometriosis often focuses on symptomatic relief, as the root cause of endometriosis cannot be treated at present.

- Reduces bleeding
  - pu huang
  - san qi
- Relieves pain
  - yan hu suo
  - tao ren
  - mo yao
- Reduces uterine tissue
  - **E zhu tea.** White turmeric is available in the form of a powder and can be mixed into hot water to make a tea. Drink it warm.
  - zao jiao ci
  - mu li
  - xia ku cao
- Qi circulation
  - chai hu
  - xiang fu
  - chi shao
- Improves blood circulation
  - chuan xiong
  - dang gui
  - dan shen
- Warms the blood
  - cinnamon
  - ginger
  - xu duan
- Anti-inflammatory
  - zhi zi
  - mu dan pi
  - gui ban
- Polyherbal formula

Gui Zhi Fu Ling Wan (GZFLW). The key ingredients include fu ling (poria cocos), bai shao (peony root), tao ren (peach seeds), gui zhi (cassia twig), and mu dan pi (moutan peony).

TABLE 6.11	Common Ingredients for Endometriosis		
Spices	**Herbs/Leaves**	**Miscellaneous**
Cinnamon (gui zhi)	Cattail pollen/Pu Huang (*Typha angustifolia*)	Pseudoginseng (san qi)
Ginger (gan jiang)	Peach seed/tao ren (*Prunus persica*)	Corydalis/yan hu suo (*Corydalis yanhusuo*)
	Mo yao (myrrh)	Oyster shell (mu li)
	White turmeric/Zedoary/e zhu (*Curcuma zedoaria*)	Turtle shell/gui ban (*Chinemys reevesii*)
	Gleditsia spine/zao jiao ci (*Gleditschiae Sinensis Spina*)	Castor oil
	Heal-all spike/xia ku cao (*Spica prunellae*)	
	Bupleurum (chai hu)	
	Cyperus (xiang fu)	
	Red peony (chi shao)	
	Cnidium (chuan xiong)	
	Tang kuei (dang gui)	
	Red sage/danshen (*Salvia miltiorrhiza*)	
	Dipsaci (xu duan)	
	Moutan (mu dan pi)	
	Gardenia (zhi zi)	

Hua Yu Xiao Zheng: The key ingredients include danshen (red sage), ba ji tian (morinda root), tian qi (Chinese ginseng), yi yi ren (coix seeds), zhe bei mu (fritillary bulb), xia ku cao (heal-all spike), bian xu (knotgrass), da huang (Chinese rhubarb), yan hu suo (corydalis), shui zhi (dried medicinal leech), pu huang (cattail pollen), and xue jie dragon's blood).

Dang Gui Shao Yao San: The key ingredients include dang gui (female ginseng), fu ling (poria cocos), chuan xiong (Szechuan lovage roots), bai zhu (white atractylodes rhizome), bai shao (peony root), and ze xie (common water-plantain).

Shao Fu Zhu Yu Tang: The key ingredients include dang gui (female ginseng), xiao hui tang (fennel), chi shao (red peony root), chuan xiong (Szechuan lovage roots), gui zhi (cassia twig), and sheng jiang (fresh ginger).

Jia Wei Xiao Yao San: The key ingredients include chai hu (Chinese thoroughwax), bai shao (peony root), fu ling (poria cocos), dang gui (female ginseng), bai zhu (white atractylodes rhizome), sheng jiang (fresh ginger), zhi zi (cape jasmine), bo he (mint), gan cao (licorice), and moutan peony (mu dan pi).

Zuo Gui Wan: The key ingredients include gui ban (turtle shell), chu di huang (Chinese foxglove root), shan yu rou (Asiatic cornelian cherry fruit), gou qi zi (wolfberry), lu jiao jiao (deer antler glue), shan yao (yam rhizome), tu si zi (dodder seeds), and niu xi (ox knee).

Therapeutic Measures

Lifestyle

Castor oil packs—soak a piece of cloth in castor oil and place on the lower abdomen. Place a clean piece of cloth on top of the castor-oil-soaked cloth and place a hot pack on top of that. Let it sit for 30 to 60 minutes before removing and cleaning the area.

Western/Other Natural Remedies

Common Recipes

Oral

Teas/Brews

Cinnamon tea. As above.

Ginger tea. As above.

Pine needle tea. Take unblemished edible pine needles. Wash and cut into small pieces. Add 2 cups of boiling water. Steep for 10 to 15 minutes. Strain and drink. Add honey to taste.

Variation #1. It is available as capsules or tablets. Pycnogenol brand is widely used.

Therapeutic Measures

Diet

- Consume foods rich in **omega-3 fatty acids**, such as salmon, sardines, mackerel, and anchovies. They are also available in the form of commercial preparations, such as capsules. Omega-3 fatty acids have been found to have an anti-inflammatory as well as pain-reducing effect on women with endometriosis.
- Consume a diet high in **vegetables** as they are rich in flavones, which inhibit aromatase, the enzyme that is responsible for converting androgens into estrogen.
- **Flaxseeds** should be incorporated into the diet as they have been found to be beneficial for estrogen-related conditions such as endometriosis.

Lifestyle

- A healthy lifestyle should be adopted, such as performing a regular and light exercise. Exercise has been found

TABLE 6.12	Common Ingredients for Endometriosis	
Spices	Herbs/Leaves	Miscellaneous
Cinnamon		Omega-3 foods (flaxseed, oily fish)
		Pine bark (*Pinus pinaster*)
Ginger		Hot pack

to reduce estrogen levels in the body and hence improve endometriosis symptoms.

There is currently no medicinal cure for endometriosis, and most treatment methods are aimed at helping patients cope with the pain and negative effects of endometriosis. The only definitive cures for endometriosis are surgical procedures.

Modern Remedies

Medical (Hormonal) Treatment

Combined Oral Contraceptive Pills

COCPs act by preventing ovulation and inhibiting follicular development. Initially, a trial of continuous or cyclic COCPs should be administered for 3 months and then continued for 6 to 12 months if there is pain relief.

Progesterone compounds (progestogens) inhibit gonadotropin secretion, which then prevents follicular development and ovulation, and subsequent endometrial thinning and atrophy. These include the following:

a. **Medroxyprogesterone (Depo Provera):** This is an injectable long-acting medication, which is given every 3 months. It is effective in pain suppression.

b. **Levonorgestrel (Mirena):** This widely used IUS contains an androgenic progestogen, LNG. LNG is slowly released from the implant placed in the womb.

c. **Contraceptive implant (Implanon/Nexplanon):** This is a tiny thin rod that is placed subcutaneously in the nondominant arm. It releases progestin hormone and can last for 3 years.

d. **Progesterone-only pill (POP/mini-pill):** It contains synthetic progesterone only (i.e., norethisterone). There is no estrogen. It is used when COCP is contraindicated.

GnRH Analogues. GnRH analogues produce a hypogonadotrophic-hypogonadic state by downregulation of the pituitary gland. This will, in turn, cause ovarian suppression.

Danazol. Danazol inhibits the mid-cycle follicle-stimulating hormone (FSH) and luteinizing hormone (LH) surges and prevents steroidogenesis in the corpus luteum. Side effects are due to the androgenic manifestations (i.e., oily skin, acne, weight gain, deepening of the voice, and facial hirsutism).

Surgery

- **Conservative surgery**—the aim is to lyse peritubal and periovarian adhesions and to destroy visible endometriotic implants that are the source of pain that may interfere with ovum transport. The laparoscopic method is the preferred conservative treatment in endometriosis ablation, and this can be performed with laser or electro-diathermy.
- **Radical surgery**—radical surgery is often considered in patients who do not respond to medication and do not have plans of starting a family. They include total hysterectomy with bilateral oophorectomy (TAH-BSO) or cytoreduction of visible endometriosis. Adhesiolysis is done to restore mobility and maintain normal intrapelvic organ balance.

Homeopathic Remedies

These include Sabina, Xanthophyllum, Cimicifuga, and Sepia.

Polycystic Ovarian Syndrome

PCOS is a common cause of infertility. It is the development of multiple cysts in the ovaries due to an imbalance of hormones in the body. It often presents as irregular menstrual cycles as well as excessive facial and body hair, acne on the face, chest, and upper back, hair loss, weight gain, skin crease darkening, and the appearance of skin tags (especially in the neck and armpit areas). There are two common hormonal imbalances that cause PCOS:

- **High androgen levels:** Androgens are a hormone commonly produced in large amounts in males. Females produce small amounts of androgen, but excessive androgen production causes the development of male traits such as male-pattern baldness. High androgen levels also cause excessive facial and body hair growth and acne. It may also prevent ovulation.
- **High insulin levels:** Insulin is a hormone that regulates glucose levels in the body. High insulin levels often occur in obese individuals, those with a family history of type 2 diabetes and individuals with unhealthy eating habits and who do not get enough exercise.

Tests include abdominal ultrasound and blood tests for androgens (testosterone and DHEA), insulin, anti-Mullerian hormone (AMH), glucose, and lipids.

Indian Natural Remedies

PCOS is mainly a kapha disorder that is classified under Yonivyapad (female genital tract disorders). The excess kapha blocks the natural reproductive channels (i.e., artava vaha srota) that courses through the female reproductive tissue. (i.e., Artava dhatu. Shukra refers to both sperm and ovum. Atrava refers to ovum.)

Common Recipes

Oral

Teas/Brews

Amla juice. Lightly pound three to four amla fruits and strain the juice. Take this juice on an empty stomach in the morning with a glass of warm water.

Arugampul juice. Take ½ cup of arugampul (without roots). Soak for a few hours. Blend with 1 cup of water. Strain and drink fresh first thing in the morning on an empty stomach.

Ashoka bark paste. Take ¼ to ½ teaspoon ashoka tree bark powder. Add little water or honey. Consume after meal.

Ashwagandha brew. Place 1 teaspoon of Ashwagandha root powder into a pot with ½ a cup of milk, ½ a cup of water, and 1 teaspoon of sugar. Boil gently until the volume reduces to about ½ a cup. Cool slightly and drink it warm.

Chitrak. Take 1 to 2 g of chitrak root powder. Mix with some honey and consume.

Cinnamon tea. Add a stick of cinnamon to a pot of hot water and allow it to steep for about 10 minutes. Add honey to taste and drink.

TABLE 6.13	Common Ingredients for Polycystic Ovarian Syndrome	
Spices	**Herbs/Leaves**	**Miscellaneous**
Cinnamon	*Asparagus racemosus* (shatavari)	Purified asphaltum (shilajit)
Fenugreek	*Tinospora cordifolia* (giloy)	Vetiveria zizanioides (usheera)
Garlic	*Terminalia belerica* (bibhitaki)	Momordica charantia (karavellaka)
Ginger	Amla (*Phyllanthus emblica*)	Zinc calx (yashad bhasma)
Long pepper (*Piper longum*)	*Symplocos racemosa* (lodhra)	*Garcinia cambogia* (vrikshamla)
	Gurmar (*Gymnema sylvestre*)	*Coccinia indica* /Ivy gourd (kunduru/kovakkai)
	Saraca indica (ashoka)	Bael fruit/ bilva
	Terminalia chebula (haritaki)	
	Cedrus deodara (devadaru)	
	Withania somnifera (ashwagandha)	
	Arugampul	
	Punarnava (*Boerhavia diffusa*)	
	Guduchi (*Tinospora indica*)	
	Chitrak (*Plumbago zeylanica*)	
Turmeric	*Azadirachta indica* (neem)	Eugenia jambolana (java plum/jamun)

Fenugreek brew. Soak a handful of fenugreek seeds in warm water overnight. Drink and consume the amber water with the swelled seeds in the morning on an empty stomach.

Giloy juice. Place a handful of giloy leaves into a blender and blend until smooth. Strain and drink. Alternatively, chew on fresh giloy leaves or consume in the form of powder.

> Variation #1. **Giloy tea.** Add dried giloy leaves or powdered giloy to a cup of boiling water and mix well. Drink it warm.

Ginger tea. Lightly pound 2 to 3 inches of fresh ginger and add to a pot with 1 cup of water. Bring to a boil and then reduce the heat, simmering gently for 10 to 15 minutes. Add honey to taste and drink. Drink three times a day after meals.

Guduchi juice. Place a handful of fresh guduchi leaves in a blender and blend until smooth. Strain and add honey to taste. Drink this daily in the morning on an empty stomach.

Gurmar brew. Gurmar is available as a powder or in the form of dried leaves. Alternatively, make gurmar brew by mixing 1 teaspoon of gurmar powder (or 1 to 2 g of dry leaves) in one cup of warm water. Add honey to taste and drink. Consume ½ hour after lunch and dinner.

Gurmar juice. Take some fresh washed leaves. Blend with a little water and make fresh juice. Consume 20 to 30 mL once or twice a day.

Gurmar leaves. Chew on one to two of fresh gurmar leaves every day.

Ivy gourd. It is cooked as a vegetable in a spicy stir-fry.

> Variation #1. Ivy gourd juice. Place one to two cut ivy gourds into a blender and blend until smooth, gradually adding up to 1 cup of water. Strain and drink.

Java plum (Jamun) juice. Take 10 to 15 washed black jamun fruits. Deseed and blend with 1 cup of water with added ¼ teaspoon of black salt and a small piece of ginger. Strain and drink. Add some honey and ice if desired.

Neem juice. Place six to eight neem leaves into a blender and blend until smooth, gradually adding up to 1 cup of water. Strain and drink.

Neem tea. Place a handful of fresh neem leaves into a pot with about 2.5 cups of boiling water. Bring to a boil before removing from the heat. Cover and allow it to steep for 5 to 10 minutes. Strain and drink it warm.

Shatavari brew. Slightly warm 120 mL of milk in a pot. Meanwhile, add 1 teaspoon of ground shatavari to a pot along with ⅛ teaspoon of cinnamon powder and a pinch of ginger powder. Pour a little milk over the powder and mix to form a paste. Slowly add the remaining milk, stirring well until no lumps remain. Add honey to taste and drink.

Turmeric tea. Take 2 teaspoons of turmeric powder into 3 to 4 cups of hot water. Stir and steep for about 5 to 10 minutes. Strain. Add honey, fresh lemon juice, or milk to taste.

Therapeutic Measures

- **Diet.** Consume a kapha-pacifying diet.
- **Enemas (Basti).** Medicated oils or decoctions are given rectally to release trapped toxins, kapha, or vata.
- **Cleansing (Virechan).** Herbs are given to induce bowel movements, which can remove toxins from the body and relieve PCOS symptoms.
- Yoga asanas and Pranayama breathing can balance the hormones and lower stress. These include:
  - Corpse pose (Shavasana)
  - Reclining butterfly pose (Supta Baddha Konasana)
  - Bharadvaja's twist (Bharadvajasana)
  - Mill churning pose (Chakki Chalanasana)

Chinese Natural Remedies

Common Recipes

Oral

Teas/Brews

False unicorn root brew. Take ¼ to ½ teaspoon dried root. Steep in hot water. Strain and consume three times a day. For tincture, take ½ to 1 teaspoon three times a day.

Ginseng tea. Place three to five slices of ginseng into a cup with hot water. Cover and steep for 5 to 10 minutes. Drink it warm.

Licorice tea. Add 1 teaspoon of ground licorice to a pot with 1 cup of boiling water. Allow it to simmer for 30 to 45 minute before straining.

Therapeutic Measures

Acupressure

- Large Intestine 11 (LI 11)
  - LI 11 is located on the outside side of the elbow crease.
- Conception Vessel 4 and 6 (Ren-4 and Ren-6)
  - Ren-6 is located one palm's width below the belly button, while Ren-4 is located 2 finger widths below Ren-6.
- Spleen 6 (SP 6)
  - SP 6 is located one palm's width above the tip of the ankle bone on the inner aspect of the foot.
- Stomach 36 (ST 36)
  - ST 36 is located one palm's width below the bottom edge of the kneecap in the depression on the outer aspect of the shinbone.

TABLE 6.14	Common Ingredients for Polycystic Ovarian Syndrome	
Herbs/Leaves	**Miscellaneous**	
Angelica sinensis (female ginseng/dong quai)	Cordyceps	
False unicorn		
Paeonia lactiflora (white peony)	*Glycyrrhiza glabra* (licorice/gan cao)	

TABLE 6.15	Common Ingredients for Polycystic Ovarian Syndrome	
Spices	Herbs/Leaves	Miscellaneous
Flaxseed	Spearmint	Apple cider vinegar (ACV)
Ginger	Vitex agnus-castus (chasteberry)	Fish oil
	Serenoa repens (saw palmetto)	Bitter gourd
	Lepidium meyenii (maca)	Ivy gourd
	Barberry/Berberine	Myo-inositol

Western/Other Natural Remedies

Common Recipes

Oral

Teas/Brews

Apple cider vinegar. Mix 1 tablespoon of ACV into 1 cup of water and drink.

Barberry tea. Take 1 to 2 teaspoons of crushed berries or 1 to 2 teaspoons of dried barberry root. Add 1 cup of hot water. Steep for 10 minutes. Strain and consume three times a day.

Bitter gourd juice. Place one to two cut bitter gourds into a blender and blend until smooth, gradually adding up to 1 cup of water. Strain and drink it.

Chasteberry tea. Refer to "Western/Other Natural Remedies" under "Heavy Periods."

Ivy gourd juice. Place one to two cut ivy gourds into a blender and blend until smooth, gradually adding up to 1 cup of water. Strain and drink it.

Maca-ginger tea. Place three to five pieces of cut ginger into a cup with boiling water. Add 1 teaspoon of Maca powder and mix well. Steep for 5 to 10 minutes and drink it warm.

Myo-inositol. It is available as a powder form. A night dose of 2 to 4 g is consumed.

Spearmint tea. Place six to eight spearmint leaves into a cup with boiling water. Cover and let sit for 5 to 10 minutes. Drink it warm. Take 2 cups of spearmint tea per day for 5 days.

Modern Remedies

There is no cure for PCOS presently, and treatment methods are aimed at helping patients to manage and treat their symptoms accordingly.

Homeopathic Remedies

These include pulsatilla, Calcarea carb, *Thuja occidentalis*, sepia, Natrum mur, and others.

Fibroids

Fibroids are most common in women ages 30 to 50.

They are growths that occur in and around the uterus and are made up of muscle and fibrous tissue. Fibroids often produce symptoms such as heavy and painful periods, abdominal pain, lower-back pain, constipation, and frequent urges to urinate. The cause of fibroids is not clear at present, but it is thought that excessive estrogen levels may play a role. It is also thought that being obese increases the risk of developing fibroids, as obesity increases the levels of estrogen in the body. There are three main types of fibroids:

- Intramural fibroids: These are the most common types of fibroids, and they develop in the muscle wall of the womb.
- Subserosal fibroids: Subserosal fibroids often develop on the outside of the uterine wall and invade the pelvis.
- Submucosal fibroids: Submucosal fibroids are often found in the muscle layer below the inner lining of the uterus. These fibroids may extend into the uterine cavity.

Uterine fibroids are benign tumors of the uterus that can grow inside the muscle layer of the uterus or outside the uterus wall or grow in the inner layer of the uterus. They are often due to estrogen dominance.

General Management

- Avoid or reduce xenoestrogen exposure. These xenohormones are endocrine disruptors that are environmental toxins and chemicals. Poor liver function can also lead to poor excretion of these biotoxins.
- Avoid synthetic body care products.
- Consume more organic foods with more fruits, vegetables, seeds, and nuts.
- Avoid or reduce red meat consumption.
- Avoid high fat, carbohydrates, and sugar intake.
- Regular exercise is important.

Indian Natural Remedies

Common Recipes

Oral

Teas/Brews

Aloe vera juice. Wash and dry an aloe vera leaf. Slit the leaf down the center. Scrape out the white gel, discarding any of the yellow gel. Cut into smaller pieces and add to a blender. Blend until smooth. Add to a fruit/vegetable smoothie or warm water or drink alone. Take one to two times a day in the week. Add some honey.

Amla juice. Lightly pound three to four amla fruits and strain the juice. Take this juice on an empty stomach in the morning with a glass of warm water. Continue for 3 months.

Ashoka bark paste. Place 25 g of ashoka bark powder into a pot with 200 mL of water. Boil slowly until the water has reduced to about 50 mL. Add 50 mL of milk and continue to boil until only 50 mL of liquid is left. Strain

TABLE 6.16 Multidisciplinary Management of Polycystic Ovarian Syndrome (PCOS)

Symptoms	Treatment/Medications	Notes
1. Irregular periods	Oral contraceptives	Oral contraceptives contain estrogen and progestin and may be used to regulate menstrual cycles. This may also reduce the long-term risk of developing uterine cancer associated with irregular or absent periods.
2. Unwanted hair growth (hirsutism) and hair loss (alopecia)	a. Medications to control excessive hair growth and loss include: • Specific types of combined oral contraceptive tablets (such as co-cyprindiol, Dianette, Marvelon, and Yasmin) • cyproterone acetate • finasteride b. Cream: eflornithine	These medications block the effects of "male hormones" (i.e., testosterone), and some also inhibit production of these hormones by the ovaries. • Cream: eflornithine can also be used to slow down the growth of unwanted facial hair.
3. Infertility	• Clomiphene citrate • Letrozole (*an aromatase inhibitor*) • In vitro fertilization (IVF) • Gonadotropins (FSHr)	Most women with polycystic ovarian syndrome (PCOS) can get pregnant following treatment. Majority can be successfully treated with a short course of tablets taken at the beginning of each cycle for several cycles. Clomiphene is usually recommended for women with PCOS who are trying to get pregnant. Clomiphene induces ovulation (i.e., it stimulates the monthly release of an egg from the ovaries). Letrozole helps to stimulate the ovaries and induces ovulation. It blocks estrogen production and increases FSH. If these are not successful, IVF treatment can be offered. There is an increased risk of multiple pregnancies (rarely more than twins) with these treatments. Gonadotropin-like recombinant follicle-stimulating hormone (FSHr) is used in anovulatory women with PCOS to prepare for intrauterine insemination.
4. Overweight	Orlistat Diet and lifestyle changes	It inhibits gastric and pancreatic lipase (an enzyme that breaks down triglyceride) in the intestine. The dietary triglycerides are not broken down into absorbable free fatty acids and instead are excreted unchanged. See under 'Obesity in Endocrine chapter'
5. High cholesterol	Statins	See under "CVS" chapter
6. Acne	Anti-acne management	See under "Acne" chapter
7. Diabetes	Metformin	Metformin is often used to treat type 2 diabetes, but it can also lower insulin and blood sugar levels in women with PCOS.
8. Others: Metabolic syndrome, Sleep apnea, Depression	Treat associated obesity, diabetes, hypercholesterolemia, hypertension	These are common in women who are overweight. Treating the associated symptoms can improve the negative emotions.

and cool. Take 20 to 30 mL in the morning to reduce menstrual blood flow.

Variation #1. Take some ashoka tree bark and add about 200 mL of water. Boil and reduce to ¼ volume. Consume 40 to 50 mL twice a day.

Beetroot mix juice. Cut a fresh beetroot into smaller cubes. Place the beetroot cubes into a blender and blend while gradually adding 1 cup of water to the blender. Strain. To the fresh beetroot juice, add 1 tablespoon of blackstrap molasses and 1 tablespoon of aloe vera. Mix and consume daily.

Black cohosh tea. Take 1 teaspoon of black cohosh into a pot with 1 cup of water. Bring to a gentle boil and allow to cook for 20 to 30 minutes. Strain and drink it warm.

Cinnamon tea. Add a stick of cinnamon to a pot of hot water and allow it to steep for about 10 minutes. Add honey to taste and drink.

Fenugreek tea. Take 2 teaspoons of fenugreek seeds. Add 1 cup water. Boil and then simmer for about 5 minutes until the water is pale yellow-brown. Strain and consume

TABLE 6.17	Common Ingredients for Fibroids	
Spices	Herbs/Leaves	Miscellaneous
Cinnamon	*Commiphora wightii* (guggulu)	Black cohosh root
Fenugreek		Milk
		Ghee
		Honey
	Lemon juice	
	Aloe vera	
	Beetroot	
	Castor oil	
	Amla	
Garlic	*Saraca asoca* (ashoka tree bark)	
Ginger	*Bauhinia variegata* (kanchanara)	
Turmeric	*Crataeva nurvala* (varun/varuna)	

the liquid. The seeds can be eaten at the same time. It can be taken once or twice a day.

Garlic. Consume two to four pips of roasted garlic and/or part of daily diet.

Ginger tea. Lightly pound about 1 to 2 inches of fresh ginger (if unavailable, use 1 to 2 teaspoons of ginger powder) and add to a cup of hot water. Allow to steep for 5 to 10 minutes. Strain and drink while warm. Add honey to taste.
Variation #1. Consume ginger as a part of daily diet.

Guggulu supplements. Guggulu is the sap produced by the Indian bdellium tree and is believed to have cholesterol-reducing properties. It is available in the form of dietary supplements. Adults can take about 25 mg of guggulu supplements every day after a meal.

Kanchanara. To make a decoction. Take 10 g of kanchanara bark powder. Add 150 mL of water. Boil and simmer until reduced to half volume. Strain into a glass bottle. To consume, take 10 to 20 mL twice a day and add ½ teaspoon of dried ginger and/or honey.

Lemon juice. Take 2 teaspoons of lemon juice. Add 1 teaspoon of baking soda to a glass of warm water. Drink it daily.

Turmeric tea. Take 2 teaspoons of turmeric powder into 3 to 4 cups of hot water. Stir and steep for about 5 to 10 minutes. Strain. Add honey, fresh lemon juice or milk to taste.

Varun. Take ½ to 1 teaspoon of varun powder and mix with honey. Consume after food.

Commercial Preparations

Kanchanara guggulu tablets. Kanchanara, guggulu, and other herbs are available in the form of commercial preparations

often as a tablet. It is often used to cleanse the lymphatic system, which is thought to be one of the causes of menstrual disorders. The herbs may also be taken with ghee, honey, or milk to form a paste.

Therapeutic Measures

Castor oil pack. Soak a thin towel or cloth in warm castor oil and place it on the abdomen. Place a hot pack on top of the oil cloth. Keep for 30 minutes. Repeat these alternate nights for 3 months.

Chinese Natural Remedies

In TCM, it is believed that fibroids are due to blood stagnation in the uterus or accumulation of dampness. Blood stagnation is often due to the estrogen dominance from the xenohormones leading to obstruction in blood flow.

Dampness is often related to poor digestion and liver function.

Several Chinese herbs regulate and balance the hormones, act as uterine tonic, and also can shrink fibroids in the uterus.

Common Recipes

Oral

Teas/Brews

Cinnamon tea. Add a stick of cinnamon to a pot of hot water and allow it to steep for about 10 minutes. Add honey to taste and drink.

Han Lian Cao. Take 9 to 30 g of han lian cao every day in the form of a decoction, paste, or juice. Alternatively, it is available in the form of commercially prepared powder or pills.

Chuan Xiong. Take 3 to 6 g of chuan xiong in the form of a decoction every day.

TABLE 6.18	Common Ingredients for Fibroids	
Spices	Herbs/Leaves	
Cinnamon	Bur reed tuber/San Leng (*Rhizoma sparganii*)	
	Ligusticum wallichii (chuan xiong)	
	False daisy (han lian cao)	
	Goldenseal root	
	Poria (*Wolfiporia extensa*)	
	Peony/Bai shao (radix paeoniae alba)	
	Moutan peony bark (*cortex moutan*)	
	Red peony root/chai shao (*radix paeoniae rubra*)	
	Female ginseng/dong quai	

San Leng. Place 3 to 9 g of san leng into a cup of boiling water and let it sit for 5 to 10 minutes. Strain and drink it warm once a day.

Goldenseal root. Take 1 teaspoon of goldenseal root or leaves. Add 2 or 3 cups of boiling water. Steep for 10 minutes. Strain and add honey or lemon to taste.

Variation #1. Consume 400 mg of goldenseal root powder every day.

Polyherbal mix. There are many combinations:

- **(Guizhi Fuling Formula):** Poria, ramulus cinnamomi, radix paeoniae rubra, radix paeoniae alba, semen persicae, and cortex moutan
- **Dong quai** polyherbal
- **Cinnamon and Poria** pills

Therapeutic Measures

Lifestyle Changes

Reduce obesity. Maintain gut health. Avoid alcohol consumption.

Hot Packs. Apply hot packs to the lower abdomen to increase blood flow.

Acupuncture. This can help small- to medium-size fibroids up to 5 cm.

- **Hegu (LI4)**—Locate the acupoint valley of harmony (LI–4 or Hegu), in the web between your thumb and index finger on your right hand. Use the left thumb and press this point for 2 minutes until sore. Repeat the same on the left hand.
- **Sanyinjiao (SP6)**—Place four fingers above the medial malleolus (inner ankle) behind the posterior edge of the tibia. It is on the spleen meridian, which is the meeting point of the liver, kidney, and spleen channels.
- **Neiguan (PC6)**—"Inner Gate" Locate this point— three finger-widths above the wrist crease, between the two tendons on the inside of the left forearm. Exert firm pressure with the thumb and hold for 5 minutes. Repeat on the other arm.
- **Guanyuan (CV4)**—"Gate of Origin." Place one hand's width below the navel. Locate this point on the conception vessel (CV) channel. It is at the intersection along the midline.
- Other points include **Zusanli (ST36), Zhongji (CV3), Qihai (CV6), Xuehai (SP10), and Zigong (MCA18).**

Western/Other Natural Remedies

Common Recipes

Oral

Teas/Brews

Apple cider vinegar. Take 2 tablespoons of apple cider vinegar and 2 tablespoons of baking soda. Add 1 glass of water. Stir and consume daily.

Black cohosh tea. Take 1 teaspoon of black cohosh into a pot with 1 cup of water. Bring to a gentle boil and allow to cook for 20 to 30 minutes. Strain and drink warm.

TABLE 6.19	Common Ingredients for Fibroids	
Herbs/Leaves	**Miscellaneous**
Dandelion (root and leaves)	*Vitex agnus-castus* (chasteberry)
Goldenseal	Omega-3 fish oil
Green tea leaf	Oregon grape root
Milk thistle	Apple cider vinegar
	Olive oil
	Lemon juice
	Evening primrose oil
	Black cohosh
	Essential oil (clary sage, thyme, and frankincense)
	Burdock root
Raspberry leaf	Castor oil

Burdock root tea. Roughly chop fresh or dried burdock root into smaller chunks. Add 2 tablespoons of the chopped root to a pot with water. Simmer for about 10 minutes. Strain and drink warm.

Variation #1. Take 1 teaspoon of dried burdock root. Add 1 cup of hot water. Steep for 10 to 15 minutes. Strain and consume three times a day.

Variation #2. Consume 10 to 25 drops of burdock root tincture three times a day. Take this for at least 3 months.

Chasteberry tea. Take 1 teaspoon of dried chasteberry or three to six crushed berries. Steep in hot water for about 10 minutes. Consume one to two times daily for a few weeks.

Variation #1. Consume 25 to 30 drops of chasteberry tincture three to four times a day.

Dandelion tea. Place dandelion roots or leaves into a pot with 1.5 cups of water. Bring to a boil and allow to simmer for about 15 minutes. Strain and drink three times a day.

Variation #1. Boil 1 teaspoon of ground dandelion root in a pot of water. Drink three to four times a day. Dandelion root is also available in tablet form.

Evening primrose. The seeds, flowers, and roots are edible. The seeds can be added to salads or smoothies. The seed oil is available as a dietary supplement.

Variation #1. Take about 2 teaspoons of dried flowers. Add 1 cup of hot water and steep for about 5 to 10 minutes. Drink twice a day.

Goldenseal root. Take 1 teaspoon of goldenseal root or leaves. Add 2 or 3 cups of boiling water. Steep for 10 minutes. Strain and add honey or lemon to taste.

Variation #1. Consume 400 mg of goldenseal root powder every day.

Green tea. Add 1 teaspoon of green tea leaves to a pot with a cup of hot water. Boil and then simmer gently for 3 to 5 minutes and strain the mixture. Add honey to taste.

Milk thistle. The seed and leaf extracts are available as powder, tablet, tea, or tincture. Steep a tea bag in a cup of hot water for 5 minutes and consume.

Olive oil and lemon mix. Take 1 tablespoon of lemon juice and 1 tablespoon of olive oil. Add 1 glass of warm water. Drink daily, first thing in the morning.

Omega-3 fish oil. Consume cold water oily fish or take omega-3 fatty acid supplements.

Oregon grape root tea. Take 2 teaspoons of dried root into a pot with 1 cup of boiling water. Bring to a boil before reducing the heat and simmer for 15 minutes. Strain and drink it warm.

Raspberry tea. Take 1 teaspoon of dried leaves. Add 1 cup of boiling water and steep for about 5 to 10 minutes. Strain and drink it warm.

Therapeutic Measures

Essential oil massage. Apply 2 drops of the essential oil (clary sage, thyme, and frankincense) on the lower abdomen and message gently. Perform this twice a day.

Modern Remedies

Choice of management would depend on the patient's reproductive wishes and contraceptive needs. Hence, the following medical management is divided as follows.

Combined Oral Contraceptive Pills

COCP consists of estrogen and progestogen and is generally given for 3 weeks. This is followed by a pill-free week in which the woman experiences a hormone withdrawal bleed. With this COCP, there is about a 50% reduction in blood loss, and there is the additional benefit of regulation of bleeding. The COCP can be *tri-cycled*—three packets are taken consecutively without the pill-free weeks. The menstrual frequency and blood loss volume are reduced. Hence, it is a preferred option for many women.

Levonorgestrel (Mirena)

This popular IUS contains an androgenic progestogen, LNG. LNG is slowly released from the IUS to act on the local endometrial environment, preventing proliferation and inducing an atrophic endometrium.

Oral and Topical Progesterone

Oral progesterone functions as an anti-estrogen by minimizing the effects of estrogen on the target cells. This causes the endometrium of the uterus to remain thin and reduce blood flow during menstruation.

Progesterone cream can also be applied on the skin.

Non-Steroidal Anti-Inflammatory Drugs

NSAIDs exert their anti-inflammatory effect through inhibition of cyclooxygenase, which is the enzyme that catalyzes the transformation of arachidonic acid to prostaglandins and thromboxane. Hence, this will reduce tissue damage at the time of menstruation and stop the prolonged menstrual bleeding.

Examples: Mefenamic acid

Tranexamic Acid

Tranexamic acid treats menorrhagia by inhibiting the activation of plasminogen to plasmin. This reduces blood clotting. It prevents fibrinolysis and blood-clot breakdown by inhibiting the endometrial plasminogen activator. It also stops the small blood vessels in the uterus lining from bleeding.

Gonadotropin-releasing Hormone (GnRH) Agonists

GnRH agonists block estrogen and progesterone production and cause a menopause-like state. Menstruation will then cease, fibroids shrink, and anemia will be less.

Example: Leuprolide acetate (Lupron subcutaneous injection) is a synthetic gonadotropin-releasing hormone.

Non-Surgical Procedures

- **Uterine artery embolization (UAE)**—this procedure is performed by a radiologist and works by blocking the blood vessels that supply the fibroids, causing them to shrink.
- **Endometrial ablation**—endometrial ablation is a procedure that uses laser energy, a heated wire loop or hot fluid in a balloon to remove uterus lining. It is mainly used to reduce heavy menstruation in patients with fibroids.

Surgery

- **Hysterectomy**—this involves the removal of the uterus (via vaginal or abdominal route or laparoscopy) and is the most effective method of removing fibroids. It is often recommended in the case of large fibroids and severe bleeding in individuals with no plans to start a family.
- **Myomectomy**—a myomectomy is a surgical procedure (via laparoscopy, hysteroscopy, or abdominal surgery) to remove fibroids from the uterus walls and is often used as an alternative to a hysterectomy. It allows individuals to have children in the future should they wish to.
- **Hysteroscopic fibroid resection**—this procedure involves the use of a hysteroscope to remove fibroids from the uterus walls. No incisions are made as the hysteroscope is introduced through the vagina and cervix into the uterus.

Homeopathic Remedies

These include *Calcarea carb* (associated heavy periods), *Thlaspi bursa pastoris* (associated prolonged periods), *Sabina officinalis* (associated clots), and *Fraxinus americana* (associated severe bearing down sensation).

Vaginal Discharge

Normal vaginal fluid is clear to translucent. It is physiological and there are changes in color, consistency, volume, and odor depending on the menstrual phase, pregnancy, breastfeeding, and during sex.

It is abnormal if there are changes in the above characteristics and if there is also associated perineal/vulvovaginal itching, redness, burning and painful urination, and foul odor of the discharge. Excessive, thick white discharge with marked perineal itching is the most common and is usually due to yeast (candida) infection.

Causes of Vaginal Discharge

- **Non-infective:** Physiological, foreign bodies (retained gauze, tampons, etc.) cervical ectopy, vulvar dermatitis, and contact/irritant dermatitis (from latex condoms or diaphragms, vaginal spermicides, or lubricants)
- **Non-sexually transmitted infection:** Bacterial vaginosis, candida infections
- **Sexually transmitted infection:** *Chlamydia trachomatis* and trichomonas vaginalis, and *Neisseria gonorrhoeae*

Risk factors include obesity, unhealthy lifestyle and diets, multiple sex partners, abortion, antibiotic overuse, associated medical conditions (like diabetes, steroid treatment, iron deficiency) intrauterine device (IUD), and oral contraceptive use.

Investigations include vaginal discharge for whiff-amine test, microscopy and culture, pH >4.5, special stains, and presence of clue cells.

General Measures for Vaginal Health

- Wash the vulva and perineum daily to keep the vagina clean. Use plain water or a mild unscented soap or hygiene wash solutions. Dab dry with a clean towel or tissue.
- Avoid bubble baths, douche, chemical-based feminine products, deodorants, feminine sprays, talc powder, or Vaseline.
- Always wash or wipe from front to back to prevent bacteria from getting into the vagina and causing an infection after passing stools.
- Moisturize the vulvovaginal area with olive oil or coconut oil if necessary.
- Use 100% cotton underwear and avoid thongs, nylon pantyhose, or tight clothing. Change often if there is profuse sweating. Undergarments must be dry and clean. Wash in hot water if they are soiled.
- Wear loose clothes during sleep and avoid wearing underwear.
- Practice good menstrual hygiene and use good quality sanitary pads.
- Eat a balanced and low-carbohydrate diet. Consume also plain unsweetened yogurt and probiotics that have *Lactobacillus acidophilus*.

TABLE 6.20	Common Ingredients for Vaginal Discharge	
Spices	**Herbs/Leaves**	**Miscellaneous**
Cumin	Nirgundi	Coconut oil
	Aloe vera	Lodhra bark
	Lady's mantle	Shatavari (Asparagus root)
		Red rice water
		Banana flowers
		Ashoka tree bark
		Dhataki flowers
Fenugreek	Neem leaves	Banyan bark
Garlic	Triphala	Yogurt
Turmeric	Guava leaves	Fig bark

- Wash the vulva and vagina, and urinate after intercourse.
- Use panty liners if discharge is heavy. Wear a sarong or lungyi if the area is inflamed and avoid intercourse.

Indian Natural Remedies

It is believed there is aggravation of kapha dosha.

Herbs and Spices

Topical

Neem (margosa) powder wash. Take some fresh washed neem leaves. Air-dry them or toast them lightly on a pan. Grind them to a powder and store in a bottle. Take 1 tablespoon of the ground neem and mix with some water. Apply in and around the vagina.

Guava leaf wash. Take a handful of guava leaves. Add 100 mL of water. Boil until the volume is reduced to 25 mL. Strain and use it as a sitz bath. Do it twice a day.

Lady's mantle leaf wash. Refer above under "Heavy Periods" to make the tea. Apply as a douche.

Banyan and fig bark wash. Take 1 tablespoon of banyan tree bark powder and 1 tablespoon of fig tree. Boil in 1 L of water and reduce to half volume. Apply as a douche.

Yogurt or coconut oil. Gently rub some yogurt or organic coconut oil on the vulva and around the vagina two or three times per day. It can also be consumed. Coconut oil is soothing and has antifungal properties against *Candida albicans*.

Fenugreek wash or tea. Take a handful of fenugreek seeds and boil in about 1 L of water. Strain and use the warm liquid to wash in and around the vagina as often as possible. It can also be consumed as an herbal tea infusion.

Triphala wash. Take about 1 tablespoon of triphala powder and boil in about 1 L of water. Strain and use the warm liquid to wash in and around the vagina as often as possible.

Shatavari (asparagus root) wash. Equal amounts of ground asparagus root mixed with honey can be applied twice a day.

Lodhra (*Symplocos racemosa*) wash. Its bark is boiled in water. Strain and use the warm liquid to wash in and around the vagina as often as possible.

Rice water wash. Extra water is added to rice that is being cooked. Drain and strain this starchy liquid. When cool, use it to wash the affected areas.

Nirgundi (Vitex negundo) wash or oil. The juice of the leaves is applied on the affected areas. The oil can also be rubbed.

Oral

Turmeric. Drink a glass of warm milk with an added teaspoonful of turmeric daily until discharge clears.

Garlic. Add more fresh garlic to the diet. Garlic capsules are also available.

Aloe vera. Drink fresh, pure aloe vera juice daily until the discharge settles.

Banana inflorescence juice. Blend or crush some banana flowers in 10 to 15 mL warm water. Add a little honey and drink the juice on an empty stomach in the morning for 2 weeks.

Banana flower dosa. To make banana flower dosai or adai, take 1 cup of rice, ¼ cup of toor dhal (yellow split pea), 2 tablespoons of black dal (urad), 1 tablespoon of chickpeas (chana dal) and 1 tablespoon of green/mung bean (moong dal). Soak overnight. Blend with some grated coconut, two red chilis, 1 teaspoon of cumin seeds, a little asafetida, and 1 cup chopped boiled banana flower. Take 2 scoops and make the pancake on a skillet.

Neem capsules. Consume neem capsules.

Ashoka bark paste. Take ¼ to ½ teaspoon ashoka tree bark powder. Add a little water or honey. Consume after meal.

  Variation #1. Place 25 g of ashoka bark powder into a pot with 200 mL of water. Boil slowly until the water has reduced to about 50 mL. Add 50 mL of milk and continue to boil until only 50 mL of liquid is left. Strain and cool. Take 20 to 30 mL in the morning to reduce menstrual blood flow.

  Variation #2. Take some ashoka tree bark and add about 200 mL of water. Boil and reduce to ¼ volume. Consume 40 to 50 mL twice a day.

Dhataki brew. Take 1 teaspoon of dried flowers. Mix with some water. Consume twice a day after meals.

Herbal red rice water. Add 1 tablespoon each of cumin and brown sugar into 1 cup of washed red rice water. Boil for 10 minutes and consume at noon.

- There are many oral and topical Ayurvedic remedies written in detail to suit the dosha type, and this information can be found under "Shweta Pradara" (meaning white discharge) or *Charaka Chikitsa Sthana*, 30th chapter, "Yoni Vyapat." This is carried out in consultation with an Ayurveda practitioner.

- Common commercial Ayurvedic formulations include:
  Lukol Himalaya tablet: Dhataki (*Woodfordia fruticosa*), shatavari (*Asparagus racemosus*), kokilaksha (*Hygrophila auriculata*), punarnava (*Boerhaavia diffusa*), and sarpagandha (*Rauwolfia serpentina*) are the main ingredients.

  Femiforte tablet: Ashoka (*Saraca indica*), triphala, vasa (*Adhatoda vasica*), jeera *(cumin seeds)*, daruharidra (*Berberis aristata*), and Amaranth (*Amaranthus spinosus*) are the main ingredients.

  Femiplex tablet: Ashoka, kankola (*Piper cubeba*), lodhra (*Symplocos racemosa*), phitkari shuddha *(Potash alum)*, triphala, and japa chhal *(Torreya nucifera)* are the main ingredients.

  Pushyanug churna: This is a polyherbal powder, which can soothe all the three doshas and is consumed with warm milk or rice water.

  V-gel Himalaya: This topical gel contains satapatri (Persian rose), triphala, and cardamon as the key ingredients.

Therapeutic Measures

Cold Hip Bath

Immerse up to hip level in a bath of icy cold water for 10 to 15 minutes. Do this twice a day. It is invigorating, improves circulation, and removes discharge.

Chinese Natural Remedies

Chinese Herbs

It is believed that abnormal vaginal discharge is a manifestation of:

- **Damp-heat in the liver channel:** This is treated with xiao yao wan formula; the key ingredients are *Angelica sinensis* root (dang gui), *Bupleurum chinense* root (chai hu), *Paeonia lactiflora* root (white peony/bai shao), *Rumex crispus* root (suan mo cao), *Silybum marianum* seed (nai ji zi), *Atractylodes* rhizome (cang zhu), *Poria-cocos* (fu ling), *Foeniculum vulgare* seed (xiao hu xiang), *Mentha* (bo he), *Althaea officinalis* root (marshmallow), *Medicago sativa* (mu xu cao), *Citrus aurantium* peel (zhi si), *Urtica dioica* (qian ma cao), and *Zingiber officinalis* (sheng jiang).

- **Dampness in the lower jiao with spleen-qi deficiency:** This is treated with gui pi tang, a spleen-qi tonic; the key ingredients include *astragalus root* (huang qi), *Codonopsis pilosula* root (dang shen), *A. sinensis* root (dang gui), *Atractylodes* rhizome (cang zhu), *Crataegus monogyna* fruit (shan zha), *Inula helenium* root (elecampane), *Poria-cocos* (fu ling), coix seed (yi yi ren), *Althea officinalis* (yao shu kui gen), *Phyllanthus emblica* (yu gan zi), and *F. vulgare* fruit (xiao hu xiang).

- **Deficiency in the liver and kidney yin:** This is treated with liu wei di huang formula: the key ingredients are *Dioscorea opposite* (shan yao), *Rehmannia glutinosa* root (shu di huang), *P. asiatica* (che qian cao), *Poria-cocos* (fu ling), *Schisandra chinensis* fruit (wu wei zi), *Polygonum multiflorum* root (he shou wu), *Elettaria cardamomum* (bai dou kou), *P. lactiflora* root (white peony/bai shao), *Scrophularia* (Xuan Shen), *Sesame indicum* (hei zhi ma), *Lycium chinense* (goji berry/gou qi zi), and *A. officinalis* root (marshmallow).

- *Steaming, washing therapy with hip bath:* The patient sits in a hip bath with a mixture of Chinese herbs in hot liquid. Before this, steaming is done.
- *Vaginal lavage or herbal douching:* This is done with various Chinese herbs to improve the vaginal pH, reduce the vaginal discharge, and kill the microorganisms.
- *Comfrey oil* extracted from comfrey (*Radix lithospermi* root) is commonly used to treat candida vaginitis. It has a high cure rate and lower-recurrence rate.

Therapeutic Measures

Acupuncture

LIV-5, HT-8, and SP-9 are useful. Commonly used acupoint injections with Chinese herbs have also been tried to decrease inflammation.

Western/Other Natural Remedies

Common Recipes

Topical (vaginal wash, vaginal suppository or pessary, douche, or Sitz bath)

Apple cider vinegar (ACV) drink, wash, or soak. Add 1 tablespoon in a glass of water to drink. The diluted solution can be applied as a wash to the affected areas. For bath, add ½ cup of the ACV into a bathtub of warm water. Garlic oil squeezed from one crushed garlic clove (or oil from one garlic pearl) can be added to the bathwater. Sit in the tub and soak for 20 minutes. Repeat once or twice a day for 5 to 7 days.

TABLE 6.21	Common Ingredients for Vaginal Discharge	
Spices	**Herbs/Leaves**	**Miscellaneous**
Persian shallot	Olive leaves	Apple cider vinegar
	Shirazi thyme	Tea tree oil
	Slippery elm (*Ulmus rubra*)	Oregano oil
	Purple coneflower/ echinacea (*Echinacea purpurea*)	Goldenseal (*Hydrastis canadensis*)
	Yarrow	Comfrey root
	Myrrh	
	Witch hazel (*Hamamelis virginiana*)	
	Sweet broom	
	Guava leaf	
	Wormwood	
	Green tea leaves	
	Blackberry	
	Blackcurrant	
	Olive leaf extract	

Tea tree oil (*Melaleuca alternifolia*) suppositories or wash. The suppository or a tampon soaked in the diluted oil can be inserted into the vagina. Two drops of the oil are mixed with 15 mL of coconut or jojoba oil. This diluted oil can also be used as a wash or rub on affected areas. Beware of its irritant effects; a forearm skin test can be tried first.

Oil of oregano. This oil from *Origanum vulgare* has antifungal properties. It is also mixed with a carrier oil and used as above.

Shirazi thyme (*Zataria multiflora*). This plant-based cream has antimicrobial effects and is used as an effective vaginal cream in Iran.

Herbal vaginal suppositories or pessaries. Various herbs such as echinacea, slippery elm, goldenseal (Hydrastis canadensis), myrrh, or yarrow can be formulated and compounded by an herbalist or homemade (using coconut oil and some essential oils and frozen).

Persian shallot (*Allium hirtifolium*). This spice plant also has antimicrobial actions.

Comfrey root, witch hazel, and goldenseal mix. Add ½ teaspoon of comfrey root and ½ teaspoon of witch hazel to 250 mL (or 2 cups) of water. Simmer for 30 minutes. Add 1 teaspoon of goldenseal. Steep for 15 minutes. Use as a vaginal douche twice a day for about 2 weeks.

Sweet broom and guava leaf wash. Take a handful of sweet broom leaves and a handful of guava leaves. Add 2 cups of boiling water. Allow to steep for 10 minutes. When cool, strain and use it as a wash.

Boric acid vaginal suppositories. This is an old remedy, and it is inserted into the vagina via an applicator for 14 days.

Oral

Wormwood (Artemisia absinthium) leaf powder. Take ½ to 1 teaspoon of dried wormwood leaves. Add 1 cup of boiling water. Steep for 5 to 10 minutes. Strain and add lemon juice and or honey to taste. It is also available as capsules.

Olive leaf extract. Consume olive leaf extract capsules once a day.

Green tea drink or wash. This can be consumed daily or applied as a wash solution as above.

Blackberry tea. Take 1 to 2 teaspoons of dried crushed blackberry leaves. Add 1 cup of hot water. Steep for 5 minutes, then strain.

Blackcurrant tea. Take 1 teaspoon of fresh chopped leaves (or 1 to 2 teaspoons of dried leaves) and add 1 cup of hot water. Steep for 5 to 10 minutes. Strain and drink.

Commercial Botanicals (Oral)

VF10 Complete Feminine Care Formula: This is a poly-botanical blend of oregano oil, olive leaf, Ceylon cinnamon, goldenseal, and caprylic acid together with vitamins (D3, pantothenic acid, and biotin) and minerals (selenium and zinc). It is available as capsules.

Therapeutic Measures

- **Hydrogen peroxide (H_2O_2) soak:** A diluted wash or bath soak can be used short-term (half-to-half mix).
- **Ozone therapy:** Ozonated water is given as a vaginal lavage for 3 days during non-menstrual days. Vaginal ozone insufflation has also been used.
- **Vitamin C:** High dose of oral vitamin C can be taken, as it has antimicrobial activity.

Modern Remedies

Bacterial vaginosis (There is an unhealthy overgrowth of anaerobic bacteria flora in the vagina and reduction in the hydrogen peroxide producing lactobacilli.)

- *Metronidazole:* Use 2 g as a single oral dose or 400 to 500 mg twice daily for 5 to 7 days or intravaginal gel (0.75%) once daily for 5 days.
- *Clindamycin:* Use intravaginal cream (2%) once daily for 7 days.

The infection often recurs, and acidic vaginal jelly (such as Relact from Kora Healthcare) may reduce relapse rates.

Vulvovaginal candidiasis

- Antifungals: Use vaginal gel or oral *imidazole* preparations (such as clotrimazole, econazole, miconazole) or oral *fluconazole* 150 mg, single dose.
- Steroid cream: It can be used if the vulva is inflamed.

Chlamydia trachomatis

- *Doxycycline:* Use 100 mg twice daily for 7 days (contraindicated in pregnancy).
- *Azithromycin:* Use 1 g orally as a single dose.

Gonorrhea

- *Cefixime:* Use 400 mg as a single oral dose.
- *Ceftriaxone:* Use 250 mg intramuscularly as a single dose.
- Referral to a genitourinary clinic is indicated due to resistant strains of the organism.

Trichomonas vaginalis

- *Metronidazole:* Use 2 g orally in a single dose or 400 to 500 mg twice daily for 5 to 7 days. Resistant strains are known to occur.
- *Tinidazole:* This is an antiparasitic drug and is effective to treat T. vaginalis.

Homeopathic Remedies

Most of these remedies do not have antifungal properties but improve the immune system to defeat the fungal or bacterial infection. They include borax, kreosotum, graphites, pulsatilla, sepia, thuja, nitric acid, natrum mur, calcarea carb, etc.

Infertility

Infertility means the failure to conceive or get pregnant for at least 1 year despite frequent unprotected intercourse.

A normal sperm count ranges from 40 to 300 million [DR1] sperms per mL of semen. A low sperm count is diagnosed if the count is less than 15 million sperms per mL or less than 39 million sperms total per ejaculation. Poor sperm motility is defined as when less than 32% [DR2] of the sperm moves effectively.

There are two types of infertility:

Primary infertility [DR3]: The woman has never conceived before, i.e., [DR4] she has had no previous pregnancies.

Secondary infertility: The woman has had a previous pregnancy but is unable to conceive again.

The causes can be due to female issues (⅓ of cases), male issues (⅓ of cases), [DR5] and combined male and female factors (⅓ of cases).

Female Causes

Ovulation problems

1. Endocrine disorders: PCOS, thyroid disease (hypothyroidism or hyperthyroidism), and hyperprolactinemia.
2. Increasing age
3. Premature ovarian failure: There is early menopause before age 40 years.

Uterus and cervix problems

1. Endometriosis
2. Uterine fibroids
3. Uterine and cervix abnormalities: Abnormal shape of uterus, polyps, benign tumors

Tubal causes

1. Tube blocks or damage from infection (pelvic inflammatory disease or sexually transmitted disease or endometriosis)
2. Previous abdominal surgery or salpingectomy
3. History of ectopic pregnancy

Others

These include unexplained infertility or recurrent miscarriage.

Male causes

1. Sexual dysfunction due to premature ejaculation. Retrograde ejaculation can occur in diabetes or spinal cord injury.
2. Sexually transmitted diseases (STDs) or urogenital infection.
3. Testicular damage (from undescended testes, infection from mumps, STD or HIV, or diabetes) or varicocele.
4. Sperm problems (sperm abnormalities, abnormal spermatogenesis, sperm motility problems, sperm transport problems, anti-sperm antibodies, and seminal plasma abnormality).

Low sperm count is the cause of about 90% of male infertility.

Combined causes

1. Substance abuse with alcohol, tobacco, and illicit drugs.
2. Occupational exposure: Radiation, pesticides, heavy metals.

3. Others include obesity, anorexia, stress, excessive sports, or exercise, underlying medical conditions, endocrine disorders, autoimmune diseases, cystic fibrosis, cancer, excessive heat from the sauna or hot tub baths or electromagnetic radiation, and medications.

General measures to improve fertility

- Well-balanced diet with sufficient dark leafy greens, asparagus, broccoli, citrus fruits, bananas, shellfish (especially oysters, eggs, garlic, walnuts, and almonds), exercise, lifestyle measures, and stress reduction are all important.
- Know when you ovulate if periods are regular. It is usually halfway. If it is a 28-day cycle, then ovulation occurs around day 14. Keep a menstrual diary.
- Lie down and lie still for at least 30 minutes or place a pillow under the pelvis so that there are better chances for the sperm to swim up to the egg.
- Use natural lubricants if required. Most oils like olive or coconut oil are safe. Chemicals in artificial lubricants can kill the sperm.
- Create romance and enjoy sex.
- Avoid vaginal sprays, douches, or scented tampons.
- Avoid overheating the scrotum from overuse of saunas, hot baths, tight clothes, placing electronic gadgets or mobile phones over the genital area.
- Avoid environmental toxins and plastics. Plastics when heated or hot can release xenohormones or xenoestrogens, which mimic estrogens that lead to endocrine disruption and reduced fertility.
- Stop oral contraceptives for at least 4 months before trying to conceive.
- Take pre-pregnancy nutritional supplements to have adequate folate, omega-3, and vitamin C.

Indian Natural Remedies

The Ayurveda approach for fertility combines diet, lifestyle, and herbs.

The *Bringhana* foods consist of *Ojas* (vitality)-enriching foods, which include organic fruits and vegetables, whole grains, cumin, saffron, honey, dates, soaked almonds or walnuts, mung beans, milk, ghee, pomegranate, etc. These are essential to build all the seven *dhatus* (tissues), including the *shukra dhatu* (reproductive tissue).

Vrishya foods are essential for shukra dhatu development, and these include asparagus, dates, broccoli, and spices (black cumin, ginger, turmeric, ajwain, fenugreek, saffron). These are aphrodisiac foods.

The main *dosha* involved in infertility is *Vata*. Ayurveda principles of management are based on practicing regular *Pankajakarma* treatments. This will lead to a healthy *Agni* and healthy *Ojas* and hence a purified body and mind. *Utharavasti* is a special medicated herbal enema administered through urethral or vaginal routes to treat male and female urogenital and reproductive disorders.

TABLE 6.22 Common Ingredients for Infertility

Spices	Herbs/Leaves	Miscellaneous
Cardamon	Shankhpushpi (*Convolvulus pluricaulis*)	Honey
Cinnamon	Guggulu (*Commiphora wightii*)	Pistachio nuts (*Pistacia vera*)
Cumin or Black cumin	Ashwagandha/Indian ginseng (*Withania somnifera*)	Ghee
Fennel	Holy basil	
	Jeevanti (*Leptadenia reticulata*)	
	Banyan tree root (*Ficus benghalensis*)	
	Bala	
	Indian abutilon (*Abutilon indicum*)	
	Punarnava (*Boerhavia diffusa*)	
Fenugreek	Shatavari (*Asparagus racemosus*)	Castor oil
Garlic	Amla (*Phyllanthus emblica*)	
Hot chillies	Aloe vera	
Mustard	Giloy/Guduchi (*Tinospora cordifolia*)	
Nutmeg	Dashamoola	Rose petal
Saffron	Jatamansi (*Nardostachys jatamansi*)	Pomegranate
Turmeric	Ashoka (*Saraca asoca/Saraca indica*)	Amla

Vata-pacifying diets and practices are essential to correct the vata imbalance.

Ayurvedic Herbs

Infertility is often related to associated or underlying issues. Hence, the treatment is directed towards eradicating the underlying cause. One herb alone is not useful and usually a combination of herbs is used to treat the organic or functional problem that caused infertility.

These herbs regulate hormone balance and menstrual cycles, improve sperm health (count, morphology, motility, and viscosity), promote sleep, reduce stress and anxiety, increase blood flow in the pelvic region, and increase energy levels so that fertility is enhanced.

Ayurvedic Herbs Used to Treat Infertility

- Ovulation disorder: Shatavari, Ashoka, Dashmoola, Aloe vera, Guggulu

- Premature ovarian failure (POF): Shatavari, Ashoka, Dashmoola, Guduchi, Jeevanti
- Blocked fallopian tubes, adhesions, and pelvic inflammatory disease: Punarnava, Guduchi
- Hormone balancing (i.e., follicle stimulating hormone [FSH] and luteinizing hormone [LH]): Shatavari, Ashwagandha, and Amalaki can effectively balance FSH and LH.
- Aphrodisiac spices: These include fenugreek and saffron.

Bala drink. Take the whole plant. Blend with little water. Extract the juice.

Ghee. Consume ghee as a part of the daily diet.

Ashwagandha. Mix 1 tablespoon of the powder in a glass of warm water and drink twice a day.

Ashoka bark paste. Take ¼ to ½ teaspoon ashoka tree bark powder. Add little water or honey. Consume after meal.
  Variation #1. Place 25 g of ashoka bark powder into a pot with 200 mL of water. Boil slowly until the water has reduced to about 50 mL. Add 50 mL of milk and continue to boil until only 50 mL of liquid is left. Strain and cool. Take 20 to 30 mL in the morning to reduce menstrual blood flow.
  Variation #2. Take some ashoka tree bark and add about 200 mL of water. Boil and reduce to ¼ volume. Consume 40 to 50 mL twice a day.

Indian abutilon. Take the whole plant. Dry and grind into powder. Consume 1 teaspoon of the powder with 1 teaspoon of honey daily for 6 months.

Jeevanti. The herbal formulation of *Leptadenia reticulata* is commonly consumed orally in tablet form.

Dashamoola. This is a polyherbal formula with 10 herbal roots. It has calming properties and is a muscle tonic. Consume 10 to 15 mL twice a day.

Shankhpushpi. Take 5 to 6 shankhpushpi (fresh blue pea) flowers. Add 1 cup of boiling water. Allow to steep for 5 to 10 minutes. Drink before bedtime.
  Variation: Mix 1 teaspoon of ground shankhpushpi into 1 cup of warm milk. Drink warm twice a day.

Guduchi juice. Place a handful of fresh guduchi leaves in a blender and blend until smooth. Strain and add honey to taste. Drink this daily in the morning on an empty stomach.

Banyan tree roots. Add 1 to 2 teaspoons of the powder into a cup of warm milk. Consume before bedtime for three consecutive nights after the end of every menstrual cycle. This is done until pregnancy.

Shukra Dhatu promoting herbs (aphrodisiacs). These include shilajit, ashwagandha, mahakalyanaka ghrita (polyherbal ghee-based formula), bhringrajasava *(Eclipta alba and other polyherbs)*, and kaunch pak (kapikacchu/ *Mucuna pruriens* with other herbominerals).

Black cumin (nigella seeds) tea. Take 1 tablespoon of nigella seeds. Crush them nicely. Add 1 cup of hot water. Steep for 10 minutes. Strain and drink.

Cinnamon. Mix 1 teaspoon of cinnamon powder in a cup of warm water. Consume daily for about 3 months. It can also be sprinkled on food.

Fenugreek tea. Take 2 teaspoons of fenugreek seeds. Add 1 cup of water. Boil and then simmer for about 5 minutes until the water is pale yellow-brown. Strain and consume the liquid. The seeds can be eaten at the same time. It can be taken once or twice a day. Consume fenugreek seeds as a part of a diet.

Pistachio nuts. Consume about 100 g of pistachio per day for 3 weeks.

Saffron. Consume about 30 g of saffron per day for 4 weeks. It can be taken with antidepressants.

Turmeric tea. Add 1 to 2 teaspoons of ground turmeric to 1 cup of hot water. Mix well and add honey to taste. Drink one to two times a day. Alternatively, lightly pound 2 to 3 inches of fresh turmeric and add to a cup of boiling water. Allow to steep for 5 to 10 minutes and strain. Add honey to taste.

Nutmeg. Mix 3 g of nutmeg powder and 3 g of sugar in a cup of milk during menses.

Garlic. Eat 4 or 5 raw garlic pips daily and then drink a cup of warm milk.

Mustard. Consume mustard paste after menses.

Holy basil. Chew three to five leaves daily followed by a cup of milk.

Fennel tea. Boil a teaspoon of fennel seeds (or fennel powder) in a pot of hot water. Strain the mixture. Drink three to four times a day.
  Variation #1. **Fennel and rose petal.** Mix 10 g of fennel seed powder and 50 g of rose petal jam. Consume this paste with a cup of warm milk every night.
  Variation #2. **Fennel and butter.** Mix 6 g of fennel powder with 2 spoons of butter and consume this paste for about 3 months.

Pomegranate. Fresh fruit or juice can be consumed. The dried seeds and bark in equal amounts can be consumed twice a day for a few weeks. Mix ½ teaspoon of this powder in a glass of warm water.

Hot chillies. Consume as part of a diet.
  Note: Some of the herbs or spices can produce the opposite effects if taken in excess.

Punarnava leaf juice. Blend or grind fresh tender punarnava leaves. Extract 1 to 2 teaspoons of juice. Add some water and consume.
  Variation #1. Blend or grind the roots to make a paste. Take 1 teaspoon and mix with milk. Consume.
  Variation #2. Take half a teaspoon of the root powder (churna). Mix with some honey and consume.
  Variation #3. Punarnava decoction. Take 1 teaspoon of the root powder (churna). Add two cups of water. Boil and reduce to ¼ volume. Take this extract and add some water to consume.

Guggulu. Adults can take about 25 mg of guggulu supplements every day after a meal.

Therapeutic Measures

Diet

Consume Ayurvedic herbs and spices to enhance fertility.

Yoga

Various poses can help towards conception. The second chakra (sacral chakra) is below the navel and related to intimacy, sexuality, and fertility. It is stimulated via various *asanas* (poses) and blood flow to the reproductive organs is increased. Also, yoga promotes relaxation and stress reduction.

Viparita Karani (leg-up-the-wall pose): This may increase the chances of conception if done immediately after sex.

Janu Shirasana (one-legged forward bend or the head to knee pose), *Paschimottanasana* (seated forward fold), *Hastapadasana* (standing forward bend,) *Bhujangasana* (cobra pose) and *Setu Bandha Sarvangasana* (bridge pose) are asanas that can increase pelvic blood flow and may improve chances of conception.

Balasana (child's pose or fetal position) and *Bhramari Pranayama* (humming bee breath) are calming and reduce stress and anxiety.

Baddha Konasana (butterfly pose): This pose can ensure a less painful delivery.

Spiritual practices

Women with reproductive issues are advised to circumambulate around the peepal tree during the early morning hours.

Chinese Natural Remedies

It is believed that infertility is due to:
- stagnation of qi and blood causing poor circulation to all organs;
- weakness in the liver or kidney qi (kidney-yang deficiency, kidney-yin deficiency);
- liver-qi stagnation; and
- heat in the organs causing problems in sperm production and mucus production in the female.

Common Recipes

Oral

Quince tea. Steam the fruits. Slice the fruit and dry it. Make the fruit into powder. Take 5 to 6 g and prepare tea.

Lilyturf root. Slice the dried root. Make it into a decoction. It can also be added to rice congee with red dates and rock sugar.

Ginger. As above.

Stinging nettle.

Lady's mantle tea. Take 5 to 10 g of lady's mantle and add 1 L of boiling water and allow it to steep for 10 to 15 minutes.

Chasteberry tea. Take 1 teaspoon of dried chasteberry and steep in hot water for about 10 minutes. Consume this as a tea drink daily for a few weeks. Capsules or tinctures are also available.

False unicorn root brew. Take ¼ to ½ teaspoon dried root. Steep in hot water. Strain and consume three times a day. For tincture, take ½ to 1 teaspoon three times a day.

Tribulus terrestris. It also regulates menstrual cycles and regular ovulation. Sexual desire, dysfunction, and libido are improved in women. It helps with PCOS. In males, it may improve sperm count and quality. It is also used in Ayurveda medicine.

Maca (*Lepidium meyenii*). Mix ¼ to ½ teaspoon of maca powder in a cup of warm milk or water and consume daily for a few months. Stop if pregnant.

TABLE 6.23	Common Ingredients for Infertility		
Spices	**Herbs/Leaves**		**Miscellaneous**
Cinnamon (Cinnamomum verum)	Stinging nettle (*Urtica dioica*)		Quince fruit (*Cydonia oblonga*)
	Lady's mantle (*Alchemilla mollis* or *Alchemilla vulgaris*)		Bitter orange/zhi shi (*Citrus aurantium*)
	Chasteberry (*Vitex agnus*)		Water plantain tuber/ze xie (*Alisma Plantain d'Eau*)
	Puncture vine/Gokshura (*Tribulus terrestris*)		Lilyturf root (*Liriope muscari*)
	Maca (*Lepidium meyenii*)		Rose flower buds (Rosa)
	Female ginseng/Dong quai (*Angelica sinensis*)		Poor man's ginseng/dang shen (*Codonopsis pilosula*)
	Asian ginseng (*Panax ginseng*)		Colla cornus cervi (deer antler gel/lu jiao jiao)
	Ginkgo biloba		
	False unicorn root (*Chamaelirium luteum*)		
	Raspberry leaf (*Rubus idaeus*)		
	Horny goat weed/yin yang huo (*Epimedium*)		
	Cynomorium/suo yang (*Cynomorium songaricum*)		
Ginger (Zingiber officinale)	Red clover (*Trifolium pretense*)		Corydalis/yan hu suo (*Corydalis yanhusuo*)

Dong Quai. It reduces bleeding due to menorrhagia and relieves PMS pain and discomfort. It also regulates hormonal levels.

Red clover. It nourishes and rejuvenates the female reproductive system. It contains isoflavone phytoestrogens and is also rich in vitamins, magnesium, and calcium. It is used to treat PMS, menopause, and infertility.

Ginkgo biloba. It increases blood flow by relaxing the blood vessels and may have aphrodisiac effects. It can interfere with blood thinners.

Red ginseng. It can improve erectile function in men and may increase sexual arousal in women. It can interfere with blood thinners.

Horny goat weed tea. Take 5 g of dried leaves or powder. Simmer in 250 mL of water. Strain and drink warm.

Red raspberry leaf. It can prevent recurrent miscarriages and help in implantation of the embryo. This tonic can be consumed as a tea drink throughout pregnancy.

Cinnamon. This spice is also used widely in traditional Chinese medicine.

There are many other herbal formulae designed to treat specific causes.

Polyherbal Formula

Ning Xia Zhong Cao Yao Shou Ce: The key ingredients include Suo Yang (cynomorium), Fu Ling (poria), Long Gu (dragon bones), Sang Piao Xiao (ootheca mantidis), and Rou Cong Rong (cistanche).

Shan Gan Ning Qing Zhong Cao Yao Xuan: It contains Shan Yao (Chinese yam), Dang Shen (codonopsis), and Fu Pen Zi (raspberry fruit).

White peony root, Bupleurum, and Dang Gui: These combinations are also used.

Therapeutic Measures

Acupuncture

It can improve and increase in vitro fertilization (IVF) success rates. It mainly decreases the stress-related hormone and increases the beta-endorphins to produce better relaxation. Blood circulation to the uterus, fertility hormonal regulation (FSH, LH, and estrogen), sperm quality and the immune system, which impact infertility, may also be improved.

The four effective acupuncture points for fertility in men and women are SP6 (Sanyinjiao), CV3 (Zhongji), CV4 (Guanyuan), and Zigong (Ex-CA1). It is started 3 months before any assisted reproductive procedure with a course of 6 to 10 treatment sessions to improve pregnancy success.

Foot or hand reflexology. Pressure on specific points on the feet or hands, which are linked to the reproductive organs, can stimulate energy flow.

Western Natural Remedies

Common Recipes

Oral

Alfalfa juice. Place a handful of fresh alfalfa into a blender and gradually add water. Blend until smooth. Drink on

TABLE 6.24	Common Ingredients for Infertility	
Spices	**Herbs/Leaves**	**Miscellaneous**
Ginger (*Zingiber officinale*)	Black cohosh (*Actaea racemosa* or *Cimicifuga racemosa*)	D-aspartic acid
		L-arginine
	Licorice (*Glycyrrhiza glabra*)	Evening primrose oil (Oenothera)
	Damiana (*Turnera diffusa*)	Alcohol
	Maca (*Lepidium meyenii*)	Apple cider vinegar
	Red clover/clover (*Trifolium pratense*)	Chocolate
	Chasteberry (*Vitex agnus*)	Oysters
	Asparagus	Vitamin E and other antioxidants
	Gingko	Pumpkin seeds
	Ginseng	Avocado
	Alfalfa	Coenzyme Q

its own or mixed with other fruit or vegetable juice. Fresh alfalfa may also be added to salads.

Asparagus. Consume it as part of the daily diet.

Black cohosh tea. Take 1 teaspoon of black cohosh into a pot with 1 cup of water. Bring to a gentle boil and allow to cook for 20 to 30 minutes. Strain and drink warm.

Chasteberry tea. Refer to "Western/Other Natural Remedies" under "Heavy Periods."

Damiana tea. Take 1 teaspoon of the dried leaves and add 1 cup of boiling water. Steep for 10 minutes. Strain and drink warm.

D-aspartic acid. It is available as supplements.

Evening primrose. The seeds, flowers, and roots are edible. The seeds can be added to salads or smoothies. The seed oil is available as a dietary supplement.

Variation #1. Take about 2 teaspoons of dried flowers. Add 1 cup of hot water and steep for about 5 to 10 minutes. Drink twice a day.

Ginger tea. Lightly pound about 1 to 2 inches of fresh ginger (if unavailable, use 1 to 2 teaspoons of ginger powder) and add to a cup of hot water. Allow to steep for 5 to 10 minutes. Strain and drink while warm. Add honey to taste.

Ginseng brew. Add 2 to 3 slices of panax ginseng to a cup of hot water and allow it to steep for 5 to 10 minutes. Drink it warm.

Licorice tea. Take 1 teaspoon of dried ground root in 1 cup of water. Boil for 5 minutes. Drain and drink warm.

Variation #1. Take a handful of licorice sticks. Wash, pound, and flatten the sticks lightly in a mortar. Put them in a saucepan of water, add a handful of raisins, and boil for about 15 to 20 minutes. Drink a cupful of this warm brew three to four times a day.

Maca. Mix ¼ to ½ teaspoon of maca powder in a cup of warm milk or water and consume daily for a few months. Stop if pregnant.

Red clover tea. Take 2 teaspoons of red clover in 1 cup of water. Boil for 5 minutes. Allow it to steep. Drink it warm.

Therapeutic Measures

Diet

Zinc-rich foods: Zinc-rich foods include oysters and pumpkin seeds. These may improve sperm count and motility and increase testosterone. Others include vitamins A, C, E, selenium-rich diets (antioxidants), vitamin B, bioflavonoids, lipoic acid, omega-3, and arginine, which also can improve sperm quantity, quality, and enhance implantation.

Aphrodisiac foods: Certain foods, plants, or spices are believed to increase sexual desire, pleasure, or performance. These include oysters, chocolate, asparagus, avocado, and ginger.

Maca: The recommended dose in commercial preparation is 1.5 to 3.5 g/day for 2 to 12 weeks.

Water: Consume sufficient water to produce adequate seminal fluid.

Coenzyme Q: It can improve sperm function and reduce excessive white cells in the seminal fluid.

Alcohol: Moderate amounts may relax the couple and create the right mood. However, excessive volumes will depress sexual function and act as a teratogen.

Apple cider vinegar: It can improve sperm count and motility by nourishing the prostate gland.

Combination products are available. They contain damiana, gingko, ginseng, vitamins, and L-arginine.

Modern Treatment

Tests in the woman include a daily basal body temperature chart (to determine ovulation), pelvic ultrasound, blood hormones to assess ovulation and pituitary function (estrogen, progesterone, gonadotropins, AMH, and prolactin). AMH levels indicate ovarian reserve, and a high level means better chances of pregnancy. Other general and specific blood or genetic tests will depend on an underlying disease.

Hysterosalpingography (HSG) is carried out by injecting a contrast into the uterus to assess the patency of the tubes and assess the cavity of the uterus. Hysteroscopy or laparoscopy are endoscopic procedures done via the cervix or navel to look at the reproductive organs.

Tests in the man include semen analysis to look at sperm count and quality, blood hormones (testosterone, DHEA, dihydrotesterone and androstenedione, and gonadotropins), scrotal or transrectal ultrasound to look at the testes, and paratesticular structures and testicular biopsy to look for abnormalities or for sperm retrieval.

Treatment for Female Infertility

General: Improve lifestyle factors (as listed under combined causes)

Specific medications

Fertility drugs to stimulate ovulation if there are ovulation problems. These include:

Clomiphene: It stimulates the pituitary to produce more gonadotropins (FSH and LH), which then stimulate the ovarian follicles, which contain the eggs. It is available as a tablet and is taken for 5 days on day 3 or day 5 after the start of the periods. Ovulation is expected to occur about 7 days after the last dose of Clomiphene. It is usually tried for 6 months. The ovulation rate is around 60% to 80%, and the pregnancy rate is about 50% within 3 months. Side effects are mild and include nausea, bloating, headaches, and hot flashes. There is a higher chance of multiple births.

Injected hormones (Gonadotropins and Gonadotropin-Releasing Hormone, GnRH): These include:

- human chorionic gonadotropin *(hCG)* to stimulate the ovaries to release an egg;
- gonadotropin-releasing hormone *(GnRH)* to stimulate the release of FSH and LH from the pituitary gland;
- gonadotropin-releasing hormone agonist *(GnRH agonist)* to prevent premature ovulation during the ovarian stimulation procedure during IVF protocol;
- gonadotropin-releasing hormone antagonist *(GnRH antagonist)* to block premature LH surge during IVF protocol; and
- human menopausal gonadotropin (hMG): This medication combines FSH and LH and stimulates the ovaries to produce eggs.

There is a risk of ovarian hyperstimulation syndrome with associated abdominal pain, tenderness, bloating, nausea, vomiting, and diarrhea.

Letrozole: This is an oral fertility drug to induce ovulation or superovulation. The side effects are similar to Clomiphene.

Metformin: This oral medication is given if there is associated PCOS.

Bromocriptine and Cabergoline: These are oral medications given if infertility is related to high prolactin levels.

Surgery: Hysteroscopic surgery or laparoscopic surgery is done for submucosal fibroids, endometrial polyps, blocked fallopian tubes, or pelvic adhesions. Laparoscopic ovarian drilling is done for PCOS if medications fail.

Treatment for Male Infertility

General: Improve lifestyle factors (as listed under combined causes).

Medications

Clomiphene, testosterone with synthetic androgens, GnRH, GnRH + HCG or anti-estrogens such as Tamoxifen, Anastrozole.

Clomiphene in males can increase testosterone and improve erectile dysfunction and sperm counts.

HCG: It can increase testosterone levels if there are low testosterone levels. It stimulates the testes to produce testosterone and sperm.

Tamoxifen: It is reported to increase sperm density and the number of live sperm, especially in severe oligospermia.

Anastrozole: It increases testosterone levels by inhibiting the aromatase enzyme, which prevents testosterone conversion to estradiol. It also improves erectile dysfunction and reduces male hypoandrogenism symptoms. Side effects include cough, bone pain, nausea, insomnia, rash, and raised liver enzymes and hemoglobin.

Surgery: These include varicocelectomy for varicocele and transurethral resection of the ejaculatory duct (TURED), an endoscopic procedure for ejaculatory duct obstruction (epididymal blockage).

Assisted reproductive technology

There are several methods to handle the egg or sperm to produce a successful pregnancy.

Sperm retrieval: There are many ways to collect sperm for fertility indications. Nonsurgical or surgical retrieval methods will be recommended by the urologist, depending on whether there is nonobstructive azoospermia or obstructive azoospermia.

Sperm preparation and processing: Several steps are involved from washing, swimming up to gradient separation to selecting the healthy, fastest-moving sperm.

Egg retrieval: Transvaginal egg (oocyte) retrieval is a minimally invasive procedure. This is done via vaginal needle aspiration and a vaginal ultrasound—transvaginal ultrasound aspiration. About 10 to 20 eggs are usually retrieved for IVF after ovarian stimulation and trigger hCG shots (medications listed above).

Intrauterine insemination (IUI): The selected sperms are inserted inside the woman's uterus via the cervix around ovulation time so that the sperm migrate to the fallopian tubes and fertilization can occur. After one cycle of IUI, the pregnancy rate is about 10% to 20% and for three to six cycles, the pregnancy rate is about 80%.

In vitro fertilization (IVF): Fertilization occurs externally. After ovarian stimulation, many mature eggs are retrieved as described above. They are then fertilized with selected sperm in a dish in the laboratory. The embryo is then implanted in the uterus.

Intracytoplasmic sperm injection (ICSI): This technique is used if there is a male infertility factor. One live sperm is injected directly into a mature egg. The pregnancy rate is around 80% to 85%. There is a small risk of egg damage during needle insertion. There is also a four times higher risk of a sex chromosome abnormality with ICSI than with natural spontaneous conception. Other risks include higher miscarriage chance, and higher learning and behavior challenges or heart defects in the ICSI-born infant.

Assisted hatching: A laser micro-hole is done in the zona pellucida, i.e., the soft shell of the early embryo just before embryo transfer. The embryo needs to hatch or come out of the zona so that it can implant on the endometrium. The zona normally will dissolve by itself. This micromanipulation may be done to ensure a better chance of embryo implantation (laser-assisted hatching).

Donor sperm or eggs: Sperm or eggs may be taken from an anonymous or known donor if the couple's own sperm or eggs cannot be used.

Surrogacy: In traditional surrogacy, the carrier woman donates her egg. The selected sperm is from the intended father or donor sperm. The pregnancy is usually established via intrauterine insemination (IUI). In gestational carrier surrogacy, the egg is not from the carrier. The egg is from the intended mother or donor or the sperm is from the intended father or donor. Pregnancy is achieved via IVF.

Homeopathic Remedies

For Females: *Pulsatilla* (for PCOS and if periods are irregular, scanty, and brief with associated infertility), *Calcarea carb* (if infertility is due to early, prolonged and profuse periods), *Abroma radix Q* (if irregular periods or dysmenorrhea), *Borax* or *Natrum phos* (if acidic vaginal discharge from a yeast infection, which can kill sperm), *Sepia* (if low sex drive or scanty periods), *Staphysagyria* (if no known cause of infertility and there is thick cervical mucus), *Natrum mur* (if fear of intercourse with sensitive genitals), etc.

For Males: *Agnus castus* (if erectile dysfunction or scanty ejaculate and associated depression), *Sepia* (if low libido), *Argentum nitricum* (if associated anxiety, hallucinations, and stress), *Conium mac* (if painful erection and ejaculation with associated nervousness), *Caladium* (if impotent with testicular itching and depression) *Lycopodium* (if genital warts, no erection, and chronic fatigue), *Anacardium orientalis* (if low libido and nocturnal emissions with anxiety), etc.

References

Heavy Periods (Menorrhagia)

Apgar, B. S., Kaufman, A. H., George-Nwogu, U., & Kittendorf, A. (2007). Treatment of menorrhagia. *American Family Physician*, *75*(12), 1813–1819. Retrieved from https://www.aafp.org/afp/2007/0615/p1813.html.

Ashoka Tree Facts and Health Benefits. (2019, August 5). *Health benefits | health benefits of foods and drinks*. Health Benefits Times. Retrieved from https://www.healthbenefitstimes.com/ashoka-tree/.

Contursi, J. (2018, November 28). *Herbs that stop heavy bleeding with fibroids*. Healthfully. Retrieved from https://healthfully.com/herbs-that-stop-heavy-bleeding-with-fibroids-6929032.html.

Health Benefits Times. (2018, December 3). *Health benefits of banana flower*. Health Benefits. Retrieved from https://www.healthbenefitstimes.com/health-benefits-of-banana-flower/.

Healthwise Staff. (2019, November 8). *Heavy menstrual periods*. Kaiser Permanente. Retrieved from https://wa.kaiserpermanente.org/kbase/topic.jhtml?docId=abo4901.

Hebbar, J. V., & Krishnamurty, M. S. (2020, August 1). *Heavy periods, menstrual bleeding: ayurvedic treatment*. Easy Ayurveda. Retrieved from https://www.easyayurveda.com/2009/09/09/heavy-periods-menstrual-bleeding-irregular-periods-ayurvedic-herbal-remedy/.

Jing Yu, J. (2021, June 23). *The cause of heavy periods [Menorrhagia]*. Sustain Health. Retrieved from https://sustainhealth.com.au/womens-health/heavy-periods/?locale=en.

Joshi, K., Soni, D., & Ranjan, A. (2019, November 29). *Dhataki*. 1mg. Retrieved from https://www.1mg.com/ayurveda/dhataki-179.

Metha, P., Tarapure, S., & Skandhan, K. P. (2018). Ayurvedic management of dysfunctional uterine bleeding: A case study. *Gynecology & Obstetrics Case Report, 04*(01), 61. Retrieved from https://doi.org/10.21767/2471-8165.1000061.

Mitchell, K. (2017, December 13). *Herbal treatments for irregular menstrual cycles*. Herbal Living. Retrieved from https://www.motherearthliving.com/gardening/plant-profile/herbal-treatments-irregular-menstrual-cycles/

Patil, A. (2017, September 10). *Heavy bleeding during periods? Save uterus with Ayurveda!* Practo. Retrieved from https://www.practo.com/healthfeed/heavy-bleeding-during-periods-save-uterus-with-ayurveda-29648/post.

Shaw, J. A. (2020, December 20). *Menorrhagia treatment & management: medical care, surgical care*. MedScape. Retrieved from https://emedicine.medscape.com/article/255540-treatment.

Shen-Nong Limited. (2007). *Chinese herbal treatment for Dysfunctional Uterine Bleeding (DUB)*. Retrieved from http://www.shen-nong.com/eng/exam/bleeding_symptoms_dub_tcm_herbal_treatment.html.

Singh, N. (2017, January 30). *Menorrhagia—6 homeopathy remedies for treating it!* Lybrate. Retrieved from https://www.lybrate.com/topic/menorrhagia-6-homeopathy-remedies-for-treating-it/3c63b127150e691633c1b13bd6c02007.

Smith, L. (2017, February 1). *What causes heavy menstrual bleeding?* Medical News Today. Retrieved from https://www.medicalnewstoday.com/articles/295202.

Times of India. (2017, July 18). *Effective Ayurveda remedies for period problems*. The Times of India. Retrieved from https://timesofindia.indiatimes.com/life-style/health-fitness/home-remedies/effective-ayurveda-remedies-for-period-problems/articleshow/59630311.cms.

TraceGains. (2012, October 31). *Menstrual problems (PMS and Menorrhagia) (Homeopathy)*. Kaiser Permanente. Retrieved from https://wa.kaiserpermanente.org/kbase/topic.jhtml?docId=hn-2241003.

Period Cramps (Dysmenorrhea)

Ahuja, A. (2018, June 7). *7 Brilliant home remedies for period pain*. NDTV Food. Retrieved from https://food.ndtv.com/health/7-home-remedies-for-period-pain-1623302.

Ashram, A. (2017, February 24). *Home remedies for menstrual cramps*. Alandi Ayurveda. Retrieved from http://ayurveda.alandiashram.org/ayurvedic-remedies/home-remedies-for-menstrual-cramps.

Blakeway, J. (2021, May 10). *Using Chinese medicine to treat menstrual cramps*. The Yinova Center. Retrieved from https://www.yinovacenter.com/blog/using-chinese-medicine-to-treat-menstrual-cramps/.

Editors of Consumer Guide. (2021, March 24). *20 Home remedies for menstrual problems*. HowStuffWorks. Retrieved from https://health.howstuffworks.com/wellness/natural-medicine/home-remedies/home-remedies-for-menstrual-problems.htm.

India Today Web Desk. (2016, December 20). *Nani ke nuske: effective home remedies for period pain*. India Today. Retrieved from https://www.indiatoday.in/lifestyle/story/nani-ke-nuskhe-effective-home-remedies-for-period-pain-358606-2016-12-20.

Mahannah, K. (2018, February 17). *The best herbs for period cramps*. Dr. Kathleen Mahannah. Retrieved from http://drkathleenmahannah.com/blog/best-herbs-for-period-cramps.

Margolin, C. (n.d.). *Stop painful menstrual cramps with Chinese herbs*. Acufinder.Com. Retrieved from https://www.acufinder.com/Acupuncture+Information/Detail/Stop+Painful+Menstrual+Cramps+with+Chinese+Herbs.

Mayo Clinic Staff. (2020, April 8). *Menstrual cramps*. Mayo Clinic. Retrieved from https://www.mayoclinic.org/diseases-conditions/menstrual-cramps/symptoms-causes/syc-20374938.

Nazario, B. (2017, April 21). *Menstrual cramps*. WebMD. Retrieved from https://www.webmd.com/women/menstrual-cramps#1.

NHS Website. (2021, May 26). *Period pain*. NHS.UK. Retrieved from https://www.nhs.uk/conditions/period-pain/.

Penman, T. (2019, September 30). *Natural remedies for menstrual cramps*. Holistic Health Herbalist. Retrieved from https://www.holistichealthherbalist.com/natural-remedies-for-menstrual-cramps/.

Shefi, E., & Schoenbart, B. (2021, March 10). *How to treat premenstrual syndrome with traditional Chinese medicine*. HowStuffWorks. Retrieved from https://health.howstuffworks.com/wellness/natural-medicine/chinese/how-to-treat-premenstrual-syndrome-with-traditional-chinese-medicine.htm.

TraceGains, Inc. (2012, October 31). *Dysmenorrhea (Painful Menstruation) (Homeopathy)*. PeaceHealth. Retrieved from https://www.peacehealth.org/medical-topics/id/hn-2220009.

WebMD (Ed.). (2020, November 3). *Caraway: Is it good for you?* WebMD. Retrieved from https://www.webmd.com/diet/caraway-good-for-you#1.

Wong, C., & Kroner, A. (2020, May 14). *How to naturally relieve menstrual cramps*. Verywell Health. Retrieved from https://www.verywellhealth.com/herbs-for-menstrual-cramps-89901.

Irregular Periods

Acupuncture Arkansas. (n.d.). *Irregular periods and Chinese medicine*. Acupuncture Arkansas. Retrieved from http://acupuncturearkansas.com/specialties-and-services/irregular-periods-and-chinese-medicine/.

All Ayurveda. (2018). *Irregular menstrual cycle*. All Ayurveda. Retrieved from https://allayurveda.com/kb/irregular-menstrual-cycle/.

DoctorNDTV. (2018, May 15). *7 best home remedies to deal with irregular periods*. Doctor.Ndtv.Com. Retrieved from https://doctor.ndtv.com/womens-health/7-best-home-remedies-to-deal-with-irregular-periods-1827217.

Ernst, H. (2019, March 7). *8 science-backed home remedies for irregular periods*. Healthline. Retrieved from https://www.healthline.com/health/womens-health/irregular-periods-home-remedies#1.

Johnson, T. (2017, April 7). *Why is my period so random?* WebMD. Retrieved from https://www.webmd.com/women/why-is-my-period-so-random.

Kumar, A. (2017, May 23). *8 homeopathic remedies for irregular menses!* Lybrate. Retrieved from https://www.lybrate.com/topic/8-homeopathic-remedies-for-irregular-menses/a9292d-39fe049f9806d3756772945586.

Kumar, D. (2018, August 21). *7 Effective home remedies for irregular periods*. NDTV Food. Retrieved from https://food.ndtv.com/health/7-effective-home-remedies-for-irregular-periods-1662651.

NHS Website. (2021, May 5). *Irregular periods*. NHS.UK. Retrieved from https://www.nhs.uk/conditions/irregular-periods/.

Sachdev, P. (2011, July 4). *Ayurvedic treatment for irregular periods*. Onlymyhealth. Retrieved from https://www.onlymyhealth.com/ayurvedic-treatment-for-irregular-periods-1303104775.

Sacred Lotus. (2021). *Irregular menses (sometimes early, sometimes late)*. Retrieved from https://www.sacredlotus.com/go/diagnosis-chinese-medicine/get/menses-irregular-symptoms-tx-obgyn-tcm.

Shen-Nong Limited. (n.d.). *Using Chinese herbs to regulate periods*. Shen-Nong. Retrieved from http://www.shen-nong.com/eng/exam/specialties_womenpms_treatment_chiherbs.html.

Wszelaki, M. (2019, March 27). *5 favorite supplements (+ recipe) for irregular cycles: A Clinician's perspective*. Hormones Balance. Retrieved from https://hormonesbalance.com/articles/5-favorite-supplements-irregular-cycles-clinicians-perspective/.

Endometriosis

Aviva Romm. (2021, March 24). *Top herbs and supplements for endometriosis*. Aviva Romm. Retrieved from https://avivaromm.com/endometriosis-herbs-supplements/.

Chen, Z., & Gong, X. (2017). Effect of Hua Yu Xiao Zheng decoction on the expression levels of vascular endothelial growth factor and angiopoietin-2 in rats with endometriosis. *Experimental and Therapeutic Medicine, 14*(6), 5743–5750. Retrieved from https://doi.org/10.3892/etm.2017.5280.

Davila, G. W. (2021, May 10). *Endometriosis treatment & management: Approach considerations, hormonal therapy, surgical intervention.* MedScape. Retrieved from https://emedicine.medscape.com/article/271899-treatment.

Duffin, J. (2018, April 4). *The best herbs for endometriosis bloating.* Endometriosis News. Retrieved from https://endometriosisnews.com/2018/04/04/endometriosis-bloating-best-herbs-peppermint-ginger-fennel/.

Flower, A., Liu, J. P., Lewith, G., Little, P., & Li, Q. (2012). Chinese herbal medicine for endometriosis. *Cochrane Database of Systematic Reviews, 05,* 1–3. Retrieved from https://doi.org/10.1002/14651858.cd006568.pub3.

Lalwani, H. (2021, January 4). *Endometriosis is treatable—Here's your guide to Ayurvedic treatment for endometriosis.* Nirogam. Retrieved from https://nirogam.com/blogs/latest-blogs/endometriosis-is-treatable-heres-your-guide-to-ayurvedic-treatment-for-endometriosis.

Pathak, N. (2021, January 11). *Endometriosis: Which medications treat it?* WebMD. Retrieved from https://www.webmd.com/women/endometriosis/understanding-endometriosis-treatment#1.

Penman, T. (2019, September 30). *How to treat endometriosis naturally.* Holistic Health Herbalist. Retrieved from https://www.holistichealthherbalist.com/how-to-treat-endometriosis-naturally/.

Planet Ayurveda. (2020, March 11). *Endometriosis Ayurvedic treatment, herbal remedies—Causes, symptoms.* Planet Ayurveda. Retrieved from https://www.planetayurveda.com/endometriosis-ayurvedic-treatment/.

Rushall, K. (2019, January 8). *Endometriosis diminished with traditional Chinese medicine.* Pacific College. Retrieved from https://www.pacificcollege.edu/news/blog/2014/09/15/endometriosis-diminished-with-traditional-chinese-medicine.

Star Homeopathy. (2020, January 7). *Star Homeopathy | Homeopathy treatment for endometriosis.* Star Homeopathy. Retrieved from https://starhomeopathy.com/endometriosis.php.

Tsai, P. J., Lin, Y. H., Chen, J. L., Yang, S. H., Chen, Y. C., & Chen, H. Y. (2017). Identifying Chinese herbal medicine network for endometriosis: implications from a population-based database in Taiwan. *Evidence-Based Complementary and Alternative Medicine, 2017,* 7501015. Retrieved from https://doi.org/10.1155/2017/7501015.

UCLA Obstetrics and Gynecology. (n.d.). *Endometriosis: What is endometriosis? Endometriosis symptoms, treatment, diagnosis.* UCLA Health. Retrieved from https://www.uclahealth.org/obgyn/endometriosis.

Polycystic Ovarian Syndrome (PCOS)

Arora, M. (2018, July 12). *PCOS Treatment in Ayurveda—Herbs, therapies, and essential tips.* FirstCry Parenting. Retrieved from https://parenting.firstcry.com/articles/pcos-treatment-in-ayurveda-herbs-therapies-and-essential-tips/.

Balance Into Health Staff. (2019, December 14). *Top 12 homeopathic remedies for polycystic ovarian syndrome or PCOS.* Balance Into Health. Retrieved from https://www.balanceintohealth.com/blog/top-12-homeopathic-remedies-for-polycystic-ovarian-syndrome-or-pcos.

Behl, M. S. (2017, September 15). *Dong Quai for PCOS: A traditional Chinese remedy for PCOS.* Sepalika. Retrieved from https://www.sepalika.com/pcos/dong-quai-pcos/.

Clossen, A. (2013, November 18). *Traditional Chinese medicine for polycystic ovarian syndrome (PCOS).* Vitality Magazine. Retrieved from https://vitalitymagazine.com/article/traditional-chinese-medicine-for-pcos/.

Mayo Clinic Staff. (2020, October 3). *Polycystic ovary syndrome (PCOS).* Mayo Clinic. Retrieved from https://www.mayoclinic.org/diseases-conditions/pcos/diagnosis-treatment/drc-20353443.

Mitha, S. (2017, December 19). *Top 5 botanical herbs for getting pregnant with PCOS.* Samina Mitha. Retrieved from http://saminamitha.com/pcos/top-5-botanical-getting-pregnant-pcos/.

Nazario, B. (2017, April 24). *What's the treatment for PCOS?* WebMD. Retrieved from https://www.webmd.com/women/treatment-pcos#1.

Office on Women's Health. (2019, April 1). *Polycystic ovary syndrome (PCOS).* Womenshealth.gov. Retrieved from https://www.womenshealth.gov/a-z-topics/polycystic-ovary-syndrome.

Pagar, A. (2020, September 3). *The ultimate list of home remedies for PCOS.* Sepalika. Retrieved from https://www.sepalika.com/home-remedies-pcos/.

Sharma, P. (2015, February 24). *Ayurvedic treatment for PCOS.* Onlymyhealth. Retrieved from https://www.onlymyhealth.com/ayurvedic-treatment-pcos-1311153324.

The Healthline Editorial Team. (2019, April 19). *Lee from America shares her secrets to thriving while living with PCOS.* Healthline. Retrieved from https://www.healthline.com/health/pcos-lee-from-america.

Watson, K., & Wilson, D. R. (2019, March 7). *30 Natural ways to help treat polycystic ovary syndrome (PCOS).* Healthline. Retrieved from https://www.healthline.com/health/womens-health/natural-treatment-pcos.

WebMD (Ed.). (n.d.). *Inositol: Overview, uses, side effects, precautions, interactions, dosing and reviews.* WebMD. Retrieved from https://www.webmd.com/vitamins/ai/ingredientmono-299/inositol.

Fibroids

Ayurwoman Ayurveda Clinic. (2019, June 30). *Fibroids in the uterus | ayurvedic herbs for fibroid.* Ayurwoman. Retrieved from https://www.ayurwoman.com.au/uterine-fibroids/.

Blakeway, J. (2021, May 10). *Self-help strategies for uterine fibroids.* The Yinova Center. Retrieved from https://www.yinovacenter.com/blog/self-help-strategies-for-uterine-fibroids/.

Chen, N. N., Han, M., Yang, H., Yang, G. Y., Wang, Y. Y., Wu, X. K., et al. (2014). Chinese herbal medicine Guizhi Fuling formula for treatment of uterine fibroids: A systematic review of randomised clinical trials. *BMC Complementary and Alternative Medicine, 14*(2). Retrieved from https://doi.org/10.1186/1472-6882-14-2.

Daily Hunt. (2021, May 4). *7 tips for treating fibroids the natural way.* Dailyhunt. Retrieved from https://m.dailyhunt.in/news/bangladesh/english/curejoy-epaper-curejoy/7+tips+for+treating+fibroids+the+natural+way-newsid-87081139.

Ellison, B. (2020, April 22). *Fibroid tumors.* Cheryls Herbs. Retrieved from https://cherylsherbs.com/blogs/faq/fibroid-tumors.

Iftikhar, N. (2019, October 30). *Shrinking fibroids with diet: Is it possible?* Healthline. Retrieved from https://www.healthline.com/health/fibroids-diet.

Iftikhar, N., & Ernest, H. (2020, July 16). *How to treat uterine fibroids yourself.* Healthline. Retrieved from https://www.healthline.com/health/fibroids-natural-treatment.

Keville, K., & Rountree, R. (2020, February 16). *Q & A: Herbs for uterine fibroids.* Motherearthliving.Com. Retrieved from https://www.motherearthliving.com/health-and-wellness/herbs-for-uterine-fibroids.

Mayo Clinic Staff. (2020, March 14). *Cystic fibrosis.* Mayo Clinic. Retrieved from https://www.mayoclinic.org/diseases-conditions/cystic-fibrosis/diagnosis-treatment/drc-20353706.

NHS Website. (2021, March 10). *Fibroids.* NHS.UK. Retrieved from https://www.nhs.uk/conditions/fibroids/.

Roy, A. (2018, May 26). *Best 5 natural ayurvedic herbs for fibroid.* WhatsCookingIndia. Retrieved from http://whatscookingindia.com/top-5-natural-ayurvedic-herbs-for-fibroid/.

Sharma, V. (2019, March 29). *Top natural homeopathic medicines for uterine fibroids.* Homeopathy at DrHomeo.com. Retrieved from https://www.drhomeo.com/uterine-fibroids/homeopathic-reme-dies-for-uterine-fibroids-treatment/.

Torres, A. (2017, March 20). *Healing uterine fibroids naturally with acupuncture and Chinese medicine.* The Curious Coconut. Retrieved from https://thecuriouscoconut.com/blog/healing-uterine-fibroids-naturally-acupuncture-chinese-medicine.

UCLA Health. (n.d.). *Fibroid treatment.* UCLA Health. Retrieved from https://www.uclahealth.org/fibroids/treatments-procedures.

Vaginal Discharge

Dharmani, V. (2017, December 1). *White discharge from vagina—Homeopathic remedies for treating it!* Lybrate. Retrieved from https://www.lybrate.com/topic/white-discharge-from-vagina-homeopathic-remedies-for-treating-it/74d46a603a0c198e5298b9651b697a57.

Ellis, M. E. (2019, November 19). *Everything you need to know about vaginal discharge.* Healthline. Retrieved from https://www.healthline.com/health/vaginal-discharge.

Nayak, B. (2020, October 26). *7 amazing Ayurvedic home remedies for white discharge.* Dr. Brahmanand Nayak. Retrieved from https://www.drbrahma.com/ayurvedic-home-remedies-for-white-discharge/.

NHS website. (2021, January 26). *Vaginal discharge.* NHS.UK. Retrieved from https://www.nhs.uk/conditions/vaginal-discharge/.

Obgyn Key. (2016, June 6). *Excessive vaginal discharge.* Obgyn Key. Retrieved from https://obgynkey.com/excessive-vaginal-discharge/.

Romm, A. (2021, March 3). *Vaginal ecology: How to keep things healthy down there.* Aviva Romm. Retrieved from https://aviva-romm.com/vaginal-ecology-down-there/.

Singh, S. (2017, October 6). *Vaginal discharge: Treatment, procedure, cost and side effects.* Lybrate. Retrieved from https://www.lybrate.com/topic/vaginal-discharge.

Spence, D., & Melville, C. (2007). Vaginal discharge. *The BMJ,* *335*(7630), 1147–1151. Retrieved from https://doi.org/10.1136/bmj.39378.633287.80.

Ullman, D. (2017, January 23). *A homeopathic perspective on women's conditions.* Homeopathic.Com. Retrieved from https://homeopathic.com/a-homeopathic-perspective-on-womens-conditions/.

Watson, S. (2020, May 28). *Vaginal discharge: What's abnormal?* WebMD. Retrieved from https://www.webmd.com/women/guide/vaginal-discharge-whats-abnormal#2.

Zelicha, K. (2020a, June 17). *Chinese medicine treating leucorrhea—Part one herbs.* Sinimed. Retrieved from https://www.sinimed.co.il/en/gynecology/chinese-medicine-treating-leucorrhea-part-one-herbs/.

Zelicha, K. (2020b, December 25). *Chinese medicine treating leucorrhea—Part two acupuncture.* Sinimed. Retrieved from https://www.sinimed.co.il/en/gynecology/chinese-medicine-treating-leucorrhea-part-two-acupuncture/.

Zhang, Q. Q., Zhang, L., Liu, Y., Wang, Y., Chen, R., Huang, Z. Y., et al. (2019). Effect of ozonated water on normal vaginal microecology and Lactobacillus. *Chinese Medical Journal,* *132*(9), 1125–1127. Retrieved from https://doi.org/10.1097/cm9.0000000000000216.

Infertility

Association for the Advancement of Restorative Medicine. (n.d.). *Red clover (Trifolium pratense).* Restorative Medicine. Retrieved from https://restorativemedicine.org/library/monographs/red-clover/.

Ayurherbs Ayurvedic Clinic Team. (2020, April 7). *How does Ayurvedic treatment for infertility work?* Ayurherbs Clinic Melbourne. Retrieved from https://www.ayurherbs.com.au/ayurvedic-treatment-for-infertility/.

Blumenfeld, Z. (2019). Fertility preservation using GnRH agonists: rationale, possible mechanisms, and explanation of controversy. *Clinical Medicine Insights: Reproductive Health,* *13,* 1–13. Retrieved from https://doi.org/10.1177/1179558119870163.

Borten, P. (2013, May 22). *Yin Yang Huo—Xian Ling Pi—Epimedium—"Horny Goat Weed."* Chinese Herbal Medicine. Retrieved from https://chineseherbinfo.com/yin-yang-huo-xian-ling-pi-epimedium-horny-goat-weed/.

Bouchez, C. (2003, October 13). *The ancient art of infertility treatment.* WebMD. Retrieved from https://www.webmd.com/infertility-and-reproduction/features/ancient-art-of-infertility-treatment.

Bovey, M., Lorenc, A., & Robinson, N. (2010, May 10). *Extent of acupuncture practice for infertility in the United Kingdom: Experiences and perceptions of the practitioners.* ScienceDirect. Retrieved from https://linkinghub.elsevier.com/retrieve/pii/S0015028210005339.

C-DAC. (2021, July 5). *Infertility management in Ayurveda.* Vikaspedia. Retrieved from https://vikaspedia.in/health/ayush/ayurveda-1/infertility.

Health Benefits Times. (2019, August 11). *Banyan tree facts and health benefits.* Health Benefits. Retrieved from https://www.healthbenefitstimes.com/banyan-tree/.

Hebbar, J. V. (2020, September 4). *Dasamoolarishtam uses, ingredients, dose, side effects, research.* AyurMedInfo. Retrieved from https://www.ayurmedinfo.com/2011/06/18/dasamoolarishtam-ingredients-uses-dose-and-side-effects/.

Indigo Herbs. (n.d.). *Bala benefits & information.* Retrieved from https://www.indigo-herbs.co.uk/natural-health-guide/benefits/bala.

Lobo, A., D'cunha, P., & Lobo, B. (2018). Effectiveness of homoeopathic treatment in female infertility. *Reproductive Medicine International,* *1*(2). Retrieved from https://doi.org/10.23937/rmi-2017/1710008.

Loike, J. D., & Masiello, D. J. (2017). Homeopathic treatment of infertility: A medical and bioethical perspective. *International Journal of Complementary & Alternative Medicine,* *5*(5). Retrieved from https://doi.org/10.15406/ijcam.2017.05.00167.

Mayo Clinic. (2019, July 25). *Infertility.* Mayo Clinic. Retrieved from https://www.mayoclinic.org/diseases-conditions/infertility/symptoms-causes/syc-20354317.

NHS Website. (2021, April 7). *Infertility.* NHS.UK. Retrieved from https://www.nhs.uk/conditions/infertility/.

Petruzzello, M. (2017, November 17). *Black cumin.* Encyclopedia Britannica. Retrieved from https://www.britannica.com/plant/black-cumin.

Puscheck, E. E. (2021, July 19). *Infertility: Practice essentials, overview, Etiology of infertility.* MedScape. Retrieved from https://emedicine.medscape.com/article/274143-overview.

Seladi-Schulman, J. (2019, February 3). *Everything you need to know about infertility.* Healthline. Retrieved from https://www.healthline.com/health/infertility.

Ten Benefits Editorial Team. (2019, October 7). *10 Benefits of Dasamoolarishtam.* Ten Benefits. Retrieved from https://tenbenefits.com/10-benefits-of-dasamoolarishtam/.

Todd, N. (2008, December 16). *Infertility treatments.* WebMD. Retrieved from https://www.webmd.com/infertility-and-reproduction/guide/understanding-infertility-treatment.

WebMD (Ed.). (n.d.). *Horny goat weed: Overview, uses, side effects, precautions, interactions, dosing and reviews.* WebMD. Retrieved from https://www.webmd.com/vitamins/ai/ingredientmono-699/horny-goat-weed.

Yarnell, E., & Abascal, K. (2009). Multiphasic herbal prescribing for menstruating women. *Alternative and Complementary Therapies,* *15*(3), 126–134. Retrieved from https://doi.org/10.1089/act.2009.15305.

Zhu, J., Arsovska, B., & Kozovska, K. (2018). Acupuncture treatment for fertility. *Open Access Macedonian Journal of Medical Sciences,* *6*(9), 1685–1687. Retrieved from https://doi.org/10.3889/oamjms.2018.379.

7

Eyes

Introduction

Eye conditions are common in both children and adults and are becoming an increasing issue due to excessive exposure to screens, leading to computer vision syndrome (CVS) or digital eye strain (DES). These are characterized by a range of symptoms such as dry eyes, blurry vision, and increased risks of short-sightedness (myopia).

Some of the eye conditions discussed are

1. Allergic conjunctivitis/allergic eyes
2. Refractive error
3. Squint
4. Preventing cataracts

Allergic Conjunctivitis/Allergic Eyes

Allergic eyes are caused by exposure to allergens in the environment. Some common allergens include pet fur, dust, and pollen. When exposed to allergens, mast cells in the eye release histamine, which causes allergic symptoms. Eye allergies produce symptoms such as swollen eyelids, eye redness, itching, burning, and tearing. Blurred vision may also occur.

Indian Natural Remedies

Common Ingredients

Common Ingredients for Allergic Conjunctivitis

Spices	Herbs/Leaves	Miscellaneous
Cardamom (Elettaria cardamomum)	Bibhitaki (Terminalia bellirica)	Milk
Coriander (Coriandrum sativum)	Cilantro (Coriandrum sativum)	Ghee
Fennel seed (Foeniculum vulgare)	Amla (Phyllanthus emblica)	Rose petal (Rosa)
Turmeric (Curcuma longa)	Haritaki (Terminalia chebula)	Castor oil (Ricinus communis)
	Green tea (Camellia sinensis)	Honey
		Lavender essential oil (Lavandula angustifolia)
		Crape jasmine (Tabernaemontana divaricata)

Common Recipes/Therapeutic Measures

Eye Compresses

Coriander seed compress. Lightly crush 1 teaspoon of coriander seeds in a small bowl. Pour hot water over the seeds and cover. Allow it to steep for 15 minutes. Strain, and soak sterile cotton balls in the liquid. Squeeze the excess fluid out, and place on closed eyelids for about 20 minutes. This may be performed two to three times a day.

Fennel compress. Place 1 teaspoon of fennel seeds in a small bowl, and pour hot water over them. Cover, and steep for 15 minutes. Strain, and soak sterile cotton balls in the liquid. Squeeze the excess fluid out, and place on closed eyelids for about 20 minutes. Repeat two to three times a day.

Cardamom compress. Lightly crush 1 teaspoon of cardamom seeds in a small bowl, and pour hot water over them. Cover, and steep for 15 minutes. Strain, and soak sterile cotton balls in the liquid. Squeeze the excess fluid out, and place on closed eyelids for about 20 minutes. Repeat two to three times a day.

Cold milk compress. Dip cotton balls into cold milk, and squeeze out any excess milk. Place on closed eyelids, and let it sit for about 10 minutes before removing.

Castor oil compress. Dip cotton balls into a bowl of castor oil, and squeeze out the excess. Place the cotton balls on closed eyelids, and let it sit for 15 minutes. Finally, remove, and wash the eyes with water.

Rose water compress. Place a cup of rose petals into a pot with 1.5 cups of water. Bring to a boil before lowering the heat and allowing it to simmer for 5 to 10 minutes. Strain the mixture, and soak sterile cotton balls in the liquid. Squeeze out any excess rose water, and place on closed eyelids. Let it sit for 15 to 20 minutes.

Green tea compress. Add 1 teaspoon of green tea leaves to a pot with a cup of hot water. Boil, and then simmer gently for 3 to 5 minutes. Soak sterile cotton balls in the liquid. Squeeze out any excess rose water, and place on closed eyelids. Let it sit for 15 to 20 minutes.

Turmeric compress. Place 1 teaspoon of turmeric into a pot with ½ cup of water. Bring to a boil, and then remove from the heat. Allow it to cool slightly. Soak sterile cotton balls in the liquid and squeeze out any excess. Place on closed eyelids for 10 to 15 minutes. Turmeric reduces inflammation and has antibacterial properties.

Eyewash/Eye Drops

Ghee. Warm a quarter cup of ghee to melt it. Allow to cool at room temperature before pouring half of the liquid into an eyecup. Place the eyecup over the eye. Tip the head back and with eyes open, immersing the eye in ghee. Keep the eyecups over the eyes for 2 minutes; blink and look around to completely immerse the eyes. Perform three to four times a week for 2 to 3 weeks.

Triphala eye wash. Triphala is made up of amla, bibhitaki, and haritaki. Add equal portions of the three ingredients into a pot with 1 cup of water. Bring to a boil, and then remove from the heat. Strain the mixture, and use the liquid to wash the eyes several times a day.

Honey eye drops. Place a drop of honey in both eyes two times a day.

Rose water eye drops. Prepare rose water as stated earlier. Place a drop of rose water into each eye two to three times a day. Rose water has astringent properties and relieves inflammation and itchiness.

Crape jasmine. Take the juice from the flowers. Use it as eye drops.

Note: Ensure that all materials and utensils are properly sterilized to avoid infections and further complications.

Ensure that the ingredients used are organic.

Therapeutic Measures

Diet
- Consume cooling herbs such as fennel tea, rose petal tea, and coriander tea—they can be drunk warm.
- Avoid dairy products.

Chinese Natural Remedies

Common Ingredients for Allergic Conjunctivitis

Herbs/Leaves	Miscellaneous
Baikal skullcap/huang qin (*Scutellaria baicalensis*)	
Balloon flower root/jie geng (*Platycodon grandiflorus; Radix*)	
Chinese angelica root /bai zhi (*Radix angelicae dahuricae*)	
Chinese foxglove root/shu dì huáng (*Rehmannia glutinosa*)	
Chinese rhubarb/dà huáng (*Rheum palmatum*)	
Chuan Xiong (*Rhizoma Ligustici Chuanxiong*)	Forsythia Fruit/Lian qiao (*Fructus Forsythiae*)
Ephedra/ma huang (*Ephedra sinica*)	Centipede/wu gong
Fang feng/Siler root (*Radix Saposhnikoviae*)	Talcum
Female ginseng/dang gui (*Angelica sinensis*)	
Great yellow gentian (*Gentiana lutea*)	
Gypsum fibrosum (shi gao)	
Japanese Catnip/Jing jie (*Herba schizonepetae*)	Gardenia fruit/zhi zi (*Fructus gardeniae*)
Liquorice/zhi gan cao (*Glycyrrhiza glabra*)	
Manchurian wild ginger/xi xin	
Notopterygium root/qiang huo (*Notopterygium Incisum Rhizoma et Radix*)	Sodium sulfate
Peony/bai shao (*Radix Paeoniae Alba*)	
Peppermint/bo he (*Mentha piperita*)	
Radix aconiti (chuan wu)	Silkworm (*Bombyx mori*)
White atractylodes rhizome/ bai zhu (*Atractylodes macrocephala*)	

Common Recipes

Oral
- Decoction for "Wind-Heat Attacking Eyes"
  - Modified "Quick Wind Dispersing Powder": Qiang huo, fang feng, jing jie, chuan xiong, chuan wu
- Decoction for "Damp-Heat in Qi Wheel"
  - Modified "Ledebouriella Powder to Unblock the Superficial": Fang feng, ma huang, da huang, sodium sulfate, jing jie, bo he, zhi zi, talcum, shi gao, lian qiao, huang qin, die geng, chuan xiong, dang gui, bai shao, bai shu, gan cao
- Decoction for "Blood Deficiency and Wind Attacking"
  - Modified "Four substance Decoction": Dang gui, chuan xiong, bai shao, shu di, fang feng, Angelica dahuria, silkworm, caltrop fruit, centipede
- Eye Wash:
  - Add 15 g of each of the following herbs to a pot with 500 mL of water: Ledebouriella root, Chinese gentian root, Manchurian wild ginger, and licorice root (gan cao). Bring to a boil, and steam the eyes over the mixture for approximately 20 to 30 minutes and blink frequently. Cool to room temperature and use as an eyewash two to three times a day.

Notes

- Wind-Heat Attacking Eyes
  - This condition presents as severe itchy eyes with a gritty, burning, or painful sensation. The inner eyelids may have a sandpaper-like rash. The eyes may be red with sticky mucus production, tearing, and blurred vision.
  - The principles of the remedy used are to disperse wind, clear the heat, activate the blood, and resolve qi stagnation in the body.
- Damp-Heat in Qi Wheel
  - This condition presents as itchy, gritty eyes with excessive tearing, and mucus. The inner eyelids may have a sandpaper-like rash. The eyes may be red with blurry vision. The patient may have a low urine volume.
  - The principles of the remedy used are to dispel dampness, clear heat, disperse the wind, and stop the itching.
- Blood Deficiency and Wind Attacking
  - This condition presents as mild to intermittent eye itching. The eyes may or may not be bloodshot.
  - The principles of the remedy are to nourish the blood, extinguish the wind, and reduce itching.

Western/Other Natural Remedies

Common Ingredients

Common Ingredients for Allergic Conjunctivitis

Herbs/Leaves	Miscellaneous
Agrimony (*Agrimonia eupatoria*)	Coconut oil
Calendula	
Chamomile flower (*Matricaria chamomilla*)	Aloe vera (*Aloe barbadensis*)
Chickweed (*Stellaria media*)	Potato (*Solanum tuberosum*)
Comfrey leaves	
Elderflower (*Sambucus canadensis*)	Tea tree oil
Eyebright (*Euphrasia officinalis*)	Teabag
Pot marigold (*Calendula officinalis*)	Saline
Witch hazel (*Hamamelis virginiana*)	Cucumber (*Cucumis sativus*)

Common Recipes

Topical

Eye Compress and Eye Wash

Cold compress. Dip sterile cotton balls in ice-cold water. Squeeze any excess fluid out, and place on closed eyelids. Let it sit for 5 to 10 minutes, and repeat two to three times a day. The cold helps to reduce inflammation and itchiness.

Chamomile compress. Place 5 to 10 dried or fresh chamomile flowers (or chamomile tea bags) into a cup. Pour boiling water over the flowers, and allow it to steep for 5 minutes. Place the tea into the refrigerator until cold. Soak sterile cotton balls in the tea, and squeeze out any excess. Place on closed eyelids for 10 to 15 minutes. Perform two to three times a day.

Witch hazel compress. Soak sterile cotton balls in witch hazel extract, and squeeze any excess out. Place on closed eyelids for 5 to 10 minutes, two to three times a day.

Comfrey leaf compress. Place a handful of fresh leaves in 1 cup of water. Boil it for 10 to 15 minutes. Place the tea into the refrigerator until cold. Soak sterile cotton balls in the tea, and squeeze out any excess. Place on closed eyelids for 10 to 15 minutes, two to three times a day.

Elderflower compress. Place a handful of fresh elderflower blossoms in a cup, and pour boiling water over it. Steep for 10 to 15 minutes before straining. Refrigerate until cold, and soak sterile cotton balls in the tea. Squeeze any excess out, and place the cotton balls on closed eyes for 15 to 20 minutes. Repeat two to three times a day.

Calendula compress. Make calendula tea by placing dried or fresh calendula petals into a cup with boiling water. Steep for approximately 5 minutes. Strain and refrigerate until cold. Soak sterile cotton balls in the tea, and squeeze any excess out. Place the cotton balls on closed eyes for 15 to 20 minutes. Repeat two to three times a day.

Agrimony compress. Place 2 to 3 teaspoons of dried agrimony into a cup with hot water. Steep for 10 to 15 minutes. Strain, and refrigerate until cold. Soak sterile cotton balls in the tea, and squeeze any excess out. Place the cotton balls on closed eyes for 15 to 20 minutes. Repeat two to three times a day.

Aloe vera juice compress. Slit an aloe vera leaf down the center, and scoop out the white gel. Discard any yellow gel. Cut the white gel into cubes, and place into a blender. Blend until smooth, and refrigerate until cold. Soak sterile cotton balls in the cold aloe vera juice, and squeeze any excess out. Place on closed eyes for 10 to 15 minutes. Repeat three to four times a day.

Cucumber. Cut two slices of cold cucumber, and place over closed eyelids. Let it sit for 5 to 10 minutes. Repeat two to three times a day.

Teabag. Refrigerate used tea bags until cold, and use them as a compress on closed eyes. Leave for 10 to 15 minutes. Use whenever the eyes begin to itch.

Potatoes. Cut two slices of a cold, raw potato, and place over closed eyelids. Let it sit for approximately 15 minutes, two to three times a day.

Eyebright eyewash. Prepare eyebright tea, and let it cool. Soak sterile cotton balls in the tea, and squeeze any excess out. Place the cotton balls on closed eyes for 15 to 20 minutes. Repeat two to three times a day.

To make the tea, take 1 to 2 teaspoons of dried eyebright. Add into 1 cup of hot water, and allow it to steep for 15 minutes. Cool until warm to the touch, and use as an eyewash three to four times a day.

Tea tree oil salve. Mix three to four drops of tea tree oil with 1 teaspoon of coconut oil. Rub this oil around the eyes, and let it sit for 20 minutes before rinsing off.

Saline eyewash. Wash the eyes with saline solution two to three times a day. Homemade saline can be made by adding ½ teaspoon of salt to 1 cup of boiled filtered water. Herbal extracts can be added to this solution if desired.

Chickweed eyewash. Take 1 to 2 teaspoons of dried herb in 1 cup of boiling water. Allow to steep for 15 to 20 minutes. Cool until warm to the touch, and use as an eyewash three to four times a day.

Chamomile eyewash. Prepare the chamomile tea. Add 3 to 4 tablespoons of fresh (or three to five dried) chamomile flowers into a cup. Pour 1 cup of boiling water over the flowers, and allow to steep for 10 minutes. Use the cool chamomile tea two to three times a day as an eyewash.

Modern Remedies

Eye Drops/Artificial Tears

Artificial tears work to increase tear volume and lubricate the eyes, providing temporary relief from irritation due to dry eyes.

Antihistamines

These medications produce competitive inhibition of histamine at the H1 receptor sites and block the effects of endogenously released histamine.

a. Azelastine eye drops: This is commonly used.

b. Emedastine difumarate (Emadine) is a relatively selective H1 receptor antagonist for topical administration.
   These eye drops are applied two to three times a day.

Mast Cell Stabilizers

Mast cell stabilizers act by inhibiting degranulation and the release of mediators such as histamine from the mast cells when exposed to specific antigens.

Example: Sodium cromoglycate drops (Nedocromil), ketotifen

It is used four times a day because it is short acting and can be used safely for many years.

Corticosteroids

Corticosteroids have antiinflammatory and immunomodulatory properties. They decrease inflammation rapidly by suppressing the migration of polymorphonuclear leukocytes and reversing increased capillary permeability.

Example: Betamethasone eye drops

If viral infection is present, steroids can make it worse. Glaucoma is another adverse occurrence. Steroid drops should be used only if other treatments fail.

Homeopathic Remedies

These include *Allium cepa* (associated eye watering and sneezing), *Euphrasia* (with inflamed eye and acrid eye discharge), *Pulsatilla* (associated with thick greenish eye discharge and relief with cold water), *Calcarea sulph* (associated yellow eye discharge), *Belladonna* (with acute inflamed

dry eyes), and *Argentum nitricum* (with copious purulent discharge).

Refractive Error

Refractive error occurs when the shape of the iris does not bend light correctly, causing blurry vision. There are four main types of refractive error:

- Myopia (nearsightedness): Myopia is when close objects are clear, but distant objects appear blurry. Myopia is usually inherited and progresses throughout childhood and the teenage years.
- Hyperopia (far-sightedness): Hyperopia is the opposite of myopia, in which close objects are blurry and distant objects are clear. Hyperopia can also be inherited.
- Presbyopia (loss of near vision with age): Past the age of 40, the lens in the eye becomes rigid and loses its focusing ability. Reading at close range becomes difficult.
- Astigmatism: Astigmatism means vision that appears slightly distorted. It causes blurred vision at all distances due to an asymmetrical curvature of the cornea.

Blue light exposure has been found to increase the risk of macular degeneration. Blue light has been found to be able to penetrate all the way to the retina and may cause damage to the light-sensitive cells there.

Indian Natural Remedies

Common Ingredients for Refractive Error

Spices	Herbs/Leaves	Miscellaneous
Black pepper (Piper nigrum)	Amla (Phyllanthus emblica)	Ground almond (Prunus dulcis)
Fennel seed (Foeniculum vulgare)	Licorice/yashtimadhu (Glycyrrhiza glabra)	Milk
Ginger	Bibhitaki (Terminalia bellirica)	Rock sugar/ mishri
	Haritaki (Terminalia chebula)	Ghee
	Bhringraj	Honey
	Coriander leaves	
	Triphala (amla + bibhitaki + haritaki)	
	Trikatu	

Common Recipes

Oral

Coriander leaf juice. Take a few sprigs of fresh coriander leaves. Blend with little water and drink.
   Variation #1. The leaves can also be ground to make fresh coriander chutney. Curry leaves may also be added.

Spice mixture. Grind black pepper and fennel seed into a fine powder. Mix 100 g of ground fennel seed, 20 g of ground black pepper, 100 g of ground almond, and 200 g of mishri. Take 1 teaspoon with milk, two times a day.

Trikatu brew. Steep equal parts of black pepper, long pepper, and ginger in a cup of hot water. Steep for about 10 to 15 minutes. Drink it warm.

Triphala and yashtimadhu powder. Mix triphala powder and yashtimadhu powder in equal proportions. Take 1 teaspoon at bedtime with some milk or water.

Variation #1. Mix 1 teaspoon of triphala powder with ghee and ½ teaspoon of honey to make a paste. Consume after each meal.

Therapeutic Measures

- **Ghee eye immersion:** Please refer to page 168 on Allergic Conjunctivitis.
  - **Bhringraj oil.** Put one to two drops of oil every night to improve vision.
- **Eye massage:** Massage around the eye with ghee to remove strain and increase blood flow to the eye muscles.
- **Eye exercises:** Perform eye exercises every day by moving the eyes in all directions. "Tratak karma" involves concentrating on a point until the eyes begin to water.
- **Palming technique:** Close both the eyes using the palms of the hands.
  - **Bhringaraj nasal drops.** Place two drops of bhringraj oil or juice mixed with water in each nostril in the morning and inhale or pull inward.

Chinese Natural Remedies

Common Ingredients for Refractive Error

Herbs/Leaves	Miscellaneous
Chrysanthemum/ju hua (*Chrysanthemum morifolium*)	Goji berry/gou qi zi (*Lycium barbarum*)
	Buddleia flower buds or mi meng hua (*Buddleja officinalis*)
Green tea leaf (*Camellia sinensis*)	Ginkgo biloba

Common Recipes

Oral

Teas/Brews

Buddleja officinalis extract. Buddleia flower bud extract is available in the form of a powder.

Chrysanthemum tea. Take a handful of dried chrysanthemum flowers into a pot with 2 cups of water. Bring to a boil, and then remove from the heat. Strain, and drink throughout the day.

Ginkgo. Ginkgo is often consumed in a sweet dessert with dried bean curd. Place five pieces of ginkgo into a pot. Add some dried bean curd (fu chuk) and approximately 2 cups of hot water. Bring to a boil, and add some rock sugar to taste. Drink the liquid, and eat the ginkgo. Alternatively, consume ginkgo in the form of an extract, available as a commercial preparation.

Goji berries. Goji berries can be consumed on their own as a snack, added to soups or consumed as tea.

Green tea. Add 1 teaspoon of green tea leaves to a pot with a cup of hot water. Boil, then simmer gently for 3 to 5 minutes and strain the mixture. Add honey to taste, and drink three to four times a day.

Therapeutic Measures

- **Eye exercises:** Perform eye exercises every day by moving the eyes in all directions.
- **Eye massage:** Massage the area around the eyes, paying special attention to the eye sockets, the bridge of the nose, the point exactly in between the eyebrows, and on the inner corners of the eyes.
  - Acupressure

Si Zhu Kong Point. It is at the outer and lateral part of the eyebrow.

Zan Zhu Point. It is at the inner and medial part of the eyebrow, near the bridge of the nose.

Western/Other Natural Remedies

Common Ingredients for Refractive Error

Spices	Herbs/Leaves	Miscellaneous
Flaxseed (*Linum usitatissimum*)	Eyebright (*Euphrasia officinalis*)	Bilberry (*Vaccinium myrtillus*)
	Indian coleus (*Coleus Forskohlii*)	Elderberry (*Sambucus canadensis*)
	Common rue (*Ruta graveolens L.*)	Chamomile

Common Recipes

Oral

- **Teas/Brews**

  Bilberry tea. Take 1.5 teaspoons of bilberry leaves into a cup with boiling water, and steep for 10 to 15 minutes. Strain, and drink it warm. Alternatively, make bilberry extract by mashing 1 teaspoon of crushed berries with 1 teaspoon of water until smooth. Take for 3 days.

  Chamomile tea. Place 5 to 10 dried or fresh chamomile flowers (or chamomile tea bags) into a cup. Pour boiling water over the flowers and allow it to steep for 5 to 10 minutes. Drink it warm.

  Elderberry tea. Take dried elderberry flowers and berries into a cup with boiling water. Allow it to steep for 15 to 20 minutes and drink it warm. Alternatively, consume elderberries in the form of an extract, available as a commercial preparation.

  Eyebright tea. Take 1 to 2 teaspoons of eyebright in 1 cup of water. Boil, and steep for 5 to 10 minutes. Strain, and drink it warm. Add honey to taste. Consume three times a day.

  Rue tea. Take 1 teaspoon of dried crushed rue leaves. Add ½ cup of boiling water. Steep for 15 minutes. Strain, and consume ½ cup a day.

- **Forskolin extract:** Forskolin is available in the form of a commercial preparation and contains about 18%

forskolin. The recommended dose for adults is about 50 mg two to three times a day.

- **Flaxseed:** Grind flaxseed into a fine powder and consume with some water. Alternatively, incorporate flaxseed into the diet.

Therapeutic Measures

- **20/20/20 rule:** Every 20 minutes of using a visual display unit (computer, TV, handphone), the individual should look at objects more than 20 feet away for at least 20 seconds. This rule should be used by people of all ages.
- **Optimal lighting:** Optimal lighting is key in reducing strain on the eyes, hence reducing the risk of worsening eyesight.
- **Nutrients:** Nutrients such as lutein and zeaxanthin (found in marigold) and carotenoids as well as astaxanthin are important for eye health because they play a role in protecting the eye against free radical damage.

Modern Remedies

Eye glasses

Prescription eye glasses are often used to correct refractive error. They do this by correcting the manner in which light is refracted onto the retina. Eyeglasses are not customizable and can cater to all types of refractive error. Presbyopia is often treated through the use of reading glasses, which makes close vision clearer.

Contact Lenses

Contact lenses are small pieces of hard or soft plastic that sits on the eyeball and corrects the refractive error.

- Soft contact lenses: Soft contacts are generally more comfortable and are used in patients with myopia, hyperopia, and mild astigmatism.
- Hard contact lenses: These are rigid contact lenses often prescribed in patients with irregular astigmatism. The lenses correct the shape of the eyeball as well as light refraction.

Surgery

- *Laser in situ keratomileusis (LASIK).* This is a laser-assisted refractive eye surgery to correct myopia, hyperopia, and astigmatism. A cutting femtolaser is used to make a flap in the outermost layer of the cornea (i.e., epithelium), then the cornea is reshaped with an excimer later, and the flap is replaced. Recovery and results occur within a few days. Chronic dry eye, halos at night, blurred vision, flap complications, or infections can occur post LASIK.
- *Photorefractive keratectomy (PRK).* It is similar to LASIK, but here, the epithelium layer of the cornea is removed. Although recovery takes about a month, PRK has a higher and longer history of success compared with LASIK.
- *Radial keratotomy (RK).* This is non-laser refractive eye surgery to correct myopia. A diamond blade is used to reshape the cornea. Complications are more compared with laser eye surgeries.

- *Automated lamellar keratoplasty (ALK).* This is non-laser refractive eye surgery to correct myopia. A microkeratome is used to make a flap and reshape the cornea. Recovery is fast, but the results are variable.
- *Intracorneal ring segments (ICRSs) or (Intacs).* This is a non-laser refractive eye surgery used to treat mild myopia and astigmatism associated with keratoconus. A small incision is made in the cornea, and then two crescent-shaped plastic rings are inserted at the outer edge of the cornea.
- *Conductive keratoplasty (CK).* This is a non-laser refractive eye surgery using radio waves via a microneedle high-frequency probe to make a ring of corneal burns to treat mild to moderate hyperopia or presbyopia after age 40.
- *Astigmatic keratotomy (AK).* This is a modified form of RK used to treat astigmatism. Tiny, precise scratches are made on the cornea to flatten the steepest part of the cornea.
  - *AK-LASIK.* The combined incisional and laser ablative surgery is used to treat high astigmatism.
- *Laser thermal keratoplasty (LTK).* This is a laser-assisted refractive eye surgery where holmium laser is used to make a ring of corneal burns (similar to CK).

Homeopathic Remedies

These include physostigma, phosphorus, *Agaricus muscarius, Ruta graveolens, Lilium tigrinum*, and others for myopia.

Strabismus/Squint

Squint is a misalignment of the eyes that is split into the following broad categories:

- *Esotropia.* Esotropia is a convergent squint characterized by one eye turning toward the inner corner of the eye, toward the nose.
- *Exotropia.* Exotropia is a divergent squint where one eye turns toward the outer corner of the eye.
- *Hypertropia and hypotropia.* Hypertropia is a squint in which one eyeball is higher than the other, whereas hypotropia is the opposite—one eyeball is lower than the other.
- *Paralytic squint.* Three cranial nerves supply the eye muscles—cranial nerves 3, 4, and 6. When these nerves get damaged, a squint and limited eye movements occur.

Indian Natural Remedies

Common Ingredients for Squint

Herbs/Leaves	Miscellaneous
Amla (*Phyllanthus emblica*)	Ghee
Bibhitaki (*Terminalia bellirica*)	Honey
Haritaki (*Terminalia chebula*)	Milk
Triphala	Carrot (*Daucus carota*)

Common Recipes

Oral

- **Triphala paste.** Mix one teaspoon of triphala powder with 1 teaspoon of ghee and 2 teaspoons of honey. Stir until it forms a paste, and consume it twice a day with milk.
- **Carrot.** Consume as part of diet.

Therapeutic Measures

- **Ghee eye drops:** Put two drops of ghee into each eye every night.
- **Eye exercise:** Perform eye exercises every day by moving the eyes in all directions. "Tratak karma" involves concentrating on a point until the eyes begin to water.
- Practice yoga and pranayama regularly.

Chinese Natural Remedies

Therapeutic Measures

Acupressure/Acupuncture

- "Huatuojiaji at C3"
  - This acupuncture point is located on the sides of the spine at C3. It is about 1.5 cm lateral to the lower border of C3.
  - The cervical C3 Huatuo is thought to innervate the eyes and may also be used as an acupressure point. This point is not usually needled and is often used with *tuina* therapy to stimulate the flow of qi.
- Small Intestine 17 (SI 17)
  - This acupuncture point is also known as tianrong, or celestial appearance. It is located on the outer aspect of the neck, behind the angle of the jaw. It is in the depression on the front border of the sternocleidomastoid muscle in the neck.
  - Massage this point for 2 to 3 minutes with the index finger if performing acupressure. It may also be used as an acupuncture point.
- Large Intestine 18 (LI 18)
  - LI 18 is also known as fu tu, or protuberance assistant. It is located on the neck, on the side of Adam's apple.
  - This point is often used in acupuncture, but needling is often shallow to avoid puncturing the jugular vein or carotid artery.
- Governing Vessel 23 (GV 23)
  - This point is known as Shangxing, or the upper star point. It is located in the midline on the top of the head, about 1.5 cm above the hairline.
- Gallbladder 8 (GB 8)
  - GB8 is also known as shuai gu, or valley lead. It is located above the apex of the ear, about 5 cm into the hairline.
  - This point is used to treat a number of conditions including visual disturbances, headaches, and migraines.
- Gallbladder 12 (GB 12)
  - GB12 is also called wangu, or completion bone. It is located in the depression behind and below the mastoid process.

Western/Other Natural Remedies

Common Ingredients for Squint

Herbs/Leaves

Eyebright *(Euphrasia officinalis)*
Lemongrass *(Cymbopogon citratus)*

Common Recipes

Oral

Teas/Brews

Eyebright tea. Take 1 to 2 teaspoons of dried eyebright. Add into 1 cup of hot water and allow it to steep for 15 minutes. Strain, and consume. Add some honey if desired.

Lemongrass tea. Cut one stick of lemongrass into smaller chunks. Place lemongrass pieces into a cup, and fill with hot water. Allow it to steep for 10 to 15 minutes before straining. Drink it warm.

Therapeutic Measures

- **Eye exercises:** Eye exercises for squint are aimed at getting the eyes to focus on the same fixed point.
  - **Pencil push-ups:** Hold a pencil at arm's length, pointing the tip away from the body. Focus on the back end of the pencil while moving it slowly toward the bridge of your nose. Keep it in focus, and stop when your vision becomes blurred.
  - **Brock string:** Attach three colored beads to a 5-foot-long string. Secure one end of the string to a stationary object, such as a chair. Space the beads out equally, and hold the other end of the string against the tip of your nose. Shift your focus from bead to bead.

Modern Remedies

Squint is often treated with a combination of patching, eyeglasses, eye drops, eye exercises, and surgery.

Patching

Patching is used in patients with a lazy eye. It is done by placing a patch over the normal eye, forcing the individual to use the lazy eye. The patch is usually worn for a set number of hours in a day to improve the lazy eye. This absolute occlusion helps the squinting eyes to see with corrected glasses, and the vision rapidly improves in that eye. The occlusion is most effective up to the age of 8 years old.

Eyeglasses

Eyeglasses are often used in children with a squint that is caused by refractive error. Refractive error is a problem with focusing light accurately on the retina due to the eye shape causing blurred vision, such as in near or far-sightedness. In some cases, eyeglasses used to correct refractive error may also cure the squint.

Eye Exercises

It is done to achieve the binocular vision and to increase the range of stereoscopic fusion preoperatively and postoperatively. Eye exercises are often used as an adjunct to other forms of squint treatment and are used to help to strengthen the eyes and encourage coordination.

Surgery

Surgery may be performed to improve the appearance of a squint and may sometimes improve judgment of depth and distance. Squint surgery involves operating on the muscles that move the eye—weak eye muscles are tightened while excessively strong eye muscles are loosened to improve the eye positioning. Absorbable stitches are used to hold the eye muscles in place.

Homeopathic Remedies

These include *Physostigma* (associated short-sightedness), *Jaborandi* (associated long-sightedness), *Gelsemium* (associated visual disturbances including blurring and diplopia), *Natrum Mur* (with eye muscle weakness and worse in bright light), and *Cyclamen* (with convergent squint and clouding vision).

Preventing Cataracts

Cataracts are blurred vision due to the clouding of the lens in the eyes, which are behind the iris and pupil. Cataracts are usually caused by aging and are more common in older people. Cataracts can occur in one or both eyes. It is the part of the eye that focuses light onto the retina to form an image. The lens is made up of water and protein. It is normally transparent, allowing light to pass through to the retina. In cataracts, the lenses become cloudy due to protein clumping causing blurred vision. The lens also adjusts the eye's focus, allowing for clear near and far-sighted vision.

Indian Natural Remedies

Common Ingredients for Preventing Cataracts

Spices	Herbs/Leaves	Miscellaneous
Turmeric *(Curcuma longa)*	Bibhitaki *(Terminalia bellirica)*	Ghee
	Haritaki *(Terminalia chebula)*	Honey
	Amla *(Phyllanthus emblica)*	
	Licorice *(Glycyrrhiza glabra)*	

Common Recipes

Oral

Pastes

Turmeric paste. Mix 3 to 6 g of ground turmeric with honey or ghee to form a paste. Consume two to three times a day.

Triphala paste. Mix 3 to 6 g of triphala powder (which contains equal amounts of amla, haritaki, and bibhitaki) with honey or ghee to form a paste. Consume two to three times a day.

Yashtimadhu (Licorice) paste. Mix 3 to 6 g of turmeric with honey or ghee to form a paste. Consume two to three times a day.

Triphala brew. Add a tablespoon of triphala powder to a cup of warm water. Mix well, and let it sit for 12 hours. Strain through a piece of clean muslin and consume.

Therapeutic measures

Amla salve. Place whole amla fruits into a blender, and blend until smooth, making about 1 L of amla juice. Add 50 g of ghee and 50 g of honey to the blended amla, and mix well. Apply to closed eyelids, and let it sit for 5 to 10 minutes before rinsing with water.

Ghee eye drops. Place two drops of ghee into each eye before bedtime every night.

Triphala eye wash. Prepare the triphala mixture as stated earlier, and strain. Use it as an eyewash two to three times a day.

Avoid rancid foods and foods rich in animal fats.

Consume larger amounts of foods high in sulfur and food rich in amino acids such as grains and legumes. Vitamin E–rich foods such as nuts and seeds may also play a role in reducing the risk of contracting cataracts.

Chinese Natural Remedies

Common Ingredients for Preventing Cataracts

Herbs/Leaves	Miscellaneous
Buddleia flower buds/mi meng hua *(Buddleja officinalis)*	Ginkgo biloba
Sophora tree flower/huai hua mi *(Styphnolobium japonicum)*	Wolfberry/goji berry *(Lycium barbarum)*
	Celosia seed/qing xiang zi *(Celosia argentea L.)*
	Chrysanthemum flower/ju hua *(Chrysanthemum morifolium)*
	Abalone shell/shi jue ming (Haliotis diversicolor)

Common Recipes

Oral

- **Gingko.** Take 1 tablespoon of fresh ginkgo leaves (or 1 teaspoon of dried leaves). Add 1 cup of hot water. Steep for 10 minutes. Strain, and consume warm. Add some honey if desired.
- **Wolfberry.** Take 1 tablespoon of dried goji berries. Soak in some warm water first, and then add 2 cups of boiling water. Steep for 3 to 5 minutes. Consume it warm. It can also be eaten as a snack or added to soups.

- **Chrysanthemum tea.** Take a handful of dried chrysanthemum flowers into a pot with 2 cups of water. Bring to a boil, and then remove from the heat. Strain and drink throughout the day.
- **Pagoda tree flower.** Dried pagoda tree flowers or buds are made into a decoction and consumed.
- **Buddleia flower buds.** Cut the flowers and buds. Boil in a pot of water for at least 20 minutes. Consume only 60 mL (or 4 to 12 g/day). Dried forms are also available.

Abalone shell. This is part of a polyherbal preparation.

Celosia seed. Take ½ teaspoon to 3 tablespoons of seeds; mix with water, and consumed as a tea.

Western/Other Natural Remedies

Common Remedies

Oral

- Consume carotene-rich foods, which are orange in color (e.g., papaya, carrots, sweet potato, pumpkin, and squash).
- Omega-3–rich foods such as salmon should be consumed regularly. They contain essential fatty acids that are beneficial to the eyes. Docosahexaenoic acid (DHA) is found in fish and is a nutrient found in large amounts in the retina.
- Eggs contain DHA and carotenoids. The carotenoids in eggs are more readily absorbed than from vegetables due to the fat content in eggs.
- Consume vitamin E–rich foods such as nuts and seeds (almonds, walnuts, and sunflower seeds). These have antioxidant properties and protect the eyes from free radical damage.

Therapeutic Measures

- Make sure to protect the eyes against ultraviolet (UV) rays from the sun, which can contribute to cataract formation in the eyes. UV light is thought to be able to oxidize protein in the eyes, hence increasing the risk of developing cataracts.
- Develop a healthy lifestyle by keeping diabetes under control and quitting smoking. Eyes should be checked frequently (once a year for unproblematic eyes).
- Reduce strain on the eyes by improving lighting in the house and limiting night driving.

Modern Remedies

Surgery

There are 3 types of cataract surgery.

1. Phacoemulsification
   A small incision is made in the eye , and a high-frequency ultrasound device is used to break the cloudy lens into pieces, which are then removed via suction.
2. Extracapsular surgery
   A longer incision is made on the side of the cornea and the cloudy core of the lens is removed in one piece. Suction is then used to remove the remainder of the lens.

The new lens is then placed behind the iris and pupil in the same location as the old lens.
   The incision is in the eye is then closed and a protective shield is placed over the eye to protect it and facilitate recovery.
3. Intracapsular surgery
   A larger incision is made compared to the extracapsular surgery. This seldom used.
4. FLACS Femtosecond laser assisted cataract surgery (FLACS) is a new form of cataract surgery.

Cataract surgery involves removing the cloudy lens in the eye and replacing it with a clear new artificial lens (intraocular lens [IOL]). A small incision is made in the eye, and a high-frequency ultrasound device is used to break the cloudy lens into pieces, which are then removed with a gentle suctioning device. The new lens is then placed behind the iris and pupil, in the same location as the old lens. The incision in the eye is then closed and a protective shield is placed over the eye to protect it and facilitate recovery. There are a number of different IOLs available:

Aspheric IOL. These IOLs have a spherical optical design, which may induce minor optical imperfections because they do not perfectly mimic the shape of the natural eye lens.

Toric IOL. Toric IOLs are used to correct astigmatism and near- and far-sightedness.

Accommodating IOL. These IOLs are designed to move forward and backward to facilitate far and near vision, such that reading glasses need not be used.

Multifocal IOL. Multifocal IOLs function in a similar manner to accommodating IOLs but provide better near vision. However, they are also more likely to cause glare or mildly blurred far vision.

Homeopathic Remedies

These include *Calcarea carbonica, Silicea, Natrum muriaticum, Calcarea fluorica, Phosphorus, Cineraria maritima, Conium, Maritima, Causticum, sulfur, Zincum sulphuricum,* and others.

References

Allergic Conjunctivitis/Allergic Eyes

American College of Allergy, Asthma & Immunology. (2014). *Eye allergies\causes, symptoms & treatment.* ACAAI Public Website. Retrieved from https://acaai.org/allergies/types/eye-allergy.

Au, A., & Grigorian, A. P. (2019, September 8). *Allergic conjunctivitis.* American Academy of Ophthalmology. Retrieved from https://eyewiki.aao.org/Allergic_Conjunctivitis.

Dabur. (n.d.). *What are eye allergies? Eye allergies meaning & definition.* Dabur.com. Retrieved from https://www.dabur.com/daburarogya/ophthalmology-eye-diseases/eye-allergies/ophthalmology-eye-diseases/eye-allergies.aspx.

Doctor NDTV. (2018, June 27). *Allergic conjunctivitis on the rise in kids and adults: 6 effective home remedies for allergic conjunctivitis.* NDTV.com. Retrieved from https://www.ndtv.com/health/allergic-conjunctivitis-on-the-rise-6-best-home-remedies-1874160.

Healy, E. (2019, May 31). *4 herbal remedies to soothe dry, itchy eyes.* NaturallySavvy.Com. Retrieved from https://naturallysavvy.com/care/4-herbal-remedies-to-soothe-dry-itchy-eyes/.

Heiting, G. (2021, June 16). *Eye allergies: Get relief from itchy, watery eyes.* All About Vision. Retrieved from https://www.allaboutvision.com/conditions/allergies.htm.

Lakshmi Ayurveda Editors. (2019, March 1). *An ayurvedic perspective of crape jasmine.* Lakshmi Ayurveda. Retrieved from https://www.lakshmiayurveda.com.au/2019/03/an-ayurvedic-perspective-of-crape-jasmine/.

Lowth, M., & Huins, H. (2017, February 28). *Allergic conjunctivitis.* Patient.com. Retrieved from https://patient.info/eye-care/eye-problems/allergic-conjunctivitis#nav-5Re.

Patel, P. (2020, March 16). *7 ways to beat seasonal allergies with Ayurveda.* Mindbodygreen. Retrieved from https://www.mindbodygreen.com/0-9869/7-ways-to-beat-seasonal-allergies-with-ayurveda.html.

Seltman, W. (2010, February 10). *How to get relief from eye allergies.* WebMD. Retrieved from https://www.webmd.com/allergies/eye-allergies#1.

Sen, P. (2017, January 19). *Eye allergies—5 homeopathic remedies for it—by Dr. Pankaj Sen.* Lybrate. Retrieved from https://www.lybrate.com/topic/eye-allergies-5-homeopathic-remedies-for-it/090e2cd08d15380e179a4c895caa6d63.

Sharma, V. (2015, September 24). *5 best homeopathic medicines for conjunctivitis.* Homeopathy at DrHomeo.com. Retrieved from https://www.drhomeo.com/homeopathic-treatment/homeopathic-medicines-conjunctivitis/.

Shen-Nong Limited. (n.d.). *Itchy eyes and Chinese medicine.* Shen-Nong. Retrieved from http://www.shen-nong.com/eng/exam/itchy_eyes.html.

Sinus & Allergy Wellness Center. (2020, October 16). *Allergic rhinitis: 6 herbal remedies to try.* Sinus & Allergy Wellness Clinic. Retrieved from https://www.sinusandallergywellnesscenter.com/blog/allergic-rhinitis-6-herbal-remedies-to-try-sinus-allergy-wellness-clinic.

Stewart, M., & Dajani, S. (2019, August 26). *Betamethasone eye drops and eye ointment (Betnesol, Vistamethasone).* Patient.com. Retrieved from https://patient.info/medicine/betamethasone-eye-drops-and-eye-ointment-betnesol-vistamethasone.

Stewart, M., & Dajani, S. (2021, April 2). *Sodium cromoglicate eye drops (Catacrom, Eycrom, Librachrom, Murine, Opticrom, Optrex, Pollenase).* Patient.com. Retrieved from https://patient.info/medicine/sodium-cromoglicate-eye-drops-catacrom-eycrom-librachrom-murine-opticrom-optrex-pollenase.

WebMD Editors. (n.d.). *Taking on eye allergies.* WebMD. Retrieved from https://www.webmd.com/eye-health/ss/slideshow-eye-allergies.

Refractive Error

Agrawal, S. (2017, April 19). *Ayurvedic treatment for myopia!* Lybrate. Retrieved from https://www.lybrate.com/topic/ayurvedic-treatment-for-myopia/8367a699fc24b6056f363f370c304bc1.

Bixler, J. E. (n.d.). *Refractive errors.* Kellogg Eye Center University of Michigan. Retrieved from https://www.umkelloggeye.org/conditions-treatments/refractive-errors.

Bjarnadottir, A. (2019, May 3). *Carrots 101: Nutrition facts and health benefits.* Healthline. Retrieved from https://www.healthline.com/nutrition/foods/carrots#plant-compounds.

Gopi, K. S. (2017, February 7). *Homoeopathy for nearsightedness or myopia.* Linkedin. Retrieved from https://www.linkedin.com/pulse/homoeopathy-nearsightedness-myopia-dr-ks-gopi.

Health Magazine. (2016, July 17). *10 ways to manage refractive errors.* Retrieved from https://www.healthmagazine.ae/health-tips-remedies/10-ways-to-manage-refractive-errors/.

National Eye Institute. (2017, January 2). *Refractive errors.* MedlinePlus. Retrieved from https://medlineplus.gov/refractiveerrors.html.

National Eye Institute. (2020, August 28). *Refractive errors.* NIE. Retrieved from https://www.nei.nih.gov/learn-about-eye-health/eye-conditions-and-diseases/refractive-errors.

Srivastava, P. K. (2016, August 2). *Ayurveda and myopia.* Lybrate. Retrieved from https://www.lybrate.com/topic/ayurveda-and-myopia/6ebfb8b475f441a82d32674748090e57.

The Johns Hopkins University. (2021). *Refractive errors.* Johns Hopkins Medicine. Retrieved from https://www.hopkinsmedicine.org/health/conditions-and-diseases/refractive-errors.

Weinberg, D. (2011, November 26). *Acupuncture for amblyopia.* Science-Based Medicine. Retrieved from https://sciencebasedmedicine.org/acupuncture-for-amblyopia/.

Squint

Brind'Amour, K. (2018, January 11). *Strabismus: Natural ways to help resolve "crossed eyes."* Dr. Axe. Retrieved from https://draxe.com/health/strabismus/.

Cyber Legend Ltd. (2014). *Small intestine SI 17.* Acupuncture.Com. Retrieved from http://acupuncture.com/education/points/small-intestine/si17.htm.

Cyber Legend Ltd. (2015a). *Large intestine LI 18.* Acupuncture.Com. Retrieved from http://acupuncture.com/education/points/largeintestine/li18.htm.

Cyber Legend Ltd. (2015b). *Shangxing.* Acupuncture.Com. Retrieved from http://www.acupuncture.com/education/points/du/du23.htm.

Doctor NDTV. (2018, March 26). *Have a squint? Get rid of it with these tips.* Doctor.Ndtv.com. Retrieved from https://doctor.ndtv.com/eyes/want-to-get-rid-of-squinted-eye-try-these-methods-1726189.

Gallbladder 12 (GB 12)—acupuncture points. (n.d.). Acufinder.com. Retrieved from https://www.acufinder.com/Acupuncture+Points/Gallbladder+12+(GB+12)/273.

Gopi, K. S. (2020, June 4). *Homeopathy for squint.* Linkedin. Retrieved from https://www.linkedin.com/pulse/homoeopathy-squint-dr-ks-gopi/.

Herbpathy. (2021). *Squint herbal treatment, prevention, symptoms, causes, cured by.* Retrieved from https://herbpathy.com/Herbal-Treatment-for-Squint-Cid4521.

Herzliya Medical Center. (n.d.). *Strabismus treatment.* Retrieved from https://hmcisrael.com/operation/strabismus-treatment/.

Jyotirmay Eye Clinic, Thane. (2018, September 5). *Eye exercises.* Jyotirmay.com. Retrieved from http://www.jyotirmay.com/eye-exercises-for-squint-treatment/.

Marcin, J. (2017, September 1). *3 eye exercises to help strabismus.* Healthline. Retrieved from https://www.healthline.com/health/eye-health/strabismus-exercises%23barrel-cards.

NHS website. (2020, January 15). *Squint.* NHS.UK. Retrieved from https://www.nhs.uk/conditions/squint/.

Prakash Nethralaya. (2021, March 13). *Ayurvedic treatment of squint or strabismus.* Ayurprakash.com. Retrieved from https://www.ayurprakash.com/diseases/eye-diseases/strabismus-squint/.

Sharma, V. (2019, March 30). *Homeopathic treatment for squint.* Homeopathy at DrHomeo.com. Retrieved from https://www.drhomeo.com/homeopathic-treatment/homeopathic-treatment-squint/.

Yin Yang House. (n.d.). *Chinese herbal and acupuncture treatment protocols for lazy eye—formulas, protocols, TCM Diagnoses.* Retrieved from https://theory.yinyanghouse.com/conditions-treated/alternative-natural-options-for-lazy-eye.

Yin Yang House. (2021a). *Huatuojiaji at C3—acupuncture point.* Retrieved from https://theory.yinyanghouse.com/acupuncturepoints/x-huatuo-c3.

Yin Yang House. (2021b). *Shuai Gu*. Retrieved from https://theory.yinyanghouse.com/acupuncturepoints/gb8.

Yoga Journal Editors. (2021). *Pranayama exercises & poses*. Yoga Journal. Retrieved from https://www.yogajournal.com/poses/types/pranayama/.

Preventing Cataracts

All About Vision Editorial Team. (2021, January 20). *Can a healthy diet prevent cataracts?* All About Vision. Retrieved from https://www.allaboutvision.com/nutrition/cataracts.htm.

Doctor NDTV. (2018a, May 21). *These amazing home remedies will help you treat cataracts*. Doctor.Ndtv.com. Retrieved from https://doctor.ndtv.com/eyes/these-amazing-home-remedies-will-help-you-treat-cataracts-1838369.

Doctor NDTV. (2018b, October 10). *Eyesight: Top 7 Ayurvedic remedies to improve eyesight*. Doctor.Ndtv.com. Retrieved from https://doctor.ndtv.com/eyes/ayurvedic-remedies-natural-remedies-eyesight-top-7-ayurvedic-remedies-to-improve-eyesight-1859254.

Frank, C. (2019, October 9). *The treatment of cataracts with Chinese medicine*. Six Fishes. Retrieved from https://sixfishes.com/2018/01/10/the-treatment-of-cataracts-with-chinese-medicine/.

Goodman, S. (2020, March 6). *Improving vision with traditional Chinese medicine*. Pacific College. Retrieved from https://www.pacificcollege.edu/news/blog/2014/09/27/improving-vision-with-traditional-chinese-medicine.

Hubbard, S. B. (2015, September 17). *9 foods that fight cataracts*. Newsmax. Retrieved from https://www.newsmax.com/health/headline/foods-fight-cataracts-nutrition/2015/09/17/id/692101/.

Mayo Clinic Staff. (2018, June 23). *Cataracts*. Mayo Clinic. Retrieved from https://www.mayoclinic.org/diseases-conditions/cataracts/diagnosis-treatment/drc-20353795.

Me and Qi. (n.d.). *Abalone shells (Shi Jue Ming) in Chinese medicine*. Meandqi.Com. Retrieved from https://www.meandqi.com/herb-database/abalone-shell.

National Eye Institute. (2019, August 3). *Cataracts*. Retrieved from https://www.nei.nih.gov/learn-about-eye-health/eye-conditions-and-diseases/cataracts.

Pacific College of Health and Science. (2020, March 6). *Acupressure points for better vision*. Pacific College. Retrieved from https://www.pacificcollege.edu/news/blog/2015/03/30/acupressure-points-for-better-vision-1.

Seltman, W. (2016, October 24). *How can I prevent cataracts?* WebMD. Retrieved from https://www.webmd.com/eye-health/cataracts/how-can-i-prevent-cataracts#1.

Sharma, V. (2019, February 15). *Effective homeopathic medicines for cataract*. Homeopathy at DrHomeo.com. Retrieved from https://www.drhomeo.com/homeopathic-treatment/homeopathic-medicines-for-cataract/.

Thompson, V. (2021, April 15). *IOLs: Choosing the best implant for cataract surgery*. All About Vision. Retrieved from https://www.allaboutvision.com/conditions/iols.htm.

TraceGains, Inc. (2012, October 31). *Cataracts (homeopathy)*. Kaiser Permanente. Retrieved from https://wa.kaiserpermanente.org/kbase/topic.jhtml?docId=hn-2208001.

Vision Source. (2014, June 25). *Is there any way to prevent cataracts?* Retrieved from https://visionsource.com/blog/prevent-cataracts/.

Wong, C., & Bull, M. (2020, April 12). *All-natural strategies to prevent cataracts as you age*. Verywell Health. Retrieved from https://www.verywellhealth.com/preventing-cataracts-naturally-89270.

Your Sight Matters. (2019, August 6). *Foods that fight cataracts*. Retrieved from https://yoursightmatters.com/foods-that-fight-cataractscid20130812ysmrm/.

8

Bones and Joints

Introduction

Some of the conditions of bones and joints discussed are:
1. Back pain
2. Fractures
3. Osteoporosis
4. Rheumatic disorders
5. Osteoarthritis (OA)
6. Cervical spondylitis

Back Pain

Back pain is a common condition because of several causes such as injury or disease affecting the:
- lower vertebrae bone (lumbar > sacral or thoracic) (e.g., fracture, OA, bone spurs, osteoporosis, scoliosis, infection, and tumor).
- discs between the vertebrae (e.g., degenerative disc disease with bulge or rupture of discs).
- muscles, ligaments (from strain, sprain, poor posture, or fall) or nerves (radicular pain, sciatica, cauda equina syndrome).
- spinal cord (spinal canal stenosis).
- adjacent pelvic internal organs (kidney infection or stones, uterus disorders), chest tumors, or aorta disease.

Risk factors include excessive physical activities/sports or occupation, old age, pregnancy, poor lifestyle, genetic predisposition, and/or underlying medical conditions.

Most backaches will resolve by 3 months.

Medical evaluation is indicated if infection (fever), tumor (weight loss), neurological deficits (leg weakness, incontinence, etc.), or persistent pain are present. Imaging for low back pain is not routinely indicated.

Indian Natural Remedies

Common Ingredients for Back Pain

Spices	Herbs/Leaves	Miscellaneous
Ajwain seed		Essential oils (clove, cumin, or lemongrass)
Cardamom		Coconut oil
Fenugreek		Honey
Garlic	*Withania somnifera* (ashwagandha)	Milk
Ginger	*Vitex negundo* (nirgundi)	Rock candy
Piper longum (long pepper)	Indian frankincense (*Boswellia serrata*)	Camphor
Turmeric	*Commiphora mukul* (guggulu)	Rock salt

Common Recipes

Oral

Teas/Brews

Ajwain tea. Place a teaspoon of ajwain seeds into a pot of water and boil it for 5 to 10 minutes. Strain the mixture, and drink warm.

Ashwagandha milk. Mix 1 teaspoon of ashwagandha in a cup of warm milk. Drink once a day at bedtime.

Cardamom-turmeric milk. Lightly crush one to two cardamom pods and place them into a cup of warm milk. Stir in a pinch of turmeric. Drink once a day before bedtime. Alternatively, add turmeric to cooked dishes as a spice.

Garlic milk. Lightly crush one to two cloves of garlic. Place in a cup, and fill with hot milk. Steep for 5 to 10 minutes before straining. Drink once a day.

Ginger–long pepper powder. Mix equal parts of ground ginger and ground long peppers. Add rock candy to the spices and mix well. Consume a teaspoon of this with a cup of warm water every night.

Ginger tea. Lightly pound about 1 to 2 inches of fresh ginger (if unavailable, use 1 to 2 teaspoons of ginger powder), and add to a cup of hot water. Allow to steep for 5 to 10 minutes. Strain, and drink while warm. Add honey to taste.

Topical Treatment

Garlic massage oil. Pour ½ cup of castor or sesame oil into a frying pan, and heat it. Add two to three lightly crushed cloves of garlic to the oil. Fry until fragrant and the garlic is lightly browned. Let it cool completely, and pour into a glass or metal container. Use this oil to massage the back.

Camphor massage oil. Place three to five pieces of camphor into a pot with ½ cup of coconut oil. Allow to boil gently for about 5 minutes before removing from the heat. Allow to cool completely and store in a glass or metal container. Use this oil to massage the back at bedtime.

Fenugreek salt. Lightly roast 100 g of fenugreek seeds. Grind to a fine powder, and mix with about 30 g of rock salt. Mix 2 teaspoons of this powder into a bowl of moderately hot water. Soak a clean piece of cotton in the mixture, and wring out any excess liquid. Place on the affected area, and let it sit until cool.

Therapeutic Measures

Diet
Diet: Consume a mainly raw diet of vegetables (tomatoes, carrot, cucumber, radish, and lettuce) and fruit. Lightly steamed or boiled vegetables may also be consumed.

Avoid fatty, fried, and spicy foods. Limit the consumption of sweetmeats, sugar, and caffeine-containing products such as tea and coffee.

Lifestyle
Yoga Poses:
- Bhujangasana (cobra pose)
- Shalabhasana (locust pose)
- Halasana (plough pose)
- Shavasana (corpse pose)
- Bharadvajasana I (Bharadwaja's twist)

Kati vasti. This is an oil retention therapy for low back pain. Warm polyherbal oil in sesame oil base is poured over a ring pool made of black gram (urad dal) paste and retained for about 20 to 30 minutes.

Chinese Natural Remedies

Causes
Qi and Blood Stagnation
- Injury or trauma to the lumbar region of the spine may cause qi and blood stasis, leading to lower back pain.
- A symptom of qi and blood stagnation is sharp fixed back pain.

Cold-Damp Exposure
- Exposure to cold and damp places for a long period leads to the accumulation of these two qualities in the body. This impairs qi and blood circulation.
- A symptom of this condition is lower back pain with a cold or heavy sensation. The pain is alleviated by warmth and may gradually worsen over time. The patient may have difficulty turning their upper body, and the pain is not relieved by lying down.

Heat-Damp Exposure
- This is due to prolonged exposure to hot, damp places. Accumulation of these qualities also causes back pains.
- This condition causes hot lower back pain, which may be present with redness and swelling. The pain may

be aggravated by rainy, hot weather and relieved by coldness and exercise.

Poor Diet
- Diets consisting of cold, raw, sweet, and fatty foods make the body "damp," causing back pains.
- In this condition, the lower back pain is sore in nature, and the patient may feel weak.

Common Ingredients for Back Pain

Herbs/Leaves	Miscellaneous
Acanthopanax root/wu jia pi (*Acanthopanax senticosus/ Eleutherococcus senticosus*)	
Cibot rhizome/gou ji (*Rhizoma Cibotii*)	
Eucommia bark/du zhong (*Eucommia ulmoides*)	Citrus (chenpi)
Myrrh (mo yao)	
Ox knee/huai niu xi (*Achyranthes bidentata*)	
Psoralea fruit/bu gu zhi (*Psoralea corylifolia fructus*)	
Rehmannia (shu di huang)	
Szechuan ox knee/chuan niu xi (*Cyathula officinalis; Radix*)	
Tang kuei (dang gui)	
Teasels/xu duan (*Dipsacus*)	Carthamus (safflower/ hong hua)

Common Recipes

Oral
Most of the aforementioned herbs are used in different combinations in the form of decoctions. They are also commercially available in the form of pills. A sensei should be consulted for an accurate and personalized set of remedies, depending on the patient's age, health status, and other information.

Therapeutic Measures
Acupressure (Topical)
- Bladder 23 (B 23) or Sea of Vitality
  This acupressure point is located in the middle of the waist, exactly between the hip bone and rib cage 2.5 inches on either side of the spine.
- Bladder 47 (B 47)
  This point is located between the second and third lumbar vertebrae, about 2.0 inches to either side of the spine.
- Bladder 18 (B 18)
  This acupressure point is found about 5 cm to the outer side of the lower border of the ninth thoracic vertebrae.
- Bladder 54 (B 54)
  This point is in the region of the sacrum, about 10 cm on the outer side of the middle sacral crest.
- Bladder 60 (B 60)
  B 60 is located on the foot, behind the outer ankle bone. It is found in the depression between the tip of the outer ankle bone and the calcaneal tendon.

- Governing Vessel 4 (GV 4)
  This point is found at the midpoint of the line joining B 23 on either side of the spine.
- **Point CV 6** (Sea of Energy point)
  Place the three fingers (i.e., index, middle, and ring finger) together just under the navel. The firm region where the ring finger is lies the CV 6 point.

Acupuncture

Acupuncture will also help with pain relief.

Western/Other Natural Remedies

Common Ingredients for Back Pain

Spices	Herbs/Leaves	Miscellaneous
Cayenne pepper	Menthol	Coconut oil
		Grated beeswax (or beeswax pastilles)
		Arnica (Arnica montana)
Clove	Willow bark	Hot pack
Turmeric	Essential oils (rosemary, lemon, bergamot, lavender, orange peel, calendula, scots pine, grapefruit, peppermint, or eucalyptus)	Cold pack

Common Recipes

Oral

Teas/Brews

Clove tea. Lightly pound three to five cloves. Place into a cup of hot water, and cover. Allow to steep for 5 to 10 minutes before straining. Drink it warm.

Turmeric tea. Add 1 to 2 teaspoons of ground turmeric to 1 cup of hot water. Mix well and add honey to taste. Drink one to two times a day. Alternatively, lightly pound 2 to 3 inches of fresh turmeric, and add to a cup of boiling water. Allow to steep for 5 to 10 minutes, and strain. Add honey to taste.

Willow bark tea. Take 2 teaspoons of willow bark into a pot with about 200 mL of water. Allow to gently simmer for about 10 minutes before removing from the heat. Strain. and add honey to taste. Drink it warm.

Topical Treatment

Cold compress. Cold packs can be used to constrict blood vessels and bring down inflammation. Wrap a cold pack in a thin towel before placing it on the skin. Place the cold pack on the skin, and leave for about 10 minutes. Repeat as necessary.

Hot compress. Hot packs may be used to reduce stiffness and hence relieve pain. Place a hot pack or warm towel on the site of pain, and leave for 10 to 15 minutes. Repeat, as necessary.

Clove oil. Lightly crush 10 to 15 cloves. Add to a pot, and pour in ½ cup of coconut oil. Gently simmer for 10 to 15 minutes. Let it cool completely and strain into a glass jar. Rub this oil over the affected area.

Capsaicin oil. Mix 3 tablespoons of cayenne pepper powder into 1 cup of coconut oil. Heat in a double boiler for about 5 to 10 minutes. Stir ½ cup of grated beeswax into the mixture and stir until it has completely dissolved. Let it cool and pour into a glass container. Rub this oil over the affected area.

Commercial Preparations

- Gels, creams, ointments, balms, roll-ons (rubefacient rubs), patches, or sprays containing capsaicin, methyl salicylate, menthol, hemp oil, or arnica are also available commercially.
- In addition, combination products that contain counterirritant analgesics (menthol, camphor, turpentine oil, oil of wintergreen/methyl salicylate, or capsaicin) mixed with essential oils (bergamot, lavender, orange peel, rosemary, lemon, calendula, scots pine, eucalyptus, and turpentine— some of the essential oils are also counterirritant) and terpineol alcohol extract are available for topical use in pain relief. Local allergic reactions should be looked out for. Examples: Perskindol, Biofreeze, Deep Heat, IcyHot

Therapeutic Measures

Chiropractic Techniques

Various spinal manipulations and adjustments are done to relieve acute back pain. Serious complications (e.g., disc herniation, nerve compression, or stroke) are rare.

Osteopathic Techniques

These include mobilization via slow and rhythmic stretching, pressure, and manipulation methods.

Modern Remedies

Oral Medication

Nonsteroidal Antiinflammatory Drugs: Analgesics

Nonsteroidal antiinflammatory drugs (NSAIDs) work by inhibiting the production of prostaglandins, which are chemicals that promote inflammation and pain. There are two prostaglandin-producing enzymes: cyclooxygenase (COX)-1 and COX-2. Both enzymes produce prostaglandins that promote inflammation and pain, but only COX-1 produces prostaglandins that protect the stomach and intestinal lining. NSAIDs block both COX-1 and COX-2 enzymes, which means that while inflammation and pain are reduced, they may cause stomach ulcers.

Examples: aspirin, celecoxib, diclofenac, ibuprofen

Muscle Relaxant

Muscle relaxants work by blocking transmission through the neuromuscular junction at nicotinic receptors, causing a decreased skeletal muscle tone. This may reduce backache by relaxing the otherwise tense muscles.

Examples: baclofen, dantrolene, metaxalone

Topical Pain Relievers

These medications are salves, creams, or ointments applied to the skin over the painful area. These work similarly to NSAIDs by inhibiting COX-1 and COX-2 enzymes, which reduces prostaglandin synthesis and sensitization of nerve endings in the peripheral tissues.

Examples: *Patches containing lidocaine* or *diclofenac sodium gel*. Counterirritants may also be added.

Physical Therapy and Support

- **Physiotherapy.** This physical therapy with various exercises and poses (some like yoga) are done to improve the range of movements, muscle strength, and function.
- **Traction.** Weights and pulleys are used to give constant or intermittent force to gradually "pull" and align the bones and joints during acute pain. There is some temporary pain relief during traction. The pain may recur after traction is off.
- **Orthotics, corsets, and belts.** These may also offer support.

Electrical Therapy

- Transcutaneous Electrical Nerve Stimulation (TENS)

  In TENS, electrode pads are placed over the area of pain. Low-frequency currents from a battery-driven gadget are given to the painful area. This blocks the incoming pain signals from the peripheral sensory nerve endings. The perception of pain is thus modified and reduced.
- Interferential Therapy (IFT)

  IFT is a type of electrical stimulation (electrotherapy) that uses medium-frequency electric currents (4000 Hz) to stimulate the muscle motor nerve fibers in deep tissues to reduce pain, swelling, and muscle spasms related to muscle, nerve, or soft-tissue injury.

  Ultrasound. It uses waves of different frequencies to heat, increase blood flow, relax the muscle, and break down scar tissue.

  Laser Therapy. Low-level laser therapy using a single wavelength of light is sometimes used by physiotherapists to treat back pain.

  Side effects include redness, discoloration, and scarring in the treated area.

Minimally Invasive Procedures

Epidural Injections

Epidural spinal injections (ESIs) and facet joint injections are done for the relief of focal chronic pain. These are minimally invasive procedures and can be done as an outpatient. Magnetic resonance imaging (MRI) of the spine is helpful to determine the site and source of pain.

Corticosteroids have an antiinflammatory effect on the tissues of the body, reducing inflammation and pain.

Steroids (dexamethasone or betamethasone) and a local anesthetic (LA; usually lidocaine, ropivacaine, bupivacaine, or mepivacaine) are injected into the epidural space via three approaches (i.e., interlaminar, caudal [sacral hiatus/tailbone opening], or transforaminal under image guidance [computed tomography [CT] or x-ray/fluoroscopy]).

With the interlaminar and caudal ESI approaches, the steroid diffuses over several spinal segments. With the transforaminal ESI (also called a nerve block), the injected steroid is more focal into one spinal segment. Prior to the steroid injection, a contrast dye is used to ensure that the medication will be in the targeted area. These medications inhibit and block nerve conduction in the area of pain. The duration of pain relief can last for several months. Spinal (lumbar) epidural injections are very safe and effective in more than 80% of patients with persistent sciatica and lumbar disc herniation. Side effects are rare, mild, and self-limiting. These include transient headaches, flushing, local increase in pain, insomnia, water retention, bleeding, infection, and hyperglycemia. Chronic use of steroid injections is not recommended as it may lead to increased functional impairment.

In facet joint pain, injections are given into and around the facet joint.

These injection treatments must be integrated with physical therapies and oral medications.

Radiofrequency Denervation

This is done for chronic low back pain if there is a good response with a diagnostic medial branch block. A CT laser-guided needle placement is done under local anesthesia. Radiofrequency waves heat the tip of the needle (to about 80°C to 90°C) to deactivate or disrupt the spinal nerve endings so that pain signals are not sent to the brain. Pain relief lasts for 6 to 12 months or even years.

In *pulsed radiofrequency,* the temperature is at 40°C. This is a nondisruptive electrical treatment to modulate and reset the nerves.

Surgery

It is seldom necessary but can be very effective. There are many types of spinal surgery for chronic back pain. The three main types are laminectomy (spinal decompression), spinal fusion, and discectomy. Others include artificial disc replacement, vertebroplasty, and foraminotomy.

Homeopathic Remedies

Depending on the symptoms in the backache patient, the remedies include *Arnica montana,* Rhus toxicodendron, Calcarea carbonica, Natrum muriaticum, Calcarea phosphorica, sulfur, Kali carbonicum, Bryonia, *Aesculus hippocastanum, Hypericum perforatum,* and others.

Fractures

Fractures are broken bones that are either completely or partially fractured in any number of ways. They are usually caused by traumatic injury or large force to a bone. There are many common types of fractures.

Stable fracture: The edges of the broken bone line up almost perfectly.

Open compound fracture: The skin is broken, and the bone may or may not be visible in the open wound.

Transverse fracture: A horizontal fracture line is known as a transverse fracture.

Oblique fracture: An oblique fracture is a bone that has been broken at an angle.

Comminuted fracture: The bone in this type of fracture is shattered—it is often broken into multiple pieces.

Indian Natural Remedies

Common Ingredients for Fracture

Spices	Herbs/Leaves/Others	Miscellaneous
Black caraway seed	Ashoka tree bark	Milk
Sesame seed	Ganglong (*Cryptolepis buchanani*)	Castor oil
	Tinospora cordifolia (*guduchi/giloy*)	Honey
Turmeric	Veld grape (*Cissus quadrangularis*)	Coconut oil

Common Recipes

Oral

Teas/Brews

Coconut Oil. Consume 1 tablespoon of coconut oil once a day. It can strengthen the bones and assist in healing.

Ganglong decoction. Make a leaf paste up to 100g. Add 200 ml milk. Consume three times per day for five days.

Giloy. Boil the giloy stem in 1 cup of milk and ginger. Strain and consume.

> Variation #1: Giloy juice. Place a handful of giloy leaves into a blender and blend until smooth. Strain and drink. Alternatively, chew on fresh giloy leaves or consume in the form of powder.

Sesame seeds. Lightly roast 1 to 2 tablespoons of sesame seeds. Consume once a day to speed up the healing process of a fracture.

Turmeric milk. Add 1 teaspoon of turmeric powder into a glass of hot milk. Drink warm once a day preferably before bedtime. Add honey to taste.

Topical Treatment

Oils and Compresses

Black caraway seed oil. Place about 2 to 3 tablespoons of black caraway seed into a pot, and add ½ cup of castor oil. Gently simmer for 5 to 10 minutes in a double boiler before removing from the heat. Place in a warm, sunny place for about 5 days before straining. To use, warm up a tablespoon of the oil and apply it to the skin over the fracture. Leave it to dry, performing three to four times a day.

Ganglong paste. Grind the leaves to make a paste. Add mustard oil. Place the mixture on a banana leave and apply it over the fracture site for 1 week or longer.

Giloy. Ground the stem into a paste and apply over the fracture site.

Veld grape. Grind the stems with some egg white to form a paste. Apply this ground paste under fracture site and bandage.

Veld grape–turmeric compress. Cut some old veld grape stems into smaller chunks, and pound into a paste. Add 1 to 2 teaspoons of ground turmeric, and mix until well combined. Place the paste into a clean piece of linen and tie it tightly. Apply this to the skin over the fracture as a compress.

Sesame seed oil. Gently warm up some sesame oil, and apply the oil to the skin over the fracture once a day.

Castor oil. Soak a clean piece of linen with castor oil, and wring out any excess oil. Wrap the piece of linen around the skin over the fracture and leave it on for one to two nights.

Coconut oil. Warm some coconut oil up, and apply it to the skin over the fracture once a day.

Ashoka tree bark paste. Take some ashoka tree bark powder. Add some water to make a paste. Apply on the fracture site.

Gandha thailam. It is an herbal medicated oil and is also available as capsules. Consume 2 to 10 drops of oil or the capsules with milk daily. It can also be applied externally to hasten fracture healing.

Notes

Natural remedies for fractures should never be used alone. It should only ever be used as an adjunct to allopathic treatment.

There are many other bone setting herbs used by traditional healers in India.

These include Bambusa arundinacea (Bamboo), Symphytum officinale (knit bone), Mesua ferrea (Nagkesar), Commiphora weighti (Guggul), Terminalia arjuna (Arjuna), Acacia arabica (Babool), Teasel (Dipsacus species), Cannabis sativa (Bhang), Piper Long (Pippali), Curcuma Longa (Tumeric), Cedrus deodara (Cedarwood), Betula utilis (Birch), Piper sarmentosum (Wild betel/Kadok), Coelogyne cristata (angel orchid), Ehretia cymosa (Murembu tree), and Pholidota articulata (rattlesnake orchid) are also used for healing fractures.

Chinese Natural Remedies

Common Ingredients for Fracture

Herbs/Leaves	Miscellaneous
Angelica sinensis (dang gui)	
Burreed tuber/San Leng (*Rhizoma sparganii*)	Dan shen (*Salvia miltiorrhiza*)
Corydalis/yan hu suo (*Corydalis yanhusuo*)	
Frankincense/ru xiang (*Olibanum gummi*)	*Glycyrrhiza glabra* (licorice root/gan cao)
Myrrh (mo yao)	*Dioscorea villosa* (wild yam)
Teasels/xu duan (*Dipsacus*)	Red peony root (chi shao)

Common Recipes

Oral

Teas/Brews

Dang gui. The dried root is boiled for 2 hours with other herbs (rehmannia, cortex moutan, ginger), which are tied in a muslin cloth and consumed as a soup or brew. Black chicken pieces may also be added.

San Leng polyherbs. It is boiled with other herbs and drunk as a brew.

Teasel tea. Take some dried teasel herb into a cup of hot water and let it sit for 5 to 10 minutes. Strain and drink it warm.

Topical

Ru xiang and **mo yao.** They are often used together as external applications to improve blood circulation to the fractured bone and heal any open wounds.

Notes

- Traditional Chinese remedies for fractures should be used only as adjunctive therapy to allopathic treatment and in the nonacute stage.
- The principle of most Chinese natural remedies in fracture healing is to promote blood circulation to the fracture site to speed up the healing process.

Western/Other Natural Remedies

Common Ingredients for Fracture

Herbs/Leaves	Miscellaneous
Arnica (Arnica montana)	
Avena sativa (oats)	Coconut oil
Boneset (Eupatorium perfoliatum)	
Catnip (Nepeta cataria)	Elemi essential oil (Canarium luzonicum)
Chamomile	Epsom salt
Comfrey (Symphytum uplandica)	
Cottonwood (Populus balsamifera or P. trichocarpa)	
Horsetail (Equisetum arvense)	Aloe vera
Urtica dioica (nettles)	Lavender oil

Common Recipes

Oral

Teas/Brews

Aloe vera juice. Slit an aloe vera leaf down the center. Scrape out the white gel, discarding any of the yellow gel. Cut into smaller pieces, and add to a blender. Blend until smooth. Add to a fruit or vegetable smoothie, or drink alone. Take one to two times a day in the week.

Boneset tea. Take ¼-½ teaspoon dried leaf and flowers. Add one cup of boiling water, allow to steep for 10-15 minutes. Consume when warm. Take maximum 3 cups per day.

Catnip tea. Place 2 teaspoons of dried catnip in a cup. Add hot water and allow it to steep for 5 to 10 minutes. Add honey to taste, and drink warm.

Catnip-chamomile tea. Place 2 teaspoons of dried catnip and 1 teaspoon of dried chamomile flowers into a cup. Pour hot water over the herbs and let sit for 5 to 10 minutes. Add honey to taste, and drink it warm.

Chamomile tea. Place some dried or fresh chamomile flowers into a cup. Pour boiling water over the flowers and allow to steep for 10 minutes. Strain, and add honey to taste. Drink it hot.

Horsetail tea. Horsetail herb is available as a dried herb. Place 1 to 2 teaspoons of dried horsetail into a cup of hot water, and let it sit for 10 to 15 minutes. Add honey to taste, and drink it warm.

Oatstraw infusion. Place about 28 g of dried oat straw into a cup, and pour boiling water over it. Cover, and let it steep overnight or for at least 4 to 6 hours. Strain in the morning, and drink warm. Drink once a day to strengthen bones.

Stinging nettle tea. Place 1 cup of fresh stinging nettle leaves in a cup. Boil 2 to 3 cups of hot water and pour over the stinging nettle leaves. Steep for 10 to 15 minutes, and drink. Alternatively, dried stinging nettle may also be purchased to make tea.

Topical

Arnica based oil or cream. This can be applied on the skin over the closed fracture site if there is bruising and swelling.

Boneset cast. The roots are finely ground and mixed with some water. Apply this paste over the fracture site and allow to dry for about 1 hour. (herbal plaster)

Cottonwood bud oil. Take fresh cottonwood buds and place them in a slow cooker. Fill with olive oil till brim and let it simmer and steep for 5 days. Strain into a clean jar to use as a salve.

It can also be steeped in alcohol such as vodka or rum for 2 to 3 weeks, then strained and used as a salve.

Lavender oil. Add two to three drops of lavender essential oils to about ½ cup of coconut oil. Massage the skin over the fracture with this oil once a day, allowing it to dry on the skin.

Elemi oil. Add two to three drops of elemi essential oils to about ½ cup of coconut oil or 50 g of cold cream. Massage the skin over the fracture with this oil or cream mixture once a day, allowing it to dry on the skin.

Epsom salt bath. Run a warm bath and add about 1 cup of Epsom salt to the bathwater.

Therapeutic measures **Pulsed electromagnetic therapy (PEMF).** Pulsed electromagnetic therapy is FDA approved. It is used to treat non-union fractures. It is applied during cast immobilization to increase healing rate.

Infrared laser light. Exposure to this light can also increase bone healing rate.

Modern Remedies

Principles of Treatment for Closed Fracture

Reduce

The goal is to oppose and align the bone fragments. The types of reduction are:

Closed reduction. Closed manipulation is suitable for all minimally displaced fractures, fractures in children, and fractures that are likely to be stable after reduction.

Methods include reduction by gravity (collar, cuff, or hanging cast), closed manipulation, and continuous traction (skin or skeletal traction).

Open reduction. This is indicated when closed reduction fails, when there is a large articular fragment that needs positioning, or presence of avulsion fractures, or arterial damage.

Methods include internal fixation. (Bone fragments may be fixed with screws, pins, nails, and metal plates.)

Hold

The aim is to prevent displacement with some restriction of movement to alleviate pain, promote soft-tissue healing, and allow free movement of the unaffected parts.

Methods include

- **Sustained traction.** Traction is applied to the limb distal to the fracture to exert a continuous pull in the long axis of the bone.
- **Cast splintage.** Plaster of Paris is used as a splint.
- **Functional bracing.** Plaster of Paris is used to prevent joint stiffness while still permitting fracture splinting and loading.
- **Internal fixation.** Bone fragments may be fixed with screws, pins, nails, and metal plates.
- **External fixation.** Bones are transfixed above and below the fracture with screws, pins, and wires; and these are then clamped to a frame or rigid bars.

Principles of Treatment for Open Fracture

Antibiotics

An initial antibiotic is given stat on arrival at emergency (based on local infection protocols, usually cloxacillin/flucloxacillin). During wound débridement, a second antibiotic is added, usually gentamicin or teicoplanin. Both antibiotics provide prophylaxis against most gram-positive and gram-negative bacteria that may have entered the wound during the time of injury. They are given intravenously for 48 to 72 hours, then switched to oral antibiotics for 7 to 10 days.

Débridement

The operation aims to render the wound free of foreign material and dead tissue, leaving a clean surgical field with a good blood supply throughout.

Stabilization of Fracture

Devices used to stabilize an open fracture include external fixators and internal fixators with plates, screws, and intramedullary nails.

Soft-Tissue Cover

A small uncontaminated wound may be sutured. In severe grades of injury, fracture stabilization is carried out. Wound cover is done using split-skin grafts, local or distant flaps if the wound is clean and viable after débridement. Both orthopedic and plastic surgeons are jointly involved.

Homeopathic Remedies

Arnica montana can reduce the initial pain and swelling. *Eupatorium perfoliatum* can set and heal the bone. *Hypericum* reduces any nerve pain. *Symphytum officinale* helps to promote callus formation. *Ruta graveolens* heals periosteal injuries, bruising and severe bone pain. *Calcarea phosphorica* helps in bone formation. *Bryonia* helps if movements aggravate bone pain.

Osteoporosis

Osteoporosis is a bone disease in which there is lowered bone mass and bone density, resulting in weak, brittle bones (increased bone fragility). It occurs because the body is losing too much bone or making too little new bone. Osteoporosis is common in adults aged 50 and older. Osteoporosis does not produce obvious symptoms. Patients often only become aware of it when they have broken a bone, notice a reduction in height, or become stooped.

Risk factors include postmenopausal women, poor lifestyle and nutrition, genetics, ethnicity (higher among Chinese and Caucasians), low-protein, high-oxalate, and high-phosphate diets, lack of sunlight, medications, and underlying medical conditions.

The bone mineral density (BMD) is measured by a test called bone DEXA scan (dual energy x-ray absorptiometry) over the lumbar spine and hips. It predicts the risk of fracture. A T-score of -2.5 or lower indicates osteoporosis. Blood and urine tests are also done to check the calcium, phosphate, vitamin D levels, and other biochemical parameters.

Indian Natural Remedies

Common Ingredients for Osteoporosis

Spices	Herbs/Leaves	Miscellaneous
Black pepper	*Ipomoea digitata* (vidari kanda)	Jaggery
Cardamom	*Withania somnifera* (ashwagandha)	Milk
Cinnamon	*Sida cordifolia* (bala)	Sesame oil
Clove	*Commiphora wightii* (guggulu)	Almond
Ginger	*Asparagus racemosus* (shatavari)	Soy sprout
Turmeric	Amla (*Phyllanthus emblica*)	Sesame seed
	Terminalia chebula (haritaki)	Honey
	Terminalia bellirica (vibhitaki)	
	Veld grapes (*Cissus quadrangularis*)	
	Tinospora cordifolia (guduchi/giloy)	

Common Recipes

Oral

Teas/Brews

Almond milk. Soak a handful of almonds overnight in warm water. In the morning, peel the almond skins off, and discard. Grind the almonds into a fine paste and mix with milk. Drink once a day.

Amla juice. Lightly pound three to four amla fruits, and strain the juice. Take this juice on an empty stomach in the morning with a glass of warm water.

Ashwagandha brew. Add 1 teaspoon of ashwagandha root powder into a pot with ½ cup of milk and ½ cup of water. Boil gently until the volume reduces to approximately ½ cup. Cool slightly and drink it warm. Add honey to taste.

Bala drink. Take the whole plant. Blend with little water. Extract the juice.

Gandha thailam. Consume 2 to 10 drops of oil or the capsules with milk daily to increase bone mass and density.

Giloy. Boil the giloy stem in 1 cup of milk and ginger. Strain and consume.

> Variation #1: Giloy juice. Place a handful of giloy leaves into a blender and blend until smooth. Strain and drink. Alternatively, chew on fresh giloy leaves or consume in the form of powder.

Guggulu supplements. It is available in the form of dietary supplements. Adults can take about 25 mg of guggulu supplements every day after a meal.

Sesame oil. Add sesame oil to dishes and salads.

Sesame seed. Soak a handful of sesame seeds in water overnight. In the morning, strain, and chew on the sesame seeds.

Shatavari. Add 2 to 5 g of shatavari powder to a glass of milk. Drink twice a day.

Shatavari-sesame. Mix one part sesame seeds with half part shatavari powder, some ground ginger, and jaggery. Consume once a day.

Shatavari–vidari kanda. Mix ½ teaspoon of shatavari powder and ½ teaspoon of vidari kanda powder. Stir into a cup of warm milk, and drink once a day

Spice milk. Place a cup of milk into a pot, and heat it up till it begins to boil gently. Add two to three cardamom seeds, one stick of cinnamon, 2 to 3 inches of fresh ginger, three to five black peppercorns, 1 teaspoon of ground turmeric, and three to five cloves. Simmer for approximately 5 minutes, then strain, and add honey to taste. Drink it warm.

Soy sprouts. Consume 1 small cup of soy sprouts every day in a salad or alone.

Triphala tea. Add ½ teaspoon of triphala powder to 1 cup of hot water. Mix well, and drink warm.

Veld grape. Take the stems. Dry and grind into a fine powder. Store in a bottle. Take ½ teaspoon and mix with some honey. Consume it daily.

Vidari kanda tea. Take ½ to 1 teaspoon of powder. Add 1 cup of water. Consume 1 to 2 times daily after a meal.

Topical treatment

- Perform self-massages once a day with sesame oil or Gandha Thailam

Notes

- Natural remedies should be used as an adjunct to allopathic treatment of osteoporosis.
- Most of the remedies above are more useful as preventive methods rather than cure.

Chinese Natural Remedies

Common Ingredients for Osteoporosis

Herbs/Leaves	Miscellaneous
Atractylodes root (cang zhu)	
Cassia bark (rou gui)	
Cassia twig (gui zhi)	
Chinese angelica (dang gui)	Chinese date (da zao)
Cibot rhizome/gou ji (*Rhizoma Cibotii*)	
Common yam root (huai shan yao)	Indian bread (fu ling)
Dried ginger (gan jiang)	
Dry rehmannia root/shu di huang	Asiatic cornelian cherry fruit (shan yu rou)
Eucommia bark/du zhong (*Eucommia ulmoides*)	
Fresh ginger (sheng jiang)	
Horny goat weed/yin yang huo (*Epimedium*)	
Largehead atractylodes root (bai zhu)	Fresh oyster shell (sheng mu li)
Licorice root (gan cao)	
Milkvetch/huang qi (*Fabaceae astragalus*)	
Mulberry mistletoe/sang ji sheng (*Taxillus chinensis*)	
Oriental water plantain rhizome or ze xie	Papaya (mu gua)
Prepared common monkshood daughter root/cao wu	
Processed rehmannia root (shu di huang)	
Stephania root/han fang ji (*Stephania tetrandra*)	
Suberect spatholobus stem (ji xue teng)	
Szechuan lovage root/chuan xiong (*Ligusticum chuanxiong*)	Black-tail snake/wu shao she (*Zaocys dhumnades*)
Teasels/xu duan (*Dipsacus*)	Psoralea fruit/bu gu zhi (*Psoralea corylifolia fructus*)
Tree peony bark (dan pi)	Barbary wolfberry fruit (gou qi chi)
Unprocessed gypsum (shang shi gao)	
White peony root (bai shao)	Unprocessed fossil fragment (sheng long ku)

Common Recipes

Oral

Decoction for Yin Deficiency of Liver and Kidney. *Modified "Liuwei DiHuang pellets"*: gan di huang, shan yu rou, huai shan yao, fu ling, dan pi, gou qi chi, and chuan duan.

These herbs are used to nourish the yin of the liver and kidneys. Dan pi is used to clear heat from the body. Chuan duan is used to strengthen the tendons and bones.

Decoction for Blood Deficiency and Excessive Dampness

Modified "Danggui Shaoyao powder": dang gui, bai shao, fu ling, bai zhu, ze xie, chuan xiong, fang ji, gui zhi, gan jiang, and gan cao.

These herbs are used to remove dampness from the body and nourish the blood, which helps to strengthen the bones.

Decoction for Retention of Dampness Because of Kidney Deficiency

Modified "ZhenWu": zhi fu pian, bai shao, sheng jiang, du ling, bai zhu, gui zhi, bu gu zhi, chuan duan, sang ji sheng, xian ling pi, and ji xue teng.

This decoction is taken to warm the qi in the body and remove any dampness from the body.

Decoction for Asthenia Syndrome of Superficies with Interior Dampness Retention

Modified "FangYi HuangQi": sheng huang qi, fang ji, sheng jiang, da zao, gan cao, gui zhi, bai shao, lang zhu, sheng long ku, and sheng mu li

This decoction aims to strengthen qi in the body by aiding digestion and absorption of food by the spleen and stomach.

Decoction for Cold in the Superficies and Heat in the Interior

Modified "Yuebi Jiashu": ma huang, cang zhu, sheng jiang, da zao, gan cao, shang shi gao, han fang ji, and mu gua.

This decoction is used to remove heat from the body, which is thought to remove pathogens and invigorate the stomach, which strengthens bones and tendons.

Decoction for Marrow Deficiency and Channels—Bi Syndrome

Modified "Yougui pellets": shu di huang, shan yao, shan zhu yu, gou qi chi, gan cao, du zhong, rou gui, zhi fu zi, wu shao she, xing ling pi, cang zhu, gou ji, and sang ji sheng.

This decoction is taken to nourish the bone marrow and improve qi and blood circulation in the body.

Other Polyherbal Formulas

Go Ji Wan. The key ingredients are Tu Si Zi (Chinese Dodder Seeds) and Bi Xie (dioscorea root).

Si Bao Dan. The key ingredients are Su Mu Jie (Sappan Wood Joint), Wu Tou (Radix Aconiti Carmichaeli), and dioscorea root.

Gou Ji Juice (Yin). The key ingredients are Xu Duan (Japanese Teasel Root), Eucommia Bark, and Hai Feng Teng (Kadsura Stem).

Western/Other Natural Remedies

Common Ingredients for Osteoporosis

Herbs/Leaves	Miscellaneous
Black cohosh	Apple cider vinegar
Boneset (*Eupatorium perfoliatum*)	Banana
	Soy products
	Yogurt
	Minerals: boron, zinc, manganese, copper, strontium, calcium, magnesium, iron, selenium, and silica supplements
	Vitamins: D3, C, and K2
	Bioactive collagen peptides (BCPs)
Dandelion	Essential oils: sage, rosemary, thyme, ginger, orange, wintergreen, cypress, fir, helichrysum, peppermint, eucalyptus, and lemongrass
Horsetail	Coconut oil
Purslane pigweed (*Portulaca oleracea*)	Pineapple
Red clover	Peanut butter
Rose hip (*Rosa canina L.*)	Fig
Rosemary	Milk

Common Recipes

Oral

Teas/Brews/Others

Apple cider vinegar (ACV). Mix 2 teaspoons of ACV into 1 cup of warm water, and drink once a day. ACV can contain calcium, potassium, and magnesium, which benefits bone health.

Banana smoothie. Cut one to two bananas into smaller chunks. Place in a blender, and blend until smooth, adding up to 1 cup of milk. Drink once a day.

Boneset tea. Take ¼-½ teaspoon dried leaf and flowers. Add one cup of boiling water, allow to steep for 10–15 minutes. Consume when warm. Take maximum 3 cups per day.

Dandelion tea. Place 2 to 3 teaspoons of dried dandelions in a cup of hot water. Cover, and let steep for 5 to 10 minutes. Add honey to taste, and drink warm.

Essential oils. Mix one to two drops of pure essential oils into 1 cup of hot water and consume once a day. This is believed to inhibit bone loss.

Figs. These can be incorporated into the diet.

Horsetail tea. Horsetail herb is available as a dried herb. Place 1 to 2 teaspoons of dried horsetail into a cup of hot water and let it sit for 10 to 15 minutes. Add honey to taste and drink it warm.

Peanut butter. This can be consumed.

Pineapple juice. Cut a pineapple into small chunks, discarding the skin. Place the chunks into a blender, and blend until smooth. Strain and drink once a day.

Purslane pigweed. The leaves can be eaten cooked or raw.

Rose hip. This can be consumed as tea or brew.

Rosemary tea. Add three to five sprigs of fresh rosemary (or 1½ teaspoons of dry rosemary leaf needles) to a cup of hot water, and steep for 10 to 15 minutes. Drink it warm.

Adequate minerals (boron, zinc, manganese, copper, strontium, calcium, magnesium, iron, selenium, and silica) and vitamins (D3, C, and K2) are essential for bone health. Too much calcium can predispose to kidney stones and may displace other minerals such as zinc, manganese, and iron. The dose of magnesium is usually about half of the calcium dose. Boron about 5 mg/day can increase bone density and estrogen level. The recommended dietary allowance for calcium and magnesium in women above 50 years is up to 1000 mg per day and up to 450 mg per day respectively.

Bioactive collagen peptides (BCPs). BCP is a type of collagen supplement made of collagen short-chain protein peptides. They are obtained by enzymatic hydrolysis from bovine sources. It is recognized by the World Health Organization (WHO) as being able to improve bone and joint health.

Therapeutic Measures

- Exercise regularly, incorporating flexibility, weight-bearing, balance, strengthening, stretching, and endurance exercises into the routine. This helps to strengthen muscles and bone.
- Quit smoking and drinking alcohol. It leads to inflammation that leaches more calcium from bone, causing more bone loss.
- Avoid sweetened and soda drinks. They contain high amounts of phosphorus, which removes calcium from bones. Sugar may also increase inflammation.
- Avoids foods that leach calcium from the bones such as caffeine, alcohol, high-oxalate foods, and aluminum (via foods and utensils).
- Avoid medications that prevent calcium absorption such as steroids and laxatives.

Modern Remedies

The use of various bone-sparing drugs is recommended.

Bisphosphonates

This medication works by inhibiting the resorption of bone by osteoclasts, which are cells that break bone down in the body. They may also have effects on osteoblasts, the cells that produce new bone. Hence they reduce the rate at which bone breaks down in the body, maintaining bone density and reducing fracture risks.

Examples: alendronate, risedronate, zoledronate (zoledronic acid).

Alendronate or risedronate can be taken daily or weekly for a duration of 3 to 5 years, or even longer for 7 to 10 years in high-risk patients with osteoporotic fragility fractures. Common side effects include dyspepsia or acid reflux and there is risk of osteonecrosis of jaw and atypical femoral fractures.

Zoledronate is long acting, most potent, and given intravenously every 1.5 to 3 years.

Selective Estrogen Receptor Modulators (SERMs)

SERMs affect bone like the hormone estrogen. It inhibits the differentiation of osteoclasts, which decreases their number and hence reduces the rate of bone breakdown and maintains bone density. They have estrogen-like effects (partial agonist) on certain organs (bone, heart, and skin) and antiestrogen effects (antagonist) on other organs (breast and uterus). It is used in postmenopausal women.

Examples: raloxifene (Evista), bazedoxifene, and ospemifene. There is risk of hepatotoxicity with these drugs.

Parathyroid Hormone

The parathyroid hormone (PTH) is naturally produced in the body and regulates the amount of calcium in bone. It works by increasing calcium release from bones. This then stimulates osteoblasts to create new bone. This medication increases bone density as opposed to just maintaining it.

Teriparatide (Forteo): It is a recombinant PTH formulation that is given subcutaneously once a day for up to 2 years. It can increase bone mass to about 13% in 2 years. Side effects include local irritation, dyspepsia, weakness, and dizziness.

Calcitonin

Calcitonin-salmon (Fortical, Miacalcin) is a hormone that decreases osteoclast activity and hence reduces postmenopausal bone loss. It is administered intranasally once a day.

Side effects include nasal irritation with cold symptoms, headache, rash, abdominal or joint pain, and swelling of feet.

Monoclonal Antibody

Humanized monoclonal antibodies are directed against the receptor activator of the nuclear factor κB ligand (RANKL). This is a key mediator of the resorptive phase of bone remodeling. It decreases bone resorption by inhibiting osteoclast activity.

Example: *denosumab (Prolia):* It is a RANKL inhibitor. It is an injection given subcutaneously every 6 months. Side effects include itching, skin blisters or peeling, hypocalcemia, muscle or joint pain, headache, gastrointestinal disturbances, and risk of osteonecrosis of the jaw.

Calcium and Vitamin D Supplements

Calcium supplements in adequate doses are often prescribed. Vitamin D3 is often given to aid in the absorption of calcium to increase new bone formation.

Hormone Replacement Therapy

This is indicated if there is premature menopause before age 40 years.

Strontium Ranelate

It increases bone formation and decreases bone resorption at the same time. It is an oral medication used in women with postmenopausal osteoporosis and who are unable to tolerate bisphosphonates. It reduces risk of vertebral fracture. Side effects include risk of thromboembolism.

Aptamers

Aptamers are small single-stranded oligonucleotides which are nonimmunogenic and target the RANKL protein. They are more promising than monoclonal antibodies but are currently still experimental.

Homeopathic Remedies

These include Calcarea carbonica, Silicea, *Calcarea phosphorica*, *Symphytum officinale*, phosphorus, *Ruta graveolens*, and *Calcarea fluorica*. Others include sulfur, *Hypericum*, and *Ammonium muriaticum* to treat the complications.

Rheumatic Disorders

Rheumatic disorders or rheumatism are conditions that affect the tendons, ligaments, bones, and muscles of the joints. Symptoms of rheumatic disease include joint pain, swelling and redness in a joint, and limited range of movements in the joint. Rheumatic disorders are often autoimmune. They are caused by the body's immune system attacking the joints. Rheumatic diseases have different types, with some common diseases being:

- OA
- Rheumatoid arthritis (RA)
- Lupus
- Ankylosing spondylosis
- Psoriatic arthritis
- Gout

Indian Natural Remedies

Common Ingredients for Rheumatic Disorders

Spices	Herbs/Leaves	Miscellaneous
Carom seed (ajwain)	Veld grape	Honey
Cinnamon	*Vitex negundo* (nirgundi)	Mustard seed oil
Coriander	*Tinospora cordifolia* (guduchi/giloy)	Milk
Cumin	Bala (*Sida cordifolia*)	Eucalyptus oil
Garlic	Vijaysar leaves	Cedarwood oil
Ginger	Castor oil leaves	Coconut oil
Piper nigrum (black pepper)	*Boswellia serrata* (shallaki)	Castor oil (eranda)
Turmeric	Ceylon leadwort/chitrak (*Plumbago zeylanica*)	Buttermilk

Common Recipes

Oral

Teas/Brews

Ajwain brew. Place a teaspoon of ajwain seeds in a cup filled with boiling water. Cover, and steep for 5 to 10 minutes. Strain and drink it warm.

Bala drink. Take the whole plant. Blend with little water. Extract the juice.

Buttermilk. Drink 1 cup of buttermilk every day to prevent flare-ups.

Coriander tea. Grind coriander seeds into a fine powder and add 1 tablespoon of this to a pot of water. Bring to a boil and reduce the heat to allow the mixture to simmer for 5 minutes. Drink once a day.

Garlic oil. Two cloves of pounded garlic with 15 mL of sesame oil can be heated and consumed daily.

Giloy. Boil the giloy stem in 1 cup of milk and ginger. Strain and consume.

Ginger tea. Lightly pound about 1 to 2 inches of fresh ginger (if unavailable, use 1 to 2 teaspoons of ginger powder), and add to a cup of hot water. Allow to steep for 5 to 10 minutes. Strain, and drink while warm. Add honey to taste.

Nirgundi decoction. Place 5 to 10 nirgundi leaves into a pot with water. Allow to boil gently for about 5 to 10 minutes before straining. Drink it warm.

Turmeric-ginger tea. Bring 2 cups of water to a boil in a pot. Add 1 tablespoon of chopped ginger and ½ teaspoon of ground turmeric. Allow to gently simmer for 5 to 10 minutes before straining. Allow to cool for about 5 to 10 minutes and stir in honey to taste. Drink it warm.

Turmeric milk. Add 1 teaspoon of turmeric powder into a glass of hot milk. Drink warm once a day preferably before bedtime. Add honey to taste.

Turmeric tea. Add 1 to 2 teaspoons of ground turmeric to 1 cup of hot water. Mix well, and add honey to taste. Drink one to two times a day. Alternatively, lightly pound 2 to 3 inches of fresh turmeric and add to a cup of boiling water. Allow to steep for 5 to 10 minutes, and strain. Add honey to taste and drink.

Veld grape. Take the stems. Dry, and grind into a fine powder. Store in a bottle. Take ½ teaspoon and mix with some honey. Consume daily.

Topical Treatment

Joint Pastes

Ginger paste. Grind fresh ginger into a smooth paste or grind a piece of dry ginger into a smooth paste, adding a little water, as necessary. Ginger powder may also be used. Mix enough ginger powder and water to make a thick paste. Apply to the joint, and let it sit for 15 to 20 minutes.

Garlic oil paste. Pound two cloves of garlic. Heat with some sesame oil. Apply this oil on the joint.

Ajwain paste. Grind ajwain seeds into a fine powder, and add some water to make a thick paste. Apply to the joint, and let it sit for 15 to 20 minutes.

Nirgundi paste. Grind 5 to 10 nirgundi leaves into a smooth thick paste. Apply to the joint, and let it sit for 15 to 20 minutes before washing it off.

Vijaysar paste. Apply a paste of the vijaysar leaves over the joint, let it sit for about 20 minutes, and then wash off.

Castor leaf and sesame oil. The castor leaf is warmed first and then smeared with sesame oil. This oiled leaf is then placed over the affected joint to reduce inflammation. It is carried out regularly.

Turmeric paste. Grind fresh turmeric into a smooth paste, or grind dry turmeric into a smooth powder, adding a little water as necessary to make a thick paste. Alternatively, mix turmeric powder with enough water to make a thick paste. Apply to the joint, and let it sit for 15 to 20 minutes before washing off.

Bala paste. Take some powder. Make a paste with little water. Apply on the joint.

Chitrak. Apply medicated oil (boiled chitrak root and sarp gandha in mustard oil) on the inflamed joints.

Ayurvedic oil massages. Several oils may be used for their antiinflammatory and pain-relieving properties. To use the oils, place some of the oil on the palms of the hands and rub together until the palms are warm. Apply to the affected joint, massaging gently but firmly for about 5 to 10 minutes. Some of the oils that may be used are:

Mustard seed oil

Castor oil

Coconut oil

Cedarwood oil

Eucalyptus oil

Sesame and garlic oil

Many commercial oils with polyherbal formulations are also available.

Examples:

mahanarayan tailam, dhanwantaram tailam, etc. for topical use

dashamoola kwatha/churna, vishwadi kashaya, etc. for oral use

Chinese Natural Remedies

Common Ingredients for Rheumatic Disorders

Herbs/Leaves	Miscellaneous
Millettia/ji xue teng *(Spatholobus suberectus)*	Bee venom
Mulberry mistletoe/sang ji sheng *(Taxillus chinensis)*	
Stephania root/han fang ji *(Stephania tetrandra)*	
Szechuan ox knee/chuan niu xi *(Radix cyathula officinalis)*	
Thunder god vine/lei gong teng *(Tripterygium wilfordii Hook F)*	Quince *(Cydonia oblonga)*

Common Recipes

Oral

Traditional Chinese medicine for the treatment of arthritis is mainly aimed at symptomatic relief.

Thunder god vine. It is available as dried herbal tea decoction or as a tablet.

Millettia stem. Prepare a decoction using ½ to 1 tablespoon of the dried powder. Alternatively, millettia stem is also available in the form of tablets.

Chuan niu xi. Take ½ to 1 tablespoon of dried root. Boil in water, and consume as a decoction.

Polyherbal formulas.

Xuan Bi Tang. The main key ingredients include xing ren (apricot seeds), fang gi (stephania roots), can sha (silkworm feces), ban xia (crow-dipper rhizome), lian qiao (forsythia fruits), yi yi ren (coix seeds), zhi zi (cape jasmine fruits), chi xiao dou (red beans), and hua shi (talc).

Duhuo Jisheng Wan. It is a polyherbal formula of seven herbs, including sang ji sheng (mulberry mistletoe), duhuo (angelica pubescens root), du zhong (eucommia bark), and fu ling (poria cocos).

Topical

Thunder god vine liniment can be applied over the painful joint.

Therapeutic Measures

Acupuncture can effectively treat symptoms of rheumatic diseases. It is thought to increase blood flow to the joints and reduce inflammation.

Bee venom acupuncture can also help.

Western/Other Natural Remedies

Common Ingredients for Rheumatic Disorders

Spices	Herbs/Leaves	Miscellaneous
Borago officinalis (borage)	Evening primrose	Cetyl myristoleate (CMO)
Cayenne pepper	Rosemary	Cajeput oil
Celery seed	Joe Pye weed *(Eutrochium purpureum)*	
	Common rue	
	Giloy	
	Stinging nettle	
	Meadowsweet	
	Pokeweed root	
	Fleabane	
Cinnamon	Willow bark	Eucalyptus
Ginger	Green tea	Apple cider vinegar

Common Recipes

Oral

Teas/Brews

Apple cider vinegar. Mix 2 teaspoons of ACV into 1 cup of warm water, and drink once a day.

Borage seed oil. They are usually available as oral supplements (as capsules) and can be taken together with standard painkillers.

Boswellia (Indian frankincense). Take boswellia extract supplements.

Variation #1. Combinations of boswellia with curcumin or boswellia with methylsulfonylmethane (MSM) are also available.

Cayenne pepper brew. Mix ¼ teaspoon of cayenne pepper into a cup of hot water. Stir well, and drink once a day.

Celery seed tea. Lightly crush ½ tablespoon of celery seeds. Steep in a cup of hot water for approximately 20 minutes. Strain the mixture, and drink.

Cetyl myristoleate (CMO). This is a natural fatty acid found in some animals (whale, cows, mice, etc.) and is available as a dietary supplement.

Cinnamon tea. Add a stick of cinnamon to 1 cup of hot water and allow to steep for approximately 10 minutes. Add honey to taste, and drink.

Ginger tea. Lightly pound about 1 to 2 inches of fresh ginger (if unavailable, use 1 to 2 teaspoons of ginger powder), and add to a cup of hot water. Allow to steep for 5 to 10 minutes. Strain and drink while warm. Add honey to taste.

Joe pye weed root tea. Take 1 ounce of dried crushed root. Add ½ L of water. Boil for 30 minutes, and drink ½ a cup every 2 hours.

Joe pye weed flower tea. Take 1 teaspoon of the dried flower. Add 1 cup of boiling water. Steep for 10 minutes.

Meadowsweet tea. Take 2 tablespoons of dried meadowsweet. Add 1 cup of hot water. Steep for 10 minutes. Strain and consume it warm.

Rosemary tea. Add three to five sprigs of fresh rosemary (or 1½ teaspoons of dry rosemary leaf needles) to a cup of hot water, and steep for 10 to 15 minutes. Drink it warm.

Rue tea. Take 1 teaspoon of dried crushed rue leaves. Add ½ cup of boiling water. Steep for 15 minutes. Strain, and consume ½ cup a day.

Stinging nettle tea. Boil 1 cup of fresh leaves in 2 to 4 cups of water. Steep for 5 to 10 minutes. Strain, and drink. The cooked leaves can be added to food.

Topical

Capsaicin. This is available as 0.025% creams or patches and can be rubbed or placed over the affected joints 2 or 3 times per day.

CMO creams. Various combination creams are available.

Examples are CMO joint health cream (with glucosamine) and Rub on Relief (CMO with multiple polyherbs like white willow extract, *Boswellia*, turmeric, arnica, calendula, peppermint oil, safflower oil, lime, lemon, plumeria, aloe vera, vitamin E, camphor, MSM, and magnesium sulfate).

Cajeput oil. Apply the oil on to the sore joint after diluting it with a carrier oil.

Stinging nettle creams. Nettle-based creams can be applied over the painful joints.

Pokeweed. Apply pokeweed root as a poultice over the affected joints.

Fleabane. Take some fresh leaves (or other parts). Pound and extract the juice. Apply the juice over the sore joints.

Modern Remedies

Disease-Modifying Antirheumatic Drugs

Disease-modifying antirheumatic drugs (DMARDs) work by slowing the progression of rheumatism and preventing permanent damage to the joints and other tissue. The exact mechanism of action remains unclear at present.

Examples: methotrexate, hydroxychloroquine, sulfasalazine

Nonsteroidal Antiinflammatory Drugs

It reduces mild to moderately severe pain. It inhibits or reduces prostaglandin synthesis by blocking COX, hence reducing the inflammatory mediators. There are two types of NSAIDs: nonselective and selective. Examples in each category are listed as follows.

Nonselective NSAIDs	Selective NSAIDs
The actions of both cyclooxygenase (COX)-1 and COX-2 enzymes are blocked to relieve pain.	The action of only COX-2 enzyme is blocked to relieve pain.
• ibuprofen (Advil, Motrin, Ibuprofen)	• celecoxib (Celebrex)
• naproxen (Aleve, Anaprox, Naprelan)	• meloxicam (Mobic)
• diclofenac (Cataflam, Voltaren)	
• ketoprofen (Actron, Orudis)	

NSAIDs, Nonsteroidal antiinflammatory drugs.

Long-Acting Corticosteroids

Steroid medication reduces inflammation and pain while also slowing the rate of joint damage.

Examples: prednisolone, intramuscular methylprednisolone

Biologicals (Biologics)

They are antibodies or soluble factors produced biologically in genetically modified cells, to inhibit various inflammatory cytokines. There are different types for different rheumatic disorders.

Tumor Necrosis Factor (TNF) Antagonists

Etanercept (Enbrel): TNF-α receptor fusion protein that binds to TNF-α.

Infliximab (Remicade): human mouse chimeric anti–TNF-α monoclonal antibody.

Adalimumab (Humira): human anti–TNF-α monoclonal antibody.

Interleukin (IL)-1 Antagonists

Anakinra (Kineret): recombinant IL-1 receptor antagonists.
Rituximab (Rituxan): monoclonal antibody to CD20 antigen.

Janus-activated kinase (JAK) inhibitors

Upadicitinib, tofacitinib, baricitinib. They inhibit JAK1 and JAK3 signaling and can improve the quality of life in RA and ankylosing spondylitis (AS). Side effects include risk of infection and venous thromboembolism.

Therapeutic Measures

Regular sports and exercises are helpful.

Regular exercises such as swimming, cycling, or running.

Physiotherapy, occupational therapy, and psychological therapy are also helpful.

Surgery

Operative treatment may be indicated at any stage of the disease if conservative treatment alone is not effective. Early on, this consists mainly of soft-tissue procedures such as synovectomy, tendon repair or replacement, and joint stabilization.

In the late rheumatoid disease, severe joint destruction, fixed deformity, and loss of function are clear indications for reconstructive surgery.

Examples of procedures would include arthrodesis, osteotomy, and arthroplasty.

Homeopathic Remedies

These include *Bryonia, Belladonna or Phytolacca* (mostly in acute disease or flare-ups), *Rhus tox* (more in chronic disease), and *Calcarea fluor* (in degenerative state). Others include *Sepia, Apis mellifica, Pulsatilla, Causticum* (potassium hydrate), *Formica, Ledum palustre, Symphytum, Berberis vulgaris, Calcarea carbonica* (oyster shell), *Arnica, Calcarea phosphoricum, Hekla lava,* and *Ruta graveolens.*

In the acute phase, the remedies can be taken every 1 to 2 hours. In the chronic phase, a low-potency remedy is taken over a few months.

There is an overlap in the remedies for rheumatoid disorders and OA, and they may be cross used.

Osteoarthritis

OA is also known as degenerative joint disease and is a common condition affecting the large joints and some small joints in the body. The joints are lined by cartilage, which protects the bones from rubbing against each other. When the cartilage breaks down, the joint bones rub against each other, resulting in pain, stiffness, and swelling. The joints most affected in OA include the knees, hips, lower back, and neck, as well as the small finger joints and the bases of the thumb and big toe.

OA is most common in adults older than 65 years. Risk factors for OA include increasing age, obesity, joint injury, joint overuse, weak muscles, and possibly genetics. Symptoms of OA are painful, swollen joints with a limited range of movement. The joint may also appear red and hot to the touch.

Indian Natural Remedies

Common Ingredients for osteoarthritis

Spices	Herbs/Leaves/Fruits
Fenugreek	*Terminalia chebula* (haritaki)
	Commiphora guggul (also called *Commiphora mukul, Commiphora wightii,* or guggulu)
	Asparagus racemosus (shatavari)
	Boswellia serrata (Indian frankincense)
	Rudraksha *(Elaeocarpus ganitrus)*
	Babool *(Acacia arabica)*
Flaxseed	*Withania somnifera* (ashwagandha)
Ginger	*Terminalia bellirica* (bibhitaki)
Turmeric	*Phyllanthus emblica* (amla/Indian gooseberry)

Common Recipes

Oral

Teas/Brews

Amla juice. Lightly pound three to four amla fruits and strain the juice. Take this juice on an empty stomach in the morning with a glass of warm water.

Ashwagandha brew. Place 1 teaspoon of ashwagandha root powder into a pot with ½ cup of milk and ½ cup of water. Boil gently until the volume reduces to about ½ cup. Cool slightly, and drink warm. Add honey to taste.

Babool Gum brew. Take 3g of Babool gum powder. Add one cup of boiling water. Steep for 5-10 minutes. Consume once a day.

Boswellia (Indian frankincense). Take boswellia extract supplements.

Variation #1. Combinations of boswellia with curcumin or boswellia with MSM are also available.

Variation #2. Combinations of Boswellia extract [Acetyl-11-keto-β-boswellic acid (AKBA)], alpinia galangal, beta caryophyllene, and collagen type 11(avian sternum) are also available.

Fenugreek brew. There are many variations of the recipe.

Variation #1. Lightly roast some handfuls of fenugreek seeds, and grind into a fine powder. Store in an airtight bottle. Mix 1 teaspoon of the powder in 1 cup of warm water. Drink in the morning on an empty stomach.

Variation #2. Soak 4 tablespoons of seeds in 300 mL of warm water overnight. Drink the amber water, and chew on the swollen seeds the next morning on an empty stomach.

Variation #3. Soak 4 tablespoons of seeds in 300 mL of warm water overnight. In the morning, place the soaked seeds into a blender and blend until smooth. Strain the mixture, and drink once a day for at least 3 months.

Flaxseed brew. Soak 2 teaspoons of flaxseed in a cup of warm water overnight. Drink the water in the morning, and chew on the flaxseeds.

Ginger tea. Lightly pound about 1 to 2 inches of fresh ginger (if unavailable, use 1 to 2 teaspoons of ginger powder), and add to a cup of hot water. Allow to steep for 5 to 10 minutes. Strain, and drink while warm. Add honey to taste.

Guggulu supplements. It is available in the form of dietary supplements. Adults can take about 25 mg of guggulu supplements every day after a meal.

Indian mallow. Take some Indian mallow leaves. Add some cumin seeds. Blend them together. Add some water. Strain, and consume regularly.

> Variation #1. Take ½ teaspoon of the powder. Mix with some warm water and honey. Consume once or twice a day after meals.

Shatavari brew. Mix ¼ or ½ teaspoon of shatavari powder with honey or milk, and take twice a day after food. If shatavari liquid extract is used, then put 30 drops into some juice or water. Consume two or three times per day.

Triphala tea. Add ½ teaspoon of triphala powder to 1 cup of hot water. Mix well, and drink warm.

Turmeric tea. Add 1 to 2 teaspoons of ground turmeric to 1 cup of hot water. Mix well and add honey to taste. Drink one to two times a day. Alternatively, lightly pound 2 to 3 inches of fresh turmeric, and add to a cup of boiling water. Allow to steep for 5 to 10 minutes, and strain. Add honey to taste and drink.

Polyherbal brews or tablets (also called decoction, *kwath*, or *kadha*)

- **Rasna Saptak Kwath (brew).** It is a decoction or a tablet made from 7 herbs *(Pluchea lanceolata, Cassia fistula, Tinospora cordifolia, Castor root, Tribulus terrestris, Cedrus deodara and Punarnava/Boerhavia diffusa)*. Equal amounts of each herb are taken. They are boiled in 8 parts of water, then reduced to ¼ volume and then strained.
- **Polyherbal Ayurvedic tablet.** *Zingiber officinale* (ginger), *Boswellia serrata*, *Withania somnifera* (Indian ginseng), *Commiphora mukul* (Indian bdellium tree), *Pluchea lanceolata* (rasna), *Oroxylum indicum* (Indian trumpet tree), and *Smilax china* (China root) —These have anti-inflammatory properties.
- **Polyherbal decoction (kadha).** Consume a decoction of Eucalyptus, Turmeric and Ginger are great for treating joint and muscle pain.

Topical

Ayurvedic oil massages such as *snehana, svedana, matra basti, mridu virechana,* and *jalaukavacharana* have been used along with oral medications to reduce the vata dosha.

Janu Basti. A ring pool of moist ground black gram (urad dal) paste is created over the affected knee joint (or other joints). Warm medicated herbal oil is poured into this ring pool and left for at least 30 minutes (oil retention therapy).

Blended polyherbal oils (thailam). Some of the common commercial thailam include Murivenna, Mahanarayana thailam, Balashwagandhadi thailam, and Dhanwantharam thailam (sesame-based oil). They reduce joint swelling and vata dosha and can also be massaged directly over the joint.

Murivenna thailam contains mainly juices of betel leaf, aloe vera, moringa leaf, onion, shatavari, pongamia, etc boiled in coconut oil base.

Dhanwantharam thailam contains mainly amla, ashwagandha, ginseng, bilva or Indian bael, bala (country mallow) and others in sesame oil base.

Polyherbal oil (homemade). Take 50 ml of sesame oil. Add 10 pips of garlic (chopped), 1 inch piece of ginger chopped, 1 teaspoon fenugreek, 5 cloves and 4 to 5 ajwain leaves (chopped). Boil for about 5 minutes. When cool, strain and store in a bottle. Apply the oil over the painful joint. Wrap a plastic sheet over the oiled joint and leave overnight. Repeat for 7 to 10 days.

Rudraksha paste. Make a paste with some Rudraksha powder and mustard oil. Apply on affected joints.

Therapeutic Measures

Meditation. Meditation is thought to improve the emotional and spiritual aspects of a person, which, in turn, can bring about physiological changes in the body such as immune response.

Panchakarma. It is very beneficial in management of osteoarthritis.

Varma therapy. This is therapy is targeted at the nerves, veins, tendons, soft tissues or ligaments, organs, and bone joints and is used commonly in several musculoskeletal conditions such as osteoarthritis of the knees, frozen shoulder, lumbar and cervical spondylosis with disc bulges, writer's cramp, foot drop, sciatica, etc.

An example is illustrated for knee osteoarthritis.

Varma Points

1. **Chippi Varmam:** Situated 6 finger breaths below Saramudichu, 3 finger breaths lateral on either side.
2. **Uppukuttri Varmam:** Situated 3 finger breaths above posterior aspect of the heel.
3. **Kuthikaal Varmam:** Situated 7 finger breaths above posterior aspect of the heel.
4. **Viruthi kaalam:** Situated between big toe and adjacent in its dorsal aspect.
5. **Komberi kaalam:** Situated 8 finger breaths above medial malleolus.
6. **Naai thalai Varmam:** Situated 3 finger breaths below knee joint.
7. **Kaal moottu Varmam:** Situated in centre of the popliteal fossa.
8. **Veeradangal:** Situated 4 finger breaths above kaal moottu Varmam.

Each varma point will be stimulated with pressure mentioned in text and may vary according to patients pirakuruthi (body constitution).
From Janani L, Manickavasaga, R. *Effectiveness of Varmam Therapy for the Management of Osteoarthritis.* 2017. *International Journal of Pharmaceutical Sciences and Research,* 42. https://doi.org/10.13040/IJPSR.0975-8232.8(12).5286-90.

Chinese Natural Remedies

In Traditional Chinese medicine, there are thought to be four types of arthritis, which are all treated differently.

Zuo Bi: This type of arthritis manifests as the affected joints becoming numb with pain that is aggravated by dampness.

Re Bi: In re bi, there is swelling, tenderness, and sharp pain in the affected joint (or joints).

Xing Bi: The joint pain in this condition moves from joint to joint. Patients are often slender in stature.

Tong Bi: Tong bi produces symptoms such as severe pain localized to one or more joints, aggravated by the cold and inactivity. Heat often relieves the pain.

Common Ingredients Osteoarthritis

Herbs/Leaves	Miscellaneous
Ginger	
Glycyrrhiza glabra (licorice/gan cao)	
Green tea leaf	Bee venom
Thunder god vine	
Tripterygium wilfordii (thunder god vine)	
Uncaria tomentosa (cat's claw)	Chicken feet broth
Wild yam (shan yao)	

Common Recipes

Oral

Teas/Brews

Cat's claw tea. Cat's claw is available as bark or powder. To make the tea, boil some water and pour it into a cup. Add one to two pieces of bark or 1 to 2 teaspoons of the powder to the water. Add a few drops of lemon juice and mix well.

Chicken feet. Simmer the chicken feet in water, ginger, and herbs for several hours. Consume.

Duhuo Jisheng Wan. It is a polyherbal formula of seven herbs, including sang ji sheng (mulberry mistletoe), duhuo (angelica pubescens root), du zhong (eucommia bark), and fu ling (poria cocos).

Ginger tea. Lightly pound about 1 to 2 inches of fresh ginger (if unavailable, use 1 to 2 teaspoons of ginger powder), and add to a cup of hot water. Allow to steep for 5 to 10 minutes. Strain, and drink while warm. Add honey to taste.

Green tea. Place 2 teaspoons of dried green tea leaves in a cup of hot water. Allow to steep for 10 to 15 minutes. Strain, and drink.

Licorice tea. Add 1 teaspoon of ground licorice to a pot with 1 cup of boiling water. Allow to simmer for 30 to 45 minutes before straining.

Wild yam. It is available as a dietary supplement.

Topical

Thunder god vine liniment can be applied over the painful joint.

Therapeutic Measures

Acupuncture helps with short-term pain relief. There are several local and distal points which are stimulated manually or via electroacupuncture.

Bee venom acupuncture is also effective.

Tai chi or qi gong exercises are also recommended.

Western/Other Natural Remedies

Common Ingredients for Osteoarthritis

Herbs/Leaves	Miscellaneous
Aloe vera	Type II collagen
Arctium lappa (burdock root)	Methylsulfonylmethane (MSM)
Arnica	Silica (orthosilicic acid)
Artemisia absinthium (wormwood)	Glucosamine and chondroitin sulfate
Common rue	Green-lipped mussel
Cottonwood (*Populus balsamifera* or *P. trichocarpa*)	Oils: cajeput, avocado and soya
Stinging nettle (*Urtica dioica*)	Bone broth or gelatin
Urtica dioica (nettles)	Apple cider vinegar
Verbena (*Verbena officinalis*)	S-adenosylmethionie (SAMe)
Willow bark	Eucalyptus oil

Common Recipes

Oral

Teas/Brews

Aloe vera juice. Slit an aloe vera leaf down the center. Scrape out the white gel, discarding any of the yellow gel. Cut into smaller pieces and add to a blender. Blend until smooth. Add to a fruit or vegetable smoothie or drink alone. Take one to two times a day in the week.

Apple cider vinegar. Mix 2 teaspoons of apple cider vinegar into 1 cup of warm water, and drink once a day.

Avocado oil and soya oil. This combination capsule is available commercially as Piascledine. Consume daily for 3 to 6 months.

Bone broth and/or gelatin. These foods are rich in collagen and can be store-bought or home-made.

Bones from grass-fed and free-range cows, pigs, lamb, or poultry (or fish) are simmered over 6 to 72 hours in a slow cooker with added tomato, vinegar, and wine (acidic medium) to make bone broth.

Gelatin is a protein and is made by boiling the bones, ligaments, tendons, and skin of cows or pigs. Seaweed (agaragar) is a nonanimal source of gelatin. Eating gelatin will increase our body collagen. Gelatin provides glycine, proline, glutamate, and lysine. (They are amino-acid building blocks for collagen.)

Commercial gelatin powders are also available. These are often added to desserts.

Rarely, histamine reactions have been reported after consuming gelatin powders.

Burdock root tea. Roughly chop fresh or dried burdock root into smaller chunks. Add two tablespoons of the chopped root to a pot with water. Allow to simmer gently for about 10 minutes before turning the heat off. Strain, and drink warm.

Chondroitin sulfate (CS). It is taken orally at doses of 800 mg to 1200 mg/day for at least 2 to 4 months before improvement is seen and can be continued up to two years.

A combination of both glucosamine and CS is generally more effective in the relief of moderately severe pain, stiffness, and swelling.

Glucosamine. It is taken orally at doses of 1500 mg/day in three divided doses.

Green-lipped mussel. It is a shellfish sourced from New Zealand waters, and it contains omega-3 fatty acid (i.e., *eicosatetraenoic acid* [ETA]), which has antiinflammatory actions. It reduces leukotrienes and prostaglandins (similar effects as fish oil). This mussel also has anti–matrix metalloproteinase (MMP) actions. MMP is an enzyme present normally in joints. MMP is increased in a joint injury; hence the anti-MMP actions of this mussel can prevent further joint damage. This mussel also contains CS and other micronutrient minerals and vitamins.

Side effects include bloating, nausea, and diarrhea.

Methylsulfonylmethane (MSM). It is a natural sulfur-containing compound found in plants (vegetables or fruit) and animals (cow's milk, meat, and seafood). It can be synthetically made as a dietary supplement. MSM has antiinflammatory properties and reduces pain. It is taken orally in doses of 500 to 8000 mg/day in three divided doses.

Common side effects include nausea and diarrhea mainly and, occasionally, swelling, fatigue, headache, and insomnia.

Rue tea. Refer to "Western /Other Natural Remedies" under "Rheumatic disorder."

S-adenosylmethionie (SAMe). It is available as a dietary supplement. The initial dose is 1200 mg per day and then maintained at 400 mg per day for approximately 3 months. It is given in 2 to 3 divided doses.

Silica. Silica or silicon is a component of bone, collagen, skin, hair, and nails. The bioavailable form is choline-stabilized orthosilicic acid. It is available as a dietary supplement. Improvements are reported to be variable.

Stinging nettle tea. Place 1 cup of fresh stinging nettle leaves in a cup. Boil 2 to 3 cups of hot water and pour over the stinging nettle leaves. Steep for 10 to 15 minutes, and drink. Alternatively, 1 to 2 tablespoons of dried nettle leaves can also be used.

Type II collagen. Type II collagen is the main component in joint cartilage, and it gives the tensile mechanical strength. Bovine (cow), chicken, or marine collagen (fish) are available as powders. It is often consumed to treat joint pain associated with many types of arthritis. Undenatured collagen (UC)-II is derived from chicken bone.

Verbena (Vervain polyherbal tea). Mix equal amounts (about 2 teaspoons) of each herb, ie vervain, peppermint, elderflower, primrose, thyme, and cowslip.

Take 2 teaspoons of this herbal mix. Add 1 cup of hot water. Steep for 10 minutes. Strain and consume warm.

Willow bark tea. Place 2 teaspoons of willow bark into a pot with about 200 mL of water. Allow to gently simmer for about 10 minutes before removing from the heat. Strain, and add honey to taste. Drink warm.

Variation #1. Topical willow bark is also available.

Topical

Joint ceramic biomagnet. It is placed over any painful joint, and it provides a deep-penetrating and strong static magnetic field to the inflamed tissues and promotes healing (e.g., Jointace Active Magnet).

Other **adhesive magnet plasters or patches** are available (e.g., Elekibans is a Japanese device). Four to six circular patches are placed over stiff and painful muscles such as the affected shoulder blades, neck, back, knees, and other joints. It can remain for 2 to 3 days. It should not be used if a pacemaker is worn.

Joint patches containing glucosamine, chondroitin, and essential oils (ginger, lavender, eucalyptus, clove, orange, fennel, and menthol) with liposomal delivery system provide deep relief for about 12 hours (e.g., Jointace Patch).

Wormwood ointment 3%. This is applied 3 times a day and helps to improve pain and mobility.

Stinging nettle cream. Cream made of stinging nettle can be applied over the arthritic joints.

Arnica gel. Apply the gel over the arthritic joints.

Cottonwood bud oil. Take fresh cottonwood buds and place them in a slow cooker. Fill with olive oil till brim and let it simmer and steep for 5 days. Strain into a clean jar to use as a salve.

It can also be steeped in alcohol such as vodka or rum for 2 to 3 weeks, then strained and used as a salve.

Vervain dressing. Place a dressing soaked in the vervain polyherbal tea directly on the arthritic joint.

Therapeutic Measures

Baths

In a bath tub of warm water, add 1 cup of Epsom salt (or salt) and about 20 drops of lavender and cajeput essential oil. Soak in for about 20 minutes.

Modern Remedies

Analgesics (Oral or Topical)

If there is mild or moderate pain without apparent inflammation, acetaminophen is given. If there is no improvement, NSAIDs, preferably selective COX-2 inhibitors (oral NSAID/COX-2 inhibitor), instead of nonselective NSAIDs, are prescribed. Narcotic analgesics such as tramadol need to be considered if NSAIDs fail.

Topical creams or gels containing NSAID (diclofenac sodium) can also be rubbed on the joint. Similarly, patches containing NSAID, capsaicin, or lidocaine can be applied to the affected joint.

Physical Therapy

Cold (icing method) or moist heat packs are also used to relieve acute or chronic joint pain, respectively. Ultrasound, physiotherapy, and braces also help.

Lifestyle Measures

Preventing obesity, reducing weight, staying physically active, strengthening, and doing aerobic exercises are important. Exercises include walking, swimming, bike riding, and doing yoga.

Eating a good diet is also important. Protein-rich foods such as meat, fish, eggs, diary, and legumes contain the amino-acid building blocks (glycine, proline, glutamate, and lysine) that make collagen. Other important bone micronutrients include calcium, vitamin D, vitamin C, vitamin E, omega 3, iron, magnesium, zinc, copper, selenium, silica, and boron.

Appropriate footwear (with shock-absorbing properties), use of assistive devices (walking sticks and tap turners), and joint braces can also help.

Intra-Articular Injections
  Corticosteroids: Intra-articular injection of corticosteroid (triamcinolone acetonide/kenalog) relieves pain via its antiinflammatory effect. Some synovial fluid may be aspirated out if the knee is swollen before the steroid is injected.
  Hyaluronic acid: Intra-articular injection of sodium hyaluronate is called viscosupplementation. This is safe and reasonably effective for symptomatic relief of mild to moderate knee OA. The onset of action is within 2 to 4 weeks, and the peak effect is around 8 weeks. Its effect lasts about 6 months. Repeat injections are necessary.
  Hyaluronic acid is present naturally in joint fluid. It acts as a lubricant and shock absorber. In OA, there is loss of hyaluronic acid resulting in joint stiffness and pain. Hyaluronic acid is often injected into the joint space to replace the amount in between joints.
  Stem cells: Autologous bone marrow–derived stem cells or allogeneic mesenchymal stem cells are injected into the knee joint with mild OA changes to improve pain and stiffness.
Surgery
  • These include: Two common surgical interventions for OA are arthroscopy and total knee replacement (TKR).
  • With arthroscopy, the surgeon flushes the joint cavity and removes broken bone or cartilage pieces. The area is flushed and flushing via endoscope).
  • Knee arthroplasty/knee replacement surgery (unicompartmental or TKR). The damaged knee joint is replaced with an artificial joint using titanium metal/metal alloys, polymers, and high-grade plastics. TKR is indicated when there is severe pain and restricted mobility. It can last for about 15 years, and there is a good quality of life. Risks may include nerve damage, infection, deep vein thrombosis in the legs, or pulmonary embolism.

Homeopathic Remedies

These include Calcarea carbonica, Bryonia alba, Ruta graveolens, Calcarea fluorica, Kali carb, sulfur, Rhus tox, Arnica, Kalmia latifolia, Apis mellifica, and Causticum.

See also under Rheumatic disorders.

Cervical Spondylosis

Cervical spondylosis is a condition common in older people, although more young adults are being affected due to strain injury or ligament stiffness from digital screen overuse and during sports. It affects the joints and discs of the cervical spine. It may be asymptomatic but may also cause symptoms such as chronic, sometimes severe, neck pain and stiffness. It is thought to be caused by several factors:

• **Bone spurs:** Bone overgrowths sometimes occur when the body attempts to strengthen the spine. This puts pressure on the spinal cord and nerves, causing pain.
• **Dehydrated spinal discs:** Between each spinal disc, there is a thick gel cushion that absorbs impact and prevents friction between the discs. Sometimes the gel inside the cushions dries up over time, causing the discs to rub against each other and cause pain.
• **Herniated discs:** Sometimes cracks develop in the spinal discs, causing leakage of the gel material from inside the cushions. This compresses the spinal cord and nerves, causing pain as well as numbness of the arm.

Indian Natural Remedies

Common Ingredients for Cervical Spondylosis

Spices	Herbs/Leaves	Miscellaneous
Garlic	*Terminalia bellirica* (bibhitaki)	Ghee
	Terminalia chebula (haritaki)	Salt
	Commiphora guggul (guggulu)	Vegetable oil
	Tinospora cordifolia (guduchi/giloy)	
	Withania somnifera (ashwagandha)	
Ginger	*Phyllanthus emblica* (amla/Indian gooseberry)	Milk

Common Recipes

Oral

Teas/Brews

Amla juice. Lightly pound three to four amla fruits and strain the juice. Take this juice on an empty stomach in the morning with a glass of warm water.

Ashwagandha brew. Place 1 teaspoon of ashwagandha root powder into a pot with ½ cup of milk and ½ cup of water. Boil gently until the volume reduces to about ½ cup. Cool slightly, and drink warm. Add honey to taste.

Giloy juice. Place a handful of giloy leaves into a blender, and blend until smooth. Strain, and drink. Alternatively, chew on fresh giloy leaves, or consume in the form of powder.

Ginger tea. Lightly pound about 1 to 2 inches of fresh ginger (if unavailable, use 1 to 2 teaspoons of ginger powder), and add to a cup of hot water. Allow to steep for 5 to 10 minutes. Strain, and drink while warm. Add honey to taste.

Guggulu supplements. Guggulu tablets should be taken with warm water or warm milk. The dosage for adults is two to four tablets four times a day.

Triphala brew. Add 1 teaspoon of triphala powder to 1 cup of warm milk. Mix well, and drink warm. Drink once a day, preferably before bedtime.

Topical treatment

Salt neck wrap. Place about 500 g of salt in a large handkerchief and heat it on a dry pan until it becomes hot but not intolerably so. Apply this on the neck for about ½ an hour every day. This is thought to relieve the pressure on the nerves.

Garlic oil. Fry some garlic in a frying pan with vegetable oil until fragrant and brown. Strain, and discard the garlic. Allow the oil to cool down completely before using it to massage the neck.

Lifestyle Measures

Yoga. Yoga helps to relax the body and mind while strengthening the spinal muscles and the core. This may relieve some of the tension on the spinal muscles, reducing pain.

Chinese Natural Remedies

It is believed that chronic neck pain with radicular signs or symptoms or myelopathy in cervical spondylosis or cervical degenerative disc diseases is due to obstruction of qi flowing and blood circulation in the neck area from pathogenic wind, cold, and dampness seeping in the neck.

Common Remedies

These are often Chinese proprietary medicines (available as tablets, capsules, or topical substances) or as polyherbal compounds.

Commercial Preparations

Jingtong granule (JG). It is an oral polyherbal medication made from seven common herbs: *Radix notoginseng* (Sanqi), *Rhizoma Radix Paeoniae Alba* (Bai Shao), *Ligustici Chuanxiong* (Chuanxiong), *Rhizoma Corydalis* (Yanhusuo), *Radix Clematidis* (Wei Ling Xian), *Radix Puerariae* (Gegen), and *Rhizoma et Radix Notopterygii* (Qiang Huo).

Compound Qishe tablet. It is a polyherbal formulation made from Radix Astragali, Muscone, Radix Stephaniae Tetrandrae, Szechuan Lovage Rhizome, Ovientvine, and Calculus Bovis Artifactus.

Jingfukang granules. It is a polyherbal formulation containing the following main ingredients: white peony root, salvia, atractylodes rhizome, chuanxiong, pueraria lobata, codonopsis, earthworm, safflower, stamen, cork, astragalus, Qianghuo, gentiana, myrrh, frankincense, Shengdi Yellow, stone cassia, peach kernel, soil turtle, Wang Buliuxing, and Wei Lingxian.

Compound Extractum Nucis Vomicae. This is a topical herbal medicine which can relieve neck pain.

Therapeutic Measures

Acupressure, Acupuncture, and Electroacupuncture

Cervical hua tou jia ji points: [JT30]

- Cervical vertebra 5
- Cervical vertebra 6
- Cervical vertebra 7

Gallbladder 20 (GB 20) and Urinary Bladder 10 (UB 10) are often stimulated simultaneously. GB 10 is located on the head, behind the auricle, just behind and above the mastoid process. UB 10 is located at the nape of the neck in the depression just within the hairline at the back of the head.

Small Intestine 3 (SI 3) is also known as the back stream and is in the depression at the base of the little finger on the back of the hand.

Lung 7 (Lu 7) is also known as Broken Sequence and is located about 5 cm below the wrist crease, on the forearm, in line with the base of the thumb.

San Jiao 5 (SJ 5) is located on the back of the forearm, about 7.5 cm above the wrist crease. It is located between the ulna and radius bones of the forearm.

Urinary Bladder 23 (UB 23) is in line with the lower border of the second lumbar vertebrae.

Western/Other Natural Remedies

Common Ingredients for Cervical Spondylosis

Spices	Herbs/Leaves	Miscellaneous
Garlic	*Harpagophytum* (devil's claw)	Ice pack
	Aloe vera	Heat pack
Ginger	Willow bark	Apple cider vinegar

Common Recipes

Oral

Teas/Brews

Aloe vera juice. Slit an aloe vera leaf down the center. Scrape out the white gel, discarding any of the yellow gel. Cut into smaller pieces, and add to a blender. Blend until smooth. Add to a fruit or vegetable smoothie, or drink alone. Take one to two times a day in the week.

Apple cider vinegar. Mix 2 teaspoons of ACV into 1 cup of warm water, and drink once a day.

Devil's claw tea. Place 1 teaspoon of devil's claw herb into a cup of hot water. Let it sit for 10 to 15 minutes. Strain, and drink. It may also be taken in the form of a capsule.

Garlic. Consume one to four cloves of fresh garlic daily.

Garlic-ginger brew. Flatten a piece of ginger and a few pips of garlic. Steep them in a glass of hot water. Drink twice a day with added honey if required.

Ginger tea. Lightly pound about 1 to 2 inches of fresh ginger (if unavailable, use 1 to 2 teaspoons of ginger powder), and add to a cup of hot water. Allow to steep for 5 to 10 minutes. Strain, and drink while warm. Add honey to taste.

Willow bark tea. Place 2 teaspoons of willow bark into a pot with about 200 mL of water. Allow to gently simmer for about 10 minutes before removing from the heat. Strain, and add honey to taste. Drink it warm.

Topical Treatments

Massage. Massages help to relax the muscles around the spine, which reduces muscle inflammation and pain.

Hot or cold packs. These can be placed on the affected joint.

Modern Remedies

Medications aim to reduce morbidity and prevent complications.

Nonsteroidal Antiinflammatory Drugs

Please refer to "Rheumatic Disorders."

Corticosteroids

Please refer to "Rheumatic Disorders."

Muscle Relaxant

Skeletal muscle relaxants are combined with other treatment modalities in painful musculoskeletal conditions. It reduces nerve impulses from the spinal cord to skeletal muscle.

Example: *methocarbamol (Robaxin)*. It is used for short term only.

Therapeutic Measures

These include physical therapy and TENS.

Surgery

Please refer to "Back Pain."

Homeopathic Remedies

These include *Kalmia latifolia* (neck pain radiating down with finger paresthesia), *Rhus Tox* (stiff painful neck from injury or overuse and relief with heat), and *Gelsemium* (neck pain with associated vertigo on walking).

References

Back Pain

Ajmera AR, Chaudhary K. *7 Ayurvedic Strategies to Alleviate Lower Back Pain*. Mindbodygreen; 2020. Available at: https://www.mindbodygreen.com/0-16683/7-ayurvedic-strategies-to-heal-lower-back-pain.html.

Allayurveda.com. *Backache*. 2018. Available at: https://allayurveda.com/kb/backache/.

Bhatia J, Hwang KO. *Herbal Remedies for Natural Pain Relief*. EverydayHealth.Com; 2016. Available at: https://www.everydayhealth.com/pain-management/natural-pain-remedies.aspx.

Bourassa P. *5 Acupressure Techniques to Relieve Lower Back Pain*. Mindbodygreen; 2018. Available at: https://www.mindbodygreen.com/articles/acupressure-for-lower-back-pain.

Chauhan M. *Ayurvedic Treatment for Back Pain—Causes, Signs and Remedies*. Planet Ayurveda; 2020. Available at: https://www.planetayurveda.com/back-pain/.

Gaeddert A. *What Chinese Herbs Are Used for Back Pain?* Acupuncture Today; 2000. Available at: https://www.acupuncturetoday.com/mpacms/at/article.php?id=27668.

Jambhekar S. *Home Remedies for Backache—Times of India*. The Times of India; 2019. Available at: https://timesofindia.indiatimes.com/life-style/health-fitness/home-remedies/home-remedies-for-backache/articleshow/38483704.cms.

Mayo Clinic. *Back Pain—Diagnosis and Treatment—Mayo Clinic*. Mayoclinic.Com; 2020. Available at: https://www.mayoclinic.org/diseases-conditions/back-pain/diagnosis-treatment/drc-20369911.

McIntosh J. *What is Causing this Pain in My Back?* Medicalnewstoday.Com; 2017. Available at: https://www.medicalnewstoday.com/articles/172943.

Morse LL, Gypson W, Guyer RD, Mazanec DJ. *Traditional Chinese medicine (TCM) and Back Pain*. SpineUniverse; 2019. Available at: https://www.spineuniverse.com/treatments/alternative/traditional-chinese-medicine-tcm-back-pain-1.

NHS website. *Treatment: Back Pain*. Nhs.Uk; 2020. Available at: https://www.nhs.uk/conditions/back-pain/treatment/.

Penman T. *Herbs for Back Pain Relief*. Holistic Health Herbalist; 2019. Available at: https://www.holistichealthherbalist.com/herbs-for-back-pain/.

Sexton S. *6 Ayurvedic Tips for Chronic Pain*. Yogainternational.Com; 2014. Available at: https://yogainternational.com/article/view/6-ayurvedic-tips-for-chronic-pain.

WebMD. *Treatments & Care*. 2005. Available at: https://www.webmd.com/back-pain/guide/back-pain-treatment-care.

Wong C, Lakhan S. *Natural Remedies for Back Pain Relief*. Verywell Health; 2020. Available at: https://www.verywellhealth.com/remedies-for-back-pain-relief-89009.

Fractures

Brazier Y. *What is a Fracture?* Medicalnewstoday.Com; 2017. Available at: https://www.medicalnewstoday.com/articles/173312.

Buckley R, Page J. *General Principles of Fracture Care Treatment & Management: Approach Considerations, Elements of Initial Fracture Management, Nonoperative Therapy*. Medscape; 2021. Available at: https://emedicine.medscape.com/article/1270717-treatment.

HealthCMi. *Acupuncture Promotes Bone Fracture Recovery*. 2008. Available at: https://www.healthcmi.com/Acupuncture-Continuing-Education-News/1893-acupuncture-promotes-bone-fracture-recovery.

Kerkar P. *Chinese Remedies for Broken Bones*. EPainAssist; 2018. Available at: https://www.epainassist.com/alternative-therapy/chinese-remedies-for-broken-bones.

Krzyżańska, L., Straburzyńska-Lupa, A., Rąglewska, P., & Romanowski, L. (2020). Beneficial Effects of Pulsed Electromagnetic Field during Cast Immobilization in Patients with Distal Radius Fracture. *BioMed Research International, 2020,* 1–8. https://doi.org/10.1155/2020/6849352

Mars B. *Herbs for Injuries and Broken Bones | Brigitte Mars*. Brigittemars.Com; 2017. Available at: https://brigittemars.com/articles/herbal-natural-remedies/herbs-for-injuries-and-broken-bones/.

Orthoinfo. *Fractures (broken bones)*. Orthoinfo.Aaos.Org; 2012. Available at: https://orthoinfo.aaos.org/en/diseases—conditions/fractures-broken-bones/.

Panda, A., & Rout, S. (2011). Puttur kattu (bandage) - A traditional bone setting practice in south India. Journal of Ayurveda and Integrative Medicine, 2(4), 174–178. https://doi.org/10.4103/0975-9476.90766.

Richey C. *7 Ayurvedic Home Remedies for Injuries and Prevention.* Gaia.Com; 2014. Available at: https://www.gaia.com/article/7-ayurvedic-home-remedies-injuries-and-prevention.

Russell S. *Trauma, Contusion, Broken Bone and Bone Healing with Herbs.* Dimmak Herbs; 2018. Available at: https://www.dimmak-herbs.com/2009/03/08/trauma-contusion-broken-bone-and-bone-healing-with-herbs/.

Wang YC, Chiang JH, Hsu HC, Tsai CH. Decreased fracture incidence with traditional Chinese medicine therapy in patients with osteoporosis: a nationwide population-based cohort study. *BMC Complement Altern Med.* 2019;19(1):42. Available at: https://doi.org/10.1186/s12906-019-2446-3.

Osteoporosis

El Wakf AM, Hassan HA, Gharib NS. Osteoprotective effect of soybean and sesame oils in ovariectomized rats via estrogen-like mechanism. *Cytotechnology.* 2013;66(2):335-343. Available at: https://doi.org/10.1007/s10616-013-9580-4.

Hebbar JV. *Triphala Churna Benefits, Ingredients, Dose, Side Effects, How to Take.* AyurMedInfo; 2017. Available at: https://www.ayurmedinfo.com/2012/03/16/triphala-churna-benefits-ingredients-dose-side-effects-how-to-take/.

Kukreja K, Mishra S, Naser S, Naser S, Naser S. *Home Remedies.* STYLECRAZE; 2020. Available at: https://www.stylecraze.com/articles/health-and-wellness/home-remedies-tips/#gref.

Levy, J. C. (2018, July 27). *Osteoporosis Treatment + 7 Natural Ways to Boost Bone Density.* Dr. Axe. https://draxe.com/health/osteoporosis-treatment/

National Institute for Health and Care Excellence. *Osteoporosis—Prevention of Fragility Fractures: Scenario: Management.* Cks.Nice.Org; 2020. Available at: https://cks.nice.org.uk/topics/osteoporosis-prevention-of-fragility-fractures/management/management/.

NHS website. *Treatment: Osteoporosis.* Nhs.Uk; 2019. Available at: https://www.nhs.uk/conditions/osteoporosis/treatment/.

Pacific College of Health Science. *TCM Solutions Osteoporosis.* Pacific College; 2014. Available at: https://www.pacificcollege.edu/news/blog/2014/11/29/tcm-solutions-osteoporosis.

Ross K. *TCM Solutions for Osteoporosis and Bone Diseases.* Acupuncture Today; 2005. Available at: https://www.acupuncturetoday.com/mpacms/at/article.php?id=30147.

Rushlau K. *New Osteoporosis Treatment Uses Traditional Chinese Herb to Prevent Bone Loss.* Www.Integrative Practitioner.Com; 2017. Available at: https://www.integrativepractitioner.com/practice-management/news/new-osteoporosis-treatment-uses-traditional-chinese-herb-prevent-bone-loss.

Russell S. *Herbs for Osteoporosis: Naturally Building Stronger Bones by Increasing Calcium and Vitamin D Absorption.* Dimmak Herbs; 2018. Available at: https://www.dimmakherbs.com/2018/01/23/herbs-osteoporosis-naturally-building-stronger-bones-increasing-calcium-vitamin-d-absorption/.

Sharma P. *Ayurvedic Cure for Osteoporosis.* Onlymyhealth; 2011. Available at: https://www.onlymyhealth.com/ayurvedic-cure-for-osteoporosis-1314359661.

The Wellbeing Team. *Can Ayurveda Treat Osteoporosis?* WellBeing Magazine; 2013. Available at: https://www.wellbeing.com.au/body/health/ayurveda-for-osteoporosis.html.

Wang YC, Chiang JH, Hsu HC, Tsai CH. Decreased fracture incidence with traditional Chinese medicine therapy in patients with

osteoporosis: a nationwide population-based cohort study. *BMC Complement Altern Med.* 2019;19(1):42. Available at: https://doi.org/10.1186/s12906-019-2446-3.

WebMD. *Osteoporosis: Treatment & Care.* 2020. Available at: https://www.webmd.com/osteoporosis/guide/osteoporosis_treatment_care.

WebMD. *Osteoporosis.* 2021. Available at: https://www.webmd.com/osteoporosis/default.htm.

White LB. *3 Natural Ways to Build Bones and Prevent Osteoporosis.* EverydayHealth.Com; 2016. Available at: https://www.everyday-health.com/columns/white-seeber-grogan-the-remedy-chicks/preventing-osteoporosis-natural-remedies/.

Zhang N, Zhang ZK, Yu Y, Zhuo Z, Zhang G, Zhang BT. Pros and cons of denosumab treatment for osteoporosis and implication for RANKL Aptamer therapy. *Front Cell Dev Biol.* 2020;8:325. Available at: https://doi.org/10.3389/fcell.2020.00325.

Rheumatic Disorders

Ambardekar N. *Rheumatic Diseases: Types, Causes, and Diagnosis.* WebMD; 2021. Available at: https://www.webmd.com/rheumatoid-arthritis/an-overview-of-rheumatic-diseases#1.

Arthritis Foundation. *Rheumatoid Arthritis: Causes, Symptoms, Treatments.* Arthritis.Org; n.d. Available at: https://www.arthritis.org/diseases/rheumatoid-arthritis.

Avicenna. *Rheumatoid Arthritis—Avicenna—Acupuncture and Herbal Chinese Medicine.* 2021. Available at: https://www.avicenna.co.uk/testimonials/rheumatoid-arthritis/.

British Homeopathic Association. *Homeopathy UK.* Homeopathy UK; n.d. Available at: https://homeopathy-uk.org/.

Dharmananda S. *An Analysis of Chinese Herb Prescriptions for Rheumatoid Arthritis.* Portland, OR: Institute for Traditional Medicine; 2000. Available at: http://www.itmonline.org/arts/arthritis.htm.

Gotter A, Carteron N. *Can Acupuncture Help Treat My Rheumatoid Arthritis?* Healthline; 2019. Available at: https://www.healthline.com/health/rheumatoid-arthritis/acupuncture#benefits.

Haskins J. *Chinese Herbal Remedy as Effective as Methotrexate for Rheumatoid Arthritis, Study Finds.* Healthline; 2018. Available at: https://www.healthline.com/health-news/chinese-herbal-remedy-as-good-as-methotrexate-for-ra-041514#1.

Mayoclinic. *Rheumatoid Arthritis—Diagnosis and Treatment—Mayo Clinic.* Mayoclinic; 2021. Available at: https://www.mayoclinic.org/diseases-conditions/rheumatoid-arthritis/diagnosis-treatment/drc-20353653.

NutritionReview.org. *Traditional Chinese Herbs for Arthritis.* Nutrition Review; 2013. Available at: https://nutritionreview.org/2013/04/traditional-chinese-herbs-arthritis/.

Ramteke R. Management of rheumatoid arthritis through Ayurveda. *J Tradit Med Clin Naturopathy.* 2016;5(2):1-4. Available at: https://doi.org/10.4172/2573-4555.1000189.

Rana S. *6 Essential Ayurvedic Herbs to Reduce Arthritis Pain this Winter.* NDTV Food; 2017. Available at: https://food.ndtv.com/food-drinks/6-essential-ayurvedic-herbs-to-reduce-arthritis-pain-this-winter-1774859.

Sharma H. *Turn to Ayurvedic Remedies for Rheumatoid Arthritis.* Onlymyhealth; 2014. Available at: https://www.onlymyhealth.com/turn-to-ayurvedic-remedies-for-rheumatoid-arthritis-1406977109.

Streit L. *10 Health Benefits of Cardamom, Backed.* Healthline; 2018. Available at: https://www.healthline.com/nutrition/cardamom-benefits.

Versus Arthritis. *Duhuo Jisheng Wan (DJW).* 2018. Available at: https://www.versusarthritis.org/about-arthritis/complementary-and-alternative-treatments/types-of-complementary-treatments/duhuo-jisheng-wan-djw/.

WebMD Editors. *CORIANDER: Overview, Uses, Side Effects, Precautions, Interactions, Dosing and Reviews*. WebMD; 2013. Available at: https://www.webmd.com/vitamins/ai/ingredientmono-117/coriander.

WebMD Editorial Staff. *What to Know About Cedarwood Essential Oil*. WebMD; 2021. Available at: https://www.webmd.com/balance/what-to-know-about-cedarwood-essential-oil.

Weil A. *Osteoporosis*. DrWeil.Com; 2019. Available at: https://www.drweil.com/health-wellness/body-mind-spirit/bone-joint/osteoporosis/.

Winchester Hospital. *Winchester Hospital*. Winchesterhospital.Org; 2021. Available at: https://www.winchesterhospital.org/.

Osteoarthritis

Arthritis Foundation. *Best Supplements for Arthritis*. Arthritis.Org; n.d.-a. Available at: https://www.arthritis.org/health-wellness/treatment/complementary-therapies/supplements-and-vitamins/supplements-for-arthritis.

Arthritis Foundation. *Osteoarthritis*. Arthritis.Org; n.d.-b. Available at: https://www.arthritis.org/diseases/osteoarthritis.

Cherney K, Wilson DR. *9 Herbs to Fight Arthritis Pain*. Healthline; 2020. Available at: https://www.healthline.com/health/osteoarthritis/herbs-arthritis-pain.

Editors of the Journal of Chinese Medicine. *The Journal of Chinese Medicine & Traditional Chinese Medicine. The J Chin Med*. n.d. Available at: https://www.jcm.co.uk/osteoarthritis-and-chinese-medicine-an-overview-of-theories-and-evidence.html%20www.healthcleveland%20.org.

Mayoclinic. *Osteoarthritis—Symptoms and Causes*. 2021. Available at: https://www.mayoclinic.org/diseases-conditions/osteoarthritis/symptoms-causes/syc-20351925.

NCBI. *National Center for Biotechnology Information (NCBI)*. n.d. Available at: https://www.ncbi.nlm.nih.gov/.

NHS website. *Osteoarthritis—Treatment and Support*. Nhs.Uk; 2021. Available at: https://www.nhs.uk/conditions/osteoarthritis/treatment/.

Olmstead CB. *Cat's Claw Potential Health Benefits*. Mercola.Com; 2018. Available at: https://articles.mercola.com/herbs-spices/cats-claw.aspx.

Patel S. *Ayurvedic Approaches to Osteoarthritis*. Chopra.Com; 2011. Available at: https://chopra.com/articles/ayurvedic-approaches-to-osteoarthritis.

Patel S. *An Ayurvedic Approach to Osteoarthritis Treatment*. Integrative Practitioner; 2012. Available at: https://www.integrativepractitioner.com/practice-management/news/an-ayurvedic-approach-to-osteoarthritis.

Pavelka K, Coste P, Géher P, Krejci G. Efficacy and safety of piascledine 300 versus chondroitin sulfate in a 6 months treatment plus 2 months observation in patients with osteoarthritis of the knee. *Clin Rheumatol*. 2010;29(6):659-670. Available at: https://doi.org/10.1007/s10067-010-1384-8.

Shiel WC, Driver CB. *Osteoarthritis Treatments, Symptoms, Definition, Cause & Diagnosis*. MedicineNet; 2021. Available at: https://www.medicinenet.com/osteoarthritis/article.htm.

Thompson D, Meara A. *13 Natural Osteoarthritis Treatments*. EverydayHealth.Com; 2017. Available at: https://www.everydayhealth.com/osteoarthritis/natural-osteoarthritis-treatments/.

Versus Arthritis. *Duhuo Jisheng Wan (DJW)*. 2018. Available at: https://www.versusarthritis.org/about-arthritis/complementary-and-alternative-treatments/types-of-complementary-treatments/duhuo-jisheng-wan-djw/.

Wang L, Wu F, Zhao L, et al. Patterns of traditional Chinese medicine diagnosis in thermal laser acupuncture treatment of knee osteoarthritis. *Evid Based Complement Alternat Med*. 2013;2013:1-8. Available at: https://doi.org/10.1155/2013/870305.

Whelan C, Minnis G. *Everything You Need to Know About Osteoarthritis*. Healthline; 2020. Available at: https://www.healthline.com/health/osteoarthritis.

Ying Yang House. *Chinese Herbal and Acupuncture Treatment Protocols for Osteoarthritis (OA)—Formulas, Protocols, TCM Diagnoses*. n.d. Available at: https://theory.yinyanghouse.com/conditions-treated/alternative-natural-options-for-osteoarthritis-oa.

Cervical Spondylitis

Delgado A, Morrison W. *Cervical Spondylosis*. Healthline; 2019. Available at: https://www.healthline.com/health/cervical-spondylosis#risk-factors.

Editors of Lybrate. *Home Remedies for Cervical Spondylosis: Procedure, Recovery, Risk & Complication*. Lybrate; 2021. Available at: https://www.lybrate.com/topic/home-remedies-for-cervical-spondylosis.

Editors of Rishikulayurshala. *Home Remedies Herbs for Neck Pain*. Rishikulayurshala.Com; n.d. Available at: https://rishikulayurshala.com/home-remedies-herbs-for-neck-pain/.

Gawas C, Kamat N, Pathrikar A, Paradkar H. Ayurvedic management of cervical spondylosis: a case study. *Int J AYUSH CaRe*. 2021;5(1):1-8. Available at: http://www.ijacare.in/index.php/ijacare/article/view/204/165.

Hebbar JV. *Triphala Churna Benefits, Ingredients, Dose, Side Effects, How To Take*. AyurMedInfo; 2020. Available at: https://www.ayurmedinfo.com/2012/03/16/triphala-churna-benefits-ingredients-dose-side-effects-how-to-take/.

Highsmith JM. *Alternative Treatments for Spondylosis*. SpineUniverse; 2018. Available at: https://www.spineuniverse.com/conditions/spondylosis/alternative-treatments-spondylosis.

Ma X. *Acupuncture.Com—Cervical Spondylosis*. Acupuncture.Com; 2015. Available at: http://www.acupuncture.com/Conditions/cervical.htm.

Mayo Clinic. *Cervical Spondylosis—Diagnosis and Treatment—Mayo Clinic*. Mayoclinic.Com; 2020. Available at: https://www.mayoclinic.org/diseases-conditions/cervical-spondylosis/diagnosis-treatment/drc-20370792.

Naser S, Wells B. *Cervical Spondylosis—Symptoms, Causes, Natural Treatments + Exercises Tips*. STYLECRAZE; 2019. Available at: https://www.stylecraze.com/articles/effective-home-remedies-to-treat-cervical-spondylosis/#gref.

Sharma H. *6 Natural Treatments for Cervical Spondylosis That Really Work!* Onlymyhealth; 2015. Available at: https://www.onlymyhealth.com/6-natural-treatments-for-cervical-spondylosis-that-really-work-1429006337.

Tanwar M. *5 Home Remedies for Neck Pain*. Practo.Com; 2021. Available at: https://www.practo.com/healthfeed/5-home-remedies-for-neck-pain-32252/post/.

Trinh K, Cui X, Wang YJ. Chinese herbal medicine for chronic neck pain due to cervical degenerative disc disease. *Spine*. 2010;35(24):2121-2127. Available at: https://doi.org/10.1097/brs.0b013e3181edfd17.

Zelman D. *Cervical Osteoarthritis: Symptoms, Treatments, Risk Factors, Diagnosis*. WebMD; 2008. Available at: https://www.webmd.com/osteoarthritis/cervical-osteoarthritis-cervical-spondylosis.

9

Skin, Hair, Nails, and Teeth

Introduction

Some of the conditions of skin, hair, and nails discussed are:
- **Skin**
  - Acne
  - Atopic dermatitis/eczema
  - Psoriasis and pruritus
  - Wound healing
  - Face and skin scrubs, moisturizers, and masks
- **Hair**—dandruff
  - Head lice
  - Alopecia (hair fall/hair loss)
- **Nails**—nail fungus
- **Teeth**—toothache
  - Dental caries

Acne

Acne is the presence of blackheads, whiteheads, and other pimples on the face. The most common locations for the breakout of acne are the face, chest, shoulders, and back. There are different forms of acne:
- **Inflammatory acne**: Inflammatory acne is more severe than non-inflammatory acne and often causes complications such as scarring or pitting of the skin. Inflammatory acne is often inflamed, red, swollen, warm to the touch, and often painful. Forms of inflammatory acne include pustules, nodules, cysts, and papules.
- **Non-inflammatory acne**: Non-inflammatory acne is a non-severe form of acne such as whiteheads and blackheads.
  - **Whiteheads**: These are small whitish-colored spots and bumps. They have white, circular centers surrounded by a red circle.
  - **Blackheads**: Blackheads are small black- or dark-colored circles that appear as slightly raised bumps. Blackheads are formed from whiteheads that open and widen. When the contents of whiteheads are exposed to air, they darken.

General Management

- Avoid frequent face washing. Once or twice a day is sufficient. Use herbal face wash or honey soap.
- Avoid comedogenic cosmetics or facial/body products that contain chemicals. Hair gels, mousse or pomades which are oil-rich can cause hairline pimples. Use natural cleansers, moisturizers for face, body, and hair.
- Avoid constant use of face masks, helmets, or mobile phones which are directly on the cheek.
- Avoid frequent change of acne remedies.
- Do not touch, pinch, or prick the pimples.
- Drink plenty of water to stay hydrated. Eat a clean diet. Adopt a healthy and holistic lifestyle.
- Change pillow covers and bed linen frequently, at least twice a week.
- Steaming the face can remove oil, dirt, and grime and open the clogged pores.
- Treat any dandruff
- Treat hormonal disorders like PCOS.

Indian Natural Remedies

In Ayurveda, the impaired *Agni* (digestive fire) causes imbalance of the *tridoshas*. *Pitta dosha* vitiation or imbalance commonly occurs, leading to penetration of *Ama* (toxins or metabolic waste) into mainly *rakta* (blood), plasma (*rasa*), and fat (*meda*) *dhatus* or tissues and blocking the *srotas* (microscopic channels). This leads to inflamed, painful and red acne. *Kapha* imbalance causes mainly oily, itchy, or cystic acne. Sour, salty, spicy, and oily foods, if eaten excessively, as well as constipation, can also trigger more acne.

Common Ingredients for Acne

Spices	Herbs/Leaves	Miscellaneous
Chandan/ sandalwood (*Santalum album*)	Tulsi (holy basil)	Chickpea (*Cicer arietinum*)
Cinnamon	Coriander leaf *Coriandrum sativum*	Bottle gourd
Coriander seed (*Coriandrum sativum*)	*Terminalia bellirica* (bibhitaki)	Carrot
Cumin	*Terminalia chebula* (haritaki)	Rose water

Spices	Herbs/Leaves	Miscellaneous
Fennel	Ashoka	Beetroot
Garlic	*Amaranthus* (amaranth)	Fruits: lemon, grape, papaya, melon, watermelon
Khus khus	*Phyllanthus officinalis* (amla)	Salt
	Picrorhiza kurroa (*kutki*)	Cedarwood oil
	Tinospora cordifolia (giloy/guduchi)	White gourd (*lauki*)
	Asparagus racemosus (*shatavari*)	Moringa (*Moringa oleifera*)
	Ashwagandha (*Withania somnifera*)	Honey
	Sadabahar / Periwinkle	Potato
	Vacha (*Acorus calamus*)	Raisins (*Vitis Vinifera*)
	Rubia cordifolia (*manjistha*)	Coconut oil
	Indian sarsaparilla/ sariva (*Hemidesmus indicus*)	Toothpaste
	Symplocos racemosa (lodhra)	Orange peel
	Mango leaf	
	Betel leaf (*Piper betle*)	
	Vetiver roots (*Chrysopogon zizanioides*)	
	Haridra (*Curcuma longa*)/wild turmeric	
	Nirgundi (*Vitex negundo*)	
	Guava leaf	
	Chirata (*Swertia chirayita*)	
	Rudraksha (*Elaeocarpus ganitrus*)	
Turmeric	*Azadirachta indica* (neem)	Cucumber (*Cucumis sativus*)

Common Recipes

Oral

Teas/Brews/Others (for internal cleansing)

Amaranth. It can be eaten as a healthy porridge.

Amla-fennel juice. Blend three to four amla fruits and 1 teaspoon of fennel seeds until smooth. Take 1 teaspoon of this mixture twice a day along with a cup of warm water.

Amla juice. Place three to four amla fruits into a blender and blend until smooth, adding some water if necessary. Take this juice on an empty stomach in the morning with a glass of warm water.

Basil-turmeric brew. Place 20 basil leaves and 2 teaspoons of turmeric into a blender and blend until it is smooth. Mix ½ teaspoon of the mixture with warm water and drink 15 to 20 minutes before a meal three times a day.

Bottle gourd juice. Skin a bottle gourd and cut the flesh into smaller pieces. Blend and puree the pieces with some water. Add a pinch of salt and drink the juice on an empty stomach.

Carrot juice. Chop three to five carrots into smaller pieces and place them into a blender. Blend until smooth, adding water if necessary. Drink once a day.

Coriander-cinnamon juice. Blend a handful of coriander leaves until smooth. Pour them into a container and add about 1 teaspoon of cinnamon powder to the juice. Mix well and take 1 teaspoon of this mixture twice a day.

Indian sarsaparilla (Sariva) tea. Add ½ to 1 teaspoon of the root powder into a cup of hot water. Cover and steep for 5 to 10 minutes. Strain and drink twice a day.

Lemon water. Add a slice of lemon to your glass when drinking water; drink seven to eight glasses per day.

Polyherb juice. Add giloy, amla, and tulsi to a blender and blend until smooth. Drink once a day.

Polyherbal powder. Place equal parts of coriander seed, fennel seed, dried basil, ground turmeric, and dried ground amla in a grinder and grind into a fine powder. Take ½ teaspoon of this powder and mix it with hot water. Consume it 15 minutes before lunch and dinner.

Raisins. Take 30 to 40 raisins. Soak them in water overnight. Crush them and consume them with the water first thing in the morning for 2 to 3 months.

Three-herb tea. Mix an equal amount of cumin seeds, coriander seeds, and fennel seeds. Steep ⅓ teaspoon of these seeds in a cup of hot water for 5 to 10 minutes. Drink at least three times a day.

Three-herbal mixture. Mix equal portions of kutki, giloy, and shatavari. Take ¼ teaspoon of the mixture two to three times a day with warm water.

Triphala brew. Add a teaspoon of triphala powder or paste to a cup of warm water. Stir until dissolved and then drink it. Drink once a day before bedtime or first thing in the morning.

Watermelon juice. Consume fresh watermelon juice.

Topical

Amaranth oil. The oil can be applied as a face mask.

Amla paste. Make a paste with amla powder or freshly ground amla and apply it to the face. Leave it on for 20 minutes and then wash it off.

Ashoka bark paste. Place 25 g of ashoka bark powder into a pot with 200 mL of water. Boil the mixture slowly until the water has reduced to about 50 mL. Add 50 mL of milk and continue to boil it until only 50 mL of liquid is left. Strain and cool. Apply to the acne.
Boil the above ashoka mixture into a thicker concoction. Add some mustard oil. Apply to the acne.

Betel leaf–turmeric juice. Blend two to three betel leaves, mix them with some fresh turmeric juice and add a few drops of pure coconut oil. Apply the mixture to the inflamed spots.

Cedarwood oil. Dilute the oil with a carrier oil. Apply the oil on the acne with a cotton bud. Leave for 20 minutes and rinse off. Repeat one to two times a week.

Chirata. Make a ground paste from the chirata plant. Apply it to the face, leave it on for 15 minutes, and then rinse it off.

Coriander leaf paste. Make fresh coriander leaf paste and add little turmeric to it. Apply it to the face, leave it on for 15 minutes, and then rinse it off

Garlic rub. Cut some slits into a clove of garlic. Rub the clove of garlic onto the acne several times a day.

Giloy paste. Place ¼ teaspoon of guduchi, ⅛ teaspoon of neem, and ⅛ teaspoon of turmeric into a grinder and grind until it forms a smooth paste. Apply the paste to the face, leave it on till the mask dries, and then rinse it off. Do this at least three times a week.

Honey. Apply pure honey or manuka honey to the face. Leave it on for 10 minutes and then wash off.
Variation #1. The honey may be mixed with a little cinnamon powder.

Indian sarsaparilla (Anantmool) paste. Make a paste from sariva root powder and apply it on acne spots. Leave it on for 20 minutes to reduce dark spots and pigmentation.

Lemon water. Squeeze the juice of two lemons into a cup, diluting with 2 teaspoons of water. Apply this to the face as a tonic. Leave it on overnight and rinse it off the next morning.

Lodhra paste. Mix equal amounts of lodhra with coriander leaves and vacha to make a paste. Apply the paste to the face and leave it on for 20 to 30 minutes.

Mango-guava leaf mask. Blend two to three guava and mango leaves until they form as smooth paste. Apply the paste to the face and leave it on for 30 minutes before rinsing it off. Repeat two to three times a day.
Guava leaves may be used alone.

Manjistha paste. Mix manjistha with honey, neem, and turmeric to make a paste. Apply the paste to the face and leave it on for 20 to 30 minutes.

Melon paste. Grind the melon into a fine paste and rub it into the skin at bedtime. Sleep with this mask on overnight and wash the face in the morning.

Neem paste. Boil 10 young neem leaves for about 2 to 3 minutes before grinding them into a thick paste. Add some rosewater to the paste and apply to the face. Leave it on till it dries.
Variation #1. Cold-pressed neem oil can also be applied over the pimples.

Rudraksha powder (churna). Take equal amounts of Rudraksha powder and manjishta powder. Mix with some honey to make a thin paste. Apply on the face. Leave for 30 minutes and then rinse off with warm water.
Variation #1. Take equal amounts of Rudraksha churna and Arjuna churna and do the same as above.
Variation #2. Make a paste with some 9-mukhi Rudraksha powder and fresh Tulsi juice. Apply on the affected skin.

Neem-turmeric-nirgundi leaf ground paste. These are mixed with sandalwood and rose water and applied on the face.

Orange peel. Grind or blend some pieces of orange peel. Mix this with some rose water and apply it to the face. Leave it on for 15 minutes and then rinse it off.

Papaya mask. Mash some ripe papaya flesh and apply it to the face. Leave it on for 20 minutes and then wash off.

Papaya-sandalwood paste. Skin ½ papaya and cut the flesh into smaller chunks. Mash the papaya flesh until smooth and add 1 tablespoon of sandalwood powder to it. Add a few drops of water if necessary. Apply the mask to the face and leave it on for 15 to 30 minutes. Repeat three to four times a day.

Potato-raisin mask. Skin and slice a potato. Place the potato and 1 tablespoon of raisins in a blender and blend until smooth. Apply the mixture to the face and wash it off once it has dried. Repeat three to four times a week.

Sadabahar-Neem leaf fresh leaf. Mix this grounded paste with some turmeric powder and rose water and apply it to the face. Allow the paste to dry and then wash it off.

Sandalwood-turmeric paste. Mix some sandalwood and turmeric with some rosewater to make a paste. Apply the paste to the face for 30 minutes and then wash it off.

Toothpaste. Apply a little toothpaste (herbal- or menthol-containing) to the acne to dry it out.

Tulsi juice. Take some fresh tulsi leaves. Wash and crush them to extract some juice. Apply the juice to the face, leave it on for 20 minutes, and then wash it off.

Turmeric mask. Make a paste from turmeric powder with some rosewater or honey, apply it to the face, leave it on for 20 minutes, and then rinse it off.

Vacha paste. Mix vacha, manjistha, and turmeric together, adding enough rose water to make a paste. Use it as a mask to cleanse the skin and clear acne.

Vetiver root–wild turmeric–amla powders. These are mixed with dried rose petals and rosewater and applied to the face.

Watermelon juice. Apply watermelon juice to the face and leave it on overnight. Rinse it off the next morning.

Therapeutic Measures

Diet and Lifestyle

- Stay hydrated by drinking enough water. Minimize the consumption of sweet, oily, processed, and refined foods. Consume more whole grains, vegetables, and fiber for regular bowel movements.

- Regular purification of the blood, liver, and gut should be done (detoxification with fasting, juicing, enemas, and herbs). *Virechana* (purgation or enema) should be done every 2 to 3 months.
- Exercise regularly to keep fit.

Chinese Natural Remedies

Common Ingredients for Acne

Herbs/Leaves	Miscellaneous
Angelic root (dang gui)	Indigo naturalis/qing dai
Chinese skullcap/huang qin *Scutellaria baicalensis)*	Honeysuckle flower/jin yin hua *(Lonicera japonica)*
Female ginseng (dong quai)	
Ginseng	
Peony root (bai shao)	Cucumber
Phellodendron/huang bo *(Phellodendri cortex)*	Egg white
Red peony (chi shao)	Goji berry
Rehmannia root (sheng di)	Aloe vera
Tree peony root (mu dan pi)	Pearl barley powder

Common Recipes

Oral

Teas/Brews/Others

Ginseng tea. Add two to four slices of ginseng to a cup. Pour boiling water over the ginseng and allow it to steep for about 10 to 15 minutes and drink.

Honeysuckle tea. Add 1 tablespoon of the flower buds to boiling water. Steep for 3 minutes and drink

Pearl barley powder: Mix pearl barley powder and some goji berries. Consume as a breakfast cereal.

- Acne caused by heat in the lungs and stomach:
  - **Symptoms**: Facial acne with oily, shiny skin. Dry mouth, red tongue, dark urine.
  - **Herbs**: Huang qin, huang bo, sheng di, and mu dan pi are helpful.
- Acne caused by phlegm stagnation and dampness:
  - **Symptoms.** Dark-red clustered acne that is present for a long period of time.
  - **Herbs**: Dang gui, bai shao, and chi shao are helpful.

Topical

Qing dai. Mix a tablespoon of qing dai powder with some cucumber juice to make a paste. Apply the paste all over the face and wash off when dry.

- **Pearl barley powder.** Mix ½ cup of pearl barley powder with two egg whites and some aloe vera gel to make a paste. Apply the paste, allow it to harden, and sleep with it overnight. Continue this every day for about 2 weeks.
- **Honeysuckle face wash.** Place a handful of dried honeysuckle flowers into a bowl and pour boiling water over them. Let mixture sit overnight and strain it in the morning. Place the liquid in a clean container and store in a cool dry place. To apply, wet a ball of cotton wool and use it on the skin as a tonic.

Therapeutic Measures

Diet

- Ensure a good balance between "cold" and "warming" foods. Cold foods include raw fruit and vegetables, as well as pressed juices, shakes, and raw salads. Warming foods include chicken, spicy food, and ginger.
- Consume adaptogen-filled supplements. Adaptogens are thought to correct imbalances in the body and relieve the nervous system's stress. Ginseng is an adaptogen.

Lifestyle

Acupuncture

CV6 (Qihai). This point is located below the navel in the midline of the abdomen.

LI11 (Quchi). This point is just at the lateral (outer) elbow crease.

LR3 (Taichong). This point is on the foot about two finger widths above the second toe.

LI4 (Hegu). This point is located in the web between the thumb and index finger.

SP10 (Xuehai): With the knee flexed, this point is located at a two-finger width above the superior medial border of the patella on the bulge of the medial portion of thigh (quadriceps) muscles.

Ashi. These points are those near injuries.

ST25 (Tianshu). This point is located at a two finger width from the side of the navel.

Cupping. This is done to reduce heat and improve blood circulation.

Western/Other Natural Remedies

Common Ingredients for Acne

Spices	Herbs/Leaves	Miscellaneous
Cinnamon	Green tea leaf	Witch hazel
	Rosemary	Honey
	Chamomile flower	Essential oils: eucalyptus, lavender, neem, tea tree, rose, geranium, blue yarrow, and calendula
	Dandelion root	Apple cider vinegar (ACV)
	Burdock root	Fig seed oil
	Basil	Rosehip oil
	Hibiscus	Baking soda
	Fig leaves	Hydrogen peroxide
	Purple coneflower/ echinacea *(Echinacea purpurea)*	Alcohol
	Milk thistle	Aspirin/salicylic acid (beta hydroxy acid, BHA)
	Pokeweed leaves	Azelaic acid
	Aloe vera	Alpha hydroxy acids (AHAs) *from plant sources*

Spices	Herbs/Leaves	Miscellaneous
		Ascorbic acid (vitamin C)
	Olive leaf extract	Trichloroacetic acid (TCA)
		Allantoin
		Phloretin
		Ferulic acid

Common Recipes

Oral

Teas/Brews/Others

Rosemary tea. Add three to five sprigs of fresh rosemary (or 1 ½ teaspoons of dry rosemary leaf needles) to a cup of hot water and steep for 10 to 15 minutes. Drink warm.

Chamomile tea. Place some dried or fresh chamomile flowers into a cup. Pour boiling water over the flowers and allow to steep for 10 minutes. Strain and add honey to taste. Drink hot.

Burdock root tea. Roughly chop fresh or dried burdock root into smaller chunks. Add 2 tablespoons of the chopped root to a pot with water. Allow to simmer gently for about 10 minutes before turning the heat off. Strain and drink warm.

Olive leaf extract. Consume olive leaf extract capsules once a day.

Green tea. Add 1 teaspoon of green tea leaves to a pot with a cup of hot water. Boil and then simmer for 3 to 5 minutes. Cool and strain the mixture. Add honey to taste and drink three to four times a day.

Dandelion root tea. Place 1 to 2 teaspoons of dandelion root into a cup of hot water and steep for 5 to 10 minutes. Strain and drink.

Milk thistle. The seed and leaf extracts are available as a powder, tablet, tea, or tincture. Steep a tea bag in a cup of hot water for 5 minutes and consume.

Bitters. Place 28 g of lavender, 1 teaspoon of dried valerian root, 2 teaspoons of dried passion flower, 1 teaspoon of dried orange peel, and half a teaspoon of dried ginger into a glass jar. Cover the herbs with just enough alcohol (e.g., vodka) to submerge the herbs fully. Seal in an airtight jar. Place the jar in a cool, dark place for 2 to 4 weeks. Shake the jar once a day. When ready, strain through a piece of muslin cloth into a clean jar and store at room temperature. To serve, mix a few drops in hot tea or water.

Topical

Allantoin based products (comfrey root extract or synthetic form). It is applied on the acne.

Ascorbic acid (Topical Vitamin C). Stable and water soluble derivatives of vitamin C i.e. tetra-isopalmitoyl ascorbic acid, magnesium ascorbyl phosphate and others are used topically and usually combined with plant or herbal ingredients.

Antioxidant combinations with Vitamin C (l-ascorbic acid), phloretin and ferulic acid creams are available.

Alcohol. Apply some alcohol directly on the acne using a cotton ball.

Aloe vera gel. Wash and dry an aloe vera leaf. Slit the leaf down the center. Discard the yellowish-green gel and keep the white gel. Place the white gel in a blender and blend until smooth. Strain the mixture. Apply this gel all over the skin. Store any balance in the fridge.

Apple cider vinegar (ACV). Dilute one part ACV with three parts water and soak a cotton pad in the solution. Squeeze out any excess liquid and apply all over the skin as a tonic.

Aspirin. Take a few aspirin tablets, crush them, and add some water to make a paste. Apply the paste onto the areas with acne. Leave it on for 15 minutes and then rinse it off. Commercial salicylic acid (0.5% to 2%) is also available and very effective.

Azelaic acid. Apply azelaic acid (15% to 20% [available as gel, foam, or cream]) on the face at night or twice a day after cleansing.

It can also be combined or alternated with salicylic acid.

Baking soda. Take a teaspoon of baking soda and a little water to make a paste. Leave it on for 20-30 minutes, and then rinse it off.

Basil mask. Grind five to eight fresh basil leaves into a smooth paste. Apply on the face and leave on for 30 minutes before washing off.

Burdock root mask. Combine and make a paste of burdock root tea with some oatmeal and a few drops of lemon juice. Apply it as an anti-acne face mask.

Burdock root tonic. Soak a cotton ball in burdock tea and apply it on the face.

Chamomile tea tonic. Place some dried or fresh chamomile flowers into a cup. Pour boiling water over the flowers and steep for 10 minutes. Soak a cotton pad in the solution. Squeeze out any excess liquid and apply all over the skin as a tonic.

Chemical peels. These include trichloroacetic acid (TCA) 25%, salicylic acid 30%, and alpha hydroxy acid (AHA) containing serum or gel.

Fig oil and blends. Mix fig seed oil with any one or two non-comedogenic plant carrier oil (rosehip oil, argan, grapeseed, jojoba, or hazelnut oil). Other essential oils such as tea tree oil, frankincense, or ylang ylang oil may also be added.

Green tea tonic. Add 1 teaspoon of green tea leaves to a pot with a cup of hot water. Boil and simmer for 3 to 5 minutes and strain the mixture. Soak a cotton pad in the solution. Squeeze out any excess liquid and apply all over the skin as a tonic.

Honey cinnamon mask. Mix 2 tablespoons of honey and 1 teaspoon of cinnamon together to form a paste. Apply to a dry clean face and leave on for 10 to 15 minutes.

Hydrogen peroxide 3%. Apply some diluted hydrogen peroxide (one-part H_2O_2 to three parts water) on the acne with a cotton ball. Leave it on for 5 minutes and wash it off.

Oils. There are several oils that are beneficial in reducing acne because of their anti-inflammatory and antibacterial properties. Wet a cotton swab with the oil and apply it on the spots. Some of the oils that may be used are eucalyptus, lavender, geranium, blue yarrow, neem, calendula, and rose. Take two or three drops of any essential oil and add nine parts of carrier oil.

Pokeweed. Apply pokeweed leaves as a poultice over the affected areas.

Purple cornflower or echinacea. Apply echinacea-based cream or ointment.

Rosemary essential oil. Dilute rosemary essential oil with a carrier oil (jujube oil) and apply.

Rosemary tonic. Add 1 ½ teaspoons of dry rosemary needles to a cup of hot water and steep for 10 to 15 minutes. Soak a cotton pad in the solution. Squeeze out any excess liquid and apply all over the skin as a tonic.

Tea tree oil. Dilute the tea tree oil with water on a 1:9 ratio. Use a cotton swab and dip into the mixture and spot treat the acne. Repeat one to two times a day. Never apply pure tea tree oil to the skin directly. It may cause excessive dryness.

Witch hazel tonic. Place 1 tablespoon of witch hazel bark into a pot with 1 cup of water. Soak for 30 minutes, then boil, and simmer for about 10 minutes. Allow to sit for another 10 minutes. Strain and store the liquid in a clean dry container. To use, soak a cotton pad in the solution. Squeeze out any excess liquid and apply all over the skin as a tonic.

Therapeutic Measures

Diet

See under general management.

Lifestyle

Face steaming. Lean over a bowl of hot water and cover the head with a towel. Stay under the towel for 15 to 20 minutes before drying the face. The steam can open the pores on the face and relieve blockages in the pores.

Hot and Cold Compress. Apply a warm compress over the face for 5 to 10 minutes, then wash the face with cold water a few times or use a cold towel compress. Repeat the process at least three times.

Modern Remedies

Benzoyl Peroxide

Benzoyl peroxide is an antibacterial agent. It works by killing bacteria. It does not affect sebum production and does not cause skin cells to shed. However, it must be used continuously. Once treatment is stopped, the acne is likely to reoccur.

Salicylic Acid

Salicylic acid increases skin cell shedding and reduces the pH of the skin with increased keratin hydration. It helps to unclog pores.

Topical Retinol Gel

Retinol prevents pimple formation. It affects the growth of cells, which causes an increased cell turnover rate, hence aiding in unclogging pores. It must be used for 8 to 12 weeks before seeing significant improvement.

Antibiotics

Systemic antibiotics may be prescribed for moderate to severe acne and inflammatory acne that is resistant to topical treatment. Tetracyclines are first-line therapy in moderate to severe acne. They act by inhibiting protein synthesis in bacteria by binding to the 30S subunit of the bacterial ribosome. They also have anti-inflammatory effects by inhibiting chemotaxis. Macrolide antibiotics are also used. They have a similar mechanism of action to tetracyclines. They bind to the 50S ribosomal subunit, but the exact mechanisms of actions are not clear.

Examples: tetracycline, doxycycline

Microneedling. This is a roller with hundreds of tiny fine needles which are run over the face to make tiny punctures. The roller can be bought as an OTC item or the procedure can be done by a dermatologist. It is done usually every 4 to 6 weeks. Complications include bleeding, bruising, infection.

Homeopathic Remedies

These include *Calcarea sulphurica, Calcarea carb, Antimonium crudum, Arsenicum iodatum, Hepar sulphuris calcareum, Kalium bromatum, Pulsatilla*, psorinum, silica, and others.

Atopic Dermatitis/Eczema

Symptoms of atopic dermatitis are often present before 5 years of age. Symptoms include scaly, dry skin; rashes that leak clear fluid; cracked and painful skin, skin creasing on the palms; and darkening of the skin around the eyes.

Infantile eczema usually first appears between the ages of 2 and 3 months, sometimes from the first week of life and up to 2 years of age; but it can continue into teens or adulthood. However, most children outgrow infantile eczema by 3 to 5 years of age.

Eczema may have a genetic predisposition, but it is often triggered by multiple factors such as strong soaps or detergents, certain fabrics, pollen and mold, animal dander, heat, sweat, or dry skin. Various medications are available to lessen flare-ups and relieve the itchiness.

Indian Natural Remedies

Common Ingredients for Eczema

Spices	Herbs/Leaves	Miscellaneous
Flaxseed	*Rubia cordifolia* (manjistha)	Vegetable shortening
Khus khus	*Asparagus racemosus* (shatavari)	Olive oil
		Tea tree oil
		Coconut oil
		Oatmeal
		Milk
		Baking soda
		Honey
		Hemp seed oil
		Epsom salt
Turmeric	Neem	Ghee

Common Recipes

Oral

Teas/Brews

Flaxseed brew. Consume 2 to 3 teaspoons of ground flax-seed with a glass of warm water. Alternatively, eat flax-seed with salads or oatmeal.

- **Manjistha-neem paste.** Place equal amounts of manjistha and neem in a blender and blend until smooth. Consume ½ teaspoon twice a day.
- **Neem tea.** Place three to five fresh neem leaves into a pot with 1 cup of water. Boil for a few minutes and then simmer for 3 to 5 minutes. Remove from the heat and strain. Drink once a day.
- **Shatavari tea.** Mix 1 teaspoon of ground shatavari into a cup of warm milk. Drink this at bedtime.
- **Turmeric tea.** Mix 1 teaspoon of turmeric into a cup of warm water and drink. Take this once a day. Alternatively, use turmeric to season cooked dishes.

Hemp seed oil. Take 1 to 2 teaspoons of the oil daily.

Topical

- **Baking soda.** Mix 1 and ½ cups of baking soda with about 1 L of water. Apply the mixture to itchy skin with a clean cotton cloth.
- **Coconut oil.** Apply coconut oil all over the affected area and cover it with a plastic wrap, leaving it for 2 to 4 hours before washing off.
- **Epsom salt bath.** Add 1 to 2 cups of Epsom salts and ½ cup of Himalayan salt into a warm bath. Soak in the bath for 30 to 45 minutes.
- **Hemp seed oil.** Take ¼ cup of hemp seed oil and add 2 teaspoons of coconut oil (other essential oils can also be added). Apply the oil to the affected area.
- **Honey.** Apply honey to the skin and leave it on for about an hour. It is thought to have antimicrobial and anti-inflammatory properties.
- **Khus khus paste.** Grind khus khus with some milk or water to make a thick paste. Apply on the affected areas.
- **Olive oil.** Apply olive oil to the itchy skin and cover with plastic wrap. Let it sit for about 2 hours before washing it off.
- **Tea tree oil.** Dilute some tea tree oil with olive oil and rub it into the affected skin several times a day. It is thought to relieve itching and soften the scaly skin.
- **Turmeric paste.** Mix ground turmeric with some water to make a smooth paste. Apply the paste to the irritated skin and leave on for about 30 minutes before washing off.
- **Vegetable shortening.** Coat the affected area with vegetable shortening and cover with some plastic wrap. Leave for 2 to 4 hours before washing. Perform once a day until the rash eases.

Chinese Natural Remedies

Common Ingredients for Eczema

Herbs/Leaves	Miscellaneous
Amur cork tree/ huang bo (Phellodendri cortex)	Coix seed Yi Yi Ren (Coix lacryma-jobi)
Dandelion root	Hawthorn berries
Glycyrrhiza glabra (liquorice/ gan cao)	Mung bean (Vigna radiata)
Hybrid tea rose	Celery
Light-yellow sophora root (ku shen)	Green apple
	Bitter melon
	Tomato (Solanum lycopersicum)
	Asian pear
	Walnut
	Rice
Lotus leaf	Kelp
Sweet apricot kernel/xing ren (Prunus armeniaca)	Egg

Common Recipes

Oral

- **Acute stage of eczema:**

  Celery salad. Cut 250 g of fresh celery and blanch in boiling water for one minute. Soak in cold water immediately. Drizzle with salt and sesame oil. Consume one to two times a day for a week.

  Coix seed porridge. It can also be cooked as a porridge or soup with rice and/or lily bulbs. Add rock sugar to taste.

  Huang bo tea. Take about 3 to 12 g of the powder once a day. Place the powder into a cup of hot water and mix well. Huang bo is also available as sliced, dried pieces of bark.

  Kelp soup. Place 15 g of soaked and cut kelp, 15 g of mung beans, 6 g of tea rose, and 9 g of sweet apricot kernels in a pot with water. Boil for 30 to 40 minutes before removing the tea rose. Drink once a day, eating the kelp, mung beans, and sweet apricot kernels. Take for 10 days.

  Ku Shen egg. Beat an egg. Soak ku shen for 30 minutes, then boil for 20 minutes, strain out the herbs, 10 g of sugar, and then slowly add the egg into the herbal mixture. Consume once a day for 6 days.

  Mung bean soup. Soak 25 g of mung beans, 25 g of coix seeds, and 10 g of hawthorn berries in water for an hour, then bring to a boil for 5 to 10 minutes. Remove from the heat and let the mixture sit for 15 minutes. Drink once a day.

- **Chronic stage of eczema:**

  Celery-pear juice. Place 100 g of celery, one tomato, and 150 g of Asian pear in a blender and blend until smooth. Drink once a day for a week.

  Mung bean and green juice. Boil 30 g of mung bean in water for 30 to 45 minutes. Juice celery, bok choy, bitter melon, and a green apple. Mix the mung bean juice with the green juice with added honey and half-lemon juice. Drink once a day for a week.

  Walnut-hawthorn Congee. Boil 9 g of hawthorn, 9 g of walnuts, and half a lotus leaf for 30 minutes. Add a handful of rice and add 2 cups of water. Cook till soft. Consume when warm.

Western/Other Natural Remedies

Common Ingredients for Eczema

Herbs/Leaves	Miscellaneous
Aloe vera	
Burning bush	
Calendula/Pot marigold (Calendula officinalis)	Coconut oil
Chamomile flower	Beeswax pastilles or pellets
Chickweed leaves	
Comfrey leaf	Epsom salt
Fenugreek	Essential oils (evening primrose oil, borage oil, sea buckthorn oil, tea tree oil, neem seed, lavender, mint, cajeput and emu oil)
Milk thistle (Silybum marianum)	Almond oil
Plantain weed/leaf (Plantago major)	Himalayan salt
Purple cornflower (Echinacea purpurea)	Allantoin
Rose/Rosehip oil (Rosa damascena)	
White cnidium (Cnidium monnieri)	Honey
Yarrow flower	Donkey milk

Common Recipes

Topical

Aloe vera gel. Slit an aloe vera leaf down the center and scoop out the white gel. Discard any yellow gel. Cut the white gel into cubes and place into a blender. Blend until smooth and refrigerate. Apply over the affected areas.

Allantoin based products (comfrey root extract or synthetic form). It is applied on the eczema.

Beeswax. Take equal amounts (2 tablespoons each) of coconut oil, beeswax pellets or pastilles and shea butter. Double boil and melt the ingredients. Pour into a container and allow it to harden. Use when required.
Variation #1. Mix a little olive oil, honey, and beeswax. Apply to the skin two to three times a day.

Burning bush. Make a paste from the bark powder and apply directly as a poultice.

Calendula salve. Place 1 to 2 tablespoons of dried calendula flowers into a cup of warm almond oil and leave for 2 to 3 weeks. Strain the mixture. Gently melt ½ cup of beeswax and add to the calendula oil. Stir in some essential oil (such as lavender) and allow it to set before using.

Chamomile tonic. As above.

Chickweed leaves: Take some fresh chickweed leaves. Add equal amounts of water and white vinegar, blanch till soft, and apply the leaves on the skin as a poultice.
Variation #1. To make a salve, take two handfuls of freshly chopped leaves. Add 1 to 1 ¼ cups of olive oil.

Warm this in a double boiler for 15 minutes. Remove and place in a jar. Allow it to steep for 24 to 48 hours. Strain and add one ounce of melted beeswax to this oil. Use this salve for the skin.

Essential Oils. To use the essential oils, dilute any one of them with some carrier oil such as almond or coconut oil before applying to the affected skin. Cover with a plastic sheet and let sit for 2 to 4 hours before washing it off.

Fenugreek paste. Grind fenugreek seed into a fine powder and add some hot water, enough to make a paste. Apply to the affected skin, leave on for 10 minutes, and rinse.

Herb salve. Place 1 tablespoon of dried comfrey leaf, 2 tablespoons of dried plantain weed/leaf, 1 tablespoon of dried calendula flowers, 1 teaspoon of dried yarrow flowers, and 1 teaspoon of dried rosemary leaves into 2 cups of almond oil. Leave for 2 to 3 weeks, shaking the jar daily. When the herbs are ready, heat ½ cup of beeswax pastilles. Strain the herbs and add the beeswax to the herbal oil. Pour them into clean containers, allow to set, and apply as needed to the irritated skin.

Rose/Rosehip oil. Apply rose/ rosehip oil in carrier oil on the eczema sites.

Plantain weed/leaf. Place a handful of fresh crushed plantain leaves in a jar. Add ½ cup of coconut oil. Place the jar in a hot water bath for about 2 hours. Add 1 tablespoon of beeswax. When cooled, pour the salve into a jar.

Purple cornflower or echinacea: Apply echinacea based cream or ointment to the eczema.

Sea salt spray: Add 1 tablespoon of Himalayan salt and a pinch of Epsom salt to a pan with 1 cup of boiled water. Add 1 to 3 drops of essential oil (lavender or mint) to the mixture and heat gently until all the salt has melted. Place into a glass jar or spray bottle and use it on the affected skin. Sea salt sprays are most effective on weeping, wet eczema.

Therapeutic Measures

Baths

Daily bathing and moisturizing should be routine.
Bath soaks should be for about 15 to 20 minutes.

Lukewarm Water Bath. Use a lukewarm bath. Sit the baby in the bath for 15 to 20 minutes to reduce itching and dehydration. Then rinse the baby gently and pat dry; and apply any moisturizer or oils while the skin is still damp

Dab baby's face with plain cool water or a moisturizer several times per day to relieve itch and dryness.

Sea Salt Bath. Home-made salt baths are effective for wet/oozing eczema. Use a few tablespoons of Himalayan salt or sea salt. Any of the above oils or essential oils (10 to 15 drops) below can be added.

Magnesium Bath. Add one cup of Epsom salts or magnesium flakes and add 10 to 15 drops of any oils/essential oils to the lukewarm bath.

Combined Magnesium and Salt Bath. A few tablespoons of Himalayan or sea salt can be added to the above magnesium bath.

Oatmeal Bath. Add ⅓ cup of ground (or instant) baby oats to the lukewarm water bath, or it can be tied in a muslin cloth or a pantyhose. (A patch test is recommended on the forearm skin if it is a first-time use. Place a small amount of oatmeal paste on the skin, leave for 15 minutes, and observe for any reaction.) Soak in the bath for 15 to 20 minutes. Rinse off with warm water and pat dry.

Chamomile Tea Bath. Soak five chamomile tea bags in a lukewarm bath for 15 minutes.

Baby products

Baby products (soaps, cleansers, baths, or moisturizers) should be chemical free and natural (i.e., free of parabens, petroleum chemicals, sulfates, artificial colors, and synthetic fragrances and steroids—these are common skin irritants). Many white soaps contain titanium.

Soaps made from donkey's milk with added oils (coconut oil, almond oil, olive oil and shea butter) can help to moisturize dry skin or eczema.

Moisturizers

These include *lavender oil, coconut oil, cocoa butter, manuka honey, chamomile, cold-pressed sunflower oil,* and *tea tree oil.*

General Measures

Humidifiers and Air Conditioning. Humidity is good for the skin. It hydrates the body and reduces inflammation and itching. During cold winters, central heating can dry the skin. Having a humidifier helps. In the hot summers, cool air conditioning or fans help reduce sweating, which can aggravate the itching.

Clothes. Use light and loose clothes made of cotton or natural, breathable fabrics. Wash them in chemical-free detergents. Air and sun winter clothes frequently to remove damp and dust mites.

Sun Bath. Allow the child to play in the morning sun naked (or just use underwear or diapers) in the backyard or garden for about 15 to 20 minutes with no sunscreen or footwear. Apply only coconut oil or preferably plain cod liver oil on the whole body. This enhances more sunshine vitamin D production!

Environment. The infant should grow and live in a clean and natural environment but not obsessively sterile. There is some truth in the germ hypothesis.

Foods. For breastfed babies who develop eczema within the first week of life, the nursing mothers should try to eliminate foods that cause reactions in the baby but not herself. There are mixed views on whether weaning foods should be introduced early or late. Babies must be offered freshly cooked meals, not "dead foods or ready-to-eat jar or pouch foods." Consume functional foods.

Nutritional Supplements. *Cod liver oil*/fermented cod liver oil: This contains the fat-soluble vitamins A, D, E, and K, which help in healing.

Probiotics. Many beneficial soil-borne microorganisms that provide friendly bacteria to the gut are lost from current farming methods and/or excessive washing. We also eat more processed foods and little or no fermented foods.

Bone broths (home-made) and gelatin-rich foods also help in healing of the gut, skin, hair, and nails.

Miscellaneous. It is helpful to clip the infant's nails short or have the infant wear cotton mittens to avoid scratching the face.

Modern Remedies

There are no definitive treatments for eczema. Treatment aims to reduce the discomfort of eczema symptoms.

Moisturizers

Moisturizers are the mainstay of treatment. Eczema may flare up because of skin becoming dry and irritated. Individuals with eczema have drier than normal skin because of an imbalance in the skin barrier. Using a moisturizer regularly can protect the skin barrier and prevent eczema flare-ups. Various fragrance and preservative-free moisturizers that replenish the skin's natural oils are available. They may be oil or water based.

Examples: Cetaphil, Eucerin, Nivea, etc.

Emulsifying Ointment

This is a mix of paraffin oils and may be used to moisturize dry skin. It leaves a thin layer of oil on the skin's surface and prevents water that is in the skin from evaporating. It should be applied to damp skin.

Topical Corticosteroids

Topical corticosteroids are used in the treatment of atopic dermatitis in both adults and children and are the mainstays of anti-inflammatory therapy. They act on a variety of immune cells, including T lymphocytes, monocytes, macrophages, and dendritic cells, interfering with antigen processing and suppressing the release of pro-inflammatory cytokines. In turn, this constricts blood vessels in the skin, hence relieving skin redness and inflammation, as well as itching.

Topical steroid strength is dependent on the class. Class 1 is super potent (i.e., clobetasol propionate) while Class 7 is the least potent (i.e., hydrocortisone). Skin atrophy can occur with prolonged use.

Topical Ectoine Creams

Ectoine is a skin protective compound that can be found naturally in bacteria, or it can be synthesized. It acts as an osmolyte and stabilizes the cell from dryness or UV light stress.

Antihistamines

If itching is profound and disturbs sleep, systemic antihistamines may be given (e.g., Piriton/loratadine, cetirizine). Topical antihistamines are not effective.

Topical Calcineurin Inhibitors

Topical calcineurin inhibitors (TCIs) are second-class anti-inflammatory drugs. They are naturally produced by *Streptomyces* bacteria and block calcineurin-dependent T-cell activation, inhibiting the production of proinflammatory cytokines and mediators of the AD inflammatory reaction. They also affect mast-cell activation and decrease both the number and costimulatory ability of epidermal dendritic cells.

This decreases the incidences of flare-ups. There is no reported evidence of an increased risk of malignancy with the use of this treatment. It does not cause skin atrophy.

Example: Tacrolimus

Topical Antimicrobials

Skin infections are common in atopic dermatitis because of a compromised physical barrier, poor immune recognition, and impaired antimicrobial peptide production. *Staphylococcus aureus* can colonize the skin in atopic dermatitis. This can trigger multiple inflammatory cascades via toxins that act as superantigens and exogenous protease inhibitors, which can further aggravate and damage the epidermal barrier and potentiate allergen penetration.

Phototherapy

Phototherapy using ultraviolet B (UVB) light may be used in severe eczema. It reduces itching, relieves inflammation, and increases the skin's ability to fend off bacteria.

Oral Small Molecules (Cytokine inhibitors)

Oral and once-a-day reversible and selective JAK1 and JAK2 inhibitors, e.g., Baricitinib is used to treat moderate to severe atopic eczema.

Homeopathic Remedies

These include calcarea carbonica, *Natrum mur, Pulsatilla, Rhus tox, Hepar sulphuris calcareum, Sulfur arsenicum album,* graphites, and others.

Psoriasis and Pruritus

Psoriasis is a skin disorder where skin cells multiply about ten times more quickly than normal skin does. This causes a build-up of skin, forming bumpy red patches with white scales. It is most commonly found on the scalp, elbows, lower back, and knees. There is also a genetic predisposition.

Symptoms of psoriasis may vary from person to person depending on the type of psoriasis they have. There are five types of psoriasis:

- **Plaque psoriasis**: This is the most common type of psoriasis and often produces symptoms such as thick red patches of skin with a white scaly layer. They are often 1 to 10 cm wider but may be larger.
- **Guttate psoriasis**: This form of psoriasis forms small red spots on the skin and is the second most common form of psoriasis. The spots are small, separate, and drop shaped. They are not as thick as in plaque psoriasis but may develop into plaque psoriasis over time. It can be triggered by strep throat, stress, skin injury, or infection.
- **Inverse psoriasis**: Inverse psoriasis often occurs in folds of skin (under the armpit or groin area). It is often red, shiny, and smooth in texture.
- **Pustular psoriasis**: Pustular psoriasis is a very severe form of psoriasis that presents as white pustules surrounded by red skin. It may cover most of the body or affect isolated body parts, such as the hands or feet.

The pustules may join together and form scales. They may cause flu-like symptoms.
- **Psoriatic arthritis**: Psoriatic arthritis is painful and causes many limitations in physical ability. There is no treatment for this and it is an autoimmune disease. It may affect the joints and quite severely affect the hands.

Pruritus is chronic itchy skin caused by a variety of factors: allergies, diabetes, pregnancy, and aging.

In this section, psoriasis and pruritus have been combined as the natural remedies and modern remedies are similar.

Indian Natural Remedies

Common Ingredients for Psoriasis and Pruritus

Spices	Herbs/Leaves	Miscellaneous
Frankincense/ru xiang (*Olibanum gummi*)	Bibhitaki (*Terminalia bellirica*)	Bitter gourd
	Haritaki (*Terminalia chebula*)	Lime
	Amla (*Phyllanthus officinalis*)	Oat
	Neem	Buttermilk
	Trivrit	Ghee
	Peepal leaf/ Aswattha	Honey
	Rudraksha (*Elaeocarpus ganitrus*)	Beeswax
		Olive oil
Sesame seed	Banana leaf	Plastic wrap
Turmeric	Cabbage (*Brassica oleracea*)	Epsom salt

Common Recipes

Oral

- Teas/Brews (as Discussed Under "Atopic Dermatitis/ Eczema")

Bitter Gourd-lime juice. Cut one to two fresh bitter gourds into smaller chunks and place in a blender. Blend and puree with a little water. Squeeze in the juice of a lime and drink once a day for at least 5 to 6 months.

Cabbage juice. Place two to three cabbage leaves into a blender and blend until smooth, adding a little water if necessary. Drink once a day.

Neem tea. Crush four to five neem leaves and add to a cup of hot water. Allow to steep for about 10 minutes. Strain and drink.

Sesame seed. Soak 15 to 20 sesame seeds in water overnight. In the morning, consume the sesame seeds and drink the water, preferably on an empty stomach.

Triphala brew. Add half a teaspoon of triphala powder to one cup of hot water. Mix well and drink it warm. Triphala powder is made up of three ingredients: amla, haritaki, and bibhitaki.

Trivrit. Boil 5 g of trivrit with 200 mL of water. Reduce to 50 mL. Consume this decoction.

Turmeric tea. Add 1 to 2 teaspoons of ground turmeric to 1 cup of hot water. Mix well and add honey to taste. Drink one to two times a day. Alternatively, lightly pound 2 to 3 inches of fresh turmeric and add to a cup of boiling water. Allow it to steep for 5 to 10 minutes and strain. Add honey to taste.

Topical

Banana leaf. Apply fresh banana leaf to the affected skin.

Buttermilk. Apply buttermilk to the skin and leave on for 30 minutes before rinsing.

Epsom salt bath. Run a warm bath and add about 1 cup of Epsom salt to the bathwater. Soak for 20 to 30 minutes.

Ghee. Coat the affected area with ghee and cover with some plastic wrap. Leave for 2 to 4 hours before washing. Perform once a day until the rash calms.

Honey mixture. Take equal amounts of honey, olive oil and beeswax. Mix them and apply on the skin lesions.

Oat bath. Run a lukewarm bath and add 1 cup of raw oats. Soak in the bath for 30 minutes to an hour to soften the plaques.

Rudraksha. Place the Rudraksha in a copper jug or pot filled with 250 ml water. Leave it overnight. Consume this water first thing in the morning on an empty stomach.

For better efficacy, add 2 grams Rudraksha powder (churna) into 250 ml of water in a copper vessel. Leave overnight and consume the next morning. Alternatively, a decoction can be made by adding 5 grams Rudraksha churna into 400 ml water and boiling till the volume is reduced to 100 ml.

Sandalwood essential oil. Add 20 drops of the essential oil to half a cup of a carrier oil. Apply on skin lesions.

Turmeric paste. Grind fresh turmeric into a smooth paste or grind dry turmeric into a smooth powder, adding a little water as necessary to make a thick paste. Alternatively, mix turmeric powder with enough water to make a thick paste. Apply on the skin lesion for 15 to 20 minutes before washing off.

Chinese Natural Remedies

- Psoriasis because of **blood heat**
  - Symptoms include an acute eruption of bright, active red lesions. They spread quickly and have an irregular pattern. They may be severely itchy and are aggravated by heat.
- Psoriasis because of **blood dryness**
  - Symptoms resemble plaque psoriasis. It is chronic with large coalescent plaques, which are thicker and more difficult to peel off with dry cracked skin. Patients may appear pale, feel dizzy, or may have poor memory.
- Psoriasis because of **blood stasis**
  - This is a chronic condition with cyclic clearance and relapse of the lesions. The lesions are dark and covered by thick hard scales. The skin may sometimes appear leathery. The lesions may appear to be cracked and are painful.

Common Ingredients for Psoriasis and Pruritus

Herbs/Leaves	Miscellaneous
Anemarrhena/zhi mu (*Anemarrhena asphodeloides*)	
Balloon flower root/jie geng (*Platycodon grandiflorus; Radix*)	
Burdock fruit/niu bang zi (*Arctium lappa*)	
Chinese peony (*Radix paeoniae lactiflorae*)	
Chinese rhubarb/da huang (*Rheum palmatum*)	
Chinese skullcap/huang qin (*Scutellaria baicalensis*)	
Chuan xiong (*Rhizoma Ligustici chuanxiong*)	
Cicada slough/chan tui (*Periostracum cicadae*)	
Fang feng/siler root (*Radix Saposhnikovia divaricata*)	
Female ginseng/dang gui (*Radix Angelicae sinensis*)	
Fructus forsythia suspensa (lian qiao)	
Gardenia fruit/zhi zi (*Fructus gardeniae*)	
Gypsum fibrosum	
Herba menthae haplocalycis (bo he)	
Herba schizonepetae tenuifolia (jing jie)	Peach seed kernel (tao ren)
Indigo naturalis/qing dai	
Japanese catnip/jing jie (*Schizonepeta tenuifolia*)	
Moutan root bark (mu dan pi)	
Poria sclerotium/Poriae cocos/ Wolfiporia extensa (fu ling)	
Radix angelicae sinensis	
Radix glycyrrhizae (liquorice)	
Radix glycyrrhizae uralensis	
Radix rehmanniae glutinosae	
Radix saposhnikoviae (fang feng)	Talcum
Radix sophorae flavescentis	
Ramulus cinnamomi cassiae (gui zhi)	
Red peony root (chi shao)	
Rhizoma atractylodis lanceae	
Rice paper pith/tong cao (*Tetrapanax papyrifer*)	
Sodium sulfate/Natrii sulfas	
White atractylodes rhizome/bai zhu (*Atractylodes macrocephala*)	

Common Recipes

Oral

- Psoriasis because of **blood heat**:
  - **Fang feng tong sheng wan** (Siler and platycodon formula): This medication clears heat and toxins from the body.

    Ingredients: *Radix saposhnikoviae (Ledebouriella), Herba schizonepetae tenuifolia, Fructus forsythia suspensa, Herba menthae haplocalycis, Ramulus cinnamomi cassiae, Rhizoma ligustici chuanxiong, Radix angelicae sinensis, Radix paeoniae lactiflorae, Radix scutellariae baicalensis, Radix platycodi grandiflora, Radix glycyrrhiza (liquorice), Rhizoma atractylodis macrocephalae, Fructus gardeniae jasminoidis,* Radix et rhizoma rhei, natrii sulfas, talcum, and gypsum fibrosum

- Psoriasis because of **blood dryness**:
  - **Xiao feng wan** (arctium formula): This medication speeds up the recovery of skin lesions.

    Ingredients: *Herba schizonepetae tenuifolia, Radix saposhnikoviae divaricata, Radix angelicae sinensis, Radix rehmanniae glutinosae, Radix sophorae flavescentis, Rhizoma atractylodis lanceae, Periostracum cicadae, Fructus arctii lappae, Rhizoma anemarrhenae asphodeloides, Radix glycyrrhizae, Medulla Tetrapanax papyrifer,* and gypsum fibrosum
- Psoriasis because of **blood stasis**:
  - **Gui zhi fu ling wan** (cinnamon and poria formula): This medication promotes blood circulation to relieve blood stasis.

    Ingredients: Cinnamon, *Poria sclerotium,* moutan root bark, red peony root, and peach seed kernel

Western/Other Natural Remedies

Common Ingredients for Psoriasis and Pruritus

Herbs/Leaves	Miscellaneous
Aloe vera	Epsom salt
Burning bush	Oat
Cayenne pepper (capsaicin)	Oregon grape (burberry)
Chickweed leaves	Apple cider vinegar
Peppermint	Tea tree oil
Verbena *(Verbena officinalis)*	Dead Sea mud or salt

Common Recipes

Topical

Aloe vera gel. As above (Refer under "Acne")

Apple cider vinegar. It is a potent disinfectant. Dilute it with water in a 1:1 ratio and apply thinly to the skin. Let dry and rinse off with water. Do not use it on open wounds.

Burning bush. Make a paste from the bark powder and apply directly as a poultice.

Cayenne pepper rub. Add 1 to 2 teaspoons of cayenne pepper to a pot with 1 cup of olive oil. Bring to a simmer for 15 to 20 minutes. Let it cool completely and place it into a clean container. Apply to the affected skin to reduce redness, pain, inflammation, and scaling.

Chickweed leaves. Refer under "Atopic Dermatitis/Eczema."

Oat bath. Run a lukewarm bath and add 1 cup of raw oats. Soak in the bath for 30 minutes to an hour to soften the plaques.

Peppermint. Apply 0.5% to 1% solution twice a day.

Sea salt spray. As above.

Tea tree oil. It can be applied topically to relieve psoriasis. Dilute with coconut oil and rub onto the affected skin. This can also provide an antiseptic function.

Sea salt spray. As above.

Verbena. Take 1 tablespoon of fresh lemon verbena leaves or 1 teaspoon of dried leaves. Add 1 cup of boiling water. Steep or simmer for 15 minutes. Strain. When cool, soak a clean cloth and apply on the skin.

Therapeutic Measures

- **Swimming in sea water or Dead Sea.** Swimming in sea water can help reduce skin inflammation. Dead Sea is even more therapeutic as it is mineral-rich especially in zinc and bromide.
  - **Dead Sea products.** Various Dead Sea products including sea salts and mud are available. The Dead Sea salts are used as bath soaks or as shampoo. The Dead Sea mud is actually fine powder which is mixed with some water and this paste is applied on skin lesions or used as a mud wrap.
- **Fish spa or fish pedicure.** The feet and lower legs are immersed in a tank of water with small fish called *Garra rufa* (or doctor fish). The fish nibble away the dead skin. However, the risks of infection and contamination outweigh the benefits.

Modern Remedies

Topical Coal Tar

Coal tar products are available as shampoo, soap, cream, ointment, and gel. It slows down skin growth and reduces inflammation, itching, and scaling.

To apply the shampoo, massage it into the scalp and leave it on for 5 to 10 minutes before rinsing out.

Topical Corticosteroids

As above.

Topical Calcineurin Inhibitors

As above.

Topical Ectoin-Based moisturizers

It forms a protective layer on the skin in psoriasis.

Vitamin D Analogues

Synthetic vitamin D3 is used in oral supplements, topical creams or lotions. It may slow skin cell growth, which can be used to treat mild to moderate psoriasis.

Examples: calcipotriene, calcitriol

Biologic Drug (Monoclonal Antibody)

This is a protein-based drug derived from living cells cultured in a laboratory. It targets specific parts of the immune system. The biologics used to treat psoriasis block the action of a specific type of immune cell, that is, T cell or block proteins in the immune system (i.e., tumor necrosis factor-alpha, TNF-alpha/interleukin 17-A, and interleukins 12 and 23). These cells and proteins are present in psoriasis and psoriatic arthritis.

These biologic drugs stop the inflammatory pathway in psoriatic disease. Examples:

TNF-alpha inhibitors: Humira (adalimumab), Enbrel (etanercept), Cimzia (certolizumab), and Simponi (golimumab)

Interleukins 12 and 23 (IL-12/23) Inhibitors: Stelara (ustekinumab)

Interleukin 17 (IL-17) inhibitors: Cosentyx (secukinumab), Taltz (ixekizumab)

T-cell inhibitors: Orencia (abatacept)

Interleukin 23 (IL-23) inhibitors: Ilumya (tildrakizumab), Tremfya(guselkumab)

These biologics can be used with other treatments such as phototherapy or used topically. They are given intravenously or intramuscularly. They can improve the Psoriasis Area and Severity Index (PASI) scores significantly in severe chronic plaque psoriasis (score of 90 or 100 up to 4 years). Biologics can also increase the risk of infections.

Anthralin

Anthralin is also used to slow skin cell growth and may also help remove scales and smooth out the skin.

Topical Retinoids

Topical retinoids are vitamin A derivatives. They may help to reduce inflammation but may cause skin irritation as a side effect. They may also increase sensitivity to sunlight.

Oral Retinoids

Acitretin is an oral second-generation vitamin A (retinoid) derivative used in severe psoriasis. Side effects include dry skin, eyes, and mouth, as well as hair loss.

Phototherapy

Phototherapy using ultraviolet light A (PUVA) or ultraviolet light B (PUVB) is given two or three times per week. It alleviates the pruritis.

Immunosuppressants

These include methotrexate and cyclosporine

General Management

- Avoid processed foods.
  - Avoid foods that trigger a flare-up.
  - Avoid extremes of cool or dry weather.

Homeopathic Remedies

These include *Arsenic album* (for silver scales), *Arsenic iodatum* (for shedding of large scales), *Graphites naturalis* (for scalp psoriasis and rough, thick nails) and *Sulfur* (with severe itching and burning).

Wound Healing

Open wounds are any injuries that break the skin's surface, leaving the tissue under the skin exposed to the environment.

General wounds are classified based on the following:

Appearance: Closed or Open wounds

There are four types of open wounds:

- *Abrasion*: Abrasions, also called scrapes, are caused by the skin being rubbed against a hard or rough surface. They are often shallow and may not bleed.
- *Avulsion:* Avulsions are caused by the skin being torn away, exposing the tissue beneath it. They are usually caused by car accidents or gunshots. They often bleed extensively.
- *Laceration*: Lacerations, also called guts, are deep tears in the skin. They are caused by sharp objects, such as knives. Deep lacerations often cause profuse bleeding and may need stitches to help them heal.
- *Puncture*: When a sharp, pointed object injures the skin, a hole is formed, causing a puncture wound.

Sterility and cleanliness: Surgical wounds are classified by the Centers for Disease Control (CDC) as:

Class 1 wounds: Clean wounds

Class 2 wounds: Clean-Contaminated

Class 3 wounds: Contaminated

Class 4 wounds: Dirty (infected)

Depth of wound

Superficial wound: Loss of epidermis

Partial thickness: Loss of epidermis and dermis

Full thickness wound: Loss of dermis, subcutaneous fat and sometimes bone)

Specific wounds

Diabetic foot ulcers

Pressure sores (ulcers)

Venous ulcers

Burns

Principles of Wound Care

These include the following:

- Stop or secure bleeding (Hemostasis)
- Clean the wound
- Apply antibiotics if indicated
- Cover or close the skin of the wound
- Regular dressings till wound heals
- Provide analgesia

Indian Natural Remedies

Common Ingredients for Wound Healing

Spices	Herbs/Leaves	Miscellaneous
Carom seeds (Ajwain)	Curry leaf	Ghee
	Gotu kola	Salt
	Trivrit	Charcoal powder (burnt coconut shells or rice husk)
	Sadabahar (Periwinkle)	*Channa striatus* (snakehead fish/ mudfish/"haruan" fish)

Spices	Herbs/Leaves	Miscellaneous
	Plantain weed/leaf	Kutaja
	Banyan leaf	Yogurt
	Ceylon leadwort/ chitrak (*Plumbago zeylanica*)	Jyotishmati
	Kanchanara (*Bauhinia variegata*)	Ashoka tree bark
	Lady's mantle	Herbal oils (Thailam): *Murivenna thailam*
	Dhataki	
	Crape jasmine (*Tabernaemontana divaricata*)	
	Mimosa pudica	
	Jalakumbhi	
	Ivy gourd leaves	
	Peepal leaf	
	Bael leaf	
	Indian abutilon/Indian Mallow (*Abutilon indicum*)	
	Rudraksha (*Elaeocarpus ganitrus*)	
Clove	Betel leaf	Limestone powder (chuna)
Garlic	*Terminalia chebula* (haritaki/kadukkai)	Oils: Tea tree and coconut
Onion	Lemon leaf	Honey
Turmeric	Amla (*Phyllanthus emblica*)	Potato

Common Recipes

Oral

Teas/Brews/Others

- **Amla tonic.** Lightly pound three to four amla fruit and extract the juice. Add a little ghee to the amla juice and drink once a day.
- *Channa striatus* **(snakehead fish/mudfish/haruan fish).** See under Chinese remedies.
- **Garlic, onion, and cloves.** These have antimicrobial and antioxidant properties and are consumed in daily foods.
- **Turmeric milk.** Mix 1 teaspoon of turmeric into a cup of warm milk. Drink warm, preferably right before bedtime.

Topical

Honey-ghee. Add equal amounts of honey and ghee to a clean bowl. Mix well and rub some over the wound. Leave on for 30 to 45 minutes before washing. Apply regularly.

- **Honey.** Apply some honey on the wound regularly and let sit for 30 to 45 minutes before washing. Honey is known to have antibacterial, antifungal, and anti-inflammatory properties.

- **Garlic.** Lightly crush a clove of garlic and apply it to the wound.
- **Onion.** Skin and cut an onion into smaller chunks. Place the onion and 2 teaspoons of honey into a blender. Blend until it forms a paste and apply it over the wound.

Ashoka tree bark. Boil the ashoka tree bark with some water. Use this water to cleanse the wounds. Then apply crushed ashoka leaves and flowers on the skin.

Bael leaves. Mix bael leaf powder with some coconut oil. Apply on the wound.

Banyan leaf paste. Take some banyan leaves. Grind with some yogurt. Apply on the wound or burn.

Carom seeds (ajwain). The ajwain seeds can be crushed and applied on the skin to treat small wounds or infections.

Charcoal or carbon ash (from burnt coconut shells or rice husk). This powder is mixed with little water and applied as a poultice.

Chitrak. Mix the root powder with some water to make a paste. Apply on the wound or ulcer. Turmeric can also be added.

Coconut oil. Apply coconut oil to the wound and cover it with a clean piece of cloth. Reapply the coconut oil about two to three times a day.

Crape jasmine. Take the milky juice of the leaves. Apply directly on the wound.

Curry leaf. Pound a few curry leaves with some water to make a paste. Apply this over mild burns or wounds. Leave it overnight. The dry paste will fall off by itself.

Dhataki flower paste. Take some dried dhataki flower powder. Mix with some coconut oil. Apply on the wound.

Gotu kola. Apply poultices or ointments containing gotu kola.

Haritaki powder. Mix Haritaki powder with a little water, enough to make a smooth paste. Apply to the wound and leave on overnight before washing.

Indian mallow. Take ½ to 1 teaspoon of the Indian mallow powder. Mix with some coconut oil to make a paste. Apply on the wound once a day.
  Variation #1. Grind the leaves, flowers, and roots; extract the juice; and add a little sesame oil. Apply on the wound or inflamed skin.
  Variation #2. Take the mimosa plant. Crush it and add some water. Apply or wash on the inflamed skin or wound.

Ivy gourd leaves. Apply the crushed leaves as a poultice.

Jalakumbhi. Extract the juice from the blended leaves and boil in some coconut oil. When cool apply on the skin lesion.

Jyotishmati. Take some seeds. Soak in water with a little turmeric for 3 hours. Make into a paste. Apply on the wound or ulcer.

Kanchanara. Mix the dried bark powder with some honey to make a paste. Apply on the wound or ulcer.

Kutaja. Take ¼ to ½ teaspoon of dried seed powder and add 2 cups of water. Boil and reduce the volume to ½ a cup. Wash the wound twice a day.

Lady's mantle. Use the tea as a wash (Take 5 to 10 g of lady's mantle, add 1 L of boiling water, and allow it to steep for 10 to 15 minutes) or apply the crushed leaves as a poultice.

Lemon leaf and betel leaf. Soak the wound in warm water infused with lemon leaves for ½ hour. Then apply a paste of ground betel leaf paste over the dry wound. Leave it overnight. The dry paste will fall off by itself.

Limestone powder. Add equal amounts of limestone powder and turmeric to a pan. Heat it gently, such that the mixture becomes warm. Apply the mixture to the wound regularly to speed up the healing process.

Rudraksha powder (churna). Make a paste with some 9-mukhi Rudraksha powder and fresh Tulsi juice. Apply on the affected wound.

Mimosa. Take the mimosa leaves. Blend to a paste. Apply on the wound or skin lesion.

Murivenna thailam. Apply this medicated polyherbal oil on the wound.

Peepal. Take 2 g of Asvattha bark powder (or 25 g of the stem park). Add 200 mL of water. Boil until liquid volume reduces to 50 mL. When lukewarm, use the solution to wash the wound
Variation #1. Sprinkle some root bark powder over the wound The root bark fine powder of Asvattha is used for dusting over the oozing skin lesions to stop secretion.

Plantain weed/leaf. Warm the leaves and add some mustard oil. Place it over the wound twice a day.

Potato. Peel a potato and mash the skin until it reaches a paste-like texture. Apply the potato skin on the open wound and wrap it with a clean piece of cloth. Leave the potato on the wound overnight, washing it in the morning with saltwater.

Sadabahar. Blend and make a fine paste of sadabahar leaves and some turmeric powder. Neem leaves may also be added. Apply to the wound two to three times per day.

Saltwater. Add 1 tablespoon of salt to a cup of hot water, mixing well until the salt has completely dissolved. Wash the wound with salt water regularly as an antiseptic.

Tea tree oil. Dilute tea tree oil by adding 3 to 5 drops of it to 2 to 3 tablespoons of water. Coconut oil is preferred over water. Mix well and apply to the wound four to five times a day. Alternatively, crush a few fresh tea tree leaves and apply them to the cut.

Trivrit. Make a fine paste with trivrit and turmeric. Apply the paste on the chronic ulcer or wound.

Turmeric paste. Mix some turmeric powder with water to make a smooth, thick paste. Apply the paste to the wound to reduce inflammation.

Chinese Natural Remedies

Common Ingredients for Wound Healing

Herbs/Leaves	Miscellaneous
Angelica dahurica (Chinese angelica/bai zhi)	
Angelica sinensis (female ginseng/dang gui)	
Astragalus membranaceus (huang qi)	
Comfrey leaf	*Channa striatus* (snakehead fish/mudfish/haruan fish)
Dandelion leaf (pu gong ying)	Sea cucumber species (*haishen* in Chinese or *gamat* in Malay)
Ginseng (ren shen)	
Goldenseal (huang Lian)	
Ligusticum striatum (chuan xiong)	
Myrrh gum (mo yao)	Cattail pollen /Pu Huang (*Typha angustifolia* or *Typha orientalis*)
Pseudoginseng (san qi)	
Purple gromwell/zi cao (*Lithospermum erythrorhizon*)	Gleditsia spine/zao jiao ci (*Gleditschiae sinensis spina*)
Red peony (chi shao)	
Rehmannia root (di huang)	
Turmeric (huang jing)	
White peony (bai shao)	

Common Recipes

Oral

- Post-Trauma Tea:
  Ingredients: san qi, dang gui, comfrey leaf, huang qi, chi shao, mo yao, and huang jin.
  Method: Place the ingredients into a pot with some water and bring to a boil. Simmer gently for about 30 minutes. Strain and drink throughout the day.
- Supplementing Tea:
  Ingredients: ginseng, di huang, dang gui, tien qi, bai shao, and chuan xiong.
  Method: Place the ingredients into a pot with some water and bring to a boil. Simmer gently for about 30 minutes. Strain and drink throughout the day.
- **Soup extracts or tablets of *Channa striatus*** (snakehead fish/mudfish/haruan fish) are consumed by postpartum women for wound healing, pain relief, and rejuvenation in many Asian communities. It is rich in arachidonic acid, glycine amino acid, and polyunsaturated fatty acid, which all are necessary for prostaglandin synthesis.
- **Sea cucumber.** It is consumed as food (raw, dried, fried, pickled, or braised with other vegetables, seafoods, or meats). It has antimicrobial, antioxidant, and anti-tumour properties. It is rich in arachidonic acid, chondroitin sulfate collagen, amino acids, and many bioactive compounds. It nourishes the qi. It also helps to rebuild cartilage and promotes wound healing. It is available commercially as a health tonic. As it has blood-thinning properties, caution has to be exercised when taking it with prescription drugs.

Tuo-Li-Xiao-Du-San. It is a polyherbal mix of four herbs *Astragalus membranaceus, Angelica sinensis, Angelica dahurica,* and *Gleditsiae sinensis spina.*

Topical

Poultice. There are many recipes using various herbs.

i. *Ingredients:* comfrey leaf, dandelion leaf, myrrh gum, and goldenseal.

Instructions: Place the ingredients into a pot with some water, bring to a boil, and then simmer gently for about 30 minutes. Strain and let cool. Soak a clean piece of cloth in the liquid and squeeze out any excess. Place the cloth directly onto the wound and let it sit for 30 to 45 minutes.

ii.
  - **Creams extracts of *Channa striatus*** (snakehead fish/mudfish/haruan fish).
  - Sea cucumber "gamat" oils and ointments: These promote wound healing.

Cattail pollen. Apply the pollen and fluff on the bleeding wound. Mix it with lard and honey and apply to scalds and burns. For inflamed wounds, mix the cattail with some honey and apply.

Gleditsia spine. Take ½ tablespoon of spine or thrones. Shimmer in vinegar. Make into a paste and apply.

Notes

- Tien Qi
  - This herb is thought to heal wounds and improve blood circulation.
- Dang Gui
  - This herb has anti-inflammatory properties, helps tonify the blood, and improves blood circulation.
- Comfrey Leaf
  - Comfrey leaf speeds up wound healing.
- Huang Qi
  - This herb improves qi circulation and hydrates and energizes the body.
- Chi Shao
  - This herb is anti-inflammatory and improves blood circulation.
- Mo Yao
  - Mo yao speeds up wound healing by improving blood circulation.
- Huang Jing
  - Huang jing is anti-inflammatory.
- Ginseng
  - Ginseng aids in the circulation of qi in the body.
- Di Huang
  - Di huang may be used fresh or prepared and is thought to fill the blood with nutrients to help to improve wound healing.
- San Qi
  - San qi is thought to improve blood circulation, hence improving wound healing.
- Bai Shao
  - Bai shao is thought to tonify the blood and relax the body.

- Chuan Xiong
  - Chuan xiong is thought to improve the circulation of qi and blood in the body.

Western/Other Natural Remedies

Common Ingredients for Wound Healing

Herbs/Leaves	Miscellaneous
Achillea millefolium (yarrow)	Apple cider vinegar (ACV)
Arnica (*Arnica montana*)	Cucumber
Burning bush	Oat
Calendula flower	Aloe vera
Cayenne pepper	Activated charcoal
Chamomile flower	Witch hazel
Chickweed	Beeswax
Cinnamon	Coconut oil
Cleavers	Cajeput oil
Cottonwood (*Populus balsamifera* or *P. trichocarpa*)	
Geranium leaf	
Goldenrod (*Solidago* spp.)	Honey
Lamb's ear (*Stachys byzantina*)	
Lavender oil	Juniper berries and leaves
Mallow leaf	
Marshmallow root	Sunflower oil
Plantain weed/leaf (*Plantago major*)	Vaseline
St. John's wort	Emu oil
Verbena (*Verbena officinalis*)	

Common Recipes

Topical

Activated charcoal poultice. Make a paste with 1 teaspoon of activated charcoal powder and little water. Apply to the wound for 10 minutes and then wash off. Repeat twice a day until the wound heals. Charcoal traps odors and toxins from wounds.

Aloe vera gel. Slit an aloe vera leaf down the middle and scrape out the white gel on the inside. Discard any of the yellowish-green gel. Cut the white gel into smaller chunks and place into a blender, blending until smooth.

Apple cider vinegar: Dab some raw undiluted ACV onto the wound and rinse off when dry.

Beeswax. Take equal amounts (2 tablespoons each) of coconut oil, beeswax pellets or pastilles and shea butter. Double boil and melt the ingredients. Pour into a container and allow it to harden. Use when required.

Variation #1. Mix a little olive oil, honey, and beeswax. Apply on the skin two to three times a day.

Helichrysum italicum essential oil. This can be applied on the wound with some carrier oil.

Burning bush. Make a paste from the bark powder and apply directly as a poultice.

Cajeput oil. Apply the cajeput oil onto the wound after diluting it with a carrier oil.

Calendula. Place 1 to 2 teaspoons of dried calendula into a pot with 1 cup of water. Bring to a boil and then remove from the heat. Allow to steep for 10 to 15 minutes. Strain and soak a clean piece of cotton in the liquid. Squeeze out any excess and place the cloth on the wound for 30 to 45 minutes every day.

Cayenne pepper rub. As above.

Chamomile. Place 1 to 2 teaspoons of dried chamomile flowers into a pot with 1 cup of water. Bring to a boil and then remove from the heat. Let steep for 10 to 15 minutes. Strain and soak a clean piece of cotton in the liquid. Squeeze out any excess and place the cloth on the wound for 30 to 45 minutes every day.

Chickweed leaves. Take some fresh chickweed leaves. Add equal amounts of water and white vinegar. Blanch till soft. Apply the leaves on the wound as a poultice. Avoid this if it is an open wound.

Variation #1. To make a salve, take two handfuls of freshly chopped leaves. Add 1 to 1 ¼ cups of olive oil. Warm this in a double boiler for 15 minutes. Remove and place in a jar. Allow to steep for 24 to 48 hours. Strain and add one ounce of melted beeswax to this oil. Use this salve for the skin.

Cinnamon paste. Add some honey to ground cinnamon to make a paste and apply to the wound, leaving it on for 30 to 45 minutes before washing off. Alternatively, add a little water to cinnamon to make a paste.

Cottonwood bud oil. Take fresh cottonwood buds and place them in a slow cooker. Fill with olive oil till brim and let it simmer and steep for 5 days. Strain into a clean jar to use as a salve. It can also be steeped in alcohol such as vodka or rum for 2 to 3 weeks, then strained and used as a salve.

Cleavers. Apply fresh crushed leaves as a poultice or the juice from the leaves on the wound.

Coconut oil. Apply the coconut oil onto the wound.

Cucumber. Thinly slice some cucumber and place it on the wound. Let it sit for 30 to 45 minutes.

Emu oil. It can be applied to minor wounds. It has pain-relieving and antioxidant effects.

Geranium leaf. Apply the bruised or crushed fresh geranium leaves on the wound as poultice.

Goldenrod. Take 1 to 2 teaspoons of dried goldenrod into a pot with 1 cup of water. Bring to a boil and then remove from the heat. Let steep for 10 to 15 minutes. Strain and soak a clean piece of cotton in the liquid. Squeeze out any excess and place the cloth on the wound for 30 to 45 minutes every day.

Helichrysum italicum **essential oil.** This can be applied on the wound with some carrier oil.

Honey. Apply honey on to the wound.

Juniper berries. Apply crushed berry juice on the wound.

Lamb's ear leaf. Take some crushed or bruised leaves and place on the wound.

Mallow leaf. Apply the crushed mallow leaves as a poultice on the wounds, bruise, or inflamed site.

Mallow leaf. Apply the bruised or crushed fresh mallow leaves and flowers on the wound.

Marshmallow root poultice: Take some fresh crushed or dried ground marshmallow root powder. Add enough hot water to form a paste and place it on the cut. Cover with a piece of clean cloth and allow to sit for 30 to 45 minutes before washing off.

Variation #1. Apply the bruised or crushed fresh marshmallow leaves on the wound.

Oat bath. Run a lukewarm bath and add 1 cup of raw oats. Soak in the bath for 30 minutes to an hour to soften the plaques.

Plantain weed/leaf. Apply fresh washed plantain leaves which have been softened in hot water, or apply the plantain pulp.

St. John's wort. Apply ready-made ointment or salve containing St. John's wort on wounds.

Sunflower oil. It has anti-inflammatory and antibacterial properties. It is applied to the wound.

Vaseline. This can be applied as a barrier dressing.

Verbena. Take 1 tablespoon of fresh lemon verbena leaves or 1 teaspoon of dried leaves. Add 1 cup of boiling water. Steep or simmer for 15 minutes. Strain. When cool, soak a clean cloth and apply on the wound.

#Variation 1. Crush fresh leaves into a pulp. Apply on the wound.

Witch hazel. Dip a piece of cotton in some witch hazel and rub over the wound, leaving to dry naturally.

Therapeutic Measures

Homeopathic polybotanicals-oil mix (e.g., Emuaid). This is a rub-on cream for minor wounds (also for bedsores, eczema, rashes, and other difficult-to-treat skin conditions). It relieves pain and has antibacterial and antifungal properties. It contains argentum metallicum (silver) with emu oil, tea tree oil, castor oil, olive oil, candelilla leaf wax, moringa seed oil (tribehenin), allantoin, ceramide 3, phytosphingosine, vitamin E, and probiotic.

Hyperbaric oxygen therapy. Hyperbaric oxygen is a daily treatment where a patient is placed in a hyperbaric chamber and the atmospheric pressure increases to above sea level. Once the desired pressure has been reached, the individual stays in the chamber for about an hour, breathing normally. The pressure increase allows oxygen to dissolve into the blood plasma at a higher rate. The increase in oxygen in the body reduces inflammation in the body's tissues and reintroduces blood flow to oxygen-starved areas. Hyperbaric oxygen promotes wound healing.

Maggot therapy. Live disinfected maggots are placed onto a non-healing wound. This will clean out the necrotic tissue and aid wound healing.

Ozone. Ozone can be administered in several ways. Ozone spray or compress is also available. Ozonated water can be applied as a spray or a compress to the wound.

Platelet-rich plasma (PRP) injections. The plasma is obtained from the patient's blood and then specially centrifuged and injected around the wound.

Red light therapy. This is a low wavelength light that can penetrate deeply into the skin and helps with wound healing via new blood vessels and collagen formation.

Stem-cell injections. Stem cells may be injected to speed up wound healing as it may stimulate the formation of blood vessels and hence bring down tissue inflammation.

Modern Remedies

Basic Treatment Principles

- Clean and wash wounds or skin ulcers with saline/saltwater, diluted hydrogen peroxide, or iodine.
- **For clean wounds**, to speed up the wound-healing process and epithelialization, various items can be used:
  - *Solcoseryl gel or ointment*: It contains a protein-free dialysate from calf blood, which improves the wound tissue utilization of glucose and oxygen.
  - *Hemoglobin spray* (Granulox): It contains purified hemoglobin derived from pig's blood. It binds oxygen from the air and increases the oxygen diffusion in the wound. It is sprayed directly on the wound after every dressing change.
  - *Hyaluronic acid (HA)-based cream, gel, or sheet dressings*: These are hydrogel dressings and are obtained from slaughtered animals (rooster comb or cow/horse joints or eyeball) or plants (*Cassia angustifolia* seed or root vegetables) or bacteria fermentation. They can also be lab made. They can be directly applied to the wound.
  - *Hydrogel dressing sheet or pad:* It contains 90% water in a hydrophilic complex polymer matrix. It is non-adherent. It keeps the superficial or partial thickness wound moist for 3 to 7 days and promotes autolytic debridement, desloughing and absorbs some exudate. It also soothes and cools by providing a moist healing milieu.
  - *Hydrocolloid gel, paste, or sheet dressing*: It contains a hydrocolloid matrix derived from gelatin, pectin, or carboxymethylcellulose. These are used in non-infected partial or full-thickness or necrotic wounds and are changed every 3 to 7 days. It also promotes autolytic debridement and absorbs some exudate.
  - *Alginate dressing* (calcium alginate): It is derived from kelp and other brown seaweeds. It is biodegradable with hemostatic properties and absorbs a lot of wound fluid. It is used on exuding wounds to promote autolytic debridement. It can have a foul smell.
  - *Films*: Transparent film dressing is used to cover a wound so that the wound healing is monitored.
  - *Cellulose dressing*: It is a natural biopolymer but is synthesized from bacterial fermentation in the *Acetobacter* species. It is used in partial thickness burns to provide a cool and moist environment.
  - *Cloth dressing (cotton crepe bandage)*: This is used for minor superficial injuries like abrasions or cuts.
  - *Artificial aquaporins*. These can promote wound healing.

- For **dirty or necrotic wounds**, the following items can be used:
  - *Fibrinolysin W/DNASE ointment* (Elase): It consists of two proteolytic enzymes, fibrinolysin and desoxyribonuclease (DNase), which debride purulent and necrotic exudates.
  - *Enzyme-debriding ointments, which contain collagenase*: The collagenase ointment contains the enzyme collagenase, which is obtained from the bacteria *Clostridium histolyticum*. The collagen enzyme will digest and break down the collagen in the necrotic tissue.
  - *Papain-urea ointments* (e.g., Debridace) are also debriding agents but are rarely used now.
  - Other chemical or biological debriding agents.
  - *Antibacterial or antiseptic ointments* such as topical silver sulfadiazine (SSD) or iodine/povidone-iodine.
  - *Foam dressings*: It is made from semi permeable polymers such as polyurethane with tiny open cells that will absorb moisture. It is useful in partial or full-thickness wounds, which are exuding and leaking especially during the inflammatory stage. It can be changed every 2 to 4 days. *Antibiotic impregnated dressings and* sprays are used to prevent infection of the wound. Foam dressings impregnated with 3% povidone-iodine or 0.5% polyhexamethylene biguanide (PHMB) provide a moist environment and also antibacterial properties. Foam sprays with silver nanoparticles also have antimicrobial actions.
  - Combination dressings:
    - The antibiotic must be applied to the wound first then the collagenase ointment.
    - The HA dressings can be combined with the antiseptic.
    - Calcium alginate dressings impregnated with manuka honey are also available.
    - Activated charcoal dressing with silver (e.g., Actisorb silver): This dressing is in a non-adherent nylon sleeve. The charcoal traps odors and toxins and together with the silver can kill bacteria.
    - Organo-hydrogel bandage dressings are derived from cellulose (obtained from discarded durian fruit husks) with added yeast and glycerol. They are used as antibacterial gel bandages or biofilms.

For chronic wounds, it is important to treat underlying problems such as diabetes, poor nutrition, immobility, etc.

Stitches/Sutures/Skin Glue

Stitches, sutures, or skin glue may be used to help a wound deeper than one-half inch to heal. There are different types of surgical sutures such as absorbable or non-absorbable sutures. Non-absorbable sutures need to be removed at a later date, whereas absorbable sutures can be left in to dissolve on their own.

Skin glue is a specific glue used to hold the skin together and does not need to be removed.

Surgical Excision or Skin Grafts

Surgical excision includes debridement or removal of unhealthy, devitalized, or non-viable tissue in the operating theater or at bedside using conventional equipment. In waterjet hydrosurgery, saline under pressure is used to debride more effectively.

Autologous skin grafts are done to close chronic non-healing or large wounds. Split-thickness graft (skin contains the epidermis layer) is usually taken from hidden areas like the outer thigh or hip area. Full-thickness graft (skin contains epidermis and dermis) is taken from donor sites such as the forearm, abdomen, area above the clavicle, or groin.

Tetanus Injection

Tetanus injections are usually routine in infancy and updated every 10 years. If the wound is deep or contains foreign objects or dirt, a tetanus injection may be necessary. It may also be given if the injections are not up to date.

Antibiotics

Antibiotics may be given to prevent or cure an infected wound.

Examples: amoxicillin, clavulanate, cephalexin, clindamycin, doxycycline

Nonsteroidal Anti-Inflammatory Drugs

Example: aspirin, celecoxib, diclofenac, and ibuprofen may be given for pain relief in painful chronic wounds or skin ulcers.

Homeopathic Remedies

These include *Bellis perennis* (for deep injuries from postoperative or accident injuries with stiffness or coldness), *Arnica montana* (with associated bruising from overexertion, trauma, and surgery), *Hypericum perforatum* (associated with severe nerve pain), *Calcarea phosphorica* (associated with slow healing of fractures and bone bruises with overlying numb or cold feeling), and *Calendula* (for superficial abrasions and cuts).

Face Scrub, Mask, and Moisturizer

Many fruits or vegetables have mask, toning, scrub, exfoliating, keratolytic and moisturizing benefits. Some also act like sunscreen. The term "moisturizer" is often used as a broad umbrella term to describe all the above benefits. The aim is to get clear, glowing, supple, and smooth skin after the dead cells are removed (exfoliated) and moisture is retained.

Fruits, vegetables, plant herbs or spices are readily available for home use in all communities. There are some ethnic differences where local products are preferred, and this will be highlighted wherever applicable.

As a rule, the "wetter or oilier plants" are suitable for dry skin.

The more "acidic" fruits or enzyme-rich plants (fruits) like pineapple or papaya are more suitable for oily skin.

Use more locally available items. It also does not make sense to use expensive fresh berries like strawberries in the tropics.

The methods are common. Soft fruits or vegetables can be mashed by hand or spoon. Some may need to be blended. Apply the mashed/blended fruit or vegetable on the face.

Alternatively, after eating a fruit or peeling a vegetable, scrape and/or rub the inner side of the fruit/vegetable peel directly onto the face. Leave this mask on for at least 20 to 30 minutes or even longer. Then wash off with alternating warm and cold water to improve the circulation.

All fresh fruits/vegetables are rich in vitamin C. Vitamin A is prevalent in the yellow-orange fruit/vegetable. Minerals like potassium, iron, and copper are more in the dark-green or red-purple fruit/vegetable. Antioxidants are more in the berries, honey, and the red-purple fruits/vegetables.

For anti-inflammatory effects, add in honey or spices like cinnamon. Others include neem leaf paste, turmeric, tea tree oil, or other essential oils.

For hydrating effects, cucumber is used. It can also treat puffiness around the eyes.

To maintain skin hydration, use natural compounds which are already present in the skin. These hydrators or humectants draw water into the outer layer of skin. Examples of humectants include glycerin, lecithin, ceramides, natural moisturizing factor (NMF) and aquaporins (AQPs). Some of these compounds are synthetically made or derived from plants or bacteria.

Emollients are moisturizers that form an oil layer on the skin surface.

Petrolatum, lanolin, mineral oil and dimethicone are common emollients.

Exfoliating or keratolytic agents soften the outer keratin layer of the skin. Examples include urea, alpha hydroxy acids (lactic/citric/glycolic acid), allantoin, coal tar, olive oil, tretinoin, acitretin, pyrithione zinc and salicylate.

Plant (Fruits and Vegetables) and Herbal Extracts Used as or in Masks/Scrubs and Moisturizers

These include aloe vera, avocado, banana, seaweed, thyme, basil, chamomile, cucumber, calendula, lavender, lemongrass, geranium, ginger, rose, jojoba, olive oil, tea tree, rosemary, dandelion, argan, sea asparagus, hibiscus, pine bark, walnut, oriental thuja (biota), red marine algae, coffeeberry, chestnut, sea buckthorn, soy, eucalyptus extract, fig, grapes, grapefruit, strawberry, pea, papaya (ripe or raw pulp), pineapple, and many more.

Others include kombucha (fermented tea beverage containing *Lactobacillus* bacteria and lactic acid).

Nanoemulsions contain various vegetable plant extracts with natural antioxidants.

Various acids such as alpha hydroxy acid (AHA), beta hydroxy acid (BHA), alpha lipoic acid (ALA), ferulic acid, azelaic acid, ascorbic acid, linoleic acid, and alguronic acid (from microalgae) are also present in plants and herbs.

Squalene is a polyunsaturated hydrocarbon antioxidant present in the skin's natural lipid barrier. It can be produced from plants (rice bran, olives, and sugarcane) or animals (from shark liver). The hydrogenated form, that is, squalane has better stability as a skincare hydrator, emollient, and moisturizer. It is also used in eczema, acne, psoriasis, and dry hair.

Sauna, Spa, and Baths

They help to deep cleanse, remove toxins, exfoliate dead cells, and invigorate the skin. They are also relaxing. They are also effective in eczema, acne, and psoriasis.

Sauna. It generates dry heat. The temperature is high around 150 to 190 degrees Fahrenheit and the humidity is low around 10% to 20%.

Spa. It generates moist heat using steam. The temperature is moderate around 110 to 120 degrees Fahrenheit and the humidity is high around 80% to 90%.

Thermal spa. This refers to thermal waters from hot springs usually.

Baths. There are many types of communal baths in different countries. The terms baths and sauna are often used interchangeably.

- **Banyan bath.** This is a Russian sauna.
- **Hammam.** This is a Turkish or Moroccan bath with Arabic roots. It uses hot steam and then exfoliative massage is done with olive oil soap or rhassoul clay by the *tellek* therapist.
- **Hanjeungmak (Hanja or Hangul).** This is a Korean sauna.
- **Onsen.** A Japanese geothermal hot spring bath, usually near volcanic areas.
- **Roman bath.** In ancient times, there were *thermae* (large bath areas) and *balneae* (small bath areas) which were mostly for public bathing, and which were also regarded as social events.
- **Sento bath.** This is a Japanese public bath house.

Toilet or Bath Soaps

They are made from oil, water, and alkali (or lye, which is usually potassium or sodium hydroxide). Soap is a salt of a fatty acids. Commonly used oils include palm oil, palm kernel oil, coconut oil, canola oil, olive oil, laurel oil and rarely tallow.

Soap is used use to cleanse and disinfect the skin. Antibacterial agents such as triclosan or triclocarban are added. Natural antibacterial or antiseptic agents include neem or turmeric. Natural emollients such as shea butter or jojoba oil can also be added. Exfoliating or scouring agents such as pumice can also be added to soap.

Artisan/Handmade or Handcrafted soaps

These contain natural ingredients which are biodegradable and environment friendly. Allergic reactions are rare. They are usually made via cold process and prolonged air-drying methods.

African black soap. It is made from roasted shea tree bark. Palm tree leaves, plantains, and cocoa pods.

Aleppo soap. It is handmade in France and Syria using noble olive and laurel oils. The process including drying takes about 9 months

Azul e branco soap (also called Blue and White soap, monkey soap, or Offenbach soap). It is made in Portugal and contains silicates.

Castile soap. It is made in Spain using olive oil previously. Now, it is made from a blend of oils including olive, coconut, sunflower seed, hemp, and jojoba.

Glycerin soap. This is a transparent soap. It contains glycerin which has not been removed. (unlike in most commercial soaps)

Herbal soaps. Various herbs or plants are added. Common western herbs include lavender, chamomile, calendula, comfrey, mint, lemon, etc. Eastern herbs include neem, aloe vera, saffron, sandalwood, turmeric, wild ginger, jasmine, etc.

Medicated soaps. Various chemical or herbal compounds are added. These have antibacterial (sulfur, neem oil), antifungal (neem), or anti-parasitic/anti-scabies properties (permethrin, sulfiram, neem oil).

Milk soaps. Goat milk is commonly used.

Neem soap. This soap contains neem oil extracts.

Ideally, all cosmetic or skincare products should contain natural and organic ingredients. They should be free of mineral oil (petroleum jelly), triclosan, aluminum, carbon black, parabens, phthalates, glycols (polyethylene glycol [PEG], propylene glycol and butylene glycol), synthetic fragrances, sulphates (sodium lauryl sulphate [SLS] and sodium laureth sulfate [SLES]), dioxanes, oxybenzone, formaldehyde, ethanolamines, retinol and many others. These compounds are carcinogenic, endocrine disruptors or allergenic.

Indian Natural Moisturizers

Bael pulp. This is applied as a paste or scrub to the face (as above).

Bakuchiol. It is a retinoid antioxidant from the seeds and leaves of the babchi plant (*Psoralea corylifolia*) found in skin care products. It has anti-aging actions.

Buttermilk/yogurt. Buttermilk is rich in lactic acid. It is present in expensive skin care products. It removes dead skin cells, speeds cell turnover, and is a moisturizer.

Coconut oil. It is a moisturizer, emollient, and makeup remover. It penetrates deep inside the pores and softens the skin. Apply on chapped hands, feet, or lips. A coconut oil head massage is used for strong and healthy hair.

Green mango. Peel and discard the skin of a green mango. Cut the pale green flesh into small cubes. Add little water to cover the cubed green mango. Simmer until soft. Mash the pulp. When cool, transfer to a bottle and refrigerate. Apply the pulp paste on the face. Leave for about 30 minutes and then rinse.

Ground chickpea flour. This is applied as a paste or scrub to the face or the body. It can be mixed with buttermilk or yogurt and/or coconut oil. A pinch of turmeric may also be added.

Ground mung bean. This is applied as a paste or scrub to the face or the body (as above).

Milk. Drinking milk can improve dry skin. It contains phospholipid and protects the skin barrier.

Orange peel. Grind or blend some pieces of orange peel. Mix with some rose water and apply on the face. Leave for 15 minutes and then rinse off.

Palmarosa oil. This essential oil is from the *Cymbopogon martini* plant and is used in skincare products

Sesame oil. It is used as above.

Chinese Natural Moisturizers

Topical

- **Ashitaba.** This is a Japanese herbal plant. It is added to skincare products.
- **Ho leaf oil.** It is used as a skin conditioner and is derived from *Cinnamomum camphora.* It can be blended with other floral or citrus oils.
- **Ho wood oil.** It is also derived from *Cinnamomum camphora* but contains more linalool and used in skincare products. It is an alternative to rosewood essential oil.
- **Pearl powder face mask.** Mix the following ingredients. ½ teaspoon pearl powder, 2 teaspoons rice or wheat bran powder, 3 teaspoons of water or milk and little oil or honey. Apply on the face. Leave for 30 minutes and then rinse it off.
  Pearl powder can also be consumed.
- **Rice water mask.** The leftover water from washing rice or from boiling rice is used to wash the face or applied as a mask. The soft-cooked rice can also be mashed with some milk and honey and applied on the face. This is mostly a Japanese skin care ritual.

Diet

Include the following: Consume mushrooms, green tea, soy, bamboo, and bird's nest.

Fermented barley and soybean formula can also be consumed as a dietary supplement or drink.

Therapeutic Measure

Chinese Face Massage (Gua Sha)

The skin of the face is scraped or rubbed using a rounded edge flat stone made from jade or rose quartz and a carrier oil, usually peanut oil, or sweet almond oil. This can help to improve circulation, reduce inflammation, and tone the face skin and muscles.

- **Japanese face massage** *(Kobido).* This is an ancient art that combines acupressure, lymphatic drainage, kneading and percussion to maintain radiant skin health.
- **Kinubiyou.** This is a Japanese face massage using a silk brush.

Western Natural Moisturizers

ALA. ALA-based creams can make the skin smooth and reduce wrinkles.

Essential oil or oil bath. Various oils are used. These include rose/rosehip oil, olive oil, sunflower seed oil, jojoba, argan, shea, sweet almond, calendula, avocado oils, carrot oil, saffron, *Helichrysum italicum,* and elemi essential oils

A few drops of any of the oils or essential oils can be added to the bath (as a bath soak) or applied to damp skin as a moisturizer after a bath.

Calendula oil can also be used for chapped lips.

Honey. Honey is beneficial for many types of skin diseases.

Oatmeal bath. Oatmeal has anti-inflammatory properties and benefits dry skin (see also under atopic dermatitis).

Postbiotics. Postbiotic skincare products contain non-living bacterial lysates.

Prebiotics. Prebiotics are added to cosmetics products including serums or moisturizers to maintain a healthy skin microbiome balance. Prebiotics are essentially foods consumed by probiotics. They feed on the good gut bacteria. Examples of prebiotic-containing foods include oat and wheat bran.

Probiotics. Probiotics that contain bacteria such as *Lactobacillus, Bifidobacterium*, and *Streptococcus* are present in skin care products. *Streptococcus thermophilus* can increase the endogenous ceramides in the skin. Face and Body Scrubs

Rose water. Moroccan rose water is a natural skin astringent and moisturizer.

Aloe vera. As above.

Oatmeal honey scrub. Mix 2 tablespoons of oats with a tablespoon of honey and a dash of water.

Olive oil and sugar Scrub. Combine ½ cup of sugar with 2 tablespoons of olive oil.

Modern Moisturizers

Moisturizers make the skin soft, smooth, supple and moist. They are classified into three categories:

Water-based moisturizers (humectants, hydrators, or hygroscopic agents). They draw water from the dermis to the epidermis. These include lactic acid, urea, glycerin, hyaluronic acid, NMF, and AQPs. Lactic acid is also an exfoliator. They are best used after a bath or shower.

Oil-based moisturizers (emollients). These are ointments, gels, or lotions that will replace the lost natural oils or fats in the skin. They include petroleum jelly, essential oils (rosehip oil, jojoba oil, etc.), vitamin E, and ceramides. Dry skin contains very low skin ceramide.

Many emollients are also humectants.

Occlusive/barrier moisturizers. These are larger molecules and tend to be water-repellant. They are physical barriers that will lock in and seal moisture into the skin and prevent water from evaporating (i.e., trans-epidermal water loss [TEWL]). Examples include lanolin, beeswax, shea butter, plant oils (coconut or olive oil), and petrolatum.

Different combinations of all or some of the three types of moisturizers are used depending on age, skin type, or climate.

Dandruff

Dandruff are dry white flakes that fall out of the hair. They are caused by skin cells that grow and die too quickly. The exact cause of dandruff is not known at present, but it is thought to be caused by a fungus known as *Malassezia*. This fungus often lives on the scalp in most healthy adults but does not cause any adverse effects. However, in some adults, *Malassezia* causes dandruff. It is thought that the immune system of these individuals overreacts to the presence of the fungus, causing dandruff.

Indian Natural Remedies

Common Ingredients for Dandruff

Spices	Herbs/Leaves	Miscellaneous
Fenugreek (methi)	Neem	Egg white
Piper nigrum (black pepper)	*Phyllanthus officinalis* (amla)	Lime
	Acacia concinna (shikakai)	Camphor
	Holy basil (tulsi)	Oils: coconut, almond, olive, sandalwood, and castor
	Reetha (*Sapindus mukorossi*)	Lemon
	Mint	Chickpea flour
	Bay leaf	Curd
	Bael leaf	Vinegar
	Avuri leaves	Baking soda
	Shikakai (*Acacia concinna*)	Salt
	Dodder leaves	

Common Recipes

Topical

- **Amla-tulsi paste.** Place three to five amla fruits into a blender and blend until smooth before pouring into a bowl. Grind 8 to 10 tulsi leaves until they form a paste and mix it with the amla paste. Apply this to the scalp and let it sit for 30 minutes. Rinse out with cold water.
- **Egg white and lime juice.** Put the whites of two eggs in a bowl and add the juice of one lime. Mix well and apply to the scalp. Let sit for half an hour before washing it out of the hair.
- **Fenugreek mask.** Soak 3 tablespoons of fenugreek seeds in water overnight. In the morning, place the seeds into a blender and blend until it forms a smooth paste. Add 1 tablespoon of fresh lemon juice to the paste and massage all over the scalp and ends of the hair. Leave it on for 30 minutes before rinsing off.
- **Neem paste.** Grind fresh neem leaves into a paste and mix it into a bowl of curd. Mix well and apply all over the scalp. Let it sit for 15 to 20 minutes before rinsing with water.

Amla, reetha, and shikakai. Soak five to six reetha pods, six to seven pieces of shikakai, and three to five amla fruits in water overnight. In the morning, transfer the herbs and the water into a pot and heat them until they come to a boil. Then remove the mixture from the heat and let it cool completely. Blend until smooth Strain the mixture, discarding the residue. Use the remaining liquid as a shampoo.
Variation #1. Shikakai powder can also be mixed with henna powder and yoghurt. Apply on the scalp for about 1 hour. When it is dry, rinse it off.
Variation #2. Take 2 tablespoons each of shikakai, reetha and neem leaf powders. Mix with a little warm water. Apply on the scalp for about an hour. When it is dry, rinse it off.

Avuri leaves. Take some avuri leaves. Dry them for a few days and grind into a powder. Add some sesame oil and apply on the scalp.

Bael leaves. Mix bael leaf powder with some coconut oil. Massage into the scalp.

Bay leaf. Mix a few crushed bay leaves with hot water. Massage into the scalp.

Black pepper. Mix ground black pepper with milk and some fresh lime juice. Rub it into the scalp and leave on for an hour.

Chickpea flour. Mix 2 spoons of flour into a bowl of curd and add half a spoon of lemon juice. Apply to the scalp and leave on for half an hour before rinsing.

Coconut oil and camphor. Mix a small amount of camphor into coconut oil, ensuring that it is smooth and free of lumps. Apply to the scalp regularly, preferably before bedtime. Keep overnight and rinse in the morning.

Coconut oil and lemon. Mix 2 tablespoons of lemon with 5 tablespoons of warm coconut oil. Apply to the scalp and leave on for 30 minutes before rinsing off. Repeat every day for 2 to 3 weeks.

Dodder leaves. Take 50 g of the dodder leaves. Add 1 L of water. Boil and then simmer till half volume. Apply the decoction onto the scalp. Leave for 30 minutes and then wash.

Neem and lemon. Grind three to five neem leaves into a paste and add the juice of half a lemon. Mix until smooth and apply to the scalp, leaving it on for 30 minutes before rinsing.

Oils. Mix some fresh lime juice with oils such as coconut, almond, sandalwood, olive, or castor oil. Massage into the scalp and leave it on for 30 minutes before rinsing off.

Reetha. Take two to three half-mashed reetha pods. Add 1 cup of water. Mash the pods in the water and boil for 30 minutes. Cool and strain using a muslin cloth. Add 1 cup of water, 2 to 3 drops of essential oil and 1 teaspoon of baking soda. Mix the ingredients and use it as a shampoo.

Shikakai oil. Take 1 cup of coconut oil and ½ cup of almond oil. Add 1 to 2 tablespoons of shikakai powder. Pour into a glass bottle. Shake and allow to steep for 1 to 2 weeks. Apply the oil on the scalp two to three times per week.

Vinegar. Mix 2 tablespoons of vinegar into 1 cup of hot water and rub into the scalp. Leave it on for half an hour before washing.

Chinese Natural Remedies

Common Ingredients for Dandruff

Herbs/Leaves	Miscellaneous
Aconite root	
Amur cork tree bark	
Anemarrhena/zhi mu (*Anemarrhena asphodeloides*)	
Caulis akebiae (mu tong)	
Chinese lovage root/gao ben (*Ligusticum striatum*)	
Chinese senega root/yuan zhi (*Polygala tenuifolia*)	
Gokshura/bai ji li (*Tribulus terrestris*)	Vitex fruit
Gypsum fibrosum (shi gao)	
Herba schizonepetae (jing jie)	
Holy basil	
Jehol ligustium rhizome	
Mulberry mistletoes/Sang ji sheng (*Taxillus chinensis*)	
Mulberry root bark	
Peony root bark	
Pine leaf (Pinus pinaster)	
Radix angelicae sinensis (dang gui)	Sour jujube seed
Radix astragali (huang qi)	
Radix glycyrrhizae (liquorice/gan cao)	
Radix ledebouriella (fang feng)	
Radix paeoniae alba (bai shao)	*Periostracum cicadae* (chan tui)
Radix rehmanniae (sheng di)	Chrysanthemum flower
Radix sophorae flavescentis (ku shen)	
Rhizoma atractylodis (cang zhu)	
Rhizoma lingustici chuanxiong (chuan xiong)	*Fructus arctii* (niu bang zi)
Rhizoma zingiberis recens (sheng jiang)	
Semen sesamum (hu ma ren)	
Tuber fleeceflower/he shou wu (*Reynoutria multiflora*)	
Yerba de tajo herb	

Common Recipes

Oral

- Decoction for Blood Deficiency with Excess Wind and Dryness:
  - Modified **"angelica root drink:"** dang gui, bai shao, chuan xiong, sheng di, bai ji li, fang feng, jing jie, he shou wu, huang qi, gan cao, sheng jiang, sour jujube seed, and polygala root

- **Indication**: Itchy scalp that looks dry and flaky, with scratches and bleeding. It is usually present in the elderly, with a pale tongue and a taut, slow pulse.
- This decoction is given to nourish the blood, lubricate dryness, and disperse excess wind in the body, as well as to stop itching.
- Decoction for Wind and Dampness Mixing with Heat:
  - Modified "*Gentiana macrophylla* root pill": dang gui, sheng di, fang feng, chan tui, zhi mu, ku shen, hu ma ren, jing jie, lang zhu, niu bang zi, shi gao, gan cao, mu tong, amur cork tree bark, and peony root bark
  - **Indication**: The scalp is itchy with scratches and may be bleeding. It may look swollen and red, with eczema-like changes or thickening. It may affect young or middle-aged adults and is aggravated by heat.
  - This decoction is given to disperse wind, remove dampness from the body, clear heat, and stop itching.

Topical

- Herbal Rinse
  - Ingredients: chrysanthemum, mulberry root bark, aconite root, jehol ligustium rhizome, pine leaf, vita fruit, yerba de tajo herb, holy basil, and mulberry mistletoes
  - Method: Place 100 g of each ingredient and process it into a coarse mixture. Store it in a container and use 150 g each time to make 1500 mL of herbal solution by decocting it. Use the decoction to wash the scalp.

Gao ben-Bai zhi hair powder. Take two equal parts of bai zhi and gao ben powder. Sprinkle in hair before bed. The next morning, comb it off.

Western/Other Natural Remedies

Common Ingredients for Dandruff

Herbs/Leaves	Miscellaneous
Burdock root	Aloe vera
Chamomile	Apple cider vinegar
Parsley	Oils and or essential oils: tea tree oil, coconut, cajeput, cedarwood and olive
Rosemary	Baking soda
Thyme	Garlic
	Mouthwash
	Lemon
	Salt

Common Recipes

Topical

Aloe vera gel. Slit an aloe vera leaf down the middle and scrape out the white gel on the inside. Discard any of the yellowish-green gel. Cut the white gel into smaller chunks and place into a blender, blending until smooth. Massage the gel onto the scalp and let sit for 30 minutes before rinsing.

Apple cider vinegar. Mix 2 tablespoons of ACV into 1 cup of warm water and rub the hair with it. Wrap the hair with a towel and let sit for 15 to 60 minutes before washing the hair. Repeat twice a week.

Baking soda. Wet the hair and rub the baking soda into the scalp. Leave on for 30 minutes before rinsing.

Burdock root. Place 2 tablespoons of burdock root into a pot with 1 cup of water. Bring it to a boil and then remove from the heat. Let it cool completely and strain. Use it as a rinse after shampooing.

Chamomile. Place 1 to 2 teaspoons of dried chamomile flowers into a pot with one cup of water. Bring to a boil and then remove from the heat. Let it steep for 10 to 15 minutes. Strain and use the liquid as a rinse for the hair.

Essential oils. Mix a few drops of the essential oil with a carrier oil (coconut oil or almond oil) and massage onto the scalp. Leave for a few minutes and then rinse off.

Variation #1. Add a few drops of the essential oil directly into the shampoo. Massage onto the scalp and rinse off.

Lemon. Massage 2 tablespoons of lemon juice onto the scalp. Wrap the hair with a towel, let it sit for 15 to 60 minutes, and then rinse it off.

Mouthwash. Use an alcohol-based mouthwash as a rinse after using normal shampoo to wash the hair.

Parsley. Place a handful of parsley into a pot with 1 cup of water. Bring to a boil and then remove from the heat. Let it cool completely and strain. Use it as a rinse after shampooing.

Rosemary. Place three to five sprigs of rosemary into a pot with 1 cup of water. Bring to a boil and then remove from the heat. Let it cool completely and strain. Use it as a rinse after shampooing.

Salt. Rub salt flakes onto the scalp and massage the scalp for 5 minutes. Then shampoo as normal and wash off.

Thyme. Place three to five stalks of thyme into a pot with 1 cup of water. Bring to a boil and then remove from the heat. Let it cool completely and strain. Use it as a rinse after shampooing.

Modern Remedies

Antifungal Shampoo (Scalp Scrubs)

Coal tar. This is an antifungal agent that works by causing the dead skin cells on the scalp to shed and slow down the growth of new skin cells.

Ketoconazole. This is an antifungal that interferes with the fungal synthesis of ergosterol, a component of fungal cell membranes. This causes the fungal cells to die.

Salicylic acid.: Salicylic acid increases the rate of dead skin cell shedding but does not slow the growth of new skin cells.

Selenium sulfide. This medication reduces scalp oil production. Selenium disulfide is an antifungal agent found in the commercial medicated shampoos for the treatment of dandruff and seborrheic dermatitis associated with the scalp with fungi of genus *Malassezia*.

Zinc pyrithione. Zinc pyrithione slows the growth of yeast by disrupting the cell membrane transport.

Homeopathic Remedies

These include *Thuja occidentalis* (when the white flakes fall everywhere with associated itching and dry hair), *Natrum muriaticum* (with associated oily scalp), *Phosphorus* (with associated hair loss), and *Kali sulphuricum* (with scalp inflammation).

Head Lice

Head lice are small blood-sucking insects that live in the hair on the head and feed off blood from the scalp. This condition is contagious and may be passed on through head-to-head contact. Lice may also be transferred through combs, headphones, and hats. Preschool and school children have the highest risk of contracting head lice as they tend to play closely together. Symptoms of head lice include extreme scalp itchiness, a sensation of things crawling on the scalp, as well as sores or scabs on the scalp from scratching.

Indian Natural Remedies

Common Ingredients for Head Lice

Spices	Herbs/Leaves	Miscellaneous
Garlic	Reetha (*Sapindus mukorossi*)	Oils: coconut, olive, and tea tree
Onion	Neem leaf (*Azadirachta indica*)	Lemon/lime
	Tulsi/Holy basil (*Ocimum tenuiflorum*)	Essential oils: clove, anise seed, lemongrass, and nutmeg
	Avuri/True indigo (*Indigofera tinctoria*)	Vinegar
		Apple
		Salt
		Baking soda
		Camphor

Common Recipes

Topical

Avuri leaves. Take some avuri leaves. Dry them for a few days and grind into a powder. Add some sesame oil and apply it onto the scalp.

Coconut oil and camphor. As above.

Garlic lime. Grind 8 to 10 cloves of garlic into a paste and add the juice of one lime, mixing to form a smooth paste. Apply this mixture to the hair and scalp. Let it sit for 30 minutes and then wash with warm water.

Lemon juice. Juice one to two lemons and cover the scalp and hair with the juice. Leave it on for 2 to 3 hours before washing out.

Neem paste. As above.

Oils. Dilute essential oils (clove, anise seed, lemongrass, tea tree, and nutmeg) with coconut or olive oil. Cover the scalp and hair thickly with the oil and cover with a shower cap. Leave it overnight and rinse in the morning.

Reetha paste. Take 1 to 2 teaspoons of reetha powder. Add ½ cup of warm water to make a paste. Apply over hair and scalp. Leave it on for 2 to 3 hours before washing it out.

Vinegar. Apply distilled vinegar all over the scalp and hair. Leave for about an hour before rinsing thoroughly.

- **Apples.** Mash one to two apples into a smooth paste and apply thickly to the hair and scalp. Leave on for an hour before rinsing out.
- **Baking soda.** Mix one part baking soda with three parts hair conditioner and apply thickly to all parts of the scalp and hair then rinse with anti-lice shampoo. Repeat every 2 to 3 days.
- **Coconut camphor.** Mix 1 tablespoon of crushed camphor with 2 tablespoons of coconut oil to make a paste. Apply this paste to the scalp and put on a shower cap. Leave it overnight. Rinse it off in the morning. Repeat the procedure three times a week.
- **Onion juice.** Skin three to five onions and place in a blender. Blend with a little water. Apply all over the scalp and hair, leaving on for 3 to 4 hours. Repeat every 3 to 4 days.
- **Salt and vinegar.** Add 3 to 5 teaspoons of salt to 2 cups of vinegar, stirring well until the salt has dissolved. Saturate the hair and scalp with the mixture and leave on for 2 to 3 hours before rinsing.

Chinese Natural Remedies

Common Ingredients for Head Lice

Herbs/Leaves
Chrysanthemum

Common Recipes

Topical

- **Chrysanthemum rinse.** Place. a handful of chrysanthemums into a pot with 2 cups of water. Bring to a boil and then reduce the heat, letting it simmer for about 30 to 45 minutes. Strain and apply the liquid all over the scalp and hair. Cover with a shower cap and let it sit for 3 to 4 hours before washing off.

Western/Other Natural Remedies

Common Ingredients for Head Lice

Herbs/Leaves	Miscellaneous
Basil	Lemon juice
Cinnamon	Common rue and rue oil
Lavender	Mayonnaise
Lemongrass	Essential oils: tea tree, and cinnamon leaf
Peppermint	Aloe vera gel
Rosemary	Apple cider vinegar
Sage	Olive oil
Soap nuts	Lemon peel
Thyme	Petroleum jelly

Common Recipes

Topical

Aloe vera gel. As above.

Apple cider vinegar. Completely soak the hair and scalp with undiluted raw apple cider vinegar. Cover the hair with a shower cap and let it sit for 3 to 4 hours before rinsing it out.

Rosemary. Place three to five sprigs of rosemary into a pot with 1 cup of water. Bring it to a boil and then remove from the heat. Cool and strain. Apply and massage the hair and scalp. Cover with a shower cap and leave on for 3 to 4 hours before rinsing it off.

- **Thyme.** Place three to five stalks of thyme into a pot with 1 cup of water. Bring it to a boil and then remove from the heat. Let it cool completely and strain. Apply it to the hair and scalp, saturating every strand of hair. Cover with a shower cap and leave it on for 3 to 4 hours before rinsing it off.
- **Petroleum jelly.** Cover the hair with a thick layer of petroleum jelly and place a shower cap over the hair. Let it sit overnight before washing out.
- **Mayonnaise.** Apply mayonnaise thickly all over the scalp and hair, and cover with a shower cap. Leave it overnight and wash it off the next morning.
- **Herbal shampoo.** Combine 2 cups of water, 10 soap nuts, 2 tablespoons of lemon peel, and 1 cinnamon stick in a pot. Bring to a boil and then simmer on low heat for about 20 minutes. Remove it from the heat and add in 1 tablespoon of thyme. It may be replaced with sage, peppermint, basil, rosemary, lavender, neem, or lemongrass. Allow to steep until cool before straining the liquid through a piece of muslin cloth. Combine the liquid with apple cider vinegar, aloe vera juice, and olive oil. To use, cover the hair and scalp completely before covering the hair with a shower cap. Let it sit for 1 to 4 hours before washing it off.

Rue oil. Take 1 tablespoon of crushed dry leaves. Add ½ cup of hot olive oil. Steep for 30 minutes or longer. Strain and store in a bottle. Apply this oil on the scalp. Alternatively, rue tea can be applied to the scalp.

Rue tea. Take 1 teaspoon of dried crushed rue leaves. Add ½ cup of boiling water. Steep for 15 minutes.

Modern Remedies

Pyrethrin and Piperonyl Butoxide

Pyrethrin and piperonyl butoxide shampoo is a pediculicide used in adults and children above 2 years old, and it kills the head lice.

It is applied on the scalp and left for about 10 minutes, then lathered with warm water, and rinsed off with a regular shampoo. This process is repeated after 7 to 10 days. A lice comb may be used to remove the dead lice and nits.

Permethrin Lotion

Permethrin (belongs to the pyrethrin class) cream can be used to treat head lice. It kills live head lice but not unhatched eggs. It may continue to kill newly hatched lice for several days after treatment. A second treatment is often necessary on day 9 to kill any newly hatched lice before they can produce eggs.

Dimethicone

This medication disrupts water homeostasis in lice and causes suffocation. It has a low risk of adverse effects. Two applications one week apart can successfully kill the head lice in about 70% cases.

This lotion is applied to dry hair that has been moistened a little. Then use a comb to run through the scalp. Rinse after 10 minutes.

Benzyl Alcohol

Benzyl alcohol prevents lice from being able to close their respiratory spiracles, hence resulting in the obstruction of the spiracles and suffocation.

This lotion is used in adults and children over 6 months old. It is applied topically as above.

Ivermectin

Ivermectin binds to chloride ion channels in the lice's muscle and nerve cells, causing increased permeability of the cell to chloride ions. This leads to cell hyperpolarization leading to paralysis and death of the lice.

It is used in severe pediculosis in adults and children above 2 years with a minimum weight of 15 kg. It is an oral tablet given as a single dose and repeated after 1 week.

Homeopathic Remedies

These include *sulfur* (associated dislike for hair washing and bath), *Eucalyptus globulus, Staphysagria,* (associated suppress emotions), and *Nux vomica* (associated with loss of appetite, pallor, and lethargy).

Alopecia (Hair Fall/Hair Loss)

Alopecia refers to hair fall or hair loss. Causes may be local (e.g., fungal infection) or systemic (e.g., anemia, malnutrition, thyroid disease, autoimmune disorder, chemotherapy, stress, or medical conditions). The quantity of hair loss varies from person to person. There is currently no cure for alopecia, but hair usually will grow back.

Indian Natural Remedies

Common Ingredients for Alopecia

Spices	Herbs/Leaves/Fruits	Miscellaneous
Carom seeds (Ajwain)	Bhringraj/Karisalai (*Eclipta prostrata*)	Oils: sesame oil, coconut oil, olive oil, almond oil
Fenugreek	Neem leaves	Yogurt
	Soapberry or soapnut/ Reetha (*Sapindus mukorossi*)	Onion
	Shikakai (*Acacia concinna*)	Flaxseed
	Brahmi (Bacopa monnieri)	Jyotishmati
	Gotu kola (*Centella asiatica*)	
	Moringa *Moringa oleifera*	
	Avuri/true indigo (*Indigofera tinctoria*)	
	Henna (Lawsonia inermis)	
	Hibiscus flowers	
	Curry leaf (*Murraya koenigii*)	
	Guava leaf	
	Shikakai (*Acacia concinna*)	
	Indian gooseberry/amla (*Phyllanthus officinalis*)	
	Sariva/Indian sarsaparilla (*Hemidesmus indicus*)	

Common Recipes

Oral

Carom seeds (Ajwain). Add some carom seeds, curry leaves, raisins, and a little brown sugar to a glass of water and boil. Drink this every day. It also prevents graying.

Topical

Amla mask. Crush five to eight amla fruits to make a paste. Apply it to the scalp and hair and leave on for 30 to 45 minutes before washing it off.

Amla and mango pulp. This is applied on the scalp for about 1 hour and then rinsed off.

Brahmi mask. Grind fresh brahmi leaves into a paste and apply all over the scalp. Let it sit for 30 minutes before rinsing off.

Bhringraj polyherbal oil. Apply the oil on the scalp. It contains mainly bhringraj plant (*Eclipta alba*) in coconut oil with other herbs including amla (*Phyllanthus emblica*), brahmi (*Bacopa monnieri*), neem (*Azadirachta indica*), kutaja *Wrightia tinctoria*, raisins (*Vitis vinifera*), giloy (*Tinospora cordifolia*), almond oil (*Prunus amygdalus*), curry leaves (*Murraya koenigii*), liquorice (*Glycyrrhiza glabra*), camphor (*Cinnamomum camphora*), kshiram or sesame milk, henna (*Lawsonia inermis*), and aloe vera extract. Herb contents vary with different brands.

Bhringraj scalp mask. Grind fresh bhringraj leaves into a paste and apply the paste all over the scalp. Let it sit for 30 minutes before rinsing it off.

Curry leaf paste. Pound or blend a handful of curry leaves with a little water to make a paste. Apply and massage it onto the whole scalp or rub it over a bald patch, leave it on for 30 minutes, and then rinse off. Do this weekly.

Fenugreek mask. Grind some soaked fenugreek seeds into a paste and apply it all over the scalp. Leave for 30 minutes and then rinse.

Flaxseed mask. Place 3 to 4 tablespoons of ground flaxseed into a pot with 3 cups of water. Bring to a boil and continue to cook until it forms a gel. Apply this gel to the scalp and hair, leaving in for 30 to 60 minutes before rinsing out.

Gotu kola mask. Grind fresh gotu kola leaves into a paste and apply all over the scalp. Let it sit for 30 minutes before rinsing off.

Guava leaf. Take a handful of guava leaves. Boil them in about 100 mL of water. Blend and massage the blended paste onto the scalp.

Henna leaves. Blend the leaves into a paste. Add some strong black tea or coffee brew. Apply on the scalp weekly. Leave for about 1 hour or more and rinse it off.

Variation #1. Karisalai leaves can also be blended together with the henna leaves. Other alternatives include adding hibiscus flower petals or beetroot juice.

Variation #2. To make a moisturizing scalp hair mask, mix henna powder with egg, yogurt, lemon juice, and/or flaxseed powder, amla powder, fenugreek powder, aloe vera gel, and shikakai powder.

Hot oil scalp treatment. Apply coconut, sesame, or olive oil all over the scalp and massage well. Take a hot towel (soaked in hot water and squeezed) and wrap round the scalp. Place a plastic wrap to retain the heat. Leave for about 15 to 20 minutes or until cool. Rinse hair with shampoo and dry. Repeat weekly or fortnightly.

Jyotishmati oil. Massage the oil onto the scalp.

Moringa mask. Grind fresh moringa leaves into a paste, adding a little water if necessary. Apply all over the scalp. Let it sit for 30 minutes before rinsing it off.

Neem paste. As above.

Onion juice. Skin three to five onions and place into a blender. Blend till smooth with a little added water. Apply all over the scalp and hair, leaving on for 3 to 4 hours. Repeat every 3 to 4 days.

Reetha. Take two to three half-mashed reetha pods. Add 1 cup of water. Mash the pods in the water and boil for 30 minutes. Cool and strain using a muslin cloth. Add 1 cup of water, 2 to 3 drops of oil and 1 teaspoon of baking soda. Mix the ingredients and use it as a shampoo.

Sariva. Mix the powder with water and make a paste. Apply the paste onto the scalp.

Soap nut rinse. Place some soap nut fruits into boiling water and let it steep for 30 minutes. Use the liquid as a rinse.

Shikakai oil. Take 1 cup of coconut oil and ½ cup of almond oil. Add 1 to 2 tablespoons of shikakai powder. Pour into a glass bottle. Shake and allow to steep for 1 to 2 weeks. Apply the oil on the scalp two to three times per week.

Shikakai rinse and mask. Steep dried shikakai in hot water for about 30 minutes. Use this liquid as a hair rinse. Alternatively, mix powdered shikakai with some water to form a thick paste. Apply the paste to the scalp and let it sit for 30 minutes before washing it off.

Shikakai wash or scalp mask. Take 10 pods of shikakai and 10 pods of reetha (deseeded). Add 2 tablespoons of fenugreek and some amla powder. Soak overnight in a pot of water. Boil the following day. Grind or blend and apply this thick liquid. Apply on the scalp.

Variation #1. Shikakai powder can also be mixed with henna powder and yogurt. Apply on the scalp.

Variation #2. Take 2 tablespoons each of shikakai, reetha and amla powder. Add in two beaten eggs and juice of two lemons. Mix with a little water. Apply this paste as a scalp mask for 1 hour. When dry, rinse it off.

Medicated herbal oils. Various home-made or commercial herbal hair oils are available. They are applied regularly onto the scalp to promote and stimulate luxuriant and black hair growth. They can also prevent premature graying of hair. Some examples of these treatment oils include the following:

- Sesame or virgin coconut oil is heated with fenugreek, black cumin, and curry leaves. When cool, pour the herbal oil mix into a clean bottle.
- Hibiscus flowers, amla, henna leaves, avuri leaves, and karisalai leaves in equal amounts (by weight) are blended into a paste and then heated with coconut oil. When cool, it is strained and poured into a clean bottle.
- Amla oil is made by heating coconut oil with fresh amla paste, juice, or dried powder.
- Commercial medicated oils include bhringraj thailam, sesame oil, and many other polyherbal oils (amla, brahmi, bhringraj, avuri, etc.). Natural vitamin E is sometimes added.

General Measures

- A healthy and stress-free lifestyle and also a diet rich in vegetables and fruit are important.
- Avoid harsh hairstyling treatments that use high heat and/or chemicals.
- Treat underlying medical conditions like anemia, psoriasis, etc.
- Massage the scalp daily for about 10 to 15 minutes.
- Detoxification (via purgation, neem oil nasya, and liver cleansers like triphala and bhringraj) are also helpful.

Chinese Natural Remedies

It is believed that hair loss is due to deficiency of kidney and liver blood flow.

Common Ingredients for Alopecia

Spices	Herbs/Leaves/Roots	Miscellaneous
	Liquorice (gan cao)	Black soybean
	Ginkgo biloba (maidenhair)	Rehmannia root
	Althaea officinalis (marshmallow root)	Privet seeds
	Eclipta/False daisy	Cordyceps
	Mulberry leaf	Lingzhi
	Cnidium	Psoralea fruit
	Cistanche	Solomon's Seal Rhizome
	Fleece flower root	Japanese Teasel Root
	Chinese angelica (*Angelica sinensis*)	Black sesame seed

Spices	Herbs/Leaves/Roots	Miscellaneous
	Dodder leaves and seeds (Cuscuta reflexa)	

Common Recipes

Topical

Dodder leaves. Take 50 g of the dodder leaves. Add 1 L of water. Boil and then simmer till half volume. Apply the decoction on the scalp. Leave it on for 30 minutes and then wash.

Fleece flower tea. Take some dry root slices. Wash and soak them for 30 minutes. Boil in 2 L of water. Simmer for 1 to 2 hours. Strain and consume.

Ginkgo rinse. Add three handfuls of dried ginkgo biloba leaves to a pot with 2 cups of water. Bring it to a boil, then remove from the heat, and strain. Cool completely before pouring it over freshly washed hair.

Liquorice root rinse. Add 1 tablespoon of liquorice root to a pot with 3 cups of boiling water. Let it simmer gently for an hour and strain. Cool completely and apply the solution to the scalp and hair.

Marshmallow root rinse. Place 3 tablespoons of dried marshmallow root in a pot with 3 cups of water. Boil for 15 minutes. Strain and let it cool completely. Add this liquid to the hair conditioner for use.

Western/Other Natural Remedies

Common Ingredients for Alopecia

Herbs/Leaves	Miscellaneous
Burdock root	Apple cider vinegar (ACV)
Calendula	
Cassia obovata (cassia)	
Chamomile	
	Essential oil: rosemary, lavender, thyme, cedarwood, and peppermint
Common couch	
Dandelion	Zinc
Equisetum arvense (horsetail)	
Lavender	
Nettle	
Parsley	Garlic oil
Peppermint	
Rosemary	Olive oil
Serenoa repens (saw palmetto)	
Symphytum officinale (comfrey)	
Thyme	
Yucca schidigera (yucca)	

Common Recipes

Topical

- **Azelaic acid.** Place several drops of the azelaic acid solution (1 ml) on the clean scalp where there is hair loss. Apply twice a day.

- **Burdock root rinse.** As above.
- **Cassia paste.** Mix powdered cassia with enough water to form a smooth paste. Apply to the hair and let it sit for an hour before washing it out.
- **Comfrey rinse.** Place 1 teaspoon of dried comfrey into a bowl with 1 cup of boiling water. Add 1 tablespoon of ACV and mix well. Cool it before pouring over freshly washed hair.
- **Chamomile rinse.** As above.
- **Dandelion rinse.** Place 1 tablespoon of the dandelion herb into a pot with 2 cups of water. Boil for 10 minutes and cool it before using as a hair rinse.
- **Essential oils.** Various oils such as lavender, rosemary, thyme, cedarwood, and peppermint oil (3%) may be used. Mix a few drops of the essential oil with a carrier oil (coconut oil or almond oil) and massage onto the scalp. Leave for a few minutes.
  Variation #1. Add a few drops of the essential oil directly into the shampoo. Massage onto the scalp and rinse off.
- **Garlic oil and steroid.** Some garlic oil from a garlic capsule is mixed with betamethasone cream and applied onto the bald spot.
- **Horsetail rinse.** Steep one-part dried horsetail herb in two-parts boiling water for 20 to 30 minutes. Let the mixture cool completely before use.
- **Lavender rinse.** Place three to five stalks of lavender into a pot with 1 cup of water. Boil it for about 10 minutes, and then cool and strain it. Use it as a rinse after shampooing.
- **Nettle mask.** Grind nettle leaves into a paste and mix it with some olive oil to make a smooth, slightly thin paste. Apply all over the scalp and leave for 30 to 60 minutes before washing it off.
- **Parsley rinse.** As above.
- **Rosemary rinse.** As above.
- **Saw palmetto rinse.** Add 3 tablespoons of dried saw palmetto to 2 cups of water in a pot. Boil, simmer, and then cool the mixture. Strain and use it as a rinse.
- **Thyme rinse.** As above.
- **Yucca** rinse: Mix powdered yucca with enough water to dissolve it completely.

Oral

- **Common couch tea.** Take 2 teaspoons of dried and sliced couch grass root in a cup of water. Boil and steep for 10 minutes. Consume three times a day
- **Zinc.:** This is taken as a dietary supplement.

Modern Remedies

There is no cure for alopecia. The available forms of treatment are often suggested to encourage more rapid hair growth but do not prevent the formation of new bald patches.

Corticosteroids

- **Intralesional corticosteroids.** Steroid injections, usually triamcinolone or hydrocortisone, are given with a tiny needle (intralesional) directly to the bald areas on the scalp. It is repeated every 4 to 6 weeks.

- **Topical steroids.** These are available in different brands, strengths, and preparations such as creams, lotions, solutions, ointments, or foam. Clobetasol propionate 0.05% under occlusion or foam type or betamethasone is usually used. About a 25% increase in hair growth may be seen.

  They work by suppressing T-cell–mediated attacks by the immune system on the hair follicles. This may reduce the rate of hair loss.

Minoxidil

Minoxidil is a potassium channel opener, which causes hyperpolarization of the cell membranes. The dilation of blood vessels and opening potassium channels encourages the influx of more oxygen, blood, and nutrients, which nourishes the hair follicles and encourages growth.

A 5% Minoxidil is applied once or twice a day to help stimulate hair on the scalp, eyebrow, and beard to regrow. It is not effective in extensive hair loss.

Intradermal Minoxidil is available as an off-label treatment. It is used alone or together with steroids for small areas of alopecia areata.

Side effects include acne, facial hair, headache, and flushing

Anthralin

Anthralin, i.e., *Dithranol cream* (0.5% to 1%) is a synthetic tar-like substance. It is not a coal tar or a steroid derivative. It cannot be used if the skin is inflamed or irritated or in cases of severe psoriasis. It helps to restore the normal rate of cell proliferation and keratinization.

It is applied to the hairless patches once a day and then washed off after a few hours or left overnight. This is continued for about 6 months and may be tried in the treatment of extensive alopecia areata. Hair growth is seen after 8 to 12 weeks. Some local irritation and brownish discoloration may occur.

Other topical medications (such as cream, gel, or solution) which promote hair regrowth.

- *Contact immunotherapy* using 2,3-diphenylcyclopropenone (DPCP) or squaric acid dibutylester (SADBE) is performed on the scalp weekly.
- *Tretinoin* (all trans-retinoic acid). It is an acid form of Vitamin A.
- *Bexarotene* 1% gel. This is also a retinoid which is used as an anti-cancer agent.
- *Spironolactone* 1% gel. It is an aldosterone receptor antagonist and decreases androgen production.
- *Finasteride.* It is a selective 5-alpha reductase inhibitor. This spray solution can treat male pattern and female pattern menopausal hair loss.
- *Tacrolimus* ointment 0.1%. This is an immunosuppressant medication.
- *Ketoconazole* 2% solution. This is an antifungal and antiandrogen medication.
- *Prostaglandin analogs.* Latanoprost ophthalmic solution can be used topically
- *Capsaicin ointment.*
- *Azelaic acid.* This is a natural acid

- **Topical combination** creams or solutions in alopecia areata.
  - Minoxidil solution 5% and steroid
  - Minoxidil and tretinoin
  - Minoxidil and dithranol
  - Minoxidil and tretinoin and azelaic acid

Oral therapy

- Inosiplex (inosine pranobex) can result in reasonable hair regrowth.
- Sulfasalazine. This is given as an oral medication for 6 months.
- Pulse steroid therapy (Prednisolone)
- Oral finasteride. Prolonged use can cause sexual dysfunction and depression
- Immunosuppressants. These include methotrexate, azathioprine, and cyclosporine.
- Baricitinib. This is a reversible JAK1 and JAK2 inhibitor. It is a tablet used in severe alopecia areata in adults.

Miscellaneous

- Phototherapy. Topical PUVA.
- Red light therapy can stimulate new hair growth.
- Laser therapy (Excimer) can stimulate new hair growth.
- Platelet-rich plasma and or stem-cell intradermal injections have also been tried.
- Cover and conceal with spray, and then touch-up or restyle.
- Wigs are commonly used for total or near-total hair loss.
- Hair transplant. Grafts with healthy hair follicles are removed from the donor scalp site and transplanted to the bald recipient site. One graft contains two or three strands of hair. Usually, 2000 to 3000 grafts are taken, which will have about 5000 to 6000 hair follicles.
- **Microneedling.** This is a roller with hundreds of tiny fine needles which are run over the affected scalp to make tiny punctures. Medications such as topical minoxidil is then applied. The roller can be bought as an OTC item or the procedure can be done by a dermatologist. It is done usually every 4 to 6 weeks. Complications include bleeding, bruising, infection.

Homeopathic Remedies

These include *Silicea* (in alopecia areata with dandruff), *Thuja* (with dry grey hair and white scaly dandruff), *Fluoric acid* (in alopecia areata), *Phosphorus* (associated hair loss due to change in climate or water and dandruff), *Natrum muriaticum* (hair loss after childbirth), and *Lycopodium* (post-menopause, childbirth, premature hair greying and hormone imbalance).

Nail Fungus

Nail fungus is caused by a fungus that grows excessively on the nails of the hands or feet. It may be caused by poor blood flow to the toes, making it more difficult for the body to fight off the fungal infection. Elderly people and immunocompromised individuals may be at a higher risk of getting a fungal infection. Symptoms of nail fungus include a white or yellow spot or patch under the nail or a discolored nail (yellow, white, green, or black). The nail may also thicken or become brittle and crumbly. If left untreated, it can become painful to put pressure on the affected nail.

Indian Natural Remedies

Common Ingredients for Nail Fungus

Spices	Herbs/Leaves	Miscellaneous
Garlic	Cedar	Lime
	Lawsonia inermis (henna)	
Turmeric	Neem	Oils: tea tree, olive, and lavender

Common Recipes

Topical

- **Cedar extract.** Soak the leaves or bark of the cedar tree in a bottle of olive oil. Store in a dark place for a week or two before use. To use, apply on the toenails and leave on to dry naturally.
- **Lime juice.** Apply fresh lime juice to the toenails and let it air dry.
- **Neem extract.** Place three to five neem leaves into a pot with 1 cup of boiling water. Add two to three cloves of garlic to the mixture. Bring to a boil, then remove from the heat, and allow it to steep until cool. Strain and apply this to the toenail.
- **Turmeric paste.** Mix powdered turmeric with enough water to make a smooth paste. Apply to the toenail and leave it on until it dries before washing it off.

   Garlic.: Crush one to two garlic clips and place it on the affected nail for 30 minutes. Repeat daily.

   Henna leaves.: Crush a few fresh leaves and apply the juice onto the toenails.

Chinese Natural Remedies

Common Ingredients for Nail Fungus

Herbs/Leaves

Radix glycyrrhizae (liquorice/gan cao)

Common Recipes

Topical

- **Liquorice:** Place 3 to 4 teaspoons of dried liquorice root in 1 cup of boiling water. Let it sit for 30 minutes. Apply the liquid to the toenails and rinse it off when it has dried.

Western/Other Natural Remedies

Common Ingredients for Nail Fungus

Herbs/Leaves	Miscellaneous
Calendula	Oils: lavender, tea tree, olive, oregano, rue
Chamomile	Mouthwash

Herbs/Leaves	Miscellaneous
Common rue	Vicks VapoRub
(Ruta graveolens L.)	
	Baking soda
	Apple cider vinegar

Common Recipes

Topical

Apple cider vinegar or vinegar. Dab some raw, undiluted ACV onto the affected nail and rinse it off when dry. Alternatively, soak the foot or hand in a small tub with one-part ACV and two-parts warm water for 20 minutes. Repeat daily.

Baking soda. Add a little water to some baking soda to make a paste. Apply on the affected nail. Leave in on for at least for 30 minutes or longer, and then rinse it off. Alternatively, place some baking soda into the shoes or socks before wearing them.

Calendula. Soak five to eight calendula leaves in 2 cups of boiling water for 30 minutes. Pour the liquid into a bowl and soak the toenails in it for a while. Let the toenails air dry completely before rinsing it off.

Chamomile. Place three to five chamomile leaves into a cup of boiling water. Let it sit for 1 to 2 hours until cool. Pour the water into a bowl and soak the toes in this liquid for a while. Allow the feet to air dry when done.

Mouthwash. Dab some mouthwash onto the affected nail and rinse it off when dry.

Oils. Many oils are used to treat nail fungus because of their antifungal properties. Paint the oils directly onto the affected nail two to three times a day, leaving to air dry.

Rue oil. Apply the oil on the affected nail. Refer to the section on Head Lice.

Vicks VapoRub. Apply a small amount of Vicks VapoRub to the affected nail one to two times a day.

Modern Remedies

Oral Antifungal Drugs

Oral antifungal drugs work by inhibiting cytochrome P450-dependent enzymes, which are enzymes involved in the synthesis of the cell membrane. New uninfected nails will grow to replace the old, infected nail.

   Examples: terbinafine, itraconazole

Topical Antifungal Creams

These creams may work better if the nails are pared thin. This facilitates the medication to penetrate the hard nail surface to reach the underlying fungus.

Medicated Nail Polish

It is painted on the infected nails and surrounding skin once a day. After 7 days, wipe the piled-on layers clean with alcohol and begin fresh applications. This is a slow process and should be done weekly for about 1 year.

   Examples: ciclopirox (Penlac)

Homeopathic Remedies

These include *Antimony crudum* (associated with distorted nails), *Graphite* (for cracked and in-grown nails with associated surrounding inflammation), and *Bufo rana* (when nails are black or blue).

Toothache

Toothache is a pain in and around a tooth that may be caused by a number of reasons, such as a decayed tooth, an abscessed tooth, a damaged filling, gum infections, or repetitive motions such as chewing or teeth grinding. Symptoms of toothache include a sharp, throbbing, or constant pain on the tooth. There may also be swelling around the tooth. There may also be fever or headache and foul-tasting exudate from the infected tooth.

Indian Natural Remedies

Common Ingredients for Toothache

Spices	Herbs/Leaves	Miscellaneous
Anise seed	Neem	Oils: clove and peppermint
Asafetida (hing)		
Carom seeds (Ajwain)		
Clove	False black pepper (*Embelia ribes*)	Olive oil
Cumin		
Frankincense/ru xiang (*Olibanum gummi*)		Catechu (*Acacia catechu*)
Garlic	Peepal	Salt
Ginger	Guava leaf	Lime
Nutmeg		
Onion	Gum arabic/ babul (*Vachellia nilotica*)	Cucumber
Piper nigrum (black pepper)		
Turmeric	Bay leaf	Mustard oil

Common Recipes

Topical

Anise seed. Place a handful of anise seeds in boiling water and let them sit for about 10 minutes. Strain and drink the liquid.

Asafetida-false black pepper mix. Take a pinch of asafetida powder and false black pepper. Make a paste and apply it onto the affected tooth.

Asafetida-lime paste. Mix ground asafetida with lime juice to make a smooth paste. Apply it to the affected tooth and leave on for 20 to 30 minutes

Bay leaf. Mix a few drops of bay leaf essential oil and some carrier oil. Take a cotton bud dipped in this diluted essential oil. Apply it on the affected tooth and hold it for a few minutes and then rinse the mouth.

Carom seeds (Ajwain). Gargle a glass of warm water mixed with salt and 1 teaspoon of ajwain.

Catechu. Gargle with catechu-based mouthwash.

Clove oil. Place 5 to 10 cloves in a container and add ½ a cup of olive oil. Cover and let it steep for 2 to 3 weeks in a dark place. When ready, strain and soak a cotton swab in the oil, squeezing out any excess. Place on the affected tooth.

Cucumber. Place a slice of room-temperature cucumber on the affected tooth and let sit for about 30 minutes.

Cumin. Grind cumin into a fine powder and apply to the affected tooth.

Garlic paste. Grind one to two cloves of garlic to form a smooth paste. Mix in a pinch of salt. Apply it to the affected tooth two to three times a day.

Ginger. Bite on a slice of fresh ginger with the affected tooth for about 30 minutes.

Guava leaf. Chew the leaves and keep in contact with the affected tooth for a few minutes.

> Variation #1. Take a handful of guava leaves add 100 mL of water, and boil until the liquid volume is reduced to 25 mL. Use the guava leaf decoction as a mouth gargle.

Gum Arabic. Chew gum arabic.

Nutmeg paste. Mix ground nutmeg powder with enough mustard oil to form a smooth paste. Apply to the sore tooth and leave it on for 20 minutes before washing.

Onion. Place a slice of raw onion on the affected tooth and let sit for about 30 minutes.

Peepal. Add 200 mL of water to 2 g of Asvattha bark powder. Boil and, once cooled, use as a daily mouthwash.

Pepper and rock salt. Mix ground black pepper and rock salt and apply the mixture directly onto the sore tooth.

Peppermint oil. Place 2 to 3 drops of peppermint oil on a cotton swab and apply it to the affected tooth.

Salt-water rinse. Stir 2 tablespoons of salt into 1 cup of hot water. Let it cool and use it to rinse the mouth.

Turmeric paste. Add just enough water to a teaspoon of ground turmeric to make a smooth paste. Add this paste to a cotton ball and apply it to the affected tooth.

Chinese Natural Remedies

Common Ingredients for Toothache

Spices	Herbs/Leaves	Miscellaneous
Ginger	*Fructus tribuli* (ji li)	Hornet's nest/ lu feng fang (*Polistes mandarinus saussure*)
Piper longum (long pepper/ bi bo)	Halitum/da qing yan	Chrysanthemum flowers

Spices	Herbs/Leaves	Miscellaneous
Piper nigrum (black pepper)	Chive	Gypsum fibrosum/ shi gao
	Chinese angelica root (dang gui)	
	Chinese wild ginger/ xi xin (*Asarum heterotropoides* or *Asarum sieboldii*)	
	Rhizoma chuanxiong (chuan xiong)	
	Rhizoma ligustici (gao ben)	
	Radix angelica dahurica (bai zhi)	
	Rhizoma et radix notopterygii (qiang huo)	
	Herba ephedrae (ma huang)	
	Wolfsbane /fu zi (*Aconitum carmichaeli*)	
	American ginseng	

Common Recipes

Topical

- **American ginseng.** Bite down on a slice of American ginseng with the sore tooth.
- **Chrysanthemum tea.** Place a handful of dried chrysanthemum flowers into a pot with 2 cups of water. Bring to a boil and then remove from the heat. Strain the liquid and drink it throughout the day.
- **Ginger.** Bite down on a slice of raw ginger over the sore tooth. Leave it on the tooth for 30 to 45 minutes before rinsing it out.
- **Halitum.** Pound the rock salt into a powder and mix it with some hot water. Use it as a mouthwash.
- **Pepper:** Bite down on two or three black peppercorns over the sore tooth.
- **Wen feng san mouthwash.** Add dang gui (6 g), xi xin (4.5 g), chuang xiong (6 g), bi bo (6 g), gao ben (6 g), bai zhi (6 g), and lu feng fang (18 g) to a pot with water. Bring to a boil and remove from the heat. Let it steep until cool before straining. To use, rinse out the mouth with half the mixture and then consume the other half.
- Modified **wen feng san.** Add qiang huo, ma huang, and chuan fu zi to the wen feng san formula above. Use it in the same way.

Therapeutic Measures

Diet

Consume kidney-strengthening food such as walnuts and wolfberries.

Western/Other Natural Remedies

Common Ingredients for Toothache

Herbs/Leaves	Miscellaneous
Calendula	
Cayenne pepper	
Chamomile flower	
Oregano	
Paracress/toothache plant (*Acmella oleracea*)	Essential oil (clove, tea tree and cajuput oil)
Peppermint leaf	
Plantain weed/leaf (*Plantago major*)	
Thyme	Salt
Yarrow	Apple cider vinegar

Common Recipes

Topical

Apple cider vinegar. Dab some raw undiluted ACV onto the sore tooth and leave it on.

Cajuput oil.: Dilute tea tree oil with some water and soak a cotton swab in it. Squeeze out the excess liquid and apply it to the sore tooth.

Calendula. Soak five to eight calendula leaves in 2 cups of boiling water for 30 minutes. Use it as a mouth rinse.

Chamomile.: Place three to five chamomile leaves into a cup of boiling water. Steep and use it as a mouth rinse.

Oregano leaf. Chew on a fresh oregano leaf using the sore tooth.

Paracress flowers. Chew on fresh paracress flowers or buds over the affected tooth.

Variation #1. Put several drops of the paracress tincture into the mouth, swish it in the mouth for about 1 minute, and then spit it out.

Variation #2. Put 1 or 2 drops onto the painful tooth or use a cotton ball to apply it to the tooth.

Variation #3. Add 1 cup of boiling water to a few flowers. Steep for 10 minutes, strain, and cool. Take 30 mL of the paracress tea and use it as a gargle.

Variation #4. Consume 20 drops of the paracress tincture before food two to three times a day.

Polyherbal essential oil (commercial). Add a few drops of the essential oil onto the cotton swab. Squeeze out the excess liquid and put this cotton ball on the painful tooth.

Tea tree oil. Dilute tea tree oil with some water and soak a cotton swab in it. Squeeze out the excess liquid and apply it to the sore tooth.

- **Yarrow paste:** Mash yarrow root or leaves into a paste. Apply to the sore tooth.
- **Thyme:** Mash some thyme into a pasty texture and place on a cotton ball. Apply it to the sore tooth.
- **Cayenne pepper:** Mix some cayenne pepper with some hot water. Dip a cotton swab into the solution and apply it over the sore tooth and gum.
- **Peppermint leaf:** Chew on a peppermint leaf using the sore tooth.

- **Plantain weed/leaf:** Mash some plantain leaf into a smooth paste, adding in a pinch of salt. Place over the sore tooth.

Alternatively, take a pinch of plantain root powder and apply it over the affected tooth and gum.

Modern Remedies

Nonsteroidal Anti-Inflammatory Drugs

Nonsteroidal anti-inflammatory drugs (NSAIDs) work by inhibiting the production of prostaglandins, which are chemicals that promote inflammation and pain. There are two prostaglandin-producing enzymes, COX-1, and COX-2. Both enzymes produce prostaglandins that promote inflammation and pain, but only COX-1 produces prostaglandins that protect the stomach and intestinal lining. NSAIDs block both COX-1 and COX-2 enzymes, which means that while inflammation and pain are reduced, they may cause stomach ulcers.

Example: aspirin, celecoxib, diclofenac, ibuprofen

Homeopathic Remedies

These include *Arnica montana* (inflammation from surgery or trauma), *Chamomilla* (hypersensitivity to pain), *Hypericum perforatum* (associated nerve pain), *Coffea cruda* (pain triggered by hot drinks), *Staphysagria* (worse when eating or drinking, especially cold drinks), and *Plantago* (for hypersensitive tooth and excessive salivation).

Dental Caries

Dental caries is an oral health problem that affects children and a large percentage of adults. It starts with the formation of a small patch of softened enamel on the tooth. It then spreads into the softer, more sensitive parts of the tooth beneath the enamel. Dental caries may also affect the roots of the teeth, causing them to become exposed because of gum recession. Dental caries is caused by the action of acids on the enamel of the tooth. Symptoms include toothache, tooth sensitivity, temperature sensitivity, visible holes in the teeth, and staining on the surface of the teeth.

Indian Natural Remedies

Common Ingredients for Dental Caries

Spices	Herbs/Leaves	Miscellaneous
Carom (ajwain) seeds	Neem leaves	Lemon
	Banyan tree	Bakul
Garlic	(Peelu tree *Salvadora persica*	Oils: Mustard, sesame seed, sunflower, and coconut
Turmeric	Neem stem	Salt

Common Recipes

Banyan roots. Chew the aerial roots.

Topical

- **Ajwain mouthwash.** Place a teaspoon of ajwain seeds into a pot of water and boil it for 5 to 10 minutes. Strain and discard the seeds. Once cooled, gargle with this solution.
- **Bakul.** Make a decoction from the tree bark. Take 1 to 2 g of bark powder and add 50 to 60 mL of hot water. Gargle with 30 to 40 mL once cooled.
  Variation #1. Chew the leaf or the unripe fruit of bakul.
- **Garlic paste.** Crush three to four cloves of garlic to make a smooth paste. Add ¼ teaspoon of rock salt. Apply it to the affected tooth and leave it on for 10 minutes before rinsing. Repeat twice a day. Alternatively, rub garlic oil onto the affected tooth.
- **Neem and peelu stem.** Chew on the end of a soft young neem stem. A peelu stem may also be used.
- **Oil pulling.** Swish oil such as sunflower, sesame seed, or coconut oil in the mouth.
- **Salt paste.** Mix ½ a teaspoon of salt with a little mustard oil and lemon juice to make a paste. Massage the gums gently with this paste for a few minutes before rinsing it out with warm water. Repeat twice a day.
- **Turmeric paste.** Mix ½ teaspoon of turmeric powder with a little mustard powder. Massage the teeth and gums with this paste. Leave on for 10 minutes before spitting it out and rinsing.

Chinese Natural Remedies

Common Ingredients for Dental Caries

Spices	Herbs/Leaves
Ginger	Ginseng
	Radix glycyrrhizae (liquorice/gan cao)

Common Recipes

Topical

- **American ginseng.** As above.
- **Gan Cao.** Chew on liquorice root every day.
- **Ginger.** As above.

Diet

Consume kidney-strengthening food such as walnuts and wolfberries.

Western/Other Natural Remedies

Common Ingredients for Dental Caries

Herbs/Leaves	Miscellaneous
Comfrey leaves	
Goldenseal	
Green tea (*Camellia sinensis*)	
Myrrh	Mastic gum (*Pistacia lentiscus*)
Sage	
Thyme	

Common Recipes

Oral

Mastic gum. Chew or suck on a piece of mastic gum.

Topical

- ***Camellia sinensis* rinse.** Place 2 to 3 teaspoons of *Camellia sinensis* herbs into a pot with 1 cup of water. Bring to a boil and then remove from the heat. Let steep until cool and strain. Use as a mouth rinse.
- **Comfrey leaf rinse.** Place a handful of leaves in a pot with 1 cup of water. Bring to a boil and then remove from the heat. Let it steep until cool and strain. Use as a mouth rinse.
- **Goldenseal rinse.** Place three to five chamomile leaves into a cup of boiling water. Steep the liquid and it use as a mouth rinse.
- **Myrrh rinse.** Place three to five myrrh leaves into a pot with 1 cup of water. Bring to a boil and then remove from the heat. Let it steep until cool and strain. Use as a mouth rinse.
- **Sage rinse.** Place three to five sage leaves into a pot with 1 cup of water. Bring to a boil and then remove from the heat. Let it steep until cool and strain. Use as a mouth rinse.
- **Thyme rinse.** Place three to five sprigs of thyme into a pot with 1 cup of water. Bring to a boil and then remove from the heat. Let steep until cool and strain. Use as a mouth rinse.

Modern Remedies

For pain relief: Use paracetamol or NSAIDs.
Surgical Procedures as Indicated
- Fillings
- Tooth extraction
- Abscess drainage
- Fluoride treatment
- Root canal treatment
- Restorative procedures (crown, implants)

Homeopathic Remedies

These include *Arnica montana, Belladonna,* and *Chamomilla* (associated toothache), and *Ferrum phosphoricum, Arsenicum album, and Merc solution* (associated gum disease).

References

Acne

Allayurveda.com(n.d.). *Acne.* allAyurveda.https://allayurveda.com/kb/acne/

Black, L. R. (2016, February 20). *These 9 Spices & Herbs For Good Skin Could Change How You Look At Cinnamon & Ginger.* Bustle. https://www.bustle.com/articles/142552-these-9-spices-herbs-for-good-skin-could-change-how-you-look-at-cinnamon

Castle, L. (2019, June 26). *Best 5 Ayurvedic herbs for acne that really work.* Well Natural Health. Retrieved from https://well.org/healthy-body/best-5-ayurvedic-herbs-for-acne-that-really-work/.

Charushila, B. (2021, March 31). *10 best Ayurvedic remedies to reduce acne at home.* StyleCraze. Retrieved from https://www.stylecraze.com/articles/10-ayurvedic-beauty-tips-for-pimples/#gref.

Chen, H. Y., Lin, Y. H., & Chen, Y. C. (2016). Identifying Chinese herbal medicine network for treating acne: Implications from a nationwide database. *Journal of Ethnopharmacology,* 179, 1–8. https://doi.org/10.1016/j.jep.2015.12.032

Cole, G. W., & Stöppler, M. C. (2020, March 11). *How to get rid of acne (pimples) causes, symptoms & home remedies.* MedicineNet. Retrieved from https://www.medicinenet.com/acne/article.htm.

EverPhi. (2019, May 31). *Fig seed oil and its amazing benefits for skin.* Everphi.Com. Retrieved from https://www.everphi.com/2019/05/31/fig-seed-oil/.

Gardner, S. S. (2002, January 15). *Understanding acne treatment.* WebMD. Retrieved from https://www.webmd.com/skin-problems-and-treatments/acne/understanding-acne-treatment#1.

Gardner, S. S. (2020, August 4). *Acne visual dictionary.* WebMD. Retrieved from https://www.webmd.com/skin-problems-and-treatments/acne/ss/slideshow-acne-dictionary.

Huizen, J. (2018, July 13). *Fifteen home remedies for acne.* Medical News Today. Retrieved from https://www.medicalnewstoday.com/articles/322455.

Luttrell, M. H. (2016, December 13). *10 Ayurvedic Remedies for Acne.* (n.d.). 10 Ayurvedic Remedies for Acne. https://www.practo.com/healthfeed/10-ayurvedic-remedies-for-acne-25877/post

Klein, E., & McDonell, K. (2020, November 4). *13 powerful home remedies for acne.* Healthline. Retrieved from https://www.healthline.com/nutrition/13-acne-remedies.

Nurse Buff. (2019, June 26). *Overnight and long-term solutions for acne that really work.* NurseBuff. Retrieved from https://www.nursebuff.com/overnight-home-remedies-for-acne/.

Saleem, A. M. (2016, December 1). *10 Ayurvedic remedies for acne.* Practo. Retrieved from https://www.practo.com/healthfeed/10-ayurvedic-remedies-for-acne-25877/post.

Sengupta, S. (2020, November 11). *Ayurveda for acne: 5 easy home remedies to get rid of acne.* NDTV Food. Retrieved from https://food.ndtv.com/beauty/ayurveda-for-acne-5-easy-home-remedies-to-get-rid-of-acne-1830115.

TCM Shanghai. (2019, November 21). *Traditional Chinese medicine for acne.* TCM Shanghai Chinese Medical Centre. Retrieved from https://www.tcmshanghai.ae/traditional-chinese-medicine-for-acne/.

TraceGains, Inc. (2012, October 31). *Acne vulgaris (Homeopathy).* PeaceHealth. Retrieved from https://www.peacehealth.org/medical-topics/id/hn-2192001.

Ware, M. (2019, November 5). *What are the benefits of chickpeas?* Medical News Today. Retrieved from https://www.medicalnewstoday.com/articles/280244#_noHeaderPrefixedContent.

WebMD Editorial Staff. (2021, May 28). *What to know about cedarwood essential oil.* WebMD. Retrieved from https://www.webmd.com/balance/what-to-know-about-cedarwood-essential-oil.

Whelan, C. (2019, January 8). *What you need to know about cedarwood essential oil.* Healthline. Retrieved from https://www.healthline.com/health/cedarwood-essential-oil#benefits.

Atopic Dermatitis

Agarwal, S. (2018, June 7). *7 effective home remedies for eczema, a dry skin condition.* NDTV Food. Retrieved from https://food.ndtv.com/health/7-effective-home-remedies-for-eczema-a-dry-skin-condition-1667410.

All Ayurveda. (2018). *Eczema.* (n.d.). allAyurveda. https://allayurveda.com/kb/eczema/

Arora, M. (2018, December 11). *Top 10 Natural Remedies for Eczema in Babies.* FirstCry Parenting. https://parenting.firstcry.com/articles/top-10-natural-remedies-for-eczema-in-babies/

Bhargava, H. D. (2020, June 18). *Eczema: What is atopic dermatitis?* WebMD. Retrieved from https://www.webmd.com/skin-problems-and-treatments/eczema/eczema-basics#1.

British Homeopathic Association. (n.d.). *Eczema.* Homeopathy UK. Retrieved from https://homeopathy-uk.org/homeopathy/how-homeopathy-helps/conditions/eczema.

Bubba Organics. (2019, December 10). *Baby Eczema|Natural Eczema Relief|Bubba Organics.* (n.d.). Natural Eczema Relief|Bubba Organics. https://www.bubbaorganics.com.au/natural-eczema-relief

Conaway, B. (2011, October 31). *Eczema: What's the best treatment for you?* WebMD. Retrieved from https://www.webmd.com/skin-problems-and-treatments/eczema/treatments-for-you.

Dallmeier, L. (2018, June 13). *20 best skincare herbs for treating eczema.* Herb & Hedgerow. Retrieved from http://www.herbhedgerow.co.uk/20-skincare-herbs-for-treating-eczema/.

Gibson, L. E. (2021, February 24). *How to treat baby eczema.* Mayo Clinic. Retrieved from https://www.mayoclinic.org/diseases-conditions/atopic-dermatitis-eczema/expert-answers/baby-eczema/faq-20450999.

Gold, G. (2014, November 3). *These 7 herbs and spices can save your skin.* EverydayHealth.Com. Retrieved from https://www.everydayhealth.com/beauty-pictures/these-herbs-and-spices-can-save-your-skin.aspx.

Heng, J. (2021, April 15). *Eczema from a Chinese medicine perspective.* Sustain Health. Retrieved from https://sustainhealth.com.au/all-other-conditions/dermatology/eczema-from-a-chinese-medicine-perspective/.

Hu, H. (2013, March 15). *TCM food therapy.* Yang-Sheng.Com. Retrieved from http://yang-sheng.com/?p=8978.

Jiva Ayurveda. (n.d.). *Eczema disease: Ayurvedic treatment for skin disease and natural remedies.* Jiva. Retrieved from https://www.jiva.com/diseases/hair-and-skin/eczema.

National Eczema Association. (2017, May 25). *Ayurvedic medicine and eczema.* Retrieved from https://nationaleczema.org/ayurvedic-medicine-eczema/.

National Eczema Association. (2017, August 22). *Traditional Chinese medicine and eczema: An interview with Xiu-Min Li, M.D.* Retrieved from https://nationaleczema.org/traditional-chinese-medicine-and-eczema/.

National Eczema Association. (2021a, June 30). *Available Eczema treatments.* Retrieved from https://nationaleczema.org/eczema/treatment/.

National Eczema Association. (2021b, July 17). *Eczema topical treatments.* Retrieved from https://nationaleczema.org/eczema/treatment/topicals/.

National Institute of Allergy and Infectious Diseases. (2017, April 19). *Eczema (atopic dermatitis).* Retrieved from https://www.niaid.nih.gov/diseases-conditions/eczema-atopic-dermatitis.

Natural On. (2015, June 24). *15 of the best herbs ever for eczema relief.* NaturalON—Natural Health News and Discoveries. Retrieved from https://naturalon.com/15-of-the-best-herbs-ever-for-eczema-relief/view-all/.

NHS website. (2019, December 9). *Atopic eczema.* NHS.UK. Retrieved from https://www.nhs.uk/conditions/atopic-eczema/treatment/.

The President and Fellows of Harvard College. (2021, July 6). *The nutrition source: Coconut oil.* Retrieved from https://www.hsph.harvard.edu/nutritionsource/food-features/coconut-oil/.

Wells, K. (2020, May 22). *7 Natural Remedies for Eczema.* Wellness Mama®. https://wellnessmama.com/remedies/eczema-remedies/

Psoriasis and Pruritus

Balfour, A. (2020, April 17). *Holistic Dermatology: 5 Tips To Heal Psoriasis & Eczema.* Mindbodygreen. https://www.mindbodygreen.com/0-12144/holistic-dermatology-5-tips-to-heal-psoriasis-eczema.html

Beyer, A. L. (2021, June 28). *Are Homeopathic Remedies for Psoriasis a Real Fix?* Greatist. https://greatist.com/health/homeopathic-remedies-for-psoriasis

Bowers, E. S., & Carson-DeWitt, R. (2019, February 19). *6 anti-inflammatory spices for psoriatic arthritis: Turmeric, cloves, and more.* EverydayHealth.Com. Retrieved from https://www.everydayhealth.com/hs/psoriatic-arthritis-management-treatment/anti-inflammatory-spices/.

Butler, D. F. (2020, March 3). *Pruritus and systemic disease treatment & management: Medical care, surgical care, consultations.* Medscape. Retrieved from https://emedicine.medscape.com/article/1098029-treatment.

Doctor NDTV. (2018, October 16). *Ditch the ointments and try these amazing Ayurvedic remedies for psoriasis.* Doctor.Ndtv.Com. Retrieved from https://doctor.ndtv.com/skin/ayurveda-for-psoriasis-ditch-ointments-try-these-ayurvedic-remedies-for-psoriasis-1933011.

Goodless, D., & Gallagher, C. (2019, November 3). *Treating psoriasis with traditional Chinese medicine.* Verywell Health. Retrieved from https://www.verywellhealth.com/chinese-herbs-for-psoriasis-2788381.

Hecht, M. (2019, March 7). *10 easy home remedies for rashes.* Healthline. Retrieved from https://www.healthline.com/health/home-remedies-for-rashes.

Jailman, D. (2021, June 21). *Your skin, pruritus, and itching.* WebMD. Retrieved from https://www.webmd.com/skin-problems-and-treatments/guide/skin-conditions-pruritus.

Jaliman, D. (2019, June 25). *The basics of psoriasis.* WebMD. Retrieved from https://www.webmd.com/skin-problems-and-treatments/psoriasis/understanding-psoriasis-basics#1.

McLeod, J. (2022, June 27). *Natural Itch Relief.* Farmers' Almanac. https://www.farmersalmanac.com/natural-itch-relief-12209

Md(Ayu), H. J. V. (2019, October 26). *41 Natural Home Remedies For Itching And Pruritus.* Easy Ayurveda. https://www.easyayurveda.com/2016/09/15/home-remedies-for-itching-and-pruritus/

Md(Ayu), R. Y. S. (2019, October 26). *41 natural home remedies for itching and pruritus.* Easy Ayurveda. Retrieved from https://www.easyayurveda.com/2016/09/15/home-remedies-for-itching-and-pruritus/.

Nall, R. (2019, June 24). *How can Ayurveda treat psoriasis?* Medical News Today. Retrieved from https://www.medicalnewstoday.com/articles/316937.

National Psoriasis Foundation. (2020a, January 10). *Natural treatment options for psoriasis and psoriatic arthritis.* (n.d.). Natural Treatment Options for Psoriasis and Psoriatic Arthritis. https://www.psoriasis.org/integrative-approaches-to-care/

National Psoriasis Foundation. (2020b, October 1). *Biologics for psoriasis treatment.* Retrieved from https://www.psoriasis.org/biologics/.

Natural On. (2016, November 10). *Top 15 herbs that push psoriasis out of your space!* NaturalON—Natural Health News and Discoveries. Retrieved from https://naturalon.com/top-15-herbs-that-push-psoriasis-out-of-your-space/view-all/.

NHS website. (2019, September 25). *Psoriasis.* NHS.UK. Retrieved from https://www.nhs.uk/conditions/psoriasis/treatment/.

Nystul, J. (2021, April 15). *How to get rid of dry skin (and prevent it, too!).* One Good Thing by Jillee. https://www.onegoodthingbyjillee.com/remedies-for-dry-itchy-skin/

Patel, S. (2018, January 23). *Psoriasis—Top Ayurvedic remedies for it!* Lybrate. Retrieved from https://www.lybrate.com/topic/psoriasis-top-ayurvedic-remedies-for-it/e815f757cf2065c0e988a9964643e519.

Sharma, V. (2019, March 28). *7 best homeopathic medicines for psoriasis*. Homeopathy at DrHomeo.com. Retrieved from https://www.drhomeo.com/homeopathy-for-skin/psoriasis-and-its-homeopathic-treatment/.

Shen-Nong Ltd. (2005). *Treating skin itchiness by Chinese herbal remedies*. Shen-Nong. Retrieved from http://www.shen-nong.com/eng/exam/treating_skin_itchiness_by_chinese_herbal_remedies.html.

Shen-Nong Ltd. (2006). *Skin itchiness and Chinese medicine*. Shen-Nong. Retrieved from http://shen-nong.com/eng/exam/skin_itchiness_chinese_medicine.html.

TCM Simple. (n.d.). *Traditional Chinese medicine treatment for psoriasis*. Tcmsimple.Com. Retrieved from https://www.tcmsimple.com/psoriasis.php.

Times of India. (2019, August 21). *Best home remedies for psoriasis*. The Times of India. Retrieved from https://timesofindia.indiatimes.com/life-style/health-fitness/home-remedies/best-home-remedies-for-psoriasis/articleshow/10102733.cms.

Usedom, E. (2019, December 20). *Indigo naturalis for psoriasis*. Learnskin. Retrieved from https://www.learnskin.com/articles/indigo-naturalis-for-psoriasis.

Visser, M. (2013, February 19). *4 herbal remedies to relieve itchy skin*. Growing Up Herbal. Retrieved from https://growingupherbal.com/4-herbal-remedies-to-relieve-itchy-skin/.

Wiginton, K. (2021, June 22). *Psoriasis treatments: How to get rid of psoriasis*. WebMD. Retrieved from https://www.webmd.com/skin-problems-and-treatments/psoriasis/understanding-psoriasis-treatment#1.

Wound Healing

Advanced Tissue. (2018, September 18). *Open wound 101: Understanding the types and treatments*. Retrieved from https://advancedtissue.com/2018/09/open-wound-101-understanding-the-types-and-treatments/.

Ahamed, S., Rao, H., Akhtar, M., Ahmad, I., Hayat, M. M., Iqbal, Z., & Rahman, N. (2011). Phytochemical composition and pharmacological prospectus of Ficus bengalensis Linn. (Moraceae)—a review. *Journal of Medicinal Plants Research*, 5(28), 6393–6400. Retrieved from https://doi.org/10.5897/JMPR11.455.

Ambardekar, N. (2021, April 21). *Understanding tetanus—prevention*. WebMD. Retrieved from https://www.webmd.com/children/vaccines/understanding-tetanus-prevention.

Anand, R. (2016, December 3). *Wounds—How Ayurvedic remedies can help in healing them?* Lybrate. Retrieved from https://www.lybrate.com/topic/wounds-how-ayurvedic-remedies-can-help-in-healing-them/5ee1d549fea179ff0ebe8563e799c913.

Braza, M. E., & Fahrenkopf, M. P. (2020). *Split-thickness skin grafts*. StatPearls Publishing. Retrieved from https://www.ncbi.nlm.nih.gov/books/NBK551561/.

Brooks, J., Cowdell, F., Ersser, S. J., & Gardiner, E. D. (2017). Skin cleansing and emolliating for older people: A quasi-experimental pilot study. *International Journal of Older People Nursing*, 12(3), 1–9. Retrieved from https://doi.org/10.1111/opn.12145.

Burgess, L. (2020, January 10). *Dry skin: Seven home remedies*. Medical News Today. Retrieved from https://www.medicalnewstoday.com/articles/319555.

Cherney, K., & Radusky, R. (2020, November 4). *10 natural dry-skin remedies to DIY*. EverydayHealth.Com. Retrieved from https://www.everydayhealth.com/skin-and-beauty/natural-skin-remedies.aspx.

Chouhan, D., Dey, N., Bhardwaj, N., & Mandal, B. B. (2019). Emerging and innovative approaches for wound healing and skin regeneration: Current status and advances. *Biomaterials, 216*, 119267. https://doi.org/10.1016/j.biomaterials.2019.119267

Daley, B. J. (2020, April 24). *Wound care treatment & management*. MedScape. Retrieved from https://emedicine.medscape.com/article/194018-treatment.

deLemos, D. M. (2021, March 29). *Skin laceration repair with sutures*. Up To Date. Retrieved from https://www.uptodate.com/contents/skin-laceration-repair-with-sutures.

Elkaim, Y. (2018, June 29). *9 healing herbs and spices hiding in your kitchen*. Yuri Elkaim. Retrieved from https://yurielkaim.com/healing-herbs-and-spices/.

Elvis, A., & Ekta, J. (2011). Ozone therapy: A clinical review. *Journal of Natural Science, Biology and Medicine, 2*(1), 66. Retrieved from https://doi.org/10.4103/0976-9668.82319.

Fazal, F., Mane, P. P., Rai, M. P., Thilakchand, K. R., Bhat, H. P., Kamble, P. S., et al. (2014). The phytochemistry, traditional uses and pharmacology of Piper Betel. linn (Betel Leaf): A pan-asiatic medicinal plant. *Chinese Journal of Integrative Medicine*. Retrieved from https://doi.org/10.1007/s11655-013-1334-1.

Gallagher, G. (2019, September 10). *What is pearl powder and can it benefit your skin and health? Healthline*. Retrieved from https://www.healthline.com/health/pearl-powder#how-its-used.

Goolsby, J. (2020, September 29). *How Fermented Foods Heal Your Body & Mind*. Mindbodygreen. https://www.mindbodygreen.com/0-5634/12-Ways-Fermented-Foods-Heal-Your-Body-Mind.html

Health Benefits Times. (2019, July 28). *Health benefits of Doctorbush (Plumbago zeylanica)*. Health Benefits. Retrieved from https://www.healthbenefitstimes.com/doctorbush-plumbago-zeylanica/.

Herbpathy.com. (n.d.). *Tabernaemontana divaricata herb uses, benefits, cures, side effects, nutrients*. Herbpathy. Retrieved from https://herbpathy.com/Uses-and-Benefits-of-Tabernaemontana-Divaricata-Cid4935.

Herman, T. F. & Bordoni, B. (2022, May 4). *Wound classification*. StatPearls Publishing. Retrieved from https://pubmed.ncbi.nlm.nih.gov/32119343/.

Lawrence, R. (2016, January 6). *Natural moisturizers hidden in your kitchen*. The Times of India. Retrieved from https://timesofindia.indiatimes.com/life-style/beauty/Natural-moisturisers-hidden-in-your-kitchen/articleshow/35716670.cms.

Lenger, K. (2018). Wound healing according to biochemical laws by highly potentized homeopathic remedies containing magnetic photons. *International Journal of Applied Science—Research and Review, 5*(4), 1–8. Retrieved from https://doi.org/10.21767/2394-9988.100081.

McCarthy, C. (2017, February 21). *Parents: How to manage injuries at home—and when you need to go to the doctor*. Harvard Health. Retrieved from https://www.health.harvard.edu/blog/parents-how-to-manage-injuries-at-home-and-when-you-need-to-go-to-the-doctor-2017022111222.

Mohd, S. M. A., & Manan, M. J. A. (2012). Therapeutic potential of the haruan (*Channa striatus*): From food to medicinal uses. *Malaysian Journal of Nutrition, 18*(1), 125–136. Retrieved from https://pubmed.ncbi.nlm.nih.gov/23713236/.

Pangestuti, R., & Arifin, Z. (2018). Medicinal and health benefit effects of functional sea cucumbers. *Journal of Traditional and Complementary Medicine, 8*(3), 341–351. Retrieved from https://doi.org/10.1016/j.jtcme.2017.06.007.

Peace Health. (2012, October 31). *Surgery and recovery support (Homeopathy)*. Retrieved from https://www.peacehealth.org/medical-topics/id/hn-2259000.

Rana, S. (2018, June 7). *7 effective home remedies to heal open wounds*. NDTV Food. Retrieved from https://food.ndtv.com/health/7-effective-home-remedies-to-heal-open-wounds-1817835.

Reader's Digest Editors. (2021, May 7). *10 healing herbs and spices*. The Healthy. Retrieved from https://www.thehealthy.com/food/10-healing-herbs-and-spices-2/.

Roddick, J. (2018, September 17). *Open wound*. Healthline. Retrieved from https://www.healthline.com/health/open-wound#types.

Russell, S. (2017, March 14). *Using herbs for faster post surgery healing*. Dimmak Herbs. Retrieved from https://www.dimmakherbs.com/2010/03/14/using-herbs-for-faster-post-surgery-healing/.

Shedoeva, A., Leavesley, D., Upton, Z., & Fan, C. (2019). Wound Healing and the Use of Medicinal Plants. *Evidence-Based Complementary and Alternative Medicine, 2019*, 1–30. https://doi.org/10.1155/2019/2684108

Singhal, H. (2021, July 1). *Wound infection medication: Antibiotics*. MedScape. Retrieved from https://emedicine.medscape.com/article/188988-medication.

Syed, Y. H., Khan, M., Bhuvaneshwari, J., & Ansari, J. A. (2013). Phytochemical investigation and standardization of extracts of flowers of *Woodfordia fruticosa*; a preliminary study. *Journal of Pharmaceuticals and BioSciences, 1*(4), 134–140.

TraceGains, Inc. (2020). *Injuries (Homeopathy)*. Kaiser Permanente. Retrieved from https://wa.kaiserpermanente.org/kbase/topic.jhtml?docId=hn-2237002.

Whitechurch, D. (2019, January 28). *Ancient beauty secrets of pearl powder (10 anti aging benefits)*. Teelixir. Retrieved from https://teelixir.com/blogs/news/ancient-beauty-secrets-pearl-powder-10-anti-aging-benefits.

Xue, F. (2020, November 18). *5 ancient Chinese beauty secrets for better skin*. Byrdie. Retrieved from https://www.byrdie.com/ancient-chinese-beauty-secrets.

Zhang, X. N., Ma, Z. J., Wang, Y., Li, Y. Z., Sun, B., Guo, X., Pan, C. Q., & Chen, L. M. (2016). The four-herb Chinese medicine formula Tuo-Li-Xiao-Du-San accelerates cutaneous wound healing in streptozotocin-induced diabetic rats through reducing inflammation and increasing angiogenesis. *Journal of Diabetes Research, 2016*, 5639129. Retrieved from https://doi.org/10.1155/2016/5639129.

Dandruff

Chaudhary, A. (2019, May 20). *Simple Ayurvedic Remedies for Dandruff*. Onlymyhealth. https://www.onlymyhealth.com/ayurvedic-remedies-for-dandruff-1310360537

Gardner, S. S. (2002, March 1). *The basics of dandruff*. WebMD. Retrieved from https://www.webmd.com/skin-problems-and-treatments/understanding-dandruff-basics.

Gelman, L. (2017, February 8). *14 healthy home remedies in your spice rack*. The Healthy. Retrieved from https://www.thehealthy.com/home-remedies/home-remedies-spice-rack/.

Gope, A. (2020, February 5). *Benefits & uses of avuri or Neeli | Indigofera tinctoria*. The Indian Med. Retrieved from https://theindianmed.com/benefits-uses-of-avuri-or-neeli-indigofera-tinctoria/.

Koganti, S. (2021, June 15). *Neem oil for dandruff: 7 ways it works*. STYLECRAZE. Retrieved from https://www.stylecraze.com/articles/ways-in-which-neem-oil-can-reduce-dandruff/.

Oliver, K. (2015, November 25). *How to get rid of dandruff—9 natural remedies*. Dr. Axe. Retrieved from https://draxe.com/beauty/how-to-get-rid-of-dandruff/.

Saleem, A. M. (2021, November 26). *5 natural home remedies and Ayurvedic treatment for dandruff*. Practo. Retrieved from https://www.practo.com/healthfeed/5-natural-home-remedies-and-ayurvedic-treatment-for-dandruff-31073/post.

Sengupta, S. (2018, August 9). *Ayurveda for dandruff: 5 home remedies to beat dandruff naturally*. NDTV Food. Retrieved from https://food.ndtv.com/beauty/ayurveda-for-dandruff-5-home-remedies-to-beat-dandruff-naturally-1897357.

Shen-Nong Limited. (2005). *Itchy scalp and Chinese medicine*. Shen-Nong. Retrieved from http://www.shen-nong.com/eng/exam/itchy_scalp.html.

Stanescu, A. R. (2017, June 15). *Traditional Chinese Medicine – Dandruff*. Vitality Magazine. https://vitalitymagazine.com/article/traditional-chinese-medicine-dandruff/

Tadimalla, R. T. (2021, July 19). *Can dandruff cause hair loss?* STYLECRAZE. Retrieved from https://www.stylecraze.com/articles/can-dandruff-cause-hair-loss/.

WebMD Editors. (2014). *Bael uses, side effects, and more*. WebMD. Retrieved from https://www.webmd.com/vitamins/ai/ingredient-mono-164/bael.

Wong, C., & Jelic, S. (2021, May 11). *14 natural ways to get a better night's sleep*. Verywell Health. Retrieved from https://www.verywellhealth.com/natural-ways-to-help-you-sleep-88230.

Head Lice

American Academy of Dermatology Association. (n.d.). *How to get rid of head lice when treatment fails*. Aad.Org. Retrieved from https://www.aad.org/public/diseases/a-z/head-lice-fails.

Anthis, C. (2014, September 30). *Lice home remedies using herbs*. Herbal Academy. Retrieved from https://theherbalacademy.com/lice-home-remedies-using-herbs/.

Bhargava, H. D. (2017, April 14). *What's the treatment for lice?* WebMD. Retrieved from https://www.webmd.com/skin-problems-and-treatments/lice-treatment.

Buchanan, A. (2015, August 19). *Six alternative ways to eliminate nits*. The Telegraph. Retrieved from https://www.telegraph.co.uk/news/health/children/11812132/Six-alternative-ways-to-eliminate-nits.html.

Marlowe, M. (2021, November 30). *How to Wash Laundry Infested With Lice*. The Spruce. https://www.thespruce.com/removing-head-lice-from-clothes-2146206

Mrunal, M. (2020, May 29). *15 Home Remedies for Head Lice in Kids*. FirstCry Parenting. https://parenting.firstcry.com/articles/15-home-remedies-for-head-lice-in-children/

Ontario College of Homeopathic Medicine Admin. (2019, August 11). *Homeopathy remedies for head lice*. OCHM. Retrieved from https://ochm.ca/homeopathy-remedies-for-head-lice/.

Pathak, N. (2021, June 22). *Treating and preventing a head lice infestation*. WebMD. Retrieved from https://www.webmd.com/children/ss/slideshow-lice-overview.

Ponmani, P. T. (2019, December 23). *Head lice remedy with homeopathy*. Schwabe India. Retrieved from https://www.schwabeindia.com/blog/diseases/329-head-lice-remedy-with-homeopathy.

Prakashan, P. (2017, April 13). *How to get rid of head lice: 7 natural home remedies to treat head lice*. India News, Breaking News | India.Com. Retrieved from https://www.india.com/lifestyle/how-to-get-rid-of-head-lice-7-natural-home-remedies-to-treat-head-lice-2026711/.

Price, A. (2017, April 23). *How to get rid of lice: 8 natural remedies*. Dr. Axe. Retrieved from https://draxe.com/health/how-to-get-rid-of-lice/.

Tadimalla, R. T. (2021, April 2). *How to get rid of head lice and eggs prevention tips*. STYLECRAZE. Retrieved from https://www.stylecraze.com/articles/home-remedies-to-get-rid-of-nasty-head-lice/#gref.

Venkateshwaran, R. (2019, October 21). *5 top hair uses, benefits & side effects of indigo powder (avuri) for grey hair & hair Growth*. Wildturmeric. Retrieved from https://www.wildturmeric.net/indigo-powder-for-hair-uses-benefits-side-effects/.

Alopecia

Alsantali, A. (2011). Alopecia areata: A new treatment plan. *Clinical, Cosmetic and Investigational Dermatology, 4*, 107. Retrieved from https://doi.org/10.2147/ccid.s22767.

American Academy of Dermatology Association. (n.d.). *Do you have hair loss or hair shedding?* Retrieved from https://www.aad.org/public/diseases/hair-loss/insider/shedding.

Basu, S. (2020, August 24). *Bhringaraj: Benefits for hair, uses, dosage, formulations, and side effects.* Netmeds. Retrieved from https://www.netmeds.com/health-library/post/bhringaraj-benefits-for-hair-uses-dosage-formulations-and-side-effects.

Bhargava, H. D. (2020, September 10). *Alopecia areata.* WebMD. Retrieved from https://www.webmd.com/skin-problems-and-treatments/guide/alopecia-areata#1.

Blakeway, J. (2021, May 10). *Hair loss: How Chinese medicine can help.* The Yinova Center. Retrieved from https://www.yinovacenter.com/blog/hair-loss-how-chinese-medicine-can-help/.

Charushila B., C. (2021, February 17). *20 herbs for hair growth and how to use them.* STYLECRAZE. Retrieved from https://www.stylecraze.com/articles/7-wonder-herbs-that-will-make-your-hair-grow-longer/#Yucca.

De, H. (2018, February 16). *Ayurvedic remedies for hair loss and regrowth.* Femina.In. Retrieved from https://www.femina.in/beauty/hair/ayurveda-for-hair-loss-79150.html.

Dr Batra's Doctors. (2021, June 4). *5 best homeopathic medicines for hair loss.* Dr Batra's™. Retrieved from https://www.drbatras.com/5-best-homeopathic-medicines-for-hair-loss.

Doctor NDTV. (2018, January 11). *5 best Ayurvedic remedies to reverse hair loss.* Doctor.Ndtv.Com. Retrieved from https://doctor.ndtv.com/living-healthy/5-best-ayurvedic-remedies-to-reverse-hair-loss-1798804.

Gallagher, G. (2019, October 25). *What you need to know about the health benefits of Bhringraj oil.* Healthline. Retrieved from https://www.healthline.com/health/bhringraj-oil.

Parmar, R. (2021, June 2). *12 wonderful health benefits of Bhringraj oil.* PharmEasy Blog. Retrieved from https://pharmeasy.in/blog/12-wonderful-health-benefits-of-bhringraj-oil/.

McDermott, A. (2018, June 15). *19 herbal remedies for hair growth.* Healthline. Retrieved from https://www.healthline.com/health/herbs-for-hair-growth.

Pioneerthinking.com. (2022, July 6). *Herbs and Spices That Help Prevent Hair Loss.* Pioneer Thinking. https://pioneerthinking.com/herbs-and-spices-that-help-prevent-hair-loss/

Rajapet, M. (2021, February 22). *12 effective Ayurvedic remedies for hair fall and hair regrowth.* STYLECRAZE. Retrieved from https://www.stylecraze.com/articles/10-effective-ayurvedic-tips-for-hair-growth/#gref.

Sayee, A. (2021a, February 16). *5 Chinese herbs that may help in treating hair loss.* STYLECRAZE. Retrieved from https://www.stylecraze.com/articles/chinese-herbs-that-help-in-treating-hair-loss/#gref.

Sayee, A. (2021b, June 28). *20 herbs for hair loss that stimulate hair growth.* STYLECRAZE. Retrieved from https://www.stylecraze.com/articles/herbs-that-prevent-hair-loss/#gref.

Nail Fungus

Ayushology. (2017, December 13). *How to treat nail fungus infection at home naturally?* Ayushology.Com. Retrieved from https://ayushology.com/homemade-remedies/how-to-treat-nail-fungus-infection-at-home-naturally/.

Booth, S. (2016, October 13). *What are fungal nail infections?* WebMD. Retrieved from https://www.webmd.com/skin-problems-and-treatments/fungal-nail-infections#1.

Dewan, L. (2016, June 1). *Quick Ayurvedic remedies for toenail fungal infection (foot care for monsoon).* Boldsky.Com. Retrieved from https://www.boldsky.com/health/disorders-cure/2016/quick-ayurvedic-remedies-for-toenail-fungal-infection-foot-care-101993.html.

Jailman, D. (2020, August 31). *How to handle toenail fungus.* WebMD. Retrieved from https://www.webmd.com/skin-problems-and-treatments/ss/slideshow-toenail-fungus.

Letha. (2012, May 16). *Nail fungus.* Asian Health Secrets. Retrieved from https://www.asianhealthsecrets.com/nail-fungus/.

Manneh, E. (2021, April 29). *How to treat toenail fungus, according to a podiatrist.* The Healthy. Retrieved from https://www.thehealthy.com/foot-care/treat-toenail-fungus-podiatrist/.

McDermott, A. (2021, February 18). *Try one of these 10 home remedies for toenail fungus.* Healthline. Retrieved from https://www.healthline.com/health/home-remedies-for-toenail-fungus#snakeroot-extract.

Natural On. (2015, April 4). *12 of the best anti-fungal herbs on the planet.* NaturalON—Natural Health News and Discoveries. Retrieved from https://naturalon.com/12-of-the-best-anti-fungal-herbs-on-the-planet/view-all/.

Sharma, V. (2019, March 30). *Homeopathic remedies for nail fungus, infection, toenail fungus.* Homeopathy at DrHomeo.Com. Retrieved from https://www.drhomeo.com/nail/homeopathic-remedies-for-nail-fungus/.

Smith, M. (2019, March 25). *5 Antifungal Spices You Should Always Use.* Doug Kaufmann's Know the Cause. https://knowthecause.com/5-anti-fungal-spices-you-should-always-use/

Stanescu, A. R., & Stanescu, A. R. (2018, January 24). *Chinese Herbal Medicine for Fungal and Yeast Infections.* Vitality Magazine. https://vitalitymagazine.com/article/chinese-herbal-medicine-for-fungal-and-yeast-infections/

UHN Staff. (2020, June 30). *6 home remedies for toenail fungus.* University Health News. Retrieved from https://universityhealthnews.com/daily/aging-independence/6-top-home-remedies-for-toenail-fungus/.

Toothache

British Homeopathic Association. (2021). *Dental problems.* Homeopathy UK. Retrieved from https://homeopathy-uk.org/homeopathy/how-homeopathy-helps/conditions/dental-problems.

Dabur. (n.d.). *One of the best Ayurvedic companies in India.* Retrieved from https://www.dabur.com/?aspxcrrorpath=/article.aspx.

Frisbee, E. (2003, June 3). *An Overview of Toothaches.* WebMD. https://www.webmd.com/oral-health/guide/toothaches

Gajendran, D. (2015, November 7). *10 soothing acupressure points to relieve toothache.* Modern Reflexology. Retrieved from https://www.modernreflexology.com/acupressure-points-to-relieve-toothache/.

Gallagher, J. (2010, July 1). *Natural toothache remedy for immediate toothache relief.* LearningHerbs. Retrieved from https://learningherbs.com/remedies-recipes/toothache-remedy/.

Gopi, K. S. (2020, September 5). *Homeopathic remedies for nail fungus.* Homeopathy360. Retrieved from https://www.homeopathy360.com/2017/10/14/homoeopathic-remedies-for-nail-fungus/.

Krishnamoorthy, G. (2017, March 10). *Tooth ache—5 Ayurvedic remedies that can help you.* Lybrate. Retrieved from https://www.lybrate.com/topic/tooth-ache-5-ayurvedic-remedies-that-can-help-you/2493aa7e9d5e6aa6749d4d4b142bff69.

Lin, S. (2017). *12 home remedies to relieve tooth pain naturally.* Dr Steven Lin. Retrieved from https://www.drstevenlin.com/11-home-remedies-relieve-tooth-pain-naturally/.

Nunez, K. (2020, September 23). *What You Need to Know About the Medicinal Benefits of the Toothache Plant.* Healthline. https://www.healthline.com/health/toothache-plant

NDTV Food. (2018, June 4). *4 Natural home remedies for toothache.* Retrieved from https://food.ndtv.com/health/4-home-remedies-for-a-tooth-ache-thats-driving-you-crazy-1419426.

Sheldon O. (2019, December 8). *Got a toothache? Try these 7 acupressure points!* Baba-Mail. Retrieved from http://www.ba-bamail.com/content.aspx?emailid=28830&readmore=true.

Snyder, M. C. S. (2021, April 9). *Cinnamon for Gums: Does It Help Treat Toothaches?* Healthline. https://www.healthline.com/nutrition/cinnamon-for-gums

TraceGains, Inc. (2012, October 31). *Dental support (Homeopathy).* Kaiser Foundation. Retrieved from https://wa.kaiserpermanente.org/kbase/topic.jhtml?docId=hn-2217001.

The-Crankshaft Publishing. (2021). *Tooth pain (treatment of pain with Chinese herbs and acupuncture) Part 1.* What-When-How.Com. Retrieved from http://what-when-how.com/treatment-of-pain-with-chinese-herbs-and-acupuncture/tooth-pain-treatment-of-pain-with-chinese-herbs-and-acupuncture-part-1/.

Wilson, K. (2015, February 15). *9 herbal remedies for a toothache.* Herbal Academy. Retrieved from https://theherbalacademy.com/9-herbal-remedies-for-a-toothache/.

Xing, C. (2017, July 28). *Traditional Chinese medicine has answers for toothache.* Www.Theepochtimes.Com. Retrieved from https://www.theepochtimes.com/traditional-chinese-medicine-has-answers-for-toothache_2274414.html.

Dental Caries

Ameen, N. (2018, February 11). *Ayurvedic Remedies for Cavity and Tooth Decay.* Conscious Health. https://conscioushealth.net/ayurvedic-remedies-for-cavity-and-tooth-decay/

Bg, G. (2017, August 1). *Tooth decay—6 ways Ayurveda can help.* Lybrate. Retrieved from https://www.lybrate.com/topic/tooth-decay-6-ways-ayurveda-can-help/6489834328edbaaf7a96d8d0ba011e17.

Brennan, D. (2020, August 28). *Health benefits of cloves.* WebMD. Retrieved from https://www.webmd.com/diet/health-benefits-cloves#1-2.

British Homeopathic Association. (2021). *Dental problems.* Homeopathy UK. Retrieved from https://homeopathy-uk.org/homeopathy/how-homeopathy-helps/conditions/dental-problems.

Dental Health Foundation. (2022, April 12). *Dental Caries (Tooth Decay).* https://www.dentalhealth.ie/adult-oral-health/terms/dental-caries-tooth-decay/

Doctor NDTV. (2018, August 8). *14 home remedies to get rid of cavities.* Doctor.Ndtv.Com. Retrieved from https://doctor.ndtv.com/teeth/home-remedies-for-cavities-1895792.

EdgeWater Dental. (2018, June 20). *Six simple ways to heal tooth decay and reverse cavities.* Retrieved from https://www.edgewaterdental.ca/blog/six-simple-ways-to-heal-tooth-decay-and-reverse-cavities/.

Glowatz, E. (2017, November 16). *The Chinese Herb That Fights Cavities Naturally.* Medical Daily. https://www.medicaldaily.com/chinese-herb-fights-cavities-naturally-422355

Gupta, S. (2016, June 2). *Ayurvedic treatment for dental diseases.* Practo. Retrieved from https://www.practo.com/healthfeed/ayurvedic-treatment-for-dental-diseases-17811/post.

Holly, H. (2013, December 23). *How I reversed tooth decay naturally: Claiming your power to heal your body.* Chinese Reflexology with Holly Tse. Retrieved from https://chinesefootreflexology.com/how-i-reversed-tooth-decay-naturally-claiming-your-power-to-heal-your-body/.

Mavity, J. (2016, August 26). *5 herbs that help stop tooth decay|Basmati.* Basmati.Com. Retrieved from https://basmati.com/2016/08/26/5-herbs-help-stop-tooth-decay.

Mayo Clinic Staff. (2017, July 19). *Cavities/tooth decay.* Mayo Clinic. Retrieved from https://www.mayoclinic.org/diseases-conditions/cavities/symptoms-causes/syc-20352892.

Procter & Gamble. (2021). *What are dental caries? Treatments, signs, and symptoms.* Oral-B. Retrieved from https://oralb.com/en-us/oral-health/conditions/cavities-tooth-decay/what-are-dental-caries/.

Ullman, D. (2017, January 24). *Homeopathy and dentistry keep you smiling.* Homeopathic.com. Retrieved from https://homeopathic.com/homeopathy-and-dentistry-keep-you-smiling/.

Xing, C. (2017, July 28). *Traditional Chinese medicine has answers for toothache.* www.Theepochtimes.Com. Retrieved from https://www.theepochtimes.com/traditional-chinese-medicine-has-answers-for-toothache_2274414.html.

10

Central Nervous System

Introduction

Some of the conditions of neurology discussed are:
1. Epilepsy/seizures
2. Insomnia (see under "Mental Health" chapter)
3. Headaches
4. Dyslexia
5. Developmental delay
6. Hypotonia (floppy child)
7. Speech delay
8. Attention-deficit hyperactivity disorder (ADHD)
9. Autism
10. Cerebral palsy
11. Dementia
12. Stroke
13. Parkinson's disease

Epilepsy/Seizures

Epilepsy is a chronic and usually long-term disorder characterized by recurrent seizures. A person is diagnosed with epilepsy when they have had two unprovoked seizures not caused by any reversible medical conditions such as low blood sugar or alcohol withdrawal. Epileptic seizures may be caused by brain injury, brain tumors, infections, genetics, or a high fever, but the cause is often unknown. Trigger factors include light, noise, fever, sleep deprivation, and alcohol intake. Epilepsy often affects a person's safety and may impair their ability to carry out everyday activities. It may also affect their self-esteem and hence social interactions. There are a number of types of seizures:
- Partial Seizures
  Simple partial seizure: Symptoms include involuntary twitching of the limb muscles, vision changes, vertigo, and unusual tastes or smells. The individual often remains conscious.
  Complex partial seizure: Complex partial seizures produce similar symptoms to simple partial seizures, but consciousness is altered or lost for a period. The individual may carry out repetitive movements, such as walking in circles or staring blankly.
- Generalized Seizures
  Absence seizure: This type of seizure includes staring blankly and a brief loss of consciousness.

Myoclonic seizure: Symptoms may include twitching or jerking of the limbs.
Tonic-clonic seizure: Tonic-clonic seizures are severe seizures with symptoms such as loss of consciousness, shaking and jerking of the body, incontinence, and an unusual sensation (aura) before the seizure begins.

Tests include electroencephalogram (EEG), imaging (computed tomography [CT], magnetic resonance imaging [MRI] brain or other specialized scans like Functional MRI (fMRI), positron emission tomography (PET), single-photon emission computerized tomography (SPECT), blood tests (infection and metabolic and genetic tests, including epilepsy gene panels) and neuropsychological evaluations.

Indian Natural Remedies
Common Ingredients for Epilepsy

Spices	Herbs/Leaves	Miscellaneous
Garlic/lehsun (Allium sativum)	Ashwagandha (Withania somnifera)	Honey
	Brahmi (Bacopa monnieri)	Milk
	Shankhpushpi (Evolvulus alsinoides)	
	Tulsi/holy basil	
	Vacha/sweet flag (Acorus calamus)	
	Jyotishmati/intellect tree (Celastrus paniculatus)	
	Jatamansi (Nardostachys jatamansi)	
	Shatavari (Asparagus racemosus)	
	Giloy/guduchi (Tinospora cordifolia)	
	Kantakari (Solanum surattense)	
	Ash gourd (Benincasa hispida)	
	Banyan leaves	
	Licorice/yashtimadhu	

Common Recipes

Oral

Teas/Brews

Ash gourd juice. Blend to make 1 cup fresh juice. Add 1 to 2 teaspoons of licorice powder. Drink once daily.

Banyan leaf extract. Take 10 drops of the leaf extract three times a day.

Brahmi juice. Blend a handful of fresh brahmi leaves with a little water. Drink 5 to 10 mL of the juice with 1 teaspoon of honey every day.

Garlic milk. Blend ½ cup milk and ½ cup water with 4 to 5 garlic cloves. Boil this mixture until it is ½ of its original volume. Take it once a day.

Holy basil tea. Place 2 to 5 fresh holy basil leaves into a cup of hot water. Cover and steep for 5 to 10 minutes before drinking. Alternatively, chew 3 to 5 leaves.

Jyotishmati seeds. Boil the seeds in one cup of water for about 5 minutes. Consume.

  Variation #1. Chew on 10 to 12 seeds every morning on an empty stomach. Wash the seeds down with a cup of water.

  Variation #2. Add 3 to 5 drops of jyotishmati oil to 1 cup of milk. Consume at night or on an empty stomach, especially for children.

Polyherbal mix. Mix together 3 g of jatamansi, 3 g of shatavari, 5 g of brahmi, and 5 g of guduchi. Add ¼ of the mixture to ½ cup of water. Drink twice daily.

  Variation #1. Mix equal amounts of shankhpushpi powder and vacha. Add about 3 g of honey to the mixture to make a paste. Consume this mixture twice a day.

Shankhapushpi. Take equal quantities of shankhpushpi powder with vacha. Consume 3 g with honey twice daily.

Vacha brew. Lightly pound 1 g vacha root. Add 1 cup of boiling water. When cool, add some honey and drink.

Therapeutic Measures

Kantakari nose drops. Place 2 drops of fresh kantakari juice into each nostril.

Medicated enemas (basti). Enemas with medicated oils are detoxifying and may reduce seizure frequency.

Diet

Avoid hot, spicy, pungent, fried, and sugary foods and also stimulant beverages.

Eat a healthy and well-balanced diet with more vitamin B, magnesium, and omega-3 rich foods. Include seeds such as ash gourd or flax seeds and nuts.

Consume cow's milk and ghee. Drink coconut water.

Lifestyle

Keep a regular daily routine (dinacharya). Stay safe and stress-free. Prevent accidents and avoid overexcitement. Engage in activities to relax and strengthen the mind.

Do a head and foot massage with sesame oil daily. Add a few drops of frankincense essential oil.

Take Epsom salt baths.

Use alternating hot and cold compresses at the back of head and neck.

Avoid constipation. Take isabgol if required.

Yoga

The following asanas are helpful.

Shashankasana (rabbit pose)

Kapotasana (pigeon pose)

Camatkarasana (wild thing pose or flip dog pose)

Pranayama

Breath control with deep breathing exercises can help.
Example Bhramari Pranayama (bumblebee breath)

Meditation

• Refer to the "Introduction" chapter.

Chinese Natural Remedies

Common Ingredients for Epilepsy

Herbs/Leaves	Miscellaneous
Bupleurum	Jujube fruit
Cassia bark	
Ginger root	
Ginseng	
Licorice root	
Peony root	
Pinellia root	
Skullcap root	

Common Recipes

Oral

• **Teas/Brews**

  Ginseng tea. Add about two to four slices of ginseng to a cup. Pour boiling water over the ginseng and allow it to steep for about 10 to 15 minutes.

  Licorice tea. Place 3 to 5 g of licorice herb into a cup with boiling water. Let steep for 5 to 10 minutes before straining and drinking.

• **Herbal formula.** A mixture of bupleurum, peony root, cassia bark, jujube fruit, ginger root, and pinellia root is consumed in the form of a decoction. Skullcap root, ginseng, and licorice root are sometimes added.

Acupuncture (Topical)

• **Gallbladder 20 (GB 20/Feng Chi)**
  This point is located at the top of the sternocleidomastoid muscle in the neck.

• **Governing Vessel 20 (GV 20/DU 20/Bai Hui)**
  GV 20 is located on the highest point on the head.

• **Extra Head/Neck 1 (EX-HN 1/Si Shen Cong)**
  This is located on four points around the topmost part of the scalp, with imaginary lines dividing the scalp into four equal quadrants.

• **Extra Head/Neck 3 (EX-HN3/Yin Tang)**
  This point is located between the eyebrows.

- **Governing Vessel 26 (GV 26/DU 26/Shui Gou)**
  GV 26 is located between the upper lip and nose about one-third of the way below the bottom of the nose.
- **Pericardium 6 (PC 6/Nei Guan)**
  This is located on the palm side of the wrist, three finger widths below the wrist crease.
- **Large Intestine 4 (LI 4/He Gu)**
  LI 4 is located in the middle of the webbing between the thumb and the second finger.
- **Stomach 36 (ST 36/Zu San Li)**
  This point is located on the outside of the leg below the knee. It is about four finger widths below the knee in the depression on the outer leg.

Western/Other Natural Remedies

Common Ingredients for Epilepsy

Herbs/Leaves
Burning bush *(Dictamnus albus)*
Essential oils: lavender, vetiver, Roman chamomile, sandalwood, marjoram, and cedarwood
Floating pennywort *(Hydrocotyle ranunculoides)*
Groundsel *(Senecio vulgaris)*
Lily of the valley *(Convallaria majalis)*
Mistletoe *(Viscum album)*
Mugwort *(Artemisia vulgaris)*
Valerian *(Valeriana officinalis)*

Common Recipes

Oral

Teas/Brews

Burning bush tea. Take 2 to 3 teaspoons of dried burning bush leaves into a teapot with 2 cups of boiling water. Steep for 5 to 10 minutes and strain. Drink warm.
  Variation #1. Mix peppermint tea with burning bush bark powder.

Floating pennywort tea. Place 2 to 3 teaspoons of dried leaves into a teapot with 2 cups of boiling water. Steep for 5 to 10 minutes and strain. Drink warm.

Groundsel tea. Place 2 to 3 teaspoons of groundsel herb into a teapot with 2 cups of boiling water. Steep for 5 to 10 minutes before straining. Drink warm.

Lily of the valley tincture. Fill a jar halfway with fresh flowers. Add alcohol or vodka until full. Steep for 2 weeks. Strain. Take 10 to 15 drops and add some water to consume.

Mistletoe tea. Place 2 to 3 teaspoons of dried mistletoe into a teapot with 2 cups of cold water. Let steep overnight and strain in the morning. Consume 2 to 3 cups per day. Drink cool as heating this herb removes much of its nutrients and beneficial chemical properties.
  Variation #1. Using fresh mistletoe stems and leaves, crush and extract 25 drops of the fresh juice. Drink before bedtime or on an empty stomach in the morning.

Mugwort tea. Add some fresh mugwort into a teapot with 2 cups of boiling water. Steep for 10 to 15 minutes and strain. Drink warm.

Valerian root tea. Place 2 to 3 g of valerian root into a teapot with 2 cups of boiling water. Steep for 5 to 10 minutes and strain. Drink warm.

Essential Oils

The following oils are used: lavender, vetiver, Roman chamomile, ylang-ylang, bergamot, sandalwood, marjoram, and cedarwood.

These oils may be applied topically on the back of the neck or on the soles of the feet or inhaled via a diffuser.

Music

Listening to Mozart's Sonata 448 (Mozart K. 448) may reduce epileptiform discharges.

Note:

Generally, Traditional, Complementary and Alternative Medicine (TCAM)/ Complementary and Alternative Medicine (CAM) medications are not effective in the treatment of epilepsy, but the above herbs can help improve behaviors, memory, attention span, and sleep.

Herbal or plant stimulants like ginkgo and ginseng and caffeine-containing plants (coffee, tea, cocoa, cola, guarana, and yerba maté) and ephedrine-containing herbs (ephedra) can worsen seizures.

Herbal sedatives (chamomile, kava, passionflower, and valerian) can interact with antiepileptic drugs to promote sleep and possibly reduce seizures. St. John's wort, however, can potentially lower phenobarbitone levels in the blood via its pharmacokinetic actions in the liver.

Modern Remedies

Anti-epileptic drugs are the mainstay of treatment. There are many types and are indicated in different types of epilepsy.

Sodium Channel Blockers

Sodium channels in the body exist in three states: a resting state (sodium passes passively through the channel), an active state (sodium influx into the cell is allowed), and an inactive state (sodium is not allowed through the channel).

Sodium channel blockers stabilize sodium channels in the inactive state and prevent them from returning to the active state. This prevents the continuous and excessive firing of the axons because of the sodium influx.

Examples: carbamazepine, phenytoin, oxcarbazepine

Calcium Channel Blockers

There are three calcium channel forms in the human brain: L, N, and T. They regulate the rhythm of brain activity. Inhibiting the influx of calcium into the channels lessens the frequency of seizures. Calcium channel blockers are particularly useful in controlling absence seizures.

Examples: gabapentin, pregabalin

Gamma-Aminobutyric Acid Enhancers

Gamma-amino butyric acid (GABA) has two receptors: A and B. GABA binding to an A receptor causes a chloride influx into the cell. The influx of chloride increases the cell's negativity, which makes it more difficult to reach the action potential. This medication causes an increased rate of binding to GABA-A receptors by preventing the reuptake of presynaptic GABA.

Examples: benzodiazepine, barbiturates, propofol, valproate

Glutamate Blockers

These medications reduce the frequency of seizures by preventing the binding of glutamate to glutamate receptors. Glutamate binding to receptors causes an influx of sodium and calcium ions into the cell while simultaneously causing an outflow of potassium ions, which results in excitation of the cell.

Example: vigabatrin

Carbonic Anhydrase Inhibitors

These medications inhibit the enzyme carbonic anhydrase, causing an increase in the concentration of hydrogen ions in the cell, decreasing the pH of the cell. This causes potassium ions to move into the extracellular compartment to neutralize the pH.

Example: acetazolamide

Other Anti-Epileptic Drugs

Topiramate: has multiple mechanisms, such as GABA potentiation, glutamate α-amino-3-hydroxy-5-methyl-4-isoxazolepropionic acid (AMPA) inhibition, and sodium and calcium channel blockade.

Levetiracetam: It acts by modulation of synaptic neurotransmitter release though binding to the synaptic vesicle protein SV2A in the brain.

Rufinamide: Exact mechanism is not known, but it works via modulation of the activity of the sodium channel and, in particular, prolongation of the inactive states of the channel.

Perampanel: It is a non-competitive AMPA receptor antagonist. It specifically blocks glutamate activity at the postsynaptic AMPA receptor.

Gabapentin: It has no activity at GABA-A or GABA-B. It interacts with a high-affinity binding site in brain membranes, which has recently been identified as an auxiliary subunit of voltage-sensitive calcium channels.

Natalizumab. It is a humanized monoclonal antibody and is used in refractory focal epilepsy.

Stiripentol: It has multiple actions and has mainly GABA potentiation activity.

Status epilepticus is a medical emergency and must be treated promptly with intravenous Anti-epileptic drugs (AEDs) also called Anti-seizure medications (ASM).

Epilepsy Surgery

This may be indicated in drug-resistant epilepsy. Lesionectomy, anterior temporal lobectomy, functional hemispherectomy, and subpial resection are some of the procedures done.

Stimulation Devices (Neurostimulation or Neuromodulation)

Vagal nerve stimulator (VNS): This device is implanted under the skin in the left chest to send electrical impulses via the vagus nerve to the brain to prevent seizures. It is done by a neurosurgeon as an add-on treatment for refractory epilepsy in adults and children over 4 years old. The median seizure frequency reduction at 3 years is about 54% to 58% and 75% by 10 years. Side effects include coughing and shortness of breath.

Responsive neurostimulation (RNS) system: The NeuroPace RNS system is a closed-loop neurostimulation system to prevent seizures in adults who are refractory to anti-epileptic drugs. It is an implantable stimulator device that is placed under the scalp by a neurosurgeon. The leads are placed at the seizure focus. A median seizure frequency reduction of about 66% to 80% in 3 years is expected. Initial short-term side effects include headache, pain at implant site, and unpleasant sensations.

Homeopathic Remedies

Epilepsy may be treated with homeopathy, which can help eliminate the tendency to have seizures.

After a detailed history, different types of remedies are given based on the seizure type and the body constitution.

Cicuta: Where there are distortions of the body, cicuta is effective for grand mal seizures where the attacks of convulsion are marked by violent, distorted body shape. There is an aura and marked body arching where the head and heels touch the ground. The person is totally unconscious. The face may be blue, and the jaw is clenched. Cicuta is also one of the best herbal remedies for epilepsy following head injury.

Artemisia vulgaris: for petit mal seizures. *Artemisia vulgaris* is effective for petit mal or absence seizures in children, often triggered by strong emotions, including fear.

Stramonium: For epileptic convulsions triggered by bright light. Stramonium is effective where the convulsions arise after exposure to bright light or shining objects (photosensitivity). The consciousness is preserved, and the patient experiences jerking of muscles of the upper body part.

Cuprum met: This is effective when the seizure attack is preceded by an aura in the knee. The symptoms during the attack are clonic spasms that usually begin in the fingers or toes and soon cover the entire body. Jerking of muscles is also noticed. The triggers for the attack include fright and anger. In females, cuprum met is used for the treatment of convulsion around the time of menstruation.

Bufo rana: For epileptic fits during sleep. Bufo rana is a natural medicine for seizures during sleep. The aura is felt in the genital area. It also works well for females who have seizures or seizures during menses.

Hyoscyamus: For deep sleep following an epileptic attack. Hyoscyamus is used when deep sleep follows an epileptic fit or when other symptoms, such as picking at bedclothes, playing with hands, and muscular twitching, are present.

Other Important Medicines

For epileptic fits during fever (febrile seizures)

Belladonna and *Nux vomica* are natural medicines that are beneficial in cases of febrile seizures. Belladonna is helpful when there is fever with marked heat. The head is extremely hot with jerking of muscles. *Nux vomica* is helpful when extreme chilliness is present with seizures.

Chamomilla and *Nux vomica* help epileptic fits triggered by anger. For fits after a fright, opium and aconite may be beneficial. In cases where alcoholic drinks trigger the attack, *Ranunculus bulbosus* (Ran. B.) and *Nux vomica* are helpful.

For Epileptic Fit from Head Injury

Hypericum, nat sulph, and cicuta are recommended.

For Epileptic Fits from Brain Tumors

Medicines that are effective for seizures because of brain tumors are plumbum, cicuta, and conium.

Petit mal seizures: Artemisia, belladonna, zincum, and hyoscyamus

Clonic seizures: Agaricus and cuprum

Tonic seizures: Cicuta and plumbum

Insomnia

See "Mental Health" chapter.

Headache

There are many types of headaches, each with different causes and principles of treatment. The most common types of headaches are:

- **Tension headache.** This type of headache is the most common type of headache that happens amongst teenagers and adults. It may cause mild to moderate pain but disappears over time, producing no other symptoms.
- **Migraine headache.** There is pounding, throbbing headache usually on one side, with associated nausea, vomiting, and sound, light, or smell sensitivity. It can last from 4 hours to a few days and can occur one to four times a month. Migraine headaches without aura (visual, sensory, or motor symptoms) are more common.
- **Cluster headache.** It is the most severe form of headache with burning and piercing around or behind one eye. The eye is red and tearing and there may be ptosis (eye droop) and meiosis (small pupils). The nose is blocked.
- **Chronic daily headache.** These headaches occur every day for 15 to 30 days and for more than 3 months.
- **Sinus headache.** There is constant deep and dull pain over the forehead, cheeks, and around the nose due to sinusitis or rhinosinusitis with associated fever, runny nose, swollen face, and blocked ears.

Headaches that have associated acute neurological manifestations (like hemiplegia, speech difficulties, abnormal vision, numbness, altered consciousness, etc.) need urgent evaluation. Ear, nose, and throat (ENT) diseases (sinusitis, temporomandibular joint (TMJ) disorders, ear infections), cervical problems (trauma, spondylosis), dental, eye and heart conditions (with cardiac ischemia), which can also cause secondary headaches, should be excluded. Exertional headaches are due to strenuous sports or exercise, sex, or coughing bouts. Emotional factors, insomnia, food or alcohol indulgence and indiscretion, food allergies, fasting, dehydration, long travels or computer screen times, extreme climates (too hot or cold), menstruation, pain medication overuse, or oral contraceptives can trigger headaches.

Keep a headache diary and track the triggers.

Tests include CT/MRI of the brain, lumbar puncture, blood chemistry, and ENT, dental, eye, and cardiac evaluations when indicated.

General Management

- Avoid and prevent triggers as listed above
- Avoid bright lights and loud noises
- Place a cold compress over the forehead or a warm compress over the nape of the neck
- Practice yoga, qigong, or tai chi or do any regular exercise.

Indian Natural Remedies

Migraine is a mind-body disorder that is mainly attributed to aggravated vata dosha (vata imbalance). Vata headaches are usually due to mental stress, anxiety, poor sleep, and fatigue. It causes throbbing occipital headaches, stiff neck and shoulders, dryness, and constipation.

Kapha headaches usually occur due to nasal and sinus congestion and are associated with running nose and cough.

Pitta headaches are usually associated with dietary indiscretions (eating hot, spicy, and sour foods), hot sun exposure, and anger issues. The headaches are bitemporal and over the vertex, and there is photophobia, dizziness, burning pains, and nausea.

Common Ingredients for Headache

Spices	Herbs/Leaves	Miscellaneous
Anise (*Pimpinella anisum*)	Triphala	
Bay leaf	Haritaki/kadukkai (*Terminalia chebula*)	
Black pepper/ peppercorn	Calamus root	
Cinnamon	Aloe vera	Rock salt
Clove	Karpooravalli (*Coleus amboinicus*)	Ghee
Coriander seed	Coriander leaf	Watermelon seeds
Cumin seed	False black pepper/vidanga (*Embelia ribes*)	
Fennel seed	Rudraksha (*Elaeocarpus ganitrus*)	
Ginger	Brahmi (*Bacopa monnieri*)	Essential oils: peppermint, lavender, and clove

Spices	Herbs/Leaves	Miscellaneous
Nutmeg	Tagar (Indian valerian)	
Sandalwood (chandan)	Bhringraj leaf	Sesame oil
Sitopaladi	Ashwagandha	
True cardamom/ choti elaichi (*Elettaria cardamomum*)	Henna leaf	Coconut oil

Common Recipes

Oral

Teas/Brews

Aloe vera. Take 2 teaspoons of aloe vera gel with some water three times per day. It helps with pitta headaches.

Anise tea. Add anise to boiling water and steep for about 15 minutes. Strain the mixture before adding honey to taste. Serve it hot.

Ashwagandha. Add 2 tablespoons of ashwagandha to a glass of hot milk. Stir in 1 teaspoon of ghee and consume.

Bay leaf tea. Boil three bay leaves in 2 cups of water for about 10 minutes. Add a pinch of cinnamon. Honey or lemon juice to be added as desired.

Brahmi juice. Place a handful of the fresh brahmi leaves into a blender and add up to 1 cup of water. Blend until smooth. Add honey to taste and drink.

Coriander tea. Lightly crush 1 teaspoon of coriander seeds. Place the seeds in a cup and pour hot water over them. Let sit for 5 to 10 minutes before straining. Drink warm.

Cumin tea. Lightly crush 1 teaspoon of cumin seeds. Place the seeds in a cup and pour hot water over them. Let sit for 5 to 10 minutes before straining. Drink warm.

Ginger tea. Steep 2 to 3 inches of fresh sliced ginger in a cup of boiling water for 10 to 15 minutes. Strain and add honey to taste. Sip on the tea while it is warm.

Haritaki. Add 1 teaspoon of kadukkai (Terminalia chebula/haritaki) powder to some hot water. Consume warm before bedtime. It helps with a vata headache.

Polyspice mix. Lightly roast equal amounts of black peppercorn, false black pepper, long pepper (pipali), cloves, fennel seeds, and watermelon seeds. Grind into powder and store in an airtight bottle. Add 1 teaspoon of this powder into 1 cup of milk and consume.

Rock salt. Stir a pinch of rock salt into a cup of warm water, ensuring that it is dissolved entirely.

Sitopaladi churna. Take ½ to 1 teaspoon with some honey for sinusitis or nasal congestion.

Tagar (Indian valerian) tea. Steep 2 to 3 teaspoons of the tagar herb in a cup of boiling water for 10 to 15 minutes. Strain and sip.

Triphala. Consume this choornam with some water (especially if headaches are due to sinus or nasal congestion).

True cardamom. Chew on two to three pods of cardamom when the headache starts to become apparent.

Water. Drink plenty of warm water.

Therapeutic Measures

Topical herbs. Scalp and/or forehead.

Bhringraj. Apply bhringraj oil on the scalp.

Alternatively, it can be administered intranasally.

To make the oil, dry bhringraj leaves in the sun for 2 to 3 days. Add the dried leaves to sesame or coconut oil. Place in the sun for another 2 to 3 days until the oil color becomes green.

Variation #1. Add dried bhringraj leaf powder to hot coconut oil or sesame oil. Let it steep till the oil color is green.

Henna. Blend the henna leaves with a little water. Squeeze out the juice and apply on the forehead, temple, and/or the scalp.

Cinnamon paste. Grind cinnamon sticks into a fine powder. Add just enough water to make a paste and apply it to the forehead. Let sit for 20 to 30 minutes before washing off.

Cinnamon-cardamom paste. Mix 1 tablespoon each of cinnamon and cardamom powder. Add 1 tablespoon of warmed sesame oil. Mix and apply on the forehead. Let sit for few hours and then wash off.

Karpooravalli paste. Using three to five fresh karpooravalli leaves, add enough water to make a paste. Blend or use a pestle and mortar to form a paste. Apply the paste/juice on the forehead.

Sandalwood paste. Mix sandalwood powder with just enough water to make a smooth paste and apply it to the forehead. Let sit for 20 to 30 minutes before washing off.

Ginger paste. Mix ginger powder with just enough water to make a smooth paste and apply it to the forehead. Let sit for 20 to 30 minutes before washing off.

Nutmeg paste. Mix nutmeg powder with some water and apply the paste on the forehead. Leave for a few hours and then rinse off.

Coriander leaf. Grind or pound some fresh coriander leaves to make a paste. Apply this paste on the forehead for 30 minutes, then rinse off.

Essential oil therapy. Place one to two drops of peppermint, lavender, or clove oil to the temples.

Calamus root oil. Massage the warm oil over the neck and nape.

Coconut oil. Massage some coconut oil on the scalp, especially over the vertex for pitta headaches.

Cloves. Lightly crush five to eight cloves and place in a clean piece of cotton cloth. Tie the cloth up and sniff the cloves when a headache begins to become apparent.

Panchakarma therapy

- Nasya (Nasal medications)

Ghee nose drops. Melt 1 tablespoon of ghee. Place 3 to 5 drops of the still-warm ghee into each nostril to relieve headaches.

Sesame oil. Place 4 to 5 drops of warm sesame oil in each nostril daily and inhale the oil deeply. Continue daily until the migraine attack is relieved. This helps vata headaches.

Other herbs: bhringraj oil, brahmi in ghee, or others.
Can be administered intranasally.

- ***Whole-body or head-an-feet oil massage (oleation or snehana).*** This is relaxing, soothing and stress-reducing. Various medicated oils are used. Warm coconut or sesame oil alone on the scalp and soles can also help.
- ***Sweating therapy (swedana).*** Sweating is induced via herbal steam baths to eliminate toxins.
- ***Buttermilk takradhara.*** Buttermilk with medicinal herbs is poured in a thin steady stream over the mid-forehead.
- ***Aromatherapy (dhoomapana).*** Inhale in the vapors of burning sandalwood or cardamon, or use the essential oils via a diffuser to relax and reduce mental tension and stress.
- ***Basti (rectal enemas).*** Warm sesame oil or ghee and herbal decoctions are introduced into the rectum for vata headaches. Coffee enemas are also used. They can be self-administered at home.

Ncti pot and salinc. This is to clear nasal congestion in kapha headaches.

Steam inhalation with eucalyptus. This also is for airway decongestion.

Rudraksha. Wear a 5 or 7 mukhi (face) Rudraksha as a bracelet or a *mala* (necklace) to calm the nervous system and decrease stress.

Yoga

Do asanas (physical poses), *pranayama* (controlled breathing), *kriya* (cleansing techniques), meditation, and relaxation techniques.

- Perform the brahmari pranayama (honey bee). Place the index fingers on the tragus of both ears to cover both ears. Inhale and exhale while chanting "om."
- The asanas include:
  - Bridge pose
  - Prasarita padottanasana or the wide-legged forward bend pose
  - Child's pose (balasana)
  - Downward facing dog/downward dog pose (adho mukha svanasana)
  - Apanasana wind relieving pose (this helps to release gas or wind)

Diet

Consume vata-pacifying foods for vata headaches. These should be sweet, sour, salty and with adequate fats. Avoid bitter, pungent, astringent, cold, dry, stale, or preserved foods. Eat meals on time and avoid unnecessary fasting. Warm milk should be taken before bedtime.

Consume pitta-pacifying foods for pitta headaches. Eat cooling foods like cucumber, watermelon, and dates. Drink plenty of water or cooling fruit juices and coconut water.

Chinese Natural Remedies

In traditional Chinese medicine (TCM), it is believed that migraine is due to an external invasion or an internal disruption.

The external invasion is due to external heat, dampness, wind, and cold. Wind is the most common external invasion (wind-heat, wind-cold, or wind-damp), and it disturbs the qi and blood harmony (as in flu or colds).

The internal disruption is due to liver, spleen, and kidney disorders with associated intrinsic factors like genetics, poor diet, stress, and emotional factors that can result in liver-fire, heart-fire, and stomach-fire, which may then result in the following syndromes:

- *Excessive liver yang energy/liver yang rising.* There is agitation, anger, dizziness, headache, insomnia, and heat intolerance as in hypertension.
- Kidney Yang Deficiency
- *Blood stagnation/blood stasis.* There is focal headache, memory deficit, attention deficit, and dry skin with history of head trauma.
- *Deficiency of blood and qi.* There is fatigue, lethargy, pallor, and heaviness in the head and eyes.
- *Combination syndromes* can also occur. Damp phlegm blockage or accumulation occurs due to excess oily, sugary, or dairy foods

Common Remedies for Headache

Spices	Herbs/Leaves/Flowers	Miscellaneous
Ginger	Gingko	Scorpion
	Sichuan lovage rhizome (*Rhizoma ligustici chuanxiong*)	
	White peony root (*Radix paeoniae alba*)	
	Red peony root (*Radix paeoniae rubra*)	
	Chinese angelica (*Radix angelicae sinensis*)	
	Dahurian angelica root (*Radix angelicae dahuricae/Angelica dahurica*)	
	Manchurian wild ginger (*Herba asari*)	
	Gambir (*Uncaria gambir*)	
	Safflower (*Flos carthami*)	
	Cyathula root (*Radix cyathulae*)	
	Yanhusuo (*Rhizoma corydalis*)	
	Licorice root (*Radix glycyrrhizae*)	
	Honeysuckle (*Lonicera japonica*)	
	Chasteberry/man jingzi (*Vitex trifolia*)	
	Chinese foxglove root (*Rehmannia radix*)	

Common Recipes

Oral

Teas/Brew/Others

Chuanxiong polyherbal formulae. The key ingredient is Sichuan lovage rhizome (*Rhizoma ligustici chuanxiong*), and it is combined with many of the various herbs listed above to make more than 20 polyherbal formulae.

Ginkgo tea. Boil 2 cups of water. Add 1 tablespoon of dried ginkgo leaves. Boil for 5 minutes and then steep for another 10 minutes. Strain and consume with honey if desired.

Naoxintong capsule (NXTC). The key ingredients include Chinese red sage (danshen), *Radix astragali*, leech, scorpion, and others.

Tian Ma Gou Teng. The key ingredients include *Gastrodia rhizome*, abalone shell, gambir, Chinese skullcap root, cyathula root, *Poria cocos*, gardenia fruit, *Polygonum multiflorum*, eucommia bark, *Loranthus parasiticus, and* Chinese motherwort.

Toutongning capsule. The main herbs include *Smilax glabra, Gastrodia rhizome*, Chinese angelica, *Polygonum multiflorum*, Sichuan lovage rhizome, siler root, gypsum, *Acorus calamus,* and medicinal scorpion.

Yang-Xue-Qing-Nao granules (YXQN). The key ingredients include Chinese angelica, Sichuan lovage rhizome, white peony root, *Rehmannia radix*, cassia seed, corydalis, gambir, and *Spatholobus suberectus.*

Other commonly used single herbs include: lilyturf root, figwort root, and Chinese foxglove root.

Therapeutic Measures

Acupressure or Tui Na (Topical) and Acupuncture

This can help in chronic migraine prevention.

- Lung 7 (LU 7)

  LU 7 is located on the inner corner of the styloid process of the radius bone. It can be found by interlocking the thumbs and forefingers of both hands. The tip of the index finger marks the location of LU 7.

- Large Intestine (LI 4)

  LI 4 is found on the highest point of the webbing between the thumb and the forefinger.

- Lung 9 (LU 9)

  LU 9 is located on the inner wrist along the wrist crease in line with the bottom of the thumb.

- An Mien/SJ 17

  This point is located on the head and can be found by feeling the base of the skull in the depression directly behind the ear. Massage this point gently but firmly for 15 to 20 minutes with two fingers.

- Spleen 6 (SP 6)

  SP 6 is located a palm width above the inner ankle bone.

- Stomach 36 (ST 36)

  ST 36 is found one palm width below the bottom edge of the kneecap on the outer side of the leg. It is located in the depression between the shin and the leg muscle.

Chinese Herbal Enemas or Coffee Enemas

These are done at home on a regular basis. The cooling herbs used include *Rehmanniae radix, Scrophulariae radix, Ophiopogonis radix*, etc.

Western/Other Natural Remedies

Common Ingredients for Headache

Herbs/Leaves	Miscellaneous
Black cohosh	Passionflower
Butterbur	Peppermint
Feverfew	Cayenne pepper
Hops	CBD oil (cannabis)
Meadowsweet	Rose water
Snowdrop (Galanthus woronowii)	
Valerian	
White willow bark	Black coffee

Common Recipes

Black cohosh tea. Place 1 teaspoon of black cohosh into a pot with 1 cup of water. Bring to a gentle boil and allow to cook for 20 to 30 minutes. Strain and drink warm.

Butterbur tea. Place 1 to 2 teaspoons of butterbur root into a cup of hot water. Steep for 3 to 5 minutes before straining. Drink warm. Alternatively, consume butterbur extract, which is available commercially. Take 50 to 75 mg twice a day.

> Variation#1. Soak 1 teaspoon of dried butterbur root in 1 cup of water overnight or for 10 to 12 hours. Boil and then simmer for 5 minutes. Strain and consume. Add honey as desired.

Cayenne pepper. Add 1 teaspoon of cayenne pepper and some lemon juice to a cup of hot water. Drink warm. Cayenne pepper can also be added to foods during cooking.

CBD oil. This can provide relief in cluster headaches.

Coffee. Drink black coffee with no added sugar or milk.

Feverfew tea. Place 1 tablespoon of fresh or dried feverfew leaves in a cup. Pour 1 cup of boiling water over the herbs and let steep for 30 to 60 minutes. Strain and drink warm.

Hops tea. Place 1 to 2 teaspoons of dried hops flowers into a cup of boiling water. Cover and let sit for 10 to 15 minutes. Strain and drink warm before bedtime.

Meadowsweet tea. Add 1 cup of hot water to 2 tablespoons of dried meadowsweet flowers or 4 teaspoons of fresh flowers. Steep for 10 minutes. Strain and consume warm.

> Variation#1. Bring to a boil 2 cups of water, 1 teaspoon dried meadowsweet flowers, 1 teaspoon dried rose petals, and a pinch of ground green cardamom. Steep for 10 minutes. Strain and consume warm with added honey.

Passionflower tea. Place 1 to 2 teaspoons of dried passionflower into a cup of hot water. Cover and let steep for 5 to 10 minutes. Drink warm before bedtime.

Peppermint tea. Place a handful of peppermint leaves into a pot of water. Bring to a boil and reduce the heat. Allow the mixture to simmer for 5 to 10 minutes. Strain and drink twice a day.

Rose water. Take 2 or 3 cups of fresh rose petals and place in saucepan. Add about 2 litres of distilled water or enough to cover the petals. Simmer in the saucepan for 30 to 45 minutes till the colour comes out from the petals. Cool, then strain and store in a clean bottle. Refrigerate and use for 1 month.

> Place a compress soaked in rose water on the head for about 30 to 45 minutes.

White willow bark tea. Place 1 to 2 teaspoons of dried willow bark into a pot with 2 cups of water. Allow to simmer gently for 15 minutes before straining and drinking. Alternatively, purchase white willow bark in the form of a tincture and consume three times a day.

Therapeutic Measures

Aromatherapy. Rub peppermint essential oil, 10% of menthol solution, or gel containing menthol on the forehead and temple.

Diet. Include magnesium, vitamin B, and omega-3 rich foods.

Nutraceuticals. These include the following: riboflavin/vitamin B2 (400 mg daily for 3 months), magnesium (300 to 600 mg/day), coenzyme Q (100 mg, three times per day), omega-3 fish oil, alpha-lipoic acid, and CBD oil.

Intranasal capsaicin spray (or cream). This is administered during an acute headache, and relief is obtained within 1 to 3 minutes; the effect can last for a few hours. Side effects include local sting and eye and nose watering.

Green light therapy. Green light emitting diodes (GLED) can significantly reduce the number of headache days in chronic or episodic migraine. There is about a 60% reduction in the frequency and pain intensity of headaches. The LED green lights have a specific narrow, low-intensity wavelength band and are available as strips or lamps.

Snowdrop. The plant bulb and leaves are rubbed on the forehead to relieve headache, migraine and to improve memory and focus in mild dementia.

Aromatherapy. Use essential oils like lavender, peppermint, jasmine, and rosemary. Put 5 to 10 drops in hot water and inhale or use a diffuser.

Exercise. Regular exercise like swimming and brisk walks can reduce stress.

Relaxation. This can be achieved by meditation, deep diaphragmatic or belly breathing, mindfulness, mental imagery, biofeedback, cognitive behavioral therapy (CBT), and hypnosis, hypnosis and lymphatic self-massage.

Hyperbaric oxygen therapy (HBOT). This may provide relief during an acute migraine attack.

Modern Remedies

For Acute Pain Relief

Paracetamol: This is recommended for mild to moderate headache.

Nonsteroidal Anti-Inflammatory Drugs

Nonsteroidal anti-inflammatory drugs (NSAIDs) inhibit the production of prostaglandins, which are chemicals that promote inflammation and pain. There are two prostaglandin-producing enzymes: COX-1 and COX-2. Both enzymes produce prostaglandins that promote inflammation and pain, but only COX-1 produces prostaglandins that protect the stomach and intestinal lining. NSAIDs block both COX-1 and COX-2 enzymes, which means that while inflammation and pain are reduced, NSAIDs may cause stomach ulcers.

Examples: aspirin, celecoxib, diclofenac, ibuprofen

Triptans or ditans. They are fast-acting and recommended in severe migraine within 2 hours of onset of headache. It is available as a tablet, nasal spray, or injection.

If there is nausea or vomiting, the nasal spray form is used.

Examples: sumatriptan, zolmitriptan, rizatriptan, almotriptan, eletriptan, lasmiditan, frovatriptan

Oral sumatriptan is the first drug of choice. Intranasal spray (if more than 12 years old) or subcutaneous injection can be given if there is vomiting. Other triptans can be tried if Sumatriptan does not work. Side effects of triptans include dizziness, drowsiness, dyspnea, nausea, and flushing. It must be used cautiously in heart disease or hypertension.

Ergot. Dihydroergotamine can be taken even after 2 hours of headache onset. It is available as oral form, nasal spray, or injection.

5-HT receptor agonists. These drugs bind to the receptors on the trigeminal nerve to inhibit pain.

CGRP antagonists. Calcitonin gene-related peptide (CGRP) is a substance which causes migraine pain. CGRP antagonists like rimegepant and ubrogepant can block the effects of CGRP. They are oral medications and are used to treat acute migraine with or without aura.

Steroids. Oral prednisone is used in severe or difficult-to-treat migraine as in status migraine.

Antiemetics. If there is nausea or vomiting, antiemetics such as metoclopramide or buccal prochlorperazine are given with the analgesics.

Combination medications. Aspirin, paracetamol, and caffeine are combined as a single pill are available as over-the-counter medication.

For Chronic Migraine Relief

Antidepressants. Low-dose tricyclic antidepressants (TCA), such as amitriptyline, can be given. Weight gain may occur. The selective serotonin and norepinephrine reuptake inhibitors (SNRI), such as duloxetine, may also help to prevent migraine.

Beta blockers. Propanol is a blood pressure–reducing medication and is used to prevent migraine headaches. It should be avoided if there is a history of asthma or heart disease.

Calcium channel blockers. Flunarizine helps to improve blood flow. Side effects include low blood pressure and constipation.

Anti-epileptic drugs. Medications that control seizures also help prevent migraine. These include topiramate or sodium valproate. Side effects include drowsiness and attention difficulty.

Botulinum toxin injections. Small doses of botulinum toxin A are injected over the scalp every 3 to 4 months if there is a history of more than 15 headache days per month.

CGRP inhibitors (anti-CGRP therapies). Humanized monoclonal antibodies, such as erenumab (Aimovig), galcanezumab (Emgality), epitinezumab (Vyepti), fremanezumab (Ajovy). They are injected every 1 or 3 months using a pen device.

Side effects include hypertension and constipation.

Atogepant is available as an oral tablet..

Neuromodulation. Peripheral neuromodulation (via peripheral nerve stimulation of the occipital nerves or auriculotemporal nerves) or central neuromodulation (via implanted bilateral suboccipital stimulators) can be effective in the treatment of chronic migraine.

Lifestyle management. Stress and sleep management are important aspects of general management.

Decongestants

Decongestants may be helpful in sinus headaches as they help unblock the sinuses by constricting the blood vessels. This, in turn, reduces inflammation, relieving the headache. Examples: oxymetazoline, pseudoephedrine

Homeopathy

Homeopathic remedies for migraine include belladonna (sudden throbbing head fullness with associated photosensitivity and audiophonia), *Natrum muriaticum* (with photosensitivity, relief with sleep and darkness, and triggers with sun, menses, emotions, or eye strain), *Nux vomica* (with indigestion or dyspepsia from food or alcohol excess), *Coffea cruda* (with insomnia and overactive brain), bryonia (associated nausea and vomiting; relief with lying still and being quiet alone), *Gelsemium* (pain below the head and at the nape, often with stress trigger), *Ignatia* (with emotional upsets and face or neck twitching), silicea (with more right-sided headaches starting from back to front and worse with the cold), sepia (more left-sided headaches, worse with meal skipping, being indoors, and premenstrual or menopausal times), *Sanguinaria* (more right-sided headache from back to front, worse with missing meals and food allergies, relief with passing wind, burping, vomiting, and sleep), and others (*Lycopodium clavatum*, *Iris versicolor*, etc.).

Dyslexia

Dyslexia is a common learning difficulty that manifests as slow reading, writing, and spelling skills, reversal of alphabets or mirror image writing, poor or inconsistent spelling skills, and difficulty in planning and organizing.

Dyslexia is often treated through the use of extra educational support from schools, and children with dyslexia may be taught specialized techniques to help them overcome and cope with dyslexia. Natural or traditional remedies may help some aspects of learning only.

Indian Natural Remedies

Common Ingredients for Dyslexia

Herbs/Leaves
Brahmi *(Bacopa monnieri)*
Giloy/guduchi *(Tinospora cordifolia)*
Jatamansi *(Nardostachys jatamansi)*
Licorice (yashtimadhu)
Shankhpushpi *(Convolvulus pluricaulis)*

Common Recipes

Oral

Teas/Brews

Brahmi juice. Place a handful of the fresh brahmi leaves into a blender and add up to 1 cup of water. Blend until smooth. Add honey to taste and drink.

Brahmi tea. Place about two to three stalks of fresh brahmi leaves into a cup. Pour boiling water over the leaves and allow to steep for about 10 to 15 minutes. Add honey to taste and drink.

Giloy juice. Place a handful of giloy leaves into a blender and blend until smooth. Strain and drink. Alternatively, chew on fresh giloy leaves or consume in the form of powder.

Jatamansi brew. Add a pinch of jatamansi root powder to a cup of warm water and take twice a day.

Shankhpushpi. Add 1 cup of boiling water to five to six fresh blue pea flowers. Allow to steep for 5 to 10 minutes. Drink before bedtime.

Therapeutic Measures

Yoga

Child yoga exercises help improve brain circulation, focus, and attention.

Chinese Natural Remedies

Common Remedies

There are not many remedies available for the treatment of dyslexia in TCM as it is not regarded to be a disease. However, acupuncture may help treat dyslexia and improve its symptoms. It is thought that acupuncture may improve qi circulation to the brain, hence stimulating the development and improvement of dyslexia symptoms.

Western/Other Natural Remedies

Common Ingredients for Dyslexia

Miscellaneous
Bee pollen
Oils: flaxseed and fish
Royal jelly

Common Recipes

Oral

Bee pollen. Consume bee pollen. For adults, take 3 to 5 teaspoons three times a day before meals. For children, take 1 to 2 teaspoons three times a day. Duration of treatment is 1 to 3 months. It can be repeated two to four times a year.

Fish oil. Fish oil, similar to flaxseed oil, is rich in omega-3 fatty acids and improves brain function.

Flaxseed oil. Flaxseed oil is rich in omega-3 fatty acids and is thought to increase brain function, particularly with focus and memory.

Royal jelly. Consume as food. Capsules are available. Give 5 to 10 mL daily to children over 3 years old after breakfast.

Modern Remedies

There is currently no known way of treating dyslexia, and most treatments are specific educational approaches and techniques to help children with dyslexia process written information better.

Reading Programs

Reading programs aim to teach children with dyslexia to link alphabets with the way they sound and comprehend. These programs are made up of a few components such as fluency, text comprehension and vocabulary, and phonics. Some schools may also have individual education plan (IEP) teams to tailor a more structured education plan for children with dyslexia.

Occupational Therapy

Occupational therapy helps with penmanship and hand-eye coordination activities.

Homeopathic Remedies

These include *Baryta carbonica* and *Lycopodium clavatum* (associated lack of confidence, poor focus and memory), *Causticum* (for associated speech difficulties, using wrong words or mispronouncing when speaking), *Ammonium carbonicum* (for mathematical difficulty), *Cannabis* (associated cognitive difficulties), *Thuja occidentalis* (for reading and writing difficulties and slow speech), and *Kali bromatum* and hydrogen (writing difficulties with word omission and reversal).

Developmental Delay

There are a number of forms of developmental delay, such as language or speech delays, vision problems, motor-skill delays, social- and emotional-skill delays, and poor cognitive skills. Delays occurring in many or all of these areas is called global developmental delay. This may occur because of a number of factors, such as genetic defects, fetal alcohol syndrome, intrauterine infections, or medical problems during pregnancy or developing soon after birth. At times, there may be no apparent cause.

Indian Natural Remedies

Common Ingredients for Developmental Delay

Spices	Herbs/Leaves	Miscellaneous
Turmeric	Brahmi *(Bacopa monnieri)*	Milk
	Jatamansi *(Nardostachys jatamansi)*	Honey
	Shankhpushpi *(Convolvulus pluricaulis)*	Sesame seed oil
	Shatavari *(Asparagus racemosus)*	
	Ashwagandha *(Withania somnifera)*	
	Gotu kola *(Centella asiatica)*	
	Vacha *(Acorus calamus)*	
	Holy basil (tulsi)	

Common Recipes

Oral

Teas/Brews

Brahmi extract. Pound fresh brahmi and extract 20 mL of the juice. Consume once a day. Alternatively, mix brahmi powder with shatavari and ashwagandha powder. Consume this once a day.

Gotu kola juice. Place 8 to 10 fresh gotu kola leaves into a blender and blend until smooth. Add a little water if necessary. Drink once a day.

Holy basil tea. Place two to five fresh holy basil leaves into a cup of hot water. Cover and steep for 5 to 10 minutes before drinking. Alternatively, chew three to five leaves.

Jatamansi brew. Add a pinch of jatamansi root powder to a cup of warm water and take it twice a day.

Shankhpushpi brew. Mix 1 teaspoon of ground shankhpushpi into one cup of warm milk. Drink warm twice a day.

Shatavari brew. Mix 3 to 5 g of shatavari powder into a cup of milk. Drink once a day. Alternatively, mix equal amounts of shatavari powder and honey, stirring until smooth. Consume once a day.

Turmeric brew. Stir 1 to 2 teaspoons of turmeric into a cup of warm milk. Drink once a day.

Vacha tea. Place 1 to 2 teaspoons of vacha herbs into a cup of hot water. Steep for 5 to 10 minutes. Strain and drink warm.

Topical

- **Sesame oil massage.** Massage the scalp and bottom of the feet with sesame oil once a day.

Chinese Natural Remedies

Common Ingredients for Developmental Delay

Herbs/Leaves	Miscellaneous
Acorus (shi chang pu)/vacha	
Ginkgo leaf *(Ginkgo biloba)*	
Ginseng	Reishi mushroom/lingzhi *(Ganoderma lucidum)*
Salvia divinorum	

Common Recipes

Oral

Teas/Brews

Acorus (vacha) tea. Place 1 to 2 teaspoons of acorus/vacha herbs into a cup of hot water. Steep for 5 to 10 minutes. Strain and drink warm.

Ginkgo tea. Boil 2 cups of water. Add 1 tablespoon of dried ginkgo leaves. Boil for 5 minutes and then steep for another 10 minutes. Strain and consume with honey if desired.

Ginseng tea. Place two to four slices of ginseng into a cup of hot water. Cover and steep for 5 to 10 minutes. Strain and add honey to taste. Drink warm.

Reishi mushroom. It is often cooked as food (stewed or sauteed) or added to soups. It is added as a food supplement in various formulations

Salvia tea. Take 1 tablespoon of washed fresh salvia leaves. Chop them and add to 2 cups of boiling water. Simmer for 5 to 15 minutes. Add honey or milk. Drink warm.

Western/Other Natural Remedies

Common Ingredients for Developmental Delay

Herbs/Leaves	Miscellaneous
Green tea leaf	
Lemon balm	
Rhodiola (Rhodiola rosea)	Broccoli (Brassica oleracea)
Rosemary	Coconut oil
Sage	Walnut

Common Recipes

Oral

Teas/Brews

Broccoli. Consume as part of diet.

Coconut oil. Consume 1 teaspoon of coconut oil once a day.

Green tea. Place 1 to 2 teaspoons of green tea leaves into a cup of boiling water and steep for 10 minutes. Strain and drink warm.

Lemon balm tea. Place 1 tablespoon of dried lemon balm leaves (or 2 tablespoons of fresh leaves) into a cup of boiling water. Let sit for 10 to 15 minutes before straining. Add honey to taste and drink warm.

Rhodiola root tea. Finely chop about 5 g of *Rhodiola rosea* root. Place into a clean container and pour 1 cup of boiling water over it. Let steep for 4 hours. Strain and drink ⅓ cup three to five times a day.

Rosemary tea. Place three to five sprigs of rosemary in a cup of boiling water. Cover and let steep for 5 to 10 minutes. Drink warm.

Sage tea. Place 3 to 5 sage leaves in a cup of boiling water. Cover and let steep for 5 to 10 minutes. Drink warm.

Walnuts. Snack on walnuts throughout the day

Modern Remedies

Similar to treatment for dyslexia, the treatment for developmental delay is not curative but aims to help children to progress and develop to their full potential. Treatment plans often depend on each child's individual needs.

Early Intervention Services

Early intervention services are currently the main treatment method and include:

Speech and language therapy. This can help children with speech and language development difficulties. Speech and language therapy aims to help children gain better control over the muscles of the mouth or encourage communication. It may also be used to help children with severe disabilities to learn to use communication devices.

Occupational therapy. This helps children with developmental delays to improve skills necessary for daily living, such as fine motor skills and cognitive skills.

Physiotherapy. It aims to help children to improve their gross and fine motor skills as well as coordination and strength.

Behavior therapy. It can help children cope with disability by encouraging healthy forms of communication as well as stopping negative behavioral traits such as aggression because of frustration or poor tolerance.

Homeopathic Remedies

These include *Calcarea carb* (in an obese child with a big head, delayed walking, and slow tooth eruption), *Calcarea phos* (in a thin child with developmental delay, delayed dentition, poor digestion, and frequent nursing), and *Baryta carb* (for delayed walking, talking, and reading with normal growth).

Hypotonia (Floppy Child)

Hypotonia refers to a low muscle tone. It is often diagnosed at birth or may occur later. It is often related to issues with the brain, nerves, muscles, or spinal cord of the baby. In a baby or infant, this manifests as the child feeling limp when carried or as poor head control. There may be associated feeding difficulties, a poor cry, delayed motor milestones, slow or abnormal gait, joint hyperextensibility, and easy fatigability.

There are a number of causes of hypotonia, such as brain damage from a lack of oxygen immediately before or after birth, metabolic or genetic disorders, severe infections, spinal cord injury, or cerebral palsy.

Tests depend on the underlying suspected cause. Often, extensive metabolic-genetic tests are done in the absence of trauma or infection.

Natural remedies are seldom helpful.

Physical therapy can often improve the child's motor muscle strength and movements. Occupational therapy and speech therapy can also help with coordination, fine motor skills, activities of daily living, communication, feeding, and breathing.

Indian Natural Remedies

Common Ingredients for Hypotonia

Herbs/Leaves	Miscellaneous
Ashwagandha (Withania somnifera)	Milk
	Cow colostrum (vitamins, minerals and protein-rich)
	Kollu (horse gram)

Common Recipes
Oral
Teas/Brews

Ashwagandha brew. Add 1 teaspoon of ashwagandha root powder into a pot with half cup of milk and half cup of water. Boil gently until the volume reduces to about ½ a cup. Cool slightly and drink warm. Add honey to taste.

Colostrum. It is nutrient-dense and also enhances the immune system. It is available as a powder and can be taken with water or milk.

Kollu. The grains are soaked and then cooked until soft. They are added to soups or mixed with rice or curries and help strengthen muscles.

Chinese Natural Remedies

Common Ingredients for Hypotonia

Herbs/Leaves
Cordyceps
Eleuthero *(Siberian ginseng)*
Green tea leaf
Jiaogulan *(Gynostemma)*

Common Remedies
Oral
Teas/Brews

Cordyceps supplement. Cordyceps supplements are available as commercial preparations, often as capsules.

Green tea. Place 1 to 2 teaspoons of green tea leaves into a cup of boiling water and steep for 10 minutes. Strain and drink warm.

Jiaogulan tea. Place 1 to 2 teaspoons of dried jiaogulan into a cup of boiling water. Cover and let steep for 10 to 15 minutes. Strain and drink warm.

Siberian ginseng. Place about 1 tablespoon of thinly sliced Siberian ginseng into a cup of boiling water. Cover and let steep for 5 minutes. Add honey to taste. Drink warm and consume the soaked roots.

Western/Other Natural Remedies

Common Remedies

Common Ingredients for Hypotonia

Mitochondrial cocktail: Vitamins (megavitamin doses of various B vitamins, C, and E), alpha lipoic acid, coenzyme Q10/ubiquinol, creatine monohydrate, phosphatidylserine (PS), acetyl L-carnitine (ALCAR), glycerophosphocholine (GPC)

Nootropic nutraceuticals that can boost BDNF (brain-derived neurotrophic factor).

Nutraceuticals, Plants, Herbs, and Foods
Omega-3 rich foods (fish oils, walnuts), vitamin D, creatine, phosphatidylserine, acetyl-L-carnitine and S-adenosylmethionine (SAM), Arctic root *(Rhodiola rosea)*, resveratrol, zinc, taurine
Probiotics

Oral
Refer to table above

Therapeutic Measures
Physical Interventions & Exercise
- Swaddle the baby whenever possible as it is thought to help to improve muscle tone. The baby resists swaddling, hence building muscle tone.
- Lie the baby on their tummy on the floor, with the head to one side. Using toys or noise, encourage the baby to lift their head. This helps to improve muscle tone in the baby's head and neck.
- Encourage an older child to join activities that build overall muscle strength, such as swimming or gymnastics.
- Ensure that the child engages in physical activity, such as going on walks or playing games involving obstacle courses.

Aromatherapy
Use lavender or peppermint essential oil.

Modern Remedies

Treatment for hypotonia depends on the underlying cause, but if the underlying cause cannot be accurately diagnosed, treatment is often focused on improving muscle function.

Physiotherapy

Physiotherapy for hypotonia aims to improve posture as well as coordination to make up for the low muscle tone in the body. It is also used to strengthen the muscles around joints to provide better stability.

Occupational Therapy

Occupational therapy focuses on teaching children skills needed in day-to-day activities, such as fine motor skills, self-care skills, and cognitive skills.

Speech and Language Therapy

Speech and language therapy encourages communication and may also be used to assess the child's swallowing and feeding. This can help identify swallowing difficulties and provide the necessary treatment to improve feeding difficulty.

Speech Delay

Speech development in children varies greatly from child to child. However, there are red flags:
- By 12 months, the infant does not use gestures, such as pointing or waving.
- By 18 months, the child has problems imitating sounds and understanding simple verbal requests, as well as preferring gestures over vocalization.
- By 2 years, the child only imitates speech and actions and does not produce phrases or words spontaneously.

They may not be able to follow simple directions and only make certain sounds or words repeatedly.

Indian Natural Remedies

Common Ingredients for Speech Delay

Spices	Herbs/Leaves	Miscellaneous
Black pepper (Piper nigrum)	Brahmi (Bacopa monnieri)	Amla (Phyllanthus emblica)
Malabar leaf/tejpat (Cinnamomum tamala)	Sweet flag/vacha (Acorus calamus)	Brahmi oil
		Almond
		Sugar candy
		Butter/ghee/egg yolk

Common Recipes

Oral

Almond, black pepper, sugar candy paste. Mix seven almonds with a pinch of black pepper and grind until they form a fine paste. Add a little sugar candy to this paste and consume once a day in the morning, preferably on an empty stomach.

Amla. Consume a fresh amla fruit, taking care to chew it slowly and completely.

Black pepper butter paste. Grind black peppercorn into a fine powder and mix it into butter. Consume 1 teaspoon every morning on an empty stomach.

Brahmi juice. Place a handful of fresh brahmi leaves into a blender and add up to 1 cup of water. Blend until smooth. Add honey to taste and drink.

Cinnamomum tamala. Place this herb under the tongue and leave for 30 minutes every day.

Egg yolk. Consume more egg yolk.

Vacha tea. Place 1 to 2 teaspoons of vacha herbs into a cup of hot water. Steep for 5 to 10 minutes. Strain and drink warm.

Chinese Natural Remedies

Common Remedies

Acupuncture is thought to be an effective method to improve speech disorders. The following organs are thought to affect speech:

- Weakness of the lungs is thought to cause speech delays and disorders.
- Lung weakness is thought to sometimes be caused by a digestive system disorder.
- The spinal cord is also stimulated to ensure proper nourishment of the nerves as they develop.

Western/Other Natural Remedies

Common Remedies

Omega-3 rich foods including salmon, flaxseeds, or supplements (with DHA-EPA) may be helpful.

Miscellaneous

- Switch off the television or other gadgets. Noise is a distraction for the child in developing language skills.
- Teach the child sign language to relieve frustration at the lack of communication and encourage them to communicate their wants and needs.
- Play with the child and introduce them to simple words and names of objects.
- Use simple picture flashcards to teach the child new words.
- Put a cotton ball on the table or floor and give the child a straw. Get the child to blow through the straw to move the cotton ball. This develops the oral muscles necessary for speech.
- Allow the child to use straws to drink as it helps to strengthen mouth muscles.

Modern Remedies

Speech Therapy

Speech therapy can be used to encourage children with speech delay to verbally communicate more readily and more effectively.

Attention-Deficit Hyperactivity Disorder

ADHD most commonly affects children and teenagers but can also continue into adulthood. ADHD is the most common mental disorder in children, causing hyperactivity and difficulty controlling impulses. These children may also have trouble focusing, causing problems with school and home life.

ADHD is more common in boys and is often diagnosed in the early school years when the child is found to have trouble paying attention.

Children with ADHD tend to be vata dominant as babies. They are also picky eaters, overactive, imaginative, exploratory, curious, and adept at multitasking. When there is vata imbalance, the child becomes disruptive and oppositional in a learning situation.

There is often a strong family history of ADHD indicating a high heritability. ADHD behaviors often occur in many intellectual disability disorders (such as fragile X syndrome, tuberous sclerosis, Klinefelter syndrome, Williams syndrome, etc.).

ADHD has also been associated with comorbid disorders such as anxiety, depression, autism, bipolar disorder, obesity, and substance abuse.

The discussion on natural treatments below will be grouped collectively for all ethnic groups.

The herbs listed above are various herbs from Indian, Chinese, and Western traditional remedies. There is not a vast amount of information available on each form of traditional medicine, and a combination of all of the above, including diet and nutrition (see Section 8.2), can be tried to treat ADHD.

Natural/Alternative Remedies

Common Ingredients for Attention-Deficit Hyperactivity Disorder

Herbs/Leaves	Miscellaneous
Brahmi (*Bacopa monnieri*)	Epsom salt
Giloy/guduchi (*Tinospora cordifolia*)	Chamomile flower
Gingko (*Ginkgo biloba*)	Red clover blossom
Ginseng	Passionflower
Gotu kola (*Centella asiatica*)	Green oat/milky oat seed (*Avena sativa*)
Holy basil (tulsi)	Pine bark and pine needle (*Pinus pinaster*)
Kava root (*Piper methysticum*)	
Lemon balm (*Melissa officinalis*)	Lavender
Licorice root	
Rudraksha (*Elaeocarpus ganitrus*)	
Skullcap	Phosphatidylserine
St. John's wort	Multivitamins, multiminerals
Valerian	Omega-3 fish oil

Common Remedies

Oral

Teas/Brews

Brahmi juice. Place a handful of fresh brahmi leaves into a blender and add up to 1 cup of water. Blend until smooth. Add honey to taste and drink.

Chamomile tea. Place some dried or fresh chamomile flowers into a cup. Pour boiling water over the flowers and allow to steep for 10 minutes. Strain and add honey to taste. Drink it hot.

Giloy juice. Place a handful of giloy leaves into a blender and blend until smooth. Strain and drink. Alternatively, chew on fresh giloy leaves or consume in the form of powder.

Ginseng tea. Add about two to four slices of ginseng to a cup. Add hot water over the ginseng. Steep for about 10 to 15 minutes.

Gotu kola juice. Place 8 to 10 fresh gotu kola leaves into a blender and blend until smooth. Add a little water if necessary. Drink once a day.

Holy basil tea. Place two to five fresh holy basil leaves into a cup of hot water. Cover and steep for 5 to 10 minutes before drinking. Alternatively, chew three to five leaves.

Lavender tea. Add 2 to 3 teaspoons of dried lavender flowers to 1 cup of hot water. Steep for 10 to 15 minutes before straining. Drink it warm before bedtime.

Lemon balm tea. Place 1 tablespoon of dried lemon balm leaves (or 2 tablespoons of fresh leaves) into a cup of boiling water. Let sit for 10 to 15 minutes before straining. Add honey to taste and drink warm.

Licorice tea. Add 1 teaspoon of ground licorice to a pot with 1 cup of boiling water. Allow to simmer for 30 to 45 minutes before straining.

Passionflower tea. Add 1 teaspoon of dried passionflower to a cup of hot water. Cover and steep for 5 to 10 minutes. Strain and drink warm.

Pine needle tea. Wash unblemished edible pine needles and cut into small pieces. Add 2 cups of boiling water. Steep for 10 to 15 minutes. Strain and drink. Add honey to taste. Variation #1. It is available as capsules or tablets. The Pycnogenol brand is widely used.

Red clover blossom tea. Place 2 to 3 teaspoons of dried red clover blossoms into a cup and pour boiling water over it. Let sit for 10 to 15 minutes before straining. Drink warm.

Rudraksha. Place the Rudraksha seeds in a copper jug or pot filled with 250 ml water. Leave it overnight. Consume this water first thing in the morning on an empty stomach.

St. John's wort tea. Place 2 tablespoons of St. John's wort in a teapot with about 6 cups of hot water. Cover and let steep for 3 to 10 minutes before straining. Add a little honey to taste. Drink warm.

Valerian root tea. Those who have severe anxiety may use about 600 mg of valerian root. Valerian root is available commercially in doses of about 200 mg, which may be brewed as a tea.

Supplements

Omega-3 fish oil. Adequate amounts of EPA and DHA should be consumed.

Phosphatidylserine. It should be given in the morning for a trial period of 1 month.

Multivitamin-multimineral. Vitamin A, vitamin D, zinc, and magnesium are often found to be deficient in children with ADHD.

Therapeutic Measures

Diet and Nutrition

Avoid cold foods, as the digestive system is cool in a vata-dominant child. Consume warm and sour foods.

Types of Diets

- **Gluten-free casein-free (GFCF) diet:** GFCF diets are gluten- and casein-free diets, in which "normal" foods are substituted with gluten-free substitutes, such as gluten-free bread, waffles, chicken nuggets, and muffins. Butter may be substituted with ghee and coconut oil. Calcium and other nutritional supplements may be necessary when implementing a GFCF diet.

- **Specific-carbohydrate diet (SCD), gut and psychology syndrome (GAPS) diet, and paleo diets:** These diets are grain free but allow certain carbohydrates such as certain beans and nuts, fruits, vegetables, and yogurt. More protein should be consumed, along with extra virgin coconut oil and lemongrass.

For more information, read *Nourishing Hope: Using Food and Nutrition to Improve Autism and ADHD* by Julie Matthews.

A structured calm and warm environment is essential to maintain balance.

Play soothing music.

Refrain from excessive simulation before bedtime.

Epsom salt bath: Epsom salt baths are useful in helping the child relax.

Yoga Poses

There are functional changes and improvements in the prefrontal cortex (for executive function) hippocampus (for memory process) and amygdala (for emotional well-being).

It is self-calming and self-improving.

The following asanas are helpful.

- Vrikshasana (tree pose)
- Setu bandhasana (bridge pose)
- Marjaryasana/bitilasana (cat-cow pose)
- Bhujangasana (cobra pose)
- Shavasana (corpse pose)
- Adho mukha svanasana (downward facing dog)
- Viparita shalabhasana (superman pose)
- Tadasana (mountain pose)
- Simhasana (roaring lion pose)

Pranayama
- Breath control with deep breathing exercises can help during meltdowns and tantrums.

Meditation and mindfulness
Miscellaneous

Rudraksha. Children can wear Rudraksha beads as a bracelet or a *mala* (necklace) to improve focus, attention and concentration.

- Refer to the "Introduction" chapter.

Therapy Programs

Behavior Modification Therapy

Behavior modification therapy is an effective treatment for ADHD children. It may improve the child's behavior and self-control and raise self-esteem. Behavioral therapy teaches the child and their parents skills and strategies to cope with school and day-to-day activities, as well as how to better build relationships. Some behavioral modification therapy programs may be aimed at teaching the child coping methods, while others focus on both the children and the parents.

Modern Remedies

Medication for ADHD is not curative and is often taken to help children with ADHD focus better, be less impulsive, and learn new skills. Some medications are to be taken daily, while others only need to be taken on school days. Breaks from the medication are sometimes taken for the doctor to determine whether it is still required.

Stimulant Medications

Stimulants are central nervous system medications that block the reuptake of dopamine, a neurotransmitter. It is also thought to be responsible for blocking some of the metabolic enzymes that absorb loose dopamine. Dopamine is responsible for motivation and may also help in movement and emotional response. Stimulant medication is divided into two main types:

- Methylphenidate: Methylphenidate comes in the form of short-acting or long-acting drugs. Short-acting drugs need to be taken two to three times a day, while longer-acting drugs need only be taken in the morning, with the medication released slowly throughout the day.

Examples (shorter acting): Ritalin, Focalin, methylin
Examples (longer acting): Ritalin-SR, Metadate-ER, Concerta, Daytrana patch
- Amphetamine: This medication is also split into shorter- and longer-acting drugs.
Examples (shorter acting): Adderall, Dexedrine
Examples (longer acting): Adderall-XR, Vyvanse

Non-Stimulant Medication

Non-stimulant medications block norepinephrine receptors in the brain, which causes an increase in norepinephrine production. This increases attention while controlling hyperactivity and impulsiveness.

Examples: Strattera, Tenex

Autism

Autism is a neurobehavioral condition that impairs social interactions as well as language and communication skills. There is a wide range of symptoms, leading to this condition being called autism spectrum disorder (ASD). ASD ranges in severity from a mild handicap to a disability requiring institutional care. Children with autism may have trouble interacting with others and understanding how others think and feel.

Children with autism may perform repetitive movements such as rocking or pacing. They may have self-injurious tendencies and sometimes may not notice the goings-on in their surroundings. In some cases, children with autism may develop seizures. Autism often causes a degree of cognitive impairment, but unlike other typical cognitive impairments, they have uneven skill development. This means that while children with autism may struggle with social interactions, they may have unusually developed skills in other areas such as drawing, music, or math.

Natural/Alternative Remedies

Indian Natural Remedies

In Ayurveda, autism is a behavioral disorder. It is classified under *unmada* where there is a defect in the neuro-psychological system and abnormality in the digestive system and metabolic pathways for many reasons. Some of these described include prenatal psychological stress, genetic deficiencies, incompatible foods, and defective child-rearing practices. This results in impairments (deviations and distortions) in the intellect, mind, awareness, memory, behavior, learning, and socialization.

Principles of Management

Consanguineous marriages are prohibited in Ayurveda. Preconception counseling should be done. Prenatal and perinatal recommendations should be carried out by the parent at the time of intercourse and conception. The mental health, diet, and activities of the pregnant mother plays an important role in the physical and mental health of the child.

The principles of treatment of Ayurveda are:

Samsamana. Dosha pacifying therapies.

Panchakarma or samshodhana. Bio cleaning therapy.

Nidana parivarjana. Prevention of causes.

Pathya ahara vihara. Proper diet and lifestyle to improve the *agni* or the digestive power of the autistic child.

Although most are plant-based herbs, some Ayurvedic medicines contain heavy metals, such as mercury, lead, and arsenic, which are reported to be inactive elements. Often, preservatives in Ayurvedic medications are not listed.

Common Ingredients for Autism

Spices	Herbs/Leaves	Miscellaneous
	Amla (*Phyllanthus emblica*)	Lakshadi kuzhambu (polyherbal medicated oils)
	Jatamansi (*Nardostachys jatamansi*)	Korosanai
	Nutgrass galingale rhizome/ mushta (*Rhizoma cyperi*)	Pomegranate juice
	Brahmi (*Bacopa monnieri*)	
	Ashwagandha (*Withania somnifera*)	
	Shankhpushpi (*Clitoria ternatea*)	
	Gotu kola (*Centella asiatica*)	

Common Recipes

Oral

Ashta choornam. This polyherbal is given twice a day.

Ashwagandha brew. Mix 1 teaspoon of ashwagandha powder into a cup of warm milk. Add honey to taste.

Brahmi tea. Place about two to three stalks of fresh brahmi leaves into a cup. Pour boiling water over the leaves and allow to steep for about 10 to 15 minutes. Add honey to taste and drink.

Gotu kola tea. Steep a teaspoon of fresh or dried gotu kola leaves in a cup of hot water for about 10 to 15 minutes. Drink warm.

Korosanai. Mix a little korosanai with some breast milk and place it on the infant's tongue on Day 10 of life to improve the voice.

Pomegranate juice. Blend the pomegranate until smooth. Strain if required. Consume fresh.

Shankhpushpi tea. Add 1 cup of boiling water to five to six shankhpushpi (fresh blue pea) flowers. Allow to steep for 5 to 10 minutes. Drink before bedtime.

  Variation #1. Mix 1 teaspoon of ground shankhpushpi into one cup of warm milk. Drink warm twice a day.

Therapeutic Measures

Diet

A vegetarian or vegan diet is recommended. Processed food should be avoided.

Lifestyle

Yoga Poses

- Vrikshasana (tree pose)
- Bitilasana (cow pose)
- Adho mukha svanasana (downward facing dog pose)
- Marjaryasana (cat pose)
- Matsyasana (fish pose)
- Bhekasana (frog pose)
- Salabhasana (locust pose)
- Baddha konasana (butterfly pose)

Pranayama

- Breathing exercises include simha pranayama (lion's breath), and bhramari pranayama (bumblebee breath).

Panchakarma (Detoxification)

Panchakarma treatment is given for a duration of 3 to 5 weeks. Oral medications are also given.

- *Abhyangam* with *lakshadi kuzhambu* (a medicated herbal oil) can reduce restlessness and impulsivity in children with autism.
- *Takra dara.* Herbal buttermilk with amla, jatamansi, and mushta.
- *Basti.* Dhanavantaram mizhagu paku (medicated enema).

Massage. See below under Panchakarma.

This can be done with panchakarma treatment. Essential oil massage can also be done using gotu kola, sandalwood, and lavender.

Meditation

- Refer under "Introduction" chapter.

Sound therapy. This includes music therapy and recitation of mantras.

Chinese Natural Remedies

Common Ingredients for Autism

Spices	Herbs/Leaves	Miscellaneous
Ginger	Ginseng	Poria cocos
	Angelica sinensis	Chen pi
	Glycyrrhiza glabra	

Polyherbal Formula

Ukgansangajinpibanha (UGSJB) granule. This is a Korean polyherbal formula made up of nine herbs: (1) chuan xiong (*Cnidium officinale*), (2) bai zhu (*Atractylodes japonica*), (3) ban xia (*Pinellia ternata*), (4) chen pi (*Citrus unshiu*), (5) dang gui (*Angelica gigas*), (6) fu ling (*Poria cocos*), (7) chai hu (*Bupleurum falcatum*), (8) diao gou teng (*Uncaria sinensis*), and (9) gan cao (*Glycyrrhiza glabra*). This can help improve core symptoms of autism and the ratings in various autism rating scales. It helps with insomnia, night crying, nervousness, or anger in children.

Ukgansan. This is a Korean polyherbal formula which consists of *Angelicae gigantis radix, Atractylodis rhizoma white, Bupleuri radix, Poria, Cnidii rhizoma, Uncariae ramulus et uncus,* and *Glycyrrhizae radix.*

Jiawei Wendan decoction. This contains *Bambusa tuldoides, Citrus aurantium, Glycyrrhiza uralensis, Citrus reticulata, Acorus gramineus, Alpinia oxyphylla, Codonopsis* *pilosula, Pinellia ternata, Alpinia oxyphylla,* and *Zingiber officinale.*

Modified Ying Huo decoction. The ingredients are *Morinda officinalis, Rehmannia glutinosa, Poria cocos, Cinnamomi cortex, Asparagus cochinchinensis, Ophiopogon japonicus,* and *Schisandra chinensis.*

Supplemented Lizhong decoction. This contains *Panax ginseng, Glycyrrhiza uralensis, Zingiber officinale, Schisandra chinensis, Prunus mume,* and *Atractylodes macrocephala.* This decoction modulates the gut microbiota.

Therapeutic Measures

Acupressure Points

These include HT7, GV17, GV24.5, GB13, GB19, LR3, PC6, KI3, KI4, LR4, LU9, ST36, SP3, and SP6.

Commonly used acupressure points in autism: GV20, GV24, and EX-HN1

GV 20 (Governing Vessel 20) is also known as the hundred convergences. It is located at the top of the head, exactly halfway on an imaginary line drawn from ear to ear. Massage this point with your fingers for 1 to 2 minutes to relieve hypertension.

GV 24 (Governing Vessel 24) is midway between the AHL and GV 23. GV 24 is located 0.5 *cun* directly above the midline of the anterior hairline. It is the meeting point of the governor vessel, the foot-*taiyang* meridian, and the foot-*yangming* meridian.

EX-HN1 (sishencong). (Ex-HN-1 Four Alert Spirit SISHENCONG Acupuncture Points) A group of four points, each located 1 *cun* from → Du-20 (anterior, posterior, and lateral

Scalp acupuncture has also been used.

Scalp acupuncture will be performed in all participants by using six fixed points at GV24 (Shen Ting), GV20 (Bai Hui), and EX-HN1 (Si Shen Cong) in a total of 24 sessions for 12 weeks.

Western Natural Remedies

Common Ingredients for Autism

Miscellaneous

Multivitamin/multimineral
Omega-3 fish oil
Phosphatidylserine
Probiotics

Therapeutic Measures

Diet

Biomedical diet. These include many special diets (see below) and nutritional supplements that may improve autism symptoms.

Types of Diets

* GFCF diet: As below.
* Dairy-free diet: No dairy milk or milk products are to be taken by the child. Soy products are to be limited to about once a week, and cow's milk may be replaced with almond milk.
* SCD, gut and GAPS diet, and paleo diet: As above.
* Sugar-free diet: Sugar is thought to worsen autism symptoms and hence should be removed from the diet.
* Yeast-free diet: This is a low carb or low glycemic index diet.
* Other dietary information: Fish should be cut from the diet for at least 3 months because of its high mercury (leading to metal toxicity) levels. Small fish, such as anchovies, may be consumed. To reduce levels of yeast in the body, carbohydrates should be reduced, and protein intake should be increased.
* Nutritional supplement. These include:
* *Multivitamins/multiminerals.* Ensure that the child is given sufficient supplements such as vitamins A, C, E, D, and B complex (especially B6, B12, and folate). Minerals include mainly magnesium, calcium, and zinc.
* *Probiotics.* These should contain at least 10 million CFU.
* *Omega 3 fish oils.*
* *Antioxidants.*
* *Others.* These include phosphatidylserine, citicoline, and B12. They should be tried for 1 month to look for any improvements.
* *Digestive enzymes.* These include amylase (to break down carbohydrates), protease (to break down protein), and lipase (to break down fats).
* *Chelation.* Chelation is defined as the bonding of ions to metals. It is believed that toxicity in the body is one of the causes of autism. Toxins include heavy metals, organic pollutants, and chemicals.

It can be nutritional chelation or chemical chelation. Nutritional chelation using food items includes reishi mushrooms, coriander, etc. Chemical chelation involves using various compounds, such as DMSA (given orally or as enema), EDTA, or alpha-lipoic acid.

For more information, read *Nourishing Hope: Using Food and Nutrition to Improve Autism and ADHD* by Julie Matthews.

* **Homeopathy:** In Mike Andrews's book *Homeopathy and Autism Spectrum Disorder: A Guide for Practitioners and Families*, he writes about the homeopathic treatments identified by Dr. Barvalia for different categories of ASD symptoms:

The following remedies are given based on the symptom pattern:

* **Sensory pattern:** asarum, borax, carcinosin, *China officinalis, Nux vomica,* opium, phosphorus, stramonium, and theridion.
* **Kinetic state and stereotype:** aurum metallicum, belladonna, *Cina maritima, Tarentula hispanica,* stramonium, tuberculinum, medorrhinum, and *Nux vomica.*
* **Regressive state:** baryta carbonica, *Bufo rana, Hyoscyamus niger,* and zincum metallicum.
* **Core remedies:** carcinosin, natrum muriaticum, medorrhinum, and tuberculinum bovinum.

- **Hyperbaric oxygen:** Hyperbaric oxygen is a daily treatment in which a patient is placed in a hyperbaric chamber and the atmospheric pressure increases to that above sea level. Once the desired pressure has been reached, the individual spends about an hour in the chamber resting and breathing normally. The pressure increase allows oxygen to dissolve into the blood plasma at a higher rate. The increase in oxygen in the body can reduce inflammation in the body's tissues and reintroduce blood flow to oxygen-starved areas. Hyperbaric oxygen can benefit patients with ASD as they can have high levels of inflammation as well as oxygen-starved areas in the body. Hence, hyperbaric oxygen therapy can improve overall functioning and interactive behaviors.
- **Stem cells:** Stem-cell therapy for autism is presently experimental. Stem cells are thought to decrease tissue inflammation and hence alleviate autism symptoms as well as improve interaction skills. Mesenchymal stem cells offer better efficacy.
- **Antifungal treatment:** Antifungal treatment can help eradicate overgrowth of *Candida albicans*, a yeast-like fungus in the body, may contribute to worsening autism symptoms. Both natural remedies and modern antifungal medication may be prescribed in patients with autism.
- **Natural remedies:** *Tinospora cordifolia* (giloy/guduchi), virgin coconut oil, *Arctostaphylos* (uva ursi), and garlic.
- **Antifungal medications:** nystatin, amphotericin B, Diflucan, and Nizoral.

Therapy Programs

Non-pharmaceutical treatments aim to improve ASD symptoms via individualized behavioral and educational interventions, including behavioral and developmental programs, cognitive behavioral therapies, occupational therapies, sensory integration therapies, sleep management, and communication facilitation and neuromodulation (including transcranial magnetic stimulation, TMS).

Treatment/Therapy

1. Early Intervention Program (EIP)
   Speech therapy
   Occupational therapy
   Applied behavioral analysis (ABA)
   Sensory integration therapy (SIT)
   Music therapy
   Special pre-school/school
   Social skills training and communication training
   The Treatment and Education of Autistic and related Communication Handicapped Children (**TEACCH**) Program
   The Son-Rise Program
   iBASIS-VIPP (British Autism Study of Infant Siblings-Video Interaction to Promote Positive Parenting). This is a pre-emptive social engagement and social

development intervention program for at-risk infants during the first two years of life. This can significantly reduce the diagnosis of autism after age 2.

1. Biomedical Treatment
   Biomedical Diets. These are prescribed depending on the results of IgG food intolerance tests. Generally, they are casein-free (milk-free), gluten-free (wheat-free), soy-free, egg-free, and sugar-free diets.
   Other diets: yeast-free, ketogenic, modified Atkins, paleo, SCD, GAP, low oxalate, low salicylate, Feingold, phenol-free, etc.
   Nutritional Supplements: omega-3 fish oil, probiotics, multivitamins and multiminerals, antioxidants, digestive enzymes, others
2. Activities and Participation Therapy Approaches
   Feeding clinic
   Hydrotherapy/swimming
   Hippotherapy (horse riding)
   Child yoga
   Acupuncture
   Varma therapy/tuina/massage
   Chelation (nutritional and chemical)
   Sports (cycling, trampoline)
3. Others
   HBOT
   Advocacy and support groups
   Stem cells
   Disability registration
   Others: Fecal fat transplant (fecal microbiota transfer)
   Transcranial magnetic stimulation (TMS)

Occupational therapy (OT). Occupational therapy helps individuals work on their cognitive, physical, motor, and social skills. The goals of OT are to improve day-to-day skills and allow patients to become more independent. OT for children with autism focuses on play skills, learning strategies, and selfcare techniques.

Applied behavior analysis (ABA) therapy. ABA is a therapy focused on the science of behavior and learning. It helps individuals understand how behavior works and how the environment affects it, as well as how learning occurs. ABA therapy programs may help with improving interactive (communication and language) skills, memory, attention, social skills, and focus, as well as reducing problem behaviors.

ABA is a flexible form of therapy made to suit the needs of different individuals in different environments (school, home, or the general community). It emphasizes the importance of everyday life skills and involves both individual and group teachings. ABA therapy uses positive reinforcement as its main strategy and encourages the use of meaningful and positive behavior change. It teaches the individual about antecedents (causes of a behavior) and consequences (the effects of a behavior).

Sensory integration therapy (SIT). Sensory integration therapy aims to provide the individual with sensory stimulus to improve attention, focus, and cognitive functioning. It also aims to decrease repetitive disruptive behavior. In this form of therapy, the child is stimulated in a certain way: wearing a weighted vest or wristbands or putting a body sock on the child.

Picture exchange communication system (PECS). It is a form of therapy aimed at helping the child develop communication skills before they can master verbal or expressive language. A series of images printed on cards are made available to the child so that they may select the picture that best represents what they wish to communicate. It helps children who struggle with processing language to understand activities better and to know what to expect, hence allowing them to feel less frustrated.

The Treatment and Education of Autistic and related Communications Handicapped Children (TEACCH) method. This structured teaching aims to provide meaningful interactions in activities, independence, flexibility, and self-assurance.

The Son-Rise Program. The Son-Rise Program is based on the premise that a child's basic learning takes place within a safe, fun, and social environment. The parents or therapist enter the child's world to create a meaningful reciprocal relationship and not force the child to conform to the parents' or therapist's world. It is a flexible program that can be tailored to the individual needs of each child.

Biomedical diets. Gut and brain genes are interconnected. Eating the right foods and removing specific foods can improve the gut flora and microbiome, change genetic expression, and hence improve brain function.

Feeding clinic. The speech therapist is the key person in the team to work with the parents on the child who is a picky eater. Different food varieties, textures, tastes, and volume are introduced. Behavioral therapy is also incorporated.

Aquatherapy (hydrotherapy) and swimming. This fun and playful therapy can improve balance, focus, attention, and body awareness.

Hippotherapy. Horse riding for the disabled, including those with autism, can improve sensory regulation, social and communication skills, motor coordination, balance, and muscle tone.

Child yoga. It can improve focus, attention, balance, body awareness, social skills, and sleep.

Acupuncture. It can improve social and communication skills. Scalp acupuncture is usually used.

Varma therapy. Gentle massage is done to activate the varma points to improve brain function.

Tuina massage. This is a deep massage that can reduce stress and some stereotypic behaviors.

Chelation. This process is used to eliminate toxic heavy metals in the body, which may take 2 to 12 months. Different routes and different methods are used. Oral, rectal, and transdermal routes are preferred to the intravenous routes.

Nutritional chelation should be tried first before chemical chelation. In nutritional chelation, the goal is to increase metal or toxin excretion in the stools or urine by consuming more fiber or psyllium, water (at least 3 L/day), and unprocessed whole foods so as to evacuate the bowels one to three times per day and pass a lot of urine. Stool softeners can be tried.

Various nutraceuticals are used. Some of these include multivitamins (especially vitamins C and E), multiminerals (zinc, magnesium, and selenium), peptides/amino acids (glutathione, L-glycine), herbs (garlic, cilantro, and uva ursi), probiotics, and others.

Chemical chelation is carried out usually with (dimercapto succinic acid) (DMSA), alpha lipoic acid, and N-acetyl-cysteine (NAC).

Modern Remedies

There is no cure for autism, but early diagnosis and intervention can help children to improve social and communication skills, as well as education development.

Educational Approaches

Educational approaches for autistic children vary depending on each child's individual needs and how they are affected by autism. Generally, interventions focus on improving the most important aspects of the child's development:

- Communication skills—Communication therapy aims to encourage the child to communicate, such as through the use of pictures.
- Social interaction skills—This form of therapy aims to help children develop the ability to understand the emotions of others and how to respond appropriately.
- Imaginative play skills—This encourages the child's use of imagination.
- Academic skills—This intervention aims to help a child to develop the skills necessary to progress with their education, such as comprehension, reading, writing, and math.

Drugs

Pharmaceutical treatments are used as adjunctive therapies to reduce ASD symptoms like aggression, anxiety, depression, hyperactivity, stereotypic, self-harm behavior, insomnia, and seizures.

These include risperidone, haloperidol, methylphenidate, aripiprazole and melatonin. Memantine has been used as adjunctive treatment in autism patients > 18 years old with associated anxiety and agitation. Anti-epileptic drugs are used if indicated.Anti-epileptic drugs are used if indicated.

Cerebral Palsy

Cerebral palsy (CP) is a non-progressive disorder that affects posture, balance, movement, and muscle tone. CP may be congenital or acquired, occurs before age 2, and is due to prenatal, perinatal, and postnatal factors. There are four main types: spastic, dystonic, ataxic, and mixed.

The most commonly diagnosed form of cerebral palsy is spastic cerebral palsy, which is characterised by stiff, tight muscles in the arms and legs. Over time, this often causes limbs to be bent into rigid, fixed positions. This makes mobility difficult and often causes pain.

The severity of cerebral palsy varies from person to person. It may or may not cause intellectual impairment. Comorbidities can affect every system.

Indian Natural Remedies

Common Ingredients Cerebral Palsy

Spices	Herbs/Leaves	Miscellaneous
Ginger	Ashwagandha (Withania somnifera)	Amla (Phyllanthus emblica)
Turmeric	Brahmi (Bacopa monnieri)	Sesame seed
	Guggulu (Commiphora mukul)	

Common Recipes

Oral

Teas/Brews

Amla juice. Pound three to five amla fruit, extracting the juice. Drink the juice once a day in the morning, preferably on an empty stomach.

Ashwagandha brew. Stir 1 teaspoon of ashwagandha paste into a cup of warm milk and drink once a day.

Brahmi juice. Place a handful of fresh brahmi leaves into a blender. Blend and puree with a little water and drink once a day.

Ginger tea. Place two to three pieces of fresh sliced ginger into a cup of boiling water. Cover and steep for 10 to 15 minutes. Strain and drink.

Guggulu supplements. It is available as a polyherbal supplement.

Sesame seeds. Soak a handful of sesame seeds in water overnight. In the morning, strain and chew on the sesame seeds.

Turmeric tea. Stir 1 teaspoon of turmeric into a cup of warm water or milk. Drink warm once a day.

Chinese Natural Remedies

Common Ingredients for Cerebral Palsy

Spices	Herbs/Leaves
Ginger	Astragalus root

Common Recipes

Oral

Teas

Astragalus tea. Place two to four slices of astragalus root into a cup of hot water. Steep for 5 to 10 minutes before straining and drinking.

Ginger tea. Lightly pound 1 to 2 inches of cut ginger and add to a cup of hot water. Steep for 5 to 10 minutes. Strain and drink.

Therapeutic Measures

- **Acupuncture:** Acupuncture along the spine and neck can help relieve symptoms of cerebral palsy.

Scalp acupuncture has been widely used to treat motor dysfunction in children with cerebral palsy in China.

Scalp acupuncture using Jiao's motor area (equivalent to the precentral gyrus) and the Sishencong (EX-HN1) acupoint are used to treat motor dysfunction in children with CP.

Tongue acupuncture is also sometimes used. It can improve swallowing and speech.

- **Qi gong:** Qi gong is a form of energy exercise aimed at improving the coordination of body posture, movement, breathing, and meditation. It is thought to be highly beneficial for health and may alleviate symptoms of cerebral palsy.
- **Tuina:** Tuina is a form of Chinese massage therapy often used in conjunction with acupuncture. It uses a combination of finger movements on acupressure points and is thought to alleviate cerebral palsy symptoms.

Western/Other Natural Remedies

Common Ingredients for Cerebral Palsy

Miscellaneous

Apple cider vinegar (ACV)

Epsom salt

Essential oil: peppermint

Omega-3 fish oil

Common Recipes

Topical

- **Essential oil therapy.** Dilute peppermint oil with a carrier oil such as almond or olive oil. Apply the oil to the joints and muscles for increased blood flow to the areas and pain-relieving properties.
- **Apple cider vinegar.** Apply ACV topically to the joints and muscles as it is thought to reduce muscle spasticity that occurs because of cerebral palsy.
- **Fish oil.** Fish oil is omega-3 fatty acid rich, which can have anti-inflammatory properties. This improves the neural connections and communication between the brain and the muscles. Examples of fish-oil-rich foods include salmon, walnuts, and flaxseed oil.
- **Epsom salt bath.** Add ½ a cup of Epsom salts to a warm bath and soak for 30 to 45 minutes. This can reduce muscle pain and inflammation caused by cerebral palsy.

Modern Remedies

Cerebral palsy (CP) is a complex condition, and treatment is often a combination of drug therapy and other forms of complementary therapy. There is no definite cure for CP.

Cerebral Palsy Management

Neurorehabilitation must be holistic and with functional goals.

1. Body Structures Therapy Approaches
   Physiotherapy/neurodevelopmental therapy (Bobath therapy)

Occupational therapy
Botox/phenol injections (for focal spastic)
Braces (orthoses/splints/casting)
Electrical stimulation
Fitness training
Massage
Acupuncture
Oral motor treatment
Pressure care
Sensory processing/sensory integration therapy (SIT)
Strength training
Stretching

2. Activities Therapy Approaches
Communication training
Conductive education
Constraint-induced movement therapy (CIMT)
Dysphagia management (safe swallow)
Drooling—scopolamine patches/Botox injections into salivary glands/oral glycopyrrolate
Goal directed training
HABIT (bimanual training)
Home programs/early intervention prog (EIP)
Hydrotherapy
Hippotherapy
Speech language therapy
Sports therapy

3. Environmental Therapy Approaches
Assistive technology (Robotic-assisted/Lokomat)
Alternative and augmentative communication (GoTalk, Proloquo2Go)
Equipment/seating
Orthotics/splints/ankle foot orthoses/braces
Seating and mobility devices

4. Others
Medications (Baclofen/Sinemet/Artane/others)
HBOT
NeuroSuit/TheraSuit
Stem cells
Drugs (baclofen/Sinemet/Artane/others)
Nutrition
Disability registration (Social Services)
Advocacy/support groups

Orthopedic surgery and neurosurgery: tenotomy, tendon lengthening, tendon transfer, myotomy, neurectomy, osteotomy
SEMLS//ITB/DBS/scoliosis surgery
- **GIT** (fundoplication for reflux, PEG percutaneous endoscopic gastrostomy, submandibular gland relocation for drooling)
- **Eye:** Squint surgery
- **Bladder:** catheterization, bladder augmentation, Botox instillation

Medications for Hypertonia (Spasticity and Dystonia)

- *Baclofen.* It is a skeletal muscle relaxant and a GABA-B agonist and reduces the excitatory neurotransmitters. It relieves muscle spasticity and improves movement, speech, and swallowing.
- *Dopaminergic drug.* This medication increases dopamine levels in the body, which relieves muscle rigidity or dystonia. Example: carbidopa-levodopa (Sinemet).
- *Anticholinergic drugs.* These include trihexyphenidyl (Artane) and benztropine, which can reduce dystonia. Glycopyrrolate (Cuvposa or Robinul) reduces drooling.
- *Tizanidine.* It is a skeletal muscle relaxant that decreases spasticity by inhibiting the presynaptic motor neurons and also reduces the excitatory neurotransmitters.
- *Dantrolene/Dantrium.* It is a skeletal muscle relaxant that decreases spasticity by blocking the release of intracellular calcium.
- *Benzodiazepine.* It is a relaxant that enhances the effects of at the GABA receptors. This drug also has sedative, anti-convulsant, and muscle-relaxant effects on the patient. Diazepam is usually used.
- *Botulinum toxin-A* is used to treat focal spasticity in the limbs or in drooling. It is injected into the spastic muscles or salivary glands.

Medications for Seizures

- Diazepam/Valium is often used to prevent seizures as it has sedative and anticonvulsant properties. It also functions as a muscle relaxant.
- Valproate is commonly used to treat seizures.
- Refer to chapter on epilepsy for other anti-epileptic drugs.

Other Medications

- Laxatives or stool softeners for constipation, anti-reflux medications
- Sleep medication
- Pain medication
- Antidepressants
- Nutritional supplements
- Bone density medication (for osteoporosis)

Surgery

Multidisciplinary assessments and teams are required to achieve functional goals.

For hypertonia

- *Tendon surgery (tenotomy, tendon lengthening, and tendon transfer).* Tight tendons are cut to relieve spasticity in a tenotomy. Commonly, percutaneous needle hip adductor tenotomies and tendo-Achilles tenotomies are done. Other types will depend on the functional goal.
- *Myotomy.* The tight muscle is cut or released.
- *Neurectomy.* The nerve is cut to relieve spasticity. A selective obturator neurectomy is usually done with an adductor tenotomy or release to treat severe scissoring of legs to facilitate perineal hygiene.
- *Intrathecal baclofen (ITB) pump.* The pump implant is placed in the abdomen and delivers metered doses of baclofen into the spinal CSF to relieve spasticity in the muscles.

- *Selective dorsal rhizotomy (SDR)*. In this neurosurgical procedure, about 30% to 50% of the dorsal roots of the sensory spinal nerves are cut via a L5-S1 laminectomy to decrease spasticity in spastic diplegia type of CP.
- *Orthopedic selective spasticity-control surgery (OSSCS)*. This is a Japanese procedure for selective reduction of specific muscle hypertonia.
- *Single-event multilevel surgery (SEMLS)*. Orthopedic surgery is done to treat contractures and deformities from untreated spasticity.
- *Deep brain stimulation*. This neuromodulation therapy, especially thalamic stimulation, is effective for hyperkinesia and/or dystonia. The GPi stimulation works better for opisthotonus and tongue protrusions.
- *Reconstructive surgery*. This is done mostly for upper limbs for deformed joints.
- *Scoliosis surgery*. This may be done in an ambulatory CP patient if indicated.

For Feeding

- Nasogastric tube feeding, button or PEG feeding, and fundoplication are done when indicated.

Others

- These include squint (strabismus) surgery and bladder procedures.

Dementia

Dementia is a cognitive disorder which cause problems with thinking, reasoning, and memory. It occurs when the parts of the brain responsible for memory, decision making, learning, and language become damaged or diseased. Common causes of dementia include Alzheimer's disease, vascular disorders, traumatic brain injuries, nutritional deficiency, mental disorders, and long-term alcohol or drug use. There may also be a genetic association or risk factor.

Age-related memory loss (memory lapse or simple forgetfulness or absentmindedness) is usually due to lack of focus and is not progressive unlike dementia which usually gets worse over time.

Dementia is not a curable disease, but certain remedies can provide protective benefits to the brain and potentially help to reduce the risk of getting dementia. There are three stages of dementia:

- **Stage 1:** Stage 1 dementia is the onset. It involves short-term memory loss, disorientation, confusion, forgetfulness, mood changes, and anxiety. This stage may last from 2 to 4 years.
- **Stage 2:** Stage 2 dementia causes restlessness, reduced memory, hallucinations, muscle spasms, incoherence, and irritability. This may last from between 2 and 10 years.
- **Stage 3:** Stage 3 dementia is marked by seizures, difficulty swallowing, incontinence, skin infections, and head injuries. This stage lasts from 1 to 3 years.

Tests for dementia include cognitive tests, imaging (CT or MRI brain or CT angiography), EEG, blood tests (thyroid function tests, B12 levels, genetic tests, routine biochemistry and blood counts) and lumbar puncture if indicated.

General measures to improve memory and intellect

Foods. Avoid or minimize alcohol, sugar, processed foods, refined carbohydrates, and meats. Consume more leafy green vegetables, fruit, teas, fats, and foods that are anti-inflammatory and antioxidant rich.

Plant herbs and nutraceuticals can prevent dementia or its progression.

There are various herbs, nutraceuticals, or drugs that can boost BDNF. These include ashwagandha *(Withania somnifera)*, gotu kola *(Centella asiatica)*, bacopa *(Bacopa monnieri)*, curcumin *(Cucurma longa)*, ginseng *(Panax ginseng)*, lion's mane mushroom *(Hericium erinaceus)*, ginkgo *(Ginkgo biloba)*, cordyceps *(Cordyceps militaris)*, magnolia bark *(Magnolia officinalis)*, Arctic root *(Rhodiola rosea)*, resveratrol, zinc, taurine, and lithium.

Other nootropic nutraceuticals include omega-3, fish oil, Vitamin D, curcumin, creatine, resveratrol, phosphatidylserine, acetyl-L-carnitine, and SAMe.

Physical exercises. Do regular yoga, *taichi*, *qigong* or any aerobic sport or exercise to improve brain circulation. Avoid sitting too long.

Mental exercises (Brain training and Brain Workouts). Engage in crossword puzzles, Sudoku, chess, mobile apps with memory games, learn a new language, activity, skill, art, craft or a hobby. Do something new, challenging and satisfying.

Routine Habits. Maintain a regular daily routine for activities of daily living (meal, bath or toilet times) and medication times. Maintain lists or timetable for activities or chores .Keep the home simple, organized, clutter-free and daily use or important items within sight and in the same place.

Memory joggers/Reminders. Develop associations or mnemonics (via pictures, stories, rhymes, aloud repetitions, visualization, flash cards, sticky notes, etc). Associate people's names with some funny traits or type it on the mobile phone.

Social connectivity. Avoid solitude and have an active social life with family and friends. Engage in humor and laughter.

Sleep. Ensure adequate sleep for at least 7 to 9 hours.

Stress relievers. Engage in regular meditation and mindfulness.

Medical disorders. Identify and treat underlying health conditions.

Pro-dementia medications. Avoid anticholinergic drugs that are used as antipsychotics, anti-depressants, anti-Parkinson drugs, overactive bladder drugs, anti-epilepsy drugs, anti-asthma or anti-vertigo medications. Their long-term use can lead to higher risk of dementia.

Improved vision. This may prevent dementia.

Indian Natural Remedies

There are many herbs that are brain tonics and help to enhance memory and intellect.

Common Ingredients for Dementia

Spices	Herbs/Leaves	Miscellaneous
Cinnamon	Brahmi (*Bacopa monnieri*)	Ashoka seeds (*Saraca indica*)
	Gotu kola (*Centella asiatica*)	Celery
	Bhringraj leaves	Jyotishmati oil
	Jyotishmati seeds (*Celastrus paniculata*)	Jatamansi (*Nardostachys jatamansi*)
	Mulethi (*Glycyrrhiza glabra*)	
	Vacha (*Acorus calamus*)	
	Shatavari (*Asparagus racemosus*)	
	Methi leaves (*Trigonella foenum-graecum*)	
	Jatamansi (*Nardostachys jatamansi*)	
	Shankhpushpi (*Convolvulus pluricaulis/ Convolvulus prostratus*)	
Turmeric	Ashwagandha (*Withania somnifera*)	Coconut oil

Common Recipes

Oral

Teas/Brews

Ashwagandha brew. Place 1 teaspoon of ashwagandha root powder into a pot with ½ cup of milk and ½ cup of water. Boil gently until the volume reduces to about ½ a cup. Cool slightly and drink warm. Add honey to taste.

Celery juice. Cut two to three stalks of celery into small pieces. Place in a blender and blend until smooth, adding a little water if necessary. Drink once a day.

Cinnamon tea. Lightly crush one to two cinnamon sticks. Add the cinnamon to 1.5 cups of hot water and cover. Let sit for 10 to 15 minutes before straining. Drink warm.

Coconut oil. Take 1 tablespoon of coconut oil three times a day.

Gotu kola juice. Place 8 to 10 fresh gotu kola leaves into a blender and blend until smooth. Add a little water if necessary. Drink once a day.

Jyotishmati seeds. Boil the seeds in 1 cup of water for about 5 minutes. Consume all.

Variation #1. Chew on 10 to 12 seeds every morning on an empty stomach and then wash them down with a cup of water.

Variation #2. Add 3 to 5 drops of jyotishmati oil to 1 cup of milk. Consume at night or on an empty stomach. This can be given to children.

Methi. Use the fresh leaf greens in curries or salads or mixed into flatbread dough.

Polyherbals.

- Combine bhringraj and ashwagandha. This is particularly good for Alzheimer's disease.
- Combine equal parts ashoka bark root powder and brahmi powder. Add 1 teaspoon of this mixture to 1 cup of milk. Drink twice a day.
- Combine the rhizomes of vacha (*Acorus calamus*), brahmi (*Bacopa monnieri*), gotu kola (*Centella asiatica*), and *Rauwolfia serpentina*.
- Combine shankhpushpi powder (5 g), gotu kola leaf powder (5 g), almonds (2 pieces, ground) and elaichi (1 piece, ground). Add 1 glass of milk and boil. Consume daily for 6 months.
- Combine equal amounts of shatavari root, shankhpushpi, gotu kola, and *Glycyrrhiza glabra* ground powders. Boil 1 teaspoon of this mixture in milk.
- Chew ashoka seeds with a piper betel leaf for 2 to 4 weeks.
- Combine equal amounts of gotu kola leaf, *Nardostachys jatamansi* (jatamansi) whole plant, and vacha root (*Acorus calamus*) powders. Mix with a little honey and consume.

Shankhpushpi. Add five to six fresh blue pea flowers to 1 cup of boiling water. Allow to steep for 5 to 10 minutes. Drink it before bedtime.

Shatavari. Take 1 teaspoon of shatavari root powder with milk every day.

Turmeric tea. Add 1 to 2 teaspoons of ground turmeric to 1 cup of hot water. Mix well and add honey to taste. Drink one to two times a day. Alternatively, lightly pound 2 to 3 inches of fresh turmeric and add to a cup of boiling water. Allow to steep for 5 to 10 minutes and strain. Add honey to taste.

Therapeutic Measures

Yoga Asanas to Improve Memory

These include bhramari pranayama (bee breathing), sarvangasana (shoulder stand pose), padmasana (lotus pose), paschimottanasana (seated forward bend pose), padahastasana (standing forward bend pose), and halasana (plough pose).

Chinese Natural Remedies

Common Ingredients for Dementia

Herbs/Leaves

Angelica dahurica
Chinese club moss
Chinese skullcap (*Scutellaria baicalensis*)
Gingko (*Ginkgo biloba*)
Ginseng
Lion's mane mushroom
Salvia

Common Recipes

Oral

Teas/Brews

Angelica. It is usually part of a polyherbal formula.

Chinese club moss tea. Add 2 to 3 teaspoons of dried club moss to a cup with boiling water. Let steep for 15 to 20 minutes before straining. Drink it warm.

Chinese skullcap. Add 1 tablespoon of dried skullcap to 2 cups of boiling water. Steep for 15 minutes. Strain and add honey to taste.

Ginkgo tea. Place three to five fresh ginkgo leaves into a cup of boiling water. Steep for 10 to 15 minutes before drinking.

Ginseng tea. Add about two to four slices of ginseng to a cup. Add hot water over the ginseng. Steep for about 10 to 15 minutes.

Lion's mane mushroom. It can be cooked and eaten.

Salvia tea. Chop 1 tablespoon of washed fresh salvia leaves. Add to 2 cups of boiling water. Simmer for 5 to 15 minutes. Add honey or milk. Drink warm.

Therapeutic Measures

Lifestyle. Engage in mental challenging games like mahjong or chess. Engage in tai chi or qigong physical exercises.

Acupressure points for acupuncture for memory and concentration. These include the following points at:
- DU20 ban hui. Meeting of hundred (over the vertex).
- EX 6 si shen gong. Four spirit alert.
- LU 9 influential point of blood vessels (at wrist).
- GB 39 influential point of brain marrow (at ankle near lateral malleolus).

Western/Other Natural Remedies

Common Ingredients for Dementia

Herbs/Leaves/Fruits/Seeds	Misc.
Bilberry	
Blueberries	Lithium orotate
Lemon balm	Zinc
Pine needle	Taurine
Rhodiola rosea	SAMe
Rosemary	Omega-3 fish oil
Saffron (Crocus Sativus)	
Sage	Resveratrol
Snowdrop (Galanthus woronowii)	

Common Recipes

Oral

Teas/Brews

Bilberry tea. Add 1½ teaspoons of bilberry leaves into a cup with boiling water and steep for 10 to 15 minutes. Strain and drink it warm. Alternatively, make bilberry extract by mashing 1 teaspoon of crushed berries with 1 teaspoon of water until smooth. Take for 3 days.

Lemon balm tea. Place 1 tablespoon of dried lemon balm leaves (or 2 tablespoons of fresh leaves) into a cup of boiling water. Let sit for 10 to 15 minutes before straining. Add honey to taste and drink warm.

Other nutraceuticals. These include omega-3 fish oil, choline, SAMe, resveratrol, taurine, and zinc. There are mixed views about whether small doses of lithium orotate can prevent dementia progression.

Phosphatidylserine. It is available as supplements. It should be given in the morning for a trial period of 1 month.

Pine needle tea. Wash unblemished edible pine needles and cut into small pieces. Add two cups of boiling water. Steep for 10 to 15 minutes. Strain and drink. Add honey to taste.

Variation #1. It is available as capsules or tablets. The Pycnogenol brand is widely used.

Rhodiola root tea. Chop finely about 5 g of *Rhodiola rosea* root. Add 1 cup of boiling water. Let steep for 4 hours. Strain and drink ½ a cup three to five times a day.

Rosemary tea. Add three to five sprigs of fresh rosemary (or 1½ teaspoons of dry rosemary leaf needles) to a cup of hot water and steep for 10 to 15 minutes. Drink warm.

Sage tea. Place three to five sage leaves in a cup of boiling water. Cover and let steep for 5 to 10 minutes. Drink warm.

Snowdrop. The plant bulb and leaves are rubbed on the forehead to improve memory and focus in mild dementia

Saffron tea. Take a pinch of saffron. Add 1 cup of boiling water. Steep for 10 minutes. Strain and consume. Add a lemon slice and a sweetener if desired.

#Variation 1. Saffron threads can be added to rissoto and paella (preferbaly soaked in hot water first).

Therapeutic Measures

Music therapy. Listening to music or singing songs can help improve the mood, reduce stress and anxiety in patients with Alzheimer's disease. It can be personalized. A low tone of 40 Hz sine wave sound source may be helpful in some.

Occupational therapy. Engage in colouring or art, crossword puzzles, look at old photos, watch old favourite movies, etc.

Diet. Consume a diet rich in fatty fish, green leafy vegetables, berries and moderate red wine.

Modern Remedies

Cholinesterase Inhibitors

This medication inhibits the action of acetylcholinesterase, an enzyme that breaks down acetylcholine in the brain. Acetylcholine is a neurotransmitter responsible for communication between nerve cells. Raising acetylcholine levels can temporarily stabilize and improve dementia symptoms.

Examples. Galantamine (Razadyne) and *Rivastigmine* (Exelon) for mild to moderate Alzheimer's.

Donepezil (Aricept) for any severity of Alzheimer's.

Memantine

Memantine is thought to block the current flow through channels of N-methyl-d-aspartate (NMDA) receptors by binding to the NMDA receptors, temporarily relieving symptoms of dementia.

Biologics and Human Monoclonal Antibodies

Aducanumab, gantenerumab, and donanamab are promising immunotherapies being used in the treatment trials of Alzheimer's disease to reduce the buildup of beta amyloid plaques to improve cognition and memory. Side effects include headache and "amyloid-related imaging abnormalities (ARIA) such as cerebral edema."

Melatonin

Take melatonin 1-3 mg. Good quality sleep can improve dementia.

Stroke

A stroke occurs when a blood vessel to the brain carrying oxygen and nutrients becomes blocked by a clot or ruptures. A part of the brain then cannot get the necessary blood and oxygen, causing a section of the brain to die. Symptoms of a stroke include sudden numbness or weakness in the face, arms, or legs, especially on one side of the body. There may be sudden confusion, dizziness, and problems speaking or seeing in one or both eyes. There are two main types of stroke: ischemic or hemorrhagic.

- **Ischemic stroke** is caused by a blood clot that develops at a fatty plaque within a blood vessel. Another cause of the stroke is when a clot forms in the heart, dislodges, and travels to the brain.
- **Hemorrhagic stroke** occurs when a weakened blood vessel bursts.
- Causes and contributing factors include metabolic syndrome (hypertension, hypercholesterolemia, and diabetes), obstructive sleep apnea, smoking, alcohol or illicit drug abuse, family history, obesity, physical inactivity, oral contraceptive use, and associated medical conditions like kidney disease or heart conditions.

Investigations include CT, MRI, MRA, cranial Doppler ultrasound, CT contrast angiogram, blood tests (blood counts, lipids, glucose, and thrombophilia screen), cardiac evaluation (ECG and cardiac ultrasound with Doppler), and sometimes a lumbar puncture.

Indian Natural Remedies

Common Ingredients for Stroke

Spices	Herbs/Leaves	Miscellaneous
Garlic		Pomegranate
Ginger	Gotu kola (Centella asiatica)	Coconut oil
Turmeric	Ashwagandha (Withania somnifera)	Carrot

Common Recipes

Teas/Brews

Ashwagandha brew. Add 1 teaspoon of ashwagandha root powder into a pot with ½ cup of milk, and ½ cup of water. Boil gently until the volume reduces to about ½ cup. Cool slightly and drink warm. Add honey to taste.

Carrot juice. Chop three to five carrots into smaller pieces and place them in a blender. Blend until smooth, adding water if necessary. Drink once a day.

Coconut oil. Consume 1 tablespoon of coconut oil once a day.

Garlic. Consume one to four cloves of fresh garlic daily.

Ginger tea. Place 2 to 3 pieces of fresh sliced ginger into a cup of boiling water. Cover and steep for 10 to 15 minutes. Strain and drink it.

Gotu kola juice. Place 8 to 10 fresh gotu kola leaves into a blender and blend until smooth. Add a little water if necessary. Drink once a day.

Pomegranate. Consume pomegranate.

Turmeric brew. Stir 1 to 2 teaspoons of turmeric into a cup of warm milk. Drink once a day.

Chinese Natural Remedies

Mild stroke involves attack of meridians and blood vessels and there is no loss of unconsciousness. In a severe stroke, there is an attack of zang-fu organs with loss of unconsciousness.

Prodrome of Stroke: Causes and Patterns	Polyherbal Treatment Recommendation
Pattern of ascendant hyperactivity of liver yang	Tian ma gou teng decoction modified
Pattern of phlegm qi deficiency and blood stasis	Bu yang huan wu decoction modified
Pattern of phlegm turbidity and stagnation	Ban xia bai zhu tian ma decoction modified
Pattern of kidney deficiency and blood stasis	Liu wei di huang wan decoction modified

Meridian Stroke Pattern	Polyherbal Treatment Recommendation
Pattern of wind-phlegm obstructing the meridians	Hua tan tong luo decoction modified
Pattern of qi deficiency and blood stasis	Bu yang huan wu decoction modified
Pattern of wind-stirring due to yin deficiency	Zhen gan xi feng decoction modified and yu yin xi feng decoction modified
Pattern of phlegm-heat the fu-organ	Xing lou cheng qi decoction modified

A common type of ischemic stroke is *qi* deficiency along with blood stasis syndrome. (QDBS).

Common Ingredients for Stroke

Spices	Herbs/Leaves	Miscellaneous
Ginger	Asian ginseng	Earthworm (Pheretima aspergillum)
	Ginkgo (Ginkgo biloba)	Scorpion (Buthus martensii)
	Chinese motherwort (Leonurus japonicus)	
	Baikal skullcap	
	Dong quai (Angelica sinensis)	
	Dang shen (Codonopsis pilosula)	
	Kudzu (Pueraria montana/ Pueraria lobata)	

Common Recipes

Oral

Teas/Brews

Commercial Polyherbal formula. For ischemic stroke with QDBS syndrome, the following formula are given to invigorate *qi* and yin and activate blood circulation: *Buyang Huanwu* granules (BHG): contain seven herbs: *Radix astragali, Paeoniae radix rubra, Angelicae sinen-*

sis, Persicae semen (peach kernel), Lumbricus, Cnidii rhizoma, and *Carthami flos.*

Yangyin Tongyao granules (YTG): contain six herbs: *Radix astragali, Radix rehmanniae, Ligustici chuanxiong rhizoma, Puerariae lobatae radix,* hirudo, and *Dendrobii caulis.*

Naoxintong capsules (NXTC): contain 16 herbs: Radix astragali, Paeoniae radix rubra, Angelicae sinensis, Persicae semen (peach kernel), frankincense *(Boswellia carterii),* myrrh *(Commiphora myrrha), Cinnamomum cassia, Morus alba, Radix salviae miltiorrhizae, Ligusticum chuanxiong,* hirudo *(Whitmania pigra),* Carthami flos, Achyranthes bidentata (ox knee), Caulis spatholobi, scorpion *(Buthus martensii),* and pheretima *(Pheretima aspergillum).*

Dang shen–ginger tea. Place 3 to 4 teaspoons of dang shen herb into a pot with 5 to 6 cups of water. Lightly smash 5 to 8 inches of ginger root and add to the pot. Bring to a boil and then reduce the heat, allowing to simmer for 1 to 1½ hours. Strain and drink warm.

Dong quai tea. Place 1 to 2 teaspoons of dried dong quai herb in a pot with a cup of boiling water. Bring to a boil, then reduce the heat, and simmer gently for about half an hour. Strain and drink.

Ginger tea. Lightly pound 1 to 2 inches of cut ginger and add to a cup of hot water. Steep for 5 to 10 minutes. Strain and drink.

Ginkgo tea. Place 3 to 5 fresh ginkgo leaves into a cup of boiling water. Steep for 10 to 15 minutes before drinking

Ginseng tea. Add about two to four slices of ginseng to a cup. Add hot water over the ginseng. Steep for about 10 to 15 minutes.

Motherwort tea. Place 1 to 2 teaspoons of dried chopped motherwort herb in a cup of boiling water. Cover and steep for 5 to 10 minutes. Drink warm.

Skullcap tea. Place 1 to 2 teaspoons of dried chopped skullcap in a cup of boiling water. Cover and steep for 5 to 10 minutes. Drink warm.

Therapeutic Measures

Acupuncture

The principal acupuncture points include Baihui (GV 20), Neiguan (PC 6), Weizhong (BL 40), Sanyinjia (SP 6), Shuigou (GV 26), Quchi (LI 11), Zusanli (ST 36), Waiguan (TE 5), Hegu (LI 4), Yanglingquan (GB 34), and Huantiao (GB 30).

The supplementary points for mainly upper limb hemiplegic involvement include Shousanli (LI 10) and Jianliao (TE 14).

The supplementary points for mainly lower limb hemiplegic involvement include Taichung (LR 3) and Xuanzhong (GB 39).

The supplementary points for mouth or tongue deviation include Jiache (ST 6) and Dicang (ST 4).

The motor area of Jiao's scalp acupuncture point is specifically used to treat motor dysfunction after stroke.

Tuina massage of the meridians can help with motor recovery.

Fuming-washing therapy. Vapor from a boiling decoction is applied on the affected limb to reduce pain and stiffness.

Intravenous therapy. Intravenous puerarin is given in acute stroke.

Western/Other Natural Remedies

Common Ingredients for Stroke

Herbs/Leaves
arnica (*Arnica montana*)
Burdock root
Cramp bark
Goldenrod (*Solidago spp.*)
Lady's mantle
Lavender
Mistletoe
Nettles
Rosemary
Sage
Shepherd's purse
Sweet marjoram (*Origanum majorana*)
Thyme
Viola odorata
Walnut leaf

Common Recipes

Oral

Teas/Brews

Rosemary tea. Add three to five sprigs of fresh rosemary (or 1½ teaspoons of dry rosemary leaf needles) to a cup of hot water and steep for 10 to 15 minutes. Drink warm.

Sage tea. Place three to five sage leaves in a cup of boiling water. Cover and let steep for 5 to 10 minutes. Drink warm.

Stroke recovery herbal tea. Add arnica flowers (20 g), lady's mantle (30 g), goldenrod (10 g), mistletoe (10 g), and shepherd's purse (20 g) to a pot with 5 to 6 cups of boiling water. Steep for 15 minutes and strain. Add honey to taste and sip throughout the day.

Variation #1. Add arnica flowers (20 g), shepherd's purse (20 g), mistletoe (10 g), rosemary (20 g), and sage (20 g) to a pot with 5 to 6 cups of boiling water. Steep for 15 minutes and strain. Add honey to taste and sip throughout the day.

Variation #2. Add nettles (20 g), burdock root (20 g), shepherd's purse (20 g), *Viola odorata* (210 g), and walnut leaves (20 g) to a pot with 5 to 6 cups of boiling water. Steep for 15 minutes and strain. Add honey to taste and sip throughout the day.

Thyme tea. Place three to five thyme leaves into a cup of hot water and let steep for 5 to 10 minutes. Add honey to taste and sip throughout the day.

Modern Remedies

Ischemic Stroke

Tissue Plasminogen Activator via Intravenous Injection
An injection of tissue plasminogen activator (tPA) is given through a vein in the arm. This drug is a thrombolytic

agent, which means that it restores blood flow by dissolving the blood clot in the brain. It does this by activating plasminogen, which forms a product called plasmin. Plasmin can dissolve blood clots by breaking cross-links between fibrin molecules, which provides structural stability in blood clots.

Emergency Endovascular Procedures
- Medication may be administered directly to the brain via a long tube called a catheter sent into the brain by an artery in the groin. Thrombolytic agents are then administered to dissolve the blood clot.
- A catheter may also be inserted and a stent retriever maneuvered into the blocked vessel in the brain. The blood clot is then removed using the stent. This procedure is often indicated in patients with large blood clots and may be used in conjunction with intravenous tPA.

Hemorrhagic Stroke
Surgery
- Surgical clipping is a procedure in which a tiny clamp is placed at the base of the aneurysm to stop blood flow. This prevents the aneurysm from bursting, causing further complications.
- Endovascular embolization involves inserting a catheter into the brain through an artery in the groin. Tiny detachable coils are then maneuvered into the brain, which fills the aneurysm and blocks off blood flow. This causes the blood to clot.
- A small aneurysm may be removed if it is in an accessible part of the brain and if removal of the tissue in that area does not cause a large loss in brain function.

Homeopathic Remedies

These may include *Arnica montana*, belladonna, causticum, plumbum, *Lachesis*, *Crotalus horridus*, baryta carbonica, etc.

Parkinson's Disease

Parkinson's disease (PD) is a loss of nerve cells in the part of the brain called the substantia nigra that produces dopamine. It produces symptoms such as muscle rigidity, changes in speech and gait, and tremors. There is currently no cure for Parkinson's disease, and medication is mostly aimed at alleviating symptoms and making day-to-day activities more manageable. The loss of brain cells in Parkinson's is thought to be caused by a number of factors such as genetics, environmental factors, and medication, as well as cerebrovascular disease.

Indian Natural Remedies

Common Ingredients for Parkinson's Disease

Spices	Herbs/Leaves	Miscellaneous
Turmeric	Brahmi (*Bacopa monnieri*)	Kapikachhu/cowhage (*Mucuna pruriens*)

Common Recipes
Oral
Teas/Brews
Brahmi juice. Take a handful of fresh brahmi leaves and blend with a little water. Drink 5 to 10 mL of the juice with 1 teaspoon of honey every day.

Cowhage. Cowhage seed may be consumed in the form of a powder and may contain levodopa or L-dopa, which can alleviate symptoms of Parkinson's.

Turmeric tea. Add 1 to 2 teaspoons of ground turmeric to 1 cup of hot water. Mix well and add honey to taste. Drink one to two times a day. Alternatively, lightly pound 2 to 3 inches of fresh turmeric and add to a cup of boiling water. Allow to steep for 5 to 10 minutes and strain. Add honey to taste.

Chinese Natural Remedies

The main symptom patterns in Parkinson's disease are yin deficiency of kidney and liver, deficiency of qi, deficiency of blood, blood stasis and internal-wind stirring, and phlegm heat and internal-wind stirring.

Common Ingredients for Parkinson's Disease

Herbs/Leaves
Cat's claw (*Uncaria rhynchophylla*)
Female ginseng/dong quai (*Radix angelica sinensis*)
Ginkgo (*Ginkgo biloba*)
Green tea leaf
Licorice/gan cao (*Radix glycyrrhizae*)

Common Recipes
Oral
Teas/Brews
Cat's claw tea. Boil some water and pour it into a cup; add 1 to 2 pieces of cat's claw bark. Steep for 5 to 10 minutes before straining and drinking.

Dong quai tea. Place 1 to 2 teaspoons of dried dong quai herb in a pot with a cup of boiling water. Bring to a boil, then reduce the heat, and simmer gently for about half an hour. Strain and drink.

Ginkgo tea. Place three to five fresh ginkgo leaves into a cup of boiling water. Steep for 10 to 15 minutes before drinking.

Green tea. Place 1 to 2 teaspoons of green tea leaves into a cup of boiling water and steep for 10 minutes. Strain and drink warm.

Licorice tea. Add 1 teaspoon of ground licorice to a pot with 1 cup of boiling water. Allow to simmer for 30 to 45 minutes before straining.

Yi Gan San. This is a polyherbal formula (restrain-the-liver powder). It contains Dang Gui, Fu Ling, Gou Teng, Chuan Xiong, Bai Zhu, and Gan Cao and Chai Hu.

Therapeutic Measures

Acupuncture

It can improve balance and gait.

The acupuncture point commonly used is LR3. Others include GV20, GB34, EX-HN1, GB20, LI11, ST36, and KI3.

LR3. It is located on the dorsum of the right foot in the hollow between the big toe and second toe.

GV 20 (Governing Vessel 20) is also known as the hundred convergences. It is located at the top of the head, exactly halfway on an imaginary line drawn from ear to ear.

GB34. It is located on the lateral aspect of the lower leg, in the hollow anterior and inferior to the head of the fibula.

EX-HN1. These are four points located around the vertex (i.e., 1 finger breadth from GV20).

GB20. Gallbladder 20 is located at the nape of the neck below the occiput, just lateral to the trapezius muscle.

LI 11. This point is located at the elbow. With the elbow flexed, the point is at the end of the transverse crease at the midpoint between the lateral epicondyle of the humerus and LU5 (radial side of biceps).

ST36. It is located at the tibialis anterior muscle four finger breadths below the patella and one finger breadth lateral from the anterior crest of the tibia.

KI3. It is located in the hollow between the tip of the medial malleolus and tendoachilles on the medial aspect of the foot.

Diet

Consume kidney-strengthening food such as walnuts and wolfberries.

Western/Other Natural Remedies

Common Ingredients for Parkinson's Disease

Miscellaneous
Apple cider vinegar
Blueberry
Celery and celery seed
Fish oil

Common Recipes

Oral

- **Fish oil.** Fish oils are high in omega-3 fatty acids, which are thought to help to protect the brain against Parkinson's disease. Some foods high in omega-3 fatty acids are salmon, mackerel, and walnuts.
- **Blueberries.** Blueberry extract is rich in antioxidants and phytonutrients and can have protective effects against Parkinson's disease.
- **Celery juice.** Cut two to three stalks of celery into smaller pieces. Blend with little water until smooth. Stir a teaspoon of honey into the juice and drink before bedtime.
- **Apple cider vinegar.** Mix 2 teaspoons of apple cider vinegar into 1 cup of warm water and drink once a day.

Modern Remedies

Carbidopa-Levodopa

This medication contains levodopa, a chemical that passes into the brain to be converted into dopamine. It is combined with carbidopa, which prevents levodopa from conversion into dopamine outside of the brain.

Dopamine Agonists

Dopamine Agonists mimic the effects of dopamine on the brain by binding to dopamine receptors and activating them.

Examples: pramipexole, rotigotine

Anticholinergics

Anticholinergics block the action of acetylcholine in the brain, a neurotransmitter responsible for signals being passed from the brain to the muscles. It is thought that blocking acetylcholine receptors increases the activity of the neurons responsible for movement.

Examples: benztropine, trihexyphenidyl

Monoamine Oxidase B Inhibitors

These drugs prevent the breakdown of dopamine in the brain by inhibiting the enzyme monoamine oxidase B (MAO B). This prolongs the effects of dopamine in the brain and relieves Parkinson's symptoms.

Examples: selegiline, rasagiline, safinamide

Deep Brain Stimulation Surgery

Subthalamic nucleus deep brain stimulation (STN-DBS) is a form of neuromodulation via stereotactic surgery. It is very effective for dyskinesias and dopaminergic medication reduction in Parkinson's disease. It improves quality of life. Side effects can include infection, headache, seizure, poor focus or memory, or stroke. Stimulation of the thalamus or globus pallidus interna (GPi) are also done.

Ablative or Lesioning surgery

Radiosurgical or ultrasound thalamotomy, subthalamotomy, or pallidotomy are permanent "destructive or ablative" surgeries which are seldom done now for PD, although they are effective.

Stem Cells

Fetal stem cells have also been injected into the corpus striatum.

References

Epilepsy/Seizures

Epilepsy. (n.d.). allAyurveda. https://allayurveda.com/kb/epilepsy/.

Chauhan, M. (2019, March 2). *Ayurvedic treatment of epilepsy.* Planet Ayurveda. Retrieved from https://www.planetayurveda.com/library/epilepsy/.

Cherney, K. (2019, August 23). *Natural treatments for epilepsy: Do they work?* Healthline. Retrieved from https://www.healthline.com/health/natural-treatments-epilepsy.

Cheuk, D. K., & Wong, V. (2014). Acupuncture for epilepsy. *Cochrane Database of Systematic Reviews*. Published. Retrieved from https://doi.org/10.1002/14651858.cd005062.pub4.

Dereyan, A. (2015, December 23). *Top 5 natural epilepsy treatments.* Pharmacy Times. Retrieved from https://www.pharmacytimes.com/view/top-5-natural-epilepsy-treatments.

Epilepsy Foundation Eastern Pennsylvania. (n.d.). *Treatment options.* EFEPA Epilepsy Foundation Eastern Pennsylvania. Retrieved from https://www.efepa.org/living-with-epilepsy/treatment-options/.

Epilepsy Foundation of America. (n.d.). *Neuromodulation devices.* Epilepsy Foundation. Retrieved from https://www.epilepsy.com/learn/treating-seizures-and-epilepsy/neuromodulation-devices.

Epilepsy Society. (2021, June 28). *Epilepsy treatment.* Retrieved from https://epilepsysociety.org.uk/about-epilepsy/treatment#.XIK17y17EfE.

Healthcare Medicine Institute. (2014, May 7). *Acupuncture synergizes epilepsy relief.* HealthCMi. Retrieved from https://www.healthcmi.com/Acupuncture-Continuing-Education-News/1306-acupuncture-synergizes-epilepsy-relief-new-finding.

Mayo Clinic Staff. (2021, March 31). *Epilepsy.* Mayo Clinic. Retrieved from https://www.mayoclinic.org/diseases-conditions/epilepsy/diagnosis-treatment/drc-20350098.

Pacific College of Health and Science. (2019a, February 21). *TCM for epilepsy and seizure disorders.* Pacific College. Retrieved from https://www.pacificcollege.edu/news/blog/2014/12/25/tcm-for-epilepsy-and-seizure-disorders.

Pacific College of Health and Science. (2019b, February 21). *The benefits of TCM and acupuncture for epilepsy.* Pacific College. Retrieved from https://www.pacificcollege.edu/news/blog/2015/01/18/the-benefits-of-tcm-and-acupuncture-for-epilepsy.

Sharma, V. (2019, May 4). *Top homeopathic remedies for epilepsy treatment.* Homeopathy at DrHomeo.Com. Retrieved from https://www.drhomeo.com/epilepsy/homeopathic-remedies-for-epilepsy/.

Sirven, J. I. (2021, January 21). *What is epilepsy?* Epilepsy Foundation. Retrieved from https://www.epilepsy.com/learn/about-epilepsy-basics/what-epilepsy.

Spinella, M. (2001). Herbal medicines and epilepsy: The potential for benefit and adverse effects. *Epilepsy & Behavior, 2*(6), 524–532. Retrieved from https://doi.org/10.1006/ebeh.2001.0281.

Venkateswara Ayurveda Nilayam Ltd. (n.d.). *Ayurvedic treatment and medicine for epilepsy.* Ayuraarogyam. Retrieved from https://ayuraarogyam.com/Others/Epilepsy.

Winger, J. (2018, August 31). *8 essential oils for sleep.* The Prairie Homestead. Retrieved from https://www.theprairiehomestead.com/2014/03/essential-oils-sleep.html.

Zamponi, N., Passamonti, C., Cesaroni, E., Trignani, R., & Rychlicki, F. (2011). Effectiveness of vagal nerve stimulation (VNS) in patients with drop-attacks and different epileptic syndromes. *Seizure, 20*(6), 468–474. Retrieved from https://doi.org/10.1016/j.seizure.2011.02.011.

Insomnia

Fry, A. (2020, September 18). *Treatments for insomnia.* Sleep Foundation. Retrieved from https://www.sleepfoundation.org/insomnia/treatment.

Lamoreux, K. (2020, July 27). *Everything you need to know about insomnia.* Healthline. Retrieved from https://www.healthline.com/health/insomnia.

WebMD Editors. (2003, May 31). *Understanding Insomnia treatments.* WebMD. Retrieved from https://www.webmd.com/sleep-disorders/understanding-insomnia-treatment.

Headache

Addison, N. (n.d.). *Herbs and Spices to Soothe Headaches.* MiND-FOOD. https://www.mindfood.com/article/herbs-and-spices-for-headaches/

Ahuja, A. (2018, August 20). *Home remedies for headaches: 10 natural ways to treat headaches.* NDTV Food. Retrieved from https://food.ndtv.com/health/10-natural-home-remedies-for-headaches-that-actually-work-1215616.

Calabro, S., & Craig, C. W. (2009, February 23). *Herbal remedies for headache and migraine relief.* EverydayHealth.Com. Retrieved from https://www.everydayhealth.com/headache-migraine/herbal-remedies.aspx.

Daining, C. (2015, March 14). *15 herbs for headaches.* Scratch Mommy. Retrieved from https://scratchmommy.com/15-herbs-for-headaches/.

Glaser, A. (2020, October 4). *9 pressure points for headaches you need to know.* Migraine Again. Retrieved from https://www.migraine-again.com:443/pressure-points-for-headaches-and-nausea/.

Happe, S., Peikert, A., Siegert, R., & Evers, S. (2016). The efficacy of lymphatic drainage and traditional massage in the prophylaxis of migraine: A randomized, controlled parallel group study. *Neurological Sciences, 37*(10), 1627–1632. Retrieved from https://doi.org/10.1007/s10072-016-2645-3.

Iftikhar, N. (2019, March 15). *CGRP migraine treatment: Could it be right for you?* Healthline. Retrieved from https://www.healthline.com/health/migraine/cgrp-migraine#cost.

Kubala, J. (2018, February 4). *18 remedies to get rid of headaches naturally.* Healthline. Retrieved from https://www.healthline.com/nutrition/headache-remedies.

Maharishi Ayurveda Staff. (2021). *Ask the expert: Headaches.* Maharishi Ayurveda. Retrieved from https://www.mapi.com/ayurvedic-knowledge/stress/ayurvedic-headache-relief.html.

Martin, L. F., Patwardhan, A. M., Jain, S. V., Salloum, M. M., Freeman, J., Khanna, R., et al. (2020). Evaluation of green light exposure on headache frequency and quality of life in migraine patients: A preliminary one-way cross-over clinical trial. *Cephalalgia, 41*(2), 135–147. Retrieved from https://doi.org/10.1177/0333102420956711.

Memorial Sloan Kettering Cancer Center. (2019, October 24). *Acupressure for pain and headaches.* Retrieved from https://www.mskcc.org/cancer-care/patient-education/acupressure-pain-and-headaches.

Pacific College of Health and Medicine. (2020, March 7). *Don't let headaches interfere with your life: Chinese medicine can help.* Pacific College. Retrieved from https://www.pacificcollege.edu/news/blog/2015/03/23/dont-let-headaches-interfere-your-life-chinese-medicine-can-help.

Sengupta, S. (2018, April 21). *5 Ayurvedic foods and remedies to relieve headache.* NDTV Food. Retrieved from https://food.ndtv.com/food-drinks/5-ayurvedic-foods-and-remedies-to-relieve-headache-1840787.

Shefi, E., & Schoenbart, B. (2021, April 1). *How to treat headaches with traditional Chinese medicine.* HowStuffWorks. Retrieved from https://health.howstuffworks.com/wellness/natural-medicine/chinese/how-to-treat-headaches-with-traditional-chinese-medicine.htm.

Shen-Nong Limited. (2006). *How Chinese medicine understands headache disorders.* Shen-Nong. Retrieved from http://www.shen-nong.com/eng/exam/headaches_chinese_medicine_understands.html.

T. (2020b, February 21). *15 Herbs for Headaches-.* The Homestead Garden. https://www.thehomesteadgarden.com/15-herbs-for-headaches/.

WebMD Editors. (2002, March 27). *Headache basics.* WebMD. Retrieved from https://www.webmd.com/migraines-headaches/migraines-headaches-basics#2.

WebMD Editors. (2007, January 1). *Headache treatment options and remedies*. WebMD. Retrieved from https://www.webmd.com/migraines-headaches/understanding-headache-treatment-medref#1.

Child Dyslexia

Cures Decoded Staff. (n.d.). *Home remedies and herbs for dyslexia*. CuresDecoded. Retrieved from https://www.curesdecoded.com/conditions/dyslexia/80.

Davis Dyslexia Association International. (n.d.). *Dyslexia is not a disease*. Dyslexia.Com. Retrieved from https://www.dyslexia.com/question/dyslexia-is-not-a-disease/.

Fernandes, S. B. (n.d.). *Case histories of acupuncture dyslexia*. Effects of Acupuncture on Challenged Children. Retrieved from http://acupunctureonchallenged.blogspot.com/p/case-histories-of-acupuncture-dyslexia.html.

Gillis, M. (2021, June 21). *Treating dyslexia*. Smart Kids. Retrieved from https://www.smartkidswithld.org/getting-help/dyslexia/treating-dyslexia/.

Herbpathy. (n.d.). *Dyslexia herbal treatment, prevention, symptoms, causes, cured by*. Herbpathy: Make Life Healthy. Retrieved from https://herbpathy.com/Herbal-Treatment-for-Dyslexia-Cid4573.

Kumar, R. (2016, February 11). *10 best homeopathic medicines for dyslexia*. Homeopathica. Retrieved from https://homeopathica.com/10-best-homeopathic-medicines-for-dyslexia/.

Mayo Clinic Staff. (2017, July 22). *Dyslexia*. Mayo Clinic. Retrieved from https://www.mayoclinic.org/diseases-conditions/dyslexia/symptoms-causes/syc-20353552.

NHS website. (2018a, August 15). *Dyslexia management*. NHS UK. Retrieved from https://www.nhs.uk/conditions/dyslexia/living-with/.

NHS website. (2018b, October 10). *Dyslexia*. NHS UK. Retrieved from https://www.nhs.uk/conditions/dyslexia/.

Sharma, V. (2019, February 21). *Top homeopathic medicines for developmental delay*. Homeopathy at DrHomeo.Com. Retrieved from https://www.drhomeo.com/developmental-delay/developmental-delay-and-homeopathy/.

Sharma, A., Gothecha, V., & Ojha, N. (2012). Dyslexia: A solution through Ayurveda evidences from Ayurveda for the management of dyslexia in children: A review. *AYU (An International Quarterly Journal of Research in Ayurveda)*, 33(4), 486. Retrieved from https://doi.org/10.4103/0974-8520.110521.

Shirole, T. (2019, December 28). *Dyslexia—causes, symptoms, diagnosis, treatment*. Medindia. Retrieved from https://www.medindia.net/patients/patientinfo/dyslexia.htm.

Tayde, S. (2017, March 6). *Treating 'learning & mental disabilities' with herbal medicines*. Dalmia HealthCare. Retrieved from https://dalmiahealth.com/treating-learning-and-mental-disabilities-with-herbal-medicines/.

The Tole Acupuncture and Herbal Medical Centre Sdn Bhd. (n.d.). *Dyslexia treatment*. The Tole. Retrieved from https://www.thetole.org/DyslexiaBrainTreatmentCure.html#.XIK33S17EfE.

WebMD Editors. (n.d.). *Common vitamins and supplements to treat dyslexia*. WebMD. Retrieved from https://www.webmd.com/vitamins/condition-1160/dyslexia.

WebMD Editors. (2017, April 12). *What are the treatments for dyslexia?* WebMD. Retrieved from https://www.webmd.com/children/understanding-dyslexia-treatment#1.

Child Developmental Delay

Blakeway, J. (2021, May 10). *Brain power: Using chinese medicine to stay focused*. The Yinova Center. Retrieved from https://www.yinovacenter.com/blog/brain-power-using-chinese-medicine-to-stay-focused/.

Colquhoun, J. (2019, March 1). *11 herbs that will help make your memory, focus and brain work better than ever*. FOOD MATTERS®. Retrieved from https://www.foodmatters.com/article/11-herbs-that-boost-your-brain-power.

Kelsey, L. (n.d.). *Enhance brain function and learning with traditional Chinese medicine*. Acufinder.Com. Retrieved from https://www.acufinder.com/Acupuncture+Information/Detail/Enhance-+Brain+Function+and+Learning+with+Traditional+Chinese+Medicine.

Khalsa, K. P. S. (2019, August 7). *Five great Ayurvedic herbs for the mind and memory*. Banyan Botanicals. Retrieved from https://www.banyanbotanicals.com/info/blog-banyan-vine/details/five-great-ayurvedic-herbs-for-the-mind-and-memory/.

Maharishi AyurVeda Staff. (n.d.). *Seven keys to unlock your brain power this spring*. Maharishi AyurVeda. Retrieved from https://www.mapi.com/ayurvedic-knowledge/brain-power/ayurvedic-brain-power-tips.html.

Riley Children's Health. (2016, June 9). *Developmental delay*. Retrieved from https://www.rileychildrens.org/health-info/developmental-delay.

Stuart, A. (2007a, September 25). *Developmental delays in young children*. WebMD. Retrieved from https://www.webmd.com/parenting/baby/recognizing-developmental-delays-birth-age-2#1.

Stuart, A. (2007b, September 25). *Spotting developmental delays in your child: Ages 3–5*. WebMD. Retrieved from https://www.webmd.com/parenting/recognizing-developmental-delays-your-child-ages-3-5#1.

Therapies For Kids Staff. (2021, April 1). *Developmental delay*. Therapies for Kids. Retrieved from https://therapiesforkids.com.au/developmental-delay-2/.

Turner, L. (2018, January 1). *10 Best herbal nootropics for cognitive function and enhancement*. Better Nutrition. Retrieved from https://www.betternutrition.com/features/herbal-nootropics/.

Wong, C., & Kelly, C. (2020a, February 3). *7 best herbs and spices to help improve your brain health*. Verywell Mind. Retrieved from https://www.verywellmind.com/best-herbs-and-spices-for-brain-health-4047818.

Wong, C., & Kelly, C. (2020b, February 3). *7 best herbs and spices to help improve your brain health*. Verywell Mind. Retrieved from https://www.verywellmind.com/best-herbs-and-spices-for-brain-health-4047818.

Hypotonia

Cristol, H. (2018, January 26). *What is hypotonia?* WebMD. Retrieved from https://www.webmd.com/baby/hypotonia-floppy-infant-syndrome#2.

Dorfman, K. (2013, November 7). *The Impact of Nutrition on Children with Low Muscle Tone | Day 2 Day Parenting*. Day 2 Day Parenting. https://day2dayparenting.com/impact-nutrition-children-low-muscle-tone/.

Dynamic Solutions. (2020, December 7). *Treating children with hypotonia with physical and occupational therapy*. Dynamic Solutions: Pediatric Therapy. Retrieved from https://www.dynamicsolutionstherapy.com/2020/12/07/treating-children-with-hypotonia-with-physical-and-occupational-therapy/.

Fratkin, J. K. (2007, September 1). Treating infants and small children with Chinese herbal medicine. *Acupuncture Today*, 8(9). Retrieved from https://www.acupuncturetoday.com/mpacms/at/article.php?id=31576.

Herbpathy. (n.d.). *Hypotonia herbal treatment, prevention, symptoms, causes, cured by*. Herbpathy: Make Life Healthy. Retrieved from https://herbpathy.com/Herbal-Treatment-for-Hypotonia-Cid4697.

Immel, J. (2019). *Flabby muscles/poor tone (muscle hypotonia) health remedies*. Joyful Belly School of Ayurveda. Retrieved from https://www.joyfulbelly.com/Ayurveda/symptom/Flabby-muscles-Poor-tone/899.

NHS website. (2018, October 3). *Hypotonia treatment*. NHS UK. Retrieved from https://www.nhs.uk/conditions/hypotonia/treatment/.

The Royal Children's Hospital Melbourne. (2018, September). *Low muscle tone*. Retrieved from https://www.rch.org.au/kidsinfo/fact_sheets/Low_muscle_tone/.

Young, R. M. (2019, April 12). *Acupuncture for kids, children*. Red Tent Health Centre. Retrieved from https://redtent.com.au/therapies/acupuncture/acupuncture-chinese-med-for-children/.

Speech Delay

Adams, C. (2019, October 1). *Herbs treat children with learning and behavior issues*. Heal Naturally. Retrieved from https://www.realnatural.org/herbal-medicine-treats-children-with-learning-and-behavioral-problems/.

Agrawal, M. (2017, April 21). *Effective home remedies for speech problems*. InlifeHealthCare. Retrieved from https://www.inlifehealthcare.com/effective-home-remedies-for-speech-problems/.

Bang, M., Lee, S. H., Cho, S. H., Yu, S. A., Kim, K., Lu, H. Y., et al. (2017). Herbal medicine treatment for children with autism spectrum disorder: A systematic review. *Evidence-Based Complementary and Alternative Medicine, 2017*, 1–12. Retrieved from https://doi.org/10.1155/2017/8614680.

Hartnett, J. K. (2019, November). *Delayed speech or language development (for parents)*. Nemours Kidshealth. Retrieved from https://kidshealth.org/en/parents/not-talk.html.

Herbpathy. (n.d.). *Speech disorder herbal treatment, prevention, symptoms, causes, cured by*. Herbpathy: Make Life Healthy. Retrieved from https://herbpathy.com/Herbal-Treatment-for-Speech-Disorder-Cid4519.

Mansfield, B. (2021, July 16). *10 speech therapy ideas to do at home (support your therapy with at-home practice)*. Your Modern Family. Retrieved from https://www.yourmodernfamily.com/helping-a-toddler-with-a-speech-delay-activity-ideas/.

McLaughlin, M. R. (2011). Speech and language delay in children. *American Family Physician, 83*(10), 1183–1188. Retrieved from https://www.aafp.org/afp/2011/0515/p1183.html.

Santos-Longhurst, A. (2019, May 9). *What is speech therapy?* Healthline. Retrieved from https://www.healthline.com/health/speech-therapy.

The SLP Solution. (2019, July 11). *How to help a late talker*. Speech and Language Kids. Retrieved from https://www.speechandlanguagekids.com/speech-delay-help/.

Upadhyay, K. (2017, January 31). *Speech disorders—how Ayurveda can help you?* Lybrate. Retrieved from https://www.lybrate.com/topic/speech-disorders-how-ayurveda-can-help-you/313579c5d166f64a81415917f063d504.

Attention-Deficit Hyperactivity Disorder

Centers for Disease Control and Prevention. (2020, September 4). *Parent training in behavior management for ADHD*. Retrieved from https://www.cdc.gov/ncbddd/adhd/behavior-therapy.html.

Hirning, T. (2015, November 16). *The SCD, GAPS, and paleo diets: How they compare and how they may help your patients*. The Great Plains Laboratory, Inc. Retrieved from https://www.greatplainslaboratory.com/articles-1/2015/11/13/the-scd-gaps-and-paleo-diets-how-they-compare-and-how-they-may-help-your-patients.

Matthews, J. (2008). *Nourishing hope for autism: Nutrition and diet guide for healing our children [perfect paperback]* (3rd ed.). Healthful Living Media. Retrieved from https://www.amazon.com/Nourishing-Hope-Autism-Nutrition-Paperback/dp/0981655807.

NHS website. (2021, March 25). *Attention deficit hyperactivity disorder (ADHD)*. NHS.UK. Retrieved from https://www.nhs.uk/conditions/attention-deficit-hyperactivity-disorder-adhd/treatment/.

Raman, R., & Arnarson, A. (2019, October 31). *7 Emerging benefits of bacopa monnieri (Brahmi)*. Healthline. Retrieved from https://www.healthline.com/nutrition/bacopa-monnieri-benefits.

Sitnikova, T. (2015, March 24). *12 Herbs that help stop ADHD*. NaturalON Natural Health News and Discoveries. Retrieved from https://naturalon.com/12-herbs-that-help-stop-adhd/view-all/.

Story, C. M. (2019, February 19). *Herbal remedies for ADHD*. Healthline. Retrieved from https://www.healthline.com/health/adhd/herbal-remedies#green-oats.

WebMD Editors. (2004a, July 1). *Non stimulants and other ADHD Drugs*. WebMD. Retrieved from https://www.webmd.com/add-adhd/adhd-nonstimulant-drugs-therapy.

WebMD Editors. (2004b, July 1). *Stimulant medications for ADHD*. WebMD. Retrieved from https://www.webmd.com/add-adhd/adhd-stimulant-therapy#1.

WebMD Editors. (2008a, September 18). *Attention deficit hyperactivity disorder (ADHD)*. WebMD. Retrieved from https://www.webmd.com/add-adhd/childhood-adhd/attention-deficit-hyperactivity-disorder-adhd#1.

WebMD Editors. (2008b, October 10). *Vitamins & supplements for ADHD*. WebMD. Retrieved from https://www.webmd.com/add-adhd/childhood-adhd/vitamins-supplements-adhd.

Windermere, A. (2020, July 15). *Should you try the GFCF (Gluten-Free CaseinFfree) diet?* HealthCentral. Retrieved from https://www.healthcentral.com/article/should-you-or-your-child-try-the-gfcf-glutenfree-caseinfree-diet.

Autism

Andrews, M. (2014). *Homeopathy and autism spectrum disorder: A guide for practitioners and families* (1st ed.). Singing Dragon. Retrieved from https://www.amazon.com/Homeopathy-Autism-Spectrum-Disorder-Practitioners/dp/1848191685.

Association for Science in Autism Treatment. (2019, August 1). *Sensory integrative therapy (Sensory Integration, SI, or SIT)*. ASAT: Association for Science in Autism Treatment. Retrieved from https://asatonline.org/for-parents/learn-more-about-specific-treatments/sensory-integrative-therapy-sensory-integration-si-or-sit/.

Autism Research Institute. (n.d.). *Implementing special diets*. Retrieved from https://www.autism.org/implementing-special-diets/.

Autism Speaks. (n.d.-a). *Applied behavior analysis (ABA)*. Retrieved from https://www.autismspeaks.org/applied-behavior-analysis.

Autism Speaks. (n.d.-b). *Occupational therapy (OT)*. Retrieved from https://www.autismspeaks.org/occupational-therapy-ot-0.

Autism Speaks. (n.d.-c). *Treatments for autism*. Retrieved from https://www.autismspeaks.org/treatments-autism.

Chunkath, S. R. (2018, July 15). *Ayurveda cure for autism*. The New Indian Express. Retrieved from https://www.newindianexpress.com/lifestyle/health/2018/jul/15/ayurveda-cure-for-autism-1842419.html.

Kaylene, K. (2018, February 1). *Everything you need to know about PECS*. Autistic Mama. Retrieved from https://autisticmama.com/pecs-picture-exchange-communication-system/.

Lee, S. H., Shin, S., Kim, T. H., Kim, S. M., Do, T. Y., Park, S., et al. (2019). Safety, effectiveness, and economic evaluation of an herbal medicine, Ukgansangajinpibanha granule, in children with autism spectrum disorder: A study protocol for a prospective, multicenter, randomized, double-blinded, placebo-controlled, parallel-group clinical trial. *Trials, 20*(1), 434. Retrieved from https://doi.org/10.1186/s13063-019-3537-7.

Matthews, J. (2008). *Nourishing hope for autism: Nutrition and diet guide for healing our children [perfect paperback]* (3rd ed.). Healthful Living Media. Retrieved from https://www.amazon.com/Nourishing-Hope-Autism-Nutrition-Paperback/dp/0981655807.

McKeny, P. T., Nessel, T. A., & Zito, P. M. (2021). *Antifungal antibiotics*. StatPearls Publishing. Retrieved from https://www.ncbi.nlm.nih.gov/books/NBK538168/.

Morales-Brown, L. (2020, September 3). *What to know about chelation therapy*. Medical News Today. Retrieved from https://www.medicalnewstoday.com/articles/chelation-therapy.

National Autistic Society. (2020, August 20). *Strategies and interventions*. (n.d.). Autism.Org.Uk. https://www.autism.org.uk/advice-and-guidance/topics/strategies-and-interventions.

Pranaji, S. (2014). *Autism and varma therapy: A parent's guide*. Persatuan Siddha Varma Kalai Malaysia.

Riordan, N. H. (2020). *Stem cell therapy for autism*. Stem Cell Institute. Retrieved from https://www.cellmedicine.com/stem-cell-therapy-for-autism/.

Sakulchit, T., Ladish, C., & Goldman, R. D. (2017). Hyperbaric oxygen therapy for children with autism spectrum disorder. *Canadian Family Physician, 63*(6), 446–448. Retrieved from https://www.ncbi.nlm.nih.gov/pmc/articles/PMC5471082/.

Unlock Food Canada. (2019, March 26). *Autism and nutrition*. Unlock Food. Retrieved from https://www.unlockfood.ca/en/Articles/Childrens-Nutrition/Health-Conditions/Autism-and-Nutrition.aspx.

WebMD Editors. (2002, April 1). *Autism*. WebMD. Retrieved from https://www.webmd.com/brain/autism/understanding-autism-basics#1.

WebMD Editors. (2008, September 9). *Gluten free/casein free diets for autism*. WebMD. Retrieved from https://www.webmd.com/brain/autism/gluten-free-casein-free-diets-for-autism#1.

Cerebral Palsy

Cerebral Palsy Treatment Hospital Staff. (2015, June 25). *Traditional Chinese Medicine Treatment of Cerebral Palsy*. (n.d.). Cerebral Palsy Treatment Hospital. https://cerebralpalsychina.wordpress.com/2015/06/25/traditional-chinese-medicine-treatment-of-cerebral-palsy/.

Charaka The Speciality Ayurveda. (n.d.). *Cerebral palsy (CP)*. Charaka. Retrieved from http://charaka.org/cerebral-palsy/.

Chauhan, M. (2020, March 11). *Ayurvedic treatment of cerebral palsy*. Planet Ayurveda. Retrieved from https://www.planetayurveda.com/library/cerebral-palsy/.

Healthcare Medicine Institute. (2020, June 20). *Acupuncture alleviates cerebral palsy*. HealthCMi. Retrieved from https://www.healthcmi.com/Acupuncture-Continuing-Education-News/1763-acupuncture-alleviates-cerebral-palsy.

Jansheski, G. (2020, February 29). *Cerebral palsy treatment*. Cerebral Palsy Guidance. Retrieved from https://www.cerebralpalsyguidance.com/cerebral-palsy/treatment/.

NHS website. (2020, October 19). *Cerebral palsy treatment*. NHS. UK. Retrieved from https://www.nhs.uk/conditions/cerebral-palsy/treatment/.

Patwa, J. V. (2015, September 11). *Living with cerebral palsy*. Lybrate. Retrieved from https://www.lybrate.com/topic/ayurveda-helps-in-cerebral-palsy-cerebral-palsy-refers-to-a-group-of-neurological-disorders-that-app-8600/d8eb357da59139f03f0e42e0d0fddb1c.

Peterson, B. (2018, February 7). *Natural remedies for cerebral palsy symptoms*. Cerebral Palsy Group. Retrieved from http://cerebralpalsygroup.com/natural-remedies-cerebral-palsy-symptoms/.

Sanger, T. D. (2019). Deep brain stimulation for cerebral palsy: Where are we now? *Developmental Medicine & Child Neurology, 62*(1), 28–33. Retrieved from https://doi.org/10.1111/dmcn.14295.

Sharan D. (2017). Orthopedic surgery in cerebral palsy: Instructional course lecture. *Indian Journal of Orthopaedics, 51*(3), 240–255. Retrieved from https://doi.org/10.4103/ortho.IJOrtho_197_16.

Staughton, J. (2020, September 22). *13 Natural ways to help with cerebral palsy*. Organic Facts. Retrieved from https://www.organicfacts.net/home-remedies/cerebral-palsy.html#fish-oil.

Stern, K. A. (n.d.). *Treatment for cerebral palsy*. Cerebralpalsy.Org. Retrieved from https://www.cerebralpalsy.org/about-cerebral-palsy/treatment.

Wang, J., Shi, W., Khiati, D., Shi, B., Shi, X., Luo, D., et al. (2020). Acupuncture treatment on the motor area of the scalp for motor dysfunction in children with cerebral palsy: Study protocol for a multicenter randomized controlled trial. *Trials, 21*(1), 29.

Warmbrodt, R. (2020, March 29). *Homeopathy treatment for cerebral palsy*. Cerebral Palsy Guidance. Retrieved from https://www.cerebralpalsyguidance.com/cerebral-palsy/treatment/homeopathy/.

WebMD Editors. (2017, April 24). *What is cerebral palsy? What causes it?* WebMD. Retrieved from https://www.webmd.com/children/guide/understanding-cerebral-palsy-basic-information#1.

Yin Yang House. (n.d.). *Tam healing and tong ren therapy for cerebral palsy*. Retrieved from https://theory.yinyanghouse.com/treatments/tongren-treatment-of-cerebral-palsy.

Dementia

Alzheimer's Drug Discovery Foundation. (2016, June 1). *Cinnamon & your Brain*. Cognitive Vitality. Retrieved from https://www.alzdiscovery.org/cognitive-vitality/ratings/cinnamon.

Bhowmik, D. (n.d.). *Traditional Indian memory enhancer herbs and their medicinal importance | Abstract*. Traditional Indian Memory Enhancer Herbs and Their Medicinal Importance. https://www.scholarsresearchlibrary.com/abstract/traditional-indian-memory-enhancer-herbs-and-their-medicinal-importance-5272.html.

Cohen, P. (2015, March 30). *The MIND diet: 10 foods that fight Alzheimer's (and 5 to avoid)*. CBS News. Retrieved from https://www.cbsnews.com/media/mind-diet-foods-avoid-alzheimers-boost-brain-health/.

Farooqui, A. A., Farooqui, T., Madan, A., Ong, J. H. J., & Ong, W. Y. (2018). Ayurvedic medicine for the treatment of dementia: Mechanistic aspects. *Evidence-Based Complementary and Alternative Medicine, 2018*, 1–11. Retrieved from https://doi.org/10.1155/2018/2481076.

Gaeddert, A. (2003, April 1). The herbal approaches to treating memory loss, dementia, and alzheimer. *Acupuncture Today, 4*(4). Retrieved from https://www.acupuncturetoday.com/mpacms/at/article.php?id=28184.

Group, E. (2015, October 5). *5 Herbs and spices for dementia*. Dr. Group's Healthy Living Articles. Retrieved from https://explore.globalhealing.com/herbs-spices-for-dementia/.

Gunnars, K., & Arnarson, A. (2020, February 12). *Top 10 evidence-based health benefits of coconut oil*. Healthline. Retrieved from https://www.healthline.com/nutrition/top-10-evidence-based-health-benefits-of-coconut-oil#TOC_TITLE_HDR_2.

Gandhi, B. (n.d.). *10 Foods that prevent dementia & Alzheimer's*. Mindbodygreen. https://www.mindbodygreen.com/0-7613/10-foods-that-prevent-dementia-alzheimers.html.

Harvard Health Publishing. (2014, July 16). Worried about your memory? Take action. Health Harvard Edu. https://www.health.harvard.edu/mind-and-mood/worried-about-your-memory-take-action.

Jenarius, R. G. (2018, July 4). *9 yoga asanas that can boost memory power and keep degenerative diseases at bay*. IndiaTimes. Retrieved from https://www.indiatimes.com/health/tips-tricks/9-yoga-asanas-that-can-boost-memory-power-and-keep-degenerative-diseases-at-bay-348654.html.

Lin, Z., Gu, J., Xiu, J., Mi, T., Dong, J., & Tiwari, J. K. (2012). Traditional Chinese medicine for senile dementia. *Evidence-Based Complementary and Alternative Medicine, 2012*, 1–13. Retrieved from https://doi.org/10.1155/2012/692621.

Mayo Clinic Staff. (2021, April 6). *Can music help someone with Alzheimer's?* Mayo Clinic. Retrieved from https://www.mayoclinic.org/diseases-conditions/alzheimers-disease/expert-answers/music-and-alzheimers/faq-20058173.

Wegerer, J. (2021, May 1). *The benefits of ashwagandha, a natural way to fight Alzheimer's*. Alzheimers.Net. https://www.alzheimers.net/ashwagandha-for-alzheimers.

NHS website. (2020, July 2). *What are the treatments for dementia?* NHS.UK. Retrieved from https://www.nhs.uk/conditions/dementia/treatment/.

Rao, R. V., Descamps, O., John, V., & Bredesen, D. E. (2012). Ayurvedic medicinal plants for Alzheimer's disease: A review. *Alzheimer's Research & Therapy, 4*(3), 22–31. Retrieved from https://doi.org/10.1186/alzrt125.

Rosenbloom, C. (n.d.). *10 foods that can help fight dementia*. Chatelaine. https://www.chatelaine.com/health/foods-that-fight-dementia/.

Salamon, M. (2018, March 20). *Dementia treatments: Medication, therapy, diet, and exercise*. WebMD. Retrieved from https://www.webmd.com/alzheimers/dementia-treatments-overview#1.

Sumner, I. L., Edwards, R. A., Asuni, A. A., & Teeling, J. L. (2018). Antibody engineering for optimized immunotherapy in Alzheimer's disease. *Frontiers in Neuroscience, 12*. Retrieved from https://doi.org/10.3389/fnins.2018.00254.

Susannah, S. (2021, September 2). *How to make pine needle tea (benefits & pine tea recipe)*. HealthyGreenSavvy. Retrieved from https://www.healthygreensavvy.com/pine-needle-tea-how-make-benefits/.

Teitelbaum, J. (2016, November 1). *7 Powerful ways to protect your brain and prevent dementia*. Better Nutrition. Retrieved from https://www.betternutrition.com/conditions-and-wellness/ways-prevent-dementia/.

WebMD Editors. (2006, February 3). *Dementia*. WebMD. Retrieved from https://www.webmd.com/alzheimers/types-dementia#1.

William, A. (2019, July 7). *How celery juice helps Alzheimer's, dementia & memory issues*. Medical Medium. Retrieved from https://www.medicalmedium.com/blog/how-celery-juice-helps-alzheimers-dementia-memory-issues.

Wong, C., & Kelly, C. (2020, February 3). *Herbs and spices to help improve your brain health*. Verywell Mind. Retrieved from https://www.verywellmind.com/best-herbs-and-spices-for-brain-health-4047818.

Yan, H., Li, L., & Tang, X. C. (2007). Treating senile dementia with traditional Chinese medicine. *Clinical Interventions in Aging, 2*(2), 201–208. Retrieved from https://www.ncbi.nlm.nih.gov/pmc/articles/PMC2684515/.

Stroke

American Heart Association. (n.d.). *Types of stroke*. Stroke.Org. Retrieved from https://www.stroke.org/en/about-stroke/types-of-stroke.

Greger, M. (n.d.). *How your spice rack could stop you having a stroke, you can cut your blood pressure with.........* Algoa fm. https://www.algoafm.co.za/kaycee-rossouw/how-your-spice-rack-could-stop-you-having-a-stroke-you-can-cut-your-blood-pressure-with.

Mdhealthonline. (2020, August 25). *Caulis Spatholobi: An Herb Of Many Purposes–From Blood Flow To Immune Systems*. (n.d.). MDhealthonline. https://mdhealthonline.com/blog/caulis-spatholobi-an-herb-of-many-purposes-from-blood-flow-to-immune-systems/.

Meenal D., M. (2018, April 28). *Ayurvedic treatment for stroke*. Nirogam. Retrieved from https://nirogam.com/ayurvedic-treatment-for-stroke/.

Mercola, J. (2011, March 2). *Common spice curcumin, protects and rebuild brain cells after stroke*. Stroke. (n.d.). Mount Sinai Health System. https://www.mountsinai.org/health-library/condition/stroke.

Narsaria, R. (2019, April 18). *Homeopathic medicine, treatment and remedies for Dementia*. MyUpchar. Retrieved from https://www.myupchar.com/en/disease/dementia/homeopathy.

Nutrition Review. (2013, April 22). *Herbal support for speedy recovery after stroke, heart attack and surgery*. Retrieved from https://nutritionreview.org/2013/04/herbal-support-speedy-recovery-stroke-heart-attack-surgery/.

TCM Simple. (2021). *Chinese medicine treatment for stroke*. Tcmsimple.Com. Retrieved from https://www.tcmsimple.com/stroke.php.

The Healthline Editorial Team. (2019, June 1). *Complementary and alternative treatments for stroke*. Healthline. Retrieved from https://www.healthline.com/health/stroke/alternative-treatments.

Wang, Y., Zhang, L., Pan, Y. J., Fu, W., Huang, S. W., Xu, B., et al. (2020). Investigation of invigorating qi and activating blood circulation prescriptions in treating qi deficiency and blood stasis syndrome of ischemic stroke patients: Study protocol for a randomized controlled trial. *Frontiers in Pharmacology, 11*. Retrieved from https://doi.org/10.3389/fphar.2020.00892.

WebMD Editors. (n.d.). *Diagnosis & treatment*. WebMD. Retrieved from https://www.webmd.com/stroke/guide/stroke-treatment-care.

Zhong, L. L. D., Kun, W., Shi, N., Ziea, T. C., Ng, B. F. L., Gao, Y., et al. (2020). Evidence-based chinese medicine clinical practice guideline for stroke in Hong Kong. *Chinese Medicine, 15*(1). Retrieved from https://doi.org/10.1186/s13020-020-00397-9.

Parkinson's Disease

Axe, J. (2018, April 17). *Parkinson's disease natural treatment & remedies —in 5 steps*. Dr. Axe. Retrieved from https://draxe.com/health/parkinsons-disease-natural-treatment-remedies/.

Essa, M. M., Manivasagam, T., Thenmozhi, A. J., Dhanalakshmi, C., & Khan, M. A. S. (2016). Food and Parkinson's Disease. In *Spices and Parkinson's Disease* (pp. 59–75). Nova Science Publishers, Inc. Retrieved from https://squ.pure.elsevier.com/en/publications/spices-and-parkinsons-disease.

Groiss, S. J., Wojtecki, L., Südmeyer, M., & Schnitzler, A. (2009). Deep brain stimulation in Parkinson's disease. *Therapeutic Advances in Neurological Disorders, 2*(6), 20–28. Retrieved from https://doi.org/10.1177/1756285609339382.

Group, E. (2015, December 14). *5 Herbs and spices for parkinson's disease*. Dr. Group's Healthy Living Articles. Retrieved from https://explore.globalhealing.com/5-herbs-and-spices-for-parkinsons-disease/.

Halpern, M. (2017, June 30). *Parkinson's disease (kampavata): Understanding the Ayurvedic approach*. California College of Ayurveda. Retrieved from https://www.ayurvedacollege.com/blog/parkinson/.

Homepage. (n.d.). *Be the cure for Parkinson's*. Parkinson's UK. Retrieved from https://www.parkinsons.org.uk.

Mayo Clinic Staff. (2020, December 8). *Parkinson's disease diagnosis and treatment*. Mayo Clinic. Retrieved from https://www.mayoclinic.org/diseases-conditions/parkinsons-disease/diagnosis-treatment/drc-20376062.

Mumal, I. (2018, July 25). *Chinese compound helps reduce levodopa-induced dyskinesia, eases motor symptoms in Parkinson's, study finds.* Parkinson's News Today. Retrieved from https://parkinsonsnews-today.com/2018/07/25/parkinsons-disease-chinese-compound-with-levodopa-eases-motor-symptoms/.

NHS website. (2019a, May 9). *Parkinson's disease causes.* NHS.UK. Retrieved from https://www.nhs.uk/conditions/parkinsons-disease/causes/.

NHS website. (2019b, May 9). *Parkinson's disease treatment.* NHS. UK. Retrieved from https://www.nhs.uk/conditions/parkinsons-disease/treatment/.

Nutrition house Canada. (n.d.). *Parkinson's disease (PD).* Retrieved from https://www.nutritionhouse.com/Library/WellnessItem.aspx?ID=63974.

WebMD Editors. (n.d.). *Treatment & care.* WebMD. Retrieved from https://www.webmd.com/parkinsons-disease/guide/parkinsons-treatment-care.

Weil, A. (2016, November 15). *Cat's claw: An herbal treatment for parkinson's disease?* DrWeil.Com. Retrieved from https://www.drweil.com/vitamins-supplements-herbs/herbs/cats-claw-an-herbal-treatment-for-parkinsons-disease/.

11
Mental Health

Introduction

The following common mental health disorders are discussed:
1. Anxiety disorders
2. Depression
3. Schizophrenia
4. Insomnia

Various amino acids are precursors in the synthesis of different brain neurotransmitters which regulate mental health, emotions, behavior, memory, attention, learning, and sleep.

These amino acids include L-theanine, L-glutamine, L-tyrosine, L-tryptophan/5HTP, D-phenylalanine, and GABA.

The brain's excitatory neurotransmitters include acetylcholine, biogenic amines (dopamine, norepinephrine, epinephrine, serotonin, and histamine), and glutamate. The inhibitory neurotransmitter is GABA.

Dopamine and norepinephrine are synthesized from tyrosine. Serotonin is synthesized from tryptophan. Histamine is synthesized from histidine.

Neurotransmitter deficiency can cause various mental health problems. For example, low serotonin level is associated with phobias, panic attacks, social anxiety, mental chatter, intrusive thoughts, and insomnia. Low GABA levels are associated with symptoms of anxiety or panic attacks. However, the validity of a food frequency questionnaire (FFQ) in estimating amino acid intake is low to moderate.

Neurotechnology tools like functional near-infrared spectroscopy (fNIRS) can be screening tools to differentiate between different mental health disorders like depression, schizophrenia, and bipolar disorder.

Wearable neurotechnology and Articifical Intelligence (AI) to decode one's thoughts is in development. However, the NeuroRights Foundation protects and ensures human rights and privacy.

Organic brain syndromes can mimic mental health conditions and they must be carefully excluded with appropriate investigations.

General Management: Diet, Lifestyle, and Environmental Modification

- Take vitamin and mineral supplements such as folic acid; vitamins B6, B12, and D; and magnesium. Some of these may help in the methylation pathway. Omega-3 fatty acids and virgin coconut oil may also benefit.
- Environmental toxicity must be minimized and mitigated via toxic-free practices. Food, water, soil, and air must be clean. Cellular health via immune, hormonal, and mitochondrial pathways must not be poisoned so that mental health is normal.
- A 5-HTP amino acid supplement may also help.
- Eat whole foods and/or functional foods that are anti-inflammatory, antioxidant, and rich in vitamin B (especially folate in dark-green leafy vegetables and lentils and B$_{12}$ in animal foods only). Avoid refined carbohydrates, sugars, and processed foods.
- Quit smoking, alcohol, caffeinated beverages, and recreational drugs. They overstimulate the nervous system, disrupt sleep, and cause higher stress and anxiety levels. Avoid substance abuse.
- Reduce social media time. Excessive screen time is disruptive to the nervous system. Make real friends. This can also reduce cyberbullying.
  - Live a life of purpose
- Engage in sports and outdoor activities. Do regular light exercise, especially in the open air. Even a gentle walk is therapeutic. This can boost endorphin production and reduce feelings of anxiety for a few hours after exercising.
- Sit down. Do meditation, relaxation, abdominal breathing techniques, or guided visualization.
- Practice yoga. Choose one that suits best. Pranayama yoga is the practice of controlling the breath. It helps to calm the mind, reduce stress and anxiety, and improve body health.
  - Common types of pranayama yoga are nadi shodhana, kapalabhati pranayama, and bhastrika pranayama.
  - Ujjayi pranayama: It is also known as ocean/hissing breath and is performed by filling the lungs completely while slightly contracting the throat and breathing through the nose.
  - Alternate/same-side nose breathing: This is a breathing technique involving breathing through one or alternate nostrils.
- Ensure good sleep hygiene. Set a proper routine for bedtime and stop using electronics one hour before bedtime.

- Virtual reality. This is being explored as a tool to improve mood, reduce anxiety, and improve overall emotional well-being, especially in the elderly.

Support and Psychotherapies

- Counselling sessions, social rehabilitation, and support groups are also beneficial. Increase social interaction with young people or at places of worship or clubs.
- Cognitive behavior therapy (CBT): This form of psychotherapy is the most effective. It helps to modify thinking, feeling, and behavior. It combines "cognitive therapy" and "behavior therapy" so that a person has healthy thoughts and behaviors.
- Other forms of psychotherapy include talk therapy, psychodynamic or psychoanalytic therapy (for long-standing unresolved issues with a focus on the past and unconscious thoughts), interpersonal therapy (for relationship issues), dialectical therapy (learn coping skills, mindfulness, and crisis coaching), family therapy, couple therapy, and humanistic therapy(client-centered therapy for a better sense of self, i.e., self-actualization with focus on the present and future and on the conscious thoughts). All these types can be done as an individual, a group, a family, or a couple.

Anxiety Disorders

Anxiety is a normal aspect of life that occurs with stress. Anxiety disorders, however, involve worry or fear that is not temporary. The anxiety may not go away and may interfere with daily activities and social interactions. It may also worsen over time. There are several types of anxiety disorders:

- **Generalized anxiety disorders.** Symptoms include feeling restless and on edge, fatigue, difficulty focusing, irritability, increased muscle tension, and sleep problems.
- **Panic disorders.** People with panic disorders often suffer recurrent panic attacks. These attacks may be brought on by a trigger, such as an object or a particular situation. Symptoms include an increased or pounding heartbeat, sweating, trembling, shortness of breath, feelings of impending doom, and a lack of control. These people tend to avoid situations they worry might bring on an attack, which often leads to a progression to other problems such as agoraphobia.
- **Phobia-related disorders.** A phobia is an intense fear of a specific object or situation. The fear felt is often disproportionate to the amount of danger the object may cause. They may actively avoid the object or situation, which may lead to other social complications. Social phobia, now called social anxiety disorder (SAD) starts in childhood. There is a persistent and intense fear of being observed or negatively assessed in performance or social situations leading to poor school performance and social isolation.

Indian Natural Remedies

Common Ingredients for Anxiety

Spices	Herbs/Leaves	Miscellaneous
Ginger	Brahmi (Bacopa monnieri)	Baking soda
	False daisy/bhringraj (Eclipta prostrata)	Essential oils: vetiver, lavender, rose, and frankincense
	Jatamansi (Nardostachys jatamansi)	Milk
	Ashwagandha (Withania somnifera)	Honey
	Vacha (Acorus calamus)	Rudraksha (Elaeocarpus ganitrus)
	Kava (Piper methysticum)	

Common Recipes

Oral

Teas/Brews/Others

Ashwagandha milk. Mix 1 teaspoon of ashwagandha in a cup of warm milk. Drink once a day at bedtime. Alternatively, take ashwagandha in the form of a capsule or a liquid extract.

Brahmi tea. Place about two to three stalks of fresh brahmi leaves into a cup. Pour boiling water over the leaves. Steep for about 10 to 15 minutes. Strain and add honey.

False daisy tea. Place 2 teaspoons of dried false daisy herbs in a cup of hot water. Steep for 5to 10 minutes. Strain and add honey. Drink warm.

Ginger tea. Lightly pound 1 to 2 inches of cut ginger and add to a cup of hot water. Steep for 5 to 10 minutes. Strain and drink.

Jatamansi brew. Add a pinch of jatamansi root powder to a cup of warm water and take it twice a day.

Kava tea. Place 1 to 2 teaspoons of kava root in a cup of hot water. Steep for 5 to 10 minutes before straining. Drink it warm.

Vacha tea. Place 1 to 2 teaspoons of vacha herbs into a cup of hot water. Steep for 5 to 10 minutes. Strain and drink warm.

Therapeutic Measures

Essential oil aromatherapy. Essential oils such as lavender, vetiver, jasmine, rose, etc. have calming properties and may help to reduce feelings of anxiety and stress. Dilute a few drops of the chosen essential oil with some water and add the mixture to a humidifier/diffuser. If a humidifier is not available, sprinkle some of the essential oils on clothes or bed sheets.

Ginger-baking soda or Epsom salt bath. Fill up a warm bath and add some crushed or sliced ginger about 3 to 5 inches long. Add in about ½ cup of baking soda (or Epsom salt) and mix with a hand until it dissolves. Get into the bath and soak for 30 to 45 minutes.

Meditation. Refer to details under *Introduction*.

Yoga. Various asanas can help boost GABA levels and reduce anxiety. These include: child's pose (Balasana), corpse pose (Savasana), easy pose (Sukhasana), shoulderstand (Salamba Sarvangasana), downward-facing dog pose (Adho Mukha Svanasana), butterfly pose (Baddha Konasana), upward-facing dog pose (Ūrdhva Mukha Svānāsana), and standing forward fold pose (Uttanasana).

Sudarshan kriya yoga. It is a type of rhythmic breathing technique that promotes deep mental relaxation, improves mental clarity and promotes overall good health.

Rudraksha. Wear a 5 or 7 mukhi (face) Rudraksha as a bracelet or a *mala* (necklace) to calm the nervous system and decrease stress.

Chinese Natural Remedies

Common Ingredients for Anxiety

Herbs/Leaves	Miscellaneous
Cynomorium/suo yang (Cynomorium songaricum)	
Dang gui root	
Ginkgo (Ginkgo biloba)	Jujube date
Ginseng	
Glycyrrhiza glabra (liquorice root/gan cao)	
Polygonum root	Polyrhachis ant
Rehmannia root	Longan (Dimocarpus longan)
Reishi	

Common Recipes

Oral

Teas/Brews

Ginkgo dessert. Ginkgo is often consumed in a sweet dessert with dried bean curd. Dried beancurd is not known to have any benefit to mental health, however. Place five pieces of ginkgo into a pot. Add some dried bean curd (fu chuk) and approximately 2 cups of hot water. Bring to a boil and add some rock sugar to taste. Drink the liquid and eat the ginkgo. Alternatively, consume ginkgo in the form of an extract, which is available as a commercial preparation.

Ginseng tea. Add about two to four slices of ginseng to a cup. Add hot water over the ginseng. Steep for about 10 to 15 minutes.

Liquorice tea. Add 1 teaspoon of ground liquorice to a pot with 1 cup of boiling water. Allow to simmer for 30 to 45 minutes before straining.

Longan. It can be consumed daily as tea or soup.

Therapeutic Measures

Acupressure

- Hall of impression
  - This point is in the midline of the face exactly between the eyebrows.
- Heavenly gate point
  - This point is located in the upper depression of the ear at the tip of the innermost hollow.
- Shoulder well point
  - This point is found in the middle of the shoulder muscle. It can be massaged by pinching the middle of the shoulder muscle between a finger and thumb.
- Union valley point
  - This point is located in the middle of the webbing between the thumb and index finger.
- Great surge point
  - This point is on the top of the foot about two to three finger widths above the intersection of the big and second toe.
- Inner frontier gate point
  - This point is on the inner forearm about three-finger widths below the wrist crease.

Acupuncture

This needling technique can also reduce stress and anxiety. It regulates the *xing* (physical body), restores qi, and balances *shen* (mind and spirit) so that emotional health is maintained.

Tai chi. It can also boost GABA levels and allay anxiety.

Aromatherapy

Ho wood essential oil is relaxing, reduces stress and anxiety, and can improve emotional and mental wellbeing.

Western/Other Natural Remedies

Common Ingredients for Anxiety

Spices	Herbs/ Leaves/ Flowers	Miscellaneous
Dried orange peel	St John's wort (Hypericum perforatum)	Valerian root (Valeriana officinalis)
	Rosemary	Maca root (Lepidium meyenii)
	Dried lavender flower	Phosphatidylserine
	Chamomile flower	Essential oils (geranium, etc)
	Passionflower (Passiflora)	GABA supplements
	California poppy	Amino acid supplements (L-theanine, L-glutamine, L-tyrosine, L-tryptophan/5HTP, D-phenylalanine)
	Catnip	Griffonia simplicifolia seeds (5-HTP extract)
	Pulsatilla	
	Saffron (Crocus Sativus)	
	Rose/Rosehip oil (Rosa damascena)	
	Verbena (Verbena officinalis)	
Ginger	Thyme	Arctic root (Rhodiola rosea)

Common Recipes

Oral

Teas/Brews/Others

Arctic root tea. Add 1 to 2 teaspoons of dried Arctic root to a cup and cover. Allow to steep for 5 to 10 minutes. Strain and drink it warm.

Bitters recipe. Place 28 g of lavender, 1 teaspoon of dried valerian root, 2 teaspoons of dried passion flower, 1 teaspoon of dried orange peel, and ½ teaspoon of dried ginger into a glass jar. Cover the herbs with just enough alcohol (e.g., vodka) to submerge the herbs fully. Seal tightly and store the jar in a dark, cool place for 2 to 4 weeks. Shake the jar once a day. When ready, strain through a piece of muslin cloth into a clean jar and store at room temperature. To serve, mix a few drops in hot tea or water. It may also be consumed as a tincture.

California poppy. It can be combined with hawthorn and magnesium.

Chamomile tea. Place some dried or fresh chamomile flowers into a cup. Pour boiling water over the flowers and allow to steep for 10 minutes. Strain and add honey to taste. Drink hot.

Ginger tea. As above.

Maca root tea. Place 1 to 2 teaspoons of maca powder into a cup of hot water and mix well. Drink it warm.

Psilocybin. This is a psychedelic compound isolated from magic mushrooms. It gives immediate and long-term positive effects.

Rosemary tea. Add three to five sprigs of fresh rosemary (or 1 ½ teaspoons of dry rosemary leaf needles) to a cup of hot water and steep for 10 to 15 minutes. Drink it warm.

Saffron tea. Take a pinch of saffron. Add 1 cup of boiling water. Steep for 10 minutes. Strain and consume. Add a lemon slice and a sweetener if desired.

　#Variation 1. Saffron threads can be added to rissoto and paella (preferbaly soaked in hot water first).

St John's wort. Place 2 tablespoons of St John's wort in a teapot with about 6 cups of hot water. Cover and let steep for 3 to 10 minutes before straining. Add a little honey to taste. Drink it warm.

Thyme tea. Add one to two sprigs of dried thyme to a cup of hot water. Steep for 10 to 15 minutes. Drink it warm.

Valerian root tea. Those who have severe anxiety may use about 600 mg of valerian root. Valerian root is available commercially in doses of about 200 mg, which may be brewed as a tea.

Verbena tea. Take 1 tablespoon of fresh lemon verbena leaves or 1 teaspoon of dried leaves. Add 1 cup of boiling water. Steep or simmer for 15 minutes. Strain and consume warm with a desired sweetener.

Therapeutic measures

Supplements

Amino acid supplements. L-theanine, L-glutamine, L-tyrosine, L-tryptophan/5HTP, and D-phenylalanine can help.

Griffonia simplicifolia seeds are rich in 5-HTP.

Aromatherapy or massages with essential oils. Read under "Insomnia."

GABA supplements. These can be given via the sublingual route.

Lifestyle measures. Camping Office refers to working outdoors and surrounded by nature or in a rural setting to achieve a low stress environment.

Phosphatidylserine. It is available as a supplement. It should be given in the morning for a trial period of 1 month.

Cognitive behavior therapy and other general measures (listed earlier).

Modern Remedies

Psychotherapy

Psychotherapy is often considered a key aspect of treatment for anxiety. It can alleviate symptoms of anxiety and is often made up of two segments: psychodynamic psychotherapy and supportive expressive therapy. They focus on anxiety as an extension of feelings about important relationships. There is another form of therapy called CBT, which teaches individuals about behavioral relaxation techniques and restructuring of their thinking patterns to help them control their anxiety and reduce incidences of anxious thoughts. CBT is recommended as a long-term standard treatment for anxiety disorders.

Online CBT or internet-delivered supportive therapy has been particularly useful for SAD since an office visit is often an anxiety-triggering situation.

Selective Serotonin Reuptake Inhibitors

Serotonin is a neurotransmitter in the brain responsible for feelings of happiness and contentment. Patients suffering from anxiety may have a lack of serotonin. Selective serotonin reuptake inhibitors (SSRIs) relieve anxiety and depression symptoms by blocking the reuptake of the chemical serotonin in the brain. This means that there is more serotonin left available, which boosts mood. The onset of action is 2 to 6 weeks. They are not habit-forming. Side effects include fatigue, headaches, dry mouth, nausea, blurred vision, erectile dysfunction, and weight gain.

Examples: citalopram, paroxetine, sertraline, fluvoxamine.

Serotonin-Norepinephrine Reuptake Inhibitors

Serotonin-norepinephrine reuptake inhibitors (SNRIs) increase the levels of serotonin and norepinephrine in the brain. This is done by inhibiting their reuptake similar to the action of SSRIs. This is useful in helping to boost the moods of the patient suffering from anxiety and depression. The onset of action is also long like the SSRIs. Side effects include high blood pressure, constipation, nausea, and fatigue.

Example: venlafaxine, duloxetine.

Benzodiazepines

These are sedative drugs and are often used for short-term treatment of anxiety or as an add-on medication to other anxiety medications. They are effective in promoting muscle relaxation and relieving physical symptoms of anxiety. They are habit-forming.

Examples: alprazolam, lorazepam, diazepam.

Tricyclic Antidepressants

Tricyclic antidepressants are often preferred over the long-term use of benzodiazepines. However, there are significant side effects such as dry mouth, hypotension, and constipation.

Example: amitriptyline, imipramine, nortriptyline.

Beta Blockers

Although these are used to treat hypertension, it decreases the effects of norepinephrine so that physical symptoms of anxiety are relieved.

Example: propranolol.

Pulsed electromagnetic therapy (PEMF). PEMF therapy is used to modify the neurochemical circuits to increase serotonin, dopamine and melatonin and reduce the stress hormones.

Homeopathic Remedies

These include *Arsenicum album, Calcarea carb, Argentum nitricum, Ignatia, Gelsemium, Lycopodium,* kali phosphoricum, *Pulsatilla, Stramonium,* and silica.

Depression

Depression is an increasingly common mood disorder. It causes severe symptoms that may negatively affect day-to-day activities and social relationships. A diagnosis of depression is made when the symptoms have been present for at least two weeks. There are a few different forms of depression:

- **Persistent depressive disorder:** This is also known as dysthymia and is a depressed mood lasting more than 2 years. Patients may experience bouts of major depression with less severe symptoms, but the symptoms must have lasted for at least 2 years to be considered a persistent depressive disorder.
- **Psychotic depression:** This form of depression occurs when a person has depression with some symptoms of psychosis, such as delusions or hallucinations. Psychosis often revolves around themes such as poverty, guilt, or illness.
- **Seasonal affective disorder:** Seasonal affective disorder is the onset of depression during the winter when there is a reduction in the amount of natural sunlight. This depression is generally relieved by spring and summer.
- **Postpartum depression:** Postpartum depression is a severe form of anxiety and depressive symptoms experienced by women after giving birth. They experience major depression during and after pregnancy, with feelings of extreme sadness, anxiety, and fatigue.

General Management

- Exclude medical conditions that are commonly associated with depression. Example: thyroid disorders, epilepsy, dementia, post-stroke, ischemic heart disease, multiple sclerosis, and endocrine disorders. Do basic blood investigations.
- Exclude also other comorbid psychiatric conditions. Example: anxiety.
- Look also for medications that are known to cause depression.
- Differential diagnoses include bipolar disorder.
- Refer further under "Introduction & General Management: Mental Health Disorders."

Indian Natural Remedies

Common Ingredients for Depression

Spices	Herbs/Leaves	Miscellaneous
Cardamom seed	Brahmi (*Bacopa monnieri*)	Rose petal
	Shankhpushpi (*Convolvulus pluricaulis*)	Apple, banana
	Jatamansi (*Nardostachys jatamansi*)	Milk
	Ashwagandha (*Withania somnifera*)	Honey
	Pudina (peppermint)	Avocado leaves (*Persea americana*)
	Holy basil (tulsi)	Coconut oil
	Sage	Seeds: Sesame seeds and Pumpkin seeds
		Rudraksha (*Elaeocarpus ganitrus*)

Common Recipes

Oral

Teas/Brews/Others

Apple milk. Add some honey to warm milk, stirring until warm. Eat an apple and drink the milk with it.

Ashwagandha. Add 2 tablespoons of ashwagandha to a glass of hot milk. Stir in 1 teaspoon of ghee. Drink twice a day.

Banana. Eat at least five bananas a day, gradually decreasing the number to 1 in time.

Brahmi juice. Place a handful of the fresh brahmi leaves into a blender and add up to 1 cup of water. Blend until smooth. Add honey to taste and drink.

Brahmi tea. Place about two to three stalks of fresh brahmi leaves into a cup. Pour boiling water over the leaves. Steep for about 10 to 15 minutes. Add honey to taste and drink.

Cardamom brew. Grind two green cardamom seeds into a fine powder. Stir the powder into a cup of hot water. Drink warm at least twice a day.

Coconut oil. Consume 1 tablespoon of coconut oil once a day.

Holy basil tea. Place two to five fresh holy basil leaves into a cup of hot water. Cover and steep for 5 to 10 minutes before drinking. Alternatively, chew three to five leaves.

Jatamansi brew. Add a pinch of jatamansi root powder to a cup of warm water and take it twice a day.

Pudina tea. Place three to five pudina leaves into a cup and add some hot water. Cover and steep for 5 to 10 minutes. Strain and drink warm.

Pumpkin seeds. Snack on pumpkin seeds throughout the day.

Rose petal tea. Place three to five fresh rose petals into a cup and pour boiling water over it. Steep for 5 to 10 minutes then strain. Add honey and drink it warm.

Sesame seeds. Lightly roast 1 to 2 tablespoons of sesame seeds. Sprinkle over any salad, vegetables, or porridge.

Tulsi and sage. Place two to three fresh tulsi leaves and two to three fresh sage leaves into a cup and add boiling water to it. Steep for 5 to 10 minutes and strain. Drink twice a day.

Therapeutic Measures

- Warm some fresh avocado leaves up in a pan and place them on the forehead.
- A warm immersion bath can relieve stress and symptoms of depression.
- Practice yogic asanas such as halasana, paschimottanasana, and savasana.
  Notes
  Home remedies for depression should be used as adjunctive therapy to allopathic treatment.

Rudraksha. Wear a 5 or 7 mukhi (face) Rudraksha as a bracelet or a *mala* (necklace) to calm the nervous system and decrease stress.

Chinese Natural Remedies

- There are two main causes of depression in traditional Chinese medicine:
  - **Qi deficiency:** This produces symptoms such as a pale tongue, eyelids, and skin. Sadness is the predominant emotion.
  - **Qi excess:** Symptoms of qi excess depression are chest distension, flank pain, nausea, poor appetite, moodiness, and excessive sighing. Anger is the predominant emotion in this cause of depression. It may be caused by overwork.
- Emotions are further thought to relate to specific organs:
  - **Liver:** The liver is thought to oversee creativity and intuition. It is thought that a stressed or unhealthy liver leads to depression with a lack of motivation and direction. This causes feelings of being overwhelmed and indecisive.
  - **Lungs:** The lungs are thought to play a role in developing a sense of self. Unhealthy or weak lungs cause the urge to withdraw from social interactions, as well as to feel vulnerable and extremely sensitive. It may also cause feelings of isolation and disconnection, leading to constant crying.
  - **Spleen:** The spleen is responsible for a heightened mental capacity, helping individuals make decisions and work through problems. Unhealthy spleens cause excessive worry and overthinking. It also causes a lack of concentration. It causes a tendency to stress eat.
  - **Kidneys:** The kidneys are thought to be responsible for memory, ambition, and willpower. It is thought that overly hot/cold kidneys cause emotions such as despair and fear with a loss of libido.

Common Ingredients for Depression

Herbs/Leaves	Miscellaneous
Arctic root (Rhodiola rosea)	Ginkgo (Ginkgo biloba)
Ginger (sheng jiang)	
Ginseng	
Glycyrrhiza glabra (liquorice root/ gan cao)	
Mimosa bark/he huan pi (Albizia julibrissin)	
Mint	
Poria	Sour date
White peony root (bai shao)	

Common Recipes

Oral

Teas/Brews/Others

Arctic root tea. Add 1 to 2 teaspoons of dried Arctic root to a cup and cover. Allow to steep for 5 to 10 minutes. Strain and drink it warm.

Bai shao tea. Place three to five pieces of dried bai shao into a cup and add boiling water. Cover and steep for 5 to 10 minutes before straining. Drink warm once a day.

Ginger tea. Lightly pound about 1 to 2 inches of fresh ginger (if unavailable, use 1 to 2 teaspoons of ginger powder) and add to a cup of hot water. Allow to steep for 5 to 10 minutes. Strain and drink while warm. Add honey to taste.

Ginkgo dessert. Ginkgo is often consumed in a sweet dessert with dried bean curd. Dried beancurd is not known to have any benefit to mental health, however. Place five pieces of ginkgo into a pot. Add some dried bean curd (fu chuk) and approximately 2 cups of hot water. Bring to a boil and add some rock sugar to taste. Drink the liquid and eat the ginkgo. Alternatively, consume ginkgo in the form of an extract, which is available as a commercial preparation.

Ginseng tea. As above.

Liquorice tea. Place 1to 2 teaspoons of dried liquorice herb into a cup of boiling water. Cover and steep for 5 to 10 minutes. Drink before bedtime.

Mimosa bark tea. Take ½ to 1 tablespoon of dried bark powder. Add boiling water. Cover and steep for 5 minutes. Strain and drink warm.

Mint tea. Place three to five fresh mint leaves into a cup and add boiling water. Cover and let steep for 5 to 10 minutes. Strain and drink warm.

Western/Other Natural Remedies

Common Ingredients for Depression

Herbs/Leaves	Miscellaneous
Chamomile flower	Lemon balm
Lavender flower	Omega-3 fatty acids
Rose/Rosehip oil (Rosa damascena)	
Rosemary	S-S-adenosylmethionine (SAMe)
Saffron	Lily of the valley essential oil

Herbs/Leaves	Miscellaneous
Saffron *(Crocus Sativus)*	
St John's Wort (Hypericum perforatum)	Apple cider vinegar
Valerian root	Psilocybin
Verbena *(Verbena officinalis)*	

Common Recipes

Oral

Teas/Brews/Others

Apple cider vinegar. Mix 2 teaspoons of apple cider vinegar into 1 cup of warm water and drink once a day. ACV contains calcium, potassium, and magnesium.

Chamomile tea. Place some dried or fresh chamomile flowers into a cup. Pour boiling water over the flowers. Steep for 10 minutes. Strain and add honey to taste. Drink hot.

Lavender tea. Place 2 to 3 teaspoons of lavender buds into a cup and pour some boiling water over it. Let sit for 3 to 5 minutes and strain. Drink warm.

Omega-3 fatty acid. These supplements may help relieve symptoms of depression.

Psilocybin. This is a psychedelic compound isolated from magic mushrooms. It gives immediate and long-term positive effects.

Rosemary tea. Add 3 to 5 sprigs of fresh rosemary (or 1 ½ teaspoons of dry rosemary leaf needles) to a cup of hot water and steep for 10 to 15 minutes. Drink warm.

S-adenosylmethionine (SAMe). It is available as a dietary supplement. It is given for about 3 months daily in 3 divided doses. Alternatively, it can be given as an injection for 1 month.

Saffron tea. Add three to five strands of saffron to a cup of hot water and cover. Steep for 5 to 10 minutes before straining. Drink it warm.

St John's Wort tea. As above. Place 2 tablespoons of St John's wort in a teapot with about 6 cups of hot water. Cover and let steep for 3 to 10 minutes before straining. Add a little honey to taste. Drink it warm.

Verbena tea. Take 1 tablespoon of fresh lemon verbena leaves or 1 teaspoon of dried leaves. Add 1 cup of boiling water. Steep or simmer for 15 minutes. Strain and consume warm with a desired sweetener.

Therapeutic Measures

Aromatherapy

Use lily of the valley or rose/rosehip essential oil via a diffuser. Take five drops of lily of the valley essential oil and add sweet almond oil as a carrier oil.

Therapeutic Measures

Psychological Approaches

Psychotherapeutic interventions. These include cognitive behavior therapy, interpersonal therapy, family therapy, and couple Therapy.

Psychosocial interventions. These include counseling, case management, prevention of relapse, care coordination, community support via religious or group activities, motivational support, and psychotherapy.

Reminiscence therapy. This therapy is to help people with depression and dementia recollect and remember people, places, and events in their lives via family or work pictures.

Mental health apps. Only appropriate, well-researched or evidence-based mental health apps should be downloaded. *Brightside* and *Cerebral* can connect the users to psychiatrists who can prescribe antidepressant medications. Other popular apps like *BetterHelp, Talkspace,* and *Ginger* can connect with a licensed therapist via phone, text, or video. Digital mental health and digital psychiatry are growing fields and may be suitable in crisis situations or for mild disorders whilst waiting for in-person care appointments.

Light therapy (SAD lamp). This is useful in seasonal affective disorder and augments pharmacotherapy. In this light-based treatment, a light box filters out nearly all UV light and mimics sunlight. A SAD lamp with a brightness of 10,000 lux can improve energy levels, mood and help with winter depression, i.e., seasonal affective disorder (SAD). A bright sunny day has a brightness of at least 100,000 lux and ordinary home lighting gives less than 10,000 lux.

Sleep deprivation treatment. Sleep deprivation for one or more nights can have antidepressant and mood-improving effects.

Animal or pet therapy. Caring, stroking, or petting an animal, especially dogs, can release endorphins from the brain and ease depression.

Massage therapy. Various types of massage can improve mood, sleep and mind, and relieve physical pains and aches.

Touch therapy. Gentle touch techniques like Reiki or simply intuitive touching from head to feet may also be soothing, calming, and healing.

Neuromodulation

Electroconvulsive therapy (ECT). It is very effective and safe, especially in drug-resistant epilepsy. An electrical stimulation is applied to the brain via scalp electrodes under general anesthesia to produce a generalized seizure lasting for about 1 minute. Side effects include muscle aches and headaches. Each treatment is repeated two or three times per week for a total of 6 to 12 treatments.

Repetitive transcranial magnetic stimulation (rTMS). Rapidly alternating magnetic fields are used to stimulate specific areas of the brain. There is no seizure produced. Side effects include headaches and muscle twitches and pain or discomfort at the site of stimulation. It is given four to five times per week for a total of 4 to 6 weeks.

Deep brain stimulation (DBS). DBS of the subcallosal cingulate (SCC) gives good and sustained antidepressant effects in treatment-resistant depression.

Vagal nerve stimulation. An implant device is placed on the chest to provide electrical stimulation of the vagus.

Transcranial direct current stimulation (tDCS). This is a non-invasive and non-convulsive treatment (unlike

ECT) which is promising. Two surface scalp electrodes are placed, and low amplitude electric current (usually 1 to 2 mA) is given to alter the membrane potential of the neurons and change the depolarization rate.

Pulsed electromagnetic therapy (PEMF). PEMF therapy is used to modify the neurochemical circuits to increase serotonin, dopamine and melatonin and reduce the stress hormones.

Modern Remedies

Selective Serotonin Reuptake Inhibitors (SSRIs). As above.
Serotonin-Norepinephrine Reuptake Inhibitors (SNRIs). As above.
Tricyclic Antidepressants. As above.

Tetracyclic Antidepressants

Tetracyclic antidepressants work by inhibiting the reuptake of norepinephrine and 5-HT. They have anti-histaminergic and anticholinergic effects on the body.

Example: maprotiline.

Monoamine Oxidase Inhibitors

Monoamine oxidase inhibitors (MAOIs) work by inhibiting the action of an enzyme called monoamine oxidase. This enzyme breaks down monoamines. Inhibiting the breakdown of monoamines means that more neurotransmitters are available, hence boosting mood.

Example: phenelzine, isocarboxazid.

Atypical Antidepressants

Atypical antidepressants are a group of relatively new antidepressants that do not fit the above categories. They affect serotonin, norepinephrine, and dopamine levels in the body and help to regulate moods.

Example: bupropion, mirtazapine.

Homeopathic Remedies

These include arsenicum album (associated diarrhea, indigestion, fear, and panic attacks); natrum muriaticum (stoical with a strong sense of duty and inability to cry); *Sepia* (usually in females who are silent, sad, and solitary); and *Ignatia* (associated loss or grief). Others are baryta carb and alumina.

Schizophrenia

Schizophrenia is a severe chronic mental disorder that often affects the individual's daily life and social relationships. The individual often thinks, feels, and behaves differently. Symptoms of schizophrenia begin between the ages of 16 and 30. Chronic latent parasitic infections such as Toxoplasmosis have been linked with schizophrenia.

There are three main types of schizophrenia symptoms:

Positive symptoms: This type of schizophrenia symptom involves psychotic behavior not usually seen in healthy people. They may seem out of touch with reality, with symptoms such as hallucinations, delusions, agitated body movements, and unusual thoughts.

Negative symptoms: Negative symptoms involve disruption of normal emotion and behavior such as reduced emotion in the tone of voice and facial expression. Patients may also experience reduced pleasure in everyday activities and a lack of motivation as well as a desire to speak.

Cognitive symptoms: Cognitive symptoms of schizophrenia are more subtle but often involve changes in memory and thoughts. Symptoms include poor comprehension ability and inattention.

Another old but useful classification identifies four types: *paranoid* schizophrenia; *catatonic* schizophrenia (this is a medical emergency where the patient shuts down physically, mentally, and emotionally); *schizoaffective* (disordered thoughts and mood); and *undifferentiated* (vague symptoms like noncommunication, paranoia, or lack of motivation in self-care).

Indian Natural Remedies

Common Ingredients for Schizophrenia

Spices	Herbs/Leaves	Miscellaneous
Saffron	*Rauwolfia serpentina*	Ghee
Sandalwood	Jatamansi (*Nardostachys jatamansi*)	Passionflower
	Brahmi (*Bacopa monnieri*)	Oils
	Ashwagandha (*Withania somnifera*)	Sesame
	Guggulu (*Commiphora wightii*)	Cow urine
	Rhubarb root	
	Gotu kola (*Centella asiatica*)	
	Bhringraj (false daisy/ *Eclipta prostrata*)	
	Tulsi (holy basil)	
	Shankhpushpi (*Clitoria ternatea*)	

Common Recipes

Oral

Teas/Brews/Others

Ashwagandha brew. Place 1 teaspoon of ashwagandha root powder into a pot with ½ cup of milk, and ½ cup of water. Boil gently until the volume reduces to about ½ cup. Cool slightly and drink warm. Add honey to taste.

Brahmi juice. Place a handful of the fresh brahmi leaves into a blender and add up to 1 cup of water. Blend until smooth. Add honey to taste and drink.

Brahmi polyherbal-ghee mix. Take brahmi 50 g, jatamansi 50 g, ashwagandha 50 g, shankhpushpi 50 g and make a paste. Boil ghee 100 mg and then add this herbal paste. Cook for ½ hour. Cool and filter. Consume 1 teaspoon of this mix twice a day.

Brahmi tea. Place about tow to three stalks of fresh brahmi leaves into a cup. Pour boiling water over the leaves. Steep for about 10 to 15 minutes. Add honey to taste and drink.

Cow urine potion. Cook cow urine with about 3 kg of ghee and 200 g of a herbs-spice mix (asafetida, dark salt, black pepper, long pepper, and dried ginger). Consume 1 to 2 tablespoons of this mixture every day.

False daisy tea. Place 2 teaspoons of dried false daisy herbs in a cup of hot water. Steep for 5 to 10 minutes. Strain and add honey. Drink warm.

Gotu kola tea. Steep a teaspoon of fresh or dried gotu kola leaves in a cup of hot water for about 10 to 15 minutes. Drink warm.

Guggulu supplements. It is available in the form of dietary supplements. Adults can take about 25 mg of guggulu supplements every day after a meal.

Holy basil tea. Place two to five fresh holy basil leaves into a cup of hot water. Cover and steep for 5 to 10 minutes before drinking. Alternatively, chew three to five leaves.

Jatamansi brew. Add a pinch of jatamansi root powder to a cup of warm water and take it twice a day.

Passionflower tea. Add 1 teaspoon of dried passion flower to a cup of hot water. Cover and steep for 5 to 10 minutes. Strain and drink warm.

Polyherbal and herbomineral compounds (various types are commercially available) are administered as:

churna (fine powder);

kwatha/kashayam (decoction with added ghee, milk, water, oil, or jaggery);

vati (as pills);

asava or arishta (fermented preparation with 3% to 10% alcohol);

bhasma/rashausadhies (calcined or ash preparations);

ghrita preparation (preparation in cow ghee); and

oil formulation.

Rhubarb root tea. Place about 20 g of dried crushed rhubarb root into a pot and add about 1 L of water. Boil and then simmer gently for 10 to 15 minutes. Strain and drink one cup before the two main meals of the day.

Saffron. Put a few strands of saffron into milk and boil. Drink in the morning.

Sesame seed. Soak a handful of sesame seeds in water overnight. In the morning, strain, and chew on the sesame seeds.

Variation #1. Lightly roast 1 to 2 tablespoons of sesame seeds. Sprinkle over any salad, vegetables, or porridge.

Tulsi tea. Cut three to five fresh tulsi into strips and place in a cup. Pour boiling water over the leaves and cover. Let steep for 5 to 10 minutes before straining. Drink warm.

Therapeutic measures

Panchakarma and psychotherapy. The above oral herbal treatments are also combined with panchakarma (five elimination treatments of the vitiated doshas) and satt-vavajaya chikitsa (Ayurvedic psychotherapy with a psychosomatic and spiritual approach) to treat the unmada (psychosis). They can be used alone or combined with lower doses of modern antipsychotic drugs.

Medicated enemas. It is thought that enemas with ghee or oil may help cleanse the body and mind of toxins. For severe schizophrenia, medicated enemas using gotu kola and jatamansi may be used.

Spiritual and yogic therapies (such as mantra, meditation, visualizations, pranayama, and yoga) blended with herbal medicine, diet/nutrition, aromatherapy, and color therapy together with some modern medicines can provide more holistic healing.

Chinese Natural Remedies

Common Ingredients for Schizophrenia

Herbs/Leaves	Miscellaneous
Bitter orange *(Citrus aurantium)*	
Chinese rhubarb *(Rheum palmatum)*	Ginkgo *(Ginkgo biloba)*
Liquorice *(Radix glycyrrhizae preparata)*	
Pinellia tuber *(Pinellia ternata)*	
Poria cocos mushroom	
Young tangerine peel *(Pericarpium citri reticulatae)*	

Common Recipes

Oral

- **Wendan** Decoction
  - Radix *glycyrrhizae preparata,* poria cocos, *Citrus aurantium, Pericarpium citri reticulatae,* and *Pinellia ternata.*

This decoction is available in the form of a commercial preparation.

Chinese rhubarb tea. Place about 1 to 2 teaspoons of coarsely chopped dried Chinese rhubarb herb into a cup with boiling water. Cover and steep for 3 to 5 minutes before straining. Drink warm once a day before bedtime.

Ginkgo dessert. Ginkgo is often consumed in a sweet dessert with dried bean curd. Dried beancurd is not known to have any benefit to mental health, however. Place five pieces of ginkgo into a pot. Add some dried bean curd (fu chuk) and approximately 2 cups of hot water. Bring to a boil and add some rock sugar to taste. Drink the liquid and eat the ginkgo. Alternatively, consume ginkgo in the form of an extract, which is available as a commercial preparation.

Western/Other Natural Remedies

Common Ingredients for Schizophrenia

Miscellaneous

Glycine

Omega-3 fish oil supplements

Vitamin B9 (folic acid)

Common Recipes

Oral

- Vitamin B9 (folic acid) levels are low in patients suffering from schizophrenia. Taking vitamin B9 (folic acid) supplements may help to reduce symptoms.
- Take omega-3 fatty acid supplements.

- Glycine is an amino acid found to boost brain function. Some studies have found that high doses of glycine may boost the efficacy of antipsychotic drugs.

Therapeutic Measures

- A gluten-free diet can potentially reduce schizophrenia symptoms.
- Cognitive behavior therapy, i.e., cognitive restructuring therapy, is also useful.

Modern Remedies

Typical Antipsychotics (First-Generation or Conventional Antipsychotics)

Typical antipsychotics block the dopamine D2 receptors in the dopaminergic pathway of the brain. This means that the dopamine released does not have as much of an effect on the brain.

Examples: chlorpromazine, haloperidol, fluphenazine, perphenazine, thioridazine, trifluoperazine, molindone, and loxapine.

Atypical Antipsychotics (Second-Generation Antipsychotics)

Their mechanism of action is not clear. It is believed they act more on the serotoninergic receptors 5-HT2A than the dopaminergic receptors to rebalance serotonin and dopamine. They provide better control of the negative symptoms, thoughts and lower relapse rates.

Examples: clozapine, quetiapine, olanzapine, asenapine, cariprazine, aripiprazole, brexpiprazole, risperidone, ziprasidone, paliperidone.

Paliperidone palmitate is also available as a long-acting injection. It is given initially monthly then every 3 monthly for acute and maintenance treatment in schizophrenia.

Side effects include extrapyramidal symptoms (EPS), which result in stiffness, bradykinesia, tremors, and loss of facial expression. Tardive dyskinesia (involuntary body movements) is also another side effect. These are lesser with atypical antipsychotics than the typical drugs. However, the atypical antipsychotics cause more metabolic syndrome side effects (with hyperglycemia, hypercholesterolemia, and weight gain) and loss of libido. Clozapine can cause leukopenia (low white cell count).

Muscle Relaxants

Benzodiazepines are indicated in the catatonic type to relax the muscles and manage anxiety issues.

Antidepressants and Mood Stabilizers

These are combined with antipsychotic drugs in the schizoaffective type.

Methotrexate

Although methotrexate is used as an anti-cancer drug or in autoimmune diseases, it is now being used as an add-on medication in schizophrenia or in the schizoaffective type to improve the positive symptoms of schizophrenia (delusions, hallucinations, and repetitive movements).

Homeopathic Remedies

These include phosphorus, natrum muriaticum, sulphur, *Pulsatilla, Lycopodium clavatum, Thuja occidentalis* (feelings of being under superhuman power), *Lachesis muta* (in paranoid type), *Hyoscyamus niger* (for delusion of being poisoned), and *Anacardium orientale* (for auditory hallucinations). Others include *Cannabis indica* and kali bromatum.

Insomnia

Insomnia is a sleep disorder where one has difficulty in falling asleep or staying asleep throughout the night. It is acute if it lasts for a few days or weeks. It is a chronic disorder if sleeplessness occurs at least three nights a week for three months or more. It results in excessive daytime sleepiness, fatigue, low energy, irritability, and poor focus and alertness. Immune health is also affected.

1. Insomnia also can be classified as primary (if there is no known cause) and secondary (because of an associated health problem).

Common causes and risk factors include poor lifestyle, overeating, stress, night or rotating shift work, jet lag, anxiety, underlying medical conditions (like asthma, diabetes, heart failure, hyperthyroidism, etc.), pain (from cancer, acid reflux, arthritis, etc.), mental health disorders (depression, anxiety, grief, anger or trauma), menopause, old age, substance abuse (alcohol, nicotine, caffeine, and recreational drugs), obstructive sleep apnea, gadget overuse, restless leg syndrome, and worms in children. Teenagers have "forward-placed sleep cycle" because their biological clocks are pushed later and they cannot wake up early.

Medication-induced insomnia is also an important cause. Several medications, which are very effective for treating a medical condition, can also cause sleep disturbances as adverse reactions. These are:

Antidepressants such as SSRIs. The altered levels of serotonin in the body from the drug mechanism itself alter the sleep-wake cycle, which can lead to decreased sleep quality and daytime somnolence.

Antihypertensive Drugs. Beta blockers used in hypertension and/or cardiac arrhythmias have associated links with night awakenings/sleep disturbances and even nightmares. The hormone melatonin is altered and causes irregular sleep.

Alpha Blockers. Alpha blockers used also in hypertension and enlarged prostate in males can cause a decrease in rapid eye movements (REM). REM is normal in a deep state of sleep, so when reduced, it causes poor sleep function.

ACE Inhibitors. ACE inhibitors used in hypertension and other heart diseases can cause hyperkalemia, which can lead to muscle cramps, tension, or pain that could lead to sleep interruption and disturbances.

Statins. Statins reduce high cholesterol levels. A common side effect is muscle pain/soreness, which can keep a person awake throughout the night because of hyperkalemia. There is also an increased rate of Alzheimer's disease.

Anti-Arthritis Drugs. Glucosamine is combined with chondroitin to reduce joint pain. Its side effects include heartburn, headaches, and constipation/diarrhea. These can interrupt sleep or rest.

Anti-Epileptic Drugs. Anti-epileptic drugs control muscle spasms and seizures. However, the benzodiazepine group of drugs can decrease the sleep onset time, cause more night awakenings, daytime sleepiness, and sedation.

Antihistamines. The first-generation H1 antagonist is commonly used for allergies like blocked or runny nose and watery, itchy eyes. It also blocks the neurotransmitter acetylcholine, resulting in lethargy, fatigue, and drowsiness.

Diet Pills for Obesity. Some diet pills, which are appetite suppressants, contain high doses of concentrated caffeine. They stimulate the central nervous system and block adenosine and keep the person awake and alert.

Therapeutic Measures

Diet

- Avoid saturated or high-fat foods, spicy foods, and eating large meals before bedtime.
- Avoid late dinners. Eat the evening meal about 4 hours before bedtime.
- Drink a glass of warm milk with some honey at bedtime or supper.
  Malted beverages (e.g., Horlicks) are also a good alternative.
  Variation #1. Consume a warm milkshake with blended banana and some honey.
- Eat tryptophan-rich foods such as banana, turkey, and oats
- Avoid excessive fluid intake to reduce bathroom visits.
- Avoid skipping dinner as it can cause hunger pangs in some, resulting in tossing and turning or staying more alert without acquiring deep slow-wave sleep.
- Optimum intake of vitamins (especially vitamin Bs) and minerals (magnesium, zinc) are essential for calming effects and relaxation.

Exercise

- Keep fit and active with daily exercises, yoga, or sports for at least 20 to 30 minutes/day on most days of the week. This will improve sleep quality, quantity, and the amount of deep slow-wave sleep.
- Beware of excessive sports that can cause muscle fatigue, pain, or insomnia.

Lifestyle

- Limit or omit coffee, alcohol, and cigarettes. Caffeine can stay in the body for up to 12 hours. Drink decaffeinated coffee beyond lunchtime if necessary. Alcohol can lead to frequent night awakenings, nightmares, and bathroom visits. Reduce the number of cigarettes for 4 hours before sleep and omit at least 30 to 45 minutes before bedtime.
- Avoid overstimulation at bedtime from excessive screen time from gadgets or watching horror films. Stop for at least 30 minutes to one hour before bedtime.
- Feet, ear, or head/scalp, and face self-massage with or without essential oils can also help.
- Avoid night or rotating shift work if possible.

Sleep Hygiene

- A warm bath or Epsom salt bath soaks for 20 minutes before bedtime can be relaxing.
  Variation # 1. Soak feet in warm water or with some Epsom salt for about 20 minutes before bedtime. Wipe feet dry and massage the soles with essential oil if desired.
- Sleep at a regular time every night. Wake up at a regular time.
- Have a bedtime ritual. For example, after dinner and bath, read a book or engage in storybook time with the children, listen to soothing music, say prayers, meditate, or chant mantras.
- Breathing exercises can help.
- Use comfortable loose cotton or flannel nightclothes or pajamas. These are natural moisture-wickers.
- Avoid or limit afternoon naps or siesta. If required, it should not exceed 45 minutes in adults. Walk or move around after lunch to avoid postprandial sleepiness. For some, a short power nap for 10 to 20 minutes can improve productivity. Young infants or toddlers should have at least two daytime naps.
- Make peace before bedtime if there was any quarrel between spouses or partners or family.

Bedroom Environment

- The room must be cool and adequately ventilated. It should not be too hot, cold, dry or humid. Air conditioners and humidifiers can be both helpful when natural ventilation is not possible.
- Avoid light pollution. The room must be dark or dim with a small night light if necessary. Avoid flickering blue or red lights from computers. Switch off the television and unplug from all mobile devices at least one hour before sleep. Use adequate blinds, curtains, or blackout shades for windows especially if there are streetlights. An eye mask can also be helpful. Wearing wraparound glasses with an amber-tinted lens for about 2 hours before sleep may block the blue light and promote sleep.
- Avoid noise pollution. Use earplugs if necessary. Television should not be placed in the bedroom. If there is external or environmental noise from road traffic, people or barking dogs, try distracting with white noise from the sound of the whirring fan or air conditioner. White noise can also help babies and young children calm and settle them quickly to sleep.

- Wearables such as smart devices (earbuds or wristband devices) can give information on sleep time or depth of sleep (deep or light sleep). Headphones with music can help some fall asleep faster. However, long-term use of earbuds or headphones can lead to ear wax accumulation and hearing loss.
- Sleep trackers (from Fitbit or Oura) can measure sleep efficiency, total sleep time and total wake time.
- The bedroom color tones should be soft, muted, and soothing.
- Essential oils via a diffuser can be used if preferred. For some, these odors can disturb sleep.
- Soft toys like teddy bears or bolsters and leg pillows are comforting for some.
- Allergens from bedding, carpets, curtains, or toys can also affect sleep. They should be clean and of natural or eco-friendly materials.
- Pets may be comforting for some although they can be a source of allergens.
- Sleeping on the floor is a cultural practice and does not affect sleep quality.
- Special mattresses are mostly not required unless there is a medical indication. A ripple mattress is helpful when there is a painful bedsore.
- Special pillows (made of memory foam, cotton, feather, down, latex, water, or buckwheat) are also generally not necessary unless there is a medical need. Head and neck support are essential during sleep. Sleeping without a pillow can also be beneficial for some.
- Avoid looking at the clock if you are unable to sleep. Cover it or move it away if necessary. Get out of bed, listen to music, read a book, or watch a movie until sleepy.

Indian Natural Remedies

Sleeplessness can be caused by imbalances in vata, pitta, or kapha dosha.

In *vata-related disorders,* the mind is overactive with too many thoughts and emotions. It is difficult to relax, settle, and fall asleep or sleep is light and restless. One wakes up tired.

In *pitta-related sleep disorders,* there is no problem settling in to sleep, but there is night awakening during the small hours of the morning with the inability to return to sleep for many hours. This tends to occur in those with emotional stress or trauma.

In *kapha-related sleep disorders,* there is long and deep sleep, but there is lethargy and exhaustion on waking and during the daytime.

Common Ingredients for Insomnia

Spices	Herbs/Leaves	Miscellaneous
Black seed (Nigella sativa)	Mimosa	
Cardamom	Sarpagandha (Rauwolfia serpentina or Indian snakeroot)	Coconut oil

Spices	Herbs/Leaves	Miscellaneous
Cumin	Jatamansi (Nardostachys jatamansi)	Rudraksha (Elaeocarpus ganitrus)
Fenugreek	Shankhpushpi (Convolvulus pluricaulis)	Banana
Khus khus (poppy seed)	Vacha (Acorus calamus)	
Nutmeg	Ashwagandha/Indian ginseng (Withania somnifera)	Honey
Saffron	Amla	
	Brahmi	
	Indian sorrel (Oxalis corniculata)	
	Bhringraj leaves	

Common Recipes

Oral

Amla. Consume 15 to 20 mL amla juice before going to bed.

Anise. Drink a glass of warm milk with some honey and anise at bedtime.

Ashwagandha. Take ready-made ashwagandha powder (choornam) 5 g and mix with sugar and ghee and consume twice a day after meals. Alternatively, mix 1 teaspoon of the powder into a cup of warm milk and drink it before bedtime.

Black seed. Drink a glass of warm milk with some honey and black seed at bedtime.

Brahmi. It is available as tablets and can be mixed with a glass of warm milk. It can also be consumed as brahmi juice or tea.

Cardamon. Mix a pinch of ground green cardamom with warm milk.

Cumin seed and banana paste. Gently fry cumin seed and grind into a fine powder. Mix 1 to 2 teaspoons of the ground cumin seed with a ripe banana, mashing until it makes a paste. Consume this paste before bedtime to induce sleep.

Fenugreek. Add some fenugreek powder to warm water or milk.

Indian sorrel. Take about 15 g of sorrel leaves. Wash and crush them to extract the fresh juice. Add some water or buttermilk. Consume before bedtime.

Variation #1. Take 1 tablespoon of sorrel juice and mix with 1 tablespoon of castor oil. Massage the mixture on the forehead.

Jatamansi. Take ¼ to ½ teaspoon jatamansi powder. Mix with little honey. Consume after food before bedtime. It can also be taken twice a day.

Khus khus. Take a tablespoon of khus khus and brown it lightly with little ghee in a saucepan. Add a glass of milk. Drink it warm with some honey.

Khus khus Almond milk (Thandai). Take a handful of soaked and peeled almonds, 1 tablespoon of soaked white poppy seeds and blend with little water (or milk). Add this to the saucepan and 2 cups of milk, some rock sugar, 1 tablespoon ghee, 1 teaspoon of cardamon powder (green cardamon) and a pinch of saffron or turmeric. Boil, then simmer and consume it warm.

Mimosa. Take 1 teaspoon of mimosa leaves. Grind to make a paste. Add a cup of water and boil. Strain and consume at bedtime for 2 to 4 weeks.

Moonmilk. This milk is consumed at bedtime. Boil 1 cup of milk (or diary-free milk) and then simmer. Blend or whisk in a pinch of ground nutmeg and ½ teaspoon each of cinnamon, ground ginger, and ashwagandha and lastly add in little virgin coconut oil and some honey.

Nutmeg. Mix a pinch of ground nutmeg with warm milk and consume.

Polyherbal formulations (containing ashwagandha, shankhpushpi, jatamansi, and sarpagandha) are believed to be more effective than single herbs because of their synergistic effects from a different mechanism of actions. Examples: Sleepcap, Calmtone, Sunidra, etc.

Another polyherbal tablet is Sarpagandha Ghan Vati which contains largely Sarpagandha with small amounts of Hyoscyamus niger, Jatamansi root powder and Cannabis sativa with some added Piper longum roots. It is consumed about 2 hours before sleep. Side effects include nasal congestion and dry mouth.

Saffron. Boil some saffron threads in milk. Drink it warm.

Sarpagandha-cardamom powder. Grind cardamom seeds into a fine powder. Mix some cardamom powder with sarpagandha powder. Consume before bedtime.

Shankhpushpi. Take 3 to 5 g of shankhpushpi ground powder per day before or after a meal, in two divided doses. Consume with a glass of warm water. Do not take on an empty stomach.

Variation #1. Take five to six fresh blue pea flowers. Add 1 cup of boiling water. Allow to steep for 5 to 10 minutes. Drink before bedtime.

Vacha. Place 1 to 2 teaspoons of vacha herbs into a cup of hot water. Steep for 5 to 10 minutes. Strain and drink warm.

Topical

- Massage the body with coconut oil before bedtime to relax and induce sleep.

For vata-related sleep disorders, choose gentle exercises like yoga, walking, swimming, or tai chi. Since vata is cold and dry, eat foods that are warm, moist, and oil-enriched. It is also helpful to eat a vata-balancing diet, which is sour, salty, and sweet. Eat three warm cooked meals of moderately heavy texture and added fats with the large meal at noon. Eat dinner before 7 pm and sleep before 10 pm or 9.30 pm. A warm bath with rose oil essence can calm the mind or rub the rose essential oil on the skin after the bath.

For pitta-related sleep disorders, choose cooling exercises that do not cause overheating like swimming or walking in shaded areas. It is helpful to eat pitta-pacifying foods, which are sweeter, more bitter and astringent. Consume sweet,

juicy fruits. Eat foods and drinks at room temperature and not steaming or boiling hot. Have a glass of warm milk during the afternoon snack. Do not skip or delay meals. Eat a large evening meal. Use rose or vetiver/khus essential oils to pacify pitta dosha at bedtime.

For kapha-related sleep disorders, wake up before 6 a.m. or avoid coffee. Consume a kapha-pacifying diet. Avoid cold, sweet, and heavy desserts. Exercise vigorously during the kapha time of the morning (6 a.m. to 10 a.m.). Also, take deep breaths during exercise and throughout the day. Use a myrrh (commiphora myrrha) or henna (lawsonia inermis) essential oil to pacify kapha dosha at bedtime.

Oil Massages

Abhyanga: This is a full-body massage with medicated warm herbal oils based on the dosha and/or the medical condition. Do daily self-massage with a dosha-pacifying oil.

Vata-pacifying oils include sesame and olive oils. Adding herbs like shatavari, ashwagandha, bala, and other herbs can help a person with high vata dosha to be calmer and more grounded.

Pitta-pacifying oils include coconut, sunflower, and neem oils. Blend in herbs like brahmi, shatavari, guduchi manjistha, and liquorice to cool the mind and body.

Kapha-pacifying oils include almond, corn, sesame, or combination oils and with added herbs like chitrak (Plumbago zeylanica), punarnava (Boerhavia diffusa), calamus/vasambu (Acorus calamus), and rosemary to decrease kapha.

Padabhyanga (foot massage): This refers to a foot massage with the above oils.

Shirodhara oil massage with brahmi oil is helpful in moderate to severe insomnia.

Ear oiling (karna pratisaranam). Our ears are connected to our doshas, especially vata dosha. *Prana vata/vayu* (the air life force) present in the ears is also connected and flows into the bone layer (asthi dhatu) and the nerve layer (majja dhatu). Daily ear oiling promotes calmness, grounding, and good sleep.

Henna oil: Massage henna oil on the scalp and body. Rinse off.

Bhringraj. Apply bhringraj oil on the scalp.

Alternatively, it can be administered intranasally.

To make the oil, take bhringraj leaves dry in the sun for 2 to 3 days. Add the dried leaves in sesame or coconut oil. Dry in the sun again for another 2 to 3 days till the oil color becomes green.

Variation #1. Add dried bhringraj leaf powder to hot coconut oil or sesame oil. Let it steep till the oil color is green.

Miscellaneous

- *Vastu shastra* is an ancient science of architecture for a positive-energy home. Ideally, the bedroom should be in a south-west direction. Any sleeping direction is good except the head must not be in the north. Head in the south is said to be the best direction for good sleep quality. Avoid mirrors in front of the bed.

- Universal **mantras** like "om" or "gayatri mantra" can be chanted or heard via YouTube.
- Meditation and mindfulness are also helpful for sleep health.
- **Yoga poses** for sleep include legs up against the wall (viparita karani), cat stretch (marjariasana), child pose (shishuasana), butterfly pose (baddha konasana), forward bend with hand-to-foot pose (hastapadasana), corpse pose (savasana), etc.
- *Sudarshan kriya yoga.* It is a type of rhythmic breathing technique that promotes better sleep and overall good health.

Rudraksha. Wear a 5 or 7 mukhi (face) Rudraksha as a bracelet or a *mala* (necklace) to calm the nervous system and decrease stress.

Chinese Natural Remedies

It is believed that insomnia is due to an imbalance of yin and yang. During the day, *yang* is more dominant to keep us alert. At night, *yin* is more dominant as it is quiet, cool, and rejuvenating.

Unlike the Western classification system, TCM identifies more than five TCM pattern differentiations in insomnia, the most common being deficiency of both heart and spleen. Analysis of the tongue and pulse also provides diagnostic information. Tongue features such as red tongue, pale tongue, and different types of coating and pulse features (fine pulse is the commonest type in insomnia) can indicate a deficiency or excess qi states. Sleep-related symptoms (such as excessive dreaming, dizziness, half-sleep, restless sleep, waking up with a start, shallow sleep, etc.) and non-sleep-related symptoms (such as palpitations, bitter taste, constipation, poor appetite, etc.) are also included to define insomnia etiologies, pattern differentiations, and specific TCM remedies.

The following are associated with sleep disorders:
- Liver fire (hotness)
- Liver and gallbladder damp heat
- Heart fire
- Heart qi deficiency
- Spleen qi deficiency

Deficiency of both heart and spleen qi is due to overwork, stress, and overthinking. This leads to heart dysfunction and then blood deficiency. There is inadequate blood flow to the brain, spleen, and intestines. This results in poor food digestion and assimilation and a lack of nutrients. There is easy arousal from sleep or difficulty falling back to sleep with associated headache, dizziness, and forgetfulness.

Sleep onset difficulty is due to excessive fire.

Liver qi stagnation is due to chronic stress and depression. This will lead to excessive fire, which will rise to affect the heart and spirit. Hence, the affected person cannot sleep.

Liver and gallbladder disorders are associated with frequent fearful awakening, sighing, nervousness, and timidity.

Common Ingredients for Insomnia

Herbs/Leaves/Roots	Miscellaneous
China root	Chrysanthemum flower
Chinese senega roots/yuan zhi (*Polygala tenuifolia*)	Dried Longan
Green tea leaf	Honokiol (extract from magnolia bark)
Jujube	Oyster shell
Lily bulb	
Lilyturf root /Mai Dong (*Liriope muscari* or *Radix Ophiopogonis*)	Lotus flowers
Liquorice (gan cao)	Bamboo shavings
Valerian	Passionflower
White peony root (bai shao)	Chamomile

Common Recipes

Oral

Teas/Brews

Chamomile tea. Place some dried or fresh chamomile flowers into a cup. Pour boiling water over the flowers and allow to steep for 10 minutes. Strain and add honey to taste. Drink it hot.

Chrysanthemum tea. Take a handful of dried chrysanthemum flowers. Add 2 cups of water. Boil and then remove from the heat. Strain and drink throughout the day.

Dried longan. It can be consumed daily as tea or soup.

Green tea. Place 1 to 2 teaspoons of green tea leaves into a cup of boiling water and steep for 10 minutes. Strain and drink it warm.

Lilyturf root. Slice the dried root. Make it into a decoction (or tea).

Liquorice tea. Place 1 to 2 teaspoons of dried liquorice herb into a cup of boiling water. Cover and steep for 5 to 10 minutes. Drink before bedtime.

Lotus tea. Take 2 teaspoons of dried lotus flowers (petals and stamen) with 2 cups of hot water. Steep for 5 minutes. Add ½ teaspoon of fresh lotus seeds if desired. Drink thrice a day.

Magnolia bark. Take ¼ cup of peeled magnolia bark twigs. Rinse the bark. Place in a pot. Add 8 cups of water. Soak for 30 minutes. Boil and then simmer to reduce the final volume to about 2 cups. Strain and consume before bedtime.

Oyster shell. It is consumed as part of a polyherbal formula.

Passionflower tea. Place 1 to 2 teaspoons of dried passion flower into a cup of hot water. Cover and let steep for 5 to 10 minutes. Drink it warm before bedtime.

Valerian tea. Mix ½ teaspoon (2 to 3 g) of dried valerian root in a cup of hot water. Cover and steep for 10 to 15 minutes. Consume 30 minutes to 2 hours before sleep.

White peony root tea. Take 1 tablespoon of the dried white peony root. Add 1 cup of water. Boil for 10 minutes. Strain and drink.

Polyherbal formulae

- **Hange-koboku-to.** This is a Japanese formula with 5 herbs including magnolia bark.
- **Saiboku-to.** This is a Japanese formula with 10 plant extracts including magnolia bark.

Therapeutic Measures

Diet

Yin-and-yang foods: Consume more yin foods such as soy, fruits, vegetables, and water. Yang foods are high in fat, protein, and salts, which can lead to sleep difficulties.

Herbs

- Consume lily bud, dried longan, spinal date seed, or bo zi ren herb as part of the daily diet.
- Consume soup daily using dan shen (red sage), yu zhu (Solomon's seal), and lian zi (lotus seed).
- Use *Albizia julibrissin* (mimosa/he huan pi) flowers as herbal teas to balance qi and promote sleep. It is associated with heart and liver meridians.
- *Rose bud* herbal tea also balances qi and promotes sleep.
- *Gui pi tang* and *an shen bu nao ye* are herbs given for deficiency of both spleen and heart and associated dizziness.
- *Suan zao ren* is an herb that promotes blood flow to the heart and liver and calms the liver.
- For liver qi stagnation, the herbs *xiao yao wan* and *zhen zhu feng* are useful for stress- or depression-related insomnia. The herbs *bao he wan* and *jian pi wan* are recommended for indigestion-related insomnia.

Acupressure, Acupuncture, and Massage

It regulates the yin yang and promotes blood flow/qi (energy) to promote mental health and sleep. The following points are stimulated.

- **Triple warmer meridian.** Calming the triple warmer meridian helps to restore healthy sleep patterns. This meridian controls our fight, flight, or freeze response.
  This meridian starts from the tip of the ring finger along the outside corner of the nail and passes between the knuckles of the fourth and fifth fingers onto the wrist.
- **Pericardium 6 (P6/Inner Gate/Nei Guan)**
  Massage the nei guan (P 6 point, which is three-finger breadths below the wrist in between the two tendons. It is associated with the inner forearm.)
- **Shi Mien**
  This is located on the base of the foot, located by drawing an imaginary line from the inner ankle bone to the sole of the foot. This point is directly in front of the heel.
- **Shen men (Heavenly Gate/Divine Gate point)**
  It is in the upper one-third ear at the apex of the triangular fossa). Gently twirl or twist both the upper ears with the thumb at the back and index finger in front using both hands at the same time in an anticlockwise manner for about 1 minute (about 20 times).
- **Heart 7 (H7/Shen Men)**
  H7 is located in line with the base of the little finger on the wrist crease on the outer corner of the upturned hand. Stimulate this point for about 20 seconds to soothe the mind.
- **An Mien /SJ 17**
  This point is located on the head and can be found by feeling at the base of the skull in the depression directly behind the ear. Massage this point gently but firmly for 15 to 20 minutes with two fingers.
- **Bai hui** (GV 20)
  It is a point on the Governor Vessel. It is on the highest place of the head where all the yang meridians meet. The D20 point at the vertex/midline of a line between the ears, same as the crown chakra.
  Massage bai hui points to facilitate qi circulation and dissipate the heat build-up in those areas

Auricular therapy using magnetic pearls. This can improve the quality and quantity of sleep among the elderly.

Foot reflexology. Pressure on various points on the feet is applied usually with the fingers and sometimes with a special stick.

Tai chi. This is an ancient form of exercise and is described as "meditation in motion."

Feng shui is an ancient system that aligns the furniture items with the flow of chi. Some basic feng shui in the bedroom layout may be helpful to promote sleep such as placing the bed centrally and not in line with the door, avoiding seeing mirrors, keeping all drawers or doors closed when not in use, and avoiding clutter.

Western/Other Natural Remedies

Common Ingredients for Insomnia

Herbs/Leaves/Seeds	Miscellaneous
California poppy (*Eschscholzia californica*)	Lavender flower
Catnip (*Nepeta cataria*)	Honey
Cowslip	White grape
Griffonia simplicifolia seeds (5-HTP extract)	GABA (Gamma-Aminobutyric Acid)
	Griffonia simplicifolia seeds (5-HTP extract)
Hops (*Humulus lupulus*)	Apple cider vinegar
Lady's mantle	CBD oil
Lemon balm leaf (*Melissa officinalis*)	Kava root (*Piper methysticum*)
Little-leaf linden leaf (*Tilia cordata*)	Passion flower (*Passiflora incarnata*)
Magnolia bark (*Magnolia officinalis*)	Epsom salts
Pulsatilla	Essential oils: lavender, cedarwood, rose, jasmine, geranium, etc.
St. John's wort	Tart cherries
Valerian root	Chamomile flower
Verbena (*Verbena officinalis*)	Nobiletin
Wild Black Cherry (*Prunus serontina*)	Celery

Common Recipes

Oral

Teas/Brews/Others

Apple cider vinegar brew. Mix 2 tablespoons of raw apple cider vinegar with ¼ to 1 cup of water. Add honey to taste and drink before bedtime.

California poppy tea. Any above-ground part of the California poppy plant may be used to make tea (stems, leaves, flowers). They may also be used dry or fresh. Place a handful of fresh herbs into a teapot and fill with 2 cups of water. Cover and steep for 10 to 15 minutes before straining. Add honey to taste and drink warm before bedtime.

California poppy tincture. Using 50% alcohol, place the herbs into a glass jar and fill up with alcohol. The ratio of dried herb to alcohol is 1:5, while the ratio of fresh herb to alcohol is 1:2. Cover tightly and let sit in a cool, dark place for 3 to 4 weeks. To use, take 30 to 60 drops four times a day. If awakened at night and unable to sleep alternatively, place a dropperful of the tincture under the tongue.

Catnip tea. Place 2 teaspoons of dried catnip herb into a cup of boiling water. Cover and steep for 5 to 10 minutes before straining and drinking.

CBD (cannabidiol) oil. It can be taken about 1 hour before bedtime to promote good sleep.

Celery juice. Cut two to three stalks of celery into smaller pieces. Blend with little water until smooth. Stir a teaspoon of honey into the juice and drink before bedtime.

Chamomile tea. Place 1 to 2 teaspoons of dried chamomile flowers in a cup of boiling water, letting it steep for 10 to 15 minutes. Strain and add honey to taste. Drink warm before bedtime.

Cowslip-herbal mix tea. Take 50 g of cowslip, 10g of St. John's, 10 g of hops plant and 25 g of lavender flowers. Make a mixture of all the herbs. Take 1 teaspoon of this dry herb mix into 250 mL of hot water. Steep for 5 to 10 minutes.

Griffonia simplicifolia seeds. 5-HTP extract is obtained from the seeds.

Hops tea. Place 1 to 2 teaspoons of dried hops flowers into a cup of boiling water. Cover and let sit for 10 to 15 minutes. Strain and drink warm, before bedtime. It is available usually in combination with valerian and passionflower.

Kava root. Place 1 to 2 teaspoons of kava root in a cup of hot water. Steep for 5 to 10 minutes before straining. Drink it warm.

Lady's mantle tea. Take 5 to 10 g of lady's mantle and add 1 L of boiling water and allow it to steep for 10 to 15 minutes. Strain and consume. Alternatively, some leaves can be kept under the pillow.

Lavender tea. Add 2 to 3 teaspoons of dried lavender flowers to 1 cup of hot water. Steep for 10 to 15 minutes before straining. Drink it warm before bedtime.

Lemon balm tea. Place 1 tablespoon of dried lemon balm leaves (or 2 tablespoons of fresh leaves) into a cup of boiling water. Let sit for 10 to 15 minutes before straining. Add honey to taste and drink warm.

Linden tea. Boil the flowers or buds and let it steep for 10 to 15 minutes. Strain and drink.

Magnolia bark tincture. Cut dried magnolia bark into smaller segments and place the magnolia bark into a clean dry container. Add 50% alcohol and seal the jar. Place the jar in a cool, dark place for 3 to 4 weeks. To use, strain, and take 30 to 60 drops a day. The ratio of herbs to alcohol is 1:5.

Nobiletin. This is available as powder supplements. A combination of nobiletin and melatonin is also available which can improve the sleep-wake cycle.

Passion flower tea. Place 1 to 2 teaspoons of dried passion flower into a cup of hot water. Cover and let steep for 5 to 10 minutes. Drink it warm before bedtime.

Polyherbs. *Commercial* preparations contain various herbs such as valerian root, passion flower, lemon balm, and Tilia cordata.

Sleep cocktail. Mix 1 cup each of tart cherry juice and white grape juice. Add in valerian root tincture (½ dropper) and little CBD oil. Consume before bedtime.

St John's wort. Place 2 to 3 teaspoons of St John's wort fresh flowers in 1 cup of hot water. Cover and let steep for 5 minutes. Strain and add a little honey to taste. Drink warm.

Tart cherry juice. Take sips from 1 cup of the juice about 1 to 2 hours before sleep.

Verbena tea. Take 1 tablespoon of fresh lemon verbena leaves or 1 teaspoon of dried leaves. Add 1 cup of boiling water. Steep or simmer for 15 minutes. Strain and consume warm with a desired sweetener.

Valerian tea. Mix ½ teaspoon of dried valerian root (or 2 to 3 g teaspoon) in a cup of hot water. Cover and steep for 10 to 15 minutes. Consume 30 minutes to 2 hours before sleep. It can also be taken as capsules/tablets 300 to 600 mg before bedtime. It may be more effective if taken continuously for at least 4 weeks instead of on and off.

Wild black cherry juice. Take 30 mL of fresh black cherry juice 2 hours before sleep.

Therapeutic Measures

Diet

GABA (Gamma-Aminobutyric Acid) Supplements. These may promote relaxation and sleep. Side effects include nausea, poor appetite, drowsiness and weakness. It can interact with barbiturates and benzodiazepines.

Minerals and Vitamins. Take adequate oral magnesium (300 to 400 mg/day for adults) and vitamin B (especially B3 and B6) to relax muscles and reduce stress.

Amino acids that promote sleep include glycine, L-theanine, and tryptophan (5-HTP or 5-hydroxytryptophan is the derivative of tryptophan and it is used by the body to make melatonin). They are available as supplements or found in foods.

Examples of L-theanine–rich foods include green tea and mushroom, and tryptophan-rich foods include nuts, seeds, eggs, dairy products, turkey, and red meat.

Melatonin-rich foods include various grains (barley, rolled oats), vegetables (sweet corn, asparagus, broccoli, olives, and tomato), fruit (tart cherries, grapes, strawberry), and nuts and seeds (pistachio, almond, peanut, walnut, flaxseed, mustard seed).

Side effects of tryptophan supplements include headaches, nausea, and a serious disorder called eosinophilia-myalgia syndrome.

Combination Sleep Aids. These combine GABA, 5-HTP and melatonin. Some propriety brands include Dream Water, Sleep Shot and Sleep Powder.

Lifestyle

Epsom salt bath. Run a warm bath and add ½ cup of Epsom salts (magnesium sulphate). Soak in the bath for about 30 to 60 minutes to relax the body and induce good-quality sleep. Lavender essential oils may also be added to the bath.

Aromatherapy/Essential oils. Many oils, used singly or in combination, can be relaxing and promote deep sleep. These include lavender, rose/rosehip oil, jasmine, sandalwood, citrus, bergamot, lemon balm, peppermint, chamomile, cedarwood, geranium, ylang-ylang, and vanilla. It can be rubbed or massaged at the wrists, temples, neck, and soles of the feet or dropped onto the pajama collar or on the pillow cover. An aromatherapy diffuser can also be used. Beware of allergic reactions.

Sleep position. Sleeping on the left side, i.e., left lateral position, is believed to give better sleep quality via better blood circulation and increased elimination of stools. Sleeping prone (on the tummy) is not advised.

Hypnotherapy. This method uses the power of suggestion to bring desirable and positive changes in the patient under hypnosis.

Bowen therapy. This is a gentle hands-on and non-manipulative technique that uses rolling movements to stimulate the soft tissues and release both physical and emotional pain in insomnia and other conditions.

Weekend camping. Preliminary studies have shown that weekend camping under the night sky can promote earlier sleep onset and reset the body's circadian rhythms with a rise in salivary melatonin levels.

Baby Dream Machine. This is a sleep device which promotes quality and quantity sleep in children from 3 months old to 12 years old, via 5 mechanisms. ie night light, red light (to increase melatonin secretion), pink noise (via sound machine), cool-mist humidifier and aromatherapy (with organic natural essential oils).

Modern Remedies

Relaxation Training

This form of treatment teaches individuals suffering from insomnia about muscle relaxation to relax the body and induce sleep. Breathing exercises, mindfulness, meditation, and guided imagery may also be taught as a part of relaxation training.

Stimulus Control

Stimulus control teaches individuals how to form an association between sleeping and the bedroom by restricting the types of activities carried out in the bedroom, for example, only going to the bedroom when the individual feels sleepy and leaving the bedroom if they are unable to sleep for 20 minutes or more.

Cognitive Behavioral Therapy

CBT teaches individuals behavioral changes such as a regular bedtime routine and time. It works to remove negativity and worries regarding sleep and associate it instead with rational and healthy thoughts.

Biofeedback Therapy

This method is often used together with relaxation training so that one is more aware of one's physical stress response and how to control the stress response.

Pulsed electromagnetic therapy (PEMF)

PEMF pillows or pads are used to modify the neurochemical circuits to increase serotonin , dopamine and reduce the stress hormones. PEMT can increase melatonin and improve sleep quality.

Later School Start Time

This is suitable for teenagers who tend to have a "forward-placed sleep cycle" and cannot wake early.

Sedatives and Hypnotics

Benzodiazepine Hypnotics

This form of medication binds to benzodiazepine receptors on the GABA receptor complex in the body, enhancing its activity. The enhancement of GABA activity in the brain leads to increased feelings of drowsiness, allowing the individual to fall asleep or maintain sleep. It is habit-forming and should not be used long term. Examples: diazepam, alprazolam, flurazepam, quazepam, and estazolam.

Non-Benzodiazepine Hypnotics: This form of medication works similarly to benzodiazepine hypnotics but has different chemical structures to benzodiazepines. Examples: zolpidem (Ambien), zopiclone (Imovane), and zaleplon (Sonata).

Melatonin and Melatonin Receptor Agonist

Melatonin is a hormone responsible for regulating our sleep-wake cycles. Melatonin receptor agonists are analogues of melatonin that bind to the melatonin receptors, causing increased feelings of drowsiness and helping to induce sleep. Side effects include headache, dizziness, and nausea. Melatonin in a dose of 0.1 to 3 mg is usually sufficient. The fast-release and slow-release formulas are both available. It is safe to use for short term for 3 months or less. It can interact with anti-platelet drugs, anticoagulants, and anti-hypertensive drugs.

Ramelteon: It is a melatonin receptor agonist.

Selective Serotonin Reuptake Inhibitor Class

Trazodone. It is an antidepressant medication and is also used as a sleep aid.

Alpha-2 Antagonist

Mirtazapine (RemeronSolTab) is an orally disintegrating tablet that is taken sublingually.

Orexin Receptor Antagonist

Lemborexant (Dayvigo) may help patients who have difficulties with sleep onset and/or sleep maintenance.

CBD (Cannabidiol) Oil

This is from the marijuana or hemp plant. It helps to improve sleep quality by increasing NREM sleep. A dose of 25 to 175 mg is recommended.

Homeopathic Remedies

These include arsenicum album (in the anxious person or in the overthinkers who have difficulty falling asleep); aconite (if fear of sleep and death); alumina (if slow and dull in the morning because of light sleep and frequent night awakening); baryta carb (frequent awakening with nightmares); *Nux vomica* (insomnia because of overeating or overindulgence); *Coffea cruda* (for light sleepers with noise sensitivity and inability to get into a deep sleep); aurum metallicum (if early morning awakening at 4 or 5 a.m. with the inability to return to sleep, usually in depression); *Staphysagria* (early morning awakening with anger and daytime sleepiness); belladonna (if bad dreams waken one up and unable to return to sleep); *Lycopodium* (if no dreams and associated indigestion), calcarea carb (if associated physical fatigue and muscle weakness), *Cina* for worms in children, *Rhus tox* for restless leg syndrome, causticum if associated bedwetting soon after sleep, *Pulsatilla* etc.

Take the remedy about one hour before bedtime. It can be repeated just before lying in bed or if there is night awakening.

References

Yoga Guy. (2020, December 29). *11 types of pranayama breathing techniques with instructions*. Yogic Logic. Retrieved from https://yogiclogic.com/types-of-pranayama/.

Anxiety Disorders

Anxiety and Depression Association of America (ADAA). (n.d.). *Treatment*. ADAA. Retrieved from https://adaa.org/find-help/treatment-help.

Anxiety and Depression Association of America (ADAA). (2019, July). *Medication options*. ADAA. Retrieved from https://adaa.org/find-help/treatment-help/medication-options.

Kecskes, A. A. (2019, February 21). *Anxiety disorders and traditional Chinese medicine*. Pacific College. Retrieved from https://www.pacificcollege.edu/news/blog/2014/10/04/anxiety-disorders-and-traditional-chinese-medicine.

Khalsa, K. P. S. (2020, October 30). *How adaptogenic herbs reduce stress*. Better Nutrition. Retrieved from https://www.betternutrition.com/features/adaptogenic-herbs-for-stress/.

Mental Health Food Admin. (2017, October 1). *12 Herbal remedies for depression and anxiety*. Mental Health Food. Retrieved from https://mentalhealthfood.net/13-herbs-for-treating-depression-and-anxiety/.

mindbodygreen. (2020a, August 25). *Why My Anxiety Led Me To Chinese Medicine*. https://www.mindbodygreen.com/0-8282/why-my-anxiety-led-me-to-chinese-medicine.html

Mischke, M. (2021, July 3). *Cultivating calm*. Banyan Botanicals. Retrieved from https://www.banyanbotanicals.com/info/ayurvedic-living/living-ayurveda/health-guides/the-channel-of-the-mind/cultivating-calm/.

Okada, C., Iso, H., Ishihara, J., Maruyama, K., Sawada, N., Tsugane, S., & JPHC FFQ Validation Study Group (2017). Validity and reliability of a self-administered food frequency questionnaire for the JPHC study: The assessment of amino acid intake. *Journal of Epidemiology*, *27*(5), 242–247. Retrieved from https://doi.org/10.1016/j.je.2016.06.003.

Pitko, C. (2015, January 8). *A basic intro to alternate nostril breathing*. DoYou. Retrieved from https://www.doyou.com/a-basic-intro-to-alternate-nostril-breathing/.

Prakash, P. (2017, April 10). *6 Natural herbs for anxiety to calm you down*. NDTV Food. Retrieved from https://food.ndtv.com/food-drinks/6-natural-herbs-for-anxiety-to-calm-you-down-1674389.

Rana, S. (2017, August 28). *5 Ayurvedic herbs you can use to fight stress and calm your mind*. NDTV Food. Retrieved from https://food.ndtv.com/health/5-ayurvedic-herbs-you-can-use-to-fight-stress-and-calm-your-mind-1742290.

Scullion, E. (2020, April 8). *Top homeopathy remedies for relieving anxiety*. Homeopathy Healing. Retrieved from https://www.homeopathy-healing.com/top-homeopathy-remedies-for-relieving-anxiety/.

The National Institute of Mental Health Information Resource Center. (2018, July). *Anxiety disorders*. NIH. Retrieved from https://www.nimh.nih.gov/health/topics/anxiety-disorders/.

Thorne, T. (2017, March 16). *3 Common kitchen herbs and spices for anxiety and depression*. Green Med Info. Retrieved from https://www.greenmedinfo.com/blog/3-common-kitchen-herbs-and-spices-anxiety-and-depression.

WebMD Editors. (2003, February 2). *Anxiety disorders*. WebMD. Retrieved from https://www.webmd.com/anxiety-panic/guide/anxiety-disorders#1.

White, A. (2019, March 29). *What are some homeopathic options for treating anxiety?* Healthline. Retrieved from https://www.healthline.com/health/homeopathy-for-anxiety.

Depression

Anxiety and Depression Association of America (ADAA). (n.d.). *Treatment*. ADAA. Retrieved from https://adaa.org/understanding-anxiety/depression/treatment.

Cohen, J. (n.d.). *Ayurvedic herbal home remedies for depression*. Streetdirectory. Retrieved from https://www.streetdirectory.com/travel_guide/110846/depression/ayurvedic_herbal_home_remedies_for_depression.html.

Farkas, T. (2017, May 10). *Chinese herbs for depression unclog your qi—Beliefnet*. Depression Help. Retrieved from https://www.beliefnet.com/columnists/depressionhelp/2017/10/chinese-herbs-depression.html.

Li, M., Yao, X., Sun, L., Zhao, L., Xu, W., Zhao, H., et al. (2020). Effects of electroconvulsive therapy on depression and its potential mechanism. *Frontiers in Psychology*, *11*, 80. Retrieved from https://doi.org/10.3389/fpsyg.2020.00080.

Maharishi AyurVeda Staff. (2021). *Ten ways to beat the blues: Ayurvedic recommendations for emotional health*. Maharishi AyurVeda. Retrieved from https://www.mapi.com/ayurvedic-knowledge/emotional-support/ten-ayurvedic-tips-for-beating-depression.html.

Mayo Clinic Staff. (2017, February 8). *Light therapy*. Mayo Clinic. Retrieved from https://www.mayoclinic.org/tests-procedures/light-therapy/about/pac-20384604.

Mental Health Food Admin. (2017a, September 1). *5 Ways to spice up your mental health*. Mental Health Food. Retrieved from https://mentalhealthfood.net/5-ways-to-spice-up-your-mental-health/.

Mental Health Food Admin. (2017b, October 1). *12 Herbal remedies for depression and anxiety*. Mental Health Food. Retrieved from https://mentalhealthfood.net/13-herbs-for-treating-depression-and-anxiety/.

Natural On. (2016, December 4). *7 Herbs and spices that can treat depression naturally*. NaturalON—Natural Health News and Discoveries. Retrieved from https://naturalon.com/7-herbs-and-spices-that-can-treat-depression-naturally/view-all/.

NHS website. (2021, February 26). *Treatment—clinical depression*. NHS.UK. Retrieved from https://www.nhs.uk/mental-health/conditions/clinical-depression/treatment/.

NYU Langone Hospitals. (n.d.-a). *Depression in adults*. NYU Langone Health. Retrieved from https://nyulangone.org/conditions/depression-in-adults.

NYU Langone Hospitals. (n.d.-b). *Therapy for depression in adults*. NYU Langone Health. Retrieved from https://nyulangone.org/conditions/depression-in-adults/treatments/therapy-for-depression-in-adults.

Patel, A. (2016, November 13). *14 Effective homeopathic remedies for depression—Natural Homeopathic Clinic*. Natural Homeopathic Clinic. Retrieved from http://www.naturalhomeopathicclinic.co.uk/14-effective-homeopathic-remedies-for-depression/.

Positivity, P. O. (2018b, August 16). *10 Essential Spices That Help Fight Depression*. Power of Positivity: Positive Thinking & Attitude. https://www.powerofpositivity.com/spices-fight-depression/

Rana, S. (2018, June 1). *How to get rid of depression: 5 Herbal remedies that could help*. NDTV Food. Retrieved from https://food.ndtv.com/health/5-herbal-remedies-for-depression-know-what-could-help-1683655.

Schimelpfening, N. (2020, December 15). *The 5 major classes of antidepressants*. Verywell Mind. Retrieved from https://www.verywellmind.com/what-are-the-major-classes-of-antidepressants-1065086.

TCM Simple. (2021). *Chinese medicine treatment for depression—TCM simple*. Tcmsimple.Com. Retrieved from https://www.tcmsimple.com/depression.php.

The Chalkboard Editorial Team. (2019, January 18). *The Two Types of Depression According To Traditional Chinese Medicine*. The Chalkboard. https://thechalkboardmag.com/understanding-depression-types-traditional-chinese-medicine

National Institute of Mental Health (2021). Eating Disorders. Retrieved December 13, 2021, from https://www.nimh.nih.gov/health/topics/eating-disorders.

The National Institute of Mental Health Information Resource Center. (2018, February). *Depression*. NIH. Retrieved from https://www.nimh.nih.gov/health/topics/depression/.

University of Manchester. (2019, February 5). *Healthy diet can ease symptoms of depression*. ScienceDaily. Retrieved from https://www.sciencedaily.com/releases/2019/02/190205090511.htm.

Villines, Z. (2019, November 15). *Homeopathic treatments for anxiety: What to know*. Medical News Today. Retrieved from https://www.medicalnewstoday.com/articles/327011.

Voderholzer, U. (2003). Sleep deprivation and antidepressant treatment. *Chronobiology and Mood Disorders, 5*(4), 366–369. Retrieved from https://doi.org/10.31887/dcns.2003.5.4/uvoderholzer.

Schizophrenia

Balkrishna, A., & Misra, L. N. (2017). Ayurvedic plants in brain disorders: The herbal hope. *Journal of Traditional Medicine & Clinical Naturopathy, 6*(2), 1–9. Retrieved from https://doi.org/10.4172/2573-4555.1000221.

Busti, A. J. (2015, August). *Common Chinese herbal supplements used in the treatment of schizophrenia*. Evidence-Based Medicine Consult. Retrieved from https://www.ebmconsult.com/articles/herbal-natural-medicine-schizophrenia-psychiatry.

Casarella, J. (2016, August 31). *Schizophrenia treatment: Types of therapy and medications*. WebMD. Retrieved from https://www.webmd.com/schizophrenia/schizophrenia-therapy#1.

CCA Students. (2009, September 21). *Ayurvedic & Western approaches to the treatment of schizophrenia (by Rubén Vega, MA)*. California College of Ayurveda. Retrieved from https://www.ayurvedacollege.com/blog/schizophrenia/#Ayurevedic_Interpretation_of_Schizophrenia_and_other_Psychotic_Disorders.

Chaudhry, I. B., Husain, M. O., Khoso, A. B., Husain, M. I., Buch, M. H., & Kiran, T., et al. (2020). A randomized clinical trial of methotrexate points to possible efficacy and adaptive immune dysfunction in psychosis. *Translational Psychiatry, 10*(1), 415. Retrieved from https://doi.org/10.1038/s41398-020-01095-8.

Cleveland Clinic. (n.d.). *Schizophrenia: Symptoms, causes, treatments*. Retrieved from https://my.clevelandclinic.org/health/diseases/4568-schizophrenia.

CureJoy Editorial. (2018, January 11). *Natural remedies to help tackle schizophrenia*. CureJoy. Retrieved from https://curejoy.com/content/natural-treatment-for-schizophrenia/.

Farah, F. H. (2018). Schizophrenia: An overview. *Asian Journal of Pharmaceutics, 12*(2), 77–87. Retrieved from https://www.researchgate.net/publication/326922790_Schizophrenia_An_Overview.

Frankenburg, F. R. (2020, September 17). *Schizophrenia treatment & management: Approach considerations, antipsychotic pharmacotherapy, other pharmacotherapy*. MedScape. Retrieved from https://emedicine.medscape.com/article/288259-treatment.

Guzman, F. (2019, June 27). *First-generation antipsychotics: An introduction*. Psychopharmacology Institute. Retrieved from https://psychopharmacologyinstitute.com/antipsychotics/first-generation-antipsychotics/#Neuroleptics.

Kiefer, D. (2018, August 15). *Complementary and alternative treatments for schizophrenia*. Healthline. Retrieved from https://www.healthline.com/health/schizophrenia/alternative-treatments.

Ma, X. (n.d.). *Schizophrenia*. Acupuncture.Com. Retrieved from http://www.acupuncture.com/Conditions/schizo.htm.

Mental Health Daily. (2015, January 23). *7 Natural remedies for schizophrenia to help reduce symptoms*. Retrieved from https://mentalhealthdaily.com/2014/03/28/7-natural-remedies-for-schizophrenia-to-help-reduce-symptoms/.

Oberai, P., Gopinadhan, S., Sharma, A., Nayak, C., & Gautam, K. (2016). Homoeopathic management of Schizophrenia: A prospective, non-comparative, open-label observational study. *Indian Journal of Research in Homoeopathy, 10*(2), 108–118. Retrieved from https://doi.org/10.4103/0974-7168.183877.

Rathbone, J., Zhang, L., Zhang, M., Xia, J., Liu, X., & Yang, Y. (2005, October 19). *Chinese herbal medicine for schizophrenia*. Cochrane. Retrieved from https://www.cochrane.org/CD003444/SCHIZ_chinese-herbal-medicine-for-schizophrenia.

Rogers, J. (2017, January 8). *12 Natural remedies for schizophrenia*. Natural Alternative Remedy. Retrieved from https://www.naturalalternativeremedy.com/12-natural-remedies-for-schizophrenia/?__cf_chl_managed_tk__=pmd_ffbce6aaad468a5cc8641c1bd53584536ffd9c03-1627093312-0-gqNtZGzNAuKjcnBszQiO.

Sharma, V. (2019, March 29). *Top 7 natural homeopathic medicines for schizophrenia*. Homeopathy at DrHomeo.Com. Retrieved from https://www.drhomeo.com/schizophrenia/homeopathic-remedies-for-schizophrenia/.

Singh, V. J. (2019, January 3). *Herbal remedies for schizophrenia, ayurvedic treatment—causes & symptoms*. Chandigarh Ayurved &

Panchakarma Centre. Retrieved from https://www.chandigarhay-urvedcentre.com/blog/herbal-remedies-for-schizophrenia/.

Insomnia

Alternative Medicine for Health. (2019). *Insomnia herbal remedy is good for health*. alternativemedicineforhealth.blogspot. Retrieved from http://alternativemedicineforhealth.blogspot.com/2015/02/insomnia-herbal-hemedy-is-good-for.html.

Berkheiser, K. (2019, October 21). *The 6 best bedtime teas that help you sleep*. Healthline. Retrieved from https://www.healthline.com/nutrition/teas-that-help-you-sleep.

Bhargava, S. (2020, June 26). *Suffering from insomnia? 6 Yoga poses for deep sleep*. Swirlster.Ndtv.Com. Retrieved from https://swirlster.ndtv.com/wellness/suffering-from-insomnia-6-yoga-poses-for-deep-sleep-2252749.

Birla, S. (2016, March 11). *How to sleep better naturally with spices*. Sepalika. Retrieved from https://www.sepalika.com/sleep/how-to-sleep-better/.

Breus, M. J. (2020, April 28). *Our Definitive List Of The 15 Best Sleep Supplements & Aids**. (n.d.). The 15 Best Sleep Supplements & Aids of 2022. https://www.mindbodygreen.com/articles/supplements-for-sleep/

British Homeopathic Association. (n.d.). *Insomnia*. Homeopathy UK. Retrieved from https://homeopathy-uk.org/homeopathy/how-homeopathy-helps/conditions/insomnia.

Chauhan, V. (2016, January 22). *Complete list of ayurvedic home remedies + herbs for insomnia*. AyurvedaNextDoor. Retrieved from http://ayurvedanextdoor.com/herbs-for-insomnia/.

Cherney, K. (2019, September 30). *What the principles of Feng Shui and Vastu Shastra say about sleep direction*. Healthline. Retrieved from https://www.healthline.com/health/best-direction-to-sleep.

Cirino, E. (2018, May 24). *5 Pressure points for sleep*. Healthline. Retrieved from https://www.healthline.com/health/pressure-points-for-sleep.

Cronkleton, E. (2018, August 17). *8 Home remedies for insomnia*. Healthline. Retrieved from https://www.healthline.com/health/healthy-sleep/insomnia-home-remedies.

de Bellefonds, C. (2021, May 28). *How acupuncture can optimize sleep patterns and free you from insomnia*. Healthline. Retrieved from https://www.healthline.com/health/acupuncture-for-sleep.

Fry, A. (2020, September 18). *Treatments for insomnia*. Sleep Foundation. Retrieved from https://www.sleepfoundation.org/insomnia/treatment.

Gao, S. (2017, March 1). *Traditional Chinese medicine tricks to help you sleep better*. Culture Trip. Retrieved from https://theculture-trip.com/asia/china/articles/traditional-chinese-medicine-tricks-to-help-you-sleep-better/.

Goodman, S. (2020, March 6). *Acupuncture for insomnia and sleep disorders*. Pacific College. Retrieved from https://www.pacificcol-lege.edu/news/blog/2014/10/03/acupuncture-for-insomnia-and-sleep-disorders.

Kafeel, B. (2011, September 20). *Ayurveda - Ayurvedic Treatment | Ayurveda Remedies | Ayurvedic Cure*. (n.d.). Onlymyhealth. https://www.onlymyhealth.com/alternative-therapies/ayurveda

Lamoreux, K. (2020, July 27). *Everything you need to know about insomnia*. Healthline. Retrieved from https://www.healthline.com/health/insomnia.

Maharishi Ayurveda Staff. (2021a). *Understanding kapha dosha*. Maharishi Ayurveda. Retrieved from https://www.mapi.com/ayurvedic-knowledge/doshas/kapha.html.

Maharishi Ayurveda Staff. (2021b). *Understanding pitta dosha*. Maharishi Ayurveda. Retrieved from https://mapi.com/blogs/articles/understanding-pitta-dosha.

Maharishi Ayurveda Staff. (2021c). *Understanding vata dosha*. Maharishi Ayurveda. Retrieved from https://mapi.com/blogs/articles/understanding-vata-dosha.

Marshall, L. (2017, February 1). *Can't get to sleep? A wilderness weekend can help*. CU Boulder Today. Retrieved from https://www.colorado.edu/today/2017/02/01/cant-get-sleep-wilderness-weekend-can-help.

MedicineNet Editorial Staff. (2021, June 11). *Pulsatilla*. MedicineNet. Retrieved from https://www.medicinenet.com/pulsatilla/supplements-vitamins.htm.

Merton, A. (2021, January 20). *10 Natural herbs for sleep*. PlushBeds. Retrieved from https://www.plushbeds.com/blog/sleep-aids/10-natural-herbs-for-sleep/.

Mischke, M. (2021, July 3). *Balancing insufficient sleep*. Banyan Botanicals. Retrieved from https://www.banyanbotanicals.com/info/ayurvedic-living/living-ayurveda/health-guides/an-ayurvedic-guide-to-balanced-sleep/balancing-insufficient-sleep/.

Neel, A. B. (n.d.). *10 Types of meds that can cause insomnia*. AARP. Retrieved from https://www.aarp.org/health/drugs-supplements/info-04-2013/medications-that-can-cause-insomnia.html.

Osmun, R. (2021, June 24). *12 Natural herbs for sleep*. Eachnight. Retrieved from https://eachnight.com/sleep/12-natural-herbs-for-sleep/.

Pacific College. (2019, January 8). *Oriental medicine lays insomnia to rest*. Pacific College. Retrieved from https://www.pacificcollege.edu/news/blog/2014/08/06/oriental-medicine-lays-insomnia-to-rest.

Piper, R. (2012, May 21). *10 Sleep Tips Inspired By Chinese Medicine*. (n.d.). Mindbodygreen. https://www.mindbodygreen.com/0-4879/10-Sleep-Tips-Inspired-By-Chinese-Medicine.html?fbclid=IwAR1V7tBPKHq7S_W3_9AKHnCKzeFCx9FGAhXw0pfno5GJSdh488_qfV_9M0w

Rana, S. (2017, November 28). *6 ayurvedic herbs to induce sound sleep: From Brahmi to Ashwagandha and More!* NDTV Food. Retrieved from https://food.ndtv.com/health/6-ayurvedic-herbs-to-induce-sound-sleep-from-brahmi-to-ashwagandha-and-more-1751154.

Sagrani, R. (2016, January 8). *How to treat insomnia with ayurveda*. Ayurvedic Wellness Centre Sydney. Retrieved from https://ayurvedic-wellnesscentre.com.au/how-to-treat-insomnia-with-ayurveda-2/.

Tchi, R. (2020, September 29). *Signs of blocked qi in your home (and in your life)*. Know feng shui. Retrieved from https://www.know-fengshui.com/signs-of-blocked-feng-shui-qi-in-your-home/.

The Association of Traditional Chinese Medicine & Acupuncture UK. (n.d.). *Acupuncture for insomnia*. ATCM. Retrieved from http://www.atcm.co.uk/disease/insomnia.

The Healthline Editorial Team. (2020, July 23). *Treating insomnia*. Healthline. Retrieved from https://www.healthline.com/health/insomnia-treatments#medication.

WebMD Editors. (2003, May 31). *Insomnia treatments*. WebMD. Retrieved from https://www.webmd.com/sleep-disorders/understanding-insomnia-treatment.

Yeung, W. F., Chung, K. F., Poon, M. M. K., Ho, F. Y. Y., Zhang, S. P., Zhang, Z. J., Ziea, E. T. C., & Wong Taam, V. (2012). Prescription of Chinese Herbal Medicine and Selection of Acupoints in Pattern-Based Traditional Chinese Medicine Treatment for Insomnia: A Systematic Review. *Evidence-Based Complementary and Alternative Medicine, 2012*, 1–16. https://doi.org/10.1155/2012/902578

Yeung, W.-F., Chung, K.-F., Poon, M. M.-K., Ho, F. Y.-Y., Zhang, S.-P., & Zhang, Z.-J., et al. (2012). Prescription of Chinese herbal medicine and selection of acupoints in pattern-based traditional Chinese medicine treatment for insomnia: A systematic review. *Evidence-Based Complementary and Alternative Medicine, 2012*, 1–16. Retrieved from https://doi.org/10.1155/2012/902578.

12
Cancer

Introduction

Cancer is a name given to a group of diseases where abnormal cells divide without control and have no specific function. It arises because of changes to genes controlling cell division, which then allows the cells to evade the immune system and ignore signals that stop cells from dividing. There are several causes (etiologies) for this:

Non-modifiable Causes
- Genetics
- Old age

Modifiable Causes
- Carcinogenic exposures such as tobacco smoke and alcoholic beverages
- Radiation such as x-ray radiation and ultraviolet (UV) rays

Based on a recent statistic, there were approximately 18 million new cases of cancer worldwide in 2018; of these, 4 million cases were lung and breast cancers. Moreover, there were an estimated 9.6 million deaths from cancer worldwide in 2018; and lung, colorectal, stomach, and liver cancers account for more than 4 in 10 (44%) of all deaths.

There are more than 100 types of cancer, and below are some of the common types of cancer that will be discussed:
- Breast cancer
- Lung cancer
- Colorectal cancer
- Brain cancer
- Prostate cancer
- Leukemia

General Principles in Cancer Management

General principles in the management of cancer that will be discussed are as below:
1. Nutrition
2. Exercise and energy medicine
3. Pain relief
4. Social and spiritual wellbeing
5. Immune boosters (refer to the chapter on Immune Boosters)

Nutrition (Cancer-Fighting Foods)

Cancer patients will usually experience loss of appetite, vomiting, and/or difficulty of swallowing. When feeding is not possible, alternative methods such as nasogastric feeding tube, gastric feeding tube (G-tube), nasojejunal feeding tube, and total parenteral nutrition (TPN) are used. They need to have a well-balanced diet; and below are some nutrition tips:
- Vegetarian/vegan diet is recommended.
- Advise taking dairy-free and sugar-free products.
- Eat more foods that are fresh, natural, whole, unrefined, and unprocessed such as brown rice, rolled oats, etc.
- Consume three to four servings of high antioxidant foods daily such as:
  - Amla (Indian gooseberries): 261500 ORAC value per cup
  - Ashwagandha: 8487 ORAC value per cup
  - Ling zhi (Reishi mushroom): 9244 ORAC value per cup
  - Goji berries: 3290 ORAC value per cup
  - Wild blueberries: 13427 ORAC value per cup
  - Cranberries: 8983 ORAC value per cup
- There are many phytoactive anti-cancer compounds (flavonoids, alkaloids, carotenoids, phenolic acids, terpenes, lectins, saponins etc) which are present in all plant parts (including roots, fruits, leaf, flower, seeds, stem, stamen, or bark) in every country. The list of anti-cancer regional plants is exhaustive and is beyond the scope of this book.

Note: Oxygen radical absorbance capacity (ORAC) value is used to measure the antioxidant content of different foods.

Exercise and Energy Medicine

Exercise is important for the well-being of cancer patients. It can improve their physical and emotional states by building muscle mass and improving mood, respectively. These exercises include:
- Aerobic exercise: It is an exercise that focuses on strengthening the cardiovascular system. Some of the exercises that can be carried out are brisk walking, jogging, and cycling. It is recommended to exercise daily for at least 30 minutes. For patients that feel fatigued easily, 10 minutes of exercise three times daily is suggested.

- Yoga: It is an exercise that originated from India that is believed to work by balancing the body, mind, and spirit. It combines a series of postures with meditation and rhythmic breathing. It helps patients to cope with anxiety, stress, and side effects caused by cancer treatments such as fatigue, pain, and insomnia.
- Qi gong: It is an exercise that originated from China that is believed to work by using energy (qi). There are two types of qigong: internal—which combines slow movements, meditation, and rhythmic breathing—and external, in which energy (qi) from a qi gong master is being transferred to the body. It helps in treating emotional distress in cancer patients.
- Tai chi: It is an exercise that originated from China that is believed to work by ensuring a smooth flow of energy (qi) within the body. It is a form of qigong that uses slow movements, meditation, and rhythmic breathing. It helps to strengthen muscles and improve flexibility and the sense of well-being.

Pain Relief

Pain experienced by cancer patients as a result of the cancer and its treatments can be unbearable. Hence, relieving this pain is crucial for a better quality of life. Some pain-relief medications are as below:

- Nonsteroidal anti-inflammatory drugs (NSAIDs): These reduce inflammation and relieve pain. A commonly used NSAID for cancer pain is ketorolac.
- Topical pain relievers: These work similarly to NSAIDs. Examples of topical pain relievers are capsaicin, lidocaine patch, and diclofenac sodium gel.
- Corticosteroids: These reduce inflammation and relieve pain. An example of corticosteroid that can relieve pain is dexamethasone.

Refer to the previous chapter for more information.

Social and Spiritual wellbeing

Cancer patients may feel depressed, anxious, and emotionally distressed while coping with the disease. Hence, various methods can be used to maintain a healthy mental state, such as:

- Building a strong connection with family and friends by spending more time with them. Activities that can be done together include going on a picnic, taking a vacation, and having meals together.
- Joining local or international cancer support groups as a platform to share experiences with others. Most cancer support groups also provide peer counselling that could help patients with their concerns.
- Join organizations, such as Cancerfly that help patients to get employment and business opportunities, which then solve their financial issues.
- Religious and spiritual beliefs also play an important role in helping patients cope with cancer. For example, prayers have been reported to help increase B-lymphocytes, hence boosting the immune system to fight against cancer.

Immune Boosters

Refer to the Chapter on Immune Boosters.

Traditional Complementary Alternative Medicine

Several foods are reported to have cancer-preventive and cancer-curing properties. These will be discussed under various ethnic groups:
1. Indian remedies
2. Chinese remedies
3. Western remedies

Indian Natural Remedies

Herbs and Spices

There are various foods including herbs and spices used in Indian remedies that have anti-cancer properties:

- **Cardamom.** It contains high amounts of antioxidants that are useful in preventing cancer. Research has shown that it also contains compounds that can strengthen the immune system.
- **Garlic.** It contains selenium and allitridium, which both have anti-cancer properties.
- **Amla (Indian gooseberries).** It contains high amounts of antioxidants and polyphenols such as flavonoids and tannins. These substances are proven to have both cancer-preventive and cancer-curing properties.
- **Turmeric.** It contains curcumin, which is reported to be useful against cancer. This substance can inhibit the proliferation of cancer cells and induce apoptosis of cancer cells.
- **Ashwagandha (Indian ginseng).** It contains several anti-cancer properties such as withanolides and withaferin. Some studies have shown that it works by shrinking tumor size in fibrosarcoma and cervical cancer.

Miscellaneous

There are several treatments of cancer:

- **Siddha medicine.** It is a commonly practiced traditional medicine system in India. It uses various combinations of herbs and metals to treat cancer. For example:
  - *Rasagandhi mezhugu* **(RGM) formulation.** It is made up of 38 types of herbs and inorganic substances including heavy metals. It is widely used in Southern India to treat all types of cancer. A study has shown that chloroform extract from RGM can stimulate apoptosis of cancer cells in cervical cancer.
  - *Nilavembu kudineer* **(NK).** It is also called kalmegh or kalmegha in Ayurveda. It is used to treat lymphoma, prostate cancer, colorectal cancer, and liver cancer.
  - *Swarna bhasma* **(SB).** It mainly contains gold nanoparticles, and results have shown that it can shrink tumor size of various cancers.
  - *Heerak bhasma.* It contains diamond ash nanoparticles and is used to treat various cancers.

- *Navrattan kalp amrit ras.* It contains the calcined ash of several precious gemstones and metals like sapphire, emerald, ruby, pearl, cat's eye, gold, silver, zinc, and iron. It is used to treat various cancers.

Chinese Natural Remedies

Herbs

- *Ren shen (ginseng).* It is a root of a plant commonly used in traditional Chinese medicine. It promotes apoptosis of cancer cells and inhibits angiogenesis of tumour. An experimental result has shown that the diameter of lung adenoma is decreased by 23% after using ren shen (ginseng).
- *Ling zhi (reishi mushroom).* It is a type of mushroom that has been used traditionally to treat cancer and other diseases. It enhances the immune system and inhibits the growth of cancer cells.
- *Ban zhi lian.* It is a herb that is reported to have benefits in the treatment of cancer. A study has shown that usage of ban zhi lian can reduce the risk of skin tumors.
- *Zeng sheng ping.* This is a polyherbal formula with six types of plants: *Sophora tonkinensis, Polygonum bistorta, Prunella vulgaris, Sonchus brachyotus, Dictamnus dasycarpus,* and *Dioscorea bulbifera.* Studies have shown that it can reduce the incidence of tongue squamous-cell carcinoma approximately by 30% and esophageal squamous-cell carcinoma roughly by 12%.
- *Liu wei di huang wan.* It is a herbal formula consisting of six types of plants: *Rehmannia glutinosa, Cornus officinalis sieb,* common yam rhizome, *Alisma orientalis,* tree peony bark, and poria cocos. Results have shown that it contains anti-cancer properties that can prevent lung pulmonary adenoma by 50%.
- *Xia ku cao.* Dried spikes of this plant are reported to be useful in the treatment of several hormonal-dependent cancers as it contains anti-estrogen properties.
- *Sea cucumber*: It is a marine creature used in traditional Chinese medicine. Studies have shown that it contains fatty acids and saponins, which inhibit metastasis by stimulating apoptosis of cancer cells. It also contains frondoside A, which is believed to be effective in the treatment of breast, colon, lung, liver, prostate, and skin cancer.

Miscellaneous

- **Sabah snake grass.** It is a plant commonly found in Malaysia and Thailand. It is traditionally used to treat snakebites and has been reported to have cancer-curing properties. It is recommended to consume 50 to 300 leaves of sabah snake grass (depending on cancer stage) daily.
- *Qi xing zhen (cactus bleo).* It is a type of cactus; and the leaves contain cancer-curing compounds such as terpenoid, carotenoid, and ethyl acetate.
  Results from a study have shown that it contains high amounts of antioxidants and has a cytotoxic effect on nasopharyngeal cancer cells.

Western Natural Remedies

Herbs and Spices

- **Red clover.** It is a type of plant commonly found in Asia, Europe, and North America. It contains a cancer-preventive compound known as a flavonoid, which is rich in antioxidants. Caution: it contains isoflavones (estrogen agonist). Hence, patients with hormone-sensitive cancers should not consume it.
- **Periwinkle.** It is a type of plant that contains anti-cancer compounds such as vinblastine, vincristine, vindesine, and vinorelbine. Currently, these compounds are also used in chemotherapy.
Refer to the section on chemotherapy to read more.
- **American paw paw.** It is a fruit commonly found in Native America that contains a compound known as annonaceous acetogenin. This compound is reported to slow down the growth of tumors as well as enhance the effect of chemotherapy and radiation therapy.
- **Essiac.** It is a herbal mixture that originated from Canada. It is usually consumed as a tea and contains:
  - Burdock root, which helps in promoting blood circulation and eliminating toxins.
  - Rhubarb root, which is traditionally used in Chinese medicine and helps by eliminating toxins in the colon.
  - Sheep sorrel, which contains high amounts of antioxidants and vitamins, including vitamin A, B complex, C, D, E, and K
  - Slippery elm bark, which contains high amounts of antioxidants and helps to eliminate toxins in the colon

Juices

There are several juices believed to help in the treatment of cancer:
  (Note: use a slow-juicing machine that operates at 72 to 80 revolutions per minute.)
- Lemon juice, including the skin, which contains D-limonene, which can delay the progression of cancer and expression of tumor markers.
- Mangosteen juice, including the skin (pericarp), as the skin contains substances with anti-cancer properties, such as anthocyanins, xanthones, and procyanidins.
- Fresh papaya juice, including stems and leaves. Add some crude black molasses for taste.
- Beetroot, carrot, and wheatgrass juice. It is recommended to consume four glasses per day.

Miscellaneous

- **Grape seed extract.** It is commonly taken as a supplement. It contains anticancer substances such as phenolic acids and flavonoids. Studies have shown that it reduces breast tumor size in rats and also induces apoptosis of leukemia cancer cells.
- **Apricot seed.** It contains a compound known as amygdalin, which is believed to be effective in the treatment of cancer. Caution: Amygdalin can be converted into cyanide in the body. Hence, consuming large amounts of apricot seeds might cause cyanide poisoning.

- **Broccoli sprout.** It is a type of vegetable that contains an anti-cancer compound known as sulforaphane. Studies have shown that this compound can prevent the formation of lung and colon cancers. Moreover, it can inhibit the growth of breast cancer cells.
- **Naringenin.** This dietary supplement from citrus fruits also has antioxidant and anticancer properties. It inhibits some cancers (breast, colorectal, ovarian, etc.) via several mechanisms.
- **Olive leaf extract.** This dietary supplement also has antioxidant and anticancer properties. It inhibits some cancers via its apoptotic and anti-proliferative effects.
- **Others.** Oral Extracts of Mushroom, Bromelain, Milk Thistle, Quercetin, Graviola, Curcumin-Piperine, Green tea, Boswellia, Phloretin, Nobiletin and Hydrogen rich water. These have anti-cancer and anti-inflammatory effects.
- Dietary flavonoids are plant polyphenols which have antioxidant and anti cancer effect. Their subclasses are Flavones (luteolin, apigenin), Flavonols (myricetin, quercetin), Flavanones (naringenin, hesperidin), Catechins or Flavanols (gallocatechin, epicatechin, morin), Isoflavones (genistein, daidzein), anthocyanidins (pelargonidin, cyanidinc), and Phloretin.
- **Diet:** Consume a low carbohydrate, high fibre and high protein diet. The Warburg diet is based on eating a carbohydrate-restricted diet or a ketogenic diet. Cruciferous vegetables are beneficial.

Therapies

Several alternative therapies are available. Some of these strategies/therapies listed below are integrated with standard chemotherapy regimes.

1. Hyperthermia
2. Cryotherapy
3. Ozone therapy
4. Hydrogen peroxide therapy
5. Hyperbaric oxygen therapy
6. Detoxification therapy
7. Gerson therapy
8. Homeopathy
9. Bioresonance therapy
10. Ganoderma therapy
11. Special infusions

Hyperthermia

Hyperthermia is a cancer treatment widely used in Germany. The heat is generated via radiofrequency, microwave, ultrasound, or magnets. It is usually used in combination with radiation therapy and chemotherapy. There are several types of hyperthermia:

a. Local hyperthermia works by heating up the tumor area only. Various methods can be used such as:
- High-intensity-focused ultrasound (HIFU): A tiny needle-like device will be placed over the tumor area to be heated with ultrasound.
- Radiofrequency ablation (RFA): A tiny needle-like device is used to heat the tumor area with a high-energy radio wave. This method is commonly used as an alternative treatment for cancer that cannot be surgically removed, and it can also be used with chemotherapy.

b. Regional hyperthermia works by heating a larger region of the body. There are several methods such as:
- Regional perfusion: Blood from a specific region of the body is withdrawn into a heating device. Then, the heated blood will be circulated back to heat the specific area. It can be used with chemotherapy to treat sarcomas and melanomas of the limbs.
- Deep-tissue hyperthermia: A device is placed on the surface of the specific region. Then, microwave energy or radiofrequency is given off to heat the region.
- Continuous hyperthermic peritoneal perfusion (CHPP): Heated chemotherapy drugs are used to heat up the peritoneal cavity. This method is mainly used during a surgical procedure for peritoneal cancer.

c. Whole-body hyperthermia: This is for metastatic cancer. It works by increasing the body temperature to 105°F to 107°F (37°C to 38°C). This can be done by giving patient interferon alpha, attenuated virus, or mistletoe artificially once a week. Other reported methods to induce fever include wrapping the patient with heating blankets and placing the patient in a large incubator (thermal chamber).

Cryotherapy

In cryotherapy, cancer cells are frozen using liquid nitrogen and sometimes argon gas. This works by using extreme cold to damage cancer cells. It can be used to treat skin cancer by applying liquid nitrogen onto the tumor area using a cotton swab or directly spraying on it. Then, the frozen tumor will start scabbing off by itself. For other tumors (within the body), a cryoprobe containing liquid nitrogen or argon gas is used to reach the tumor. Then, the body will start breaking down the frozen tumor naturally. Currently, it is mainly used to treat retinoblastoma, liver cancer, early-stage skin cancer, early-stage prostate cancer, and precancerous conditions such as cervical intraepithelial neoplasia (CIN). The side effects of this therapy depend on the type of cancer. For example, in the treatment of skin cancer, the patient may experience scarring of skin and loss of sensation because of injured nerves. In the treatment of CIN, the patient may experience bleeding, cramping, and pain.

Ozone Therapy

Ozone therapy supplies a high amount of oxygen to cancer cells, preventing tumor hypoxia. In this therapy, the patient's blood is withdrawn to mix with ozone (O_3) gas. Then, it is infused back into the patient's circulation. It is important to oxygenate tumors as hypoxic tumors tend to grow more aggressively and are resistant to chemotherapy and radiation therapy. Hence, this therapy is reported to be effective when used in combination with chemotherapy and radiation therapy.

Hydrogen Peroxide Therapy

Hydrogen peroxide therapy works similarly to ozone therapy by creating a high-oxygen-content environment. In this therapy, hydrogen peroxide (H_2O_2) is administered to the body to destroy cancer cells. However, this therapy is believed to have a high risk as a high concentration of H_2O_2 can be fatal.

Hyperbaric Oxygen Therapy

Pressurized oxygen therapy can kill cancer cells in association with chemotherapy and radiation therapy.

Detoxification Therapy

This therapy is believed to treat cancer by eliminating toxins in the body, and it can be carried out using several ways:

- **Coffee enema.** In this method, cooled coffee is filled into an enema bag. Then, it is administered into the rectum to stimulate bowel and liver detoxification.
- **Water fasting.** In this method, patients need to stop consuming food and drink only large amounts of water, preferably distilled water, for 1 to 2 days (for water-fasting beginners). This method is also believed to treat cancer by stimulating autophagy, which is a self-renewal process that breaks down older cellular components.

Gerson Therapy

This is a therapy originating from Germany that requires patients to follow a strict diet regimen known as the Gerson diet. It is believed to work by boosting the immune system, balancing sodium and potassium levels in the blood, and eliminating toxins in the body. This diet includes:

- Drinking 15 to 20 pounds of organic fruits and vegetable juices every hour about 13 times a day. The juice should be freshly prepared every hour using a masticating juicer with a separate hydraulic press or a two-step juicer.
- Consuming full plant-based meals made from organic and whole products three times daily, such as salads, baked potatoes, Hippocrates soup, and cooked vegetables.
- Taking supplements such as potassium compound, Lugol's solution, vitamin B12, pancreatic enzymes, and thyroid supplements.
- Inducing detoxification by having up to five coffee enemas daily.

Homeopathy

It is a widely used therapy originating from Germany. It is believed that the body can be treated using the concept of "like with like" (natural substances matching symptoms of diseases). For example:

- *Phytolacca*, carcinosinum, and *Conium maculatum* are used in treatment of breast cancer.
- *Thuja*, carcinosinum, medorrhinum, *Cantharis*, *Conium*, and *Sabal serrulata* are used in the treatment of prostate cancer.
- Aurum metallicum is a powerful antioxidant

Bioresonance Therapy

This is a therapy originating from Germany that can be used to detect cancer accurately from an early stage. It transmits electromagnetic waves into the body using a device. The wave pattern will change in the presence of a tumor, and a device is used to detect the changes. It is also believed to be effective in treating cancer by interfering with communication between cancer cells.

Ganoderma Therapy

This is a therapy that uses a type of fungus known as *Ganoderma lucidum*, reishi mushroom or ling zhi. It is usually taken in capsule form and as a supplement because of its cancer-preventive properties. Some studies have shown that it contains compounds with high antioxidants and can enhance the activity of natural killer (NK) cells. It is believed to be effective in the treatment of breast cancer, prostate cancer, and colorectal cancer. For example, a study has shown that the tumor size of colorectal cancer is reduced after being treated with *Ganoderma lucidum* for a year.

Maitake mushroom is also used in ganoderma therapy as it has properties similar to reishi mushroom. Studies have shown that it activates the activity of NK cells and induces apoptosis of cancer cells. It is believed to be effective in the treatment of breast cancer, lung cancer, and myelodysplastic syndromes (MDS).

Special Infusions

They are used as off-label treatments. There may be more risks than benefits and some are not FDA-approved.

These include:

- Intravenous vitamins, minerals and anti-oxidants. High dose Vitamin C and glutathione are often used. Others include Vitamin B including pyridoxine.
- Intravenous methylsulfonylmethane (MSM) infusion is given for pain relief.
- Intravenous Anti-glycolytic agents (natural or synthetic) such as quercetin, phloretin, oxamic acid, and dichloroacetate can inhibit glycolysis so that adenosine triphosphate (ATP) energy generation is reduced and cancer cells will die.
- Injectable Mistletoe. Subcutaneous route is more commonly used than the intravenous route. It can slow the progression of cancer.

- Intravenous Selenium. It can prevent or decrease cancer metastases.
- Intravenous Vitamin B17 (also called amygdalin). The natural form of B17 is found in apricot kernel, bitter almond and other nuts. Laetrile is the synthetic form of B17. B17 may provide some pain relief and boost immunity. There is risk of adulterated or contaminated products. Cyanide poisoning is higher with oral B17.
- Intravenous Curcumin. Although cucurmin is a powerful antioxidant, fatal allergic reactions can occur with the injectable form.
- Metabolic interventions. Insulin -induced and/or fasting hypoglycemia are done to starve the cancer cells of glucose so as to correct the metabolic dysregulation and decrease cancer cell proliferation.

Modern Management and Treatment

Management includes specific diagnostic tests and various treatments. These tests will depend on the type of cancer:
- Breast cancer: Ultrasound, mammogram (film-screen mammography, digital mammography, and 3D mammography), and biopsy are widely used. Computed tomography (CT) and magnetic resonance imaging (MRI) scans are rarely used.
- Lung cancer: Chest x-ray, CT scan of the thorax, sputum cytology, bronchoscopy, and lung biopsy.
- Colorectal cancer: Colonoscopy and colorectal biopsy, blood for carcinoembryonic antigen (CEA), Endorectal ultrasound, PET-CT scan, MRI.
- Brain cancer: CT scan, MRI, lumbar puncture, and brain biopsy (transrectal prostate biopsy and MRI-guided transperineal fusion biopsy).
- Prostate cancer: Ultrasound and prostate biopsy (transrectal prostate biopsy and MRI-guided transperineal fusion biopsy.
- Leukemia: Complete blood count and bone marrow aspiration.
  (Note: A whole-body PET (positron emission tomography) scan is sometimes required for metastatic cancers.)
  Treatments that will be discussed are as follows:
1. Surgery
2. Chemotherapy
3. Radiotherapy & Radiosurgery
4. Immunotherapy

Surgery

Surgery performed also depends on the organ involved. The following cancer is discussed:

Breast Cancer

Surgery is considered as the primary treatment for breast cancer. The surgeries that are commonly carried out are:
1. Lumpectomy, where only a part of the breast is removed.
2. Mastectomy, where the entire breast is removed. Once it reaches an advanced stage, it tends to spread to surrounding lymph nodes. Hence, lymph nodes might need to be removed depending on the situation. The two main types of surgery for lymph nodes removal are sentinel lymph node biopsy (SLNB) and axillary lymph node dissection (ALND).

Lung Cancer

Surgery is commonly used to treat non-small-cell lung cancer (NSCLC). Rarely, surgery is used for small-cell lung cancer (SCLC) unless diagnosed at an early stage. Surgeries that can be carried out include:
1. Pneumonectomy, where an entire lung is removed. This might be needed if the tumor is near to the center of the chest.
2. Lobectomy, where the affected lobe is removed. This procedure is preferred for NSCLC if it can be done.
3. Segmentectomy (wedge resection), where only a part of a lobe is removed. This procedure is preferred for the patient who cannot withstand lobectomy.
4. Sleeve resection, which is used to treat cancers in large airways. This procedure can also preserve more lung function compared to pneumonectomy.
5. Video-assisted thoracic surgery (VATS), which can be used to treat early-stage lung cancer that is confined to the outer part of the lung. This procedure is guided by a tiny video camera.

Colorectal Cancer

Surgery is usually done using laparoscopy. Hence, only small incisions are needed to carry out the procedure. The surgeries done are:
1. Partial colectomy, where part of a colon is removed and the remaining parts are joined through anastomosis.
2. Ileocolectomy, where the ileum is removed.
3. Abdominoperineal resection, where the anus, rectum, and sigmoid colon are removed.
4. Proctosigmoidectomy, where the rectum and sigmoid colon are removed.
5. Total abdominal colectomy, where the entire colon is removed.

Brain Cancer

Surgery that is usually done is craniotomy. There are several types of craniotomies:
1. Awake craniotomy, which is performed for removal of any intra-axial tumors near the motor and language cortex.
2. Extended bifrontal craniotomy, which is performed for removal of tumors that cannot be removed by minimally invasive procedures. This is usually used to treat meningiomas, esthesioneuroblastoma (olfactory neuroblastoma), and malignant skull-base tumors.
3. Minimally invasive supraorbital craniotomy, which is performed by making small incisions within the eyebrow. This is usually used to treat skull-base tumors, pituitary tumors, and Rathke's cleft cysts.
4. Retro-sigmoid craniotomy (keyhole craniotomy), which is performed by making incisions behind the ear, hence

providing access to cerebellum and brainstem. This is usually used to treat acoustic neuromas (vestibular schwannomas), meningiomas, skull-base tumors, and metastatic brain tumors.

5. Orbitozygomatic craniotomy, which is performed by making an incision in the scalp (behind the hairline) and removing the bone that forms the contour of orbit and cheek. This is usually used to treat craniopharyngiomas, pituitary tumors, and meningiomas.

Prostate Cancer

The following types of surgery can be done:

1. Radical prostatectomy, which is the most commonly used procedure for prostate cancer. However, it can be used only if the cancer has not spread elsewhere. There are several types of radical prostatectomy:
   - Open radical prostatectomy, which is performed by making an incision at the lower abdomen (retropubic surgery) or between scrotum and anus (perineal surgery).
   - Laparoscopic radical prostatectomy, which is more commonly used as it is less invasive than the open approach.

- Robotic-assisted radical prostatectomy, which uses a robotic surgery system (da Vinci surgical system) to remove the prostate with great precision.

2. Transurethral resection of the prostate (TURP), which is performed to relieve urinary symptoms by removing the inner part of the prostate using a ureteroscope.

Leukemia

Surgery plays a limited role in the treatment of leukemia as it is usually widely spread throughout the body. However, splenectomy may be done for chronic lymphoid leukemia (CLL) if there is massive spleen enlargement.

Chemotherapy

Chemotherapy destroys cancer cells and prevents them from multiplying further. However, in this process, normal healthy cells can also be destroyed. There are several types of chemotherapy medications available, as listed below. Various combinations are used in cancer protocols

Cytotoxic Drugs

Type	Mechanism of Action	Group	Example and Indication
Alkylating agents	Interferes with transcription and replication of deoxyribonucleic acid (DNA)	Nitrogen mustards	Cyclophosphamide (commonly used), chlorambucil, ifosfamide, melphalan Used mainly in breast cancer, ovarian cancer, Hodgkin lymphoma, chronic lymphocytic leukemia (CLL), neuroblastoma, Wilms tumor, soft-tissue sarcoma, and rhabdomyosarcoma
		Nitrosourea	Lomustine, carmustine Used mainly in brain cancer because of its lipid-soluble property that can cross the blood-brain barrier
		Platinum compounds	Cisplatin, carboplatin Used mainly in ovarian cancer, breast cancer, testicular cancer, bladder cancer, and cervical cancer Note: Cisplatin may cause serious nephrotoxicity, so strict hydration regimens are needed.
		Others	Busulfan Used mainly in chronic myeloid leukemia (CML)
Antimetabolites	Inhibits dihydrofolate reductase (DHFR) enzyme and depletes intracellular tetrahydrofolate	Folate antagonist	Methotrexate Used mainly in breast cancer, head and neck cancer, osteogenic sarcoma, non-Hodgkin lymphoma, bladder cancer, and immunosuppression Note: high-dose regimens must be followed with folinic acid.
	Interferes with deoxyuridine monophosphate (dTMP) synthesis	Pyrimidine pathway antagonist	Fluorouracil Used mainly in colorectal cancer and other solid tumors
	Inhibits DNA by incorporating thiopurine analogues into the DNA structure	Purine pathway antagonists	Mercaptopurine, thioguanine Used mainly in childhood acute lymphocytic leukemia (ALL) and acute myeloid leukemia (AML) Note: may cause myelosuppression, immunosuppression, and hepatotoxicity

Type	Mechanism of Action	Group	Example and Indication
Anti-cancer antibiotics	Inhibits topoisomerase II	Anthracyclines	Doxorubicin Used mainly in breast cancer, ovarian cancer, soft-tissue sarcoma, and Hodgkin and non-Hodgkin lymphoma Note: may cause cardiotoxicity, alopecia, myelosuppression, and stomatitis
			Daunorubicin Used mainly in acute myeloid leukemia (AML), acute lymphocytic leukemia (ALL), chronic myeloid leukemia (CML), and Kaposi sarcoma.
	Interferes with ribonucleic acid (RNA) polymerase and topoisomerase II and inhibits transcription of DNA	Others	Dactinomycin or actinomycin D Used in various pediatric cancers
	Functions like an alkylating agent once activated	Others	Mitomycin Used mainly in superficial bladder cancer, gastric cancer, breast cancer, non-small-cell lung cancer (NSCLC), and head and neck cancer (in combination with radiotherapy) Note: may cause hemolytic-uremic syndrome and lung fibrosis
	Causes fragmentation of DNA chains	Others	Bleomycin Used mainly in germ-cell cancer Note: may cause pulmonary fibrosis
Plant derivatives	Acts on microtubules as mitotic spindle poison, resulting in inhibition of mitosis	Taxane (from yew tree):	Paclitaxel Used mainly in breast cancer, ovarian cancer, lung cancer, and other solid tumors Note: may cause myelosuppression and peripheral neuropathy Docetaxel (semi-synthetic analogue of Paclitaxel): used in hormone-refractory prostate cancer and other solid tumors.
	Inhibits tubulin polymerization, resulting in mitotic arrest	Vinca alkaloid	Vincristine Used mainly for Hodgkin and non-Hodgkin lymphoma and acute lymphoblastic leukemia in children Note: may cause myelosuppression, peripheral neuropathy, and alopecia
	Inhibits topoisomerase enzyme, resulting in DNA damage	Topoisomerase inhibitor	Etoposide Used mainly in germ-cell cancer, lung cancer, Hodgkin and non-Hodgkin lymphoma, and gastric cancer Note: may cause alopecia and myelosuppression
			Topotecan Used as second-line therapy for advanced ovarian cancer
			Irinotecan Used in colorectal cancer

Hormone Antagonists

Type	Mechanism of Action	Group	Example and Indication
Hormone antagonists	Inhibits transcription of estrogen-responsive genes by competing with endogenous estrogen for estrogen receptors	Anti-estrogen drugs	Tamoxifen Used mainly in hormone-dependent breast cancer Note: may cause amenorrhea, hot flashes, and weight loss

Type	Mechanism of Action	Group	Example and Indication
	Suppresses synthesis of estrogen from androgen in the adrenal cortex	Aromatase inhibitors	Anastrozole, letrozole Used mainly in breast cancer in postmenopausal women
	Acts on various steps of the androgen receptor signaling pathway within the tumor	Non-steroidal androgen receptor inhibitor	Enzalutamide Used in metastatic castration resistant prostate cancer

Monoclonal Antibodies (Targeted Therapy)

Type	Mechanism of Action	Group	Example and Indication
Monoclonal antibodies	Lyses B-cells by binding to CD20	Anti-CD20	Rituximab Used mainly in lymphoma (given with other chemotherapy drugs)
	Inhibits angiogenesis by neutralizing vascular endothelial growth factor (VEGF) Inhibits BRAF V600E mutation	Anti-VEGF	Bevacizumab, Aflibercept Used mainly in colorectal cancer Encorafenib(anti-BRAF) is used in colorectal cancer together with Cetuximab
	Binds to human epidermal growth factor receptor 2 (HER2)	Anti-EGF (anti -HER2)	Trastuzumab (Herceptin), pertuzumab, ado-trastuzumab emtansine Used mainly in HER2-positive breast cancer and metastatic breast cancer
	CD-4 inhibitor		Palbociclib (for estrogen-receptor-positive ER + progesterone-receptor-positive PR + HER-negative breast cancer patients
	PARP inhibitor (poly-ADP ribose polymerase)		Olaparib for metastatic HER2-negative breast cancer patients with BRCA1 or BRCA2 mutation

Examples of Combination Chemotherapy: FOLFIRI = Folinic acid + fluorouracil + irinotecan together with Aflibercept in relapsed colorectal cancer

New immunomodulatory agents. They include Chimaeric Antigen Receptor T(CAR-T) cells, immune-checkpoint inhibitors, CAR-Natural Killer Cells (CAR-NK), Epigenetic-modifying drugs, Bispecific T-cell engagers (BiTES) and Antibody-Drug Conjugates (ADCs). They have been used mostly in non-Hodgkin's lymphoma.

Radiotherapy

Radiation therapy is used in high doses to kill and destroy cancer cells. The types of particles used in radiotherapy are as follows:

- Photon: This particle is commonly used in treating most cancers. However, it can radiate to surrounding normal tissues, leading to many side effects.
- Electron: This particle is mainly used to treat skin cancer as it is unable to radiate to deeper tissues.
- Proton: This particle can radiate precisely on the cancer area without affecting surrounding tissues. Hence, it causes fewer side effects compared to photons. It is used

in external-beam radiation therapy to treat certain cancers such as brain cancer, head and neck cancer, eye melanoma, pediatric cancer, lung cancer, base-of-skull tumor, pituitary gland tumor, and spine tumor.

There are two main types of radiation therapy:

- Internal Radiation Therapy
  1. *Brachytherapy*: A solid form of radiation (e.g., capsules and seeds) is administered and implanted into the targeted part of the body through a catheter. It is 3D image guided and will start emitting radiation for a period depending on the type of implants. This can be used for the early stage of cervical cancer using caesium-137.
  2. *Systemic therapy*: A liquid form of radiation source is administered through oral or intravenous route. This liquid will then travel throughout the body to kill cancer cells by emitting radiation. For example, in thyroid cancer, radioisotope iodine-131 is administered orally; and in prostate cancer, radioisotope lutetium-177 is administered through an intravenous route.
- External-Beam Radiation Therapy

This therapy emits radiation using a machine, and it only targets the part of the body with cancer cells, sparing surrounding normal tissues. There are several types of external-beam radiation therapy:

1. *3D conformal radiation therapy*: This therapy is commonly used. It uses high doses of radiation without damaging normal tissues, with the help of a CT scan, MRI scan, and PET scan.

2. *Intensity-modulated radiation therapy (IMRT)*: This therapy is like 3D conformal radiation therapy, but it uses smaller beams (fewer than 10 fixed-beam angles), and the strength of radiation can be controlled to give higher doses to specific parts of cancer tissue.

3. *Image-guided radiation therapy (IGRT)*: This therapy is a type of IMRT but with higher accuracy. This is because imaging scans can be used during radiation.

4. *Stereotactic radiosurgery (SRS)*: This non-invasive therapy uses focused, targeted, high-energy radiation to treat small tumors in the brain and spinal cord usually. One high dose (5-30 Gy), is given for brain and spinal cord tumors or less than five treatment sessions are given for other tumors. This radiation dose is delivered via a linear accelerator (Cyberknife), gamma knife unit (Gamma Knife)or proton beams.

   Stereotactic body radiotherapy (SBRT). This is used in the treatment of extracranial tumours.

   Stereotactic radiotherapy: In this therapy, the external beam radiation is delivered in smaller doses (about 2 Gy) over several treatment sessions. There is more time for the surrounding healthy tissues to heal between the treatment sessions.

5. *Volumetric arc therapy (VMAT)*: This novel therapy delivers radiation dose in many beam directions at the tumor. The dose is continuous and dynamic from an arc trajectory as the gantry machine rotates so that the surrounding tissues or organs around the tumor are relatively spared. The radiation delivery time is less compared to IMRT.

6. *Tomotherapy*: This novel therapy is a single integrated system that combines treatment planning, CT-guided positioning of the patient, and treatment delivery of a helical radiation beam in thin slice volumes.

7. *Intraoperative radiation therapy (IORT)*

   In intraoperative radiation therapy (IORT), a high dose of radiation is used to remove tissues surrounding the tumour area to prevent any microscopic cancer residues in the body. This is usually used during surgical removal of cancer such as breast cancer, colon cancer, brain cancer, and metastases of the spine. It can also be used in combination with external-beam radiation therapy (EBRT) as a postoperative cancer treatment.

Immunotherapy

Immunotherapy uses the immune system to recognize cancer cells as foreign cells so that they will attack and destroy cancer cells. This therapy is mainly used in end-stage cancer patients for prolongation of life. Currently, few immunotherapies are in clinical trials:

Autologous Immune Enhancement Therapy

This therapy enhances the innate immune system and is widely used in Japan. In this therapy, about 60 mL of the patient's blood will be withdrawn weekly. Then, NK cells and cytotoxic T lymphocytes (CTL) cells will be isolated from the blood sample. After 2 weeks of culture, activation, and expansion, billions of cells are obtained. These cells are then infused back into the body to fight against cancer. This is important as a cancer patient generally has very low NK cell and CTL cell counts, which cause cancer to progress rapidly. This cycle will be repeated every 2 to 3 months for about six consecutive cycles. This therapy does not cause many significant side effects compared to other cancer therapies as the cells introduced are from the patient's blood.

Dendritic Cell Vaccine

To prepare this vaccine, dendritic cells (DCs) are isolated from the patient's blood. Then, these cells are exposed to tumor antigen obtained through biopsy (patient's tumor) or from tumor antigen bank. Once the vaccine is prepared, it is injected directly into the tumor or intravenously into the body to trigger a stronger immune response against cancer cells. An example of a vaccine currently used in the United States is Sipuleucel-T for the treatment of prostate cancer.

References

American Cancer Society, Inc. (2016, May 3). *Hyperthermia to treat cancer*. Cancer.Org. Retrieved from https://www.cancer.org/treatment/treatments-and-side-effects/treatment-types/hyperthermia.html.

American Cancer Society, Inc. (2019a, October 1). *Non-small cell lung cancer surgery | Lung cancer surgery*. Cancer.Org. Retrieved from https://www.cancer.org/cancer/lung-cancer/treating-non-small-cell/surgery.html.

American Cancer Society, Inc. (2019b, October 1). *Surgery for small cell lung cancer*. Cancer.Org. Retrieved from https://www.cancer.org/cancer/lung-cancer/treating-small-cell/surgery.html.

American Cancer Society, Inc. (2020a, January 8). *Cancer vaccines and their side effects*. Cancer.Org. Retrieved from https://www.cancer.org/treatment/treatments-and-side-effects/treatment-types/immunotherapy/cancer-vaccines.html.

American Cancer Society, Inc. (2020b, January 8). *Cancer vaccines and their side effects*. Cancer.Org. Retrieved from https://www.cancer.org/treatment/treatments-and-side-effects/treatment-types/immunotherapy/cancer-vaccines.html.

American Institute for Cancer Research. (2021, January 26). *Cancer prevention*. Retrieved from https://www.aicr.org/cancer-prevention/.

Antonacci D, B. M. (2014). Anticancer Effects of Grape Seed Extract on Human Cancers: A Review. *Journal of Carcinogenesis & Mutagenesis, s8*(01). https://doi.org/10.4172/2157-2518.s8-005.

Barrett, S. (2004, November 6). *BioResonance tumor therapy*. Quackwatch. Retrieved from https://quackwatch.org/related/Cancer/bioresonance/.

Bollinger, T. (2015, May 7). *The anti-cancer properties of sea cucumber (video)*. The Truth About Cancer. Retrieved from https://thetruthaboutcancer.com/anti-cancer-properties-of-sea-cucumber/.

Breastcancer.org. (2020, December 14). *Mammography technique and types*. Retrieved from https://www.breastcancer.org/symptoms/testing/types/mammograms/types.

Butterfield, L. H. (2013). Dendritic cells in cancer immunotherapy clinical trials: Are we making progress? *Frontiers in Immunology*, *4*(454), 1–7. Retrieved from https://doi.org/10.3389/fimmu.2013.00454.

Cancer Research UK. (n.d.). *Yoga and cancer*. Retrieved from https://www.cancerresearchuk.org/about-cancer/cancer-in-general/treatment/complementary-alternative-therapies/individual-therapies/yoga.

Cancer Research UK. (2019, August 22). *Worldwide cancer statistics*. Retrieved from https://www.cancerresearchuk.org/health-professional/cancer-statistics/worldwide-cancer#heading-One.

Cassileth, B. (2010, September 21). *Red clover (Trifolium pratense)*. Cancer Network. Retrieved from https://www.cancernetwork.com/view/red-clover-trifolium-pratense.

Chan, C. L. W., Wang, C. W., Ho, R. T. H., Ng, S. M., Chan, J. S. M., Ziea, E. T. C., & Wong, V. C. W. (2012). A systematic review of the effectiveness of qigong exercise in supportive cancer care. *Supportive Care in Cancer*, *20*(6), 1121–1133. Retrieved from https://doi.org/10.1007/s00520-011-1378-3.

Chertoff, J. (2020, May 28). *10 Aerobic exercise examples: How to, benefits, and more*. Healthline. Retrieved from https://www.healthline.com/health/fitness-exercise/aerobic-exercise-examples.

Choudhari, A. S., Mandave, P. C., Deshpande, M., Ranjekar, P., & Prakash, O. (2020). Phytochemicals in Cancer Treatment: From Preclinical Studies to Clinical Practice. *Frontiers in Pharmacology*, 10. https://doi.org/10.3389/fphar.2019.01614

Coothankandaswamy, V., Liu, Y., Mao, S. C., Morgan, J. B., Mahdi, F., Jekabsons, M. B., et al. (2010). The alternative medicine pawpaw and its acetogenin constituents suppress tumor angiogenesis via the HIF-1/VEGF pathway. *Journal of Natural Products*, *73*(5), 956–961. Retrieved from https://doi.org/10.1021/np100228d.

Das, S., Das, M., & Paul, R. (2012). Swarna Bhasma in cancer: A prospective clinical study. *AYU (An International Quarterly Journal of Research in Ayurveda)*, *33*(3), 365–367. Retrieved from https://doi.org/10.4103/0974-8520.108823.

Dunkin, M. A. (2008, October 22). *Super foods for optimal health*. WebMD. Retrieved from https://www.webmd.com/food-recipes/antioxidants-your-immune-system-super-foods-optimal-health.

Edwards, R. (2018, January 16). *Broccoli sprouts: One of nature's top cancer-fighting foods*. Dr. Axe. Retrieved from https://draxe.com/nutrition/broccoli-sprouts/.

Gerson Institute. (2021, May 18). *The Gerson therapy*. Retrieved from https://gerson.org/the-gerson-therapy/.

Jiao, L., Bi, L., Lu, Y., Wang, Q., Gong, Y., Shi, J., & Xu, L. (2018). Cancer chemoprevention and therapy using Chinese herbal medicine. *Biological Procedures Online*, *20*(1), 1–14. Retrieved from https://doi.org/10.1186/s12575-017-0066-1.

Jockers, D. (2021, April 28). *5 day water fast: What to expect on the healing journey*. DrJockers.Com. Retrieved from https://drjockers.com/water-fast/.

Jung, N. C., Lee, J. H., Chung, K. H., Kwak, Y. S., & Lim, D. S. (2018). Dendritic cell-based immunotherapy for solid tumors. *Translational Oncology*, *11*(3), 686–690. Retrieved from https://doi.org/10.1016/j.tranon.2018.03.007.

Lumlerdkij, N., Tantiwongse, J., Booranasubkajorn, S., Boonrak, R., Akarasereenont, P., Laohapand, T., & Heinrich, M. (2018). Understanding cancer and its treatment in Thai traditional medicine: An ethnopharmacological-anthropological investigation. *Journal of ethnopharmacology*, 216, 259–273. https://doi.org/10.1016/j.jep.2018.01.029

Moen, I., & Stuhr, L. E. B. (2012). Hyperbaric oxygen therapy and cancer—a review. *Targeted Oncology*, *7*(4), 233–242. https://doi.org/10.1007/s11523-012-0233-x

National Cancer Institute. (2018, May 1). *External beam radiation therapy for cancer*. Retrieved from https://www.cancer.gov/about-cancer/treatment/types/radiation-therapy/external-beam.

National Cancer Institute. (2019, January 8). *Radiation therapy for cancer*. Retrieved from https://www.cancer.gov/about-cancer/treatment/types/radiation-therapy#TRT.

National Cancer Institute. (2021a, May 5). *What is cancer?* Retrieved from https://www.cancer.gov/about-cancer/understanding/what-is-cancer.

National Cancer Institute. (2021b, June 17). *Hyperthermia to treat cancer*. Retrieved from https://www.cancer.gov/about-cancer/treatment/types/hyperthermia.

National Cancer Institute. (2021c, June 21). *Cryosurgery to treat cancer*. Retrieved from https://www.cancer.gov/about-cancer/treatment/types/surgery/cryosurgery.

OncoLink Team. (2020, July 9). *Vaccine therapy for cancer: The basics*. OncoLink. Retrieved from https://www.oncolink.org/cancer-treatment/immunotherapy/vaccine-therapy-basics.

Paddock, C. (2008, December 31). *Grape seed extract kills cancer cells in lab*. Medical News Today. Retrieved from https://www.medicalnewstoday.com/articles/134311#1.

Riyasdeen, A., Periasamy, V. S., Paul, P., Alshatwi, A. A., & Akbarsha, M. A. (2012). Chloroform Extract of Rasagenthi Mezhugu, a Siddha Formulation, as an Evidence-Based Complementary and Alternative Medicine for HPV-Positive Cervical Cancers. *Evidence-Based Complementary and Alternative Medicine, 2012*, 1–10. https://doi.org/10.1155/2012/136527

Semyonova, G. (2019, September 27). *Bio-informational therapies in supportive treatment of malignant tumors*. Cancer Tutor. Retrieved from https://www.cancertutor.com/bio-informational-therapies/.

Sharma, R., Martins, N., Kuca, K., Chaudhary, A., Kabra, A., Rao, M. M., & Prajapati, P. K. (2019). Chyawanprash: A traditional Indian bioactive health supplement. *Biomolecules*, *9*(5), 161–185. Retrieved from https://doi.org/10.3390/biom9050161.

Skwiot, S. (2018, September 18). *Can apricot seeds treat cancer symptoms?* Healthline. Retrieved from https://www.healthline.com/health/can-apricot-seeds-treat-cancer#nutrients.

Smith, L., Gordon, D., Scruton, A., & Yang, L. (2016). The potential yield of Tai Chi in cancer survivorship. *Future Science OA, 2*(4), FSO152. Retrieved from https://doi.org/10.4155/fsoa-2016-0049.

The Johns Hopkins University. (n.d.-a). *Craniotomy*. Johns Hopkins Medicine. Retrieved from https://www.hopkinsmedicine.org/health/treatment-tests-and-therapies/craniotomy.

The Johns Hopkins University. (n.d.-b). *Robotic prostatectomy*. Johns Hopkins Medicine. Retrieved from https://www.hopkinsmedicine.org/health/treatment-tests-and-therapies/robotic-prostatectomy.

Thomson, B. (2013). *Beat cancer . . . like i did twice!! with no chemotherapy or radiation*. Barry Thomson. Retrieved from https://www.happyherbshop.com.au/products/book-defeat-cancer-like-i-did-twice-with-no-chemotherapy-or-radiation-by-barry-thomson.

Tinsley, G. (2018, March 31). *6 benefits of Reishi mushroom (plus side effects and dosage)*. Healthline. Retrieved from https://www.healthline.com/nutrition/reishi-mushroom-benefits#section3.

Whitlock, J., & Wosnitzer, M. (2021, March 29). *What to expect on the day of your prostate surgery*. Verywell Health. Retrieved from https://www.verywellhealth.com/prostate-surgery-in-detail-3157328.

13

Immune Boosters

General Information

When the immune system is enhanced and activated, the body will ward off and fight various microbes. This can be achieved in several ways.

Nutrition (Functional or Bioactive Foods with Phytonutrients)

Plant-based diets support good immune health. Eat more fruits and vegetables rich in different **antioxidants** and with high oxygen radical absorbance capacity (ORAC) value.

Examples:

- Flavonoid-, iron-, folate-, and B12-rich foods include dark-green leafy vegetables (such as spinach, Bok choy, spring greens, watercress, moringa leaves, kale, watercress, dates, black raisins, etc.).
- Carotene-rich foods are orange in color (like papaya, carrots, sweet potato, pumpkin, and squash).
- Lycopene-rich foods are usually red in color (like cooked tomatoes, watermelon, red peppers, red cabbage, pink grapefruit, and mamey sapote).
- Anthocyanin-rich foods are purple-blue in color (like beet and blueberry).
- Quercetin-rich foods include apples, grapes, red onions, leafy vegetables, broccoli, tea, and red wine.
- Omega-3-rich foods include cold-water oily fish (salmon, mackerel, herring, anchovies, sardines, and tuna); krill oil; seeds (flaxseed, walnut, chia seed, hemp seeds and sacha inchi); edamame beans; kidney beans; algae/algal oil; perilla oil; rapeseed oil; purslane and brussels sprouts. Nuts and seeds (almonds, cashews, pistachios, walnuts, and foxnuts) are also antioxidant rich.
- Turmeric and dark chocolate are also antioxidant rich.
- **Probiotics and prebiotics** and **fermented foods** maintain good gut health.
- **Protein** intake of about 20% of the diet is essential to provide the building blocks (amino acids) to make immune cells and fight infections. Sprouted grains are rich in amino acids.

Colostrum, usually of bovine origin, is protein-rich with bioactive compounds such as growth factors (insulin-like growth factors I and II), immunoglobulins, enzymes, cytokines, and hormones.

Vitamins that boost immunity include vitamins C, E (antioxidants), B6 (it supports biochemical pathways), A (it protects mucosal and epithelial integrity), and D (there are vitamin D receptors on the immune cells). Vitamin-C-rich fruits include citrus fruits (orange, lemon, and grapefruit); kiwi; guava; and Indian gooseberry (amla). Vitamin-A-rich foods include cod liver oil, eggs, carrots, sweet potatoes, and pumpkins. Vitamin-D-rich foods include cold fatty fish, egg yolks, and liver. Vitamin-E-rich foods include almonds, sunflower seeds, avocado, wheat germ oil, and leafy green vegetables.

Minerals that boost immunity include iron-rich foods (dark green leafy greens as listed above, eggs, liver, red meat), zinc-rich foods (mussel, oyster, chickpea, and watermelon seeds); selenium-rich foods (brazil nuts, broccoli, barley, and sardine); and potassium- and magnesium-rich foods (banana). Shilajit (black asphaltum) has more than 84 minerals and contains fulvic acid. It is an antioxidant and immune booster with anti-inflammatory properties.

Polyporus polyherbal. This is a mushroom mix (polyporus, shitake and ganoderma) and also astragalus, poria, and coriolus.

Royal jelly. This is a bee product superfood that is rich in B-vitamins, trace minerals, specific major royal jelly proteins (MRJPs) and unique fatty acids.

Nutritional supplements (nutraceuticals). Multivitamin-multimineral or individual supplements are necessary in restrictive diets, picky eating, or chronic illness.

Meals. Well-balanced meals are important.

Breastfeeding is the best.

Avoid refined and processed foods, sugar-rich drinks and foods, alcohol, and excessive caffeine.

Eating on time is important.

Drink plenty of fluids to stay hydrated. Take frequent sips of hot water (of tolerable temperature).

Intermittent fasting or calorie restriction can provide health benefits. It can activate the lymphocyte-dependent killing of cancer cells and decrease autoimmunity.

Herbs and spices also boost the immune system.

Ginger, garlic, ginseng, green tea, and many spices/herbs are ingested in different ways amongst Asians.

- Consume ginger tea or turmeric in tea or milk.
- Drink green tea.
- Consume a spoonful of honey with crushed fresh garlic or eat two to three pips of lightly roasted garlic.
- Drink warm lemon water upon waking. This can also be mixed with turmeric, ginger, honey, and little salt.
- Boil some pounded ginger, coriander seeds, and cinnamon in a pot of water. Strain and drink the brew.
- Boil or steep crushed lemongrass *(Cymbopogon citratus)* bulbs in a pot of hot water. Add crushed ginger and/or pandanus leaves (screwpine), the latter for flavor.
- Boil or steep crushed lemongrass *(Cymbopogon citratus)* bulbs in a pot of hot water with added crushed, fresh turmeric and ginger. Simmer for about 10 to 15 minutes, cool, and strain. It can be drunk hot or cold.
- Blend some turmeric (preferably fresh), a few peppercorns, tamarind juice and some added palm sugar. Simmer for about 10 to 15 minutes. Cool, filter and store in glass bottles. It can be drunk hot or cold.
- Soak a few holy basil (tulsi) or mint (karpooravalli) leaves in a glass of water overnight and drink in the morning. Alternatively, their leaves can be washed and chewed.
- Cook foods with various Indian spices such as turmeric, mustard seeds, black cumin, coriander, fenugreek, fennel, asafetida, pepper, cloves, cinnamon, curry leaves, garlic, and ginger.
- Western herbs and spices include sage leaf, thyme, oregano, rosemary, and peppermint leaf.
- Consume herbs like *ashwagandha* (Indian ginseng), *triphala* (Phyllanthus emblica/amla, Terminalia chebula/haritaki and Terminalia bellerica/bibhitaki), *giloy* (Tinospora cordifolia) *brahmi* (Bacopa monnieri), gale of the wind/keelanelli/bhumi amla *(Phyllanthus niruri)*, *neem* (Azadirachta indica), saffron, *echinacea, andrographis, astragalus, black elderberry, AHCC* (active hexose-correlated compound, which is a Basidiomycetes medicinal mushroom extract), reishi mushrooms, milk thistle, liquorice, osha root *(Ligusticum porteri)*, or cordyceps.
  Immune Boosters

Regular consumption of polyherbal-spice decoctions/brews ("kadha") can boost immunity and also help in detoxification, digestion, metabolism, respiratory health and anti-aging.

Commercial polyherbs are also available.
Examples:

- *Chyawanprash* (Ayurvedic formulation of rejuvenating herbs which are sour, sweet, pungent, bitter, and astringent blended in ghee, sesame oil, cane sugar and honey)
- A mix of amlakai, grape seed extract, bhumi amlakai and bovine colostrum.
  Sleep of good quality and quantity is important.

Stress must be managed well. Prayer, meditation, rest, relaxation, laughter, sports, sex, social connectivity, and having pets also help.

Exercise, **sports, yoga (or qigong or tai chi), and breathing** techniques must be done regularly and preferably outdoors to strengthen the immune system. Adequate playtime for children is also essential.

Sun exposure in the morning is also helpful.

Hygiene and cleansing practices (detoxification) are also important. Taking regular or daily body baths as well as washing of hands, hair, and brushing of teeth are important. Oil pulling or oil swishing on waking for about 15 to 20 minutes with one tablespoon of coconut or sesame oil in the mouth removes bad bacteria from the mouth and teeth (oral cavity). Tongue scraping on waking also removes bad bacteria and toxins. Ice-cold baths or swimming are invigorating and can reduce inflammation. Daily or regular bowel movements or enemas help to maintain good gut health and may prevent cancers and other diseases. *Nasya* (nasal) oil application helps to cleanse and soothe the upper respiratory passages. Three to five drops of sesame oil (or medicated oil) are put into each nostril via a dropper or finger whilst the head is tilted. This is then sniffed or inhaled inwards a few times and may be done weekly.

Natural Antivirals

Colloidal silver. It blocks enzymatic reactions so that the virus cannot utilize oxygen, thus killing the virus.

Elderberry (Sambucus nigra). Its extract binds with the spikes of the viral protein, hence killing the virus before entering healthy cells.

Echinacea (Echinacea purpurea). The flowering tops and roots have antiviral properties.

Garlic. It contains allicin and alliin, which are effective against viruses, bacteria, and fungi.

Green tea (Camellia sinensis). It contains catechin type of flavonoid, which blocks enzymes in the virus so that it cannot multiply.

Olive leaf (Olea europaea). It contains elenolic acid and calcium elongate, which have antiviral properties.

St John's wort (Hypericum perforatum). It contains hypericin and pseudohypericin, which have antiviral properties.

Pau d'arco (Tabebuia impetiginosa). The inner bark of an Amazon tree contains quinoids that bind with viral deoxyribonucleic acid (DNA) or ribonucleic acid (RNA) so that viral replication does not occur.

Epilogue

From Sushruta (circa 600 BC), health was not only a state of physical well-being but also mental, brought about and preserved by the maintenance of balanced humor, good nutrition, proper elimination of bodily waste, and a pleasant, contented state of body and mind.

An ounce of prevention is better than a pound of cure.

References

Alexander, H. (2019, November 4). *5 benefits of a plant-based diet*. The University of Texas MD Anderson Cancer Center. Retrieved from https://www.mdanderson.org/publications/focused-on-health/5-benefits-of-a-plant-based-diet.h20-1592991.html.

Anthony, K. (2019, May 25). *Phytonutrients*. Healthline. Retrieved from https://www.healthline.com/health/phytonutrients.

Boyers, L. (n.d.). *9 All-Natural Antivirals To Kick Illness To The Curb*. Mindbodygreen. https://www.mindbodygreen.com/0-8990/6-allnatural-antivirals-to-kick-illness-to-the-curb.html.

Harvard Health. (2021, February 15). *How to boost your immune system*. Retrieved from https://www.health.harvard.edu/staying-healthy/how-to-boost-your-immune-system.

Kubala, J. (2019, October 21). *15 Impressive herbs with antiviral activity*. Healthline. Retrieved from https://www.healthline.com/nutrition/antiviral-herbs.

Mikstas, C. (2020, October 27). *Phytonutrients*. WebMD. Retrieved from https://www.webmd.com/diet/guide/phytonutrients-faq#1.

Pal, D., Sahu, C., & Haldar, A. (2014). Bhasma: The ancient Indian nanomedicine. *Journal of Advanced Pharmaceutical Technology & Research, 5*(1), 4. Retrieved from https://doi.org/10.4103/2231-4040.126980.

Schend, J. (2020, April 30). *15 foods that boost the immune system*. Healthline. Retrieved from https://www.healthline.com/health/food-nutrition/foods-that-boost-the-immune-system.

Wellness Team. (2020, December 4). *8 vitamins & minerals you need for a healthy immune system*. Health Essentials from Cleveland Clinic. Retrieved from https://health.clevelandclinic.org/eat-these-foods-to-boost-your-immune-system/.

Wood, A. (2020, April 25). *10 spices to protect your immune system*. ASMALLWORLD. Retrieved from https://www.asmallworld.com/explorer/articles/10-spices-protect-immune-system.

Glossary/Appendix of Common Natural Ingredients

Indian Spices, Herbs, and Leaves

Indian Natural Ingredients

Ingredients	Mechanism of Action and Health Benefits
Achar or pickle	Achar is prepared by using ingredients such as oil, salt, condiments or spices, and dry chili powder along with a vegetable or unripe fruit. They contain several essential vitamins (C, A, and K), minerals (potassium, iron, and calcium), and antioxidants.
	It has immune-boosting and hepatoprotective properties.
	It can improve digestion by promoting growth of healthy gut bacteria and also reduce the risk of gastric ulcers.
	Achar containing vinegar may help in increasing insulin sensitivity and lowering blood sugar. It also supports eye and bone health.
	Overall, it is safe. However, almost all types of achar contain a high salt content which can increase the risk of hypertension.
	Nagdeve, M. (2021, July 21). 7 surprising benefits of pickles. *Organic Facts*. https://www.organicfacts.net/health-benefits/other/health-benefits-of-pickles.html
Aerva lanata	Other names: *Bui, Polpala*
	Aerva lanata is a wild weed by the wayside. It contains flavonoids, alkaloids, tannins, steroids (β-sitosterol), saponins, polysaccharides, and terpenes (α-amyrin). Quercetin (a flavonoid) and butelin (a terpene) are the main compounds that can decrease oxalate synthesis.
	It has nephroprotective, antilithogenic, antiasthma, antiinflammatory, antimicrobial, analgesic, antioxidant, and immunomodulatory activities.
	It is used to treat kidney stones, sore throat, cough, diarrhea, indigestion, gonorrhea, and wounds.
	Bitasta, M., & Madan, S. (2016). *Aerva lanata*: A Blessing of Mother Nature. *Journal of Pharmacognosy and Phytochemistry*, 5(1), 92–101.
Agnimantha *Premna integrifolia*	Other names: *Wind killer, Arani, Arni, Headache tree*
	Agnimantha contains flavonoids, alkaloids, glycosides, tannins, steroids, and phenolic compounds. The leaves, bark, stem, and roots are used.
	It has astringent, carminative, digestive, antipyretic, and antiinflammatory actions.
	It is used to treat asthma, bronchitis, and fevers.
	It can also help in indigestion, constipation, flatulence, and diabetes. It is used in rheumatism.
	It also helps in neuralgic pain.
	It is often added to various Ayurvedic tonic formulations like *Dasamula* and *Chayawanprash*.
	Health Benefits Times. (2019, July 3). Agnimantha facts and health benefits. *HealthBenefitstimes.com*. https://www.healthbenefitstimes.com/premna-integrifolia/
Allspice	Other names: *West Indian bay leaf, pimento*
	Read under "*Bayleaf*"
	Lang, A. B. (2021a, September 24). Allspice—A unique spice with surprising health benefits. *Healthline*. https://www.healthline.com/nutrition/allspice

Ingredients	Mechanism of Action and Health Benefits
Aloe vera	Other names: *Aloe barbadensis, Aloe*

Aloe has more than 400 species. *Aloe barbadensis,* also called *Aloe vera,* is the most common variety. It contains about 75 active constituents including lignin, anthraquinone (aloin and emodin), fatty acids, triterpene, saponins, salicylic acids, and amino acids.

Aloin and emodin have analgesic, antibacterial, and antiviral properties. The terpenoid lupeol has antiseptic and analgesic properties, and the fatty acids have antiinflammatory properties. Salicylic acid is also responsible for its antiinflammatory and antibacterial activities.

It contains antioxidants (β-carotene, vitamins C and E), vitamin B12, folic acid, and choline. It also provides enzymes (cellulase, lipase, amylase, and bradykinase) and minerals (calcium, chromium, copper, selenium, magnesium, manganese, potassium, sodium, and zinc). The enzymes help in the breakdown of sugars and fats.

It is commonly used in treating wounds, as a moisturizer and protection against UV radiation, managing blood sugar levels, and treating constipation. It can also treat gastric ulcers and acid reflux.

Side effects include skin irritation, abdominal cramps, and diarrhea.

Surjushe, A., Vasani, R., & Saple, D. (2008). Aloe vera: A short review. *Indian Journal of Dermatology, 53*(4), 163–166. https://doi.org/10.4103/0019-5154.44785

Fanous, S. (2020, August 28). 7 amazing uses for Aloe vera. *Healthline.* https://www.healthline.com/health/7-amazing-uses-aloe-vera

Amaranth *Amaranthus*	Other names: *Rajgira, Ramdana, Indian spinach, Chinese spinach, African spinach, Bush greens, Choulayee*

Amaranth seeds, leaves, and roots are edible. There are many species. There are two common types of amaranth: green amaranth and red amaranth. The green amaranth leaves are more nutritious. Although amaranth is sometimes referred to as pigweed, it is very different from purslane which is also called pigweed. Amaranth contains antioxidants including vanillic acid, gallic acid, and p-hydroxybenzoic acid. It is rich in protein, fiber, minerals (iron, magnesium, manganese, phosphorus, zinc, calcium, selenium, and copper), and vitamins (folate and B6). The seeds can be eaten as a cereal. It is a gluten-free, nutrient-dense, and alkaline superfood.

Amaranth has antioxidant, antiinflammatory, glucose-lowering, immune-boosting, and antiallergy properties. It blocks the production of immunoglobulin E (IgE) antibodies.

It can lower cholesterol and blood glucose as well as help with weight loss. It can also maintain skin health.

Overall, it is safe.

Link, R. (2018, January 6). Amaranth: An ancient grain with impressive health benefits. *Healthline.* https://www.healthline.com/nutrition/amaranth-health-benefits

WebMD Editors. (2011). *Amaranth.* WebMD. https://www.webmd.com/vitamins/ai/ingredientmono-869/amaranth

Amla *Phyllanthus emblica*	Other names: *Amlakai, Indian gooseberry, Zee phyu thee*

Amla has several bioactive phytochemicals most of which are polyphenols (ellagic acid, chebulinic acid, quercetin, gallic acid, chebulagic acid, apigenin, luteolin, corilagin, etc.). Others include various glycosides (flavone, flavonol, and phenolic glycosides) and tannins (emblicanin A & B, phyllaemblicin B, and puniggluconin). It is very rich in vitamin C (600% to 800% of dietary value (DV). It also contains calcium, iron, and antioxidants (flavonoids, phenols, and tannins).

It has antioxidant and antiinflammatory properties. It also has glucose-lowering, antiplatelet, and anticancer effects.

It is a powerful superfood, immune booster, and rejuvenator. It is very beneficial for heart, digestive, liver, and skin health. It regulates blood sugar and lipids (lowers triglyceride and low-density lipoprotein [LDL] cholesterol and increases high-density lipoprotein [HDL] cholesterol) by improving endothelial function. It can prevent hair loss.

It may support kidney health and prevent kidney stones. It decreases urinary oxalate and increases urinary excretion of magnesium and potassium.

Due to its antiplatelet properties, it can thin the blood and prevent normal blood clotting. It should be avoided by women who are pregnant, breastfeeding, or trying to conceive.

Ingredients	Mechanism of Action and Health Benefits

Deesh, P. (2018, August 30). 10 wonderful benefits of amla powder: A powerful superfood. *NDTV Food*. https://food.ndtv.com/health/10-wonderful-benefits-of-amla-powder-a-powerful-superfood-1654043.

Shoemaker, M. S. (2020, October 15). Indian gooseberry: Benefits, uses, and side effects. *Healthline*. https://www.healthline.com/nutrition/indian-gooseberry

Anise
Pimpinella anisum

Other name: *Aniseed*

Anise or aniseed is from the Apiaceae family (like parsley, celery, and carrots). It has a licorice taste. The leaves can be added as a garnish to salads, soups, or stews. The seeds are added to cakes, pastries, breads, or biscuits. Anisi aetheroleum is the oil made from anise. The oil is used as a flavoring agent or a preservative in foods and also as a fragrance enhancer in soaps or perfumes.

The essential oils in anise contain the following compounds, mainly trans-anethole, estragole, methyl cacol, y-hymachalen, para-anisaldehyde, coumarins, and terpenes. Anise has antiinflammatory, antimicrobial, and antiseptic properties from the tannins compounds. It is rich in minerals (calcium, manganese, iron, copper, zinc, selenium, magnesium, and potassium), vitamins (A, C, E, and Bs), and monounsaturated fats (omega-3 and omega-6 fatty acids).

It is a carminative and improves digestive health. It is an appetite stimulant. It reduces nausea and is used as aromatherapy in palliative care. It also has a laxative effect.

It may also promote lactation and reduce menstrual pain via its estrogen-like effects. It can help with bone loss in menopause.

It is a diuretic and can treat kidney and bladder stones, urinary tract infections (UTIs), and decrease edema.

The seeds also have analgesic properties and can be used to treat migraine. Its sedative effects can improve sleep. It may have neuroprotective effects in degenerative brain disorders.

It is an expectorant and antispasmodic. It helps with coughs, sore throat, and lung congestion.

It is cardioprotective and can reduce high blood pressure and cholesterol, as well as improve cardiac contractility. It can also prevent atherosclerosis. It also can maintain blood sugar.

It may protect against cancers.

Side effects include rare allergic reactions. It can mimic the effects of estrogen in the body, which can worsen symptoms of certain hormone-sensitive conditions.

Link, R. (2018, October 15). 7 health benefits and uses of anise seed. *Healthline*. https://www.healthline.com/nutrition/anise#TOC_TITLE_HDR_10

Arjuna
Terminalia arjuna

Arjuna is a potent herbal heart tonic with cardioprotective actions. It improves coronary artery blood flow and prevents myocardial ischemic injury. It is rich in antioxidants and contains triterpenes (arjunic acid, aminoglycosides, arjunone, arjunolic acid, etc.), polyphenols, (flavonol, flavones), and phytosterols (cardenolide steroids). It contains minerals (magnesium, zinc, copper, and calcium). The triterpenes mostly have cardioactive properties. The tannins and flavonoids have more anti-cancer properties. The bark has hemostatic properties.

It balances pitta and kapha doshas.

It can be used to treat heart disease, angina, control high blood pressure, and lower cholesterol levels. It may also lower blood sugar.

It is also used in earaches, dysentery, sexually transmitted diseases (STDs), and diseases of the urinary tract.

It can also stimulate osteoblasts to increase bone formation and reduce bone resorption. It helps in bone fracture and wound healing.

Overall, it is very safe. It should be avoided by women who are pregnant, breastfeeding, or trying to conceive. High doses can cause stomach upsets and hepatotoxicity.

eMedicine Health Editors. (2021, June 14). Terminalia: Uses, side effects, dose, health benefits, precautions & warnings. *EMedicineHealth*. https://www.emedicinehealth.com/terminalia/vitamins-supplements.htm

Kumar, S. (2013). Chapter 39—Effect of *Terminalia arjuna* on cardiac hypertrophy [E-book]. In S. K. Maulik (Ed.), *Bioactive food as dietary interventions for cardiovascular disease* (1st ed., pp. 673–680). San Diego: Academia Press. https://doi.org/10.1016/B978-0-12-396485-4.00036-0

Ingredients	Mechanism of Action and Health Benefits
Arugampul *Cynodon dactylon*	Other names: *Dhoob, Durva, Vinayagar grass, Bermuda grass, Scutch grass, Rumput minyak.* Arugampul is widely used in Ayurvedic medicine and also as a religious offering. It contains more than 65% chlorophyll. It is high in alkaloids and flavonoids. It also contains several minerals (including potassium, manganese, calcium, and phosphorus), vitamins, and fiber. It has antibacterial, antiviral, immune-boosting, alkalizing, and detoxifying properties. It aids digestive health; lowers acidity; and can treat acid reflux, gastritis, and stomach ulcers. It reduces hunger pangs and helps with weight loss. It also detoxifies and cleanses the liver. It can eliminate bad breath and make the gums and teeth healthy. It can prevent kidney stones, regulate blood sugar, and treat anemia. It can treat skin conditions including fungal infections and eczema. It can treat polycystic ovary syndrome, menorrhagia, and dysmenorrhea. It can also improve lung congestion, cough, cold, and asthma. Overall, it is safe. Side effects include headache, nausea, stomach upset, constipation, and fever. Health Benefits Times. (2018, August 9). Bermuda grass facts and health benefits. *HealthBenefitstimes.com*. https://www.healthbenefitstimes.com/bermuda-grass/ TheIndianMed. (2020, July 17). Amazing arugampul benefits that will interest you! *The Indian Med.* https://theindianmed.com/amazing-arugampul-benefits-that-will-interest-you/
Asafetida *Ferula assa-foetida*	Other names: *Hing, heeng, perungayam, stinking gum* Asafetida is a milky latex or gum oleoresin derived from the roots or rhizomes of the ferula plant. When dried, it becomes a hard and dark brown resinous gum. The strong pungent odor is due to its sulfur content. There are two types of asafetida: the white or red variety. The dried gum is ground and blended with rice flour or wheat flour to mask the sulfur odor and also as an anticaking agent. It contains flavonoids which have antioxidant, antimicrobial, and diuretic effects. It is widely used in savory Indian cuisine especially dals as a flavor and carminative. It enhances digestion, promotes flow of bile, and prevents flatulence. It can help in irritable bowel syndrome (IBS). Asafetida can stimulate the production of progesterone, which increases blood flow to the uterus and regularizes periods. It can also help in bronchitis and kidney stones. Overall, it is safe. Side effects include allergic reactions, excessive gas, diarrhea, seizures, and headache. WebMD Editors. (2010). Asafoetida. *WebMD*. https://www.webmd.com/vitamins/ai/ingredient-mono-248/asafoetida
Ashoka tree *Saraca asoca*	Other names: *Sorrowless tree, Asoka tree, Sita Ashoka tree, Sita Ashok, Asoca* Ashoka means "remover of sorrows." It is a sacred tree. The bark, seeds, flowers, and leaves of Ashoka contain flavonoids (anthocyanin pigments), tannins, and glycosides. The bark also has phytosterols (phytoestrogens) that can stimulate the endometrium lining of the uterus and ovaries. It pacifies the pitta and kapha doshas. It has antiinflammatory, astringent, analgesic, diuretic, and stone-dissolving properties. It is a uterine tonic. It helps with several menstrual problems (including heavy menstrual bleeding, dysmenorrhea, amenorrhea, and premenstrual syndrome [PMS]) and also in endometriosis and menopause. It is also used for infertility. It can calm the nerves and is also helpful in insomnia. It can treat skin conditions such as eczema, acne, and psoriasis. It enhances skin complexion. It can increase urination and help with kidney stones. Overall, it is safe. Overconsumption can lead to stomach upset and heavy uterine bleeding. Ashoka Tree Facts and Health Benefits. (2019, August 5). Health Benefits|Health Benefits of Foods and Drinks. *HealthBenefitstimes.com*. https://www.healthbenefitstimes.com/ashoka-tree/ Dabur. (n.d.). Ashoka. *Dabur.com*. https://www.dabur.com/?aspxerrorpath=/article.aspx

Ingredients	Mechanism of Action and Health Benefits
Ashwagandha *Withania somnifera*	Other names: *Indian ginseng, Winter cherry, Indian stallion weed, Shui Qie* Withanolides (A to Z) are the major constituents in ashwagandha, of which Withaferin-A is the most important. Somniferin is another constituent which has anxiolytic and sedative effects. It controls the stress hormones (cortisol and adrenaline) which will reduce anxiety and stress. It also has γ-aminobutyric acid (GABA)-mimetic properties. This will induce sleep. It also has several broad-spectrum phytochemicals which have neuroprotective, antistress, adaptogen, cardioprotective, antiinflammatory, antimicrobial, antidiabetic, and immunomodulatory properties. It boosts brain function including memory, mood, and reaction time. It can also lower blood sugar. It is also a uterine tonic and is useful in recurrent miscarriages. It can increase testosterone levels as well as improve sperm count and motility. It may also increase muscle mass and strength. Long-term side effects are unknown. Large doses of ashwagandha may cause stomach upset, diarrhea, and vomiting and rarely, liver problems. WebMD Editors. (n.d.). Ashwagandha. *WebMD*. https://www.webmd.com/vitamins/ai/ingredientmono-953/ashwagandha
Athimathuram *Glycyrrhiza glabra*	Other names: *Liquorice, Licorice, sweet root, Chinese liquorice root, zhi gan cao, gan cao, or Yashtimadhu, Mulethi, Glycyrrhizae radix* Liquorice root contains glycyrrhizin, a triterpene glycoside which has a sweet taste and has several phytoactive properties. It also contains flavonoids (glabrene and glabridin) which are gastroprotective. It has antiinflammatory, analgesic, antiviral, antimicrobial, antitussive, antiallergic, antioxidant, and anticancer actions. It enhances the effects of endogenous steroids in asthma. It also has skin-brightening effects. It also has laxative and memory-stimulant effects. It is widely used as a flavoring agent in the food and beverage industry. It is also used to treat sore throats, tonsillitis, bronchitis, and asthma. It is used to treat Gastro intestinal tract (GIT) conditions including acid reflux indigestion, flatulence, colic *Helicobacter pylori* infection, gastritis, peptic ulcer, and hepatitis. It can also help reduce menstrual cramps (dysmenorrhea). It is also used in dementia, epilepsy, and attention deficit disorder with hyperactivity (ADHD). It can be used topically for eczema, mouth sores, and dental caries. Overall, it is safe. Prolonged use can cause hypertension, hypokalemia from the cortisol excess. Deglycyrrhizinated licorice is also available. It can interact with diuretics, steroids, statins, antihypertensives, and blood thinners. It should not be used in pregnancy as it can affect the development of the fetal brain. Licorice Root. (n.d.). NCCIH. https://www.nccih.nih.gov/health/licorice-root LICORICE: Overview, uses, side effects, precautions, interactions, dosing and reviews. (n.d.). *WebMD*. https://www.webmd.com/vitamins/ai/ingredientmono-881/licorice El-Saber Batiha, G., Magdy Beshbishy, A., El-Mleeh, A., M. Abdel-Daim, M., & Prasad Devkota, H. (2020). Traditional uses, bioactive chemical constituents, and pharmacological and toxicological activities of *Glycyrrhiza glabra* L. (Fabaceae). *Biomolecules*, 10(3), 352. https://doi.org/10.3390/biom10030352
Avuri *Indigofera tinctoria*	Other names: *True indigo, Indigo naturalis, Qing Dai, Ban Lan Gen, Ban Lan Gen, Da Qing Ye, Chinese Indigo, Indigo, Indigo Naturalis, Isatis indigotica, Isatis root* Indigo naturalis is an herb made from extracts of stems and leaves of several plants that contain indigo including *Baphicacanthus cusia, Indigofera tinctoria, Isatis tinctoria, Polygonum tinctorium, Isatis indigotica,* and *Strobilanthes cusia.* It is used widely in traditional Chinese medicine (TCM) (known as Qing Dai) and Ayurvedic medicine (known as Avuri). The natural compounds present include indigotin, alkaloids (tryptanthrin), indirubin, flavonoids (nimbosterol), iso-indigotin, and indole glycoside.

Ingredients	Mechanism of Action and Health Benefits
	It has antiinflammatory, antimicrobial, hemostatic, anticonvulsant, and anticolitis properties.

It is used to treat inflammatory bowel disorders including ulcerative colitis.

In TCM, Isatis root or indigo is used to treat upper airway infections.

It can be used in the treatment of skin disorders such as acne and psoriasis.

It stimulates hair growth, prevents premature graying of hair, and moisturizes the hair and scalp. It can treat scalp infections and dandruff.

It is also used to stop bleeding hemoptysis and nosebleeds.

Overall, it is safe. Side effects can include gastric upset, allergic rash, liver dysfunction, headache, and dizziness.

Gope, A. (2020, February 5). Benefits & uses of avuri or neeli|Indigofera Tinctoria. *The Indian Med*. https://theindianmed.com/benefits-uses-of-avuri-or-neeli-indigofera-tinctoria/

Sugimoto, S., Naganuma, M., Kiyohara, H., Arai, M., Ono, K., Mori, K., et al. (2016). Clinical efficacy and safety of oral qing-dai in patients with ulcerative colitis: a single-center open-label prospective study. *Digestion*, *93*(3), 193–201. https://doi.org/10.1159/000444217

Usedom, E. (2019, December 20). Indigo naturalis for psoriasis. *Learnskin*. https://www.learnskin.com/articles/indigo-naturalis-for-psoriasis

Venkateshwaran, R. (2019, October 21). 5 top hair uses, benefits & side effects of indigo powder (avuri) for grey hair & hair growth. *Wildturmeric*. https://www.wildturmeric.net/indigo-powder-for-hair-uses-benefits-side-effects/

Axlewood
Anogeissus latifolia

Other names: *Dhawa, Dhawra, Dhau, India Gum, Gum Ghatti, Bakli, Baajhi*

Axlewood is a small to medium tropical tree.

Gum ghatti is the tree exudate which is used as an emulsifier and thickener in the food and pharmaceutical industry. It is rich in tannins.

It has antiseptic, antiinflammatory, immune-boosting, and antidiabetic actions.

The seed, root, bark, and gum are used to treat fevers, cough, colds, diabetes, skin disorders, wounds, stomach ache, diarrhea, hemorrhoids, snake bites, and scorpion stings.

Mahalakshmi, S. N., & Prashith, K. T. R. (2020). An inclusive review on ethnobotanical uses of *Anogeissus latifolia* (Combretaceae) in India. In *Nature and medicine: Traditional uses, chemistry and bioprospecting of natural* (1st ed., Vol. 4, pp. 38–51). India: PS Scientific Publications.

Bael fruit
Aegle marmelos

Other names: *Bilwa, Bilva, Vilvam, Bel, Bengal Quince*

Bael fruit contains phenolic compounds, flavonoids, coumarins, carotenoids, and β-carotene. It has several minerals (including potassium, calcium, magnesium, zinc, copper, and iron), vitamins (C, A, and riboflavin), and dietary fiber. Limonene is a major component of the bael fruit flavor and has anticancer properties. Bael fruit is not the same as wood apple, although they have similar health benefits.

It has antioxidant, antiinflammatory, antibacterial, antiviral, antifungal antiulcer, blood detoxifying, and purifying properties. It is cooling and can stop bleeding.

It is used for the treatment of digestive issues (constipation, dysentery, chronic diarrhea, IBS, peptic ulcer, hemorrhoids, and stomach pain). It can be used for skin diseases and fever as well.

It can lower blood sugar and cholesterol, as well as support heart health and diabetes.

It can also be used for asthma.

Overall, it is safe. Allergic reactions are rare. Gas and bloating can occur with overconsumption.

Charoensiddhi, S., & Anprung, P. (2008). Bioactive compounds and volatile compounds of Thai bael fruit (*Aegle marmelos* (L.) Correa) as a valuable source for functional food ingredients. *International Food Research Journal*, *15*(3), 287–295. http://ifrj.upm.edu.my/15%20(3)%202008/06.%20Suvimol%20C.pdf

Mathur, M., Soni, D., & Kanodia, L. (2019, August 30). Bael. *1mg*. https://www.1mg.com/ayurveda/bael-96

WebMD Editors. (2014). Bael. *WebMD*. https://www.webmd.com/vitamins/ai/ingredientmono-164/bael

Wong, C., & Syn, M. (2020, September 29). Bael fruit nutrition facts and health benefits. *Verywell Fit*. https://www.verywellfit.com/the-health-benefits-of-bael-fruit-89602

Ingredients	Mechanism of Action and Health Benefits
Bakul *Mimusops elengi*	Other names: *Spanish cherry, medlar* Bakul flowers, fruit, seed, and bark are used for medicinal purposes. The leaves contain tannins and sterols, while the flowers contain mannitol, glycoside, and β-sitosterol. It has cooling, astringent, tonic, antiworm, and insect-repellent activities. It also has an antilithogenic effect. It is a cardiac tonic and can strengthen the heart muscle. It is used to treat disorders of the oral cavity including inflamed gums, gingivitis, mouth ulcers, and dental caries. It helps with headaches and anxiety. Baliga, M. S., Pai, R. J., Bhat, H. P., Palatty, P. L., & Boloor, R. (2011). Chemistry and medicinal properties of the Bakul (*Mimusops elengi* Linn): A review. *Food Research International, 44*(7), 1823–1829. https://doi.org/10.1016/j.foodres.2011.01.063
Bala *Sida cordifolia*	Other name: *Flannel weed* Bala contains ephedrine, pseudoephedrine, norephedrine, vasicinol, and alkaloids (vasicinone and vasicine). Ephedrine has amphetamine-like properties. It balances the three doshas. It has antiinflammatory, bronchodilatory, diuretic, immune-boosting, and blood-purifying properties. It supports respiratory health. It decongests the nose and dilates the airway. It is used to treat cough, asthma, bronchitis, and lung congestion. It can also help rheumatism, strengthen the bones, joints, and muscles. It can also increase the overall strength and stamina. It can also be used in obesity, bleeding piles, and wound healing. It can treat male and female infertility. It increases sperm count and motility. It helps in premature ejaculation and erectile dysfunction. It can also treat UTIs. Side effects include signs of sympathetic overstimulation. It should not be used with other stimulant drugs. Indigo Herbs. (n.d.). Bala benefits & information. *Indigo Herbs*. https://www.indigo-herbs.co.uk/natural-health-guide/benefits/bala WebMD Editors. (2015). Sida cordifolia. *WebMD*. https://www.webmd.com/vitamins/ai/ingredient-mono-837/sida-cordifolia
Banana flower *Musa* spp.	Other name: *Banana blossom* Banana flowers contain antioxidants (isoquercetin, catechin, and tannins), β-sitosterol, saponin, and other phenolic compounds. It is rich in vitamins (A, C, and E), minerals (potassium, magnesium, iron, copper, calcium, and phosphorus), and fibers (soluble and insoluble). It has antiinfective (from the ethanol content), antiaging, laxative, and immune-boosting properties. It may have anticancer properties. It can maintain uterine health. It can also increase progesterone levels which will decrease excessive menstrual bleeding. It can also help treat anemia, prevent bacterial infections, ulcers, and constipation. It can lower blood sugar and cholesterol, as well as regulate blood pressure. It prevents constipation in pregnant mothers and can also increase breast milk production in lactating mothers. Overall, it is safe. Health Benefits Times. (2018, December 3). Health benefits of banana flower. *HealthBenefitstimes.com*. https://www.healthbenefitstimes.com/health-benefits-of-banana-flower/
Banyan tree *Ficus benghalensis*	Other names: *Banyan, Banyan fig, Bengal fig (Ficus benghalensis)* Banyan tree is a sacred tree in Hinduism and Buddhism. It is also called a "wish fulfilling tree." The banyan tree (banyan fig) and the sacred fig (*Ficus religiosa*) are not the same but are related as they are under the same *Ficus* genus. The banyan tree root, bark, leaves, and latex have extensive medicinal uses. It contains polyphenols, flavonoids (rutin), terpenoids (friderin and β-sitosterol), and coumarins. It is rich in minerals (including potassium, magnesium, and phosphorus), fatty acids, and fiber. It has antioxidant, antibacterial, antiseptic, astringent, and immune-boosting properties. It is an aphrodisiac. It can treat premature ejaculation, improves male vitality and the sperm count.

Ingredients	Mechanism of Action and Health Benefits

Mechanism of Action and Health Benefits

It helps women with menstrual problems and with recurrent miscarriages. It also strengthens the uterine muscles during the pregnancy.

It reduces the absorption of glucose from the blood. It can be used in diabetes and hypercholesterolemia.

It can prevent dental caries, gum disease, and bad breath. It also moisturizes the skin and maintains healthy hair and vision. It can treat kidney stones.

No side effects have been reported.

Ahamed, S., Rao, H., Akhtar, M., Ahmad, I., Hayat, M. M., Iqbal, Z., et al. (2011). Phytochemical composition and pharmacological prospectus of *Ficus bengalensis* Linn. (Moraceae)—a review. *Journal of Medicinal Plants Research, 5*(28), 6393–6400. https://doi.org/10.5897/JMPR11.455

Health Benefits Times. (2019, August 11). Banyan tree facts and health benefits. *HealthBenefitstimes.com*. https://www.healthbenefitstimes.com/banyan-tree/

Barberry
Berberis spp.

Other names: *Common barberry, European barberry or barberry or Berberis vulgaris, Indian barberry or Berberis aristata, Fu Niu, Daruharidra*

There are more than 500 species in the genus Berberis. *B. vulgaris* is well known and its fruits have been used to make rice dishes. *B. aristata* is an Indian species.

The major active compounds in Barberry include berberine, oxycontin, palmatine, bervulcine, berbamine, columbamine, jatrorrhizine, coptisine, and berbamine. Berberine is a natural alkaloid which is also found in various flowering plants like *Berberidaceae, Hydrastis canadensis,* and *Coptis rhizomes.*

Berberine has antibacterial, antiviral, antiinflammatory, antioxidant, antidiarrheal, antispasmodic, antiplatelet, immunomodulatory, and antiosteoporotic activities. It can also relieve the discomfort or pain in UTI.

It also has antidiabetic, antiobesity, and hepatoprotective properties. It can reduce blood sugar and LDL-cholesterol levels. It reduces the secretion of leptin which is an appetite-stimulating hormone. It also inhibits the enzyme lipoprotein lipase which increases fat storage, decreases hepatic gluconeogenesis, and decreases insulin resistance by modulating the gut microbiota. It is a cholagogue.

It is used in the treatment of diabetes, liver disease, gallstones, obesity, and polycystic ovarian syndrome (PCOS).

It is used to treat cough, diarrhea, jaundice, skin diseases, syphilis, chronic rheumatism, and urinary disorders.

It is also used to treat heart failure, heavy menstrual periods, eye infection, and stomach swelling.

It may also be able to reduce the risk of cancer and has potential to be used for cancer treatment.

Berberine is neuroprotective and may be used in the treatment of neurodegenerative diseases such as Alzheimer disease (AD), Parkinson disease (PD), and Huntington disease.

Overall, it is safe. It should also be avoided by pregnant and breastfeeding women. It should not be used in infants or children under 12. Side effects include gastric upsets, constipation, dizziness, headache, hypoglycemia, and excessive sweating.

Chander, V., Aswal, J. S., Dobhal, R., & Uniyal, D. P. (2017). A review on Pharmacological potential of Berberine; an active component of Himalayan *Berberis aristata*. *The Journal of Phytopharmacology, 6*(1), 53–58. http://www.phytopharmajournal.com/Vol6_Issue1_08.pdf

Health Benefits Times Editors. (2017, July 6). Indian barberry facts and health benefits. *HealthBenefitstimes.com*. https://www.healthbenefitstimes.com/indian-barberry/

Drugs.com. (n.d.). Barberry. *Drugs.com*. https://www.drugs.com/npc/barberry.html

Zarei, A., Changizi-Ashtiyani, S., Taheri, S., & Ramezani, M. (2015). A quick overview on some aspects of endocrinological and therapeutic effects of *Berberis vulgaris* L. *Avicenna Journal of Phytomedicine, 5*(6), 485–497. https://www.ncbi.nlm.nih.gov/pmc/articles/PMC4678494/

Basil
Ocimum spp.

Basil belongs to the mint (Lamiaceae) family. There are about 20 types of basil, the common ones being:
- Sweet basil (Italian basil or *O. basilicum*),
- Thai basil (*O. thyrsiflora*),
- Holy basil (tulsi or *O. sanctum* or *O. tenuiflorum*). Read more under "Tulsi",
- Lemon basil (*O. citriodorum*),
- Purple basil (*O. basilicum*).

Ingredients	Mechanism of Action and Health Benefits

It has culinary and medicinal uses. The essential oils in basil contain monoterpenes derivatives (camphor, limonene, 1, 8-cineole, linalool, geraniol) and phenylpropanoid derivatives (eugenol, methyleugenol, chavicol, estragole, methyl-cinnamate). It also contains β-carotenes, flavonoids, and magnesium.

It has antibacterial, antioxidant, antiinflammatory, analgesic, antitussive, glucose-lowering, immune-boosting, stress-lowering, calming, detoxifying, and anticonvulsant effects. It may also have anti-cancer properties. Holy basil can lengthen telomeres and promote longevity.

It can relieve cough and sore throat, as well as loosen phlegm in lung conditions.

It is used in the treatment of nausea, loss of appetite, stomach aches or gripes, gas and bloating, diarrhea, and constipation.

It can lower blood pressure and cholesterol.

It maintains kidney health. It reduces uric acid levels and can prevent kidney stones. It can be used in mild kidney failure.

It can promote hair growth and prevent dandruff.

It maintains eye health and can prevent age-related macular degeneration.

Sweet linalool basil is used in skin care products.

It can also help in diabetes, fevers, infectious diseases, headaches, acne, warts, dandruff, head lice, infertility, menorrhagia, depression, and epilepsy. It can also promote lactation. It is also used to treat worm infestation and insect bites.

It rarely can cause hypoglycemia. Estragole present in basil can increase the risk of liver cancer. It can interact with blood thinners.

Mattison, L. D. (2021, June 25). Your guide to all the different types of basil. *Taste of Home*. https://www.tasteofhome.com/collection/types-of-basil/

Poonkodi, K. (2016). Chemical composition of essential oil of *Ocimum basilicum* L. (Basil) and its biological activities—an overview. *Journal of Critical Reviews*, 3(3), 56–62. http://www.jcreview.com/fulltext/197-1572429367.pdf

RxList Editors. (2021, June 11). Basil. *RxList*. https://www.rxlist.com/basil/supplements.htm

Bay leaf
Laurus nobilis

Other names: Refer below

There are different types of bay leaves. The common ones are as follows:

Indian bay leaves (tejpat),
Indonesian (daun salam or Cassia leaf),
European bay leaves (laurel bay or sweet bay),
West Indian bay leaf (allspice or pimento).

Bay leaf and its essential oil are used for medicinal and culinary purposes. It contains alkaloids, flavonoids, tannins, glycosides, lauric acid, linolenic acid, and saponins. It also contains vitamins (C and A) and minerals (potassium, iron, magnesium, and calcium).

It has antioxidant, antiinflammatory, antimicrobial, analgesic, wound healing, diuretic, anticonvulsant, and insecticide properties.

It supports digestive and oral health. It can stimulate bile flow, relieve gas and bloating, and constipation. It maintains healthy gums and prevents gum bleeding.

It can lower blood glucose, improve insulin sensitivity, and increase HDL cholesterol.

It can also prevent migraine headaches.

Overall, it is safe. It may cause drowsiness. The leaves must be removed after cooking and not eaten.

Ordoudi, S. A., Papapostolou, M., Nenadis, N., Mantzouridou, F. T., & Tsimidou, M. Z. (2022). Bay Laurel (Laurus nobilis L.) Essential Oil as a Food Preservative Source: Chemistry, Quality Control, Activity Assessment, and Applications to Olive Industry Products. *Foods, 11(5)*, 752. https://doi.org/10.3390/foods11050752

WebMD Editors. (2016). Bay leaf. *WebMD*. https://www.webmd.com/vitamins/ai/ingredient-mono-685/bay-leaf

Bearberry
Arctostaphylos uva-ursi

Other name: *Uva ursi*

Bearberry contains tannins and glycosides (arbutin). The arbutin is converted into hydroquinone, which has antiinflammatory effects. The leaves and berries can be used to make herbal tea.

It also has antiseptic, antimicrobial, astringent, and diuretic functions.

It is widely used to treat UTIs and renal calculi. It can also treat STDs, diabetes, and poor vision.

Ingredients	Mechanism of Action and Health Benefits

Although it should not be used in children, it has been tried in autism children to treat unhealthy gut flora.

It is also added to skin care products as a skin-lightening agent.

Overall, it is safe. Side effects may include vomiting, nausea, tinnitus, or shortness of breath.

Danahy, A. (2021, March 9). Does uva ursi work for urinary tract infections? *Healthline*. https://www.healthline.com/nutrition/uva-ursi#side-effects-and-safety

de Arriba, S. G., Naser, B., & Nolte, K. U. (2013). Risk assessment of free hydroquinone derived from arctostaphylos uva-ursi folium herbal preparations. *International Journal of Toxicology*, *32*(6), 442–453. https://doi.org/10.1177/1091581813507721

WebMD Editors. (n.d.). Uva Ursi. *WebMD*. https://www.webmd.com/vitamins/ai/ingredientmono-350/uva-ursi

Betel leaf
Piper betel

Other names: *Paan patta or paan ka patta, Betel, Betel Pepper, Betle Pepper, Pan, Sireh, Betel Vine (This is not to be confused with Piper sarmentosum [wild betel/kadok])*

Betel leaf contains essential oil and active constituents such as chavicol, betel phenol, eugenol, terpene, and campene. It also contains essential nutrients including minerals (iodine and potassium) and vitamins (A, B1, B2, and nicotinic acid).

It helps reduce high blood pressure, lower cholesterol levels, and promotes wound healing.

It is an antiparasitic agent, astringent, carminative, and stimulant. It also has antibacterial, antimicrobial, and immunomodulatory actions. Its antioxidant and antiinflammatory properties are helpful in treatment and management of asthma.

Copious or prolonged consumption of betel leaves can be associated with oral cancer or allergic reactions.

Fazal, F., Mane, P. P., Rai, M.P., Thilakchand, K. R., Bhat, H. P., Kamble, P. S., et al. (2014). The phytochemistry, traditional uses and pharmacology of *Piper betel*. linn (betel leaf): a pan-asiatic medicinal plant. *Chinese Journal of Integrative Medicine*. Published. https://doi.org/10.1007/s11655-013-1334-1

Raina, K. (2019, April 30). *Benefits and side effects of betel leaf (Paan)*. FirstCry Parenting. https://parenting.firstcry.com/articles/magazine-benefits-and-side-effects-of-betel-leafpaan/

Bhringraj
Eclipta alba
Eclipta prostrata

Other names: *False daisy, Karisalankanni, Yerba de tago, Gunta kalagaraku, Guntagalagaraku*

The bioactive constituents of bhringraj are wedelolactone, β-amyrin, luteolin-7-O-glucoside, luteolin, stigmasterol, alpha-terthienyl-methanol, β-amyrin wedelic acid, ecliptine, alkaloids, and saponin. The flavonoids present mainly, luteolin, have antioxidant effects. False daisies are also rich in vitamins (E and D) and minerals (iron, magnesium, and calcium).

In TCM, it helps nourish the liver and kidneys, cool the blood, and stop bleeding.

It has anticancer, antiinflammatory, hepatoprotective, antibacterial, and antiseptic properties.

It can be used for indigestion, constipation, and urinary infections. It is helpful in treating chronic respiratory infections and coughs by forcing out any remaining phlegm or mucus.

Mixing it with shampoo can help in hair growth, premature hair loss or thinning, and dandruff.

The carotene content in the leaves of false daisy can improve vision. It can also help treat anemia, lower sugar levels, and prevent miscarriage.

It may cause chills, genital itching, and dryness. In TCM, it should be taken with caution in spleen, stomach, and kidney deficiency with cold. In high doses, it can cause stomach irritation, vomiting, and nausea.

Health Benefits Times. (2018, May 21). False daisy facts and health benefits. *HealthBenefitstimes.com*. https://www.healthbenefitstimes.com/false-daisy/

Parmar, R. (2021, June 2). 12 wonderful health benefits of Bhringraj oil. *PharmEasy Blog*. https://pharmeasy.in/blog/12-wonderful-health-benefits-of-bhringraj-oil/

Bibhitaki
Terminalia bellirica

Other names: *Belleric myrobalan, Vibhitaki, Baheda, Todikai*

The active constituents present in bibhitaki include β-sitosterol, gallic acid, ellagic acid, ethyl gallate, galloyl glucose, and chebulagic acid. Other compounds include terpenoids (bellericacid and chebulagic acid), saponin (bellericoside and bellericanin), and tannins.

It has antioxidant, hepatoprotective, antimicrobial, antidiabetic, and angiogenic properties. It also has antithrombotic (thrombolytic) and wound-healing activities.

It is useful in treatment of hepatitis, bronchitis, asthma, cough, hoarseness of voice, dyspepsia, piles, diarrhea, eye diseases, and scorpion stings.

Ingredients	Mechanism of Action and Health Benefits

Ingredients

Mechanism of Action and Health Benefits

It can reduce high blood pressure, control cholesterol levels, and weight loss. It also helps improve immune system function. It may reduce the risk of cancer.

Excess consumption can lead to dry skin and constipation. It should also not be used during pregnancy or lactation period.

Gupta, A., Kumar, R., Kumar, S., & Pandey, A. K. (Eds.). (2017). Pharmacological aspects of *Terminalia belerica*. In *Molecular biology and pharmacognosy of beneficial plants* (pp. 52–64). Delhi: Lenin Media Private Limited.

Bitter cumin
Centratherum anthelminticum

See under "Cumin"

Bitter gourd
Momordica charantia

Other names: *Bitter melon, Karvellaka, Karela, Pavaikkari*

Bitter gourd is rich in antioxidants (charantin, epicatechin, gallic acid, and chlorogenic acid), flavonoids, and other polyphenols. Compounds present including charantin, (a steroidal saponin agent with insulin-like properties) and polypeptide-p have antidiabetic effects. It also contains high amounts of vitamins (A, B1, B2, B3, B9, C, and E), minerals (potassium, calcium, zinc, magnesium, phosphorus, and iron), and dietary fiber.

It is known for its medicinal properties including antidiabetic, anticancer, antiinflammation, antivirus, and cholesterol-lowering effects.

It regulates blood sugar. It may be used in the treatment of malaria. It can also help in weight loss.

Side effects include diarrhea, vomiting, vaginal bleeding, uterine contractions, abortion, and liver damage. It can be dangerous if taken with insulin as it lowers blood sugar.

Joseph, B., & Jini, D. (2013). Antidiabetic effects of *Momordica charantia* (bitter melon) and its medicinal potency. *Asian Pacific Journal of Tropical Disease, 3*(2), 93–102. https://doi.org/10.1016/s2222-1808(13)60052-3

Black Cumin
Nigella sativa

See under "Cumin"

Black gram
Vigna mungo

Other names: *Urad, uzhunnu parippu, ulundu paruppu, black lentil, black dhal*

Black gram is a black lentil which is a high protein (25 g/100 g) pulse. The leaves are edible. The dried black seeds can be whole or split, with skin or hulled, unroasted or roasted. It has a low glycemic index (GI), high fiber (soluble mucilaginous polysaccharides), and high saponins. It is rich in minerals (calcium, iron, copper, and potassium) and vitamins (B1, B6, and folate). It also contains isoflavones (genistein, glycitein, daidzein, and formononetin) which help with menopausal syndrome and osteoporosis.

It is consumed in many ways in Indian cuisine. The soaked seeds are cooked as dal and vada or together with rice are fermented to make dosa and idli. The roasted and ground flour is made into a porridge, papadam, or added to other flours.

The unroasted ground flour acts as a poultice for abscesses as it has astringent and cooling properties.

It can help with obesity and diabetes. It can increase feelings of satiety and lower total cholesterol. It inhibits α-amylase which slows carbohydrate absorption hence reducing postprandial blood glucose levels.

It has laxative effects and can prevent constipation.

Excessive consumption can cause flatulence.

Black-jack
Bidens pilosa
Bidens leucantha

Other names: Bidens, Beggar's tick, Vawkpuithal

Bidens is a weed used as folk medicine in Northeast India and Africa. The roots, leaves, flowers, and seeds are edible. It is rich in iodine.

It is also eaten as a fresh or cooked vegetable.

It has antimicrobial (from presence of flavonoids and polyacetylene compounds), antioxidant, antiinflammatory, astringent, antidiabetic, and anticancer properties. It acts on all mucous membranes.

It can treat benign prostatic hypertrophy and UTIs. It can excrete uric acid from the blood and helps in gout.

It can also treat sore throat, cough, cold, gastritis, diarrhea, and vaginal infections.

Side effects include skin irritation or allergy from the sap of the plant.

Ingredients	Mechanism of Action and Health Benefits
Black nightshade *Solanum nigrum*	Other names: *Maṇattakkāḷi or Manathakkali keerai, Makoy or Makoi, Kakamachi, Petit morel* The active compounds present in black nightshade are organic acids (acetic acid, tartaric acid, malic acid, and citric acid), glycoalkaloid (solanine), saponins, and steroidal saponin (solanigrosides). It has antitumor activity due to the presence of solanine. The antimicrobial effects are mainly due to the saponins. Black nightshade is different from the deadly nightshade *(Atropa belladonna)*. It has antioxidant, antiinflammatory, hepatoprotective, sedative, and narcotic effects. The leaves are often cooked and eaten as a vegetable. It can treat stomach irritation, intestinal cramps, and spasms. Fresh crushed leaves or its juice may also be used as poultice to treat swellings, deep abscesses, burns, ulcers, hemorrhoids, and psoriasis. The raw leaves or unripe fruit if eaten can cause nausea, vomiting, or headache. Atanu, F. O., Ebiloma, U. G., & Ajayi, E. I. (2011). A review of the pharmacological aspects of Solanum nigrum Linn. *Biotechnology and Molecular Biology Review*, 6(1), 1–7. https://academicjournals.org/journal/BMBR/article-full-text-pdf/0E4825611574 WebMD Editors. (n.d.). BLACK NIGHTSHADE: Overview, Uses, Side Effects, Precautions, Interactions, Dosing and Reviews. *WebMD*. https://www.webmd.com/vitamins/ai/ingredientmono-821/black-nightshade
Black pepper *Piper nigrum*	Black pepper is rich in alkaloids (piperine, chavicine, piperidine, and piperettine), tannins, flavonoids, and cardiac glycosides. The piperine has antioxidant activity and improves degenerative brain diseases (AD and PD). Black pepper also has high amounts of vitamins (A, B1, B2, B5, B6, C, E, and K), minerals (calcium, magnesium, manganese, phosphorus, potassium, zinc, and selenium), and fiber. It has antioxidant, antiinflammatory, and detoxifying effects. It can enhance the absorption of curcumin and β-carotene. It is used to treat chronic indigestion, obesity, sinusitis, lung congestion, vertigo, and arthritic disorders. It may also improve blood sugar control and help lower cholesterol levels. It may also improve gut health and increase the absorption of essential nutrients like calcium and selenium. Excess consumption of black pepper may lead to burning sensations in the throat or stomach. It may enhance the absorption of drugs and should be used with caution in combination with certain medications. Ganesh, P., Kumar, R. S., & Saranraj, P. (2014). Phytochemical analysis and antibacterial activity of Pepper (*Piper nigrum* L.) against some human pathogens. *Central European Journal of Experimental Biology*, 3(2), 36–41. https://www.scholarsresearchlibrary.com/articles/phytochemical-analysis-and-antibacterial-activity-of-pepper-piper-nigrum-l-against-some-human-pathogens.pdf Meixner, M. (2019, March 21). 11 science-backed health benefits of black pepper. *Healthline*. https://www.healthline.com/nutrition/black-pepper-benefits#1.
Bottle gourd *Lagenaria siceraria*	Other names: *Sorakka/Suraikkaai/Sorakaya, Lauki, Ghiya, Kaddu, Dudi/Dudhi, Calabash* Bottle gourd contains triterpenoid cucurbitacins, sterols, flavonoids, and saponins. It is rich in vitamins (K, C, riboflavin, thiamine), minerals (calcium, zinc, iron, magnesium, and manganese), and fiber. The antioxidant properties are due to its high vitamin C content. It is low in saturated fats and cholesterol. It also contains a lot of water. Hence, it is cooling and hydrating and can relieve UTI. Its water content helps in treating diarrhea and also hydrates the skin so that wrinkles appear reduced. The high fiber content is useful in treating constipation. It also helps with weight loss. It also helps in lowering blood sugar levels and high blood pressure. It contains choline which is important in mental health conditions like depression or stress. It can reduce uric acid levels and also edema in the lower limbs. It also helps to reduce liver inflammation. Bottle gourd has a bitter taste and if eaten raw, it can cause diarrhea, nausea, vomiting, discomfort, gastric ulcers, and duodenitis. Excessive consumption can also lead to hypoglycemia. NDTV Food. (2018, March 28). 7 incredible benefits of drinking bottle gourd (Lauki) juice. https://food.ndtv.com/food-drinks/7-incredible-benefits-of-drinking-of-bottle-gourd-lauki-juice-1452828 Shukla, L. (2018, September 14). Bottle gourd juice benefits, uses and side effects. *MyUpchar*. https://www.myupchar.com/en/tips/lauki-juice-benefits-and-side-effects-in-hindi

Ingredients	Mechanism of Action and Health Benefits
Brahmi *Bacopa monnieri*	Brahmi is a super brain food with active bacosides A and B and brahmi as the main saponin compounds which have antioxidant properties. Others include nicotine and herpestine. It has antiepileptic, antiinflammatory, cardiotonic, digestive aid, and possibly anticancer effects. It can improve memory, concentration, attention, visual processing, and intellect. It can reduce anxiety, ADHD, and stress. It gives restful sleep. It may also help reduce blood pressure. Side effects include allergic reactions, nausea, stomach cramps, and diarrhea. It should also be avoided by pregnant women. Raman, R., & Arnarson, A. (2019, October 31). 7 emerging benefits of Bacopa monnieri (Brahmi). *Healthline*. https://www.healthline.com/nutrition/bacopa-monnieri-benefits
Buttermilk	Buttermilk contains calcium (22% of the DV), sodium (16% of the DV), riboflavin (29% of the DV), vitamin B12 (22% of the DV), and pantothenic acid (13% of the DV). Riboflavin improves liver function and helps in detoxification. It is also a good source of phosphorus and vitamins D and K2. These nutrients help in maintaining bone strength and preventing degenerative bone diseases like osteoporosis. It may be digested easily compared to other dairy products as the lactose is broken down by the bacteria. It has antidiabetic and cholesterol-lowering effects. It may have antiinflammatory effects that can help reduce periodontitis and oral inflammation (due to radiation therapy, chemotherapy, or Crohn's disease). It reduces acidity, prevents dehydration, and can help cool the body. As it has a high sodium content, caution needs to be exercised in those with heart problems. Rarely, allergy reactions may occur in those who are lactose intolerant. Some symptoms include upset stomach, diarrhea, and gas. Negi. (2020, August 26). 10 amazing health benefits of buttermilk (Chaas). *Amritsr: The Maharaja of Indian Cuisine*. https://amritsruae.com/blog/health-benefits-of-buttermilk/ Panoff, L. (2019, October 28). Is buttermilk good for you? Benefits, risks, and substitutes. *Healthline*. https://www.healthline.com/nutrition/buttermilk
Cabbage *Brassica oleracea*	Cabbage can vary in colors (including white, green, and purple-red) and leaves can be smooth or wrinkled. It is rich in fibers (soluble and insoluble), antioxidants (kaempferol, sulforaphane, and polyphenols), phytosterols, vitamins (K1, C, and β-carotene), and minerals (zinc, potassium, calcium, and manganese especially in the purple-red cabbage). It has antiinflammatory and antioxidant properties. It supports digestive health and prevents constipation. It supports heart health. It can reduce blood pressure and LDL cholesterol (especially the purple-red cabbage). It can also strengthen the bones. Side effects include the presence of goitrogens which blocks the transport of iodine to the thyroid leading to potential hypothyroidism. It can interact with blood thinners. Kubala, J. (2017, November 4). 9 impressive health benefits of cabbage. *Healthline*. https://www.healthline.com/nutrition/benefits-of-cabbage#TOC_TITLE_HDR_2 Ware, M. (2017, November 2). The health benefits of cabbage. *MedicalNewsToday*. https://www.medicalnewstoday.com/articles/284823#nutrition
Camphor *Cinnamomum camphora*	Other names: *Kampfer, Karpoora, Karpuram, Camphora* Camphor oil is extracted from the camphor tree wood and it has a menthol-like fragrance. It is now mostly synthesized from turpentine oil. It is a terpenoid and has antiinflammatory and antimicrobial properties. It acts as a counterirritant and is applied to painful joints or skin rash. It is commonly used in coughs and colds and is a topical ingredient in many mentholated ointments such as Vicks VapoRub and helps to improve airway congestion. Camphor oil can be applied to hair to treat head lice. It is unsafe to use camphor directly and products containing more than 11% camphor should not be used. It may cause minor side effects such as redness and irritation when used topically. It should also not be used directly on broken or injured skin as it could be toxic. Any contact with eyes should also be avoided. Camphor products should be avoided when pregnant or breastfeeding.

Ingredients	Mechanism of Action and Health Benefits

Mechanism of Action and Health Benefits

Cronkleton, E., & Carter, A. (2019, August 8). How to use camphor safely: Benefits and precautions. *Healthline*. https://www.healthline.com/health/what-is-camphor

Panesar, G. (2017, August 30). 8 incredible benefits of camphor: Pain killer, sleep inducer and more. *NDTV Food*. https://food.ndtv.com/health/8-incredible-benefits-of-camphor-pain-killer-sleep-inducer-and-more-1648410

Caraway
Carum carvi

Other name: *Jeera beej*

Caraway contains active compounds such as carvone, limonene, linalool, and carveol. It is rich in antioxidants (lutein and zeaxanthin) and fiber. It is also rich in vitamins and minerals especially vitamin A, magnesium, iron, and calcium. It is often added as a spice to breads or sauerkraut.

It has antiinflammatory and immunomodulatory properties.

It reduces cholesterol, blood glucose, indigestion, and flatulence, increases bowel movements, and promotes weight loss. It may also help treat asthma, constipation, bloating, and menstrual cramps.

Caraway oil may cause allergic reactions and gastric upsets. Pregnant and breastfeeding women and those with diabetes should not consume caraway.

Black caraway actually refers to kalonji or nigella seeds.

Keshavarz, A., Minaiyan, M., Ghannadi, A., & Mahzouni, P. (2013). Effects of *Carum carvi* L. (Caraway) extract and essential oil on TNBS-induced colitis in rats. *Research in Pharmaceutical Sciences*, 8(1), 1–8. https://www.ncbi.nlm.nih.gov/pmc/articles/PMC3895295/#__ffn_sectitle

WebMD Editors. (2020, November 3). Caraway: Is it good for you? *WebMD*. https://www.webmd.com/diet/caraway-good-for-you#1

Cardamom

There are three types of cardamom:

Green *(Elettaria cardamomum)*,

Black *(Amomum subulatum)*,

White (bleached version of the green cardamom).

Green cardamom (*Elettaria cardamomum*)

Other names for *Green cardamom: Small cardamom, True cardamom, Elaichi, Ellakay*

Green cardamom is the commonest type. The bioactive constituents are alkaloids, steroids, terpenoids, phenols, glycosides, and tannins. The active ingredients in the essential oil contain cineole, terpenes, limonene, and linalool. It contains fiber, potassium, calcium, magnesium, phosphorus, and iron. It is used widely in Indian desserts (as a flavoring agent) and in curries (as a spice).

It has antioxidant, antiinflammatory, antimicrobial, anticonvulsant, and diuretic properties.

It can lower blood pressure, relieve bad breath, promote weight loss, help with metabolic syndrome, and prevent fatty liver.

The essential oil may help in epilepsy.

It may also have cancer-fighting properties.

Overall, green cardamom is safe.

Black cardamom (*Amomum subulatum*)

Other names for *Black Cardamom: Big Elaichi, Kali Elaichi, Karuppu elakkay.*

There are two main species of black cardamom: *Amomum subulatum* (for Indian cuisine) *and Amomum chao-ko* (for Chinese cuisine). Black cardamom is used in Indian meat-based curries and not for desserts.

The main active ingredient in black cardamom present is monoterpenoids (eucalyptol, geraniol, and geranyl acetate).

It has antibacterial, antiinflammatory, antioxidant, detoxifying, immune-boosting, antiaging, and antidepressant effects. Its essential oil is rich in vitamin C and manganese which are beneficial for hair growth and skin problems (acne and black spots).

Both types can be used in the treatment of respiratory disorders (asthma, whooping cough, lung congestion, bronchitis, and pulmonary tuberculosis). It also helps reduce the risk of chronic diseases such as heart disease, rheumatoid arthritis, cancer, and even some neurodegenerative diseases.

Overconsumption of black cardamom can cause respiratory problems, skin problems, gallstones, hyperactivity, and mouth ulcers.

Health Benefits Times Editors. (2018, July 20). Black Cardamom health benefits. *HealthBenefitstimes.com*. https://www.healthbenefitstimes.com/black-cardamom/

AromaWeb Editor. (n.d.). Cardamom essential oil uses and benefits. *Aroma Web*. https://www.aromaweb.com/essential-oils/cardamom-oil.asp

Ingredients	Mechanism of Action and Health Benefits
	Berry, J., & Carter, A. (2019, October 2). What are the health benefits of cardamom? *MedicalNewsToday*. https://www.medicalnewstoday.com/articles/326532
	Streit, L. (2018, August 8). 10 health benefits of cardamom, backed. *Healthline*. https://www.healthline.com/nutrition/cardamom-benefits
Carom seeds *Trachyspermum ammi*	Other names: *Ajwain, Omam, Ajowan, Ajwain imam, Bishop's weed, Thymol seeds, Ajowan caraway*

It contains the active ingredients i.e., thymol and carvacrol which have antimicrobial, antibiotic, and antiinflammatory properties. They are also rich in fiber, minerals (potassium, calcium, iron, and phosphorus), antioxidants (limonene, pinene, and terpinene), and nicotinic acid. The antioxidants along with the minerals help in hair growth, improving the immune system, and reducing the risk of chronic diseases.

It improves digestion and hyperacidity, as well as helps in weight loss. It also reduces cholesterol levels. It can be used as a mouthwash to maintain good oral hygiene. It can also relieve the pain and swelling in arthritis.

Consumption of ajwain should be avoided by pregnant or breastfeeding women as it has potential to cause birth defects or miscarriage.

Carom seeds (ajwain) are different from celery seeds (ajmoda/ajmod/radhuni). Celery seeds are from *Trachyspermum roxburghianum* (also known as *Carum roxburghianum*/Indian celery) or the related *Apium graveolens*. Ajmoda is stronger than ajwain in kindling the Agni digestive fire and eliminating toxins).

Brennan, D. (2020, September 2). Health benefits of ajwain. *WebMD*. https://www.webmd.com/dicenet/health-benefits-ajwain#1

Staughton, J. (2020, July 29). 18 best health benefits of carom seeds (ajwain). *Organic Facts*. https://www.organicfacts.net/carom-seeds.html

Cassia seed *Cassiae semen*

Other names: *Juemingzi, Senna, Cassia, Amaltas, Fan Xie Ye, Alexandrian senna*

The species names in the genera *Cassia* and *Senna* are often not precise.

Basically, *Senna* is from the *Cassia species* leaves and seed pods. There are more 330 Cassia species, of which about 300 have been moved to the genus Senna.

In United same, the common name Senna also refers to senna from *Cassia angustifolia, Cassia senna, Cassia acutifolia, Senna alexandrina, Sennae Folium (senna leaf), Sennae Fructus, (senna fruit), and Tinnevelly senna or Indian senna.*

Purging senna is from Cassia fistula (other names: Indian Laburnum, Golden Shower tree, Amaltas, Sarakondrai (an Indian Cassia) and is used in Ayurvedic medicine.

Chinese senna or cassia refers to *Cassia obtusifolia* and *Cassia tora* species. Cassia gum is an extract from the seeds of Chinese senna and is used as a thickening agent.

Senna or Cassia fruit (seed pods) seems to be gentler than Senna leaf.

Both "Senna pod" and "Senna leaf" are nonprescription laxatives.

Cassia seed is the dry and mature seed of the tree of the *Cassia* genus of *Leguminosae* family. The above listed species are used as laxatives.

However, adulterants or substitutes from the seeds of *Cassia occidentalis,* Cassia *sophera, Cassia auriculata* (Avartaki/Avarampoo/Avaram senna), or other Cassia species may occur.

Cassia contains various bioactive compounds including anthraquinones (includes rhein glycosides), sennosides, volatile oils, and sterols. The dried fruit pulp is the medicinal component although the leaf, root, and seeds are also used.

It has antibacterial, antifungal, antipyretic, analgesic, antiinflammatory, expectorant, emetic, purgative, and antidepressant properties. It has a cooling effect and is used as an antipyretic to decrease inflammation and heat of the body in chest or throat.

In Ayurvedic medicine, Cassia pacifies all the three doshas. In TCM, Cassia covers the large intestine and liver meridians. It dissipates liver heat, dispels evil wind, lubricates intestines, and helps in liver detoxification.

It is used to treat fever, skin diseases, constipation, obesity, digestive problems, respiratory problems, diabetes, and worm infestation.

It also helps in reducing blood lipids, glucose, and regulates blood pressure. It may also help in improving sleep and weight loss.

Side effects include diarrhea, abdominal cramps nausea, low blood pressure, low blood sugar, and liver damage.

Ingredients	Mechanism of Action and Health Benefits
	Basu, S. (2021, March 19). Amaltas: benefits, uses, formulations, ingredients, method, dosage and side effects. *Netmeds*. https://www.netmeds.com/health-library/post/amaltas-benefits-uses-formulations-ingredients-method-dosage-and-side-effects
	Gope, A. (2020, February 14). Health benefits of Cassia fistula|Sarakondrai. *The Indian Med*. https://theindianmed.com/health-benefits-of-cassia-fistula-sarakondrai/
	Trust Herb. (2021, February 1). 5 health benefits of Amaltas. *Trust The Herb*. https://trustherb.com/health-benefits-of-amaltas/
	Basu, S. (2022, January 7). Cassia auriculata: Incredible health benefits and medicinal uses of Avartaki. *Netmeds*. https://www.netmeds.com/health-library/post/cassia-auriculata-incredible-health-benefits-and-medicinal-uses-of-avartaki
Castor oil *Ricinus communis*	The oil extracted from the *Ricinus communis* plant seeds contains triglycerides (ricinoleic acid, oleic acid, linoleic acid, and stearic acid). The triglycerides help maintain skin moisture, cleanse the skin, improve skin health, and make the skin smoother. The ricinoleic acid present also helps boost hair growth, improve blood circulation, and balance hormones.
	It is used as a laxative in constipation.
	It has antimicrobial and antiinflammatory properties. It helps soothe joint ache and reduce acne formation. It is used in many skincare products particularly facial creams and oils.
	Castor oil can cause allergic reactions such as skin rashes, swelling, and itching.
	Kandola, A., & Wilson, D. R. (2018, June 28). Benefits of castor oil for the face and skin. *MedicalNewsToday*. https://www.medicalnewstoday.com/articles/319844
	New Directions Aromatics Editors. (2017, August 29). Castor oil—Benefits & uses for hair care, skin care, and pain relief. *New Directions Aromatics*. https://www.newdirectionsaromatics.com/blog/products/all-about-castor-carrier-oil.html
Catechu *Acacia catechu*	Other names: *Khair, Khedira, Heartwood extract, Black cutch, Cutch, Dark cutch, Mimosa catechu, Black catechu, Pale catechu*
	Catechu is an herbal plant. There are two types, i.e., black catechu and pale catechu with different bioactive compounds. However, their wood and leaves have the same medicinal uses.
	It contains catechin, an antioxidant flavonol, which is the tannic juice or boiled extract of *Acacia catechu*. Catechin is also present in other medicinal plants.
	It has astringent and hemostatic properties.
	It is used to treat gastrointestinal tract (GIT) conditions (gum diseases, mouth ulcers, diarrhea, colitis, dysentery, hemorrhoids, and indigestion), sore throat, and wounds.
	It is also used as a flavor in foods and drinks.
	Emedicinehealth. (2021, June 14). Catechu: Uses, side effects, dose, health benefits, precautions & warnings. *emedicinehealth*. https://www.emedicinehealth.com/catechu/vitamins-supplements.htm
Cedarwood *Cedrus atlantica* *Cedrus deodara*	There are many species of cedarwood, the common ones being *Cedrus atlantica* (atlas cedarwood) and *Cedrus deodara* (Himalayan cedarwood).
	Cedarwood oil is an essential oil which is used in cosmetics and medicine. The main bioactive compound present is terpenes (cedrene, cedrol, and thujopsene).
	It has antiinfective and insect-repellent properties.
	It stimulates hair growth by regulating sebum production. It can treat hair loss, dandruff, scalp eczema, and acne.
	The oil can also reduce pain over inflamed joints from rheumatism and also in fractures.
	It can reduce stress and anxiety, as well as promote sleep via aromatherapy.
	It also has antidiabetic effects.
	Overall, it is safe. It may cause skin irritation.
	WebMD Editorial Staff. (2021, May 28). What to know about cedarwood essential oil. *WebMD*. https://www.webmd.com/balance/what-to-know-about-cedarwood-essential-oil
	Whelan, C. (2019, January 8). What you need to know about cedarwood essential oil. *Healthline*. https://www.healthline.com/health/cedarwood-essential-oil#benefits
Ceylon leadwort *Plumbago zeylanica*	Other name: *Chitrak*
	Plumbago roots contain various bioactive ingredients including plumbagin, maritinone, and glucosides. The roots and leaves are used. It balances the kapha and vata doshas. It also stimulates the digestive fire (*Agni*).
	It has digestive, carminative, and detoxifying properties. It also supports liver function and breakdown of fats and sugar. It can help in maintaining optimal body weight. It is to treat piles.
	It has antifertility effects and can be used for birth control.
	It can improve appetite and digestion.
	It can also be used to loosen phlegm in lung congestion, chronic bronchitis, and sinusitis.

Ingredients	Mechanism of Action and Health Benefits

Side effects include heavy periods and burning sensation in the mouth and stomach.

Health Benefits Times. (2019, July 28). Health benefits of doctorbush (Plumbago zeylanica). *Health-Benefitstimes.com*. https://www.healthbenefitstimes.com/doctorbush-plumbago-zeylanica/

Nile, S. H., & Park, S. W. (2014). Biologically active compounds from *Plumbago zeylanica*. *Chemistry of Natural Compounds*, *50*(5), 905–907. https://doi.org/10.1007/s10600-014-1112-8

WebMD Editors. (n.d.). Ceylon leadwort. *WebMD*. https://www.webmd.com/vitamins/ai/ingredient-mono-1612/ceylon-leadwort

Chickpea
Cicer arietinum

Other names: *Garbanzo beans, Chick pea, Chana, Bengal gram, Egyptian pea*

Chickpeas are rich in bioactive compounds including saponins, carotenoids (β-carotene). It contains minerals (manganese, magnesium, copper, phosphorus, potassium, and iron), vitamins (folate and choline), protein, and fiber.

It has antiinflammatory and antioxidant properties.

It supports digestive health. It aids in weight loss by promoting fullness and increasing appetite-reducing hormones. It may prevent colon cancer and IBS.

It can help lower blood sugar and blood pressure, and reduce the risk of cardiovascular disorders.

It also promotes bone, muscle, and skin health.

It improves body metabolism, memory, muscle control and helps in brain and nervous system function.

Side effects include flatulence.

Elliott, B. (2018, May 7). 8 great reasons to include chickpeas in your diet. *Healthline*. https://www.healthline.com/nutrition/chickpeas-nutrition-benefits

Ware, M. (2019, November 5). What are the benefits of chickpeas? *MedicalNewsToday*. https://www.medicalnewstoday.com/articles/280244#_noHeaderPrefixedContent

Chicory
Cichorium intybus

Other names: *Coffeeweed, Blue sailor's succory or Succory or Blue sailors or Wild succory, Witloof, Hindbeh, Hinduba, Kasani*

Chicory is a coffee alternative. It has a coffee taste but does not contain caffeine. The roots are roasted, ground, brewed (alone or together with ground coffee beans), and consumed as a hot beverage. The leaves can be eaten as a salad.

Chicory contains mainly inulin fiber (fructo-oligosaccharide which acts as a prebiotic to promote healthy intestinal flora) and also β-carotene. It also contains chicoric and chlorogenic acids which can increase insulin sensitivity and improve blood sugar control.

Chicory is a digestive tonic.

It can stimulate bile flow from the gallbladder and also bowel movements (as it has some laxative effects). It can prevent gallstones. It also stimulates appetite. It may increase uric acid excretion in the urine.

It can help lower fat deposition in nonalcoholic fatty liver disease.

Overall, it is safe. Gastric upsets or allergic reactions may occur.

Streit, L. (2019, November 14). 5 emerging benefits and uses of chicory root fiber. *Healthline*. https://www.healthline.com/nutrition/chicory-root-fiber

WebMD Editors. (2010). Chicory. *WebMD*. https://www.webmd.com/vitamins/ai/ingredientmono-92/chicory

Chirata
Swertia chirayita

Other names: *Bitter stick, Kairata, Swertia chirata, Indian Gentian, Yin Du Zhang Ya Cai*

There are many *Swertia* species. All parts of the Chirata herbal plant have extensive medicinal purposes. It contains several bioactive compounds including glycosides, alkaloids and xanthones, chiratol, swertanone, amarogentin, and more. Chirata has a very bitter taste.

It has antiinflammatory, antiseptic, antitussive, carminative, laxative, hepatoprotective, antidiabetic, blood purifying, diuretic, antipruritic, astringent, anticancer, and antihelminthic actions.

It can treat GI disorders (constipation, indigestion, gas, loss of appetite, intestinal worm infestation, cholecystitis, hepatitis), skin disorders (scabies, eczema, acne, skin rash), respiratory disorders (cough, cold, and asthma), diabetes, fevers, infections, and anemia. In diabetes, it stimulates the pancreatic beta cells to produce more insulin. It is reported to be effective in liver cancer.

Overall, Chirata is safe. It should not be used in pregnancy. It can interact with antidiabetic drugs.

ScienceDirect. (n.d.). Swertia chirayita—An overview.*ScienceDirect*. https://www.sciencedirect.com/topics/agricultural-and-biological-sciences/swertia-chirayita

RxList. (2021, June 11). Chirata: Health benefits, side effects, uses, dose & precautions. https://www.rxlist.com/chirata/supplements.htm

Ingredients	Mechanism of Action and Health Benefits
Chyawanprash	Chyawanprash is an Ayurvedic health supplement made of several herbs and minerals. The formulation contains about 50 medicinal herbs and their extracts and also spices (cinnamon, clove, and cardamom). Amla is the base ingredient. Ghee and honey are also added. It has a fruit jam-like consistency with a sweet, sour, and spicy taste.

Chyawanprash is an Ayurvedic health supplement made of several herbs and minerals. The formulation contains about 50 medicinal herbs and their extracts and also spices (cinnamon, clove, and cardamom). Amla is the base ingredient. Ghee and honey are also added. It has a fruit jam-like consistency with a sweet, sour, and spicy taste.

It is a metabolic tonic to boost vitality and strength. It has antiaging, detoxifying, and immune-boosting properties.

It also promotes excellent health and longevity.

Its key ingredients include amla *(Phyllanthus emblica)*, ashwagandha *(Withania somnifera)*, bala *(Sida cordifolia)*, brahmi *(Bacopa monnieri)*, guduchi *(Tinospora cordifolia)*, gokshura *(Tribulus terrestris)*, pippali *(Piper longum)*, and shatavari *(Asparagus racemosus)*.

Side effects may include gastric upsets and hyperglycemia.

Sharma, R., Martins, N., Kuca, K., Chaudhary, A., Kabra, A., Rao, M. M., et al. (2019). Chyawanprash: a traditional Indian bioactive health supplement. *Biomolecules*, 9(5), 161–185. https://doi.org/10.3390/biom9050161

Cinnamon
Cinnamomum spp.

Other names: *Dar chini, Twak patra (Cinnamomum cassia)*

Despite the confusing terms "cinnamon" and "cassia," the following are important species of cinnamon in the genus Cinnamomum.

There are two main types of cinnamon:

Ceylon cinnamon or true cinnamon *(Cinnamomum zeyanicum or Cinnamomum vera)* and Cassia cinnamon.

Cassia cinnamon includes
- Indonesian cinnamon *(Cinnamomum burmannii*, also called *Korintje* or *Java cinnamon)*,
- Vietnamese Cassia, also called Vietnamese cinnamon or Saigon cinnamon *(Cinnamomum loureiroi)*,
- Chinese cinnamon or Chinese cassia or Cassia twig or Cinnamon twig or *Gui Zhi* or *Roi Gui* *(Cinnamomum aromaticum* also called *Cinnamomum cassia, Cinnamomum ramulus, Cinnamoni Cortex, Cinnamomi Cortex)*.

Ceylon cinnamon sticks have wafer-thin layers of bark which are hand-made into rolls.

Cassia cinnamon sticks consist of thick and hard layers of rolled bark. Both ground powders are difficult to distinguish.

Cinnamon is high in antioxidants (i.e., cinnamaldehyde, eugenol, and linalool). It also contains cinnamophilin which is a thromboxane A2 receptor antagonist. It also contains coumarins (lowest in Ceylon cinnamon).

It has antimicrobial, antiviral, antiinflammatory, analgesic, sedative, anticonvulsant, and immunosuppressive effects.

The "insulin-potentiating factor" can lower blood glucose and cholesterol. Cinnamon has been found to boost metabolism, suppress appetite, promote toxin excretion, and aid in reducing weight.

Cinnamon also has anticoagulant actions. It inhibits thromboxane A2 receptors, which causes platelets in the blood to clot. This reduction in clotting thins the blood and reduces blood clots in menstrual flow.

It can increase sperm production. It lowers insulin levels and blood sugar in women with PCOS so that fertility, ovulation, and pregnancy chances are better.

It is used to treat toothaches, bad breath, indigestion, diabetes mellitus, sore throat and colds, and menstrual cramps. It purifies blood. It is a good health tonic.

Overall, it is safe. Heavy use can cause stomach irritation, allergy, bleeding risk, liver injury, and cancer risk from the coumarins. It should also be avoided by pregnant and breastfeeding women.

From the TCM perspective, Chinese cinnamon or Gui zhi is obtained by sun drying the twigs of cinnamon. It is red-brown or brown. It covers the meridians of heart, lung, and bladder. It expels cold and warms the meridians.

It is often used to promote urination. It can treat rheumatoid arthritis, joint pain, irregular menstruation, amenorrhea, and dysmenorrhea. It is also helpful in relieving GI cramps.

It can improve cardiac function and edema. It also treats dizziness, fever, aversion to cold, cough, and phlegm.

Overall, it is safe. Excessive use can cause adverse reactions such as sweating, tiredness, weakness of the limbs, palpitations, dizziness, eye swelling, dry mouth, oliguria, and burning sensation of the urethra.

Ingredients	Mechanism of Action and Health Benefits

Medical Health Guide Editors. (2011). Cinnamon herbal medicine, health benefits, side effects. *Medical Health Guide*. http://www.medicalhealthguide.com/herb/cinnamon.htm

Chinese Herbs Info. (2021, March 31). *Gui Zhi (Cinnamon Twig, Ramulus Cinnamomi, Cassia Twig)*. https://www.chineseherbsinfo.com/the-benefits-and-side-effects-of-gui-zhi-cinnamon-twig

Citronella oil

Other names: *Ceylon Citronella, Cymbopogon nardus, C. afronardus, Cymbopogon validus, Andropogon nardus*

Citronella oil is an essential oil from the *Cymbopogon* grass family (above species).

Lemongrass *(Cymbopogon citratus)* is in the same family but it is not used to make citronella oil. Lemongrass is used widely in Asian cuisine.

Citronella oil has also appetite stimulant effects, diuretic, antihelminthic, and antispasmodic effects.

Citronella oil is used in mosquito repellants and applied on the skin.

It is used in perfumes, fragrances, soaps, or cosmetics.

It is also an edible flavoring in foods and beverages.

Overall, it is safe.

emedicine*health*. (2021, June 14). Citronella oil: Uses, side effects, dose, health benefits, precautions & warnings. https://www.emedicinehealth.com/citronella_oil/vitamins-supplements.htm

Citrullus colocynthis

Other names: *Indrayan, Indravaruni, Colocynth Bitter apple, Bitter cucumber, Wild gourd, Vine of Sodom, Egusi, Abu Jahl, Kadu Hanzal, Alhandal*

Colocynth is a creeping vine plant with bitter fruits that grows in arid conditions. Although it is a toxic plant, extracts from the fruit, seeds, leaves, stem, and roots can be used. The seed and roots are least toxic. The fruit powder is also used. It is widely used in Ayurvedic and Iranian medicine and homeopathy to treat many ailments. It balances pitta and kapha doshas.

It contains glycosides, essential oils, fatty acids, flavonoids, and alkaloids. The cucurbitacins are mucosal irritants and cause side effects.

It has antidiabetic (especially root powder), antiinflammatory (fruit and seeds), analgesic, lipid-lowering, blood purifying, detoxifying, and strong purgative (fruit pulp) actions. It also has abortifacient, antiepileptic, and hair growth-promoting effects.

It can treat diabetes, joint pains, and rheumatism. Topical colocynth is effective in neuropathic pain in diabetic neuropathy.

It is also used in constipation, hemorrhoids, coughs, colds, and asthma.

Side effects include acute toxic colitis with bloody diarrhea, kidney and liver failure.

Hussain, A. I., Rathore, H. A., Sattar, M. Z., Chatha, S. A., Sarker, S. D., & Gilani, A. H. (2014). *Citrullus colocynthis* (L.) Schrad (bitter apple fruit): A review of its phytochemistry, pharmacology, traditional uses and nutritional potential. *Journal of Ethnopharmacology, 155*(1), 54–66. https://doi.org/10.1016/j.jep.2014.06.011

Clove
Syzygium aromaticum

Other names: *Laung, Lavang, Ding xiang, Clavo, Clou de girofle*

Clove is rich in antioxidants (eugenol). It is high in manganese which promotes bone mass and also acts as an antioxidant. It is also an excellent source of fiber, vitamin K, potassium, and β-carotene. The carotene present can be converted into vitamin A, which can improve eyesight.

It also contains antiinflammatory, antiulcer, and hepatoprotective properties.

It reduces the risk of developing diabetes, heart disease, and cancers. It also kills bacteria and parasites. It can benefit oral health.

Eugenol present can interact with blood-thinning medication. High consumption of clove can lead to hypoglycemia and bleeding risk.

Brennan, D. (2020, August 28). Health benefits of cloves. *WebMD*. https://www.webmd.com/diet/health-benefits-cloves#1-2

Link, R., & Arnarson, A. (2020, March 12). 8 surprising health benefits of cloves. *Healthline*. https://www.healthline.com/nutrition/benefits-of-cloves#_noHeaderPrefixedContent

Ingredients	Mechanism of Action and Health Benefits
Coconut oil *Cocos nucifera*	Other names: *Copra oil, Coconut palm oil, Thengai ennai, Nariyal tel* Coconut oil contains 80% to 90% saturated fats which are high in medium chain triglycerides (MCT) which contain healthy fatty acids. These are mainly lauric acid (47%), caprylic acid (7%), capric acid (5%), and smaller amounts of myristic and palmitic acids. There are trace amounts of mono-unsaturated and polyunsaturated fats. Cold-pressed coconut oil has antibacterial, antimicrobial, antioxidant, and antiinflammatory properties. It also contains vitamins E and K. It reduces inflammation and itchiness, as well as prevents infections. It is used on the skin, hair, teeth, or nails or consumed. The lauric acid has antibacterial and antiyeast properties. The MCT are converted to ketones which improve brain function in many neurological disorders such as epilepsy and AD. It can have protective effects on the brain against dementia. It improves dental health. It moisturizes the skin and hair. It also promotes wound healing. Ingestion of too much coconut oil can lead to nausea. Other side effects may include headache, dizziness, fatigue, swollen glands, joint or muscle pain, stomach upset, chills, and rashes. Gunnars, K., & Arnarson, A. (2020, February 12). Top 10 evidence-based health benefits of coconut oil. *Healthline.* https://www.healthline.com/nutrition/top-10-evidence-based-health-benefits-of-coconut-oil#TOC_TITLE_HDR_2 The President and Fellows of Harvard College. (2021, July 6). Coconut oil. *The Nutrition Source.* https://www.hsph.harvard.edu/nutritionsource/food-features/coconut-oil/
Coconut water	Other name: *Thengai taṇṇīr* Coconut water is a fresh liquid that is inside a young green coconut of 6 to 7 months of age before the inside of the coconut matures and ripens into a thick kernel. One coconut fruit can produce about 200 to 250 mL of coconut water. It is a natural and nutritious beverage with low calories. It is rich in several minerals (sodium, potassium, magnesium, calcium, and manganese). It is usually used to quench thirst or as an oral rehydration solution during acute diarrhea. It also has antioxidant properties. It can also lower blood sugar, increase insulin sensitivity, and lower blood cholesterol and triglycerides. It can lower blood pressure. It also has antithrombotic activity and reduces the risk of blood clots. It may also prevent, break down, and flush out kidney stones. It relieves the burning sensation during urination. The presence of potassium and magnesium can reduce muscle and intestinal cramps. Overall, it is safe. It may cause allergy reactions or stomach upset in certain people. In excess amounts coconut water can increase the potassium levels in blood which can lead to kidney problems and irregular heartbeat. Spritzler, F. (2018, September 6). 8 science-based health benefits of coconut water. *Healthline.* https://www.healthline.com/nutrition/8-coconut-water-benefits Zelman, K. (2010, September 23). The truth about coconut water. *WebMD.* https://www.webmd.com/food-recipes/features/truth-about-coconut-water
Coriander *Coriandrum sativum*	Other names: *dhania, dhanya, Malli* Coriander, like cilantro, is derived from the same plant. However, it has more minerals (manganese, iron, magnesium, selenium, and calcium) and less vitamins (A, B9, C, E, and β-carotene) compared to cilantro. The leaves are used widely in Indian cuisine. Coriander leaves and seeds are high in antioxidants (terpenes, quercetin, and tocopherols). These have antiinflammatory, antibacterial, antimicrobial, antiparasitic, anticancer, immune-boosting, carminative, cardioprotective, brain-boosting, and anticonvulsant effects. Cineole (a terpene) and linoleic acid (polyunsaturated omega-6 fatty acid) in coriander have antirheumatic and antiarthritic activities. It protects gut health and balances pitta. It is used to treat diarrhea, IBS, and indigestion. It is an appetite stimulant. It has diuretic properties and helps in removal of kidney stones. It may also reduce blood sugar, blood pressure, and cholesterol levels. It can improve skin problems such as dermatitis, acne, sun tan, and dry skin. It can also help cough and loosen phlegm from kapha imbalance. Side effects include rare allergic reactions.

Ingredients	Mechanism of Action and Health Benefits

Asgarpanah, J., & Kazemivash, N. (2012). Phytochemistry, pharmacology and medicinal properties of *Coriandrum sativum* L. *African Journal of Pharmacy and Pharmacology*, 6(31), 2340–2345. https://doi.org/10.5897/AJPP12.901

Panoff, L., & Bjarnadottir, A. (2019, September 17). 8 surprising health benefits of coriander. *Healthline*. https://www.healthline.com/nutrition/coriander-benefits

WebMD Editors. (2013). CORIANDER: Overview, uses, side effects, precautions, interactions, dosing and reviews. *WebMD*. https://www.webmd.com/vitamins/ai/ingredientmono-117/coriander

Crape jasmine

Tabernaemontana divaricata

Other names: *Crepe jasmine or Pinwheel flower, Tagar plant*

Crape jasmine contains alkaloids (voachalotine, voaharine, and voalenine), flavonoids, and phenols. The flowers are mostly used for prayers and poojas. The plant is grown more for ornamental than medicinal purposes.

It has antiinfective and wound-healing properties. The flower juice can be used as eye drops in eye infections, and the leaf sap for wound healing.

Garden Plants. (n.d.). Crape Jasmine benefits. *gardenplants.com*. https://gardenplants.comparespecies.com/en/crape-jasmine-benefits/model-791-7

Herbpathy.com. (n.d.). Tabernaemontana divaricata herb uses, benefits, cures, side effects, nutrients. *Herbpathy*. https://herbpathy.com/Uses-and-Benefits-of-Tabernaemontana-Divaricata-Cid4935

Lakshmi Ayurveda Editors. (2019, March 1). An Ayurvedic perspective of crape jasmine. *Lakshmi Ayurveda*. https://www.lakshmiayurveda.com.au/2019/03/an-ayurvedic-perspective-of-crape-jasmine/

Cumin

There are various types of cumin, often with similar names, appearances and often mistaken for each other but they are unrelated species and spices and with different flavors.

Cumin (Cuminum cyminum). Other names: common cumin, cumin, plain jeera, jeera, zeera, or kala jeera. It is black in color.

Bitter cumin (Centratherum anthelminticum).

Other names: *Purple fleabane, Kali jeeri, Kalijiri, Kala jeera, Kaali jeer, Karbi jiri, Karba jeera, Kattu seeragam.*

Cumin (common cumin) or Jeera: It is used in everyday Indian cooking as a "tadka or tempering culinary spice" and has great medicinal properties.

Cumin seeds stimulate pancreatic enzyme secretions and can be effective at preventing vomiting. It is used to treat indigestion, menstrual, and postpregnancy problems. It also stimulates lactation.

Side effects include allergic reactions, upset stomach, vomiting, or constipation.

Bitter cumin contains more than 120 active compounds including fatty acids, sterols, sesquiterpene lactones, and flavonoids. The presence of flavonoids is responsible for its antiinflammatory effects.

Bitter cumin has antioxidant, antidiabetic, antiviral, antibacterial, antimicrobial, and anthelmintic activities. It also possesses anticancer, diuretic, and antifilarial (elephantiasis) effects. It is often combined with ajwain (carom seed) and methi (fenugreek) for weight loss.

It is used for cough, wound healing, and treatment of vitiligo. It is also effective against parasitic intestinal worms in children and malaria.

Unrelated to common cumin are:

1. *Black cumin (Nigella sativa).*

    Other loose or interchangeable names: *black seed, kalonji, black onion seeds, Nigella seeds, kala jeera, kalo jiro, karum jeerum, black caraway, Roman coriander*. It is totally unrelated to the common cumin, although it is often referred to as black cumin. It belongs to the onion family.
    Carum bulbocastanum is black cumin or black caraway *(other name: Krishna jeera)*
    Nigella sativa is kalonji

2. *Fennel seeds*. Other names: *perunjeeragam, saunf*. It appears to resemble cumin and is named as a type of jeera, but is also unrelated to Cumin. Read more under *"Fennel."*

3. *Shahi jeera*. Other names: *Syahi jeera, Shah jeera, Indian caraway*. It is mainly used in masala tea (spiced tea) or garam masala (a polyspice blend). There are two types of Shahi jeera, *Bunium Bulbo Castrum* and Bunium Persicum, and they resemble cumin.

4. *Caraway seeds*. Other names: *Meridian fennel, jeera beej, cake seeds, vilayati jeera, and Indian caraway*. Read more under "Caraway."

Black cumin (Kalonji) seeds and oil contain quinine compounds of which thymoquinone is the highest. It has antiinflammatory, antibacterial, antiparasitic, vasodilator, immunomodulatory, and anticancer activities.

Ingredients	Mechanism of Action and Health Benefits
	It also cleanses and purifies the genitourinary tract in men and uterus in women. It also can increase fertility.
	Kalonji is very effective and can reduce the risk of calcium oxalate kidney stone formation. It helps with weight loss, gas and bloating, indigestion, hemorrhoids, diarrhea, and constipation. It can also treat respiratory problems including nasal congestion, runny nose, sneezing, and swelling of the nasal passages, allergies, cough, lung congestion, asthma, and bronchitis.
	It relaxes the smooth muscles of blood vessels and causes vasodilatation. It acts like a calcium channel blocker to dilate blood vessels in hypertension.
	Petruzzello, M. (2017, November 17). Black cumin. *Encyclopedia Britannica*. https://www.britannica.com/plant/black-cumin
	Paydar, M., Moharam, B. A., Wong, Y. L., Looi, C. Y., Wong, W. F., Nyamathull, S., et al. (2013). *Centratherum anthelminticum* (L.) Kuntze a potential medicinal plant with pleiotropic pharmacological and biological activities. *International Journal of Pharmacology*, 9(3), 211–226. https://doi.org/10.3923/ijp.2013.211.226
Curry leaf *Murraya koenigii*	Other names: *Curry patta, Kadi patta, Karuvepillai/Garupillai/Karvapalle, Daun kari*
	Curry leaves contain carbazole alkaloids which have antiinflammatory, antibacterial, and anticancer properties. Linalool is the compound in the leaf that gives it aroma and antioxidant activity. Mahanimbicine is another carbazole alkaloid.
	It is used to treat inflamed or itchy skin. It stimulates hair growth, prevents premature graying, and treats the dandruff. It also promotes wound healing in mild burns.
	It also reduces cholesterol, blood glucose, and can promote weight loss. It has a mild laxative effect and it is useful for digestive problems. It can relieve morning sickness and nausea.
	It has no known side effects but can be allergic in certain people.
	Kubala, J., & Marengo, K. (2020, March 20). 9 benefits and uses of curry leaves. *Healthline*. https://www.healthline.com/nutrition/curry-leaves-benefits
Custard apple *Annona squamosa*	Other names: *Cherimoya, Sugar apple, Sweetsop*
	The bioactive compounds in custard apple include phenolic compounds, flavonoids (epicatechin, catechin, and epigallocatechin), kaurenoic acid, carotenoids (lutein) and fatty acids (including linoleic acid and oleic acid). It is also rich in fiber, vitamins (C and B6), and minerals (magnesium and potassium). The flavonoids have anticancer effects.
	It has antioxidant, antiinflammatory, and immunomodulatory properties.
	It can improve eye health and reduce the risk of macular degeneration and cataracts.
	Vitamin B6 present helps in creation of neurotransmitters which can regulate mood and lower the risk of depression.
	Custard apple supports heart health. It can also lower blood pressure, cholesterol, and the risk of stroke and heart disease. It can regulate blood glucose and improve insulin levels.
	It also aids in digestion and supports bowel movements.
	Custard apples (mainly seeds and peel) contain a toxin called annonacin that can affect the nervous system and brain. Overconsumption can lead to a specific type of PD.
	Streit, L. (2021, April 7). 8 surprising benefits of cherimoya (custard apple). *Healthline*. https://www.healthline.com/nutrition/cherimoya#TOC_TITLE_HDR_8
Danti *Baliospermum montanum*	Other names: *Wild castor, Wild croton*
	Danti is a blood purifier. It is rich in tannins.
	The roots and seeds are mainly used. It has antipyretic, analgesic, antiinflammatory, antihelminthic, and strong purgative actions. The leaves can be used in bronchitis and asthma.
	It is used to treat constipation, hemorrhoids, jaundice, and rheumatism.
Dashamoola	Other name: *Dasamoolarishtam*
	Dashamoola is a liquid polyherbal Ayurvedic medicine containing more than 50 herbs. The main 10 potent root herbs include: Indian bael *(Aegle marmelos)*, Agnimantha *(Premna serratifolia)*, Gambhari *(Gmelina Arborea)*, Shyonaka *(Oroxylum indicum)*, Patala *(Stereospermum suaveolens)*, Brihati *(Solanum indicum)*, Shalparni *(Desmodium gangeticum)*, Kantakari *(Solanum xanthocarpum)*, Gokshura *(Tribulus terrestris)*, and Prishniparni *(Uraria picta)*.
	It is an excellent health tonic that improves general wellbeing and vitality, especially vata disorders including anemia, fatigue, and sexual weakness.
	It has antiinflammatory, antimicrobial, antiaging, and adaptogenic properties.

Ingredients	Mechanism of Action and Health Benefits
	It improves women's fertility, conception, and postnatal health.
	It also improves sperm count and quality.
	It is also used for osteoporosis, rheumatism, as well as digestive and respiratory disorders.
	Overall, it is safe. It can cause gastric upset in high doses. It is not recommended in pitta-related disorders.

Ten Benefits Editorial Team. (2019, October 7). 10 benefits of dasamoolarishtam. *Ten Benefits*. https://tenbenefits.com/10-benefits-of-dasamoolarishtam/

Dhataki
Woodfordia fruticosa

Dhataki flower is used in Ayurvedic medicine. It contains alkaloids, flavonoids, phytosterols, and glycosides. It balances kapha and pitta.

It has astringent, antiinflammatory, and antimicrobial properties.

It is used to treat menorrhagia and leucorrhea (white vaginal discharge).

It can assist in wound healing and skin problems (including acne and sunburn).

It may help in asthma and in removal of excess mucus from the respiratory tract. It can also reduce diarrhea.

Overall, it is safe. Overconsumption may cause delirium.

Joshi, K., Soni, D., & Ranjan, A. (2019, November 29). Dhataki. *1mg*. https://www.1mg.com/ayurveda/dhataki-179

Syed, Y. H., Khan, M., Bhuvaneshwari, J., & Ansari, J. A. (2013). Phytochemical investigation and standardization of extracts of flowers of Woodfordia fruticosa; a preliminary study. *Journal of Pharmaceuticals and BioSciences*, *1*(4), 134–140.

Dill
Anethum graveolens

Other name: *Aneth*

Dill is rich in antioxidants (flavonoids, terpenoids, and tannins) which are important in gut, heart, and brain health. It also contains vitamin C. The d-limonene in the terpenes may also have antimicrobial, antiinflammatory, and anticancer properties. It also contains calcium, phosphorus, magnesium, manganese, and copper which are important for bone health. Other nutrients include zinc, iron, magnesium, potassium, riboflavin, folate, and vitamin A.

It may also have cholesterol-, triglyceride-, and glucose-lowering effects. It is used to treat colic in children and digestive problems.

The essential oils in dill have antibacterial properties especially against *Staphylococcus aureus* and *Klebsiella pneumoniae*.

It is considered safe for consumption. Rarely, allergic reactions may occur.

McGrane, K., & Hatanaka, M. (2020, February 4). All you need to know about dill. *Healthline*. https://www.healthline.com/nutrition/dill

Drumstick
Moringa oleifera

Other names: *Shigru, Sohanjna, Shobhanjana, Akshiva, Sahijana*

Moringa phytonutrients include tannins, sterols, terpenoids, flavonoids, saponins, anthraquinones, and alkaloids. It also contains anticancer agents (glucosinolates, moringine isothiocyanates, glycoside compounds, and glycerol-1-9-octadecanoate). It contains vitamins (A, B1, B2, B3, B6, B9, and C), minerals (calcium, potassium, iron, magnesium, phosphorus, and zinc), and fiber.

It also has antioxidant, antiinflammatory, hepatoprotective, antidepressant, antidiabetic, antibiotic, and antibacterial properties.

It has higher iron content than spinach, hence can be used as a treatment for anemia. It also has a higher calcium content than milk. It is also high in protein.

It is valuable in treating digestive problems (constipation, gastritis, and ulcerative colitis). It can help in weight loss and prevent colon cancer.

Its seed oil has cholesterol-lowering effects.

Drumsticks may also help in wound healing. It can reduce the risk of developing stones in the kidneys, bladder, or ureters by decreasing oxalate production.

It should not be taken alongside thyroid, blood pressure, and diabetic medicines.

Cadman, B., & Wilson, D. R. (2020, January 2). What makes moringa good for you? *MedicalNewsToday*. https://www.medicalnewstoday.com/articles/319916#_noHeaderPrefixedContent

Gopalakrishnan, L., Doriya, K., & Kumar, D. S. (2016). Moringa oleifera: a review on nutritive importance and its medicinal application. *Food Science and Human Wellness*, *5*(2), 49–56. https://doi.org/10.1016/j.fshw.2016.04.001

Ingredients	Mechanism of Action and Health Benefits
Elephant foot yam *Amorphophallus* *paeoniifolius*	Other name: *Suran* Elephant foot yam contains phytonutrients which include isoflavones, flavonoids, quercetin, terpenoids, and steroids. The isoflavones can improve the skin health and prevent skin problems like pigmentation, sagging, and roughness. Elephant foot yam is rich in fiber, omega-3 fatty acids, β-carotene, and vitamins C, B6, and A. It also contains several minerals including phosphorus, calcium, zinc, and magnesium. It has antiinflammatory, antitumor, antiaging, and anticoagulant properties. Elephant foot yam is used as an expectorant and anticatarrhal agent. It is used for bronchitis and asthma. It can also help in liver disorders, hemorrhoids, vomiting, abdominal pains, dyspepsia, fistula and spleen enlargement. Suran is used for edema, urinary disorders, acute rheumatism, toothache, boils, amenorrhea, and elephantiasis. It is also used for weight loss. Elephant foot yam juice may cause side effects such as vomiting, nausea, diarrhea, and headache. Health Benefits Times Editors. (2019, August 19). Elephant Yam facts and health benefits. *HealthBenefitstimes.com*. https://www.healthbenefitstimes.com/elephant-yam/
False black pepper *Embelia ribes*	Other names: *Vidanga, Vaividang, Vavding* Vidanga has antibacterial, antiinflammatory, detoxifying, carminative, digestive, laxative, antihelminthic, and contraceptive actions. It is used to treat indigestion, nausea, vomiting, flatulence, and constipation. It can also help in obesity. Side effects include diarrhea and hyperacidity. It should not be taken by women who are trying to conceive. Healthbenefitstimes. (2019, July 26). False black pepper facts, health benefits. *HealthBenefitstimes.com*. https://www.healthbenefitstimes.com/false-black-pepper/
Fennel *Foeniculum vulgare*	Other names: *Perunjeeragam, Saunf* Fennel seeds (and also caraway seeds) belong to the carrot family. However, their tastes are different. Fennel has a sweeter and licorice taste. Fennel seeds and caraway seeds can be substituted in cooking. Fennel seeds and bulbs have culinary and medicinal benefits. Fennel seeds have bioactive aromatic essential oils which include anethole, estragole, and fenshone mainly and some limonene, α-pinene, and camphor which give antioxidant, antiinflammatory, analgesic, antimicrobial, anticancer, and estrogenic effects. Fixed oils include tocopherols (vitamin E), oleic acid, and petroselinic acid. The leaves and seeds also contain flavonoids (quercetin and kaempferol compounds). The seeds also contain minerals (calcium, iron, magnesium, and manganese) more than the leaves. The manganese present is important for enzyme activation, metabolism, cellular protection, bone development, blood sugar regulation, and wound healing. Fennel is used as a mouth freshener. As a carminative, it improves digestive health, indigestion, and chronic constipation. The oils in fennel seeds promote the production of gastric enzymes in the stomach. Oral fennel and fennel-based vaginal creams improve menopausal symptoms. It promotes lactation. It can relieve menstrual pain. It is also an insect repellant. Fennel should not be consumed during pregnancy as high doses may have toxic effects on fetal cells. It may also interact with other medications including estrogen pills and certain cancer medications. Avoid fennel during pregnancy as it can stimulate the uterus. Kubala, J., & Arnarson, A. (2019, September 27). 10 science-based benefits of fennel and fennel seeds. *Healthline*. https://www.healthline.com/nutrition/fennel-and-fennel-seed-benefits

Ingredients

Mechanism of Action and Health Benefits

Fenugreek

Trigonella foenum-graecum

Other names: *Methi, Methika*

The fenugreek husk has higher polyphenols. It contains furostanolic saponins which increase testosterone by blocking aromatase and 5-alpha reductase enzymes. It is rich in fiber, several minerals (sodium, iron, manganese, and magnesium), and B vitamins.

It contains phytoestrogens. It acts as an estrogen receptor modulator, balances the female hormones, and prevents estrogen dominance in the body. It can also reduce follicle-stimulating hormone (FSH) and luteinizing hormone (LH) levels. It can also reduce menstrual cramps and pains (dysmenorrhea). It also eliminates toxins and excessive mucus in the pelvic tissue.

It can improve libido and low testosterone levels in women. It promotes breast milk production.

It can increase testosterone levels, sexual arousal, libido, and sperm count in men.

It is also used to treat digestive problems such as heartburn, gastric ulcers, and colitis. It also contains galactomannan, a water-soluble compound that has been found to reduce cravings. It slows glucose absorption and increases insulin sensitivity. It helps in weight loss.

It boosts metabolism. It can reduce blood glucose and cholesterol levels, as well as lower blood pressure. It prevents platelet aggregation and reduces risk of thrombosis (clot). It is used in diabetes and hypertension.

It may have anticancer properties.

Side effects include rarely allergic reactions and nasal congestion.

Marcene, B. (2020, July 4). 11 amazing health benefits of fenugreek. *Natural Food Series*. https://www.naturalfoodseries.com/11-fenugreek-benefits/

Huizen, J. (2019, January 31). Is fenugreek good for you? *MedicalNewsToday*. https://www.medicalnewstoday.com/articles/324334

Fox nut

Euryale ferox

Other names: *Makhana, Makhaa, Gorgon fruit, Prickly water lily*

Makhana (fox nut) is the seed derived from water lilies, not lotus. It is a superfood rich in minerals (including calcium, iron, magnesium, and phosphorus), vitamins, and fiber.

It is rich in antioxidants (chlorogenic acid, epicatechin, and gallic acid).

It has astringent properties.

It has high protein content with antiaging amino acids (cystine, glutamine, methionine, and arginine).

It can support heart health. It regulates blood sugar, blood pressure, cholesterol, triglycerides, and weight loss.

Overall, it is safe. Excessive consumption can cause bloating, flatulence, and constipation.

Link, R. (2021, May 5). 6 interesting makhana benefits. *Healthline*. https://www.healthline.com/nutrition/makhana-benefits

Mathur, M., Soni, D., & Kanodia, L. (2019, December 11). Makhana. *1mg*. https://www.1mg.com/ayurveda/makhana-144

Galangal

Ginger, turmeric, and galangal are closely related rhizomes and belong to the *Zingiberaceae* family. They belong to the *Zingiber, Curcuma, and Alpinia* genus, respectively. They are aromatic and spicy underground rhizomes and used extensively in Asian cuisine and as herbal remedies.

There are four main varieties and species of galangal/galanga (with other similar names):

- *Alpinia galanga* (Greater galangal, laos, Thai ginger, lengkuas),
- *Alpinia officinarum* (Lesser galangal),
- *Kaempferia galanga* (Kencur, black galangal, Sand ginger, Karchoor, Chandramallika, Sugandh wacha, Aromatic ginger, Resurrection lily),
- *Boesenbergia rotunda* (Chinese ginger or fingerroot).

Galanga has antiinflammatory, antimicrobial, antioxidant, analgesic, carminative, sedative, wound-healing, antiangiogenic, anticancer, insect-repellant, and vasorelaxant actions. The main bioactive constituents include ethyl p-methoxycinnamate, ethyl cinnamate, kaempferide, kaempferol, and more.

It is used to treat fever, cough, colds, headaches, indigestion, intestinal gas, wounds, skin disorders, arthritis, and rheumatism.

Ingredients	Mechanism of Action and Health Benefits
Sharp-leaf Galangal *Alpinia oxyphylla*	*A. oxyphylla* is rich in polyphenol antioxidants. It helps to treat diabetes mellitus, heart disease, and dementia. Other names: Yi Zhi *Ren, Bitter cardamom, Black cardamom* It covers the spleen and kidney meridians. It tonifies the spleen and kidneys. It is warm in nature. It is used in kidney deficiency states which present with enuresis, urinary incontinence, and excessive seminal discharge. It can also treat diarrhea. Kumar A. (2020, May 10). Phytochemistry, pharmacological activities and uses of traditional medicinal plant *Kaempferia galanga* L.—an overview. *Journal of Ethnopharmacology, 253*, 112667. ScienceDirect. https://www.sciencedirect.com/science/article/abs/pii/S0378874119341339
Gambhari *Gmelina arborea*	Other names: *Gambhara, Gumhar, Gmelina, Yamane, White teak, Goomar teak, Malay beechwood, English beechwood, Kashmir Tree* The whole plant, i.e., leaves, fruits, flowers, bark, seeds, and roots of Gambhari are used. They have various bioactive compounds which include flavonoids, iridoids, flavone glycoside, sterols, and lignans that have antioxidant, antiinflammatory, analgesic, wound-healing, antidiabetic, laxative, gastroprotective, digestive, antihelminthic, diuretic, cardiotonic, nervine tonic, and aphrodisiac actions. It can also promote hair growth. It is used to treat GI disorders (such as constipation, hemorrhoids, colitis, stomach ulcers, and intestinal worm infestation), skin disorders, hair loss, vaginal discharge, fevers, diabetes, heart disease, vertigo, and poor memory. Warrier, R. R., Priya, S. M., & Kalaiselvi, R. (2021). *Gmelina arborea*—an indigenous timber species of India with high medicinal value: a review on its pharmacology, pharmacognosy and phytochemistry. *Journal of Ethnopharmacology, 267*, 113593. https://doi.org/10.1016/j.jep.2020.113593 Arora, C., & Tamrakar, V. (December 2017). *Gmelina arborea*: chemical constituents, pharmacological activities and applications. *International Journal of Phytomedicine, 9*(4), 528. DOI:10.5138/09750185.2149
Gambir *Uncaria gambir*	Other names: *Gambier, Cat's claw, Hook vine, Gou Teng, Uncaria* spp. *Refer to "Cat's claw"* under Chinese Natural ingredients. Gambir is a resin from the *Uncaria gambir* plant. It has astringent properties. It is used as a catechu (tannin substance) when chewing betel leaf and areca.
Gandha thailam	Other name: *Gandha thaila* It contains sesame oil as the base oil with sesame seeds (soaked initially in water and then in milk), licorice root decoction and other herbs, oil, and milk. It has analgesic, antiinflammatory, and antiedema effects. It supports bone and joint health. It accelerates fracture healing and also joint and ligament injury healing. It strengthens ligaments, tendons, joints, and bones. It increases bone mass and density in osteoporosis, as well as prevents bone degeneration. It improves joint flexibility. It can prevent recurrent joint dislocation. It can be taken internally (oral use) or used externally (for massage). *Ayurmedinfo*. (2012, April 23). Gandha thailam uses, dosage, side effects, ingredients, reference. https://www.ayurmedinfo.com/2012/04/23/gandha-thailam-uses-dosage-side-effects-ingredients-reference/amp/
Garcinia *Garcinia cambogia*	Other names: *Malabar tamarind, Kudampuli, Vrikshamla* Common species: *G. cambogia* (Vrikshamla)*, G. atroviridis* (asam gelugur/asam keping), and *G. indica* (kokum). Garcinia fruit's rind contains hydroxycitric acid (HCA), which has been found to increase metabolism and also acts as an appetite suppressant. It has antiinflammatory, antianxiety, and antidepressant properties. It is used for weight loss, lower cholesterol, improve rheumatism, and even relieve intestinal problems. Malabar tamarinds can be taken in the form of tea, supplements, or it can be added to food. Side effects of garcinia include nausea, vomiting, diarrhea, and possible hepatotoxicity. Large doses can lead to an increase in brain serotonin, weight loss, and testicular atrophy.

Ingredients	Mechanism of Action and Health Benefits

Raina, R. (2021). Chapter 58—*Garcinia cambogia* [E-book]. In P. Verma, I. Taku, J. Malik, & R. Gupta (Eds.), *Nutraceuticals: Efficacy, safety and toxicity* (2nd ed., pp. 975–990). London: Academic Press. https://doi.org/10.1016/B978-0-12-821038-3.00058-6

WebMD Editors. (2020, November 10). Health benefits of Garcinia cambogia. *WebMD*. https://www.webmd.com/diet/health-benefits-garcinia-cambogia#1-2

Garlic
Allium sativum

Garlic contains more than 30 bioactive organo-sulfur compounds (OSCs). Allicin is degraded into DAS, DADS, and DAT i.e., diallyl sulfide, diallyl disulfide, and diallyl trisulfide, respectively, and also methyl allyl trisulfide vinyldithiins and ajoenes.

Other OSCs include S-allyl cysteine, S-allyl cysteine sulfoxide, and S-allyl mercaptocysteine.

The OSCs can fight viruses, bacteria, fungi, and parasites. They are like powerful antibiotics and are effective against the Campylobacter bacteria and others.

It is rich in antioxidants, flavonoids, enzymes, vitamins (B1, B2, B6, A, and C), and minerals (calcium, zinc, selenium, potassium, copper, manganese, and phosphorus).

Garlic contains alliin, which activates to allicin once the garlic has been pounded or crushed. Allicin is a chemical that has been found to reduce inflammation and has antioxidant properties. Aged black garlic has higher antioxidant activity compared to fresh and commercial garlic. One clove of garlic weighs approximately 3 g and has about 25 to 50 mg of allicin.

Preventive use of garlic can decrease the frequency of colds. It is cardioprotective after a heart attack or in diabetic cardiomyopathy. It also reduces high cholesterol levels, high blood pressure, and has antiplatelet aggregation activity. It is widely used in the treatment of atherosclerosis, coronary heart disease, and hypertension.

It can improve egg and sperm quality.

It has anticancer properties that may also reduce prostate, breast, intestinal, and lung cancer risks and also malignant brain tumors like glioblastoma.

Allicin can suppress hunger pangs as well as boost metabolism and hence aid in weight loss.

Allergic reactions to garlic can cause a burning sensation in the mouth or stomach, heartburn, gas, nausea, vomiting, body odor, and diarrhea. Garlic when applied to skin may cause skin irritation.

Newman, T., & Butler, N. (2017, August 18). What are the benefits of garlic? *MedicalNewsToday*. https://www.medicalnewstoday.com/articles/265853

Ghee

Other name: *Clarified butter*

Ghee is made from cow's milk or buffalo's milk. It is a good source of vitamins A, C, D, and K. This helps improve skin health and hair growth. It is also rich in vitamin E which has antioxidant properties. It has antiinflammatory and immunomodulatory properties. It is often added to ayurvedic herbs and cooked together. Ghee is also used in medicated oils as part of nasya (intranasal medications) in panchakarma therapy.

It can lower the risk of cancer, arthritis, heart diseases, and cataracts. It is also rich in omega-3, which helps lower LDL cholesterol levels.

It is a nourishing food which nourishes the uterus and growing fetus.

In the GI tract, ghee reduces the pH. In the small intestine, ghee improves the absorption ability.

It can help in improving bone strength. It also helps weight loss.

The risks of consuming too much ghee includes possibility of heart disease and weight gain.

Brennan, D. (2020, September 30). Ghee: Is it good for you? *WebMD*. https://www.webmd.com/diet/ghee-good-for-you#1

Railton, D., & Olsen, N. (2018, December 5). Is ghee more healthful than butter? *MedicalNewsToday*. https://www.medicalnewstoday.com/articles/321707

Giloy
Tinospora cordifolia

Other names. *Guduchi, Amrita*

Giloy or guduchi contains many bioactive constituents like tinosporin, tinosporaside, cordifolide, phenylpropene disaccharides cordifolioside A, B, and C, palmitine, choline, isocolumbin, tembetarine, berberine, terpenes, magnoflorine, and giloin. It is also rich in calcium and phosphorus.

It is a powerful antioxidant and is regarded as the ayurvedic root of immortality. It has antidiabetic, antimicrobial, antifungal, anticancer, antipyretic, antiinflammatory, antiallergy, antispasmodic, immunomodulatory, and antiaging properties. Giloy increases FSH and LH levels.

It also has antilithogenic and anticrystallization effects and prevents formation of calcium oxalate kidney stones.

Ingredients	Mechanism of Action and Health Benefits

In dengue fever, it can reduce the fever, improve the platelet count, and strengthen the immune system. It also removes toxins, purifies blood, and reduces blood sugar.

Its roots have strong emetic properties and are also used for bowel obstruction. It also treats various digestive ailments including hyperacidity, colitis, worm infestations, loss of appetite, abdominal pain, constipation, and vomiting.

It fights coughs and colds. It improves clarity of vision. It can reduce dark spots and wrinkles on the face. As an adaptogen, it can decrease stress and anxiety. It is also useful in diabetes.

It can promote collagen synthesis and osteoblast activity and is used to treat bone fractures and gout.

Overconsumption of giloy can cause constipation. There is risk of hypoglycemia if taken with diabetic medications. It should not be taken by pregnant or breastfeeding women.

Sharma, P., Dwivedee, B. P., Bisht, D., Dash, A. K., & Kumar, D. (2019). The chemical constituents and diverse pharmacological importance of *Tinospora cordifolia*. *Heliyon*, *5*(9), e02437. https://doi.org/10.1016/j.heliyon.2019.e02437

Ginger
Zingiber officinale

Other names: *Shunthi, Sunthi, Adarak*

Ginger has many bioactive compounds, mainly phenolic (gingerols, shogaols, paradols) and terpene compounds. The medicinal benefits are largely due to the phenolic compounds. It is also rich in chromium, zinc, magnesium, and potassium.

It has antiinflammatory, antimicrobial, antioxidant, cardiovascular protective, respiratory protective, antiemetic, carminative, digestive stimulant, antiobesity, blood-thinning, and immune-boosting properties. Ginger can aid circulation of energy in the body.

It can constrict the blood vessels by thinning the blood, hence reducing menstrual blood flow. It also increases the cell and antibody-mediated immune response.

It is used in several conditions such as digestive problems (nausea, wind, heartburn, flatulence, bloating, indigestion, colic, cramps), cold and flu, travel sickness, menstrual pain and heavy periods, morning sickness, arthritis, migraines, poor circulation, hypercholesterolemia, hypertension, and pain relief. Mild side effects including heartburn, diarrhea, burping, and stomach discomfort. It may cause skin irritation. In moderate amounts, it is safe in pregnant and lactating women. High doses of ginger might worsen some heart conditions and slow blood clotting.

Dried ginger (*sonth/saunth/sukku*) has less gingerol and more shogaols but it still has significant medicinal benefits.

Cassoobhoy, A. (2020, September 11). Health benefits of ginger. *WebMD*. https://www.webmd.com/diet/health-benefits-ginger#1

Fletcher, J. (2020, January 3). Why is ginger good for you? *MedicalNewsToday*. https://www.medicalnewstoday.com/articles/265990

Gokshura
Tribulus terrestris

Other names: *Bindii, Kharkhasak, Gokhru, Devil's weed, Puncturevine*

The main biologically active ingredients in gokshura are saponins, flavonoids, glycosides, alkaloids, and tannins. The two saponin components (protodioscin and protogracillin) have aphrodisiac activity.

The large quantities of nitrates and essential oil in the fruits and seeds give its diuretic properties. The diuretic action is useful as an antihypertensive agent.

It has antioxidant, antiinflammatory, detoxifying, antidiabetic, and analgesic properties.

It can alleviate pain in rheumatoid arthritis and osteoarthritis. It may also have antiaging properties.

It can treat urinary disorders. It can reduce phosphate levels and lower the risk of kidney stones formation by decreasing urine phosphate levels.

It can also treat gallstones and PCOS.

It is also used in the treatment of heart ailments and reduces the risk of heart attacks, strokes, and blood clots. It may also lower blood sugar in diabetes, reduce cholesterol and triglycerides, as well as blood pressure. It can also help reduce menopausal symptoms.

It helps reduce acne, pimples, treats wounds, hives, itchiness, and skin infections.

It may also reduce the risk of AD and improve memory, reasoning, problem-solving, and other cognitive abilities.

Overconsumption of gokshura can cause diarrhea, nausea, vomiting, stomach pain, cramping, constipation, difficulty in sleeping, or heavy menstrual bleeding. It should not be used by pregnant and breastfeeding women as it can cause abnormalities or birth defects in the growing fetus. It can be excreted through breast milk to the newborn and cause severe health problems.

Ingredients	Mechanism of Action and Health Benefits
	Bharat, D. (2019, December 4). Gokshura churna: Benefits, uses, method, dosage and side effects. *Netmeds*. https://www.netmeds.com/health-library/post/gokshura-churna-benefits-uses-method-dosage-and-side-effects
	Chhatre, S., Nesari, T., Kanchan, D., Somani, G., & Sathaye, S. (2014). Phytopharmacological overview of *Tribulus terrestris*. *Pharmacognosy Reviews*, 8(15), 45–51. https://doi.org/10.4103/0973-7847.125530
Gorakhmundi *Sphaeranthus indicus*	Other names: *Mundi, Mahamundi, Shravani, East Indian Globe Thistle*
	All parts of the Mundi plant can be used. It contains flavonoids, terpenes, and eudesmenolides.
	It has antiinflammatory, antiviral, antioxidant, antidiabetic, antilipidemic, antiepileptic, anxiolytic, sedative, antitussive, and digestive actions.
	It is used to treat diabetes, cough, fevers, epilepsy, indigestion, and skin disorders.
	Little data is available on toxicity.
	Galani, V., Patel, B., & Rana, D. (2010). *Sphaeranthus indicus* Linn.: a phytopharmacological review. *International Journal of Ayurveda Research, 1*(4), 247. https://doi.org/10.4103/0974-7788.76790
Gotu kola *Centella asiatica*	Other names: *Mandukaparni, pennywort, Indian pennywort, Asian pennywort* or *marsh pennywort, Hydrocotyle asiatica*
	Gotu kola contains several triterpenoid saponins which include asiaticosides, madecassoside, and madasiatic acid (for wound healing), brahmoside and brahminoside (for brain tonic effects), and centelloside (which has diuretic action in venous hypertension) It is also rich in minerals (calcium, iron, potassium) and vitamins (A, C, and B12).
	It has potent antioxidant and antiaging effects. It is neuroprotective and can improve cognitive function, enhance short-term memory, mood, decrease stress, anxiety, and depression. It also helps with insomnia. It is a mild adaptogen.
	It also stimulates collagen formation and forms new blood vessels to promote wound healing and reduce scar formation. It also improves blood circulation, reduces fluid retention, and helps with varicose veins.
	It also has some antiinflammatory action and may relieve joint pain.
	Side effects include headache, upset stomach, and dizziness. Topical application may cause skin irritation.
	Gohil, K., Patel, J., & Gajjar, A. (2010). Pharmacological review on *Centella asiatica*: A potential herbal cure-all. *Indian Journal of Pharmaceutical Sciences, 72*(5), 546. https://doi.org/10.4103/0250-474x.78519
	Chandrika, U. G., & Prasad Kumara, P. A. (2015). Gotu Kola (*Centella asiatica*). *Advances in Food and Nutrition Research, 76*, 125–157. https://doi.org/10.1016/bs.afnr.2015.08.001
	Cronkleton, E., & Wilson, D. R. (2018, September 18). Everything you need to know about Gotu Kola. *Healthline*. https://www.healthline.com/health/gotu-kola-benefits
	Wong, C., & Dashiell, E. (2020, September 17). Benefits of the herb Gotu Kola. *Verywell Health*. https://www.verywellhealth.com/the-benefits-of-gotu-kola-89566
Guava *Psidium guajava*	Other names: *Amrood, Fan Shi Liu*
	Guava is a nutritious fruit with yellow or light green skin. The flesh can be white, yellow, or pink and has edible seeds. It contains flavonoids (quercetin, avicularin, myricetin, and kaempferol) and phenolic acid (gallic acid, catechin). It is rich in antioxidants and has immune-boosting and anticancer properties. The leaf extract has antimicrobial and dental antiplaque properties.
	The fruit is rich in vitamins (A and C), mineral (potassium), and fiber.
	It supports digestive health. Eating guava fruit regularly can prevent constipation and improve bowel movements. It can also help in weight loss. The leaf extract is used to treat diarrhea.
	It supports heart health and can lower blood sugar, blood pressure, and cholesterol.
	It can help in UTI.
	It can also help with menorrhagia and menstrual cramps.
	It maintains healthy skin, gums, and teeth.
	Brown, M. J. (2018, December 13). 8 health benefits of guava fruit and leaves. *Healthline*. https://www.healthline.com/nutrition/8-benefits-of-guavas
	Kumar, M., Tomar, M., Amarowicz, R., Saurabh, V., Nair, M. S., Maheshwari, C., et al. (2021). Guava (*Psidium guajava* L.) leaves: Nutritional composition, phytochemical profile, and health-promoting bioactivities. *Foods, 10*(4), 752. https://doi.org/10.3390/foods10040752

Ingredients	Mechanism of Action and Health Benefits
Gugglu *Commiphora wightii*	Other names: *Guggul, Gugul, Gugal, Indian bdellium-tree, Mukul myrrh tree, Commiphora mukul, Balsamodendron mukul* Gugglu (or gum gugglu) is the sap or resin produced by the Indian bdellium tree. The main species include *Commiphora wightii* and *Commiphora mukul*. Its fragrance is similar to myrrh, and it is used in the Indian incense (*dhoop*) for religious purposes. It contains various plant compounds such as steroids, essential oils, lignans, flavonoids, and amino acids. Guggul may act like estrogen in the body. The plant steroids help in lowering cholesterol levels. Antiobesity activity may be promoted by the presence of guggulsterone, a plant steroid found in gugglu. It promotes weight loss and reduces both skinfold thickness and body circumference. Guggulsterone may also be able to suppress enzymes that promote tumor growth such as esophageal, pancreatic, or prostate cancers. It is commonly used for treating antiinflammatory conditions (acne, gingivitis, arthritis, eczema, and psoriasis) and sinusitis. It is also helpful in detoxifying unhealthy tissues, reducing risk of liver disorders, and treating urinary complaints. Side effects include rash, itching, nausea, vomiting, belching, diarrhea, and headache. It should not be used in estrogen-sensitive tumors. Berkheiser, K., & Marengo, K. (2020, August 12). Guggul: Benefits, dosage, side effects, and more. *Healthline*. https://www.healthline.com/nutrition/guggul Wong, C., & Kroner, A. (2020, July 11). Guggul extract and its possible health benefits. *Verywell Health*. https://www.verywellhealth.com/the-benefits-of-guggul-89567
Gum arabic *Vachellia nilotica* *Acacia nilotica*	Other names: *Acacia gum, Gum acacia, Acacia powder, Acacia arabica, Babul, Babool, Thorn mimosa* Gum arabic or babool is a dietary soluble fiber derived from the natural hardened sap of the wild *Acacia* tree. There are many Acacia species. Gum arabic is a mixture of glycoprotein, polysaccharides, and oligosaccharides. Arabinose and ribose are the natural sugars present in gum arabic. It is often added as a thickener in various foods and beverages. It is rich in phenols (condensed tannin and phlobatannin, gallic acid, protocatechuic acid, and pyrocatechol), alkaloids, volatile essential oils, steroids, and terpenes. The tannins present in its bark, leaves, and pods have astringent properties. It supports gut health. It acts as a prebiotic and probiotic. It increases fullness, reduces hunger pangs, and helps in weight loss. It is used in the treatment of IBS, diarrhea, and intestinal pain. It maintains healthy gums and teeth (oral health) and decreases the dental plaque. It can lower cholesterol and insulin resistance in diabetes. It can treat coughs, colds, sore throat, lung congestion, and also eye inflammation. Babool can help with urinary tract disorders which are usually due to vata-pitta imbalance. It also has diuretic actions. It also reduces muscle spasm and helps in the treatment of stiff joints in fracture, dislocation and arthritis. Side effects include digestive upset, gas and bloating, and mild diarrhea. It may be used for treating cancers and/or tumors (of ear, eye, or testicles). Long-term consumption of gum arabic may cause minor adverse effects, including gas and bloating, nausea, and loose stools. Sawant, R. S., Godghate, A. G., Sankpal, S. A., Walaki, S. A., & Kankanwadi, S. S. (2014). Phytochemical analysis of bark of *Acacia nilotica*. *Pelagia Research Library*, 4(2), 22–24. https://www.researchgate.net/publication/279965233_Phytochemical_analysis_of_bark_of_Acacia_nilotica WebMD Editors. (2020). GUM ARABIC: Overview, uses, side effects, precautions, interactions, dosing and reviews. *WebMD*. https://www.webmd.com/vitamins/ai/ingredientmono-268/acacia
Gurmar *Gymnema sylvestre*	Other names: *Meshashringi, Gymnema, Gudmar* The leaves of gurmar contain triterpenoid saponins which decrease sugar cravings by blocking the taste of sweetness on the tongue. Also, gymnemic acid IV in gurmar has blood-sugar-lowering properties in diabetes. It can stimulate endogenous insulin production from pancreas. It can lower LDL cholesterol and triglycerides. It also has antiinflammatory effects. It can help in weight loss, constipation, and cough. Overall, it is safe. Possible side effects include nausea, headache, dizziness, and lightheadedness. Goodson, A. (2018, June 18). 6 impressive health benefits of Gymnema sylvestre. *Healthline*. https://www.healthline.com/nutrition/gymnema-sylvestre-benefits

Ingredients	Mechanism of Action and Health Benefits
Hairy Rupturewort *Herniaria hirsuta*	Hairy rupturewort is a flowering plant. Its active compounds include flavonoids, saponins, quercetin, and triterpenes. It can increase the magnesium content and hence inhibit calcium stone formation in the kidneys. It can also treat UTIs, joint and muscle pain in arthritis, and gout. WebMD. (n.d.). Rupturewort. *WebMD*. Retrieved November 2021, from https://www.webmd.com/vitamins/ai/ingredientmono-87/rupturewort#.
Haritaki *Terminalia chebula*	Haritaki is rich in antioxidants (vitamins C and E, glutathione, and superoxide dismutase). It also contains minerals such as magnesium, potassium, iron, and copper that are beneficial to the skin. It has antioxidant, antibiotic, antiviral, antifungal, and antiinflammatory effects. It also has immunomodulatory properties. It is used in treating knee arthritis, reducing total cholesterol, and lowering blood sugar levels. It is helpful for treating scalp infections like dandruff, itching, and hair fall. It also helps in hair growth. It is also used to treat UTI. It helps in treatment of various eye infections and vision disorders like dry eyes, watery eyes, and inflamed eyes. It is used as one of the ingredients in Triphala. Overconsumption can cause diarrhea, stomatitis, dehydration, acute fever, malnutrition, stiffness of jaw, and fatigue. When taking diabetic medications, haritaki should not be taken as it can cause hypoglycemia. It should also be avoided by pregnant and breastfeeding women. Basu, S. (2020, September 21). Haritaki: Benefits, uses, dosage, formulations, and side effects. *Netmeds*. https://www.netmeds.com/health-library/post/haritaki-benefits-uses-dosage-formulations-and-side-effects
Hemp seed **Hemp seed oil** *Cannabis sativa*	Hemp seed oil is cold-pressed from hemp seeds of the *Cannabis sativa* plant (same plant as cannabidiol [CBD] oil but different variety). It differs from CBD oil. Hemp seed oil generally does not contain the psychoactive component tetrahydrocannabinol (THC). Hemp seeds are also rich in proteins, amino acids (arginine), minerals (potassium, phosphorus, magnesium, sodium, iron, and calcium), vitamin E, and soluble and insoluble fibers. Hemp seeds are very nutritious. They contain gamma-linolenic acid (GLA), (omega-6) and alpha-linolenic acid (omega-3) fatty acids. It has antioxidant and antiinflammatory properties. Hemp seed oil can be taken orally or applied on the skin. It has soothing, moisturizing, and antiaging properties. It is part of dietary supplements, used in cooking, and is a base in moisturizers, lotions, soaps, and foods. It is used to treat eczema, acne, psoriasis, and lichen planus. It can stimulate hair growth. It is also used to treat premenopausal symptoms and menopause. It may support heart health, and lower blood pressure and cholesterol. It can also help in diabetic neuropathy. It can support digestive health. Side effects are digestive upset including loose oily stools. It can interact with blood thinners. Bjarnadottir, A. (2018, September 11). 6 evidence-based health benefits of hemp seeds. *Healthline*. https://www.healthline.com/nutrition/6-health-benefits-of-hemp-seeds Gotter, A. (2019, July 3). Hemp oil for skin. *Healthline*. https://www.healthline.com/health/hemp-oil-for-skin
Henna *Lawsonia inermis*	Henna contains lawsone, tannins, ellagic acid, quercetin, and gallic acid. It is also rich in vitamin E. It has antiinfective properties. It is largely used as a hair care product. It also has purgative, astringent, and abortifacient properties. It improves hair growth, regulates sebum production, prevents dandruff, and premature hair graying. When the plant juice is applied on the head, it can provide fast relief from headaches. Mehrotra, S. (2021, March 23). Henna benefits for hair: How to get rich auburn locks. *Healthline*. https://www.healthline.com/health/beauty-skin-care/henna-benefits-for-hair RxList. (2021, June 11). Henna: Health benefits, side effects, uses, dose & precautions. https://www.rxlist.com/henna/supplements.htm Sonya Henna Admin. (2017, March 20). Health benefits of henna. *Sonya Henna*. https://sonyahenna.com/health-benefits-henna/

Ingredients	Mechanism of Action and Health Benefits

Horseradish
Armoracia rusticana

Horseradish is a white spicy root vegetable in the mustard family with a pungent taste and odor. The main active ingredients are the glucosinolates, which break down into isothiocyanates that protect against infections, cancer, and brain disease. It is also rich in minerals (including zinc, magnesium, calcium, potassium) and vitamins (folate and vitamin C).

It has antiseptic, antibiotic, antiinflammatory, and antioxidant properties. It also has a diuretic effect.

It is used to relieve breathing issues and colds. It is also effective against bronchitis and acute sinus infections.

Too much horseradish can irritate the nose, mouth, and stomach. It can cause pain to those with digestive issues, stomach ulcers, and IBS.

Pathak, N. (2020, September 17). Health benefits of horseradish. *WebMD*. https://www.webmd.com/diet/health-benefits-horseradish#1

Streit, L. (2019, July 25). What is horseradish? Everything you need to know. *Healthline*. https://www.healthline.com/nutrition/horseradish#what-it-is

Indian abutilon
Abutilon indicum

Other names: *Indian mallow, Kanghai, Paatri, Atibala, Indian Lantern plant, Chinese Bellflower, Moon flower*

Atibala in Sanskrit means very powerful.

Indian abutilon contains β-sitosterol which has antimicrobial activities. All parts of the plant including flowers, leaves, seeds, root, and bark can be used.

It also has diuretic, laxative aphrodisiac, antidiabetic, demulcent, and antiinflammatory properties.

The flowers can increase sperm count in males. In women, it ensures regular menstruation and a healthy and safe pregnancy.

It can also treat bladder infections and gonorrhea.

It can lower blood glucose and the leaves are used to treat piles.

Health Benefits Times. (2018, July 22). Indian mallow facts and health benefits. *HealthBenefitstimes.com.* https://www.healthbenefitstimes.com/indian-mallow/

Indian coleus
Coleus Forskohlii

Other name: *Plectranthus barbatus, Forskolin, Forskohlii, Colforsin, Colforsine,*

Coleus forskolii is part of the mint family. The bioactive constituents in Indian coleus include essential oil, forskolin, abietane diterpenoids and 8,13-epoxy-labd-14-en-11-one diterpenoids.

Forskolin present can be used as a therapeutic agent for weight management (obesity). It activates adenylate cyclase and lipase enzymes, hence increasing cyclic AMP (adenosine monophosphate) and breaking down fats.

It has antimicrobial, and antispasmodic activity. It can be used as an expectorant, emmenagogue and diuretic. It may also have anticancer properties.

It can cause vasodilatation of blood vessels and contraction of the heart muscles. It can improve heart function. It is used to treat chest pain (angina), heart failure in dilated cardiomyopathy, and hypertension.

It is also improves sleep (insomnia) and is also used for convulsions, epilepsy,

It can help in respiratory disorders including asthma and bronchitis.

It is used to treat intestinal disorders (such as dysentery and constipation), spasmodic pain and abdominal colic.

It can also be used for eczema, dry eyes, preventing gray hair and in painful urination

Overall, it is safe. It should not be used in conjunction with beta-blockers, vasodilators, and/or calcium channel blockers as it can lead to hypotension.

Other side effects include fast heart rate (tachycardia), bleeding and diarrhea with high doses.

Cunha, J. P. (2017, April 14). *Forskolin (Coleus Forskohlii)*. RxList. https://www.rxlist.com/consumer_forskolin_coleus_forskohlii/drugs-condition.htm

Yashaswini, S., & Vasundhara, M. (2011). Coleus (Plectranthus barbatus) - A multipurpose medicinal herb. *International Research Journal of Pharmacy, 02*(03), 47–58. https://www.researchgate.net/publication/302513813_Coleus_Plectranthus_barbatus_-_A_multipurpose_medicinal_herb

Indian frankincense
Boswellia serrata

Other names: *Frankincense, Boswellia, Salai guggul, Sallaki, Salai, Shallaki, Kundru, Lobana, Ru Xiang, Olibanum gummi, Olibanum indicum, Indian olibanum*

There are many species of frankincense trees (also called Boswellia trees) of the genus Boswellia (family Burseraceae).

Indian frankincense or Boswellia is from *Boswellia serrata* (also called *Indian olibanum*) and Arabian frankincense is from *Boswellia sacra* and *Boswellia carterii.*

Frankincense resin is derived by tapping the frankincense (Boswellia) trees. Each tree produces a slightly different type of resin.

Ingredients	**Mechanism of Action and Health Benefits**
	Frankincense oil is prepared from hardened gum resins. The oils are also used as incense in religious rituals and in perfumes.
	The main component of frankincense oil is boswellic acid (a triterpene) which has antiinflammatory, antiinfective, and anticancer properties. The boswellic acids are the bioactive components of which acetyl-11-keto-β-boswellic acid is the most important. It blocks the 5-lipoxygenase enzyme hence reducing the inflammatory leukotrienes.
	B. carterii contains mainly α-pinene with lower amounts of limonene, myrcene, and alpha-thujene, as well as good levels of the diterpenes incensole.
	B. sacra is largely α-pinene, and has high levels of diterpenes incensole.
	Incensole acetate activates the TRPV-3 receptors in the body to create a warm feeling on the skin. It also interacts with different brain channels to produce calming and spiritual exaltation feelings.
	Frankincense (Boswellia) helps in many chronic inflammatory disorders such as rheumatoid arthritis, osteoarthritis (reduces pain and stiffness), asthma (reduces wheezing), and inflammatory bowel disease (IBD) including ulcerative disease and Crohn's disease.
	It also can reduce menstrual cramps due to its pain-relieving and antiinflammatory properties.
	It improves oral health and hygiene as well as prevents gum disease.
	It can prevent metastasis in breast, brain, and pancreatic cancers.
	Side effects include gastric upset and menorrhagia or increased menstrual flow.
	Johnson, J. (2019, October 9). What to know about boswellia. *MedicalNewsToday*. https://www.medicalnewstoday.com/articles/326599
	Petre, A. (2021, March 9). 5 benefits and uses of frankincense—and 7 myths. *Healthline*. https://www.healthline.com/nutrition/frankincense
Indian sarsaparilla *(Hemidesmus indicus)*	Other names: *Anantmool, Sariva*
	Indian sarsaparilla contains more than 40 phytoconstituents including flavonoids, terpenoids, and phenols. It mainly reduces the excess pitta in the gut and the reproductive system.
	It has antiinfective, antiinflammatory, antidiabetic, and hepatoprotective properties. It has demulcent, blood purifying, detoxifying, and cooling properties. It can be used as a general health tonic.
	It is used to treat menorrhagia.
	It can stimulate hair growth. It can also improve skin health and is used in acne and wound healing.
	Chauhan, M. (2020, March 14). Anantmool, Indian Sarsaparilla (Hemidesmus indicus). *Planet Ayurveda*. https://www.planetayurveda.com/library/anantmool-hemidesmus-indicus/
	Health Benefits Times. (2019, June 24). Health benefits of Hemidesmus indicus. *HealthBenefitstimes.com*. https://www.healthbenefitstimes.com/hemidesmus-indicus/
Indian snakeroot *Rauwolfia serpentina*	Other names: *Sarpagandha, Chandra, Chandrika, Serpina, Snakewood, SnakeRoot, She Gen Mu*
	Sarpagandha contains several bioactive compounds including alcohols, sugars and glycosides, fatty acids, flavonoids, phytosterols, oleoresins, steroids, tannins, and alkaloids (indole alkaloids and reserpine). The reserpine present helps in treatment of mild to moderate hypertension, schizophrenia, and some symptoms of poor circulation.
	It depletes the granules of dopamine, serotonin, and norepinephrine in the neuron and improves sleep. It is also used for insomnia, nervousness, and mental disorders such as agitated psychosis and insanity.
	It can also be used for snake and reptile bites, fever, constipation, feverish intestinal diseases, liver ailments, achy joints (rheumatism), fluid retention (edema), epilepsy, and as a tonic for general debilities.
	Long-term use can cause depression, nasal congestion, changes in appetite and weight, nightmares, drowsiness, and loose stools.
	Lobay, D. (2015). Rauwolfia in the treatment of hypertension. *Integrative Medicine: A Clinician's Journal*, *14*(3), 40–46. https://www.ncbi.nlm.nih.gov/pmc/articles/PMC4566472/
	RxList Editors. (2021, June 11). Indian Snakeroot: Health benefits, side effects, uses, dose & precautions. *RxList*. https://www.rxlist.com/indian_snakeroot/supplements.htm

Ingredients	Mechanism of Action and Health Benefits
Indian sorrel *Oxalis corniculata*	Indian sorrel contains various active constituents including phytosterol, flavonoids, phenols, tannins, isovitexin, and vitexin. The flavonoids present may give it its anticancer properties. It also contains vitamins (A, B9, B1, B3, and C), minerals (calcium, iron, phosphorus, magnesium, and calcium), essential fatty acids (linoleic acid, linolenic acid, oleic acid, palmitic acid, and stearic acid), and citric acid.

Indian sorrel (used more in digestive disorders) is different from sheep sorrel (Rumex acetosa, used more in respiratory disorders) or Jamaican sorrel (Hibiscus sabdariffa or roselle, used more as a beverage).

Indian sorrel also has antiinflammatory, antifungal, antiinflammatory, antimicrobial, and pain-relieving features. It can lower cortisol levels in stress states and improve sleep.

It is effective in digestive disorders including gas and bloating, indigestion, anorexia, diarrhea, dysentery, and bleeding piles.

It is also used for treating flu, fever, UTIs, sprains, and backache.

With prolonged use, it can inhibit calcium absorption in the body. Due to the high oxalate content, it should be avoided in rheumatism, gout, and kidney stones.

Basu, S. (2020, August 26). Sorrel leaves: Benefits, uses, formulation, ingredients, dosage and side effects. *Netmeds*. https://www.netmeds.com/health-library/post/sorrel-leaves-benefits-uses-formulation-ingredients-dosage-and-side-effects

Planet Ayurveda. (2019, April 5). What are the health benefits of Indian Sorrel (Oxalis corniculata)? https://www.planetayurveda.com/health-benefits-of-indian-sorrel-oxalis-corniculata/

Insulin plant
Costus igneus

Other names: *Spiral banner, Blazing Costus, Step stepping stool*

Various parts of the *Costus igneus* plant (leaves, roots, and stem) contain different bioactive compounds triterpenoids, phenols (catechin), flavonoids, and steroids which can stimulate release of insulin from the pancreas and also improve insulin resistance.

The leaves are chewed to prevent or treat diabetes.

Laha, S., & Paul, S. (2019). *Costus igneus*—a therapeutic anti-diabetic herb with active phytoconstituents. *International Journal of Pharmaceutical Sciences and Research, 10*(8), 3583-3591. https://doi.org/10.13040/ijpsr.0975-8232.10(8).3583-91

Ivy gourd
(Coccinia grandis)

Other names: *Calabacita, Kovai, Kovakkai, Tindora, Coccinia indica*

Ivy gourd is a fruit vegetable used in Indian cuisine. The leaves are also edible. It contains flavonoids, saponins, alkaloids, glycosides, and steroids. It is rich in fiber.

It has glucose-lowering, antihistamine, and anticancer properties.

It is used in diabetes.

It helps in constipation. It can also help with wound healing, eczema, and psoriasis.

The leaves can be stir-fried or added to soups.

Rxlist. (2021, June 11). Ivy gourd: health benefits, side effects, uses, dose & precautions. https://www.rxlist.com/ivy_gourd/supplements.htm

Jaggery

Other names: *Palm sugar, Palm candy crystals, Panam Kalkandu*

Jaggery is derived from sugarcane, date palm, or palmyra. Palm sugar contains minerals (calcium, iron, zinc, and potassium), amino acids, and B-vitamins (B1, B2, B3, B6, and B12). It also has a low GI. It is rich in dietary fibers that help to treat constipation and indigestion. The amino acids help in cell growth and repair.

It has antioxidant and detoxifying properties. This helps remove toxins from the respiratory tract, intestines, food pipe, lungs, and stomach. It also helps lower cholesterol levels.

It is commonly used to treat sore throat, cough, and cold. It can also help reduce body heat.

It also increases metabolism. As a replacement for sugar, it can be used for infants and toddlers.

Consumption of a large amount of panam kalkandu for a long period of time can cause weight gain and diabetes.

Siyanna. (2020, September 1). Panam kalkandam or Lump sugar Natural Cure for Cough and Cold. *NatureLoc.com*. https://healthyliving.natureloc.com/panam-kalkandam-lump-sugar-cure-cough-cold/

Ingredients	Mechanism of Action and Health Benefits

Jalkumbhi
Pontederia crassipes

Other names: *Pistia stratiotes, water hyacinth. water lettuce, water cabbage, shell flower, Jal kumbhi* (they are aquatic weeds)

Pontederia crassipes, also referred to as *Eichhornia crassipes,* is Water hyacinth (or Jal kumbhi).

Pistia stratiotes, is also called *water cabbage, water lettuce, Nile cabbage, or shellflower* (sometimes also called *Jal kumbhi*).

Jal kumbhi is a floating aquatic plant and an invasive weed found in stagnant water in tropical countries. Although whole plants can be used, mostly the leaves are used. It has medicinal properties and is a common Ayurvedic component.

The phytocontinueuts include flavonoids, alkaloids, steroids, and glycosides.

It has antidiabetic, diuretic, laxative, antimicrobial, and antifungal actions. It is cooling in nature.

It is used to treat various skin conditions (including eczema, ringworm, and skin ulcers).

It can also help in inflammation of the mouth and throat.

Gupta, R., Tripathi, P., Kumar, R., Sharma, A., & Mishra, A. (2010). *Pistia stratiotes* (Jalkumbhi). *Pharmacognosy Reviews, 4*(8), 153. https://doi.org/10.4103/0973-7847.70909

Jasmine
Jasminum sp

Other names: *Mallika, Malligai, Yutika, Yuthika, Juhi*

Jasminum officinale and *Jasminum sambac* are the common varieties for jasmine tea. *Jasminum auriculatum and Jasminum grandiflorum* are used mostly in Ayurvedic medicine.

Jasmine is rich in polyphenol antioxidants. The leaves contain jasminol, lupeol, tricanthanol, and mannitol. The flower buds contain benzyl acetate, indole, and methyl anthranilate. The essential oil from the flower is used in the perfume industry.

Jasmine tea is basically green tea leaves (or sometimes black or white tea leaves) that have been brewed, scented, or flavored with jasmine flowers. Hence, it contains caffeine.

Jasmine can regulate glucose control, help in weight loss, and can be cardioprotective.

The flowers and the roots have antilithogenic properties.

It is used to treat burning urine in UTI and kidney stones.

It also helps in wound healing, disorders of the oral cavity, and headache.

Usually drinking about 3 to 5 cups per day is safe. Caffeine and oxalates are present in green tea.

No side effects are reported.

Raman, R. (2019, April 3). 9 reasons why jasmine tea is good for you. *Healthline.* https://www.healthline.com/nutrition/jasmine-tea-benefits

Jatamansi
Nardostachys jatamansi

Other name: *Spikenard*

Jatamansi is a rare and endangered small rhizome flowering plant that grows in the high Himalayan alpines. It belongs to the valerian family. It contains phenolic compounds (protocatechuic acid, gallic acid, catechin, homovanillic acid, and syringic acid), antioxidants, terpenoids (spirojatamol, nardostachysin, jatamols A and B, and calarenol). It is a natural brain tranquilizer. It inhibits acetylcholine activity and also modulates serotonin levels. It calms the hyperactive mind and induces sleep. It is also a brain tonic and rejuvenates the brain. It is a memory enhancer.

It is used in the treatment of anxiety, stress, insomnia, epilepsy, forgetfulness, and weak memory.

It is also used for wound healing, to prevent hair loss, and remove excessive dryness and makes the skin soft and glowing.

It has emmenagogue properties. It promotes menstrual flow and reduces pain. It is useful in menopause and helps to improve mood and sleep.

Consuming large content can cause loose stool, nausea, and vomiting. It can also cause frequent urination and abdominal cramps.

Drugs.com. (2021, February 3). Jatamansi. https://www.drugs.com/npp/jatamansi.html

Hoon, M., Soni, D., & Gupta, V. (2019, August 20). Jatamansi: Benefits, precautions and dosage. *1mg.* https://www.1mg.com/ayurveda/jatamansi-175

Java Plum
Eugenia Jambolana
Syzygium cumini

Other names: *Indian black berry, jamun, jambul, mahapala, naaval pazham*

Java plum has two varieties: white (more pectin) and dark purple or black (less pectin and less calories). It is rich in anthocyanins, glucoside, ellagic acid, isoquercetin, myricetin, and kaempferol. The seeds contain an alkaloid (jambosine) and glycoside (jambolin or antimellin) which stops the diastatic conversion of starch into sugar. It is high in vitamins A and C.

It has diuretic properties and can flush out toxins from kidneys.

It can reduce excessive urination (polyuria).

Ingredients	Mechanism of Action and Health Benefits

The seed is used to manage diabetes and digestive ailments. It can protect the liver. It treats bleeding piles. The bark and leaves are used to treat high blood pressure, gum diseases, and sore throat.

Side effects include coughing and chest congestion. Dairy products should not be consumed with jamun.

Ayyanar, M., & Subash-Babu, P. (2012). *Syzygium cumini* (L.) Skeels: a review of its phytochemical constituents and traditional uses. *Asian Pacific Journal of Tropical Biomedicine*, *2*(3), 240–246. https://doi.org/10.1016/s2221-1691(12)60050-1

Health Benefits Times. (2017, December 20). Health benefits of Eugenia jambolana. *HealthBenefitstimes.com*. https://www.healthbenefitstimes.com/eugenia-jambolana/

Jeevanti
Leptadenia reticulata

Other name: *Jivanti*

Jeevanti contains flavonoids (rutin and luteolin), sterols (stigmasterol), glycosides (apigenin), and terpenes.

It pacifies mostly the vata and pitta doshas. It is a nourishing, rejuvenating, and restorative herb.

It has antioxidant, antifungal, antiinflammatory, and hepatoprotective properties.

The roots and leaves can prevent habitual or recurrent miscarriages. It is used in scanty or painful menses. It is also an aphrodisiac. It improves sperm count and fertility. It also has lactogenic effects and stimulates milk production and is used during lactation.

It can treat fevers, UTIs, and wounds.

It can lower blood pressure and prevent heart diseases.

It also helps in anxiety, depression, and insomnia.

No adverse side effects have been reported.

Chauhan, V. (2019, April 6). What are the uses and health benefits of Jivanti (Leptadenia reticulata)? *Planet Ayurveda*. https://www.planetayurveda.com/jivanti-leptadenia-reticulata/

Jute
C. olitorius

Other names: *Ewedu, ayoyo, C. capsularis, Jute mallow, Nalta jute*

Jute is commonly grown in Asia and Africa. The young leaves and fruit are edible. The leaves are cooked and eaten. It is rich in several vitamins (A, β-carotene, B1, B2, B3, and C) and minerals (iron, calcium, sodium, potassium, and phosphorus). The bark produces jute fiber.

The leaves are muciliginous and have antiinflammatory, antioxidant, laxative, diuretic, gastroprotective, anticancer, and tonic effects.

It is used to treat fevers, UTIs, hemorrhoids, ascites, stimulate appetite, diabetes, and heart disease. They may also support bone health.

Rarely, acute allergic reactions may occur.

Chan, T. (2021, November 18). What are jute leaves? Nutrition, benefits, and how to eat them. *Healthline*. https://www.healthline.com/nutrition/jute-leaves

Islam, M. M. (2013). *Biochemistry, medicinal and food values of Jute (Corchorus capsularis L and C. olitorius L.) leaf: A review* (2nd ed., Vol. 11) [E-book]. ERpublications.

Jyotishmati
Celastrus paniculatus

Other names: *Malkangani, Intellect tree, Black oil plant*

Jyotishmati contains several bioactive compounds including alkaloids (paniculatin and celastrine), tannins, flavonoids, and coumarins. It balances vata.

It has antifungal and antiarthritic properties.

It is a brain and nerve tonic. It increases the acetylcholine levels in the brain and can sharpen memory in dementia and epilepsy.

It enhances skin and hair health. It promotes wound healing. The oil is black in color and is used to treat leukoderma.

Side effects include gastric irritation.

Eng, M. (2020, August 14). 7 Celastrus paniculatus uses + side effects & dosage. *SelfHacked*. https://selfhacked.com/blog/celastrus-paniculatus-2/

Hebbar, J. V. (2020, January 22). Jyotishmati (Celastrus paniculatus) benefits, research, medicines, remedies. *Easy Ayurveda*. https://www.easyayurveda.com/2012/12/05/jyotishmati-medicinal-qualities-ayurveda-benefits-and-dose/

Ingredients	Mechanism of Action and Health Benefits
Kanchanara *Bauhinia variegata*	Kanchanara plant bark is used for medicinal purposes. It contains several bioactive compounds including sitosterol, tannins, kaempferol, and steroids. It relieves kapha and pitta doshas. It is used to treat bleeding due to menorrhagia, fibroids, or hemorrhoids. It can be used in goiter and cervical lymphadenitis. It has also wound healing and vermicide properties. It has also carminative properties. Side effects can include allergic rash and gastric upsets. Gupta, S. (2021, January 27). Kanchanara (Bauhinia variegata). *IAFA Ayurveda.* https://www.iafaforallergy.com/herbs-a-to-z/kanchanara-bauhinia-variegata/
Kantakari *Solanum xanthocarpum*	Other names: *Yellow-fruit nightshade, Solanum virginianum, Solanum surattense, Thai green eggplant (Solanum melongena), Nidigdhika* Kantakari contains flavonoids, saponins, alkaloids, and phenols. It balances vata and kapha doshas and increases the pitta dosha. It has antioxidant, antimicrobial, antiinflammatory, diuretic, and expectorant properties. It is used to treat cough, cold, sore throat, asthma, and bronchitis. It can help with intestinal problems, urinary disorders including kidney stones and epilepsy. It should be used cautiously with pitta disorders. Chauhan, V. (2019, April 6). What are the health benefits and therapeutic uses of Kantakari (Solanum xanthocarpum)? *Planet Ayurveda.* https://www.planetayurveda.com/kantakari-solanum-xanthocarpum/
Kapikachhu *Mucuna prurien*	Other names: *Cowhage, Velvet bean* Kapikachhu is rich in levodopa (L-Dopa) which is converted into dopamine, epinephrine, and norepinephrine. It contains alkaloids, phenolic compounds (gallic acid), coumarins, and steroids. It also contains several minerals including zinc, magnesium, manganese, and iron. It can stabilize all three doshas. It has analgesic properties. It is a nerve tonic. It can be used to treat PD and hyperprolactinemia. It can also help in anxiety and depression. It lowers stress and improves mood. It is an aphrodisiac. It improves male fertility and increases sperm count, quality, and testosterone. It can also enhance ovulation in females. It is also used to treat snakebites. Side effects include hypertension, agitation, nausea, bloating, vomiting, and insomnia. It contains serotonin which may cause itching. RxList Editors. (2021, June 11). Cowhage. *RxList.* https://www.rxlist.com/cowhage/supplements.htm Z Living Staff. (2018, August 30). Can Cowhage be a natural treatment for Parkinson's Disease? *Z Living.* https://www.zliving.com/health/herbs/cowhage-99696/
Karpuravalli *(Coleus amboinicus or Plectranthus amboinicus)*	Other names: *Karpooravalli, Mexican mint, Indian Borage, Mexican Mint, Indian Mint, Mexican Oregano, Spanish Thyme, Origanum vulgare, Winter majoram, Wintersweet, Wild majoram, Mountain mint, Origanum.* Karpooravalli contains thymol and carvacrol, which has expectorant properties. It also has antiviral action. It is used to treat cough, cold, sore throat, asthma, lung congestion, and bronchitis. It can also be used to treat headache, wounds, and skin diseases. Overall, it is safe. Rarely, allergic reactions may occur. Venkateshwarn, R. (2013, April 14). 15 top uses of Karpuravalli (Karpooravalli|Panikoorka|Doddapatre). *Wildturmeric.* https://www.wildturmeric.net/karpooravalli-medicinal-uses-health-benefits/ Vopecpharma. (2020, June 18). The benefits of Karpooravalli Herb—Vopecpharma.com|Vopecpharma Blogs. *Vopecpharma Blogs.* https://www.vopecpharma.com/blogs/the-benefits-of-karpooravalli-herb/
Keelanelli *Phyllanthus niruri or Phyllanthus amarus*	Other names: *Chanca piedra, Gale of the wind, Bhumi amla, Bahupatra, Bhumyamalaki, Bhumi amala, Pumi amla, Jangli Amli, Bhuiawala* The stems, leaves, and flowers of Keelanelli are used. The bioactive compounds present in keelanelli include flavonoids (quercetin, astragalin, and rutin), terpenoids (limonene and lupeol), gallic acid, and ellagitannin. The leaves alsocontain niranthin, phyltetralin, and nirtetralin.

Ingredients	Mechanism of Action and Health Benefits
	It has antimicrobial, antiviral, antiinflammatory, and diuretic properties.

It is a stone breaker plant. It can alkalinize the urine and prevent kidney stone formation. It also decreases burning sensation in UTI.

It can treat hepatitis, other causes of hepatomegaly, improve liver function, decrease jaundice, and prevent gallstones. It can also lower blood glucose.

It can also treat gastric ulcers due to *H. pylori*.

Side effects include gastric upset and diarrhea.

Bagalkotkar, G., Sagineedu, S. R., Saad, M. S., & Stanslas, J. (2006). Phytochemicals from *Phyllanthus niruri* Linn. and their pharmacological properties: A review. *Journal of Pharmacy and Pharmacology*, *58*(12), 1559–1570. https://doi.org/10.1211/jpp.58.12.0001

Fletcher, J. (2020, February 25). Phyllanthus niruri: Everything you need to know. *MedicalNewsToday*. https://www.medicalnewstoday.com/articles/phyllanthus-niruri

TraceGains, Inc. (2015, August 6). *Phyllanthus*. Kaiser Permanente. https://wa.kaiserpermanente.org/kbase/topic.jhtml?docId=hn-2146004

Khella
Ammi visnaga

Other names: Bishop's weed (*Ammi majus*), *Lady's lace, Bishop's flower, Lace flower, toothpick-plant, bisnaga, toothpick weed*

Khella is a flowering plant. The phytochemicals present in bishop's weed include pyrones, saponins, flavonoids, coumarins, and essential oils. It has antiviral, antimicrobial, antioxidant, cardiovascular, and hypotensive effects. The antimicrobial properties are from the presence of flavonoids and also from *Aspergillus amstelodami*, a fungus found in the fruit of khella. The presence of khellin and visnagin gives its antilithogenic effects.

It contains a compound called methoxsalen which is useful in treatment of skin disorders such as psoriasis, tinea versicolor, and vitiligo.

It is effective in kidney stones disease (calcium oxalate and cystine stones). It has diuretic effects, relaxes the smooth muscle (antispasmodic), and increases urinary excretion of citrate.

It has vasodilator actions, can increase HDL cholesterol, and is used for heart disorders including angina. Khellin has calcium channel blocking effects.

It has bronchodilator effects and is used in asthma.

It should not be consumed by pregnant women as it may cause uterine contractions that threaten the pregnancy. It can thin the blood and prevent normal blood clotting. Other side effects include stomach upset, constipation, dizziness, and raised liver enzymes.

Wong, C., & Bull, M. (2021, February 1). Health benefits of Bishop's Weed. *Verywell Health*. https://www.verywellhealth.com/the-benefits-of-bishops-weed-88612

Khus
Chrysopogon zizanioides

Other name: *Vetiver*

The main components in vetiver roots are sesquiterpenes and phenolic compounds in leaves. The roots contain a sesquiterpene called khusimol, which has antimicrobial and antibacterial properties.

The essential oil extracted from the roots (khus oil) has antiinflammatory, antiseptic, and antioxidant properties. It improves alertness and mental fatigue. It has soothing, calming, and grounding effects.

The essential oil is inhaled via aromatherapy (with a carrier oil) to relieve stress, insomnia, ADHD, as well as for emotional traumas, shock, and nervous disorders (hysteria, anxiety, and epileptic attacks). It can also improve breathing patterns especially if there is heavy snoring.

Khus is also applied on the skin for muscle pain and joint pain (arthritis), burns, stings, and wounds.

It is considered safe in small quantities. No reliable information regarding the safety and side effects.

Agarwal, S. (2018, July 13). 5 surprising benefits of vetiver essential oil for your body and mind. *NDTV Food*. https://food.ndtv.com/fitness/5-surprising-benefits-of-vetiver-essential-oil-for-your-body-and-mind-1686318

WebMD Editors. (2011). VETIVER: Overview, uses, side effects, precautions, interactions, dosing and reviews. *WebMD*. https://www.webmd.com/vitamins/ai/ingredientmono-695/vetiver

Khus khus
Papaver somniferum

Other name: Poppy seeds

Khus khus contains benzoic acid, furfural, and vetiverol that have health benefits. It is rich in omega-6 fatty acids, proteins, oxalates, vitamins (C and B6), and minerals (calcium, iron, magnesium, zinc, copper, and iodine). It contains linolenic acid which has antiinflammatory effects.

It is used in Ayurvedic medicines and also widely in Indian cuisine.

It has strong antioxidant properties. It relieves pain and improves immunity.

Ingredients	Mechanism of Action and Health Benefits
	It improves heart, brain, gut, kidney, and skin health. It treats insomnia, prevents kidney stone formation, improves digestion, relieves bloating and constipation, improves bone density, and treats skin and hair problems like eczema, acne, and dandruff.

Excessive use may cause pulmonary edema and death may occur if consumed with tea. It should not be consumed in pregnancy.

Firdous, H., & Marwah, S. (2017, October 6). Benefits of Khus Khus and its side effects. *Lybrate*. https://www.lybrate.com/topic/khus-khus-benefits-and-side-effects

Petre, A., & Kubala, J. (2020, July 30). 6 emerging benefits of poppy seeds. *Healthline*. https://www.healthline.com/nutrition/poppy-seeds-health-benefits

Kidney beans
Phaseolus vulgaris

There are four types of kidney beans

- Red kidney bean: This is the commonest type. Other names: *Rajma, common kidney bean, Surkh lobia*
- Red speckled kidney bean
- Light speckled kidney bean
- White kidney bean: Other names: *Safaid lobia, Cannellini beans (in Italy)*

Kidney beans are nutritious beans. They contain several bioactive compounds including isoflavones and anthocyanins (mainly pelargonidin). They are rich in proteins, minerals (iron, copper, phosphorus, potassium, and manganese), and vitamins (B1, K1, and folate). They have a low GI. They also contain resistant starch and insoluble fiber (alpha-galactosides).

However, they also contain various antinutrients including starch blockers (lectins or α-amylase inhibitors which inhibit the absorption of carbohydrates), protease inhibitors (or trypsin inhibitors which inhibits protein digestion), and phytates (which inhibit the absorption of minerals such as zinc and iron). Raw kidney beans contain a toxic protein named phytohemagglutinin.

It can lower cholesterol and blood sugar and help in weight loss.

It can prevent colon cancer.

Raw kidney beans are toxic. Cooked kidney beans can cause gas and bloating.

Arnarson, A. (2019, May 14). Kidney Beans 101: Nutrition facts and health benefits. *Healthline*. https://www.healthline.com/nutrition/foods/kidney-beans

King of bitters
Andrographis paniculata

Other names: *Green chiretta or Nilavembu, Chuān Xīn Lián*

The active ingredient present in king of bitters is andrographolides which has antiviral, antiinflammatory, and antioxidant properties. It supports normal blood flow, balances blood pressure, blood sugar, and blood lipid levels.

It is a natural immune booster making it useful in treating colds, cough, sore throat, and sinusitis.

Green chiretta is used for stomach complaints in children and as a digestive tonic. It also improves gallbladder and liver functions. It may also be effective for cancers, infections, parasitic infestations, sinus infections, cancer, rheumatoid arthritis, hepatic problems, cardiac diseases, anorexia, allergies, ulcers, and skin diseases.

In high doses, it can cause side effects such as swollen lymph glands, serious allergic reactions, and elevations of liver enzymes. It can also cause loss of appetite, diarrhea, vomiting, headache, runny nose, and fatigue.

Cheepsattayakorn, A., & Cheepsattayakorn, R. (2020). Andrographis paniculata (Green chiretta) may combat COVID-19. *Journal of Lung, Pulmonary & Respiratory Research, 7*(2), 26. https://doi.org/10.15406/jlprr.2020.07.00224

Gaia Herbs. (2019, January 21). Andrographis. https://www.gaiaherbs.com/blogs/herbs/andrographis

Kollu
Macrotyloma uniflorum

Other name: *Horse gram*

Horse gram is a legume (lentil). It contains bioactive compounds including flavonoids, alkaloids, carotenoids, terpenoids, and phenols. It is high in proteins, vitamins C, minerals (phosphorus, calcium, and iron), and fiber. It generates heat in the body.

It can help in weight loss. It can help regulate diabetes.

It can improve heart health and lower the LDL cholesterol and triglycerides.

It can help prevent kidney stones and also gallbladder stones.

It can also help in hemorrhoids, diarrhea, and constipation.

It improves bone and muscle health.

It can be used to treat the cold, cough, and asthma.

Side effects include gas and bloating and occasional allergic reactions. The presence of phytate can block the absorption of minerals.

Ingredients	Mechanism of Action and Health Benefits
	Binu, S. (2020, December 4). Horse gram: A super food in its own way. *Netmeds*. https://www.netmeds.com/health-library/post/horse-gram-super-food-way
	Link, R. (2021, February 4). Is horse gram effective for weight loss? Everything You need to know. *Healthline*. https://www.healthline.com/nutrition/horse-gram-for-weight-loss
Korosanai	Other names: *Cow's stone, Gorochana, Gorochan, Cow bezoar, Ox gall*
	It is a small, fatty, and stony concretion formed in the stomach of the cow or ox. It has astringent properties. It is believed to be a panacea or an antidote for many medical problems. It is mainly used for chronic coughs and colds, improving digestion, and overall health.
	It is usually an Indian tradition to mix a little korosanai with some breast milk and place it on the infant's tongue on Day 10 of life to improve the voice.
	Wikipedia contributors. (n.d.). Gorochana. *Wikipedia*. https://en.m.wikipedia.org/wiki/Gorochana
Kutaja *(Wrightia antidysenterica* or *Holarrhena antidysenterica)*	The seeds, bark, leaves, and flowers of the kutaja plant can be used. It contains several bioactive compounds including alkaloids (such as conessine, considine, and holarrhenine). It balances the kapha and pitta doshas.
	It has antimicrobial, astringent, anthelmintic, and diuretic properties.
	It can treat IBS, diarrhea, colic, malabsorption, and ulcerative colitis.
	It can control bleeding due to dysentery, hemorrhoids, and menorrhagia.
	It can also be used for wound healing.
	Side effects may include nausea.
	Gupta, S. (2021, May 15). Kutaja (Holarrhena antidysenterica). *IAFA Ayurveda*. https://www.iafaforallergy.com/herbs-a-to-z/kutaja-holarrhenaantidysenterica/
Kutki *Picrorhiza kurroa*	Other names: *Yellow gentian, Hu Huang Lian, Picroliv, Anjani, Karu, Katuka*
	The active constituents in kutki are picroside and kutkoside (jointly called kutkin and which also contains picroliv). These have hepatoprotective effects. The apocynin, a flavonoid in kutki, may be helpful in treating PD and hypoxia and ischemia-reperfusion injuries.
	It is a bitter herb with a cooling effect. It reduces the excessive fire and balances the pitta and kapha doshas.
	They also have strong antimicrobial, antiviral, antifungal, and antiinflammatory activities. It also has antioxidant, antibacterial, immunomodulatory, antiallergic, antianaphylactic, and antineoplastic activities. They may also have anticancer effects.
	It is strongly hepatoprotective. It improves gallbladder and liver functions by protection from toxins. It relieves anorexia, nausea, and jaundice in acute viral hepatitis. It is helpful in fatty liver and other digestive disorders (acid reflux, peptic ulcer, and constipation).
	It reduces the severity and duration of asthmatic attacks and also other coughs, colds, and flu.
	It is considered safe for most adults. However, it may be allergic to certain people leading to vomiting, rash, anorexia, diarrhea, and itching.
	Herbal Reality. (2021, March 28). *Kutki*. https://www.herbalreality.com/herb/kutki/
	Krupashree, K., Hemanth Kumar, K., Rachitha, P., Jayashree, G. V., & Khanum, F. (2014). Chemical composition, antioxidant and macromolecule damage protective effects of *Picrorhiza kurroa* Royle ex Benth. *South African Journal of Botany*, *94*, 249–254. https://doi.org/10.1016/j.sajb.2014.07.001
Lady's finger *Abelmoschus esculentus*	Other names: *Okra or gumbo, bhindi, Vendakkai*
	Lady's finger or okra contains polyphenols including flavonoids and isoquercetin, and vitamins A and C, which have antioxidant and antiinflammatory properties. It is also rich in vitamin K1, folate, and magnesium. It has some protein and fiber and is low in carbohydrates.
	The high mucilage content may help to remove toxins and improve digestive health.
	In Ayurvedic medicine, it can also prevent crystallization of minerals in the urine preventing kidney stone formation. It can also help in UTI.
	It may improve heart and brain health, control blood sugar and weight.
	Due to its high oxalate content, excessive intake may lead to oxalate kidney stones.
	Ware, M., & Olsen, N. (2019, November 6). Benefits and uses of okra. *MedicalNewsToday*. https://www.medicalnewstoday.com/articles/311977

Ingredients	Mechanism of Action and Health Benefits
Lemongrass *Cymbopogon citratus*	Lemongrass is a tropical plant with culinary and medicinal uses. It is rich in antioxidants such as flavonoids (quercetin) and phenolic acids. It contains citral, a compound that is rich with antiinflammatory activity. It also contains vitamin C, iron, and calcium.

Lemongrass is a tropical plant with culinary and medicinal uses. It is rich in antioxidants such as flavonoids (quercetin) and phenolic acids. It contains citral, a compound that is rich with antiinflammatory activity. It also contains vitamin C, iron, and calcium.

It has antimicrobial, antioxidant, and antidiabetic properties. It also has diuretic, immune-boosting and blood pressure-lowering effects.

The high vitamin C content helps in strengthening the immune system and improving from colds.

Quercetin can improve heart health by reducing LDL cholesterol levels. It can also reduce cancer growth.

It can be applied topically for skin infections.

It is effective against *Escherichia coli* which can cause food poisoning, pneumonia, and UTIs. It can also be used as an insect repellant and disinfectant.

It may also help in weight loss and also relieve premenstrual symptoms such as menstrual cramps, hot flashes, and bloating.

Overall, it is safe. To certain people it can cause skin irritation when applied topically and allergic reactions.

Brennan, D. (2020, October 7). Lemongrass: Are there health benefits? *WebMD*. https://www.webmd.com/diet/lemongrass-health-benefits#1-2

McDermott, A. (2019, August 9). 10 reasons to drink lemongrass tea. *Healthline*. https://www.healthline.com/health/food-nutrition/lemongrass-tea#antimicrobial

Lodhra
Symplocos racemosa

Lodhra contains many bioactive compounds including loturine, loturidine, colloturine, symposide, symplocososide, oleanolic acid, ellagic acid, flavonoids, glycosides, and others.

It has the property to thicken blood and it will stop bleeding. It also has antiinflammatory properties.

As it is a powerful female-friendly herb, it is widely used in gynecological and hormonal disorders such as endometriosis, polycystic ovarian disorder (PCOD), regulation of menstrual cycles, and to improve fertility. Lodhra can relax the uterine tissues, hence reducing blood flow in heavy menses (menorrhagia).

It is also used to treat blood diseases, dysentery, and epistaxis.

It has antiinflammatory and antimicrobial activities and can loosen phlegm. It is used in asthma, bronchitis, coughs, colds, and sore throat.

Side effects are rare and may include stomach upsets, constipation, and antiandrogen effects in males.

Basu, S. (2021, February 3). Lodhra: Benefits, uses, formulation, ingredients, dosage and side effects. *Netmeds*. https://www.netmeds.com/health-library/post/lodhra-benefits-uses-formulation-ingredients-dosage-and-side-effects

Long pepper
Piper longum

Other names: *Pippali, Thippili, Indian long pepper, Pipli, Pippali moola, Bi Bo, Bi Ba.*

Long pepper fruit (unripe and dried) and root *(Pippali mool)* contain a large number of alkaloids (piperine, methyl piperine, pipernonaline, and piperettine, asarinine), polyphenols (sesamin, pulviatilol, and fargesin), esters and organic acids (palmitic acid and tetrahydropiperic acid).

Its anti-cancer, antioxidant, hepatoprotective, antiplatelet, anti-hyperlipidemic, antidepressant, anti-amoebic and anti-fungal activities are due to the presence of piperine. The antioxidant properties of long pepper reduces cardiotoxicity.

It also has anti-inflammatory, immunomodulatory, antiobesity, antifertility and anti-microbial properties.

It improves blood circulation in the lungs by dilating the blood vessels. It has expectorant effects and removes phlegm in bronchitis, asthma, cough and cold.

It also helps in indigestion, reflux, stomachache, gas and bloating and bone healing.

Long pepper is also used in treatment against dengue and dengue hemorrhagic fever.

Overall it is safe. It should be with caution in pregnant and breastfeeding women.

Mango seed
Mangifera indica

The active ingredients in mango seeds are tannins and polyphenols (gallic acid, coumarins, caffeic acid, vanillin, mangiferin, ferulic acid, and cinnamic acid). These polyphenolic compounds are responsible for their antioxidant effects. It contains amino acids, dietary fiber, minerals (magnesium, potassium, phosphorus, calcium, and sodium) and vitamins (A, B6, B1, B12, C, E, and K). The amino acids present include leucine (227.27% of the DV), isoleucine (193.18% of the DV), histidine (187.50% of the DV), valine (179.92% of the DV), and threonine (115.91% of the DV).

The mangiferin and gallic acid present have cytotoxic and apoptotic activities. Mangiferin also has gastroprotective properties.

Ingredients	Mechanism of Action and Health Benefits
	The mango seed can be made into powder, oil, or butter depending on how it is processed. The oil is cold-pressed from the seeds and it is light and nongreasy with moisturizing properties similar to shea or cocoa butter.
	The dried powder can help in lowering hypertension and reducing the risk of cardiovascular problems. It also helps in lowering blood sugar levels, weight loss, removing acne, treating anemia, and lowering cholesterol levels.
	The mango seed butter can help reduce alopecia, early graying, hair loss, dandruff, sunburns, and scars. The seed powder is helpful in treating diarrhea, scurvy, throat inflammation, and cough. It also improves teeth health, prevents cavities, and ensures enamel health.
	It is generally considered safe to consume except for some people who experience headaches, dry mouth, flatulence, sleep disturbance, and flu-like symptoms.
	Lebaka, V. R., Wee, Y. J., Ye, W., & Korivi, M. (2021). Nutritional composition and bioactive compounds in three different parts of mango fruit. *International Journal of Environmental Research and Public Health,* 18(02), 741–761. https://doi.org/10.3390/ijerph18020741
	Health Benefits Editors. (2017, June 7). Mango seed facts and health benefits. *HealthBenefitstimes. com.* https://www.healthbenefitstimes.com/mango-seed/
Mango powder	Other name: *Amchur*
	This is made from the unripe and peeled green mango flesh which is dried and powdered. It is widely used in Indian cuisine and medicines. It is rich in iron and also vitamins A, C, D, B6, and β-carotenes.
	It has antioxidant properties.
	It is excellent for digestive health and is effective against diarrhea, UTIs, and dysentery. It also reduces acidity and detoxifies the body. Its benefits are similar to the mango seed powder.
	It can also improve eyesight and can prevent problems like cataract. It can improve skin health and treat acne, blackspots, and blemishes.
	Rarely, acute hypersensitivity reactions occur with ingestion of mango powder. It is safe in pregnancy.
	Singh, A. (2018, May 15). Health benefits of amchur: How to use and make amchur powder at home. *NDTV Food.* https://food.ndtv.com/food-drinks/health-benefits-of-amchur-how-to-use-and-make-amchur-powder-at-home-1851957
Manjistha *Rubia cordifolia*	Other names: *Common madder, Indian madder*
	The active compounds in manjistha include quinones (rubiadin, mollugin, and furomollugin), iridoid glycoside, and triterpenoids (rupiprasin and rubiarbonol). The quinones (mainly rubiadin) present are responsible for its hepatoprotective property.
	It also exhibits antiplatelet, antistress, antimicrobial, and antidiabetic activities. It is known as one of the best blood-purifying herbs used for breaking down blockages in the blood flow and removing stagnant blood.
	It is useful in treating skin diseases (skin redness, itching from eczema, psoriasis, and dermatitis) and diarrhea. It was also found to be effective in wound healing.
	A doctor should be consulted prior to consumption if the user has hyperacidity or gastritis. Similarly a doctor should be consulted by pregnant or breastfeeding women prior to consuming manjistha.
	Deshkar, N., Tilloo, S., & Pande, V. (2008). A comprehensive review of *Rubia cordifolia* Linn. *Pharmacognosy Review, 2*(3), 124–134. https://www.phcogrev.com/article/2008/2/3-10
	Mathur, M., Soni, D., & Kanodia, L. (2019, September 5). Manjistha: Benefits, precautions and dosage. 1mg. https://www.1mg.com/ayurveda/manjistha-156
Milk	Milk usually means dairy and from animal source (mostly cow milk and sometimes goat milk). It contains several minerals (including calcium, potassium, phosphorus, zinc, and magnesium), vitamins (D, A, B6, folate, riboflavin, and choline), proteins (whey protein and casein), and saturated fat. Milk contains L-tryptophan which converts to serotonin. It has antioxidant properties. It is a complete food. Plant-based milk types are not included.
	It promotes bone and dental health. It can lower the risk of osteoporosis, rickets, and osteomalacia. It can also reduce the symptoms of osteoarthritis.
	It also helps in wound healing, increasing muscle mass and blood clotting.
	Milk can also lower blood pressure as well as reduce the risk of stroke and heart disease.
	It can also improve mood, appetite, and sleep. Hence, it can improve depression, anxiety, and weight management.

Ingredients	Mechanism of Action and Health Benefits
	It can help in preventing colon, rectum, and breast cancer.
	Overall, it is safe. Overconsumption can increase risk of heart disease, atherosclerosis, hypercalcemia, hyperkalemia, and hormonal changes. Allergic reactions can occur with symptoms including stomach upset, diarrhea, vomiting, dizziness, and anaphylaxis.
	Kubala, J. (2018, March 18). 5 ways that drinking milk can improve your health. *Healthline*. https://www.healthline.com/nutrition/milk-benefits
	Ware, M. (2019, November 7). Health benefits and risks of consuming milk. *MedicalNewsToday*. https://www.medicalnewstoday.com/articles/296564#types_of_milk_and_milk_products
Millet *Panicum miliaceum*	Millet is a small seed grass which is a cereal grain. It is rich in protein (7%–12%), minerals (iron, phosphorus, and calcium), and fiber (15%–20%). It has a better essential amino acid profile compared to other cereals. However, it is a poor source of lysine. It contains antioxidants (tannins, polyphenols, anthocyanins, phytosterols, phytates, and pinacosanols). It is nutritionally superior to wheat or rice.
	Based on grain size they are classified as major and minor millets.
	The major millets are finger millet (ragi), pearl millet (bajra or *Pennisetum glaucum*), and sorghum (jowar).
	The minor millets are foxtail millet (kakum or *Setaria italica*), little millet (kutki), barnyard millet (sanwa), kodo millets (kodon), proso millet or common millet, fonio millet, and teff millet.
	Finger millet has the highest calcium.
	Pseudo millets include buckwheat and amaranth.
	Millet is gluten-free, nonacid forming, and nonallergenic.
	It has laxative effects. It has anticancer properties.
	It decreases the risk of cardiovascular diseases and lowers blood pressure, cholesterol, and triglycerides. It can prevent diabetes and regulate blood sugar.
	It helps in constipation and gas and bloating.
	Taylor, J. R. (2019). Sorghum and millets: Taxonomy, history, distribution, and production. In *Sorghum and millets* (pp. 1–21). https://doi.org/10.1016/b978-0-12-811527-5.00001-0
Mimosa *Mimosa pudica*	Other names: *Lajjalu, Shameplant*
	Mimosa contains several bioactive constituents including alkaloids (mimosine), tannins, mucilage, phenols, and flavonoids.
	It has antimicrobial, antiparasitic, antifungal, antidiarrhea, and anticonvulsant properties. It is also effective against *H. pylori.* It is also an adaptogen and has calming effects.
	It is used for wound healing, piles, dysentery, and uterine disorders.
	It is also used to treat insomnia and epilepsy.
	Overall, it is safe. It should not be consumed during conception as it has antifertility properties.
	Health Benefits Times. (2018, November 26). 16 health benefits of sensitive plant (Touch Me Not). *HealthBenefitstimes.com*. https://www.healthbenefitstimes.com/sensitive-plant/
	Joseph, B., George, J., & Mohan, J. (2013). Pharmacology and traditional uses of *Mimosa pudica*. *Journal of Pharmaceutical Sciences and Drug Research*, 5(2), 41–44.
	Patro, G., Bhattamisra, S. K., & Mohanty, B. J. (2016). Effects of *Mimosa pudica* L. leaves extract on anxiety, depression and memory. *Avicenna Journal of Phytomedicine*, 6(6), 696–710.
Mochras Gum *Salmalia malabarica*	Other names: *Mocharasa, gum of the silk cotton tree, kapok, red cotton tree, Indian kapok tree, red silk cotton tree, Bombax Ceiba, Ilavam Pisin, semal*
	Mochras gum is obtained from the Bombax ceiba tree. It is rich in flavonoids, tannins, triterpenoids, steroids, and saponins. The gum from the flowers is used as a thickener in commercial foods and in cosmetics.
	It is a popular male and female remedy for reproductive health. In females, it can prevent heavy menstrual bleeding and irregular periods. It can also help with excessive vaginal discharge (leukorrhea). In males, it can treat erectile dysfunction. It is an aphrodisiac and it increases libido.
	It has antiinflammatory properties.
	It is also effective for skin pigmentation and acne.
	It can also be used to treat diarrhea.
	Health Benefits Times. (2019, April 3). *Red silk cotton tree facts and health benefits*. *HealthBenefitstimes.com*. https://www.healthbenefitstimes.com/red-silk-cotton-tree/

Ingredients	Mechanism of Action and Health Benefits
Mung bean *Vigna radiata*	Other names: *Green gram, Moong, Munggo/Monggo, Maash*

Mung beans contain several bioactive compounds including flavonoids, phenolic acid, caffeic acid, and cinnamic acid. They are rich in vitamins (B1–B6, folate, and selenium), minerals (magnesium, manganese, iron, phosphorus, potassium, and copper), antioxidants (vitexin and isovitexin), and essential amino acids (including leucine, phenylalanine, lysine, and valine). Compared to other legumes, mung beans are easy to digest. Sprouted mung beans contain more protein and antioxidants as well as less calories compared to unsprouted ones.

Mung beans also contain pectin, a soluble fiber and resistant starch that can aid in digestive health and promotes regular bowel movements. It can also reduce the risk of colon cancer.

It has antiinflammatory properties.

It can reduce the risk of heart disease, chronic inflammation, and cancers.

It can help in heat stroke by helping the body hydrate.

It can improve sperm count and improve fertility. It promotes growth and development of the fetus during pregnancy as well as helps prevent neural tube defects, early birth, and termination. It helps reduce symptoms of PMS (including headache, cramps, mood swings, and muscle ache).

It lowers high blood pressure and blood sugar levels, improves HDL cholesterol levels, and helps maintain heart health.

It can suppress hunger hormones and help in release of fullness hormones (such as peptide YY [PYY], cholecystokinin, and glucagon-like peptide-1 [GLP-1]) which helps in weight loss.

Overall, it is safe. It may cause allergic reactions such as wheezing, nausea, vomiting, stomach upset, diarrhea, and itching.

Kubala, J. (2018, June 12). Essential amino acids: Definition, benefits and food sources. *Healthline*. https://www.healthline.com/nutrition/essential-amino-acids

Levy, J. C. (2019, February 4). Mung beans nutrition & its big benefits! *Dr. Axe*. https://draxe.com/nutrition/mung-beans-nutrition/

| **Murva**
Marsdenia tenacissima | Other names: *White Nishoth, Safed Nishoth, Maruvabel* |

Murva is a climbing shrub. Murva root powder contains glycosides. It has blood-purifying and antidiabetic properties. It is also effective against worms.

It is used to treat various skin disorders, diabetes, poor appetite, constipation, intestinal worm infestation, and chronic cough.

Tripathi, M., Shivhare, D., Tiwari, A., Ahirwar, P. K., Pathak, S., Chitrakoot, M. G., et al. (2014). Pharmacognostical evaluation of *Marsdenia tenacissima* Wight. & Arn. Root. *International Journal of Recent Biotechnology, 2*(3), 18-23. https://www.researchgate.net/publication/330552348_Pharmacognostical_evaluation_of_Marsdenia_tenacissima_Wight_Arn_Root

| **Mustard seed**
Brassica species | Other names: *Sarson, Sorsa, Kadugu, Katuku* |

Brassica juncea (also called Chinese mustard, Oriental mustard, Indian mustard, brown mustard, leaf mustard)

Mustard seeds and leaves are edible. The seeds are generally used as a condiment. There are three types of mustard seeds black (*Brassica nigra*), brown (*Brassica juncea*), and white mustard seeds (*Brassica sinapis alba*). Mustard oil is used widely in Indian cooking.

It contains glucosinolates, which have sulfur compounds like sinigrin and isothiocyanates. The pungent taste is due to sinigrin and it has antiinflammatory, antioxidant, and antimicrobial properties. Isothiocyanate has more anticancer properties. Other flavonoid antioxidants include carotenoids, kaempferol, and isorhamnetin. The activation of glucosinolates occurs when the seeds are disrupted during cooking or processing.

It is rich in several minerals (selenium, magnesium, manganese, calcium, and copper) and vitamins (A, C, and K). They also contain volatile oil.

Mustard seeds also contain omega-3 fatty acids which can reduce high estrogen levels and regulate the menstrual cycle. They also have antiinflammatory properties. It can enhance female fertility. Mustard oil can be used as a lubricant.

It supports digestive health and the fiber present gives it laxative effects. It has diuretic properties and can increase appetite.

It can reduce blood sugar and cholesterol levels. It may promote wound healing and decrease the symptoms of allergic dermatitis. It may prevent bacterial and fungal infections as well as cancer. It can help in migraine headaches.

Ingredients	Mechanism of Action and Health Benefits
	It strengthens skin, hair, nails, and bone.
	Consuming excessive mustard consumption can cause stomach upset including diarrhea. Raw mustard seeds contain goitrogens (isothiocyanate).
	Petre, A. (2020, January 10). Is mustard good for you? *Healthline*. https://www.healthline.com/nutrition/is-mustard-good-for-you
Myrrh *Commiphora myrrha*	Other name: *Mo Yao*
	Myrrh is a gum resin obtained from trees of the genus *Commiphora*. The dried gum is reddish brown and has a unique sweet and smoky aroma. The active constituents include limonene, curzerene, germacrene B, isocericenine, myrcenol, β-selinene, and spathulenol. It also contains minerals like calcium, magnesium, aluminum, phosphorus, chlorine, and chromium.
	It is used in religious rituals and its essential oils are used in perfumes. Its medicinal uses are similar to frankincense.
	It has antiinflammatory, pain-relieving, antioxidant, anticancer, and antiparasitic properties.
	In TCM, mo yao is categorized as an herb that invigorates the blood. It focuses on the heart, spleen, and liver Qi.
	Myrrh can help the circulation of blood in cardiovascular conditions or menstrual irregularities and treat acute pains caused by blood stagnation. It can help reduce menstrual cramps. It can also be used to treat blood stagnation when it causes certain tumors, cysts, and hardened clots. It can speed up wound healing by improving blood circulation.
	Myrrh can help relieve neuropathic pain and in the treatment of rheumatoid arthritis. It is also used for cough, asthma, indigestion, ulcers, sore throat, congestion, and hemorrhoids.
	Overuse can cause severe heart irregularities and allergic contact dermatitis. If consumed by pregnant women, it may cause miscarriage. The other side effects may include making a fever worse, heart problems, hypotension, and uterine bleeding.
	Ahamad, S. R., Al-Ghadeer, A. R., Ali, R., Qamar, W., & Aljarboa, S. (2017). Analysis of inorganic and organic constituents of myrrh resin by GC–MS and ICP-MS: an emphasis on medicinal assets. *Saudi Pharmaceutical Journal*, *25*(5), 788–794. https://doi.org/10.1016/j.jsps.2016.10.011
	Me & Qi. (n.d.). Myrrh (Mo Yao) in Chinese Medicine. *meandqi.com*. https://www.meandqi.com/herb-database/myrrh
	Nordqvist, J. (2018, May 21). Health benefits and risks of myrrh. *MedicalNewsToday*. https://www.medicalnewstoday.com/articles/267107#_noHeaderPrefixedContent
Nagkesar *Mesua ferrea*	Other names: *Nagkesara, Ceylon Ironwood, Cobra's Saffron*
	The flowers, leaves, and seed oil of nagkesar plants are used in ayurvedic medicine. It contains several bioactive compounds including coumarins (mesuarin and mammeisin), phenols, glycosides, and volatile oil.
	It has astringent, antiinflammatory, hemostatic, analgesic, antipyretic, and antimicrobial properties.
	It can be used to relieve cough and cold by removing phlegm from lungs. It is also used in asthma.
	It can be used for management of menstrual disorders (including menorrhagia and leucorrhea).
	It is used in the treatment of indigestion, dysentery, stomach irritation, and bleeding piles.
	Topical application of the oil is helpful in managing skin problems, infections and wounds and fractures.
	Overall, it is safe. Side effects include low blood sugar. The oil can cause allergies on hypersensitive skin.
	Gupta, D., Soni, D., & Ranjan, A. (2019, November 1). Nagkesar. *1mg*. https://www.1mg.com/ayurveda/nagkesar-173
	Nadpara, N. P., Vaghela, J. P., & Patel, P. B. (2012). Phytochemistry and pharmacology of *Mesua ferrea* Linn.—a review. *Research Journal of Pharmacognosy and Phytochemistry, 4*(6), 291–296.
Neem *Azadirachta indica*	Other names: *Nim, Vempu, Veppelai, Margosa, Arishth, Dogoyaro*
	Neem leaves, fruit, and the bark have more than 140 bioactive compounds. They are also rich in fatty acids (oleic, linoleic, stearic, and palmitic acids). They have antiinflammatory, antimicrobial, and antioxidant effects. Neem oil also has limonoids (nimbin, nimbidin, and nimbinin) which have antiinflammatory and antimicrobial properties. The quercetin component gives its antioxidant properties.
	Neem improves skin health in acne, eczema, psoriasis, chronic skin ulcers, and wound healing.
	It also has antidiabetic, hepatoprotective, and anticancer properties. It can decrease blood glucose significantly.

Ingredients	Mechanism of Action and Health Benefits

The seed oil contains azadirachtin that kills head lice parasites. Its antiseptic and antimicrobial activities can improve oral, dental, and hair health. It can improve the inflammation in periodontitis, gingivitis, and dandruff.

It can treat UTIs.

It has spermicidal properties and does not affect male libido.

Overall, it is safe in adults. Prolonged and excessive consumption can harm the kidneys and liver. Neem oil and neem bark when taken by mouth during pregnancy can cause miscarriage. For children, oral consumption can cause side effects including vomiting, diarrhea, drowsiness, blood disorders, seizures, loss of consciousness, coma, brain disorders, and even death.

Hallal, F. (2021, May 28). What is neem extract? Benefits, uses, risks, and side effects. *Healthline*. https://www.healthline.com/nutrition/neem

Malik, K. (2018, August 28). 10 wonderful benefits and uses of neem: A herb that heals. *NDTV Food*. https://food.ndtv.com/health/benefits-and-uses-of-neem-a-herb-that-heals-1231051

Niranjan Phal
Sterculia lychnophora

Other names: *Malva nuts, Taiwan sweet gum, Umasmango, Pang Da Hai, Hat Duoi Uoi, Makjong, Kembang semangkok*

Niranjan phal or Malva nuts (seeds) are from the *Sterculia lychnophora* or *Scaphium affine* tree. The seed is used in both Ayurvedic and Chinese medicine. It contains phenols (gallic acid), alkaloids (sterculinine), tannins, and flavonoids (quercetin). It is also rich in fiber, vitamins (B1 and B2), and minerals (iodine, iron, and calcium).

It has antioxidant, laxative, and detoxifying properties. Once soaked in water, the nut swells eight times the original size and forms a gelatinous mass.

It is cooling and detoxifying. It is used in sore throat, tonsillitis, sinusitis, dry cough, and asthma.

It helps improve bowel movements as well as relieves constipation and bloody stools. It is also used for gastric, stomach ulcers, and piles.

It can help manage irregular and heavy menstrual cycles.

It is also used for skin disorders including acne, eczema, rashes, and psoriasis.

It is added to beauty and skin care products.

Overconsumption can cause cough, watery phlegm, nausea, and swollen tongue. It should be avoided in diarrhea and abdominal pain.

Health Benefits Times. (2019, December 22). Facts about malva nuts tree. *HealthBenefitstimes.com*. https://www.healthbenefitstimes.com/malva-nuts-tree/

Sales of Agricultural Products. (2017, March 14). Health benefits of malva nut. *Linkedin*. https://www.linkedin.com/pulse/health-benefits-malva-nut-teresa-dang

Nirgundi
Vitex negundo

Other name: *Nochi*

The active ingredients in nirgundi include volatile oil, triterpenes, diterpenes, sesquiterpenes, lignan, and flavonoids. Lignan present in nirgundi may help in anticholinesterase activity.

It has antibacterial, antioxidant, antifungal, antiinflammatory, antidiabetic, anxiolytic, anticonvulsant, and antiamnesic properties.

It is also used in relieving pain in joints in both osteoarthritis of rheumatoid arthritis. It helps prevent gray hair and also maintain good quality of hair.

It is also used for the treatment of cough, asthma, fever, diabetes, eye disease, intestinal worms, skin diseases, nervous disorders, and leprosy.

Mild upset stomach may occur. Application of nochi oil or paste might cause itching or develop skin rash. It is advisable to avoid its consumption during pregnancy.

Joshi, K., Chaudhary, N., & Ranjan, A. (2021, January 22). Nirgundi: Benefits, precautions and dosage. 1mg. https://www.1mg.com/ayurveda/nirgundi-192

Ullah, Z., Ullah, R., & Ahmad, I. (2012). Phytochemical and biological evaluation of *Vitex negundo* Linn: a review. *International Journal of Pharmaceutical Sciences and Research*, 3(8), 2421. https://doi.org/10.13040/ijpsr.0975-8232.3(8).2421-31

Noni
Morinda citrifolia

Other names: *Great Morinda, Mengkudu Besar, Cheese Fruit, Indian Mulberry*

Noni contains iridoid glycosides which have antioxidant properties. It is rich in vitamin C, folate, and biotin.

It has antiaging, antiinflammatory, antitumor, antistress, antiviral, and antibacterial properties.

Noni can lower blood sugar and cholesterol. It is also used to relieve arthritic pain and gout. It also helps improve immune health as well as prevent skin and hair problems.

Ingredients	Mechanism of Action and Health Benefits
	Liver toxicity may occur if more than 750 mL/day of noni juice is consumed. Also, in view of the high potassium content, it should be avoided in people with chronic kidney disease.

Times of India. (2018, July 6). What is noni juice and its health benefits. The Times of India. https://timesofindia.indiatimes.com/life-style/health-fitness/diet/what-is-noni-juice-and-its-health-benefits/articleshow/64881447.cms

Nutmeg
Myristica fragrans

Other name: *Jaiphal*

Nutmeg is abundant in antioxidants (cyanidins, essential oils, and phenolic compounds). It contains 7% to 14% essential oils i.e., mainly pinene, camphene, and dipentene. It yields about 24% to 30% fixed oil (nutmeg butter or oil of mace) of which trimyristin is the main component.

It is rich in monoterpenes, an antiinflammatory compound which helps in reducing the risk of heart disease, diabetes, and arthritis. It also has antibacterial activity. It may also lower cholesterol levels and improve blood sugar control.

It can relieve pain, soothe indigestion, strengthen cognitive function, detoxify the body, boost skin health, and alleviate oral conditions. It can also reduce insomnia, increase immune system function, prevent leukemia, and improve blood circulation. It has mild sedative properties. It may also boost female fertility.

It contains myristicin and safrole which in large quantities or prolonged use can cause nutmeg toxicity. Tachycardia, nausea, disorientation, vomiting, agitation, hallucinations, loss of muscle coordination, organ damage, or even death may occur.

The Editors of Encyclopedia Britannica. (2008, January 9). Nutmeg. *Encyclopedia Britannica*. https://www.britannica.com/topic/nutmeg

Dilmah Tea. (2021). Nutmeg (Myristica fragrans). https://www.dilmahtea.com/herbal-infusion-tea/herbal-tea-benefits/nutmeg.html

Kubala, J. (2019, June 12). *8 science-backed benefits of nutmeg*. Healthline. https://www.healthline.com/nutrition/nutmeg-benefits#TOC_TITLE_HDR_2

Onion
Allium cepa

Onion is rich in flavonoid quercetin which protects against cataracts, cardiovascular disease, and cancer. It contains vitamins (B6, B9, and C) and minerals (manganese, potassium, magnesium, and phosphorus).

It also has OSCs that are helpful in lowering blood pressure and cholesterol levels. It also contains small amounts of iron and calcium which can help anemia. It contains sulfur compounds (S-methylcysteine) and flavonoids (quercetin) which helps to reduce blood sugar.

The anthocyanins present in onions are helpful in reducing the risk of heart disease, certain cancers, and diabetes. It is also used for the treatment of urinary disorders.

It is antiinflammatory, antifungal, antibacterial, antiseptic, antispasmodic, carminative, diuretic, expectorant, febrifuge, hypotensive, lithontriptic, stomachic, and tonic. It is also commonly used for treating running nose and eyes.

It can be used to allay tooth and gum aches. It can also be applied on skin disorders including warts, poultice, boils, bruises, and wounds.

Onion is considered safe to use by most adults. However, it may cause adverse digestive effects in some people, and raw onion can cause eye and mouth irritation.

Kumar, K. P. S., Bhowmik, D., & Tiwari, P. (2010). *Allium cepa*: A traditional medicinal herb and its health benefits. *Journal of Chemical and Pharmaceutical Research*, 2(1), 283–291. https://www.jocpr.com/articles/allium-cepa-a-traditional-medicinal-herb-and-its-health-benefits.pdf

Ware, M. R., & Hatanaka, M. (2019, November 15). Why are onions good for you? *MedicalNewsToday*. https://www.medicalnewstoday.com/articles/276714

Palmarosa oil

Other names: *Gingergrass, Indian Geranium, Rosha*

This is an essential oil derived from *Cymbopogon martinii*.

It is used widely in Ayurvedic and Chinese medicine.

The active ingredients are geraniol and geranyl acetate.

It has antiinfective, antiinflammatory, antioxidant, and antistress properties.

It is widely used in cosmetic and skincare products as well as in aromatherapy.

It can help in anxiety and stress.

Overall, it is safe.

Walters, M. (2022, January 31). The skin benefits of Palmarosa oil, plus recipes and safety tips. *Healthline*. https://www.healthline.com/health/palmarosa-oil-benefits#what-is-it

Ingredients	Mechanism of Action and Health Benefits
Papaya *Carica papaya*	Other name: *Pawpaw* Papaya is a tropical fruit. It contains carotenoids (α-carotene and β-carotene, lutein, zeaxanthin, and lycopene), vitamins (A, C, folate, K, E, and pantothenic acid), minerals (copper, magnesium, potassium, and calcium), fiber, papain enzyme, and choline. It has antioxidant, anticancer, antiinflammatory, and immunomodulatory properties. The carotenoids and vitamin A present can improve eyesight, reduce the risk of night blindness and age-related macular degeneration. The papain enzyme and fiber help to improve digestion and gut health, ensure smooth bowel movement, and prevent constipation. It maintains healthy skin and hair. It promotes wound and ulcer healing as well as moisturizes the skin and hair. It can lower blood pressure and blood sugar, reduce the risk of heart disease, diabetes, asthma, and cancers. Unripe papaya can regulate the menstrual cycle and induce menses if the periods are irregular. It can increase uterine contractions and also cause an abortion. Overall, it is safe. Rarely, there is risk of latex allergy from unripe papaya. Too much carotene can cause skin to become a little yellow or orange. Fernandes, M. (2018, February 19). Health benefits of unripe green papaya. *Medindia*. https://www.medindia.net/dietandnutrition/health-benefits-of-unripe-green-papaya.htm McDermott, A. (2018, December 4). 6 ways to use papain. *Healthline*. https://www.healthline.com/health/food-nutrition/papain Ware, M. (2017, December 21). What are the health benefits of papaya? *MedicalNewsToday*. https://www.medicalnewstoday.com/articles/275517
Parsley *Petroselinum crispum*	Other name: *Prajmoda* Parsley is a culinary herb which contains carotenoids (lutein, zeaxanthin, and β-carotene), flavonoids (apigenin and myricetin), and vitamins (K, C, A, and folate). It is antioxidant rich. It can pacify the kapha buildup which can contribute to stone formation. It supports bone health and eye health as well as can stimulate hair growth. It acts as a diuretic, promotes urination as well as can prevent UTIs and kidney stones. It improves urine pH, hence reducing the formation of kidney stones. It can improve appetite and digestion as well as prevent constipation. It can lower blood pressure, reduce blood sugar in diabetes and risk of heart disease. It can prevent cancers. It can increase menstrual flow and risk of a miscarriage. Overall, it is safe. It can interact with anticoagulants and diuretics. WebMD Editors. (2012). Parsley. *WebMD*. https://www.webmd.com/vitamins/ai/ingredientmono-792/parsley Zamarripa, M. (2019, April 5). 8 impressive health benefits and uses of parsley. *Healthline*. https://www.healthline.com/nutrition/parsley-benefits
Pashanabheda *Bergenia ligulata/* *Bergenia ciliata*	Other names: *Pakhanbed ka Beeda, Pashanabheda, Stone breaker* Pashanabheda is a bitter astringent herb. It contains tannins, bergenin, gallic acid, C-glycoside, β-sitosterol, and mucilage. The rhizome has antiinflammatory and antimicrobial effects. It can balance the tridoshas. It can dissolve kidney and urinary tract stones. It also has diuretic effects and can increase urinary flow in bladder infections and urine retention. It is cardioprotective. It is a heart tonic and supports heart health. It can regulate blood sugar. It can be applied topically to painful gums in infants during teething and also for wound healing. It can also reduce fevers. Overall, it is safe. There are no adverse effects reported. Abhay. (2020, November 4). 5 health benefits of Pashanabheda—Ayurvedic treatment. *Trust The Herb*. https://trustherb.com/health-benefits-of-pashanabheda/ Kalia, A., Verma, P., & Gauttam, V. (2014). Comparative pharmacognostical studies on three different plant sources of Pashanbhed. *Journal of Ayurveda and Integrative Medicine*, 5(2), 104–108. https://doi.org/10.4103/0975-9476.131728

Ingredients	Mechanism of Action and Health Benefits
Passion flower *Passiflora incarnata*	There are several species of passion flower. *P. incarnata* has more medicinal value. The leaves, stems, and flowers are used. It can increase the level of GABA, an inhibitory neurotransmitter in the brain which has calming and sedating effects. It is used in the treatment of stress, anxiety, insomnia, ADHD, and nervous disorders (including hysteria and seizures). The flower extract may also be used in the treatment of stomach ulcers. Generally, it is considered safe. Possible side effects include drowsiness, vomiting, nausea, rapid heartbeat, and confusion. It can interact with sedative drugs and should not be taken with barbiturates, narcotics, benzodiazepines, antihistamines, as well as blood thinners. Ashpari, Z. (2018, September 29). The calming effects of passionflower. *Healthline*. https://www.healthline.com/health/anxiety/calming-effects-of-passionflower#risks WebMD Editors. (n.d.). Passionflower. *WebMD*. https://www.webmd.com/vitamins/ai/ingredient-mono-871/passionflower
Passion fruit *Passiflora edulis*	*Passiflora edulis* is the edible variety and does not have the sedating effects of *Passiflora incarnata*. The active ingredients in passion fruit present include luteolin, apigenin, and quercetin derivatives. It contains high levels of vitamin A and vitamin C along with fiber and minerals (potassium, magnesium, calcium, and iron). It also contains vitamin B3, vitamin B6, and phosphorus. It has antioxidant, antimicrobial, antiinflammatory, antihypertensive, hepatoprotective, antidiabetic, sedative, antidepressant, and anxiolytic-like properties. The passion fruit leaf is often sliced or chopped and eaten in a sambal salad in Sri Lankan cuisine. It can also be sauteed, fried, or boiled. It can lower cholesterol levels and improve the heart. It has a low GI. It also improves digestion and prevents constipation. Contrary to some beliefs, the leaves are considered safe for consumption. People with latex allergy should be careful when consuming passion fruit as it can cause an allergic reaction. Galan, N., & Marengo, K. (2019, February 6). What are the health benefits of passion fruit? *MedicalNewsToday*. https://www.medicalnewstoday.com/articles/324383 He, X., Luan, F., Yang, Y., Wang, Z., Zhao, Z., Fang, J., et al. (2020). *Passiflora edulis*: an insight into current researches on phytochemistry and pharmacology. *Frontiers in Pharmacology, 11*(617). https://doi.org/10.3389/fphar.2020.00617
Patharchatta *Kalanchoe pinnata* *Bryophyllum Pinnatum*	Other names: *Katti Pottal, Kutti podum, Parna Beeja, Ranakalli, Akkapana* Patharchatta contains flavonoids as the main active ingredient. It has antiinflammatory, antimicrobial, analgesic, antioxidant, and antivenom properties. It is used to treat respiratory diseases (sore throat and bronchitis) and GI problems (ulcers and gastritis). It is also used to treat burns, wounds, as well as snake and scorpion bites. It can prevent kidney stone formation. It can also treat and prevent premature labor. There are no significant side effects. Fernandes, J. M., Cunha, L. M., Azevedo, E. P., Louren√ßo, E. M., Fernandes-Pedrosa, M. F., & Zucolotto, S. M. (2019). *Kalanchoe laciniata* and *Bryophyllum pinnatum*: an updated review about ethnopharmacology, phytochemistry, pharmacology and toxicology. *Revista Brasileira de Farmacognosia, 29*(4), 529–558. https://doi.org/10.1016/j.bjp.2019.01.012 Priyantha, K. M. (2020, February 7). Medicinal uses of Akkapana. *Daily Mirror Online*. https://www.dailymirror.lk/medicine/Medicinal-uses-of-Akkapana/308-182714
Peelu *Salvadora persica*	Other names: *Pilu, Miswaak, Toothbrush tree* Twigs of peelu or miswaak tree are used to clean teeth or gum. It has antimicrobial, antiplaque, and antiinflammatory properties. It can be used to treat gingivitis and bad breath as well as to reduce dental plaque formation. It is an ingredient in toothpaste. Aumeeruddy, M. Z., Zengin, G., & Mahomoodally, M. F. (2018). A review of the traditional and modern uses of *Salvadora persica* L. (Miswak): toothbrush tree of Prophet Muhammad. *Journal of Ethnopharmacology, 213*, 409–444. https://doi.org/10.1016/j.jep.2017.11.030 Haque, M. M., & Alsareii, S. A. (2015). A review of the therapeutic effects of using miswak (*Salvadora persica*) on oral health. *Saudi Medical Journal, 36*(5), 530–543. https://doi.org/10.15537/smj.2015.5.10785

Ingredients	Mechanism of Action and Health Benefits

Ingredients

Peepal
Ficus religiosa

Mechanism of Action and Health Benefits

Other names: *Pipal, Peepul, Pipul, Pippala, Asvattha, Ashvattha, Ashwattha, Bodhi tree, Bo tree, Bodhi Satva Vruksha*

Read more under "Banyan Tree"

The sacred fig (*Ficus religiosa*) and the banyan tree (banyan fig) are not the same but are related as they are under the same *Ficus* genus.

The bodhi tree (also called Bo tree, peepal pipal/peepul/pipul tree/asvattha) is a type of the sacred fig which symbolizes longevity, prosperity, and good luck. It is the tree of Lord Buddha's enlightenment. It is reported that the peepal tree emits oxygen 24 hours and more in the early morning hours compared to other trees. Both the banyan and peepal trees often grow together in temple grounds and are likened as male and female (or Yin-Yang) counterparts.

All parts of the tree have therapeutic uses, similar to the banyan tree. Tannins are the most important bioactive components.

The fruits, seeds, and leaves are laxative. The fruit can stimulate appetite and libido. The leaves are also used for constipation, jaundice, heart failure, bleeding, and fevers. The bark has astringent and aphrodisiac properties.

It also has antioxidant, antibacterial, antiseptic, digestive, laxative, detoxifying, and immune-boosting properties.

It reduces the absorption of glucose from the blood. It can be used in diabetes. It can treat heart failure. It can improve lung functions and is used in asthma.

It can prevent dental caries, gum disease, and bad breath. It can treat mouth ulcers, acid reflux, constipation, and diarrhea. It also moisturizes the skin as well as maintains healthy hair and skin. It promotes wound healing.

It can treat loss of appetite. The ripe purple fruits when eaten can stimulate digestive juices and improve appetite.

It can also reduce or treat hyperpigmentation, pruritus, eczema, and cracked heels.

Krishna, K. (2021, January 27). Peepal tree: Medicinal and therapeutic benefits, skin care and contraindications. *Netmeds*. https://www.netmeds.com/health-library/post/peepal-tree-medicinal-and-therapeutic-benefits-skin-care-and-contraindications

Anupama, A. (2018, August 12). Medicinal uses of Peepal tree. *Bimbima*. https://www.bimbima.com/ayurveda/medicinal-uses-of-peepal-tree/673/

Pistachio
Pistacia vera

Pistachios are rich in protein (especially L-arginine), antioxidants [carotenoids (including lutein, zeaxanthin), polyphenols, and tocopherols], minerals (potassium, copper, manganese, and phosphorus), vitamins (B1 and B6), and fiber. It has a low GI. It is rich in melatonin.

It can lower blood pressure, LDL cholesterol, and blood sugar. It can improve endothelium-dependent vasodilation.

It increases healthy gut bacteria and helps with constipation.

It improves eye health and may help in weight loss.

It can improve erectile function in men by increasing blood flow.

Benediktsdottir, A. (2019, October 23). 9 health benefits of pistachios. *Healthline*. https://www.healthline.com/nutrition/9-benefits-of-pistachios#2.-High-in-antioxidants

Leonard, J. (2018, August 29). What are the benefits of pistachios? *MedicalNewsToday*. https://www.medicalnewstoday.com/articles/322899

Pointed gourd
Trichosanthes dioica

Other names: *Parwal, Palwal, Parmal*

Pointed gourd is a vegetable. It contains several phytoactive compounds including flavonoids, saponins, triterpenes (cucurbitacin, etc.), tannins, and peptides (trichosanthin and lectin) which have antiinflammatory, antidiabetic, lipid-lowering, cardiotonic, laxative, and diuretic effects.

The fruit is cooked and eaten as a vegetable. The juice of the leaves can also be used.

It is used to treat diabetes.

Kumar, S., & Singh, B. D. (2012). Pointed Gourd: Botany and Horticulture. *Horticultural Reviews, 39*, 203–238. https://doi.org/10.1002/9781118100592.ch5

Ingredients	Mechanism of Action and Health Benefits
Psyllium husk	Other names: *Plantain seed, Che Qian Zi*
Plantago ovata	The genus plantago has more than 200 species. Plantain is one of them. The seeds of plantain are called psyllium. These seeds are used to produce mucilage.
Plantago asiatica	
Plantago depressa	Psyllium husk is a seed husk from Plantago ovata (which is specifically called isapagula). Psyllium is also used generically for all fibers from any of the plantago genus. Their properties cannot be differentiated.

It is highly absorbent and contains about 10% to 30% of dietary fiber. It also contains hemicellulose (arabinoxylans), fixed oil with linoleic and oleic acid esters (omega-6 and omega-9 fatty acids), phytosterols, triterpenes, aucubin (iridoid glycoside), and the alkaloids (plantagonine, indicaine, and indicamine).

The arabinoxylans present can be used in the treatment of GI problems. The fiber is helpful in the treatment of constipation, diabetes, diarrhea and loose stools, IBS, diverticulosis, and metabolic syndrome.

It is also able to help manage blood glucose levels and lower cholesterol levels reducing the risk of heart disease and cholesterol gallstones. It may contain antiobesity properties as well.

It is also a prebiotic that can improve immune system function, reduce inflammation, as well as maintain healthy tissue and cells.

Possible side effects of psyllium husk include abnormal pain and cramps, diarrhea, gas, loose tools, nausea, and vomiting.

Wikidiff Staff. (2021, June 21). Psyllium vs plantain—What's the difference? https://wikidiff.com/psyllium/plantain

Wong, C., & Kroner, A. (2020, July 8). The Health Benefits of Psyllium. *Verywell Health*. https://www.verywellhealth.com/the-benefits-of-psyllium-89068

Punarnava	Other name: *Red spiderling*
Boerhavia diffusa	The active compounds present in punarnava include flavonoid glycosides, isoflavonoids (rotenoids), steroids (ecdysteroid), alkaloids, and phenolic and lignan glycosides. It contains vitamins (B3, B2, and C) and minerals such as sodium, calcium, and iron.

Punarnavoside, a phenolic glycoside, is responsible for its antifibrinolytic activity. The anticancer and antispasmodic properties of punarnava are due to the presence of rotenoids.

It can increase protein synthesis. It also has antidepressant, antiinflammatory, antistress, immunomodulation, antihyperglycemic, and hepatoprotective properties. These properties are due to ecdysteroid that is present. It is also nephroprotective and it has diuretic actions.

Punarnava is used in the treatment of rheumatoid arthritis, fever, edema, eye problems (cataract), and stomach issues (constipation, dyspepsia, and abdominal lump). It is also used in treating cough, asthma, fever, colicky pain, skin diseases, and itching.

It is very effective against kidney stone formation.

It can improve male fertility. It is an aphrodisiac and increases male libido. It can also improve sperm count.

Some possible side effects that can be observed include the risk of increased blood pressure and allergic reactions. Punarnava is considered unsafe for children and is not advised for pregnant women.

Mishra, S., Aeri, V., Gaur, P. K., & Jachak, S. M. (2014). Phytochemical, therapeutic, and ethnopharmacological overview for a traditionally important herb: *Boerhavia diffusa* Linn. *BioMed Research International*, *2014*, 1–19. https://doi.org/10.1155/2014/808302

Pushkarmool	Other names: *Pushkar, Pushkaramul, Elecampane, Xuan Fu Hua*
Inula racemosa	Refer to "Inula flowers" under Chinese Natural Ingredients.

The *Inula racemosa* species is used more in Ayurvedic medicine. It pacifies kapha and vata doshas. It is used to treat mainly respiratory and heart diseases.

Ingredients	Mechanism of Action and Health Benefits
Queen's flower or *Lagerstroemia speciosa*	Other names: *Pride of India, Banaba* Queen's flower contains terpenes (corosolic acid), saponins, flavonoids, tannins, and anthraquinone glycosides. It has antioxidant, antimicrobial, and hepatoprotective properties. It can treat diabetes, metabolic syndrome, weight loss, and gout. Overall, it is safe. Side effects may include low blood pressure. It can interact with diabetes medications. Health Benefits Times. (2020, January 28). Health benefits of Banaba. *HealthBenefitstimes.com*. https://www.healthbenefitstimes.com/banaba/ RxList Editors. (2021, June 11). Banaba. *RxList*. https://www.rxlist.com/banaba/supplements.htm
Quinoa *(Chenopodium quinoa)*	Quinoa is a seed. It is not a cereal grain. It is a complete protein with the nine essential amino acids (unlike millet) and is fiber-rich and gluten-free. It contains vitamins (B6, folate, and E) and minerals (copper, iron, zinc, phosphorus, magnesium, and manganese). It contains flavonoid antioxidants (quercetin and kaempferol). It can regulate blood sugar and cholesterol as well as helps in diabetes and obesity. It is high in oxalates and phytates which can interfere with mineral nutrient absorption. Kubala, J. (2022, January 5). 8 evidence-based health benefits of quinoa. *Healthline*. https://www.healthline.com/nutrition/8-health-benefits-quinoa
Raisins *Vitis vinifera*	Raisins are dried grapes. It is rich in antioxidants such as polyphenols, phenols, and terpenoids (oleanolic acid). Polyunsaturated fatty acids (linoleic acid and linolenic acid), several minerals (including potassium, iron, manganese, boron, and copper), fiber, and vitamin B6 are also present. It has antiinflammatory, antibacterial, and blood-purifying properties. It is also cooling. It can improve heart health by lowering blood pressure and blood sugar levels. The rich fiber content helps in digestion and stomach problems. It can also be used in the treatment of anemia. Overall, it is safe. Side effects include weight gain, stomach upset, diarrhea, and gas and bloating. Cafasso, J. (2019, January 18). Are raisins good for you? *Healthline*. https://www.healthline.com/health/food-nutrition/are-raisins-good-for-you Greenberg, J. A., Newmann, S. J., & Howell, A. B. (2005). Consumption of sweetened dried cranberries versus unsweetened raisins for inhibition of uropathogenic *Escherichia coli* adhesion in human urine: a pilot study. *The Journal of Alternative and Complementary Medicine*, *11*(5), 875–878. https://doi.org/10.1089/acm.2005.11.875 WebMD Editorial Contributors. (2020, October 7). Raisins: Are they good for you? *WebMD*. https://www.webmd.com/diet/raisins-good-for-you#2
Rock sugar	Other names: Mishri, Kalkandu, Bing tang Rock sugar is unrefined crystalized sugar and is made from sugarcane (*Saccharum officinarum*) or palm tree sap and water solution. It is less sweet compared to table sugar. It is rich in vitamins especially B12, and minerals. It is used for culinary purposes (to sweeten beverages, brews, or desserts and add shine to braised Chinese dishes) or for medicinal purposes. Sucking a piece of rock sugar (and with some fennel seeds) helps to maintain fresh breath (after a meal), relieve cough and sore throat, and decrease mental fatigue (if drunk with warm milk at night). It can boost energy and may improve fertility. Mishri also helps stop nose bleeding, improve digestion, increase hemoglobin levels, and improve blood circulation. It has antidepressant effects and increases the production of breast milk. Excess consumption of rock sugar can lead to obesity, type 2 diabetes, cardiovascular diseases, gingivitis, and periodontitis. Boldsky. (2018, January 29). 10 health benefits of rock sugar (Mishri) you should know. *Boldsky.com*. https://www.boldsky.com/health/nutrition/2018/10-health-benefits-of-rock-sugar-mishri-you-should-know-120123.html WebMD Editors. (2020a, October 5). Rock sugar: Are there health benefits? *WebMD*. https://www.webmd.com/diet/rock-sugar-health-benefits#1-2

Ingredients	Mechanism of Action and Health Benefits
Rose petals *Rosa*	The bioactive constituents of rose petals include phenolic acids (caffeic, gentisic, salicylic, and p-coumaric), flavonoids, tannins and essential oil. Its antioxidant activity is due to the presence of flavonoids and phenols present. The anthocyanins present also help in improving urinary tract, eye health, and memory. It contains vitamins (A,C and E) and minerals (iron and calcium).

Rose petals
Rosa

The bioactive constituents of rose petals include phenolic acids (caffeic, gentisic, salicylic, and p-coumaric), flavonoids, tannins and essential oil. Its antioxidant activity is due to the presence of flavonoids and phenols present. The anthocyanins present also help in improving urinary tract, eye health, and memory. It contains vitamins (A,C and E) and minerals (iron and calcium).

It has antioxidant, cytotoxic, anti-inflammatory, analgesic and antimicrobial activities. It is applied topically, sprayed or consumed.

Rose water is made from the petals usually but can also include rosehip. It is also used to maintain skin health. It is a cleanser, toner and astringent. Rose water also helps with indigestion, gas and bloating. It has also a calming effect on the nervous system. It soothes sore throats. Rose water also soothes eye allergies and tired or dry eyes.

Rose oil or rose essential oil is extracted via steam distillation from the petals (usually *Rosa damascena*). It has more calming effect on the nervous system and is used to manage stress, anxiety, depression, headache, and increase libido. It is used in aromatherapy or in perfumes. Rose oil should not be eaten.

Rose extract does not specify which part of the rose.

It also improve the immune system. It is beneficial in treating dementia and seizures. It is also used for treating liver problems, reducing severity of allergic reactions, and improving insulin resistance

It may also reduce the risk of development of certain cancers and alleviate menstrual pain. The rose petal tea may also ease flu-like symptoms such as coughing and congestion.

Rose petals can also interact with certain medications, like blood thinners or antidepressants.

Overall, rose is safe. Rarely, allergic reactions occur.

Gotter, A. (2017, May 23). Rose Water: Benefits and Uses. Healthline. https://www.healthline.com/health/rose-water-benefits

Brennan, D. (2020, October 16). *Rose Tea: Is It Good for You?* WebMD. https://www.webmd.com/diet/rose-tea-good-for-you#1-2

Nowak, R., Olech, M., Pecio, U., Oleszek, W., Los, R., Malm, A., & Rzymowska, J. (2013). Cytotoxic, antioxidant, antimicrobial properties and chemical composition of rose petals. *Journal of the Science of Food and Agriculture, 94*(3), 560–567. https://doi.org/10.1002/jsfa.6294

Roselle
Hibiscus sabdariffa

Other names: *Jamaican sorrel, Red sorrel, Karkade, Sour Tea, Pulicha Keerai*

Roselle is a member of the Hibiscus *(Malvaceae)* family. It is rich in polyphenols, vitamin C, and iron. The fresh or dried red calyces (sepals) of the roselle flower are made as a roselle tea infusion (commonly called hibiscus tea) and consumed as a hot or cold beverage. The leaves are cooked and eaten.

It can lower LDL cholesterol, blood glucose, and blood pressure, as well as increase HDL cholesterol.

Overall, it is safe.

Da-Costa-Rocha, I., Bonnlaender, B., Sievers, H., Pischel, I., & Heinrich, M. (2014). *Hibiscus sabdariffa* L.—A phytochemical and pharmacological review. *Food Chemistry, 165*, 424–443. https://doi.org/10.1016/j.foodchem.2014.05.002

Rudraksha
Elaeocarpus ganitrus

Mechanism of Action and Health Benefits

Other names: *Wooden beggar bead, Rudraki*

Rudraksha is a fruit with several phytoactive compounds including flavonoids, triterpenoids, tannins, alkaloids (rudrakine) steroids, cardiac glycosides and elaeocapine.

Rudraksha seed has many faces or facets (*mukhi*) and they are numbered from 1 to 38. Rudrakshas with 1 to 14 mukhis are more common of which the 5- mukhi Rudraksha is the commonest. Different Rudraksha with specific mukhi is used to treat various ailments. For example, for overall good health, a 7 mukhi Rudraksha is used.

It is regarded as a spiritual fruit or seed. The inner rudraksha seeds have electromagnetic properties and emit different frequencies based on the number of mukhis. This activates the chakras.

It has anti-tussive properties and can treat sore throats, cough, cold, bronchitis and asthma.

It calms the nervous system and can help in stress, anxiety, depression, ADHD, migraine and epilepsy.

It is cardioprotective and can lower blood pressure in hypertension.

It is a blood purifier and has antiaging properties. It can treat acne, pruritis, wounds, skin hyperpigmentation and maintains skin glow.

Ingredients	Mechanism of Action and Health Benefits

It has antimicrobial, anti-inflammatory, analgesic and immune modulating properties. It can treat fevers and is used in arthritis.

Overall, it is safe and can be used at all ages.

Ashraf, A. S. (2019). RUDRAKSHA: THERAPEUTIC APPROACH IN AYURVEDA. PARIPEX - INDIAN JOURNAL OF RESEARCH, 8(6).

Jain, S. (n.d.). A REVIEW ON ELAEOCARPUS SPHAERICUS (RUDRAKSHA). PharmaTutor. https://www.pharmatutor.org/articles/a-review-on-elaeocarpus-sphaericus-rudraksha

Sadabahar
Catharanthus roseus
Lochnera rosea
Vinca rosea

Other name: *Periwinkle, Bright eyes*

Catharanthus is the genus. *Vinca rosea* (synonymous with *Lochnera rosea*), is the old name for *Catharanthus roseus or Madagascar periwinkle*. It is commonly called periwinkle.

The periwinkle plant contains many bioactive compounds which include serpentine, reserpine, ajmalicine, catharanthine, lochnerin, lochnericin, and others. The four main alkaloids vinblastine, vincristine, vinorelbine, and vindesine are used in cancer chemotherapies in leukemias, lymphomas, and neuroblastoma as it has anticancer, antimetastatic, and immune support properties.

It can regulate blood glucose in diabetes, lower blood pressure in hypertension, and remove mucus or phlegm in coughs, sore throat, asthma, bronchitis, or lung congestion. It can also treat dysmenorrhea, PCOS, acne, and promote wound healing. It has neuroprotective effects and can improve memory as well as concentration.

Side effects include constipation and low blood pressure.

Basu, S. (2021, July 2). Sadabahar: Astounding health benefits of the beautiful periwinkle flower. *Netmeds*. https://www.netmeds.com/health-library/post/sadabahar-astounding-health-benefits-of-the-beautiful-periwinkle-flower

Saffron
Crocus sativus

Saffron contains more than 150 carotenoid compounds including crocin, picrocrocin, safranal, and crocetin which have antioxidant properties. Crocin and crocetin may have antidepressant properties, protect brain cells against progressive damage, improve inflammation, reduce appetite, and aid weight loss. Antiinflammatory, anticancer, and antidepressant properties are due to the presence of kaempferol (a flavonol). It is also rich in vitamins B2, B3, and B6.

Saffron can help treat PMS symptoms, which include irritability, headaches, cravings, pain, and anxiety. It improves erectile function in men. In women, there is more arousal and lubrication.

It may also help lower blood cholesterol and prevent blood vessels and arteries from clogging, control blood sugar levels and raise insulin sensitivity, and improve memory in adults with AD. It tones the skin and enhances the complexion. In Ayurveda, it mitigates all the three doshas.

Long-term use of saffron with high doses can cause some possible side effects like anxiety, headache, sweating, nausea or vomiting, and constipation. Allergic reactions can occur.

Raman, R. (2019, January 7). 11 impressive health benefits of saffron. *Healthline*. https://www.healthline.com/nutrition/saffron#

Sandalwood
Santalum album

Other name: *Chandana*

The sandalwood tree has been used mostly in the cosmetic and furniture industry. The major active components of sandalwood include sesquiterpene alcohols, α- and β-santalols. The α-sanatol present may possess anticancerous properties.

Sandalwood has a calming and relaxation effect. Hence, it can reduce stress, depression, fear, nervous exhaustion, anxiety, discomfort, and insomnia and enhances meditation.

It also possesses abortifacient, hepatoprotective, urinary antiseptic, stomachic, antiviral, and antiherpetic activities. It may have antiinflammatory, antimitotic, antihypertensive, diuretic, antipyretic, sedative, ganglionic blocking, and insecticidal properties.

Sandalwood is very beneficial for treating gastric irritability, jaundice, dysentery, tension, and confusion, and is also used as a tonic for heart, stomach, liver, antipoison, fever, memory improvement, and as a blood purifier.

The essential oil is also used to treat psoriasis.

Although there are mixed views, sandalwood is considered safe for consumption and has a GRAS (generally recognized as safe) status.

The tree actually produces an edible nut. The essential oil should be enteric-coated and it should be mixed with milk if taken orally. Side effects include itching, nausea, stomach upset, and blood in the urine. Long-term usage may cause kidney damage.

Ingredients	Mechanism of Action and Health Benefits
	Kumar, R., Anjum, N., & Tripathi, Y. C. (2015). Phytochemistry and pharmacology of *Santalum album* L.: A review. *World Journal of Pharmaceutical Research*, *4*(10), 1842–1876. https://www.research-gate.net/publication/282638998_Phytochemistry_and_Pharmacology_of_Santalum_album_L_A_Review
	Schaefer, A. (2017, August 4). The health potential of sandalwood. *Healthline*. https://www.healthline.com/health/what-is-sandalwood#home-use
Saptaranga *Salacia chinensis*	Other names: *Saptarangi, Saptachakra, Ponkoranti, Chundan Kothala Himbutu Tea, Casearia esculenta* (Chinese salacia)
	Saptaranga is a woody shrub commonly found in India and Sri Lanka. There are different species (*S. reticulata, S. oblonga*). *Casearia* is a plant genus in the family Salicaceae.
	It contains salicinol which is a bioactive glucose-lowering compound ($\alpha\alpha$-glucosidase inhibitor).
	The stem and roots are used to treat diabetes. It prevents the absorption of sugar from foods into the blood. It can lower the HbA1C levels.
	It is also to treat obesity, asthma, gonorrhea, arthritis, and menstrual problems.
	Overall, it is safe. Side effects can include nausea, diarrhea, gas, and belching.
	WebMD. (n.d.). SALACIA: Overview, uses, side effects, precautions, interactions, dosing and reviews. *WebMD.Com*. https://www.webmd.com/vitamins/ai/ingredientmono-1106/salacia
Scallion *Allium fistulosum*	Scallion contains antioxidants including flavonoids and polyphenols. It is rich in fiber, minerals (iron and copper), and vitamins (K, B9, and C). It also contains calcium, manganese, potassium, vitamins A and B2. The vitamin K present helps in strengthening bones and lowers the risk of osteoporosis.
	It has anticancer, antiviral, antidiabetic, and antibacterial properties.
	Scallion helps in weight loss, lowering cholesterol levels, and lowering dysmenorrhea (menstrual pain). It is also used in treating headaches, colds, indigestion, and insomnia.
	It promotes production of rhodopsin, a protein vital to the retina and it prevents the chances of night blindness and also sharpens vision. It also helps improve the skin health and prevents wrinkling of skin and early aging. It improves the immune system as well.
	People who are allergic to onions are also allergic to scallions. They may experience symptoms such as vomiting, shortness of breath, itching, wheezing, or skin irritation. Medications like blood thinner or Warfarin should not be taken alongside scallion.
	Health Benefits Editors. (2018, May 14). Scallion facts, health benefits and nutritional value. *HealthBenefitstimes.com*. https://www.healthbenefitstimes.com/scallion/
Sea coconut Lodoicea maldivica	The active ingredient present in sea coconut is sterols which help boost the immune system, protects the body from infections, and lowers the risk of cardiovascular diseases.
	It has antidiabetic, aphrodisiac, hypertensive, and carminative properties.
	Sea coconut helps in improving the lungs, relieves coughing, and cools the body. It is effective against cholera, jaundice, paralysis, heart disease, and vomiting. It enhances the working of the digestive system, preventing heart diseases, and reducing fever. It is also commonly used for treating hyperdipsia, colic, edema, and acute diarrhea, as well as is used as an antidote in opium and aconite poisoning.
	Sea coconut may cause allergic reactions in certain people with symptoms such as sore throat, headache, fever, headache, rash, nausea, or vomiting.
	Herbpathy.com. (n.d.). Sea coconut herb uses, benefits, cures, side effects, nutrients. *Herbpathy*. https://herbpathy.com/Uses-and-Benefits-of-Sea-Coconut-Cid4956
Sesame seed or oil *Sesamum indicum*	Sesame seed is rich in bioactive compounds including lignans, tocopherol homologues, phenols, and phytosterols. Sesamol and sesamin, two compounds present, have antioxidant, antibacterial, and anticancer properties. It has high amounts of copper (163% of the DV), manganese, and calcium. It contains other minerals including magnesium, iron, zinc, and phosphorus. It is also a good source of dietary fiber and B-vitamins (B1, B3, and B6). Sesame seeds are used to make tahini paste, which is used to make hummus.
	There are three types:
	Brown (commonest), black, and white sesame seeds. The seeds are oil-rich. It contains polyunsaturated omega-3 and omega-6 fatty acids which are heart protective.
	The seeds and oil also have antioxidant, antimutagenic, antihepatotoxic, antiinflammatory, chemopreventive, and antiaging properties.

Ingredients	Mechanism of Action and Health Benefits
	Sesame seed can help lower blood sugar levels, cholesterol levels, and blood pressure. It may also help relieve arthritic pain, improve thyroid health, and hormone balance during menopause.
	Consumption of too much sesame seeds can cause bowel obstructions as it contains a high content of fiber. It may also cause ischemia or perforation for people with bowel obstructions.
	McCulloch, M. (2019, February 13). 15 health and nutrition benefits of sesame seeds. *Healthline*. https://www.healthline.com/nutrition/sesame-seeds
	WebMD Editors. (2020, December 9). Health benefits of sesame seeds. *WebMD*. https://www.webmd.com/diet/health-benefits-sesame-seeds#1-2
Shankhpushpi	Other names: *Clitoria ternatea (Butterfly pea flower, Blue pea flower, Asian pigeonwings, bluebellvine, Gokarna, Aparajitha, Sangu poo), Convolvulus pluricaulis*
	There is some controversy if *Shankhpushpi* is *Convolvulus pluricaulis* or *Clitoria ternatea*. In Ayurveda, *Shankhpushpi* is largely *Convolvulus pluricaulis*, although it also includes three other varieties, i.e., *Clitorea ternatea, Evolvulus alsinoides*, and *Canscora decussata. Evolvulus alsinoides* is the best source of Shankhpushpi as a nerve tonic.
	Clitoria ternatea is largely used for Indian puja or it can be used as a natural food coloring.
	Shankhpushpi contains many bioactive phytoconstituents, such as alkaloids (convolamine, convoline, convolidine, and convolvine), flavonoid (kaempferol), and phenolics (scopoletin and β-sitosterol). Its antiinflammatory activities are due to the presence of convolamine and convolvine. Convoline is responsible for its antiepileptic property. Its antifungal, antiallergic, antiaging, and hypouricemic activities are from scopoletin.
	The natural tranquilizers (glycosides, flavonoids, and alkaloids) calm the mind, reduce mental fatigue, restlessness, and promote sleep. It is an alkaloid, has GABA-mimetic or GABA-agonist properties, reduces the stress hormones, and also inhibits acetylcholinesterase activity. It is a nootropic herb.
	It has anxiolytic, antipyretic, anticonvulsant, and antinociceptive properties. Shankhpushpi is a brain tonic and improves intellect and memory. It is used in treating anxiety and different types of psychotic problems like depression and dementia.
	It has diuretic actions.
	It is also beneficial in improving digestion and treating symptoms of abdominal pain, abdominal distension, ulcerative colitis, and IBS.
	It is a uterus tonic, strengthens the uterus and prevents miscarriages.
	Due to its strong antioxidant effects, it can reduce the risk of heart-related problems (heart attacks, heart blocks, and blood clots) and lower cholesterol levels. It can also be used in treating various skin infections (like psoriasis, eczema, acne, and sunburn) and also UTIs.
	Side effects include diarrhea and hypotension.
	Balkrishna, A., Thakur, P., & Varshney, A. (2020). Phytochemical profile, pharmacological attributes and medicinal properties of *Convolvulus prostratus*—a cognitive enhancer herb for the management of neurodegenerative etiologies. *Frontiers in Pharmacology, 11*, 171. https://doi.org/10.3389/fphar.2020.00171
	Basu, S. (2020, September 15). Shankhpushpi: Benefits, uses, dosage, formulations, and side effects. *Netmeds*. https://www.netmeds.com/health-library/post/shankhpushpi-benefits-uses-dosage-formulations-and-side-effects
	Sethiya, N. K., Nahata, A., Singh, P. K., & Mishra, S. (2019). Neuropharmacological evaluation on four traditional herbs used as nervine tonic and commonly available as Shankhpushpi in India. *Journal of Ayurveda and Integrative Medicine, 10*(1), 25–31. https://doi.org/10.1016/j.jaim.2017.08.012
Shatavari *Asparagus racemosus*	Other names: *Shatawari, Satavar*
	Shatavari means "Curer of a hundred diseases" in Sanskrit.
	Shatavari contains steroidal saponins (shatavarin I–VI), flavonoids, polycyclic alkaloids, and sterols. The three main antioxidants are racemofuran, racemosol, and asparagamine A. It contains phytoestrogens.
	It also contains zinc, manganese, copper, and cobalt. It also contains trace amounts of calcium, magnesium, potassium, and selenium.
	It prevents kidney stone formation especially oxalate stones via increasing magnesium concentration in the urine.
	It promotes female reproductive health. It eases PMS and menopause symptoms. It promotes fertility and breast milk production. It helps with PCOS and can reduce uterine bleeding.
	It is an adaptogen and can help with stress, anxiety, dementia, and memory problems.
	It is used for treating upset stomach (dyspepsia), constipation, and stomach ulcers. It is also used for fluid retention, pain, cancer, diarrhea, bronchitis, tuberculosis, and diabetes.

Ingredients	Mechanism of Action and Health Benefits
	Shatavari is also used to ease alcohol withdrawal.
	Possible side effects include rashes, fast heart rate, itchy eyes and skin, difficult breathing, and dizziness. It should not be used in estrogen-sensitive tumors.
	Alok, S., Jain, S. K., Verma, A., Kumar, M., Mahor, A., & Sabharwal, M. (2013). Plant profile, phytochemistry and pharmacology of *Asparagus racemosus* (Shatavari): a review. *Asian Pacific Journal of Tropical Disease, 3*(3), 242–251. https://doi.org/10.1016/s2222-1808(13)60049-3
	Cadman, B. (2018, June 6). What are the health benefits of shatavari? *MedicalNewsToday*. https://www.medicalnewstoday.com/articles/322043
	Brennan, D. (2021, May 28). Are there health benefits of Shatavari powder? *WebMD*. https://www.webmd.com/vitamins-and-supplements/are-there-health-benefits-of-shatavari-powder
Shikakai *Acacia concinna*	Other names: *Cheeyakai, Shikai, Soap pod*
	Shikakai is used as a hair care product. The pods, leaves, and bark contain antioxidants, saponins, and vitamins (A, D, E, K, and C).
	It has antibacterial, antifungal, and antioxidant effects.
	It promotes hair growth, cleanses and nourishes the hair, prevents graying, adds shine, reduces hair loss, and removes dandruff.
	It is used as a shampoo, moisturizer, and scalp mask.
	Side effects may include eye or skin irritation.
	Basu, S. (2020, August 10). Shikakai—Incredible uses of this potent Ayurvedic herb for hair and skin. *Netmeds*. https://www.netmeds.com/health-library/post/shikakai-traditional-uses-of-this-potent-ayurvedic-herb
Shilajit	Other name: *Mineral pitch*
	Shilajit (Mumiju) is a black-brown sticky material which is produced naturally from the degradation of plants by bacteria in the high mountain rocks. It contains fulvic acid (which has strong antioxidant powers), humic acid, humins, 20% minerals (there are more than 84 minerals especially selenium), 15% protein, 5% lipids, and 5% steroids and alkaloids.
	It has neuroprotective, strong antioxidant, and antiinflammatory properties. It can decrease the tau proteins in AD and improve mitochondrial function in chronic fatigue syndrome (CFS). It can regulate the estrogen and progesterone hormones so that regular periods occur. It also has antiaging properties.
	It increases testosterone and dehydroepiandrosterone levels. It can boost libido and is used in erectile dysfunction and male infertility.
	It should not be used in iron overload conditions like thalassemia or hemochromatosis. Side effects include possible allergic reactions and contamination of the shilajit with other metals or microbes.
	Higuera, V. (2019, March 8). *Benefits of Shilajit*. Healthline. https://www.healthline.com/health/shilajit
Shilapushpa *Didymocarpus pedicellata*	Other name: *Stone flower*
	Shilapushpa contains several bioactive constituents including polyphenols (didymocarpin, chalcones, and pedicin), flavones, and polyterpenes (didymocarpene and didymocarpenol).
	It is a diuretic. It has antimicrobial, analgesic, antioxidant, antiinflammatory, and nephroprotective properties.
	It regulates calcium absorption and cleanses the urinary tract. It is used to treat renal disorders including urinary tract stones (urolithiasis), kidney stones, UTI, and gallstones.
	It is also effective for liver disorder, ulcers, and hyperlipidemia.
	Overall, it is safe. Side effects may include headache, nausea, or dizziness.
	Chaudhary, A. K. (2021). Shilapushpa. *Preserva Wellness*. https://www.preservawellness.com/herbs/shilapushp
	Mishra, P., Chaudhary, N., & Ranjan, A. (2021, January 27). Stone flower: Benefits, precautions and dosage. *1mg*. https://www.1mg.com/ayurveda/stone-flower-231
Snake gourd *Trichosanthes cucumerina*	Other names: *Patola, Pudalangai, Padwal, Chichinga, Serpent gourd*
	Snake gourd is rich in compounds including flavonoids, carotenoids, phenolic acids, and soluble and insoluble dietary fibers. It contains high levels of minerals (potassium, phosphorus, sodium, magnesium, and zinc), and vitamins (A and E).
	It also has medicinal properties such as antidiabetic, antibacterial, antiinflammatory, anthelmintic, antifebrile, gastroprotective, and antioxidant activities. It also has antimicrobial and antioxidant properties.

Ingredients	Mechanism of Action and Health Benefits
	Snake gourd is used for treating diabetes, headache, alopecia, fever, abdominal tumors, bilious, boils, acute colic diarrhea, hematuria, jaundice, and skin allergy.
	Excessive consumption of snake gourd may be harmful and toxic due to the trace minerals that are present.
	Liyanage, R., Nadeeshani, H., Jayathilake, C., Visvanathan, R., & Wimalasiri, S. (2016). Comparative analysis of nutritional and bioactive properties of aerial parts of snake gourd (*Trichosanthes cucumerina* Linn.). *International Journal of Food Science*, *2016*, 1–7. https://doi.org/10.1155/2016/8501637
Soap nuts *Sapindus mukorossi*	Other names: *Reetha/Ritha, Indian soapberry*
	Reetha is rich in saponins, alkaloids, flavonoids, and tannins. It also contains several vitamins (A, D, E, and K) and contains fatty acids (including oleic acid, tridecanoic acid, palmitic acid, and stearic acid).
	It has antimicrobial, insecticidal, and antiinflammatory properties.
	It helps moisturize the skin, improves skin health, and can be used for skin disorders (including acne, rashes, psoriasis, and eczema).
	It promotes hair growth, prevents hair fall, and can cure scalp infections and dandruff.
	It is used as an ingredient in skin and hair products.
	It can be used for snake and scorpion bites.
	Overall, it is safe. Direct contact with eyes can cause swollen eyes. Allergic reactions include rashes, itchiness, and other skin or hair problems.
	Deka, M., Soni, D., & Garcha, S. (2019, September 11). Reetha: Benefits, precautions and dosage. *1mg*. https://www.1mg.com/ayurveda/reetha-46
South Africa leaf *Veronia amygdalina*	Other name: *African Bitter Leaf*
	South Africa leaf is rich in flavonoids (luteolin, luteolin 7-O-glucosides, and luteolin 7-O-glucuronide), steroid glycosides (vernoniosides A, B, A1, A2, A3, B2, B3, and A4), sesquiterpene lactones, quercetin, caffeoylquinic acid, and β-sitosterol. Vernolide and vernodalol (which are sesquiterpene lactones) have antimicrobial activity against bacteria and fungus.
	African bitter leaf also contains fiber, vitamins (A, C, and E), and minerals (magnesium, calcium, potassium, and phosphorus).
	It has antioxidant, antiinflammatory, and antimalarial properties. The leaves also have antiallergic effects that can prevent atopic dermatitis.
	South African leaf is used in the treatment of fevers, STDs, constipation, and cough. It regulates blood sugar (via the flavonoids) and blood pressure and lowers cholesterol, hence it can prevent heart disease and reduce stroke risk.
	Bitter leaves can prevent cancer including leukemia. It is also used to treat indigestion and obesity. It aids in the detoxification process in the body and is a general tonic. It can also boost fertility.
	The leaves are considered safe for consumption and are considered nontoxic. However, large doses can cause diarrhea or purge.
	Alara, O. R., Abdurahman, N. H., Abdul Mudalip, S. K., & Olalere, O. A. (2017). Phytochemical and pharmacological properties of *Vernonia amygdalina*: a review. *Journal of Chemical Engineering and Industrial Biotechnology*, *2*(1), 80–96. https://doi.org/10.15282/jceib.v2i1.3871
Spade flower *Hybanthus enneaspermus*	Other names: *Pink ladies slipper, Orithal thamarai, Ratan purush*
	Spade flower is a shrub. It contains phenols, flavonoids, tannins, terpenes, anthraquinones, and saponins.
	It has diuretic, antioxidant, antibacterial, and antidiabetic properties.
	It is often used as a male tonic and is an aphrodisiac. It can increase testosterone levels.
	It has diuretic properties and is used in UTI. The leaves and stems have demulcent properties.
	It can also treat IBS and high blood sugar.
	Side effects include low blood sugar. It cannot be taken during pregnancy.
Spinach *Spinacia oleracea*	Spinach contains several active compounds including lutein, kaempferol, nitrates, quercetin, and zeaxanthin. It is rich in fiber, vitamins (A, C, and K1), and minerals (iron and calcium). It also contains other vitamins and minerals such as potassium, magnesium, and vitamins B6, B9, and E. The antioxidants (lutein, zeaxanthin, kaempferol, quercetin, and vitamin C) help reduce the risk of chronic diseases and cancer. Vitamin K present improves the calcium absorbance and reduces the probability of bone fracture.

Ingredients	Mechanism of Action and Health Benefits
	It has antiinflammatory, antihypertensive, and antidiabetic properties.
	Spinach helps improve skin and hair growth. The zeaxanthin and lutein help in improving the eyesight and reduce the probability of blindness. With its high fiber and water content spinach can prevent constipation and improve the digestive system function.
	It contains calcium and oxalates which can help the formation of kidney stones. Thus, spinach consumption should be limited by people who are at a high risk of developing kidney stones. Spinach is high in vitamin K1, which can interfere with blood thinners, such as warfarin.
	Gunnars, K. (2019, May 14). Spinach 101: Nutrition facts and health benefits. *Healthline*. https://www.healthline.com/nutrition/foods/spinach
Sweet potato *Ipomoea batatas*	Other name: *Sakkargand, Batata, Camote, Kamote, Apichu, Kumara, Keledek*
	Sweet potato is a root vegetable that is cultivated. The root tuber and the young leaf shoots are edible when cooked. There are many varieties and colors (orange, white, purple, red, and gold/yellow). The orange variety is the commonest and has the highest amount of β-carotene and the purple ones have more anthocyanins. It is rich in vitamins (A, C, and B6), magnesium, manganese, zinc, and fiber.
	The β-carotene (provitamin A) has antioxidant actions and maintains good vision.
	Although it is a high starch carbohydrate tuber, it has an overall low GI and is suitable in diabetics. It can also lower insulin resistance. It can help with obesity and also lower cancer risk.
	It is high in oxalates.
	Sruthi, M. (2021, October 12). What do sweet potatoes do for your body? 7 benefits, side effects. *MedicineNet*. https://www.medicinenet.com/what_do_sweet_potatoes_do_for_your_body/article.htm
Tamarind *Tamarindus indica*	Other name: *Imli, Puli or Pulee*
	Tamarind contains bioactive compounds including phenolic constituents, flavonoids, anthocyanins, and carotenoids. It is rich in B vitamins (B1, B2, and B3), minerals (magnesium, potassium, iron, calcium, and phosphorus), amino acids, and fiber. It also contains trace amounts of vitamins (C, K, B6, B9, and B5) and minerals (copper and selenium).
	Various acids including tartrate, malate (laxative effects) mainly and citrate, succinate, and quinic acid are present in the tamarind pulp. Others include reducing sugars, protein pectin, cellulose, and fiber.
	Tamarind pulp has carminative, digestive, laxative, and expectorant actions. It also acts as a blood tonic.
	It has antioxidant, antimicrobial, and antiinflammatory properties. Another compound present called lupeol (a triterpene) has antibacterial effects. It also has antifungal, antiviral, and antibacterial activities.
	The phenolic compounds can help regulate cholesterol levels. Its high magnesium content helps lower blood pressure and has antiinflammatory and antidiabetic effects.
	Tamarind is commonly used to treat diarrhea, constipation, fever, and peptic ulcers. It is also used for wound healing. It may also help lower blood sugar, weight loss, and reverse fatty liver disease.
	There are no known adverse side effects of tamarind.
	Jennings, K. (2016, July 20). What is tamarind? A tropical fruit with health benefits. *Healthline*. https://www.healthline.com/nutrition/tamarind#TOC_TITLE_HDR_2
	Rana, M., & Sharma, P. (2018). Proximate and phytochemical screening of the seed and pulp of *Tamarind indica*. *Journal of Medicinal Plants Studies*, 6(2), 111–115. https://www.plantsjournal.com/archives/2018/vol6issue2/PartB/6-2-18-823.pdf
	Muzaffar, K. (2017). Tamarind: A mini-review. *MOJ Food Processing & Technology*, 5(3), 296–297. https://doi.org/10.15406/mojfpt.2017.05.00126
Tomato *Solanum lycopersicum*	Tomato belongs to the nightshade family. It contains several phytochemicals including carotenoids (lycopene, β-carotene), flavonoids (naringenin), and phenolic acids (chlorogenic acid). It is rich in vitamins (C, K, and folate), minerals (potassium), and insoluble fibers (mainly cellulose, lignin, and hemicellulose). It also has high water content. A small amount of oxalate is also present in tomatoes but this amount does not predispose to oxalate stones.
	It has antioxidant and antiinflammatory properties.
	It can improve heart health and decrease the risk of stroke and heart attacks. It can also lower LDL cholesterol.
	Tomatoes are beneficial to skin health and help protect against sunburn. It also supports eye and lung health.

Ingredients	Mechanism of Action and Health Benefits
	It may prevent cancers in the lung, breast, prostate, and stomach.
	Overall, it is safe. Side effects may include allergic reactions. Green immature tomatoes have slightly higher solanine (a toxic alkaloid).
	Bjarnadottir, A. (2019, March 25). Tomatoes 101: Nutrition facts and health benefits. *Healthline*. https://www.healthline.com/nutrition/foods/tomatoes
	Ware, M. (2017, September 25). Everything you need to know about tomatoes. *MedicalNewsToday*. https://www.medicalnewstoday.com/articles/273031#risks
Trikatu	Trikatu is an Ayurvedic blend composed of three ingredients: long pepper (*Piper longum*), black pepper (*Piper nigrum*), and ginger (*Zingiber officinalis*) in equal amounts. These three herbs work together to ensure healthy digestion. It reduces kapha in allergies by increasing the digestive fire.
	The bioactive compounds present include vanillic acid, ferulic acid, gallic acid, piperine, and 6-gingerol give trikatu antiinflammatory properties.
	It has antioxidant, hepatoprotective, antimicrobial, anthelmintic, and antiarthritis properties. It may also have anticancer activities.
	This herbal combination alleviates gas and bloating, improves digestion, and metabolism. It also promotes weight loss. It liquifies phlegm and reduces coughs and colds. It also relieves the symptoms of rheumatoid arthritis such as joint pain, swelling, redness, and stiffness of the joints. It is also used to treat gout. It can help lower cholesterol levels and reduce the risk of heart diseases. It strengthens the immune system.
	It should not be taken if there is a history of acid reflux, gastritis, or during pregnancy.
	Sewlani, S. S., & Samuel, J. (2017, July 14). Top 10 uses of Trikatu for good health. *Medindia*. https://www.medindia.net/dietandnutrition/top-10-uses-of-trikatu-for-good-health.htm
Triphala	Triphala is a polyherbal formulation made of three plants: amla (*Phyllanthus emblica*), bibhitaki (*Terminalia bellirica*), and haritaki (*Terminalia chebula*). It contains flavonoids, polyphenols, tannins, and saponins. It is also rich in vitamins C and E.
	It has antiinflammatory, antibacterial, antimicrobial, antifungal, and antioxidant properties.
	Triphala helps in lowering cholesterol levels. It may reduce the risk of cancer and aid in weight loss. It can help to dry sebum and clean pores in acne.
	Triphala has mild laxative effects that can cause GI side effects, including gas, stomach upset, cramps, and diarrhea. It should not be taken with other medications such as antifungal, antipsychotic, anticonvulsant, and antidepressant drugs.
	Wong, C., & Kroner, A. (200–12-05). The health benefits of Triphala. *Verywell Health*. https://www.verywellhealth.com/triphala-what-should-i-know-about-it-89590
Trivrit *Operculina turpethum*	Other name: *Turpeth*
	Trivrit contains glycosides (scopoletin, turpethinic acids [A–E]), terpenoids (lupeol, betulin), alkaloids, tannins, flavonoids, saponins, steroids, coumarins, and operculinosides A–D.
	In Ayurveda, it is used to treat pitta and kapha dominant disorders and also as part of purgation (virechana) in Panchakarma treatment.
	The root powder has laxative, antiinflammatory, analgesic, antihelminthic, and antiarthritic effects.
	Turpeth helps to relieve constipation, gas and bloating and helps in IBS. It also can treat fevers, anorexia, hepatosplenomegaly, intoxication, hemorrhoids, fistula, anemia, obesity, worm infestation, pruritus, ulcers/wounds, and other skin disorders.
	Side effects include gastric irritation, abdominal pain, severe diarrhea, and dizziness.
	Health Benefits Times. (2019, July 17). Turpeth facts and health benefits. *HealthBenefitstimes.com*. https://www.healthbenefitstimes.com/operculina-turpethum/
Tulsi *Ocimum tenuiflorum*	Other names: *Holy basil, Ocimum sanctum, Tulasi, Thulasi*
	Read more under *"Basil"*
	The genus Ocimum includes several species of basil. Holy basil or Tulsi is one of them. It is a sacred herb. There are many varieties of Tulsi but the three common ones are
	• Rama Tulsi (*O. sanctum = O. tenuiflorum or green leaf tulsi or Lakshmi tulsi*).
	• Krishna Tulsi (also called *O. sanctum or purple leaf tulsi or Shyama tulsi*). This variety is most potent and with more medicinal use.
	• Vana Tulsi (*O. gratissimum*).

Ingredients	Mechanism of Action and Health Benefits
	The bioactive compounds present in tulsi include terpenes (eugenol and camphor), ursolic and rosmarinic acids, flavonoid (apigenin), lutein, and ocimumosides A and B. It contains vitamins (A, C, and K) and minerals (zinc, iron, manganese, and calcium).
	It has analgesic and antimicrobial properties from the presence of eugenol (it has a clove taste) and camphor. Camphor also gives antibacterial properties. Ursolic and rosmarinic acids are compounds with antioxidant, antiinflammatory, and antiaging properties. Apigenin is responsible for helping the body remove waste at the cellular level. Lutein is an antioxidant carotenoid that can improve eye health. Ocimumosides A and B that are present help reduce stress and balance the neurotransmitters serotonin and dopamine.
	It also has expectorant, antiemetic, antipyretic, stress reducing (adaptogen), antiasthmatic, hypoglycemic, hepatoprotective, hypotensive, hypolipidemic, and immunomodulatory actions.
	It is used in the treatment of different types of poisoning, stomachache, common colds, headaches, malaria, and heart disease. Basil can aid in the expulsion of kidney stones.
	There is a risk of low sperm count and reduced FSH and LH levels.
	Holy basil should be avoided by pregnant women or trying to get pregnant because it may affect reproductive capacity. It should also be used with caution by people taking blood-sugar-lowering medications and blood thinners. Eugenol present may cause liver damage, nausea, diarrhea, rapid heartbeat, or convulsions.
	Wong, C., & Bull, M. (2020, November 23). The health benefits of tulsi. *Verywell Health*. https://www.verywellhealth.com/benefits-of-tulsi-89591
	Yamani, H. A., Pang, E. C., Mantri, N., & Deighton, M. A. (2016). Antimicrobial activity of tulsi (*Ocimum tenuiflorum*) essential oil and their major constituents against three species of bacteria. *Frontiers in Microbiology*, 7, 681. https://doi.org/10.3389/fmicb.2016.00681
Turmeric *(Curcuma longa)*	Other names: *Haluthi, Manjal*
	Turmeric contains curcuminoids, of which curcumin is the main active ingredient. Others include demethoxy curcumin and bisdemethoxy curcumin. They have antiinflammatory and antioxidant activities and also can increase bile solubility. It contains fiber, vitamins (B6 and C), and minerals such as manganese, iron, phosphorus, and potassium.
	It can also reduce the risk of heart disease.
	It may have anticancer properties, especially against pancreatic cancer, prostate cancer, and multiple myeloma. It can be used in the treatment of depression.
	Its antioxidant properties can benefit fertility-related conditions as in endometriosis and PCOS.
	Turmeric may also be used for hay fever, high cholesterol, nonalcoholic fatty liver disease, gallstones, osteoarthritis, AD, and itching.
	Overall, it is safe. Mild side effects include stomach upset, nausea, dizziness, or diarrhea which are due to high doses.
	Gunnars, K., & Warwick, K. W. (2021, May 7). 10 proven health benefits of turmeric and curcumin. *Healthline*. https://www.healthline.com/nutrition/top-10-evidence-based-health-benefits-of-turmeric
	Ware, M. (2018, May 24). Everything you need to know about turmeric. *MedicalNewsToday*. https://www.medicalnewstoday.com/articles/306981
Turnip *Brassica rapa* subsp. *rapa*	Turnips are rich in glucosinolates, flavonoids (anthocyanins), minerals (including calcium, magnesium, potassium, and phosphorus) and vitamins (C, A, K, and folate). It contains protein and fiber and has a low GI. The glucosinolates break down into isothiocyanates and indoles which have antiinflammatory properties.
	It has antioxidant, antibacterial, and hepatoprotective properties.
	The glucosinolates present decreases the risk of certain cancers (including rectal, colon, and lung).
	It helps lower blood sugar, blood pressure, LDL cholesterol, and triglyceride levels. It can prevent constipation and also aid in weight loss.
	It can help dissolve kidney stones.
	It can be used to treat arthritis and improve bone formation.
	Overall, it is safe. Overconsumption can lead to clotting tendency, muscle cramps, muscle stiffness, and rapid heartbeat.
	Bonvissuto, D. (2019, September 20). Health benefits of turnips. *WebMD*. https://www.webmd.com/diet/benefits-turnips#2.
	Lang, A. (2019, November 22). All you need to know about turnips. *Healthline*. https://www.healthline.com/nutrition/turnip-nutrition

Ingredients	Mechanism of Action and Health Benefits
Udeechya *Pavonia odorata*	Other names: *Udichya, Hrivera, Hribera, Balaka, Sugandabala* Udeechya contains alkaloids, flavonoids, and essential oil. It balances pitta and kapha doshas. It has antimicrobial, antiinflammatory, antipyretic, demulcent, calminative, diuretic, and cooling properties. It can be used to treat menorrhagia and can stop bleeding due to nose bleeds or GI bleeding. It also helps nausea and diarrhea. It can be applied on herpes skin lesions which have a burning sensation. TabletWise.com. (2020, September 28). Udeechya. *Tabletwise.Net*. https://www.tabletwise.net/medicine/udeechya
Vacha *Acorus calamus Linn*	Other name: *Sweet flag, Vasambu, Bach or Gorabach* Vacha contains more than 145 phytonutrients including phenylpropanoids (asarone and eugenol), sterols, triterpene glycosides, triterpenoid saponins, sesquiterpenoids, monoterpenes, and alkaloids. It has anticonvulsant, antidepressant, antihypertensive, antispasmodic, antiinflammatory, immunomodulatory, cardioprotective, anticancer, and antiobesity effects. Sweet flag is used in the treatment of neurological, GI, respiratory, metabolic, kidney, and liver disorders. It is also highly effective for skin diseases (eczema) and improves skin. It calms and relaxes the brain to reduce stress and improve sleep quality and memory. Vacha is used in the treatment of hallucinations, cough, headache, dyspepsia, dysentery, and diarrhea. It is also used for detoxification and toothaches. Sweet flags may cause sleepiness when taken with other medications and can cause hypotension. It can cause allergic reactions. Certain varieties of vacha contain carcinogenic compounds. Sharma, V., Sharma, R., Gautam, D., Kuca, K., Nepovimova, E., & Martins, N. (2020). Role of Vacha (*Acorus calamus* Linn.) in neurological and metabolic disorders: evidence from ethnopharmacology, phytochemistry, pharmacology and clinical study. *Journal of Clinical Medicine, 9*(4), 1176. https://doi.org/10.3390/jcm9041176
Varuna *Crataeva nurvala*	Other names: *Mavilinkam, three-leaf caper* It contains alkaloids, flavonoids, sterols, triterpenes, saponins, glucosinolates, and tannins. It has strong diuretic properties. It has anticrystallization and antilithogenic effects. It is also a good blood purifier. It has antiinflammatory and some mild laxative properties. It can be used in gout to reduce joint pain and inflammation. It is beneficial in urolithiasis (kidney stones), UTIs, prostate enlargement, and overactive bladder. It can also reduce the cysts in polycystic ovarian disease. It can regulate menstrual cycles and also dissolve fibroids. Overall, it is safe. Electrolyte imbalances should be monitored if also on modern diuretics for hypertension. Khattar, V., & Wal, A. (20120). Utilities of Crataeva nurvala. *International Journal of Pharmacy and Pharmaceutical Sciences*, 4(4), 21–26. https://www.researchgate.net/publication/287607900_Utilities_of_crataeva_nurvala
Vegetable oil	Vegetable oil is extracted from various seeds, grains, nuts, and fruits. Most common ones are corn, canola, olive, sunflower, soybean, and peanut oil. They are rich in vitamins (A, D, E, and K). Overall, it is safe. Excess consumption can lead to hyperlipidemia. WebMD Editorial Contributors. (2021, April 6). Health benefits of vegetable oil. *WebMD*. https://www.webmd.com/diet/health-benefits-of-vegetable-oil#1
Veld grape *Cissus quadrangularis*	Other name: *Asthisamharaka, Asthisamhari* Veld grape is a creeper plant. It is rich in tannins, carotenoids, and phenols. It also contains a high content of calcium and vitamin C. It has antiinflammatory and antiworm properties. It builds bones, prevents fractures and osteoporosis. It promotes wound healing. It supports digestive health, treats gastric ulcers, bleeding piles and can help with weight loss. It relieves menstrual cramps and decreases menopausal symptoms. It can regulate blood sugar, lower triglycerides and blood pressure and support heart health. Overall, it is safe. Health Benefits Times. (2020, January 24). Health benefits of Veld Grape. *HealthBenefitstimes.com*. https://www.healthbenefitstimes.com/veld-grape/

Ingredients	Mechanism of Action and Health Benefits
Vidari kanda *Ipomoea digitata* *or* *Pueraria tuberosa*	Other name: *Giant potato* Vidari kanda is a wild yam. There are several varieties. It contains β-sitosterol, reisin glycoside, and taraxerol. It is a rejuvenating and nutritional tonic. It has antiaging properties. It supports male and female reproductive functions. It increases strength, vitality, virility, and fertility. It is an aphrodisiac. It improves sperm quantity and quality. It maintains regular menses and promotes lactation. Side effects include gastric upset, reduced blood clotting allergy, and reactions. Rauniyar, N., & Srivastava, D. (2020). Ipomoea digitata: A therapeutic boon from nature to mankind. *The Journal of Indian Botanical Society*, *100*(3 & 4), 185–191. https://doi.org/10.5958/2455-7218.2020.00039.X WebMD Editors. (n.d.). Kudzu. *WebMD*. https://www.webmd.com/vitamins/ai/ingredientmono-750/kudzu
Vijaysar *Pterocarpus marsupium*	Other names: *Malabar kino, Indian Kino Tree, Pitasara* Vijaysar has many active compounds, some which include alkaloids, carpusin, epicatechin, liquiritigenin, beta-eudesmol, propterol, tannins, resins, etc. All parts of the plant can be used. The bark has antiglycemic, antiinflammatory, and antioxidant properties. It manages blood sugar levels by preventing the damage of pancreatic cells, decreases sugar cravings, and also reduces excess fat. It promotes digestive health, increases mucin, and protects the stomach and intestines from ulcers. It has antiflatulent properties and reduces gas and bloating. It helps in IBS and ulcerative colitis. It has antibacterial, antifungal, and antiviral properties. It can treat skin inflammatory conditions and bleeding disorders. The juice from the leaves can be applied to wounds as dressing or to treat dental or gum problems. It purifies the blood and removes toxins. It also has antiaging properties. Poultices can relieve the pain in arthritis. Overall, it is a safe herb. It should not be used in constipation. Basu, S. (2020, July 15). Vijaysar: Benefits, uses, formulation, ingredients, dosage and side effects. *Netmeds*. https://www.netmeds.com/health-library/post/vijaysar-benefits-uses-formulation-ingredients-dosage-and-side-effects
Watercress *Nasturtium officinale*	Watercress is a cruciferous vegetable that grows in water and has floating roots. It is a superfood and contains bioactive compounds including carotenoids, glucosinolates, and polyphenols (flavonoids, phenolic acids, and proanthocyanidins). It is rich in vitamins (K, C, A, B1, B2, and B6) and minerals (manganese, calcium, magnesium, potassium, and phosphorus). It also contains alpha-lipoic acid, dietary nitrate, proteins, and fiber. It is low in calories. Watercress has antioxidant and antiinflammatory properties. The glucosinolates are activated to isothiocyanates (which includes sulforaphane) that protect against cancer. It can lower blood pressure (from the magnesium, potassium, calcium, and nitrate content), regulate blood sugar (from ALA), and support bone health (from vitamin K, calcium, and phosphorus). Overall, it is safe. It can interact with oral anticoagulants. Groves, M. (2018, August 6). 10 impressive health benefits of watercress. *Healthline*. https://www.healthline.com/nutrition/watercress-benefits#TOC_TITLE_HDR_4 Klimek-Szczykutowicz, M., Dziurka, M., Blažević, I., Ðulović, A., Granica, S., Korona-Glowniak, I., et al. (2020). Phytochemical and biological activity studies on *Nasturtium officinale* (Watercress) microshoot cultures grown in RITA® temporary immersion systems. *Molecules*, *25*(22), 5257. https://doi.org/10.3390/molecules25225257 Ware, M. (2019, November 4). *What to know about watercress*. *MedicalNewsToday*. https://www.medicalnewstoday.com/articles/285412
Garden cress	Other names: *Lepidium sativum* *Garden cress seeds: Halim or haleem seeds, Asaliya, Aashaliya* Garden cress is also a cruciferous herb but is grown rooted in the soil (unlike watercress). It is also used as a garnish or added to salads, soups, or sandwiches and has a similar flavor to watercress.

Ingredients	Mechanism of Action and Health Benefits
	Garden cress seeds or cress seeds are nutrient-rich with iron, folate, and antioxidant vitamins A, C, and E. It can treat anemia. Garden cress seeds act as an expectorant and helps with sore throat and cough.
	Bahl, P. M. (2021, January 30). A tiny treasure of nutrients, halim seeds can help you lose weight and gain immunity. *Health Shots*. https://www.healthshots.com/healthy-eating/superfoods/6-health-benefits-of-halim-seeds/
	RxList Editors. (2021, June 11). Garden Cress. *RxList*. https://www.rxlist.com/garden_cress/supplements.htm
Water lily *Nymphaea stellata*	Other names: *Indian blue water lily, "Blue lotus of India," Kumuda, Neel Kamal, Nilakamala, Kamala, Padma, Kumudinee, Allithamarai, Indivar*
	There are many varieties and colors of water lily. Blue is the commonest but there are also pink-, white-, and mauve-colored flowers. The *Nymphaea stellata* variety is widely used in Ayurvedic medicine. All parts of the plant can be used. It is a bitter and cooling plant which dispels heat and purges fire.
	Nymphayol is a steroid from the flower which has antidiabetic actions. It stimulates secretion of insulin in the pancreatic β-cells.
	The roots, flowers, and leaves have antiinflammatory, antidiabetic, antiaging, cardiotonic, diuretic, sedative, and aphrodisiac effects.
	It is used to treat diabetes, heart diseases, urinary tract and vaginal infections, indigestion, bleeding piles, chronic diarrhea, liver diseases, menorrhagia, infertility, cough, and sore throat.
	Maruga Raja, M., Sethiya, N., & Mishra, S. (2010). A comprehensive review on *Nymphaea stellata*: a traditionally used bitter. *Journal of Advanced Pharmaceutical Technology & Research, 1*(3), 311. https://doi.org/10.4103/0110-5558.72424
White Dammar *Vateria indica*	Other names: *Dhupa maram sarjakah or Swarjarasa, Piney varnish tree*
	The resin from the white dammar tree bark has astringent, expectorant, antibacterial, antioxidant, anthelmintic, and aphrodisiac properties.
	The oil from the seeds is used topically in rheumatic disorders.
	The resin of this tree can treat infected wounds, abscess, piles, and carbuncles. It can also treat cough, sore throat, bronchitis, and asthma.
	It helps to improve skin health (in acne and hyperpigmentation). It can treat urinary tract disorders.
	Side effects include allergic reactions.
	Mane, R. N., Gholave, A. R., & Yadav, S. R. (2020). Karyomorphology of a critically endangered species *Vateria indica* L. (Dipterocarpaceae) from India. *Cytologia, 85*(2), 123–126. https://doi.org/10.1508/cytologia.85.123
White gourd *Benincasa hispida*	Other names: *Ash gourd, Wax gourd, Winter melon, Petha, Neer Pooshnikka, Pooshnikai, Kushmanda*
	It is a large fruit i.e., white gourd and eaten as a vegetable. It is used for medicinal and religious purposes.
	The unripe fruit balances pitta. The mid-ripe fruit increases kapha. The old overripe fruit increases digestive power and helps increase digestive power.
	White gourd contains fiber, vitamins (A, B2, and C), and minerals (manganese, zinc, calcium, iron, phosphorus, and magnesium). It is also a good source of antioxidants (flavonoids and carotenoids).
	It has laxative, diuretic, digestive, sedative, and aphrodisiac properties.
	They protect the body against cell damage and certain conditions like type 2 diabetes and heart disease.
	Its high fiber and water content helps in digestion and weight loss. At the same time, it is an appetite stimulant, digestive, and tonic and can promote weight gain in the emaciated.
	The vitamins and minerals present help in hair growth, and reduce flakiness and dandruff on the scalp of hair.
	Ash gourd has detoxifying properties. It cleanses the bladder and removes urinary obstructions and kidney stones.
	It is also used on skin as a moisturizer, on sunburns, rashes, and dry skin. It can also be applied on abscesses, boils, pus, or carbuncles.

Ingredients	**Mechanism of Action and Health Benefits**
	White gourd may also be used for treating fever, jaundice, hyperthyroidism, ulcer, inflammation, and insomnia.
	It should not be consumed by people suffering from asthma, cold, or bronchitis. White gourd contains vital trace minerals and overconsumption of it may result in toxic levels of these metallic elements accumulating in the system.
	Bharat, D. (2021, July 2). Ash gourd: Health benefits, nutrition, uses for skin and hair, recipes, side effects. *Netmeds*. https://www.netmeds.com/health-library/post/ash-gourd-health-benefits-nutrition-uses-for-skin-and-hair-recipes-side-effects
	Petre, A., & Seitz, A. (2020, April 21). What is ash gourd? All you need to know. *Healthline*. https://www.healthline.com/nutrition/ash-gourd
Wood apple *Limonia acidissima*	Wood apple contains phenolic compounds, flavonoids, saponins, and phytosterols. It is rich in riboflavin and thiamin.
	It has antioxidant, antiinflammatory, laxative, cleansing, and detoxifying properties.
	It helps in digestive issues (gas and bloating, fatty liver, and weight loss).
	It supports kidney, heart, and liver health.
	Nutrition Vistas Team. (2018, June 16). 14 amazing benefits of wood apple. *Nutrition Vistas*. https://www.nutritionvistas.com/wood-apple-or-limonia-acidissima-health-benefits/

Chinese Natural Ingredients

Ingredients	**Mechanism of Action and Health Benefits**
Abalone shell *Haliotis diversicolor*	Other name: *Shi Jue Ming*
	Abalone is a large snail that belongs to the mollusc *(Haliotidae)* family. The meat is eaten as a food, and the shell contains calcium carbonate and other minerals (including zinc, magnesium, iron, copper, and chromium).
	It is cold in nature and salty. It covers the liver, kidney, and lung meridians. It calms the rising liver Yang, and clears heat.
	It can improve cataracts.
	It can remove phlegm.
	It can calm and tranquilize the mind. It can help to treat spasms, seizures, tremors, headache, dizziness, and anxiety.
	It is an assistant ingredient in Chinese polyherbal formulations.
	Me and Qi. (n.d.). Abalone shells. *meandqi.com*. https://www.meandqi.com/herb-database/abalone-shell
Agar agar *Gelidium corneum*	Other names: *Agar, China grass*
	Agar is a hydrocolloid that is mainly obtained from the cell walls of the red algae seaweed called *Gelidium* and *Gracilaria* (division Rhodophyta).
	Agar has a mixture of two polysaccharides, i.e., agarose and agaropectin. This red alga contains chlorophyll, red and blue phycoerythrins, carotenoids, lutein, and zeaxanthin. It is rich in fiber, vitamins (B2, B3, B9, and K), and minerals (magnesium, iron, iodine manganese, and calcium). It also contains amino acids, essential fatty acids (omega-3 and omega-6), and antioxidants.
	It is cold in nature. It covers the large intestine, liver, and lung meridians. It can resolve phlegm and clear heat.
	It has gastroprotective and brain developing properties.
	The high fiber content aids in weight loss and relieves constipation. Its high calcium and magnesium content helps in improving bone health and reducing the risk of osteoporosis.
	It is important to consume agar-agar only after it is dissolved in water. Otherwise, it can swell and block the esophagus. It rarely causes allergic reactions.
	Moolihai.com. (2021, April 5). Health benefits of agar agar [China Grass]. https://www.moolihai.com/benefits-of-agar-agar/
	Venkateshwaran, R. (2020, January 28). 6 top benefits & uses of agar agar (China Grass). *Wildturmeric*. https://www.wildturmeric.net/agar-agar-benefits-uses-nutrition/
Agarwood *Aquilaria sinensis*	Other name: *Chen Xiang*
	Agarwood or Chen Xiang contains about 300 active compounds including chromones, terpenoids, and flavonoids. It is warm in nature. It covers the stomach, spleen, kidney, and lung meridians. It helps dispel cold and the downward movement of Qi.

Ingredients	Mechanism of Action and Health Benefits

It has antidepressant, antiaging, antibacterial, and antifungal properties. It may also have anticancer and antidiabetic effects. Agarwood essential oil has antioxidant and antiinflammatory properties. The essential oil is also used for aromatherapy.

It is used as a carminative medicine to relieve gastric problems, coughs, rheumatism, and high fever. It can also be used to relieve pain, vomiting, and asthma. The agarwood leaves help in weight loss and tea made from the leaves can improve sleep. Agarwood is also used to reduce bad breath from oral and gum diseases.

Chen Xiang has no noted adverse effects, but it should be avoided by pregnant and nursing women.

Health Benefits Times. (2018, July 23). Agarwood facts and health benefits. *HealthBenefitstimes.com*. https://www.healthbenefitstimes.com/agarwood/

Wang, S., Yu, Z., Wang, C., Wu, C., Guo, P., & Wei, J. (2018). Chemical constituents and pharmacological activity of agarwood and aquilaria plants. *Molecules*, 23(2), 342. https://doi.org/10.3390/molecules23020342

Anemarrhena
Anemarrhena asphodeloides

Other name: *Zhi Mu*

Anemarrhena contains saponin compounds (mainly asphonin, sarasapogenin, and timosaponin) and mangiferin. It covers the lung, stomach, and kidney meridians. It is cold in nature. It expels the heat and fire.

It has antiinflammatory, antidiabetic, diuretic, and antipyretic properties.

It is used for the treatment of cough, dry throat, fever, chronic bronchitis, and pneumonia. It also dissolves phlegm.

It is used to treat hypertension.

It can treat constipation, mouth ulcers, UTIs, and menopausal symptoms.

It is used to treat lower back pain. It can also lower blood glucose by reducing the insulin resistance.

Side effects include low blood pressure. It should not be used in diarrhea and in weak spleen.

Health Benefits Times. (2020, July 21). Health benefits of anemarrhena. *HealthBenefitstimes.com*. https://www.healthbenefitstimes.com/anemarrhena/

Me and Qi. (n.d.). Anemarrhena rhizomes. *Meandqi.com*. https://www.meandqi.com/herb-database/anemarrhena-rhizome

Angelica
Angelica dahurica
A. archangelica
Angelica sinensis

Other names: *Bai Zhi (A. dahurica)*

Read more below.

The Angelica genus has many root species.

The European Angelica is *A. archangelica* (also called wild celery or Norwegian angelica) or *Angelica dahurica/Radix Angelicae, Radix Angelicae Dahuricae, Radix Angelicae Pubescentis*. The American Angelica is similar to the European Angelica. It is used to treat digestive (dyspepsia, acid reflux, and flatulence) and circulatory disorders.

It has antiinflammatory actions and can reduce body aches in flus and colds.

The Chinese Angelica is referred to as *Angelica sinensis* and is used to treat hormonal balance and women's health, digestive, and circulatory issues.

(Read under Female ginseng.)

1st Chinese Herbs. (n.d.). Angelica dahurica (Bai Zhi). https://1stchineseherbs.com/a/angelica-root/angelica-dahurica-bai-zhi/

Apricot seed
Prunus armeniaca

Other name: **Xing Ren**

Apricot seed contains amygdalin (laetrile), fatty acids (including oleic, stearic, and linoleic acids), prunasee, and amygdalase.

It is warm in nature. It covers the lung and large intestine meridians. It moistens and lubricates the intestines.

It is used to treat cough, cold, sore throat, asthma, and bronchitis.

It can also treat constipation and piles.

The essential fatty acids (omega-3 and omega-6) present can improve heart health.

It should not be used in diarrhea. The amygdalin is converted to cyanide in the body which is toxic.

Acupuncture Today. (n.d.). Apricot seed (xing ren). *acupuncturetoday.com*. https://www.acupuncturetoday.com/herbcentral/apricot_seed.php

Me and Qi. (n.d.). Apricot seeds. *meandqi.com*. https://www.meandqi.com/herb-database/apricot-seed

WebMD Editors. (n.d.). Apricot kernel. *WebMD*. https://www.webmd.com/vitamins/ai/ingredient-mono-1190/apricot-kernel

Ingredients	Mechanism of Action and Health Benefits
Areca peel *Areca catechu*	Other names: *Betel nut pericarp, Da Fu Pi* Areca peel contains alkaloids (arecaidine, arecoline, and choline), gallic acid, catechin, and tannin. It is warm in nature. It covers the intestine (small and large), stomach, and spleen meridians. It regulates the downward movement of Qi and it relieves food stagnation. It is used for acid reflux, constipation, and gas and bloating. It increases the gut peristalsis and motility. It can treat stomach ulcers. It can lower hyperlipidemia and help in weight loss. Borten, P. (2013, May 19). Da Fu Pi—Betel husk—Areca peel—"Big Abdomen Peel." *Chinese Herbal Medicine*. https://chineseherbinfo.com/da-fu-pi-betel-husk-areca-peel-big-abdomen-peel/ Me and Qi. (n.d.-b). Areca peel. *meandqi.com*. https://www.meandqi.com/herb-database/areca-peel
Ashitaba	Other names: *Angelica, Angelica keiskei, Tomorrow's leaf* Ashitaba is a perennial leafy herb grown in Japan. It is usually added to soups or salads. The dried leaf powder is consumed as tea. It contains flavonoid antioxidants. It is used to treat digestive problems like stomach ulcers, constipation gastroesophageal reflux disease (GERD). It can also lower blood cholesterol and blood pressure. It also has antiaging properties and is used as an ingredient in cosmetic and skincare products. Overall, it is safe. Rxlist. (2021, June 11). Ashitaba: Health benefits, side effects, uses, dose & precautions. https://www.rxlist.com/ashitaba/supplements.htm
Asiatic cornelian cherry fruit *Cornus officinalis*	Other names: *Shan Yu Rou, Shan Zhu Yu* Cornelian cherry has antibacterial, antifungal, hypotensive, antitumor, astringent, diuretic, hepatic, and tonic properties. It is used commonly to reduce heavy menstrual bleeding and unusually active secretions including copious sweating, excessive urine, spermatorrhea, and premature ejaculation. It is used as one of the ingredients for the "Eight Flavor Rehmannia Teapills" which improves kidney function and eliminates hot flashes. Me & Qi. (n.d.). Cornelian cherries (Shan Zhu Yu) in Chinese Medicine. *meandqi.com*. https://www.meandqi.com/herb-database/cornelian-cherries
Astragalus root *Radix Astragali*	Other names: *Milkvetch, Huang Qi* The main active compounds in Huang Qi are isoflavonoids, saponins, astragalosides I–IV, polysaccharides, and GABA. It has antibacterial, antiviral, antidiabetic, antiinflammatory, and anticancer properties. It improves Qi circulation, hydrates, and energizes the body. It is used to treat fatigue, allergies, common cold, and heart disease (including heart failure and myocarditis). Astragalus can reduce the side effects of chemotherapy such as nausea, vomiting, and diarrhea. It may also help in weight loss, proteinuria, and improve kidney function. The root is available as liquid extracts, capsules, powders, teas, and injections. Minor side effects include rash, itching, runny nose, nausea, and diarrhea. Serious side effects when given by IV include irregular heartbeat. It should be avoided in pregnancy or breastfeeding or if there is history of autoimmune disease or taking immunosuppressant drugs. Ma, X. Q., Shi, Q., Duan, J. A., Dong, T. T. X., & Tsim, K. W. K. (2002). Chemical analysis of Radix Astragali (Huangqi) in China: A comparison with its adulterants and seasonal variations. *Journal of Agricultural and Food Chemistry*, 50(17), 4861–4866. https://doi.org/10.1021/jf0202279 Meixner, M. (2018, October 31). Astragalus: An ancient root with health benefits. *Healthline*. https://www.healthline.com/nutrition/astragalus#what-it-is
Baikal *Scutellaria baicalensis*	Other names: *Chinese skullcap, Huang Qin* The Chinese skullcap contains major bioactive compounds such as flavonoids including baicalin, baicalein, wogonin, and wogonoside. It also contains amino acids, essential oils, phenylethanoid, and sterols. The flavonoids present have anticancer effects. It has antibacterial, antiviral, antimicrobial, antioxidant, anxiolytic, anticonvulsant, and neuroprotective properties. It increases the GABA neurotransmitter which calms the nervous system. It is cold in nature and clears internal heat and dries dampness. It covers the lung, heart, spleen, large intestine, and gallbladder meridians.

Ingredients	Mechanism of Action and Health Benefits

It can be used in treating respiratory infections, bronchitis, asthma, hay fever, and fever. It is also used for GI infections, liver problems (hepatitis, hepatic fibrosis, carcinoma, and jaundice), and kidney infections.

It is also used in hypertension, headache, irritability, red eyes, flushed face, seizures, epilepsy, hysteria, anxiety, and to relieve a bitter taste in the mouth. It may also be used for pelvic inflammation and sores or swelling.

Chinese skullcap may cause allergic reactions, drowsiness, fever, lung inflammation, or liver toxicity.

RxList Editors. (2021, June 11). Baikal skullcap: Health benefits, side effects, uses, dose & precautions. *RxList*. https://www.rxlist.com/baikal_skullcap/supplements.htm

Zhao, Q., Chen, X. Y., & Martin, C. (2016). Scutellaria baicalensis, the golden herb from the garden of Chinese medicinal plants. *Science Bulletin*, *61*(18), 1391–1398. https://doi.org/10.1007/s11434-016-1136-5

Balloon flower root
Platycodon grandiflorus Radix

Other names: *Jie Geng, Platycodon, Platycodi radix, Chinese bellflower, Doraji*

Platycodi radix is the root of *Platycodon grandiflorum*. The active compounds in balloon flowers include phytosterol, inulin, betulic acid, and saponins. It is warm and neutral. It covers mainly lung and also stomach meridians.

It has antiinflammatory and antimicrobial properties.

It supports respiratory health. It opens the lung and promotes the lung Qi flow, expels excess phlegm from the lung. It is used to treat cough, cold, sore throat, lung congestion, asthma, bronchitis, and lung allergy.

It may also help in treating skin conditions such as eczema, skin ulcers and wound healing. It may also reduce pain and swelling in the eye when associated with allergy in the lung.

1st Chinese Herbs. (n.d.). Jie Geng. https://1stchineseherbs.com/herbs-a-z/j/jie-geng/

Lin, P. Y., Chu, C. H., Chang, F. Y., Huang, Y. W., Tsai, H. J., & Yao, T. C. (2019). Trends and prescription patterns of traditional Chinese medicine use among subjects with allergic diseases: A nationwide population-based study. *World Allergy Organization Journal*, *12*(2), 100001. https://doi.org/10.1016/j.waojou.2018.11.001

Bamboo

Other names: *Zhu Ru, Bamboo shavings, Vanshlochan or Vamsalochan, Tabasheer*

Bamboo has many species. The *Sasa* and *Indocalamus* species (which have broad leaves), *Phyllostachys edulis, Phyllostachys bambusoides, Phyllostachys aureosulcata* are some edible bamboo species to make bamboo leaf tea or to collect bamboo shoots. *Bambusae Caulis in Taeniam* extract is from the *Phyllostachys* bamboo. *Vanshlochan* (*Bamboo manna, Bamboo silica, or Bambusa arundinacea*) is a bamboo variety used in Ayurvedic medicine and also in TCM. Vanshlocan is a silica-rich deposit or concretion that is produced and discharged at the tree joint inside the hollow stem.

It is sweet, cooling, and a stimulant.

The active constituents in bamboo shavings include phenols, triterpenoids, saponins, sterols, and lignans. Bamboo is rich in silica which is essential for skin, hair, and connective tissue health and also for digestive stimulation. Silica is an essential component in collagen. Hair contains 40% silica. Silica can also block the absorption of toxic aluminum from the gut.

It also has expectorant, antioxidant, vasodilatory, antifatigue, diuretic, and aphrodisiac effects.

It can reduce phlegm and fever, especially in children, and also soothe an upset stomach. It can treat irritability, depression, sleep disorders (insomnia), and impotence It can relieve nausea and vomiting in pregnancy.

It should be avoided by people who have spleen deficiency and cold stomach. Uncooked or raw bamboo contains taxiphyllin, a poisonous cyanide glycoside.

American Dragon. (2017). Zhu Ru—竹茹—Caulis Bambusae. https://www.americandragon.com/Individualherbsupdate/ZhuRu.html

Jun, P. (2015). Potential medicinal application and toxicity evaluation of extracts from bamboo plants. *Journal of Medicinal Plants Research*, *9*(23), 681–692. https://doi.org/10.5897/jmpr2014.5657

Barley sprouts
Hordeum vulgare

Other name: *Mai Ya*

Barley sprouts contain hordenine, a compound that can sharpen mental focus and heighten energy levels. It also has mood-boosting effects. It is rich in antioxidants, fiber, essential amino acids, vitamins (B6 and B9), and minerals (iron, calcium, potassium, magnesium, manganese, and selenium). These nutrients help lower cholesterol and decrease the risk of cardiac disease.

Ingredients	Mechanism of Action and Health Benefits
	It has antibacterial, antidiabetic, hepatoprotective, and antiaging properties.

It supports digestion, reduces food stagnation due to undigested starchy foods or grains and all types of fruits. It is also used to inhibit lactation for discontinuation of nursing.

Long-term usage may injure the kidneys. It should be used with caution by people who are taking antidiabetic drugs as they can cause hypoglycemia.

American Dragon. (2017). Mai Ya—麥芽—Fructus Hordei Germinatus. https://www.americandragon.com/Individualherbsupdate/MaiYa.html

AP News Staff. (2019, March 30). Malt makes a comeback, packing powerful nutritional benefits. *AP NEWS*. https://apnews.com/article/7f5611bcba48411fa0be522507c0a7db

Bee venom

Bee venom is a complex compound which contains antiinflammatory substances (like apamin, melittin, adolapin, phospholipase A2) and proinflammatory substances (like histamine, melittin, phospholipase A2, and mast cell degranulation peptide 401).

Bee venom acupuncture is used to treat several musculoskeletal disorders like rheumatoid arthritis, knee osteoarthritis, lumbar disc disease, adhesive capsulitis, and lateral epicondylitis.

It also helps in neurological disorders like stroke, PD, and peripheral neuropathies.

Adverse reactions include bee venom anaphylaxis.

Lee, J. D., Park, H. J., Chae, Y., & Lim, S. (2005). An overview of bee venom acupuncture in the treatment of arthritis. *Evidence-Based Complementary and Alternative Medicine, 2*(1), 79–84. https://doi.org/10.1093/ecam/neh070

Biota seeds
Platycladus orientalis

Other names: *Bai Zi Ren, Oriental thuja, Biota, Biota orientalis, Oriental arborvitae*

Biota seeds are rich in flavonoids, saponins, tannins, and vitamin C. It is sweet and neutral in nature. It covers heart, large intestine, and kidney meridians. It nourishes the heart and calms the spirit and mind. It also lubricates the intestine.

It is a healthy tonic and nourishes the Yin.

It is used to treat constipation, anxiety, insomnia, palpitations, irritability, and restlessness. It also promotes hair growth (in androgenic alopecia).

It is used to treat pain (in rheumatism or headaches), menorrhagia, and hemorrhoids.

It should not be used in diarrhea.

Me and Qi. (n.d.-b). Biota seeds. *Meandqi*. https://www.meandqi.com/herb-database/biota-seeds

Bessent, C. (2021, May 21). Biota seed to calm the spirit. *Herbsmith*. https://www.herbsmithinc.com/biota-seed-to-calm-anxious-dogs/

Bird's nest

Other name: *Edible bird's nest*

Bird's nests are made by cave swiftlets in natural caves or by farm swiftlets in urban buildings. The nests are woven with the bird's saliva and are harvested after the young birds have flown away. There are three types of nests: white, red, and golden. The latter two types are from the caves only and the natural color is from the mineral content from the cave stones.

Bird's nest is a healthy and nourishing tonic which is rich in glycoproteins, collagen, growth factors, minerals, and amino acids. It has rejuvenating and immune-boosting effects. It increases energy and decreases fatigue.

It can increase appetite and digestion. It is used in chronic dry coughs. It enhances skin health and beauty. It also improves kidney function. It can help cancer patients who are receiving radiation or chemotherapy to relieve cough, poor appetite, and fatigue.

It is safe in pregnancy after the fourth month and helps with fetal growth. It can be consumed after birth and by nursing mothers.

Side effects include allergic reactions. Fake red bird nests are tainted with dyes.

Bitter orange
Citrus aurantium

Other names: *Bigarade orange, Zhi Shi*

Bitter orange contains mainly protoalkaloids such as synephrine (p-synephrine), limonene, and octopamine (p-octopamine). It also contains furanocoumarin. It is also rich in antioxidants, i.e., citrus bioflavonoids and vitamin C.

It has antiinflammatory, antifungal, and antiviral properties.

It is commonly used to treat indigestion, nausea, constipation, heartburn, weight loss, appetite stimulation, or suppression.

It can also improve athletic performance. It also helps in weight loss.

It is also applied to the skin for pain, bruises, bedsores, and nasal congestion.

Ingredients	Mechanism of Action and Health Benefits

Overall, it is safe. It can interact with decongestants and antihypertensive medications. It should not be used in glaucoma and irregular heartbeat.

Charles, A. (2021, March 17). What is bitter orange, and does it aid weight loss? *Healthline*. https://www.healthline.com/nutrition/bitter-orange

National Center for Complementary and Integrative Health. (2020, May). Bitter orange. *NCCIH*. https://www.nccih.nih.gov/health/bitter-orange

Black atractylodes rhizome
Atractylodes lancea

Other name: *Cang Zhu*

Atractylodes contain various bioactive constituents such as sesquiterpenes (β-selinene and atractylenolide I–III), sesquiterpenoids (elemol, hinesol, and atractylone), polyethylene alkynes (atractylodin), and phytosterols (stigmasterol and β-sitosterol). Atractylone has antihepatotoxic properties, whereas stigmasterol has antinociceptive and antidiabetic activities.

Atractylodes also have anticancer, antiobesity, and antiinflammatory effects.

It can eliminate dampness, strengthen the spleen, eliminate wind, and disperse cold in order to restore a harmonious balance between Yin and Yang.

It is used to traditionally treat rheumatic diseases, digestive disorders, night blindness, and influenza.

Side effects include allergic reactions, diarrhea, fatigue, and vomiting.

Jun, X., Fu, P., Lei, Y., & Cheng, P. (2018). Pharmacological effects of medicinal components of *Atractylodes lancea* (Thunb.) DC. *Chinese Medicine*, *13*(1), 1–10. https://doi.org/10.1186/s13020 018-0216-7

Me & Qi. (2021). *Black atractylodes rhizomes (Cang Zhu) in Chinese Medicine*. https://www.meandqi.com/herb-database/black-atractylodes-rhizome

Black fungus
Auricularia polytricha

Other names: *Cloud ear fungus, wood ear*

Black fungus is a mushroom which is black or dark brown in color. When soaked in water and cooked, it has a jelly-like consistency.

It tonifies the Yin and clears heat and boosts blood circulation.

It covers the lung, liver, and stomach meridians.

It is also high in antioxidants (flavonoids and polyphenols). It is a low calorie food and rich in vitamins (B2 and B3) and minerals (iron and magnesium). It is rich in polysaccharide fiber which acts as a prebiotic. It maintains a healthy gut microbiome.

It can also lower cholesterol. It may also be hepatoprotective and neuroprotective.

Overall, it is safe. It should be washed and cooked thoroughly to remove chemical residues or kill bacteria before consumption.

Wartenberg, L. M. (2019, November 11). What is black fungus, and does it have benefits? *Healthline*. https://www.healthline.com/nutrition/black-fungus

Black sesame seeds
Sesamum indicum

Other name: *Hei zhi ma*

Black sesame contains sesamin, sesamol, and anthrasesamone F. It is rich in minerals such as copper (83% of the DV), manganese (22% of the DV), calcium (18% of the DV), magnesium (16% of the DV), and iron (15% of the DV). It contains fiber, B-vitamins (B1, B2, and B9), and other minerals (phosphorus and zinc). It is also rich in antioxidants that contribute to reducing the risk of chronic diseases and cancer.

It has antibacterial, antiinflammatory, antiaging, laxative, and anticancer properties.

Black sesame oil can prevent premature graying of hair and promotes skin health.

It is used to treat constipation and moisten the intestines to soften hard stools.

It is also used for dizziness and tinnitus.

Overall, it is safe but may cause allergic reactions, mouth ulcers, and toothaches. It should not be used in chronic diarrhea.

Sen Health. (2019, April 15). *Food in Chinese medicine: Black sesame*. Sen Health Clinic. https://www.senhealthclinic.com.au/post/blacksesame

Zhou, L., Lin, X., Abbasi, A. M., & Zheng, B. (2016). Phytochemical contents and antioxidant and antiproliferative activities of selected black and white sesame seeds. *BioMed Research International*, *2016*, 1–9. https://doi.org/10.1155/2016/8495630

Black-tail snake
Zaocys dhumnades

Other name: *Wu shao she*

The Black-tail snake covers the liver meridian. It expels and disperses dampness and wind.

It can treat seizures, spasms, and paralysis.

It also helps in rheumatism and reduces the stiffness and pain in disorders of the muscles, bones, and joints.

Me and Qi. (n.d.-b). *Black-tail snakes*. meandqi.com. https://www.meandqi.com/herb-database/black-tail-snake

Ingredients	Mechanism of Action and Health Benefits
Buddleia flower buds *Buddleja officinalis*	Other names: *Mi meng hua, Butterfly bush*

Buddleia contains flavonoids (including luteolin, apigenin, and acacetin), saponins, triterpenoids, and phenylethanolic glycosides. It is cool in nature and sweet. It covers the liver meridian. It eliminates heat in the liver channel and purges fire.

It has antioxidant, antiinflammatory, and antiviral properties.

It can also detoxify the body and acts as a tonic. It replenishes the Qi and blood.

It is used to treat corneal opacity, cataracts, swollen eyes, and light sensitivity.

It can also stimulate bile flow.

Overall, it is safe. Excessive consumption can cause vomiting, dizziness, indigestion, or numbness. It should not be consumed during pregnancy.

Chinese Herbs Info. (2021, March 31). Mi Meng Hua (Flos Buddlejae). https://www.chineseherbsinfo.com/mi-meng-hua/

Me and Qi. (n.d.). Buddleia flowers. *meandqi.com.* https://www.meandqi.com/herb-database/buddleia-flowers

Burnet root
Radix Sanguisorbae
Sanguisorba officinalis

Other names: *Great Burnet root, Sanguisorba Root, Di Yu*

Burnet root contains bioactive ingredients including terpenoids and phenolics (flavonoids, phenolic acids, and neolignans). It covers the liver, stomach, and large intestine meridians. It is cool in nature and bitter. It lowers the heat in the blood and drains damp-heat.

It has hemostatic properties. It shortens clotting and bleeding times. It can stop bleeding piles, dysentery, hematemesis, menorrhagia, and hematuria.

Me and Qi. (n.d.-b). Sanguisorba roots. *meandqi.com.* https://www.meandqi.com/herb-database/sanguisorba-root

Proven Herbal Remedies. (2021, April 18). Sanguisorba Officinalis. *Chinese Herbs Healing.* https://www.chineseherbshealing.com/proven-herbal-remedies/sanguisorba-officinalis.html

Bur Reed tuber
Rhizoma sparganii
Sparganium stoloniferum

Other name: *San Leng*

The dried rhizome of San Leng contains phenylpropanoids, alkaloids, flavonoids, and steroids. It covers the spleen and liver meridians.

It can invigorate blood, break up blood stasis, and relieve food stagnation. It moves the Qi, improves blood circulation, prevents blood stasis and clots and decreases pain.

It has analgesic properties.

It can regulate menstruation and stimulate lactation.

It should not be used in bleeding disorders.

ActiveHerb Technology, Inc. (n.d.). San Leng (Burreed Tuber, Rhizoma Sparganii, 三棱). https://www.activeherb.com/chineseherbs/sanleng.shtml

Jia, J., Li, X., Ren, X., Liu, X., Wang, Y., Dong, Y., et al. (2021). Sparganii Rhizoma: A review of traditional clinical application, processing, phytochemistry, pharmacology, and toxicity. *Journal of Ethnopharmacology, 268,* 113571. https://doi.org/10.1016/j.jep.2020.113571

Cassia twig
(Cinnamomum Cassia; Ramulus)

Other names: *Gui Zhi, Chinese cinnamon*
(Read under Cinnamon, under Indian Herb)

Cat's claw
Uncaria spp.

Other names: *Gambier, Hook vine, Gou Teng, Uncaria* spp.

Uncaria is a genus with several species.
- *U. sinensis, U. gambir, U. rhynchophylla*: grows mostly in China and Southeast Asia.
- *U. tomentosa, U. guianensis:* grows mostly in South America (called Una de Gato).

Refer also to "Gambir" under Indian Natural ingredients.

Gambir is a resin from the *Uncaria gambir* plant. It has astringent properties. It is used as a catechu (tannin substance) when chewing betel leaf and areca.

In TCM, it is cool in nature and treats the hyperactive liver Yang. It clears liver heat and expels wind. It covers the liver, pericardium, and heart meridians. The stems and thorns are used as medicine.

Cat's claw contains over 30 bioactive constituents, including alkaloids, glycosides, tannins, flavonoids, and sterol fractions. It has antiinflammatory, antioxidant, analgesic, antimicrobial, wound-healing, immune-boosting, hypotensive, contraceptive, anticancer, and adaptogen actions.

It is effective in osteoarthritis, rheumatoid arthritis, and gout.

It helps in digestive disorders such as colitis, diverticulitis, gastritis, hemorrhoids, stomach ulcers, and leaky gut syndrome. It also improves immune function and infections.

Ingredients	Mechanism of Action and Health Benefits

It can treat hypertension, anxiety, headaches, tremors, seizures, spasms, and dizziness.

It may also be used for the treatment of cancer, allergies, asthma, AIDS, allergies, herpes, and ovarian cysts.

If consumed in large amounts, the tannins present in cat's claw may cause some side effects like nausea, upset stomach, and diarrhea.

Price, A. (2017, June 14). Cat's claw benefits for immunity, digestion and chronic disease. *Dr. Axe*. https://draxe.com/nutrition/cats-claw/

WebMD. (n.d.-a). CAT'S CLAW: Overview, uses, side effects, precautions, interactions, dosing and reviews. https://www.webmd.com/vitamins/ai/ingredientmono-395/cats-claw

Cattail pollen
Typha angustifolia

Other name: *Pu Huang*

Cattail pollen contains phenolic compounds, tannins, and saponins. It is also rich in several minerals (magnesium and potassium), and vitamins (K and B6).

Cattail is also used in Western herbal medicine. The roots can be boiled and eaten or the dried roots are ground into powder and used as a thickener. The seeds, stem, stamen and pollen are also edible.

It removes Stasis and stops Bleeding. It covers the Liver, Heart and Spleen meridian. It is neutral and sweet.

It has hemostatic, analgesic, anti-inflammatory, and astringent properties. It also promotes lactation. It has also anti-cancer properties.

It is used to stop bleeding in menorrhagia (heavy menses), hematemesis (blood in vomit), hematuria (blood in urine), postpartum bleeding and bleeding wounds.

It is cardiotonic and can support heart health by lowering blood lipids and preventing clotting. It is used to treat angina and hyperlipidemia. It can also lower blood glucose and can help in diabetes.

It can treat gallstones with other polyherbs. It supports digestive health.

It is also used for wound healing and toothache.

Ghanghro, A. B., Channa, U., Ghanghro, I. H., Channa, M. J., & Lanjwani, A. H. (2015). Biochemical and Phytochemical Analysis of Typha Pollens (Cattails). *Sindh University Research Journal*, 47(3), 473–476. https://sujo-old.usindh.edu.pk/index.php/SURJ/article/download/1208/1115

Medicine Traditions Staff. (n.d.). Typha, Cattail Pollen, Pu Huang. Medicine Traditions. https://www.medicinetraditions.com/typha-cattail-pollen-pu-huang.html

Health Benefits times. (n.d.). Cattail facts and health benefits. Health Benefits Times.Com. https://www.healthbenefitstimes.com/cattail/

Caulis Spatholobi

Other names: *Spatholobus stem*, *ji xue teng*, *Vine Millettia Root*

Spatholobus stem contains flavonoids, triterpenes catechins. It is warm in nature and covers the liver meridians. It can also increase hematopoiesis. It also has anticoagulant, antioxidant, antiinflammatory, immune-modulating, and tranquilizing actions.

It activates and nourishes the blood. It is suitable in disorders of blood deficiency or blood stasis as in menstrual disorders.

It can also activate collateral blood circulation in the brain and joints. It is used in stroke and rheumatism.

It should not be used during pregnancy.

Mdhealthonline. (2020, August 25). Caulis Spatholobi: An herb of many purposes—from blood flow to immune systems. Retrieved 4 November 2021, from https://mdhealthonline.com/caulis-spatholobi-an-herb-of-many-purposes-from-blood-flow-to-immune-systems/

Celosia seed
Celosia argustea L.

Other names: *Quail grass, Velvet flower, Cockscomb, Qing xiang zi*

Celosia seed is cold in nature and it covers the liver meridian. It clears liver-fire and eliminates wind-heat. The main active constituent is celosiaol.

It can improve eye health in cataracts, blurring of vision, mild corneal opacity, and acute red eye. It can dilate the pupils.

It can improve wound healing, eczema, skin itching, and skin ulcers.

It is also used to treat dysentery, hemorrhoids, and nosebleeds.

It can also lower blood pressure.

It should not be used in eye diseases associated with liver-kidney deficiency, and glaucoma.

Proven Herbal Remedies. (2021, July 19). Celosia seeds (Qing Xiang Zi). *Chinese Herbs Healing*. https://www.chineseherbshealing.com/proven-herbal-remedies/celosia-seeds.html

Ingredients	Mechanism of Action and Health Benefits
Centipede	Other name: *Wu gong*
	Dried medicinal centipedes are warm and toxic in nature. It covers the liver meridian. It clears spasm and wind, and eliminates toxins.
	Centipede venom contains many toxins (neurotoxins and cardiotoxins) and various chemicals (serotonin, histamine, and quinoline alkaloids).
	It is used to fight incurable diseases based on the premise of "fighting deadly diseases with deadly poison."
	It is used in severe migraine, cancers, snake bites, seizures in children, tetanus facial, or limb paralysis.
	Side effects include anaphylactic reactions.
	Proven Herbal Remedies. (2021, April 20). Facts about Centipedes (Wu Gong). *Chinese Herbs Healing*. https://www.chineseherbshealing.com/proven-herbal-remedies/centipedes.html
Chicken feet	Other name: *Phoenix claws*
	Chicken feet contain about 30% cartilage which is collagen rich. Some glucosamine and chondroitin are also present. It is also rich in calcium, folate, zinc, copper, and iron.
	It nourishes the Qi.
	It can strengthen the bones, tendons, and ligaments. It can reduce pain in osteoarthritis and also help reduce bone loss in osteoporosis. It also can improve skin health.
	It also enhances fertility and strengthens kidney Qi.
	Blue, C. (2015, September 12). Chicken feet soup nourishes Qi and supports fertility. *All Eyes on China*. http://65.49.34.234/2015/09/12/chicken-feet-soup-nourishes-qi-and-supports-fertility.html
	Lang, A. (2020, October 19). Eating chicken feet: All you need to know. *Healthline*. https://www.healthline.com/nutrition/chicken-feet
Chicken gizzard membrane	Other name: *Ji nei jin*
	Gizzard is rich in vitamins, mainly the B-vitamins (B2, B3, and B12). It also contains several minerals including iron, phosphorus, and zinc. These nutrients improve blood circulation, hormone production, and improve skin and hair health.
	There are three types of chicken gizzard membranes available: "*sheng* (raw) *ji nei jin*," "*cu* (vinegar) *ji nei jin*" and "*chao* (fried) *ji nei jin*." Raw gizzard membrane is used to eliminate stagnation and stones, vinegar chicken gizzard membrane can help the liver and digestion, whereas fried chicken gizzard membrane can help relieve indigestion.
	It moves stagnant food. It is helpful for nausea, vomiting, diarrhea, moving undigested foods, and in severe indigestion.
	It can improve brain function, and increase the number of white blood cells.
	It also helps improve the immune system function and reduce the risk of heart disease.
	DeLong's Gizzard Equipment. (2018, September 25). Gizzards and their numerous health benefits. DeLong's Gizzards & Poultry Processing Equipment. https://delongs.com/gizzards-and-their-numerous-health-benefits/
	Qian, Z. (2013, November 15). TCM treasures: Chicken gizzard membrane. *Shanghai Daily*. https://archive.shine.cn/sunday/now-and-then/TCM-Treasures-Chicken-gizzard-membrane/shdaily.shtml
China root *Smilax china* *Smilax glabra*	Other names: *Chinaroot, Tufuling or Tu Fu Ling, Sarsaparilla or Sarsaparilla root (Smilax officinalis), Smilax Glabra Rhizome, Glabrous greenbrier rhizome*
	The *Smilax* genus has many species, known collectively before as *Sarsaparilla*. They are trailing vines. Sarsaparilla is actually from the genus Smilax and grows in the tropics. Its extract is widely used as a flavoring agent in beverages. *Smilax glabra* and *Smilax officinalis* are often used interchangeably.
	China root contains bioactive compounds such as saponins, glucosides, gum, flavonoids, tannins, and alkaloids.
	It removes dampness and toxicity.
	It is a carminative and an antiscrophulatic. It has detoxifying, diaphoretic, and diuretic properties. It also has antiinflammatory, antiinfective, antiviral, anticancer, antidiabetic, and anticoagulation activities.
	It can treat old syphilitic cases, psoriasis, rheumatoid arthritis, gout, enteritis, UTIs, and skin ulcers.
	It is helpful in improving muscle mass and body strength.
	Overall, it is safe but large amounts can cause stomach irritation. It should also be avoided by people with kidney problems and pregnant or breastfeeding women.

Ingredients	Mechanism of Action and Health Benefits
	Mohamad, H. S., Wenli, S., & Qi, C. (2019). Tremendous health benefits and clinical aspects of *Smilax china*. *African Journal of Pharmacy and Pharmacology*, *13*(16), 253–258. https://doi.org/10.5897/ajpp2019.5070
	WebMD. (n.d.). SARSAPARILLA: Overview, uses, side effects, precautions, interactions, dosing and reviews. https://www.webmd.com/vitamins/ai/ingredientmono-379/sarsaparilla
Chinese club moss Lycopodium	Other names: *Shi Song, Shen Jin Cao* Club moss is more of a fern than a moss. There are two main species, *Lycopodium chensis (eastern)* and *Lycopodium clavatum (western)*. The bioactive ingredients in club moss include flavonoids, alkaloids (clavatine, clavatoxine, and lycopodine), triterpenes, and polyphenolic acids. Only the *L. chensis* contains huperzine A which has neuroprotective functions. It helps attention, focus, memory, and cognition. The spores are water repellent and can be used to coat tablets. It covers the liver, spleen and lung meridians. It clears damp and wind, and warms the kidney. Both species have analgesic, antipyretic, antiinflammatory, antibiotic, and diuretic properties. It can be used to treat dementia, gas and bloating, gastric upset, rheumatism, eczema, and wound healing. It is also used to treat urinary disorders and irregular menstrual cycles. Overconsumption can lead to liver damage, nausea, dizziness, sweating, and respiratory depression. Medicine Net. (2021, June 11). Chinese club moss. https://www.medicinenet.com/chinese_club_moss/supplements-vitamins.htm Medicine Traditions. (n.d.). Lycopodium, Clubmoss, Shen Jin Cao. https://www.medicinetraditions.com/lycopodium-clubmoss-shen-jin-cao.html Misra, K., Sharma, P., & Bhardwaj, A. (2018). *Management of high altitude pathophysiology* (1st ed.). London: Academic Press. https://doi.org/10.1016/B978-0-12-813999-8.00011-2
Chinese foxglove root *Rehmannia glutinosa*	Other names: *Rehmannia root or Rehmanniae Radix, Shu Di Huáng or Sheng Di Huang* Chinese foxglove or Shu dì huáng is the root of the Rehmannia *glutinosa* plant. The main bioactive compounds present are catalpol, cerebroside, dammelittoside, melittoside, and rehmaglitin. These compounds have antiinflammatory and antifungal properties. Catalpol can also reduce elevated blood sugar, promote sex hormone production, and protect the liver from damage. It also contains high amounts of vitamins A, B, and C, amino acids, and iron. It is commonly used to treat conditions that are caused by Yin deficiency. It cools blood, clears heat, and nourishes Yin. It has anticancer, antidiabetic, antihyperlipidemic, antibacterial, antiseptic, antiaging, and antistress properties. It improves circulation to all parts of the body including capillaries and especially to the brain. It is used in many conditions including anemia, prolonged fever, night sweats, constipation, chronic kidney disease, hearing problems, blurred vision, insomnia, and irregular menstruation. Chinese foxglove can also heal injured bones, relieve arthritis pain, regulate menstrual flow, and help with urinary tract problems. Side effects include abdominal pain, diarrhea, heart palpitations, and edema. It should not be used in chronic liver disease. This herb can also cause loose bowel movements in some people and bloating. Health Benefits Times. (2020, June 28). Health benefits of Rehmannia. *HealthBenefitstimes.com*. https://www.healthbenefitstimes.com/rehmannia/ Xi'an Le Sen Bio-technology. (n.d.). *Rehmannia Glutinosa Root Extract*. Xi'an Le Sen Bio-Technology Co., Ltd. https://www.lsherb.com/plant-extract/rehmannia-glutinosa-extract.html
Chinese goldthread *Rhizoma coptidis*	Other names: *Huang lian, Coptis chinensis* Chinese goldthread is considered one of the 50 fundamental herbs of TCM. It contains several compounds including berberine, an alkaloid with antibacterial and antiinflammatory properties. Berberine also lowers lipid levels, improves heart health, bone and joint health, and is beneficial for the respiratory system. Other alkaloids present include palmatine, epiberberine, columbamine, and coptisine. Coptisine is a powerful antioxidant that can reduce the risk of heart diseases, cancer, and help relieve fever. It has antioxidant, antiinflammatory, antimicrobial, hepatoprotective, and antidiabetic properties. It is used in heart failure, diarrhea, vomiting, jaundice, digestive disorders, diabetes, and acute and chronic infections.

Ingredients	Mechanism of Action and Health Benefits
	There are no known long-term side effects of goldthread. Berberine is known to cause an increase in bilirubin which may cause brain damage in both newborns and developing fetuses. Thus, it should never be used in children, during pregnancy, or while breastfeeding. Huang lian should also be avoided by people taking diabetic medicine as it can lead to hypoglycemia.

Group, E. (2016, November 29). Health benefits of Goldthread. Dr. Group's Healthy Living Articles. https://explore.globalhealing.com/health-benefits-of-goldthread/

Wong, C., & Kroner, A. (2021, January 17). The benefits of Coptis Chinensis (Huang Lian). *Verywell Health*. https://www.verywellhealth.com/the-benefits-of-coptis-chinensis-88938

Chinese hawberry
Crataegus pinnatifida

Other names: *Chinese haw, Chinese hawthorn, Shan Zha*

The main bioactive compound in Chinese hawberry is polyphenols, which are powerful antioxidants. It also contains flavonoids, triterpenoids, steroids, sesquiterpenoids, rutin, saponins, vitexin, catechins, and several anthocyanidins.

Hawberry has antiinflammatory, hypoglycemic, antiplatelet, and antiarrhythmic effects.

It is "warm" in nature and will benefit those who have too much "cold" in their bodies due to "Yin excess" (Yin is cold in nature) or "Yang deficiency" (Yang is hot in nature).

It is cardiotonic and improves heart health. It has hypotensive and antiatherosclerotic properties. It breaks blood stasis, disrupts and dissipates clumps to invigorate the blood. It is used in the treatment of myocardial dysfunction, blood circulation problems, and atherosclerosis. It can stabilize blood pressure, dilate coronary blood vessels, decrease cholesterol levels, reduce shortness of breath, palpitations, and fatigue, and increase stamina and energy.

It also contains fiber that can help digestion by reducing constipation and acting as a prebiotic. It decreases food stagnation or food retention. It improves the digestion of meats and fatty foods.

It is also used as a therapeutic agent for cancer, cough, flu, asthma, stomach ache, rheumatic pain, nephritis, and hemorrhoids. Hawthorn also promotes healthy hair growth and skin.

It helps reduce anxiety and may also lower the risk of type 2 diabetes, and boost the immune system.

It should be avoided by those with stomach and spleen deficiency. Some people may experience mild nausea, stomach upset, fatigue, sweating, headache, dizziness, palpitations, nosebleeds, insomnia, and agitation. Chinese hawberry should not be taken alongside medications for heart, blood pressure, or cholesterol as it can affect the drugs taken.

Shoemaker, S. (2019, August 26). 9 impressive health benefits of Hawthorn Berry. *Healthline*. https://www.healthline.com/nutrition/hawthorn-berry-benefits

Venskutonis, P. R. (2018). Phytochemical composition and bioactivities of hawthorn (Crataegus spp.): Review of recent research advances. *Journal of Food Bioactives*, 4, 69–87. https://doi.org/10.31665/jfb.2018.4163

Chinese patchouli
Agastache rugosa

Other names: *Korean mint, Huo xiang*

The active compounds present include flavonoids, phenolic acids, lignana, and terpenoids. Huo xiang is considered bitter and warm, working its effects on spleen, stomach, and lungs.

Essential oil is obtained from its leaves and is rich in estragole, isomenthone, and limonene. It has antiviral, antimicrobial, antioxidant, cardiovascular, and antiinflammatory properties.

The oil can be used against angina, headache, stomach pain, morning sickness, and GI disorders.

InTCM, Korean mint is used to relieve nausea and vomiting, and cure fungal infections. It is also used in the treatment of chronic hepatitis, congestion, diarrhea, dyspepsia, hyperemesis, atherosclerosis, and splenosis (breaking off of spleen tissue).

The dried Korean mint leaves can be brewed into tea that is aromatic or used as a carminative, diaphoretic, or febrifuge.

Anupama, A. (2018, July 14). Agastache rugosa (Korean Mint) health benefits and medicinal usage. *Bimbima*. https://www.bimbima.com/herbs/korean-mint/4102/

Chinese senega root
Polygala tenuifolia

Other names: *Seneca root, Yuan Zhi*

Chinese senega contains saponins, oligosaccharide esters, and xanthon. It is warm in nature and covers kidney, heart, and lung meridians. It calms the spirit, expels phlegm from the lungs and heart.

It has antiinflammatory, antidepressant, and neuroprotective properties.

It can treat palpitations, irritability, insomnia, and restlessness. It lowers stress, anxiety, and insomnia, and releases pent up emotions.

It can treat respiratory problems including asthma and bronchitis.

Ingredients	Mechanism of Action and Health Benefits
	Side effects include dizziness and gastric upset including diarrhea.
	Me and Qi. (n.d.). Chinese senega roots. *Meaandqi.com*. https://www.meandqi.com/herb-database/chinese-senega-root
	WebMD Editors. (2014). Senega. *WebMD*. https://www.webmd.com/vitamins/ai/ingredientmono-679/senega
Chinese thorowax root *Radix bupleuri*	Other names: *Hare's Ear Root, Chai Hu* The main bioactive constituents of Chinese thorowax root are essential oils, triterpenoid saponins, polyacetylenes, flavonoids, lignans, fatty acids, and sterols. It is the root of the *Bupleurum falcatum* plant. The essential oils have antifungal and antiinflammatory properties. In TCM, *radix bupleuri* is capable of regulating the exterior and interior metabolisms, dispersing evil heat from the superficies, soothing the liver, and promoting Yang and Qi. It has anticancer, antipyretic, antimicrobial, antiviral, hepatoprotective, neuroprotective, and immunomodulatory effects. Chinese thorowax is commonly used for the treatment of fever, pain, and inflammation associated with influenza and the common cold. It can also be used as analgesics in treatment of distending pain in the hypochondriac region of the chest and against amenorrhea. It is used in the treatment of anxiety and depression. These roots in combination with other herbs can also provide relief from epilepsy. Possible side effects include intestinal gas, increased bowel movements, and drowsiness. Chinese thorowax roots should be avoided by people with bleeding disorder, autoimmune disease, and diabetes. Health Benefits Times. (2020, January 7). Chai Hu facts and health benefits. *HealthBenefitstimes.com*. https://www.healthbenefitstimes.com/chai-hu/ Yang, F., Dong, X., Yin, X., Wang, W., You, L., & Ni, J. (2017). Radix Bupleuri: A review of traditional uses, botany, phytochemistry, pharmacology, and toxicology. *BioMed Research International, 2017*, 1–22. https://doi.org/10.1155/2017/7597596
Chinese wild ginger *(Asarum heterotropoides Asarum sieboldii)*	Other names: *Xi Xin, Manchurian wild ginger, Herba Asari, Asarum, Snakeroot, Wild ginger, Asarabacca* Chinese wild ginger contains lignans, flavones, terpenes, and volatile oil. It is warm in nature and covers the heart, lung and kidney meridians. It warms the Yang and expels wind-cold and wind-damp. The Qi is moved upward to disperse the phlegm and to make nasal passages open. It is used to treat cough, cold, sinusitis, shortness of breath, headache, chronic bronchitis, asthma, constipation, rheumatism, and toothache. It can help in migraine headaches. Me and Qi. (n.d.). Wild ginger. *Meandqi.com*. https://www.meandqi.com/herb-database/wild-ginger
Chrysanthemum *Chrysanthemum morifolium*	Other names: *Ju Hua, Flos Chrysanthemi* The active compounds in ju hua are mainly volatile oils, terpenoids, polyphenols (chlorogenic acid), and flavonoids (apigenin, acacetin-7-O-β-glucoside, and luteolin). It is rich in potassium, magnesium, phosphorus, calcium, and iron. Apigenin has antiviral, antihypertensive, antibacterial, and antiinflammatory properties. It treats wind-heat syndromes with fever, headaches, and painful red or dry eyes. It releases heat and wind, and clears heat in the liver channel. As it is an excellent source of calcium, it helps in bone disorders like osteoporosis. Potassium present can help reduce the risk of hypertension, heart disease, stroke, cancer, digestive disorders, and infertility. It is also used in diabetes. It can also be used topically as an insecticide in shampoos for head lice. Chrysanthemum is considered to be safe for consumption without any known serious side effects. It rarely causes allergic reactions like sensitive skin. Brennan, D. (2020, November 12). Health benefits of Chrysanthemum tea. *WebMD*. https://www.webmd.com/diet/health-benefits-chrysanthemum-tea#1-2
Chuan Xiong *Rhizoma ligustici chuanxiong*	Chuan xiong is the dry rhizome of the Ligusticum *chuanxiong* plant. The main active compounds in ligusticum include essential oil, alkaloids, phenolic acids, and phthalide lactones. Chuan Xiong has the effects of invigorating blood and promoting Qi. It has the effects of dispelling wind and pain. It has shown vasorelaxation, antiinflammation, antioxidant, antibacterial, antinociceptive, and antiproliferative activities.

Ingredients	Mechanism of Action and Health Benefits
	It can help prevent and reduce the effects of several cardiovascular and cerebrovascular diseases including atherosclerosis, vasodilatation, myocardial ischemia, angiogenesis, and stroke. It may help in treatment and prevention of liver fibrosis.
	It is also used for fever and dental caries. It has the probability to prevent, inhibit, or halt the development of tumors.
	Large doses of Chuan Xiong can lead to dizziness, nausea, or vomiting. It should also be avoided by pregnant and nursing women.
	Ran, X., Ma, L., Peng, C., Zhang, H., & Qin, L. P. (2011). Ligusticum chuanxiongHort: A review of chemistry and pharmacology. *Pharmaceutical Biology*, *49*(11), 1180–1189. https://doi.org/10.3109/13880209.2011.576346
Cibot Rhizome *Rhizoma cibotii* *Cibotium barometz*	Other name: *Gou Ji* The bioactive compounds in cibot rhizomes include flavonoids, anthraquinones, tannins, and phytosterols. It covers the liver, kidney, bladder, and heart meridians. It is warm in nature. It removes wind and dampness and can lubricate the joints. It has analgesic and antiinflammatory properties. It can treat rheumatoid arthritis, stiff back, lower back ache, and knee pain. It also helps in frequent urination and vaginal discharge. Overall, it is safe. Eu Yan Sang Staff. (n.d.). Cibot Rhizome. *EuYanSang.com*. https://www.euyansang.com/en_US/cibot-rhizome/herb-CibotRhizome.html Proven Herbal Remedies. (2021, May 3). Cibotium Barometz (Gou Ji). *Chinese Herbs Healing*. https://www.chineseherbshealing.com/proven-herbal-remedies/cibotium-barometz.html
Cicada slough *Periostracum cicadae*	Other name: *Chan Tui* Cicada skin or molt is the exoskeleton and is shed by the cicada. It is sun dried and consists mainly of chitin (consists of polysaccharides and proteins), proteins, and other minerals, wax, and lipids. It covers the liver and lung meridians. It is cool in nature. It clears the heat and expels the wind. It has antispasmodic action. It is used to treat skin diseases including allergic problems. It is used in sore throat. Chitosan is the commercial preparation. No significant side effects have been found. Dharmananda, S. (2015). *Chantui: Use of chitin in Chinese herb formulas*. Portland, OR: Institute for Traditional Medicine. http://www.itmonline.org/arts/chantui.htm Huimin Herb Enterprise. (n.d.). Chan Tui (Cicada Slough) 4oz. https://www.herbsf.com/products/cicada-slough-chantui
Coix seeds *Coix lacryma-jobi*	Other names: *Job's tears, Chinese pearl barley* or *Yi Yi Ren* Coix seeds *(Coix lacryma-jobi)* are different from barley *(Hordeum vulgare)*. Coix seeds contain phytosterols, carotenoids, polyphenols, and spiroenone. They have more protein to carbohydrate ratio. They are rich in fiber. They are used for culinary and medicinal purposes. They can be cooked as a rice substitute. It is cold in nature and bland in taste. It covers the spleen, lung, and kidney meridians. It stimulates and strengthens the spleen and lungs, and removes heat. It also has diuretic and antiallergy properties. It is used to treat conditions with damp-heat. It makes the skin more hydrated and is used to improve skin, hair, and nail health. It reduces wrinkles and dark spots. It is used to treat eczema and acne. It is added to skin care products such as lotions and creams. It supports digestion and can be used to treat diarrhea. It is used for arthritis and UTIs. It also helps in weight loss (obesity). Overall, it is safe. Side effects include gas and bloating. Acupuncture Today. (n.d.). Coix seed (yi yi ren). *Acupuncturetoday.com*. https://www.acupuncturetoday.com/herbcentral/coixseed.php Zhu, F. (2017). Coix: Chemical composition and health effects. *Trends in Food Science & Technology*, *61*, 160–175. https://doi.org/10.1016/j.tifs.2016.12.003

Ingredients	Mechanism of Action and Health Benefits
Cordyceps *Ophiocordyceps* *sinensis*	Other names: *Caterpillar fungus, Dong Chong Xia Cao* Cordyceps contain alkaloids, gums, mucilages, phenolic compounds, flavonoids, saponins, and amino acids. They are considered as a natural energy booster in TCM. These mushrooms have antiinflammatory, antimicrobial activities, antioxidative, antiaging, and antistress properties. It is used in the treatment of arrhythmias, asthenia after severe illness, bronchitis, cancer, hyperglycemia, hyperlipidemia, hyposexuality, night sweating, renal dysfunction, and renal failure. Cordyceps are also useful in preventing asthma, depression, diabetes, fatigue, high cholesterol, and upper respiratory tract infections. These mushrooms are safe for short-term use. They can cause allergic reactions in some with mild symptoms of stomach ache, nausea, diarrhea, or dry mouth. Cordyceps should be avoided by people taking diabetes medications, anticoagulants ("blood thinners"), or anticlotting drugs. It should also not be used by children, pregnant women, or nursing mothers. Rajput, R., Sethy, N. K., Singh, V. K., Sharma, S., Sharma, R. K., Deswal, R., et al. (2016). Phytochemical and proteomic analysis of a high altitude medicinal mushroom cordyceps sinensis. *Journal of Proteins and Proteomics*, *7*(3), 187–197. https://www.researchgate.net/publication/316240578_PHYTOCHEMICAL_AND_PROTEOMIC_ANALYSIS_OF_A_HIGH_ALTITUDE_MEDICINAL_MUSHROOM_CORDYCEPS_SINENSIS Wong, C., & Dashiell, E. (2020, August 2). 4 benefits of the medicinal mushroom cordyceps. *Verywell Health*. https://www.verywellhealth.com/benefits-of-cordyceps-89441
Corydalis *Corydalis yanhusuo*	Other name: *Yan Hu Suo or Yanhusuo* The main bioactive compounds present in corydalis include alkaloids (tetrahydropalmatine, corydaline, berberine, and columbamine), anthraquinones, and steroids. It covers the heart, lung, spleen, and liver meridians. It is warm in nature. It breaks blood stagnation and moves the blood. It has analgesic and sedative properties. It can treat chest pain and also prevent stroke and heart attack. It can also reduce pain and swelling traumatic fractures. It is used to treat dysmenorrhea, amenorrhea, endometriosis, and infertility. Side effects include dizziness, fatigue, and hepatotoxicity. Acupuncture Today. (n.d.). Corydalis (yan hu suo). *acupuncturetoday.com*. https://www.acupuncturetoday.com/herbcentral/corydalis.php Lu, Y., Ma, Q., Fu, C., Chen, C., & Zhang, D. (2020). Quality evaluation of *Corydalis yanhusuo* by high-performance liquid chromatography fingerprinting coupled with multicomponent quantitative analysis. *Scientific Reports*, *10*(1), 1–10. https://doi.org/10.1038/s41598-020-61951-x Me and Qi. (n.d.). Corydalis tubers. *meandqi.com*. https://www.meandqi.com/herb-database/corydalis-tuber
Cynomorium *Cynomorium* *songaricum*	Other name: *Suo Yang* Cynomorium contains more than 30 bioactive compounds including terpenoids (ursolic acid, oleanolic acid, and acetylursolic acid), flavonoids (catechin, proanthocyanidins, quercetin, and rutin), steroids, and phenolic acids. It is warm in nature. It covers the liver, kidney, and large intestine meridians. It nourishes the blood, tonifies the kidney, and strengthens the Yang. It is an aphrodisiac. It is used to treat infertility in both men and women. It helps in erectile dysfunction and premature ejaculation. It can reduce stress and fatigue. Side effects include diarrhea. Acupuncture Today. (n.d.). Cynomorium (suo yang). *acupuncturetoday.com*. https://www.acupuncturetoday.com/herbcentral/cynomorium.php Patočka, J., & Navrátilová, Z. (2020). Cynomorium plants: bioactive compounds and pharmacologic actions. *Military Medical Science Letters*, *89*(2), 90–98. https://doi.org/10.31482/mmsl.2020.001 Proven Herbal Remedies. (2021, April 20). Cynomorium Songaricum (Suo Yang). *Chinese Herbs Healing*. https://www.chineseherbshealing.com/proven-herbal-remedies/cynomorium-songaricum.html

Ingredients	Mechanism of Action and Health Benefits
Dang shen *Codonopsis pilosula*	Other name: *Poor man's ginseng*

The active compounds present include essential oils, polysaccharides, inulin, saponins, scutellarein, resins, mucus, glycosides, alkaloids (choline and perlolyrine), and various amino acids.

It is regarded as an effective and more affordable substitute for ginseng.

It has antiinflammatory, antidiabetic, anticancer, and hepatoprotective properties.

Dang shen can reduce fatigue, and help to increase red blood cell counts and hemoglobin levels. It can also help against immune deficiency-related illnesses, including HIV infections. The roots are also used for treatment of diarrhea, vomiting, flatulence, and excessive stomach acid.

It is used for ailments associated with weakness, fatigue, poor appetite, and anemia. It is used as an herbal remedy for arthritis and other conditions of the muscles and joints.

There are no known adverse reactions of using dang shen. It has very low toxicity and can be used for a long period of time.

MD Health Online. (2021, April 7). The richness of "Poor Man's Ginseng." https://mdhealthonline.com/the-richness-of-poor-mans-ginseng/

Sturluson, T. (2018, October 25). Poor Man's Ginseng or Dang Shen herb uses and health benefits. *The Herbal Resource.* https://www.herbal-supplement-resource.com/poor-mans-ginseng-dang-shen.html

Deer antler glue
Cornu Cervi

Other names: *Lu Jiao Jiao Cervus nippon, Cervus elaphus*

Lu Jiao is a calcified deer antler and is obtained from old (dropped or killed) deer.

It is warm in nature. It covers the liver and kidney meridians. It tonifies the blood and the kidney Yang. It improves blood circulation.

It has antiinflammatory properties.

It can treat heavy bleeding due to menorrhagia or hematuria.

It can also treat impotency and hypothyroidism.

Side effects include diarrhea.

Me and Qi. (n.d.). Deer antler glue. *Meandqi.com.* https://www.meandqi.com/herb-database/deer-antler-glue

paramounttechnetwork. (2020, September 3). The role of Lu Rong (deer velvet) products in Chinese herbal medicine. Safflower Chinese Medicine Dispensary. https://safflower.com.au/the-role-of-lu-rong-deer-velvet-products-in-chinese-herbal-medicine/

Deer antler glue
(precalcined)
Cornu Cervi pantotrichum

Other names: *Lu Rong, Deer velvet*

Lu rong is precalcified antler. It is rich in several growth factors.

It is warm in nature. It tonifies and invigorates the kidney Yang. It also promotes circulation of the blood.

It has antiinflammatory, antiaging, and anticancer properties.

It is cardiotonic, and it can treat anemia.

It also has aphrodisiac properties and improves blood testosterone levels. It can also increase adrenocortex hormone. It can treat impotence, menopausal symptoms, and menorrhagia.

It can also help in wound healing.

Side effects include diarrhea.

paramounttechnetwork. (2020, September 3). The role of Lu Rong (deer velvet) products in Chinese herbal medicine. Safflower Chinese Medicine Dispensary. https://safflower.com.au/the-role-of-lu-rong-deer-velvet-products-in-chinese-herbal-medicine/

Penner, J. (n.d.). Lu Rong. *American Dragon.* https://www.americandragon.com/Individualherbsupdate/LuRong.html

Dodder seeds
Cuscuta reflexa

Other names: *Cuscuta seeds, Amarbel, Giant dodder, Tu Si Zi, Cuscuta chinensis Lam*

The *Cuscuta* genus has over 100 species. *Cuscuta reflexa* (or giant dodder) is one of them. It is a parasitic, twirling, and sprawling vine. Its seeds are rich in hydroxycinnamic acids, flavonoids (such as quercetin and kaempferol), alkaloids, tannins, and saponins. It is warm in nature and sweet in taste. It covers the liver, kidney, and spleen meridians.

It strengthens the Yin and tonifies the kidney Yang. It also nourishes the liver.

It has antioxidant, antibacterial, antiinflammatory, and immunomodulatory properties.

It improves digestion and can treat diarrhea. It is also used to treat urinary tract disorders (including urinary incontinence, nephrotic syndrome, UTIs, and enuresis).

Ingredients	Mechanism of Action and Health Benefits

It is used to treat impotence, erectile dysfunction, premature ejaculation, and improve sperm count and motility. It can also be used to improve ovulation, egg quality, and uterine hypoplasia, regulate menstruation, and prevent miscarriages.

It encourages hyaline cartilage repair, improves bone density, and prevents osteoporosis. It also improves vision and can be used for dry eyes.

Overall, it is safe. It should not be used in hard or dry stools, kidney fire, and persistent penile erection.

DePry, A. (2020, April 5). Tu Si Zi. *Mysite.* https://www.depryacupuncture.com/post/tu-si-zi

GinSen Clinics London. (2021, July 6). Benefits of Dodder Seeds (Semen Cuscutae). TCM Blog by GinSen. https://tcmblog.co.uk/benefits-of-dodder-seeds/

Me and Qi. (n.d.). Cuscuta seeds. *Meandqi.Com.* https://www.meandqi.com/herb-database/cuscuta-seeds

Earthworm
Pheretima aspergillum

Other names: *Di Long, Pheretima vulgaris, Pheretima guillelmi*

Earthworms have nutritional and medicinal values and are used in both TCM and Ayurveda and in Asian countries.

Earthworms are cold in nature. It covers the liver, lung, spleen, and bladder meridians. It clears the liver heat and lung heat.

It has antiinflammatory, antipyretic, and neuroprotective properties.

The earthworm powder extract is made by boiling worms in salted water and onion.

It is used in rheumatism/rheumatoid arthritis, epilepsy, stroke, and asthma.

Cooper, E. L., Balamurugan, M., Huang, C. Y., Tsao, C. R., Heredia, J., Tommaseo-Ponzetta, M., et al. (2012). Earthworms Dilong: ancient, inexpensive, noncontroversial models may help clarify approaches to integrated medicine emphasizing neuroimmune systems. *Evidence-Based Complementary and Alternative Medicine, 2012*, 1–11. https://doi.org/10.1155/2012/164152

Eel
Anguilla rostrata

Other names: *Japanese eel or Anguilla japonica*

(*Unagi* = freshwater eel and *anago* = saltwater eel), *Man yu*

It is a thin, long snake-like fish. There are more than 400 eel fish species.

It thrives in both freshwater and saltwater.

Eel is regarded as a stamina food in Japan and Korea. It is rich in minerals (iron, zinc, calcium, magnesium, manganese, selenium, and phosphorus) and vitamins (A, B12, and E). It is also high in proteins and omega-3 fatty acids.

It is warm in nature. It can tonify Qi, blood, and Yin. It expels wind-damp and cold, and clears damp. It covers the lung, spleen, kidney, and bladder meridians. It can also strengthen the tendons and bones.

Eel can lower cholesterol, blood sugar, and blood pressure. It can also maintain skin health and promote tissue regeneration.

Eel can treat malnutrition, general fatigue, rheumatoid arthritis, backache, and impotence.

Eels are steamed, grilled (as sushi or tempura), or pickled. Dried eel powder is also available.

Raw eel should not be consumed. The eel blood is poisonous and toxic.

M, S. (2017, June 18). Eel fish facts, health benefits and nutritional value. *HealthBenefitstimes.com.* https://www.healthbenefitstimes.com/eel-fish/

Ephedra
Ephedra sinica

Other name: *Ma Huang*

Ephedra or Ma huang contains the alkaloids, ephedrine, and pseudoephedrine. Ephedrine is an amphetamine-like compound which stimulates the nervous system and heart.

It is warm in nature and bitter. It covers the lung and bladder meridians. It clears lung heat, dispels wind cold, and enhances Qi circulation.

It is used to treat cough, cold, bronchitis, asthma, eczema, and acute nephritis.

It also promotes urination and weight loss.

Side effects include hypertension, seizures, heart attack, kidney stones formation, and sudden death. It has been banned in some countries.

Drugs.com. (2021). Ma Huang. https://www.drugs.com/npc/ma-huang.html

Me and Qi. (n.d.). Ephedra. *meandqi.com.* https://www.meandqi.com/herb-database/ephedra

Ingredients	Mechanism of Action and Health Benefits
Eucommia bark *Eucommia ulmoides*	Other names: *Rubber tree bark or Du Zhong* Eucommia bark contains several bioactive compounds including flavonoids, alkaloids, coumarin, and terpenes. It is warm in nature. It covers the liver and kidney meridians. It strengthens the kidney and liver, and calms ascending liver Yang. It strengthens ligaments, tendons, muscles, and bones. It supports bone health and can be used in osteoporosis, arthritis, backache, knee pain, and rheumatism. It can stop bleeding in menorrhagia, miscarriage, and bleeding piles. It can lower blood pressure and can treat hypertension, headache, and dizziness. Overall, it is safe. Side effects may lead to dizziness, headache, and edema. Acupuncture Today. (n.d.). Eucommia bark (du zhong). *acupuncturetoday.com*. https://www.acupuncturetoday.com/herbcentral/eucommiabark.php Huang, L., Lyu, Q., Zheng, W., Yang, Q., & Cao, G. (2021). Traditional application and modern pharmacological research of *Eucommia ulmoides* Oliv. *Chinese Medicine, 16*(1), 73. https://doi.org/10.1186/s13020-021-00482-7 Me and Qi. (n.d.). Eucommia bark. *meandqi.com*. https://www.meandqi.com/herb-database/eucommia-bark
Evodia fruit *Evodiae fructus*	Other name: *Wu zhu yu* *Evodia fructus* is the dried, unripe fruit of *Evodia rutaecarpa*. Its main bioactive components include evodiamine, rutaecarpine, evocarpine, limonin, narcissoside, rutin, and ocimene. The essential oil from wu zhu yu has antioxidant, antimicrobial, antiviral, antiparasitic, and antiinflammatory properties. Evodia fruit may also contain anticancer effects. It can settle the stomach Qi in acid regurgitation, stomach ulcers, vomiting, and diarrhea. It can also help in weight loss. It is used for headaches, hypertension, and heart failure. It can regulate the central nervous system (CNS) and homeostasis, and reduce the risk of cardiovascular diseases. It may also be used in management of AD. It can cause irregular heartbeat. It should also be avoided by pregnant and breastfeeding women. WebMD Editors. (n.d.). EVODIA: Overview, Uses, side effects, precautions, interactions, dosing and reviews. *WebMD*. https://www.webmd.com/vitamins/ai/ingredientmono-1159/evodia Li, M., & Wang, C. (2020). Traditional uses, phytochemistry, pharmacology, pharmacokinetics and toxicology of the fruit of *Tetradium ruticarpum*: A review. *Journal of Ethnopharmacology, 263*, 113231. https://doi.org/10.1016/j.jep.2020.113231
False unicorn *Chamaelirium luteum*	False unicorn is a woman's herb. It contains glycosides, saponins, and steroids. It can treat menstrual disorders, morning sickness, PCOS, menopausal syndrome, and infertility. It can also prevent miscarriages. It can help in digestive disorders, increase urine flow, and reduce water retention. Side effects include gastric upsets. Romm, A. (2010). Chapter 5—Menstrual wellness and menstrual problems. In B. Clare, J. E. Stansbury, L. Ryan, R. Trickey, L. Lee, & A. Hywood (Eds.), *Botanical medicine for women's health* (1st ed., pp. 97–185). Churchill Livingstone. https://doi.org/10.1016/B978-0-443-07277-2.00007-6 WebMD Editors. (n.d.). False Unicorn. *WebMD*. https://www.webmd.com/vitamins/ai/ingredient-mono-193/false-unicorn
Fang feng *Radix Saposhnikovia divaricata*	Other names: *Siler root, Ledebouriella* Fang feng is sweet and warm in nature. It covers the liver and spleen meridians. It dispels wind, cold, and dampness. It contains clemiscosin, fangfeng pyrimidine, adenosine, and β-sitosterol. It has antiviral, antipyretic, and antibiotic properties. It is used to treat headaches, colds, chills, convulsions, and tremors. It can also help ease body ache. It can also improve bowel movements and can treat diarrhea. Overall, it is safe. It should not be taken with Yin and blood deficiency heat patterns. 1st Chinese Herbs. (n.d.). Fang Feng. https://1stchineseherbs.com/herbs-a-z/f/fang-feng/ Acupuncture Today Staff. (n.d.). Siler Root (Fang Feng). *Acupuncture Today*. https://www.acupuncturetoday.com/herbcentral/siler.php
Fan Shi Liu *Psidium guajava*	Refer under "Guava"

Ingredients	Mechanism of Action and Health Benefits
Female ginseng *Angelica sinensis*	Other names: *Chinese angelica, dang gui, dong quai, bai zhi* Female ginseng or Dong quai contains chemical compounds including organic acids (ferulic acid, protocatechuic acid, caffeic acid, phthalic acid, and vanillic acid), phthalides, and polysaccharides. Ferulic acid has antiinflammatory effects. Ligustilide (E and Z), a major phthalide, is mainly responsible for the antiplatelet effect. It also contains phellopterin, angelic acid, and angelicotoxin. It has an intense aroma. It can expel wind and dampness, relieve pain and a stuffy nose. It is associated with the stomach and lung meridians. It has antioxidant, antiinflammatory, analgesic, antimicrobial, antipyretic, and immune-modulating properties. It also possesses anticancer, radioprotective, and neuroprotective effects. It is used to treat women's health issues to enrich blood, promote blood circulation, and treat menstrual disorders (amenorrhea and dysmenorrhea). It can also be used to treat chronic constipation of the elderly. It is used to treat colds, headaches, and rhinitis. It is used in the treatment of oral diseases including toothache. It can also be used for skin conditions like atopic dermatitis, psoriasis, and wound healing. Dang gui is also used for treating cardio-cerebrovascular disease, nervous system diseases, and nephrotic syndrome. Possible side effects include bloating, loss of appetite, diarrhea, fever, high blood pressure, and excessive bleeding. Female ginseng has anticoagulant and estrogen-like effects so it should be avoided by people with bleeding disorders, women who experience excessive menstrual bleeding, pregnant and breastfeeding women, and people with estrogen-related conditions. It should also not be taken by people with hormone-sensitive conditions such as endometriosis, uterine fibroids and breast, uterus, or ovary cancers. It can interact with birth control pills, ibuprofen, blood thinners, and lorazepam. 1st Chinese Herbs. (n.d.). Angelica Dahurica (Bai Zhi). https://1stchineseherbs.com/a/angelica-root/angelica-dahurica-bai-zhi/ Chen, X. P., Li, W., Xiao, X. F., Zhang, L. L., & Liu, C. X. (2013). Phytochemical and pharmacological studies on Radix Angelica sinensis. *Chinese Journal of Natural Medicines*, *11*(6), 577–587. https://doi.org/10.1016/s1875-5364(13)60067-9 Jeong, S. H., Kim, B. B., Lee, J. E., Ko, Y., & Park, J. B. (2012). Evaluation of the effects of Angelicae dahuricae radix on the morphology and viability of mesenchymal stem cells. *Molecular Medicine Reports*, *12*(1), 1556–1560. https://doi.org/10.3892/mmr.2015.3456 Wong, C., & Forgoros, R. N. (2020, January 8). *The health benefits of Dong Quai. Verywell Health*. https://www.verywellhealth.com/the-benefits-of-dong-quai-89448.
Figwort root *Radix scrophulariae*	Other name: *Xuan shen* Figwort roots contain harpagide, harpagoside, ajugol, aucubin, oleanolic acid, ursolic acid, cinnamic acid, verbascoside, and rehmannioside. It has antiinflammatory, antifungal, and anticancer properties. In TCM, xuan shen works on the lung, stomach, and kidneys Qi. It has a slightly salty, bitter taste, and cold properties. Figwort root can clear heat toxins, eliminate nodules, purge fire, and nourish Yin. It can be used to treat febrile diseases, hot flushes, red and swollen eyes, swollen lymph nodes (tonsils), sore throat (chronic pharyngitis), and high fever in children. It also clears heat and cools the blood. It is also used to treat chronic prostatitis, lymphadenopathy, breast hyperplasia, constipation, and thromboangiitis obliterans. Xuan shen should not be used by people with spleen and stomach weaknesses such as poor appetite or diarrhea. It should not be used with the herb, black hellebore (li lu). Acupuncture Today. (n.d.). Scrophularia (xuan shen). https://www.acupuncturetoday.com/herbcentral/scrophularia.php Chinese Herbs Info. (2021, March 31). Xuan Shen (Radix Scrophulariae or Ningpo Figwort Root). https://www.chineseherbsinfo.com/xuan-shen/

Ingredients	Mechanism of Action and Health Benefits
Five-flavor berry *Schisandra* *chinensis*	Other name: *Wu Wei Zi* Five-flavor berry or schisandra is rich in antioxidants i.e., flavonoids (hesperetin and quercetin). It has all five tastes (sweet, sour, salty, spicy, and bitter) and will cover all the Yin organs (heart, lung, kidney, spleen, and liver). It is warm in nature. It covers all the above meridians. It tonifies the kidney and heart, and calms the spirit. It is also a brain tonic. It has astringent and antiaging properties. It is an adaptogen and can increase physical and mental stamina, alertness, and libido. It can relieve premenstrual symptoms and vaginal discharge. It can treat asthma, cough, hypertension, and palpitation. It can also improve liver function, help in diarrhea, indigestion, and diabetes. Overall, it is safe. Side effects include gastric upset. Me and Qi. (n.d.). Schisandra berries. *Meandqi.com*. https://www.meandqi.com/herb-database/schisandra-berries Sun, W., Shahrajabian, M. H., & Cheng, Q. (2021). *Schisandra chinensis*, five flavor berry, a traditional Chinese medicine and a super-fruit from North Eastern China. *Pharmacognosy Communications*, *11*(1), 13–21. https://doi.org/10.5530/pc.2021.1.4
Fleeceflower root *Radix polygoni* *multiflori*	Other names: *He Shou Wu or Heshouwu, Fo-Ti root, Polygonum multiflorum* Fleeceflower root contains flavonoids, quinones, and stilbenes. It is warm in nature. It covers the liver, kidney, and heart meridians. It nourishes the liver and kidneys, and tonifies the blood. It has antioxidant, antiinflammatory, antidiabetic, and antiaging properties. It can mimic estrogen in the body. It can prevent premature graying of hair and help in depigmentation disorders. It can also treat hair loss and prevent dandruff. It promotes healthy aging and can help in diabetes, heart disease, constipation, blurring of vision, and low back ache. Side effects include hepatotoxicity, gastric upsets, and hypocalcemia. It should not be used in estrogen-sensitive tumors. Me and Qi. (n.d.). Fleeceflower roots. Meandqi.com. https://www.meandqi.com/herb-database/fleeceflower-root West, H. (2019, January 14). He Shou Wu (Fo-Ti): benefits, dosage, and side effects. *Healthline*. https://www.healthline.com/nutrition/he-shou-wu
Forsythia fruit *Fructus forsythiae*	Other name: *Lian qiao* Forsythiae fructus is the fruit of *Forsythia suspensa*. It contains terpenoids (such as oleanolic acid and betulinic acid) and phenolic compounds (pinoresinol and matairesinoside). It is cold and bitter in nature. It clears heat and eliminates toxicity of the blood. It also expels external wind and heat. It covers the lung, heart, and small intestine meridians. It has antiinflammatory, antiviral, antibacterial, and antipyretic properties. It can increase insulin secretion, and decrease blood glucose. It is often used to treat wind-heat cold-cough and skin conditions such as acne and psoriasis. It can treat obesity, fever, and headaches. 1st Chinese Herbs. (n.d.). Lian Qiao. https://1stchineseherbs.com/herbs-a-z/l/lian-qiao/ Me & Qi. (n.d.). Forsythia fruits. *meandqi.com*. https://www.meandqi.com/herb-database/forsythia-fruit
Frankincense *(Olibanum gummi)*	Other name: *Ru Xiang* Refer to the "Indian Frankincense."
Fritillary bulb *Fritillaria thunbergii bulb*	Other name: *Zhe Bei Mu* Fritillary bulb contains several bioactive compounds including alkaloids (frithunbol), terpenes, sterols, and amino acids. It is cool in nature. It covers the lung and heart meridians. It clears the lung heat and hot phlegm, and stops cough. It is used to treat sore throat, chronic bronchitis, asthma, and tonsillitis. It also disperses nodules, treat thyroid swellings (goiter), neck swellings, and breast and lung abscesses. Me and Qi. (n.d.). Fritillary bulbs. *Meandqi.com*. https://www.meandqi.com/herb-database/fritillary-bulb Proven Herbal Remedies. (2021, May 3). Fritillaria (Chuan Bei Mu). *Chinese Herbs Healing*. https://www.chineseherbshealing.com/proven-herbal-remedies/fritillaria.html

Ingredients	Mechanism of Action and Health Benefits
Gardenia fruit *Fructus gardeniae* *Gardenia augusta*	Other names: *Zhi zi, Gardeniae fructus, Gardenia augusta, Gardenia jasminoides* Gardenia fruit has many species. The chemical components present in gardenia fruit include flavonoids (crocin, chlorogenin, and ardenin), iridoids, sitosterol, ursolic acid, mannitol, and tannin. Apart from medicinal uses, it is also used as a yellow food coloring. In TCM, gardenia is considered to have a bitter taste and a cold temperature in the body. Due to this reason it is used for illness and dysfunction that stems from excessive heat. It acts directly on the blood to help cool it. It works on the heart, lungs, stomach, and liver Qi. It has analgesic, antiinflammatory, antibacterial, antioxidant, and antiviral effects. Gardenia fruit can be used to eliminate heat in the body that is manifested as irritability, sores in the mouth, or jaundice. It is also helpful for treating eye infections, itchy skin irritations like eczema, and burns. It may also help lower blood pressure, lower lipids, insomnia, and treat influenza. The fruit is used to treat nosebleeds, blood in the urine, and hematemesis. It may be used to stop hemorrhages and speed the healing of traumatic injuries. There are no known side effects of zhi zi reported but it should not be used for low appetite or loose stools related to cold. Those taking blood pressure medication should avoid or use it with caution as it can lead to hypotension. Some symptoms of allergic reactions from gardenia fruit are dizziness and fainting, and may render anesthesia ineffective (in rare cases). 1st Chinese Herbs. (n.d.). Zhi Zi. https://1stchineseherbs.com/herbs-a-z/z/zhi-zi/ Sherman, S. (2020, March 5). Gardenia's use and benefits in Chinese Medicine. *Empirical Point*. https://www.philadelphia-acupuncture.com/gardenia-chinese-medicine/
Gastrodia rhizome *Gastrodia elata*	Other names: *Tian Ma, Rhizoma Gastrodiae* Gastrodia rhizome contains more than 80 bioactive compounds including gastrodin, vanillin, β-sitosterol, and parishin. It covers the liver meridian. It pacifies and calms the liver wind to control blood pressure. It also sedates the liver Yang. It expels the liver wind to control seizures. It removes and wind-damp to relieve pain. It is neuroprotective. It is used to treat headache, dizziness, hypertension, migraine, seizures, epilepsy, stroke, and dementia. Overall, it is safe with long-term use. Acupuncture Today. (n.d.). Gastrodia (tian ma). *acupuncturetoday.com*. https://www.acupuncturetoday.com/herbcentral/gastrodia.php Me and Qi. (n.d.). Gastrodia rhizomes. *meandqi.com*. https://www.meandqi.com/herb-database/gastrodia-rhizome Zhan, H. D., Zhou, H. Y., Sui, Y. P., Du, X. L., Wang, W. H., Dai, L., et al. (2016). The rhizome of *Gastrodia elata* Blume—an ethnopharmacological review. *Journal of Ethnopharmacology*, *189*, 361–385. https://doi.org/10.1016/j.jep.2016.06.057
Gentian *Gentiana lutea* *Gentiana scabra* *Gentiana macrophylla*	Other names: *Dragon Gallbladder Herb, Bitterwort, Bitter Root* Gentiana is a large genus with more than 400 species. • *Gentiana lutea (Great yellow gentian)*. This is most common and is used in TCM, Ayurveda, and in Western herbal medicine. • *Gentiana scabra or Scabrous Gentian (Long dan cao/Japanese gentian)*. It is also used in TCM. • *Gentiana macrophylla (Qin jiao)*. It is also used in TCM. The active ingredients include flavonoids, secoiridoids, iridoids, and xanthones. It covers the liver, stomach, and gallbladder meridians. It drains the damp heat from the liver and gallbladder. It dispels wind damp, and moistens the intestine. It has antiinflammatory, antioxidant, and anticancer properties. It is hepatoprotective and also diuretic. It is a stomach tonic and increases the secretion of saliva, bile, gastric juices, and small intestinal enzyme secretions. It is traditionally used to treat loss of appetite, especially in children. It can treat jaundice, gastritis, acid reflux, and dry constipation. It can also loosen phlegm from the airway. It can be used to treat cough, sore throat, bronchitis, and sinusitis. It can be used to treat hypertension, hair loss, arthritis, fever, flank pain, and red eyes. In high doses, it can cause digestive upsets, headache, and dizziness. It should not be used in spleen and stomach deficiency cold. Proven Herbal Remedies. (2021, April 20). Gentian root. *Chinese Herbs Healing*. https://www.chineseherbshealing.com/proven-herbal-remedies/gentian-root.html Streit, L. (2020, November 3). Gentian Root: uses, benefits, and side effects. *Healthline*. https://www.healthline.com/nutrition/gentian-root#benefits

Ingredients	Mechanism of Action and Health Benefits
Ginkgo biloba	Ginkgo is derived from the ginkgo tree (maidenhair tree). It contains flavonoids which have antioxidant effects and terpenoids which improve circulation by dilating blood vessels, increasing nitric oxide, and making the platelets less sticky. It also has antiinflammatory properties. It opens the meridians so that Qi flows to all the vital organs.
	It improves brain health. It can improve blood flow to the brain and is believed to boost brain development. It can increase mental performance, attention, and memory in healthy individuals, and may decrease cognitive decline in dementia, including AD. It is also used to treat migraine, headaches, stress, anxiety, and depression, schizophrenia, and tinnitus. It is also used in stroke prevention.
	It can also improve heart health and circulation, premenstrual symptoms, and vision.
	Side effects include dizziness, headaches, stomach upsets, constipation, skin rash, and palpitations. It should not be used with anticoagulant medication, ibuprofen, or tranquilizers. The raw ginkgo nuts if consumed can be fatal.
	Hill, R. A. D. (2018, May 29). 12 Benefits of Ginkgo Biloba (plus side effects & dosage). *Healthline.* https://www.healthline.com/nutrition/ginkgo-biloba-benefits
	WebMD Editors. (n.d.). Gingko. *WebMD.* https://www.webmd.com/vitamins/ai/ingredientmono-333/ginkgo
Ginseng	Other names: Asian ginseng or Ren Shen *(Panax ginseng),* American ginseng or Xi Yang Shen *(Panax quinquefolius)*
	The Panax genus has many species. Two most common types are the American ginseng and the Asian ginseng (the latter includes or is also called the Korean, Chinese, or Japanese ginseng). The American ginseng is reported to be cooler and less stimulating.
	Panax is derived from a Greek word "panakeia," which means "all healing." Two important active compounds present in Panax are ginsenosides and gintonin. It has antioxidant and antiinflammatory properties from the presence of ginsenoside compounds. Siberian ginseng is from the root of *Eleutherococcus senticosus* and not from the Panax genus and its active compound is eleutherosides, hence it is not a ginseng.
	Ginseng helps improve brain functions like memory, behavior, mood, mental performance, and mental health. It also helps reduce stress, promote relaxation, and boost energy.
	It can boost endurance, decrease fatigue, lower blood sugar and cholesterol levels, increase insulin, reduce the risk of certain cancers (such as lip, mouth, esophagus, stomach, colon, liver, and lung cancers), and improve erectile dysfunction in men and menopause in women. It also strengthens the immune system. It causes more urination.
	Side effects may include headaches, diarrhea, and changes to blood sugar or blood pressure, sleep problems, palpitations, swollen breasts, and vaginal bleeding.
	It interacts with caffeine, alcohol, and several drugs including insulin, diabetic medications, anticoagulants, furosemide, and immunosuppressants. It should not be used for more than 2–3 months at a time.
	Ginsana. (2020, January 14). A history of Ginseng. https://www.ginsanaproducts.com/health-insights/energy-immune-system/a-history-of-ginseng/
	Semeco, A. (2018, February 28). 7 proven health benefits of ginseng. *Healthline.* https://www.healthline.com/nutrition/ginseng-benefits
	WebMD Editors. (n.d.). Panax Ginseng. *WebMD.* https://www.webmd.com/vitamins/ai/ingredient-mono-1000/panax-ginseng
Glossy privet berry *Ligustrum lucidum*	Other name: *Nu Zhen Zi*
	The phytochemical constituents of privet berry are oleanolic acid, ursolic acid, mannitol, eriodictyol, taxifolin, quercetin, nuezhenide, and ligustrosidic acid. The berry also contains minerals such as potassium, calcium, magnesium, sodium, zinc, iron, manganese, copper, nickel, and chromium.
	In TCM, nu zhen zi is considered sweet and bitter in flavor and cool in nature. It nourishes the liver and enriches the kidney.
	It has antioxidant, antimicrobial, antibacterial, laxative, antiaging, antitussive, and antitumor effects. It improves insulin resistance.
	It can be used to treat diabetes, diminished eyesight, dizziness, fever, and insomnia, and to increase immune function in cancer patients. It is also used for coronary heart disease, chronic atrophic gastritis, hepatitis, chronic bronchitis, hyperlipidemia, and poor digestion.

Ingredients	Mechanism of Action and Health Benefits
	Glossy privet berries have very low toxicity levels and should be used after consulting a doctor. It should be avoided by people with deficiency-cold in spleen and stomach, diarrhea, and deficiency of Yang. Pregnant and breastfeeding women are also advised to avoid the use of nu zhen zi. If taking diabetic medicines or insulin, the berries should be used with caution.
	Chinese Herbs Healing Editors. (2021, April 20). Chinese Privet (Ligustrum Lucidum, Nu Zhen Zi). *Chinese Herbs Healing*. https://www.chineseherbshealing.com/proven-herbal-remedies/chinese-privet.html
Green tea *Camellia sinensis*	Other names: *Chinese tea, Japanese tea, Sencha green tea*
	Green tea contains a high amount of polyphenol antioxidants. Epigallocatechin-3-gallate is a catechin, the main bioactive compound in green tea that prevents cell damage and gives its medicinal properties. The polyphenols present may also help in preventing cardiovascular diseases by lowering total and LDL cholesterol levels, lowering blood pressure, decreasing inflammation, and improving epithelial function. It also contains caffeine and L-theanine, an amino acid, both of which together act synergistically to improve brain function including performance, focus, attention, mood, and memory.
	It also contains anticancer, antidiabetic, antiobesity, and antiinflammatory properties.
	It may lower breast, prostate, and colorectal cancer risks. It may reduce the risk of dementia via its neuroprotective effects. It may also prevent diabetes, cardiovascular disease, and obesity.
	Overall, green tea is safe. People with caffeine sensitivities may experience insomnia, anxiety, irritability, nausea, or an upset stomach. Rarely, high consumption of green tea can cause liver injury.
	Gunnars, K., & Arnarson, A. (2020, April 6). 10 evidence-based benefits of green tea. *Healthline*. https://www.healthline.com/nutrition/top-10-evidence-based-health-benefits-of-green-tea#_noHeaderPrefixedContent
	Joshi, G., & Kaur, R. (2016). *Tinospora cordifolia*: A phytopharmacological review. *International Journal of Pharmaceutical Sciences and Research*, *7*(3), 890–897. https://doi.org/10.13040/IJPSR.0975-8232
Gypsum fibrosum	Other name: *Shi gao*
	Gypsum or Shi gao is prepared by powdering and heating the gypsum mineral. It is composed of calcium sulfate dihydrate. It is cold in nature and is sweet.
	It covers the lung and stomach meridians. It clears heat from the stomach and lung.
	It is used to treat high fever, cough, bleeding, toothache, and gum inflammation. It relieves thirst.
	It is used for wounds, eczema, burns, and mouth and stomach ulcers.
	It may benefit diabetes and arthritis.
	Adverse side effects are not known. It should not be used with a weak stomach and insufficient spleen Yang.
	Acupuncture Today. (n.d.). Gypsum (shi gao). *AcupunctureToday.Com*. https://www.acupuncturetoday.com/herbcentral/gypsum.php
	Me and Qi. (n.d.). Gypsum. *meandqi.com*. https://www.meandqi.com/herb-database/gypsum
Halitum	Other names: *Halite, Da Qing Yan*
	Halitum is a rock salt mineral. It is cold in nature. It covers the kidney, heart, and bladder meridians. It cools the blood and clears heat.
	It can treat inflamed and bleeding gums, toothache, inflammation in the eyes, hematemesis (stomach bleeding), and hematuria (blood in urine).
	It also improves eyesight.
	Health Wisdom Staff. (n.d.). Da Qing Yan 大青盐, Halite, Halitum. *Health Wisdom™*. https://www.healthwisdom.shop/products/da-qing-yan-halite-halitum
	TCM wiki. (2016, September 23). Halitum. https://tcmwiki.com/wiki/halitum
Han Lian Cao *Eclipta prostrata*	Other name: *False daisy*
	Refer to "Bhringraj."
Hawthorn *Crataegus*	Other name: *Shan Zha*
	It is rich in polyphenols that are powerful antioxidant compounds that include rutin, vitexin, saponins, catechins, and several anthocyanidins.
	It also has antiinflammatory properties.
	It is "warm" in nature and will benefit those who have too much "cold" in their bodies due to "Yin excess" (Yin is cold in nature) or "Yang deficiency" (Yang is hot in nature).

Ingredients	Mechanism of Action and Health Benefits
	It is cardiotonic and improves heart health. It can stabilize blood pressure, dilate coronary blood vessels, decrease cholesterol levels, reduce shortness of breath, palpitations, and fatigue, and increase stamina and energy.
	It also contains fiber that can help digestion by reducing constipation and acting as a prebiotic.
	It helps reduce anxiety and may also lower the risk of type 2 diabetes, asthma, boost the immune system, and prevent hair loss.
	In some people hawthorn can cause nausea, stomach upset, fatigue, sweating, headache, dizziness, palpitations, nosebleeds, insomnia, and agitation.
	Shoemaker, S. (2019, August 26). 9 impressive health benefits of Hawthorn Berry. *Healthline*. https://www.healthline.com/nutrition/hawthorn-berry-benefits#Side-effects-and-precautions
Heal-all spike *Spica prunellae*	Other names: *Self-heal, Prunella, Xia Ku Cao, Carpenter's weed, Brunelle*
	Spica prunellae is the spike or whole plant of *Prunella vulgaris*. It is a mint herb. It can be eaten as a salad. It contains tannins, flavonoids, oleanolic acid, and ursolic and rosmarinic acids.
	It clears the liver heat, calms liver fire, and ascendant Yang.
	It has antioxidant, antiinflammatory, antiviral, and anticancer properties.
	It can lower blood glucose, cholesterol, and triglycerides. It can be used to treat diabetes and hypertension.
	It can treat sore throats and herpes infection. It also reduces nodules and thyroid swelling (goiter). It can be used for IBD and gastroenteritis.
	It can also help in endometriosis and wound healing.
	Overall, it is safe.
	Me and Qi. (n.d.). Heal-all spikes. *meandqi.com*. https://www.meandqi.com/herb-database/heal-all-spikes
	Streit, L. (2019, June 17). Prunella vulgaris: Uses, benefits, and side effects. *Healthline*. https://www.healthline.com/nutrition/prunella-vulgaris
Ho leaf oil **Ho wood oil**	Other names: *Ravintsara essential oil (Ho leaf oil), Cinnamomum camphora linalooliferum (Ho wood oil)*
	Ho leaf oil and Ho wood oil are essential oils obtained by steam distillation from the leaves and wood of *Cinnamomum camphora* tree. This tree also produces white camphor. It is a substitute or alternative to rosewood essential oil.
	It contains mainly linalool as the active ingredient.
	It has antimicrobial effects and is used in skin care products. It also has antistress and antianxiety properties.
	It is used in acne and in various skin types. It is also used as a moisturizer and can blended with other essential oils.
	It is used in aromatherapy to relieve anxiety, depression, and improve emotional wellbeing. It can also be used as massage oil.
	It should not be used in pregnancy.
	Healthbenefitstimes. (2017, September 25). Ho leaf essential oil facts and health benefits. *HealthBenefitstimes.com*. https://www.healthbenefitstimes.com/ho-leaf-essential-oil/
Honeysuckle *Lonicera japonica*	Other names: *Jin Yin Hua or Jin Yinghua, Lonicera flower*
	Honeysuckle has many species and different parts of the honeysuckle are used to treat different diseases. The flower bud is the most commonly used. It contains saponins, terpenoids, alkaloids, alkyl glycosides, and phenylpropanoid glycosides.
	It is cold in nature. It covers the stomach, heart, and lung meridians. It clears heat, cools the blood, and removes the toxicity.
	It can treat skin sores, boils, and acne. It can also treat sore throat, tonsillitis, and headaches.
	Overall, it is safe. Side effects include gastric upset.
	Acupuncture Today. (n.d.). Honeysuckle flower (jin yin hua). *acupuncturetoday.com*. https://www.acupuncturetoday.com/herbcentral/honeysuckle_flower.php
	Me and Qi. (n.d.). Honeysuckle flowers. *meandqi.com*. https://www.meandqi.com/herb-database/honeysuckle-flowers

Ingredients	Mechanism of Action and Health Benefits

Hong Qu
Red yeast rice

Red yeast rice is made by fermenting rice with red yeast, *Monascus purpureus.*

It contains monacolin K which is the active compound (also present in statins) that lowers cholesterol levels.

It is believed that hong qu inhibits cholesterol synthesis, hence lowering cholesterol levels in the body. It is an HMG-CoA inhibitor. Hence it should not be taken together with prescription statins.

The recommended dose of red yeast rice is 1200 mg to 2400 mg/day taken orally with food. The total cholesterol level, triglycerides and "bad" LDL cholesterol reduction of about 15% to 25% occurs at about 8 weeks to 12 weeks of treatment.

Red yeast rice can reduce inflammation and reduce oxidative stress in the body.

It can also help to treat metabolic syndrome by also reducing blood glucose, insulin, and blood pressure.

It may help reduce the growth and spread of prostate cancer.

Stools may be red while on the red yeast rice. The side effects are similar to statins and include muscle pain, heartburn, bloating and gas, allergic reactions, and liver toxicity.

It may also contain citrinin contaminants, which can cause kidney failure.

It should not be taken by those who had previous heart attacks, strokes, who have diabetes, high cholesterol levels, or atherosclerosis.

Link, R. (2021, July 23). Red yeast rice: Benefits, side effects and dosage. *Healthline.* https://www.healthline.com/nutrition/red-yeast-rice#metabolic-syndrome

Hornet's nest

Other name: *Lu Feng Fang*

Commonly used species include *Nidus Vespae, Polistes mandarinus Saussure, and P. olivaceus*

Hornet's nest covers the stomach and lung meridians. It expels wind damp and wind heat and removes toxicity.

It has antiinflammatory and analgesic properties. It promotes blood clotting.

It can reduce pain in arthritis. It is also used as a wash for itchy skin conditions and skin rashes. It is used in difficult psoriasis.

It also helps in mastitis and possibly breast cancer.

It is used as a warm gargle for toothache.

Borten, P. (2013, May 29). Lu Feng Fang—Hornet Nest. *Chinese Herbal Medicine.* https://chineseherbinfo.com/lu-feng-fang-hornet-nest/

Horny goat weed
Epimedium

Other names: *Yin Yang Huo, Xian Ling Pi*

Horny goat weed contains flavonoids (including quercetin and icariin) and phytoestrogens. Icariin blocks the phosphodiesterase type 5 enzyme. It is a tonic herb and is warm in nature. It covers the kidney and liver meridians. It can tonify the kidney, eliminate dampness, and dispel wind.

It is a sexual health tonic that is used in impotence, premature ejaculation, and erectile dysfunction. It also prevents bone loss in menopausal women.

It can strengthen and cleanse the kidneys.

It is helpful in osteoporosis, rheumatism, atherosclerosis, hypertension, and hay fever. It can also protect nerves.

It has mild side effects including dizziness, tachycardia, and nosebleed. It can interact with antihypertensive medication and blood thinners. It should not be used in hormone-sensitive tumors.

Me and Qi. (n.d.). Epimedium herbs. *Meandqi.com.* https://www.meandqi.com/herb-database/epimedium-herb

Morris, S. Y. (2021, July 13). Horny goat weed: Does it work to treat erectile dysfunction? *Healthline.* https://www.healthline.com/health/erectile-dysfunction/horny-goat-weed#alternative-ed-treatments

Schwarcz, J. (2017, March 20). What is horny goat weed? *McGill: Office for Science and Society.* https://www.mcgill.ca/oss/article/health-you-asked/what-horny-goat-weed

TraceGains, Inc. (2015, May 6). Horny goat weed. *Kaiser Permanente.* https://wa.kaiserpermanente.org/kbase/topic.jhtml?docId=hn-4391000

Ilex root
Ilex asprella

Other names: *Rough-leaved holly, Plum-leaved holly*

Ilex root is bitter and has cold properties. It covers the heart and lung meridians. It improves circulation, clears stasis, and removes heat.

It is used to treat coughs and colds due to wind-heat, lung abscess, asthma, hypertension, and angina.

It can also be used for wound healing.

It can interact with anticoagulants.

Acupuncture Today. (n.d.). Ilex (mao dong qing). https://www.acupuncturetoday.com/herbcentral/ilex.php

Ingredients	Mechanism of Action and Health Benefits
Immature bitter orange *Fructus aurantii*	Other name: *Zhi Qiao* The components present in zhi qiao include p-Synephrine, hesperidin, neohesperidin, nobiletin, quinoline, narcotine, noradrenaline, tryptamine, tyramine, and N-methyltyramine. p-Synephrine is a natural stimulant like ephedra. It has antifungal properties and is used in fungal infections such as jock itch, athletes' foot, and ringworm. It also has hepatoprotective and antidiabetic properties. In TCM, immature bitter orange breaks stagnant Qi, reduces accumulation (epigastric or abdominal pain or indigestion with focal distention or gas), transforms phlegm, relieves distension (food retention in the large intestine: distention in the abdomen, constipation, or diarrhea with tenesmus), and is used in Qi tonics. Other benefits include improving digestive health, easing occasional constipation, reducing the risk of cardiovascular disorders, and wound healing. Zhi qiao may also help in weight management. Bitter orange is commonly found in weight loss medications with added caffeine and other ingredients. Synephrine can cause an increased heart rate and blood pressure and vasoconstriction. It should be avoided by women who are pregnant or nursing and people with high blood pressure or any heart issues. 1st Chinese Herbs. (n.d.). Immature fruit of bitter orange. https://1stchineseherbs.com/herbs-a-z/b/bitter-orange-fruit-immature/
Inula flowers *Inula japonica* *Inula britannica* *Inula racemosa*	Other names: *Elecampane, Xuan Fu Hua, Pushkarmool* The genus *Inula* has about 90 species. Inula flowers are rich in sesquiterpenoids (mainly sesquiterpene lactones including aponicones, alantolactone, britanin, and tomentosin), and flavonoids (luteolin and quercetagetin). It is bitter in taste and warm in nature. It covers the stomach, spleen, liver, lung, and large intestine meridians. It dissolves and disperses stagnant phlegm in the lung, enhances blood circulation, and stops vomiting. It has expectorant, bronchodilator, cardioprotective, carminative, antiemetic, and diuretic properties. It is a respiratory tonic. It can treat cough, cold, sore throat, bronchitis, and asthma. It is also used to treat heart diseases such as hypertension, hypercholesterolemia, angina, heart failure, and myocardial ischemia. It calms the digestive system and can be used for indigestion. Side effects include gastric upset and spasms with overconsumption. Acupuncture Today. (n.d.). Inula (xuan fu hua). *acupuncturetoday.com*. https://www.acupuncturetoday.com/herbcentral/inula.php Me and Qi. (n.d.). Inula flowers. *meandqi.com*. https://www.meandqi.com/herb-database/inula-flower Borten, P. (2013, May 17). Xuan Fu Hua—Inula flower—Elecampane—"Revolved, Upturned Flower." *Chinese Herbal Medicine*. https://chineseherbinfo.com/xuan-fu-hua-inula-flower-elecampane-revolved-upturned-flower/
Isatis Root	Other names: *Ban Lan Gen, Ban Lan Gen, Da Qing Ye, Chinese Indigo, Indigo, Indigo Naturalis, Isatis indigotica, Avuri* Refer to "Avuri" under Indian Natural Ingredients Isatis is used to treat common colds, sinusitis, rhinitis (upper respiratory tract infections), and salivary glands infections (parotitis). It also helps in psoriasis and diarrhea. Overall, it is safe for topical use and short-term oral use. Rxlist. (2021, June 11). Isatis: Health benefits, side effects, uses, dose & precautions. https://www.rxlist.com/isatis/supplements.htm
Japanese catnip *Schizonepeta tenuifolia*	Other names: *Nepeta, Jing Jie* Japanese catnip is warm in nature and covers the lung and liver meridians. It dispels evil wind and clears heat. It contains menthone, menthol, hesperidin, schizonodiol, cineole, and caffeic acid. It is used to treat itchy skin conditions. It can reduce inflammatory swellings. It can also stop bleeding and can treat uterine bleeding, bloody stools, and nosebleeds. It can also treat colds and flu. Side effects include acute allergic reactions. Acupuncture Today. (n.d.). Schizonepeta (jing jie). https://www.acupuncturetoday.com/herbcentral/schizonepeta.php Me and Qi. (2021). Japanese catnip. *Meandqi.com*. https://www.meandqi.com/herb-database/japanese-catnip

Ingredients	Mechanism of Action and Health Benefits
Japanese Climbing Fern *Lygodium japonicum*	Other names: *Vine-like fern, Hai Jin Sha* *Lygodium japonicum* is native to Japan. *Lygodium microphyllum, is* another species (old world climbing fern or small leaf climbing fern). Lygodium is a climbing vine which is like an invasive "weed." It contains saponins, flavonoids, coumarin, and alkaloids. It is sweet and cold, and covers the bladder and small intestine meridians. It clears heat. The dried spores have medicinal uses and act as a diuretic for kidney and urinary problems. In Indonesian folk medicine, *Lygodium microphyllum*, is used to treat kidney stones. It can also treat various skin disorders (including wounds and eczema). It can help in dysmenorrhea. It is an expectorant and can also reduce cough and colds. Acupuncture Today. (n.d.). Lygodium (hai jin sha). *Acupuncturetoday.com*. https://www.acupuncture-today.com/herbcentral/lygodium.php
Jiaogulan *Gynostemma pentaphyllum*	Other name: *Southern ginseng* Jiaogulan contains various phytochemicals including rutin, quercetin, gallic acid, saponins (gypenoside), phenols, and flavonoids. The flavonoids present have antioxidant and antiproliferative effects. It is cold in nature and covers the heart and lung meridians. Jiaogulan has antiaging, antiinflammatory, antianxiety, and detoxifying properties. It is used to treat hypertension, hypercholesterolemia, and obesity. It also improves heart function and the immune system. It is an adaptogen, increases stamina and improves memory. It can be used as a substitute for ginseng. It may also help reduce the airway inflammation in asthma. It is considered generally safe but it can cause side effects including nausea and an increase in bowel movements. The herb should be avoided in autoimmune diseases. It should also be avoided when taking anticoagulants, antiplatelet agents, insulin, or other blood-sugar-lowering medications. Wong, C., & Kroner, A. (2021, January 14). The health benefits of Jiaogulan. *Verywell Health*. https://www.verywellhealth.com/the-lowdown-on-jiaogulan-88940 Xie, Z., Liu, W., Huang, H., Slavin, M., Zhao, Y., Whent, M., et al. (2010). Chemical composition of five commercial *Gynostemma pentaphyllum* samples and their radical scavenging, antiproliferative, and anti-inflammatory properties. *Journal of Agricultural and Food Chemistry*, 58(21), 11243–11249. https://doi.org/10.1021/jf1026372
Jingtong granule (JG)	Jingtong granule is comprised of seven commonly used herbs, including *Radix notoginseng* (Sanqi), *Rhizoma Ligustici Chuanxiong* (Chuanxiong), *Rhizoma Corydalis* (Yan hu suo), *Radix Paeoniae Alba* (Bai Shao), *Radix Clematidis* (Wei Ling Xian), *Radix Puerariae* (Gegen), and *Rhizoma et Radix Notopterygii* (Qiang Huo). JG reduces local edema, congestion, and lymphocyte infiltration of inflammatory reaction, and lowering the amount of substance P. Zhu, L., Gao, J., Yu, J., Feng, M., Li, J., Wang, S., et al. (2015). Jingtong Granule: A Chinese patent medicine for cervical radiculopathy. *Evidence-Based Complementary and Alternative Medicine*, 2015, 1–9. https://doi.org/10.1155/2015/158453
Jujube *Ziziphus jujuba*	Other names: *Chinese date, Red date, Da Zao* Jujube fruits contain several antioxidants (flavonoids, polysaccharides, and triterpenic acids) and amino acids. It is rich in fiber, vitamin C (77% of the DV), and potassium (5% of the DV). It also contains vitamins A and B and minerals such as calcium, phosphorus, iron, copper, manganese, and magnesium. Chinese dates also contain bromelain, an enzyme that can reduce phlegm and mucus buildup. The fruits have antiinflammatory, antianxiety, hypolipidemic, and antimicrobial effects. The fiber can improve digestion and strengthen the lining of the stomach and intestines, decreasing the risk of damage from ulcers, injury, and harmful bacteria. It helps improve sleep, reduce the risk of chronic diseases, and certain cancers including thyroid, ovarian, cervical, breast, liver, colon, and skin. It helps improve brain function and the seed extracts may help treat dementia caused by AD. Chinese dates can also help in weight loss and detoxify blood. Overall, it is safe. Due to its high fiber content, it can be hard to digest. People suffering from intestinal parasites, bloating, tooth disease, and excessive phlegm should consult a doctor prior to consumption. It can interact with antidepressant medication venlafaxine or other serotonin-norepinephrine reuptake inhibitors.

Ingredients	Mechanism of Action and Health Benefits
	Saxena, S. (2020, October 21). Top 12 health benefits of Jujube fruit. *Medindia.* https://www.medindia.net/dietandnutrition/top-12-health-benefits-of-jujube-fruit.htm
	Shoemaker, S. (2019, August 23). What is Jujube fruit? Nutrition, benefits, and uses. *Healthline.* https://www.healthline.com/nutrition/jujube#intro
Konjac root *Amorphophallus konjac*	Other names: *Konjaku, Konnyaku potato, Snake palm, Devil's tongue, Elephant yam (not to be confused with Elephant foot yam)* It is a root vegetable that is consumed in many Asian Oriental countries. It is high in soluble fibre, glucomannan that slows digestion and regulates intestinal movements. It is also rich in minerals such as iron, calcium, magnesium and zinc. It can lower LDL cholesterol, triglycerides and blood glucose. It can help in the management of obesity, diabetes, hypercholesterolemia and constipation. It can prevent diverticular disease and piles. It is boiled and eaten or ground into flour to make shirataki noodles or snack foods. It is regarded as near-zero calorie pasta. Overall, it is safe. Excessive consumption may cause gas and bloating. There is risk of throat or intestinal obstruction due to its gummy gelatinous nature. Rarely, allergic reactions occur. McDermott, A. (2017, April 27). What Is Konjac? Healthline. https://www.healthline.com/health/konjac WebMD. (2020). GLUCOMANNAN: Overview, Uses, Side Effects, Precautions, Interactions, Dosing and Reviews. https://www.webmd.com/vitamins/ai/ingredientmono-205/glucomannan
Kudzu *Pueraria montana/ Pueraria lobata*	Other names: *Japanese arrowroot, Kakkon, Kudsu, Daidzein, Indian kudzu, Ge Gen, Gegen, Bidarikand,* Kudzu is an invasive vine. The main components present include polyphenols, isoflavonoids and glycosides. The starchy roots, flower and young leaf shoots are edible. It has antihyperlipidemic, antihypertensive, antiglycation and anti-diabetic properties. It contains puerarin which can treat and also prevent chest pain, lower LDL cholesterol, lower blood glucose and improve diabetic nephropathy. It increases circulation to the heart and brain. Intravenous puerarin injection is used in TCM to treat acute stroke or angina. It is used to treat alcoholism, alcoholic hangovers and the associated headaches and stomach upsets. It may also help with common cold, fever, menopausal symptoms and maintain mental fitness in post-menopausal women. It can also help with weight loss. It may be hepatotoxic. It should not be taken in estrogen-sensitive cancers, diabetes, and with blood thinning medicines or oral contraceptives. Panoff, L. (2021, February 8). *Kudzu Root: Benefits, Uses, and Side Effects.* Healthline. https://www.healthline.com/nutrition/kudzu-root#benefits Wong, C. (2021, July 5). *The Health Benefits of Kudzu.* Verywell Health. https://www.verywellhealth.com/the-benefits-of-kudzu-89059
Leech	Other names: *Hirudo, Whitmania pigra, Hirudo nipponica and Poecilobdella manillensis, Shuizhi* Leech is a medicinal animal. There many species with marked genetic variation. The above are some common medicinal leeches. It contains many bioactive compounds including peptides, phosphatidylcholine, pteridines, glycosphingolipids, and sterols. Hirudin is an active peptide isolated from the saliva. It has anticoagulant, antithrombotic, antiinflammatory, antiplatelet aggregation, and antiatherosclerotic actions. It is combined with other herbs to treat blood stasis disorders. It is neuroprotective in ischemic stroke with cerebral ischemia-reperfusion injury. Ma, C. J., Li, X., & Chen, H. (2021). Research progress in the use of leeches for medical purposes. *Talent of Medical Research.* Published. https://doi.org/10.12032/TMR20200207159
Licorice *Glycyrrhiza glabra* *Glycyrrhizae radix*	Other names: *Liquorice, Chinese liquorice root, zhi gan cao, gan cao, or Yashtimadhu or Athimathuram (Indian), Mulethi* See under *Athimathuram.*
Lilyturf root *Liriope muscari* *Radix Ophiopogonis*	Other names: *Dwarf lilyturf, Mai Dong, Mai Men Dong, Ophiopogon japonicus* Lily turf root contains alkaloids (lilidine and etioline), phenols, and saponins. It also contains several minerals (including iron, calcium, and phosphorus) and vitamins (C, B1, B2, and folate). It is cool in nature. It covers the stomach, lung, and heart meridians. It is used to treat stomach upset, constipation, and excessive thirst. It also helps in chronic dry cough.

Ingredients	Mechanism of Action and Health Benefits
	It can calm the mind and improve insomnia.
	It is also used in infertility and to treat hot flashes in menopause.
	Me & Qi. (n.d.). Dwarf lilyturf roots. *Meandqi.com*. https://www.meandqi.com/herb-database/dwarf-lilyturf-root
	Shahrajabian, M. H., Khoshkharam, M., Sun, W., & Cheng, Q. (2019). Lily bulbs (Bai He), A super food and A herbal remedy. *International Journal of Agriculture and Nutrition*, *1*(2), 21–23.
Longan *Dimocarpus longan*	Other name: *Long Yan Rou*
	The dried flesh of the longan fruit (after removal of outer shell and seed) is used. It contains flavonoids (quercetin), alkaloids, polysaccharides, and carotenoids. It is also rich in several minerals (magnesium, phosphorus, iron, and potassium), vitamins (C and A), antioxidants, and fiber.
	It is warm in nature and sweet in taste. It is associated with heart and spleen meridians.
	It treats blood and Qi deficiency. It also tonifies heart and spleen.
	It can improve memory, insomnia, and anxiety, and prevent forgetfulness.
	It is used to treat anemia and improve circulation. It reduces fatigue and increases energy.
	It also helps in digestion.
	Overall, it is safe. It can be consumed daily as tea or soup especially in the winter months.
	Me & Qi. (n.d.). Longans. *meandqi.com*. https://www.meandqi.com/herb-database/longan
Loquat leaf *Folium eriobotrya japonica*	Other name: *Pi pa ye*
	Loquat leaves are rich in phenolic compounds. These have antioxidant and anticancer properties.
	In TCM, loquat leaves are associated with the lung and stomach Qi. The leaves are considered to be cool and bitter. Its functions involve transforming phlegm, clearing lung heat, and harmonizing the stomach.
	It has hypoglycemic and hypolipidemic activities.
	Pi pa ye are commonly used for the treatment of nausea, vomiting, belching, hiccups, and GI distress. It also helps to stop bleeding. The leaves can be used for the treatment of skin conditions such as eczema and skin ulcers as a part of a poultice.
	Loquat leaves should not be used long term and should not exceed the maximum recommended dosage. There are no known side effects or drug interactions.
	Acupuncture Today Editors. (n.d.). Loquat leaf (pi pa ye). *Acupuncture Today*. https://www.acupuncturetoday.com/herbcentral/loquat_leaf.php
	Kubala, J. (2019, October 18). 7 Surprising benefits of loquats. *Healthline*. https://www.healthline.com/nutrition/loquats
Lotus *Nelumbo nucifera*	Other names: *Kamal kakri, Lian, Sacred lotus*
	The lotus seeds, roots, and stamen are edible. It has antiinflammatory, antioxidant, anticancer, antiviral, antispasmodic, antiobesity, and calming properties.
	The *root* is often used as food (stir-fry or soup). The root is rich in minerals (potassium and iron), vitamins (C and B), and dietary fiber. It can regulate blood pressure, reduce stress, and promote weight loss. It can also prevent constipation.
	The juice from the lotus *leaves* is used to treat diarrhea, reduce bleeding, and excessive sebum.
	Lotus *stamen* has strong astringent properties compared to the seeds. It is rich in flavonoids and phenolic acids. It is neutral in nature and has a sweet taste. It covers the heart and kidney meridians. It is used to treat excessive urination, vaginal discharge, and excessive seminal discharge.
	Lotus *seeds* are rich in proteins, vitamins (A, B, C, and E) and minerals (sodium and potassium).
	Overall, it is safe. Rarely allergic reactions can occur.
	Me and Qi. (n.d.). Lotus stamens. *meandqi.com*. https://www.meandqi.com/herb-database/lotus-stamens
	WebMD Editors. (2009). Lotus. *WebMD*. https://www.webmd.com/vitamins/ai/ingredientmono-124/lotus
Lysimachia *Herba Lysimachiae* *Lysimachia christinae*	Other names: *Gold coin grass, Jin Qian Cao*
	Gold coin grass clears damp heat from the liver and gallbladder. It is cool in nature. It is salty and sweet in taste. It can also clear kidney heat and increase urination. It is a diuretic.
	It has antiinflammatory and antibacterial effects.
	It can prevent and expel gallstones and kidney stones, and clear toxins. It inhibits urinary calcium excretion and increases urinary citrate, both of which help to reduce kidney stone formation.
	It cleanses the liver and promotes bile secretion so that the sediment in the bile duct will easily flow out.

Ingredients	Mechanism of Action and Health Benefits

Side effects include vertigo. It should not be taken during diarrhea or when taking antidiuretic medicines.

Me & Qi. (n.d.). Gold coin herb (Jin Qian Cao) in Chinese Medicine. *Meandqi.com*. https://www.meandqi.com/herb-database/gold-coin-herb

Magnolia bark
Magnolia officinalis

Other names: *Hou Po, Flos Magnoliae (Xin Yi), Magnolia liliiflora*

Magnolia bark is rich with antioxidants, mainly polyphenols. The two main compounds are magnolol and honokiol. It prevents release of the stress hormones (like adrenaline), increases GABA level, and activates the cannabinoid receptors to promote sleep.

It has antiinflammatory, antimicrobial, anticancer, and sedative effects.

It is used to treat nasal congestion, asthma, anxiety, depression, and stomach disorders. They can reduce the risk of diabetes, cancer, heart disease, and neurodegenerative diseases like AD.

Magnolia bark can also help menopausal women experiencing symptoms of sleep and mood alterations.

Generally, magnolia bark is considered safe for use. Common side effects include drowsiness, headache nausea, and vomiting.

Snyder, C. (2020, April 7). Magnolia Bark: benefits, usage, and side effects. *Healthline*. https://www.healthline.com/nutrition/magnolia-bark

Medicinal mushrooms

All medicinal mushrooms have antioxidant, antiinflammatory, immune-boosting (increased white cells and antiinflammatory cytokines), antiaging, longevity-boosting, and anticancer actions, some actions more than the other. Some are also more organ-specific. They are used to treat infections, allergies, metabolic syndromes, chronic illnesses, neurological disorders, and cancers. Mushrooms are also effective against wrinkles, sunspots, and photoaging.

The main medicinal mushrooms include the following:

Lion's Mane mushroom: (Hericium erinaceus, *Hou tou gu or Monkey head mushroom, Yamabushi-take or Mountain monk mushroom*): It has one of the highest antioxidant scores and supports brain health. It has various neurotrophic or nootropic factors (such as hericenones and erinacines which are beta-glucan polysaccharides). They are neuroprotective and can stimulate neuronal regeneration and nerve growth factor (NGF) synthesis. NGF modulates neuroplasticity and can boost brain functions like memory, mood cognition, and visual processing. It is used in autism, stroke, and neurodegenerative disorders like PD and AD (beta-amyloid is reduced in AD with lion's mane).

Cordyceps mushroom (Cordyceps sinensis, Caterpillar Fungus): The Cordyceps mushroom is a parasitic fungus and has more lung-protective and energy-boosting effects. It has cordycepin and adenosine nucleotide compounds which can increase ATP levels (the body's energy molecules) to boost physical endurance, stamina, and performance. It is used also in allergies, bronchitis, asthma, and lung disorders.

Reishi mushroom (Ganoderma lucidum, Lingzhi or Ling zhi, Reishi or Mannentake): Ganoderma has many species with many shapes and colors. It is a fungus which can also grow in hot humid climates and is now mass produced by artificial commercial cultivation. It has strong immunomodulating actions and is an excellent general health tonic for stress, sleep, and fatigue. It replenishes the Qi. It contains various bioactive compounds such as triperpenes (danoderiol, danderenic acid, ganoderic acid, and lucidenic acids) with antioxidant, antitumor, and lipid-lowering actions, ganodermin with antifungal effects, polysaccharides with antitumor actions, peptidoglycans like *G. lucidum* ganoderans A, B, and C polysaccharides with broad-spectrum biological activities, proteoglycan, GLPG) and more.

It is often mixed with other medicinal mushrooms like shiitake, maitake, Agaricus, and other herbs.

Chaga mushroom: (Inonotus obliquus, Black moss): It is a parasitic fungus which grows usually on the birch trees. It is rich in triterpenes. It supports liver and digestive health, lowers blood sugar and cholesterol, and helps in diabetes and heart conditions.

Turkey Tail mushroom: (Trametes versicolor or Coriolus versicolor): It improves the immune and lung functions.

Shiitake mushroom: (Lentinula edodes): Dried and fresh shiitake mushrooms are used a lot in Asian cuisine.

Maitake mushroom: (Grifola frondosa, Dancing Mushroom): It is a large polypore mushroom. It stimulates the immune system including the T-helper cells and natural killer cells. It also regulates blood pressure.

Ingredients	Mechanism of Action and Health Benefits

Agaricus mushroom (Agaricus brasiliensis or Agaricus subrufescens, Almond mushroom): It is used in diabetes, hypercholesterolemia, digestive disorders, and cancers.

Benzie, I. F., & Wachtel-Galor, S. (2011). *Herbal medicine: Biomolecular and clinical aspects* (2nd ed.). Boca Raton: CRC Press.

Jacob, D. (2021, April 6). What is the best mushroom to fight cancer? *MedicineNet*. https://www.medicinenet.com/what_is_the_best_mushroom_to_fight_cancer/article.htm

E.Qi.Librium Herbs. (n.d.). Medicinal Mushrooms—Cordyceps, Reishi, Shiitake, Maitake, Coriolus Versicolor. https://www.eqilibrium.net/en/medicinal-mushrooms.html

Millettia Stem
Spatholobus suberectus

Other name: *Ji Xue Teng*

Millettia is a variety of climbing vine. The stem contains a reddish-brown resin that resembles dried chicken blood. It contains phenols (mainly gallic acid), flavonoids (butin), saponins, and quinones.

It is warm in nature. It covers the liver, heart, and spleen meridians. It invigorates and tonifies the blood. It also relaxes the tendons.

It is used in arthralgia, arthritis, and backache.

It can treat menstrual disorders including dysmenorrhea, irregular periods, amenorrhea, and menorrhagia.

There are no reported side effects.

Acupuncture Today. (n.d.). Millettia (ji xue teng). *Acupuncturetoday.com*. https://www.acupunctureto-day.com/herbcentral/millettia.php

Borten, P. (2013, July 29). Ji Xue Teng—Millettia or Spatholobus root and vine. *Chinese Herbal Medicine*. https://chineseherbinfo.com/ji-xue-teng-millettia-or-spatholobus-root-and-vine/

Mimosa bark
Albizia julibrissin

Other names: *Persian silk tree, He Huan Pi, Albizia odoratissima*

Mimosa bark contains various bioactive compounds such as triterpenoid saponins (julibrosides), glycosides (budmunchiamines), saponins (albiziatrioside), and flavonoids (quercetin and isoquercetin).

It is also referred to as "Collective Happiness Bark." The leaves, seeds, and stems of the plant are used.

It covers the heart and lung meridians. It invigorates blood. It dispels liver Qi stagnation.

It has calming, antioxidant, analgesic, and antidiabetic properties.

It enhances mood. It is used in depression and anxiety. It also regulates negative emotions such as irritability, anger, and insomnia.

It supports joint health. It is used to treat bruises and pain and swelling in fractures.

Overall, it is safe. It may cause drowsiness and sleepiness.

Karuppannan, K., Priyadharshini, S. D., & Sujatha, V. (2013). Phytopharmacological properties of Albizia species: A review. *International Journal of Pharmacy and Pharmaceutical Sciences*, 5(3), 70–73.

Yin Yang House Staff. (n.d.). He Huan Pi. *Yin Yang House*. https://theory.yinyanghouse.com/theory/herbalmedicine/he_huan_pi_tcm_herbal_database

Monk fruit
Siraitia grosvenorii

Other name: *Luo han guo*

The main chemical compounds present in monk fruit are glycosides belonging to cucurbitane triterpene glycosides. Mogroside, a group of the triterpene glycosides compounds, are responsible for the sweet taste of the fruit and are powerful antioxidants.

Monk fruit has antidiabetic, anticarcinogenic, antibacterial, antitussive, and antiallergic activities.

It is used as an emollient for the treatment of dry coughs, sore throats, dire thirst, and constipation. It also promotes weight loss.

The ripe fruit extract is used commercially as a supplement and a constituent in health foods and drinks as a substitute of sugar.

Acute allergic reactions from monk fruits are rare.

Jin, J. S., & Lee, J. H. (2012). Phytochemical and pharmacological aspects of Siraitia grosvenorii, luo han kuo. *Oriental Pharmacy and Experimental Medicine*, 12(4), 233–239. https://doi.org/10.1007/s13596-012-0079-x

McDermott, A. (2017, October 12). *Why everyone's going mad for Monk Fruit*. Healthline. https://www.healthline.com/health/food-nutrition/monk-fruit-health-benefits

Moutan Peony
Paeonia suffruticosa Andr

Other names: *Tree peony bark, Mu Dan Pi*

The natural components in moutan peony include flavones, asparagine, alkaloids, paeonol, paeonoside, paeonolide, apiopaeonoside, paeoniflorin, ozypaeoniflorin, gallic acid, biotin, resins, volatile oils, and stigmasterol. The most abundant glucoside is paeoniflorin which has antiinflammatory and immunoregulatory effects.

Moutan peony bark in Chinese medicine is pungent, bitter, and a slightly cool herb. It is mainly used for heart, liver, and kidney Qi.

Ingredients	Mechanism of Action and Health Benefits
	It has analgesic, antipyretic, antibacterial, and sedative effects.
	It is used to strengthen the blood, eliminate blood stasis, remove excess heat and drain pus. It also supports proper blood circulation, promotes healthy liver function, and benefits the immune system.
	It is used in treatment of Crohn's disease and ulcerative colitis. Peony bark may also be used in management of rheumatoid arthritis and systemic lupus erythematosus as well.
	There are no known side effects of mu dan pi.
	1st Chinese Herbs. (n.d.). Mu Dan Pi. https://1stchineseherbs.com/herbs-a-z/m/mu-dan-pi/
	Chen, T. F., Hsu, J. T., Wu, K. C., Hsiao, C. F., Lin, J. A., Cheng, Y. H., et al. (2020). A systematic identification of anti-inflammatory active components derived from Mu Dan Pi and their applications in inflammatory bowel disease. *Scientific Reports*, *10*(1), 1–10. https://doi.org/10.1038/s41598-020-74201-x
Mulberry Mistletoe *Taxillus chinensis* *Loranthus parasiticus*	Other names: *Chinese taxillus herb, Sang Ji Sheng* Mulberry mistletoe contains several bioactive compounds including cardiac glycosides, alkaloids, saponins, and terpenoids.
	It covers the kidney and liver meridians. It dispels the dampness and wind. It also tonifies the kidney and liver. It also nourishes the blood.
	It can strengthen bones, ligaments, and tendons. It is used to treat rheumatism, arthralgia, and arthritis.
	It can also lower blood pressure and is used in hypertension.
	Me and Qi. (n.d.). Mulberry Mistletoe. *Meandqi.com*. https://www.meandqi.com/herb-database/mulberry-mistletoe
	Puneetha, G. K., Murali, M., Thriveni, M. C., & Amruthesh, K. N. (2014). Phytochemical screening, antioxidant and antibacterial properties of *Taxillus cuneatus* (Roth.) Danser-a hemi-parasitic angiosperm. *International Journal of Current Microbiology and Applied Science, 3*(5), 702–711.
Natto	Natto is a Japanese superfood made from fermented soybeans. It is rich in fiber. It contains manganese (134% of the DV), which is important for enzyme function in the body and other functions including blood clotting and metabolism. It is also high in vitamin C (38% of the DV), which is an antioxidant. The vitamin K2 and nattokinase enzymes present can reduce cholesterol, arterial calcification, and dissolve blood clots. Other minerals (iron, copper, magnesium, calcium, potassium, and zinc) and vitamins (B1, B6, B9, K2, and choline) are also present.
	It has antihypertensive, antiobesity, anticancer, antiplatelet, neuroprotective, and antistress effects.
	The bacteria present in natto called *Bacillus subtilis* improves gut health and digestion. Natto also reduces the risk of some types of cancer, obesity, cardiovascular disease, diabetes, and osteoarthritis.
	People who are allergic to soy should avoid natto. Hypersensitivity reactions or anaphylaxis may occur. Children with chronic allergies may experience recurrent vomiting, diarrhea, and failure to thrive.
	Benefits. (2021, January 4). Verywell Fit. https://www.verywellfit.com/natto-nutrition-facts-and-health-benefits-4781758
	Petre, A. (2017, March 31). Why natto is super healthy and nutritious. *Healthline*. https://www.healthline.com/nutrition/natto#TOC_TITLE_HDR_3
Notopterygium root *Notopterygium Incisum Rhizoma et Radix*	Other name: *Qiang huo* The main components present in qiang huo are furocoumarins, organic acids, amino acids, and β-sitosterol.
	It is believed that notopterygium root has pungent, bitter, and warm properties. It is associated with the urinary bladder and kidney Qi. It is used to disperse cold and unblock painful obstructions caused by wind/damp/cold pain.
	It has antioxidant, analgesic, and antiallergy properties.
	It helps treat conjunctivitis, colds, fevers, headaches, muscle pain (particularly in the upper back and shoulders), joint pain, and eczema caused by allergic reactions.
	Overdosing on notopterygium roots can cause nausea and vomiting. It should also not be used by those with blood or Yin deficiency.
	1st Chinese Herbs. (n.d.). Qiang Huo. https://1stchineseherbs.com/herbs-a-z/q/qiang-huo/
	Chinese Herb Info. (2021, March 31). Qiang Huo (Notopterygium Root). https://www.chineseherbsinfo.com/benefits-and-side-effects-of-qiang-huo/

Ingredients	Mechanism of Action and Health Benefits
Nutgrass galingale rhizome *Rhizoma cyperi*	Other names: *Xiāng fù, Mushta or Mustha or Mustaka or Musta, Nagarmotha or Motha, Nut grass, Cyperus rotundus, Java grass, Coco grass, Purple nutsedge* Nutgrass is a weed. Galingale rhizome is categorized as a Qi-regulating medicinal herb. It is the dried rhizome of *Cyperus rotundus species.* It has a pungent smell and a neutral taste. In TCM, it can soothe the liver, regulate Qi, and alleviate pain. It is also widely used in Ayurvedic medicine to treat fevers. It has antioxidant, antimutagenic, and neuroprotective activities. It also has antidiabetic, lipid-lowering, antiobesity cardioprotective, uroprotective, antipyretic, antiinflammatory, emmenagogue, and antidiarrheal actions. It is used to treat diabetes, atherosclerosis, UTIs, and cancers. It can ease abdominal discomfort in the stomach or flank regions and regulate the menstrual cycles to relieve painful periods. It may also be used in epilepsy and neurodegenerative disorders, such as PD. It has no known side effects. Lee, C. H., Hwang, D. S., Kim, H. G., Oh, H., Park, H., Cho, J. H., et al. (2010). Protective effect of *Cyperi rhizoma* against 6-hydroxydopamine-induced neuronal damage. *Journal of Medicinal Food*, *13*(3), 564–571. https://doi.org/10.1089/jmf.2009.1252 Traditional Chinese Medicine Wiki. (2016, September 23). Nutgrass Galingale Rhizome. *TCM Wiki*. https://tcmwiki.com/wiki/nutgrass-galingale-rhizome
Orange *Citrus sinensis*	Orange contains flavonoids, steroids, hydroxy amides, alkanes, fatty acids, coumarins, carotenoids, volatile compounds, and peptides. It also contains minerals such as potassium, magnesium, calcium, and sodium. Orange is rich in vitamin C, a powerful antioxidant which reduces the risk of developing chronic disorders or cancer. It has antibacterial, antifungal, antiparasitic, antiinflammatory, and antiproliferative activities. Orange can lower cholesterol levels, aid in weight loss, prevent cardiovascular events, and development of kidney stones. It can also improve the levels of phosphorus and calcium in bones reducing bone loss and help in preventing osteoporosis. Its essential oil is used in aromatherapy. Consumption of a large dose of vitamin C supplements at one time can cause side effects such as nausea, vomiting, diarrhea, stomach cramps, headache, and insomnia. The high acidic content of oranges can worsen the symptoms of GERD. Bonvissuto, D. (2019, July 12). Oranges. *WebMD*. https://www.webmd.com/food-recipes/health-benefits-oranges Favela-Hernández, J. M. J., González-Santiago, O., Ramírez-Cabrera, M. A., Esquivel-Ferriño, P. C., & Camacho-Corona, M. R. (2016). Chemistry and Pharmacology of *Citrus sinensis*. *Molecules*, *21*(2), 247–271. https://www.ncbi.nlm.nih.gov/pmc/articles/PMC6273684/#!po=1.21951
Oregon grape *Mahonia aquifolium* *Berberis aquifolium*	Other name: *Gong Lao Mu* The main active compound in Oregon grapes is berberine, which has antiinflammatory and antimicrobial properties. Berberine is also able to increase the levels of serotonin and dopamine which can alleviate symptoms of depression and chronic stress. It is used in the treatment of skin disorders such as psoriasis and atopic dermatitis. Oregon grapes can ease symptoms of IBS, gut inflammation, and prevent heartburn. It can also tone the uterine tissues and slow the development of fibroids. It is available orally and topically as supplements, extracts, oils, creams, and tinctures. Children and women who are pregnant or breastfeeding should avoid the use of Oregon grapes. Berberine can cross the placenta and cause contractions. Bantilan, C. (2019, October 24). What is Oregon grape? Uses and side effects. *Healthline*. https://www.healthline.com/nutrition/oregon-grapewa
Ox knee *Achyranthes bidentata*	Other name: *Huai Niu Xi* The roots, leaves, and stems of the plant are used in Chinese medicine to revitalize blood flow. The active compounds present include phytosterone, phytoecdysteroids, saccharides, and saponin. It has analgesic, antiinflammatory, antirheumatic, and diuretic effects. It may also have anticancer properties.

Ingredients	Mechanism of Action and Health Benefits
	Ox knee is used to stimulate menstruation when periods are delayed or scanty. It can also ease menstrual pain. It is also used in the treatment of canker sores, toothache, bleeding gums, and nosebleeds. It can also treat hypertension, hyperlipidemia, stroke, and back pains.
	Juice from its roots is used for toothaches, indigestion, and asthma.
	The use of huai niu xi should be avoided during pregnancy and breastfeeding. It should not be taken when experiencing diarrhea or heavy menstruation.
	Health Benefits Time. (2020, July 8). Ox Knee facts and health benefits. *HealthBenefitstimes.com*. https://www.healthbenefitstimes.com/ox-knee/
	Jiang, Z., Qian, J., Dong, H., Yang, J., Yu, X., Chen, J., et al. (2017). The traditional Chinese medicine *Achyranthes bidentata* and our de novo conception of its metastatic chemoprevention: From phytochemistry to pharmacology. *Scientific Reports*, 7(1), 1–13. https://doi.org/10.1038/s41598-017-02054-y
Oyster mushroom *Pleurotus ostreatus*	Other name: *Ping Gu*
	Oyster mushrooms contain various bioactive constituents including flavonoids, steroids, phenols, and terpenoids. It is rich in vitamins (C, B1, B2, and B3), minerals (iron, zinc, calcium, potassium, and phosphorus), and natural statins.
	It is warm in nature. It covers the stomach, kidney, and spleen meridians. It drains dampness and expels wind chill. It also strengthens blood vessels.
	It tonifies the kidney and improves kidney function. It strengthens bone, joint, muscle, and tendon.
	It also increases insulin sensitivity and lowers cholesterol in type 2 diabetes. They are more prebiotic foods.
	It is also used to treat impotency, numbness and weakness in the lower limbs.
	Rahimah, S. B., Djunaedi, D. D., Soeroto, A. Y., & Bisri, T. (2019). The phytochemical screening, total phenolic contents and antioxidant activities in vitro of white oyster mushroom (*Pleurotus ostreatus*) preparations. *Open Access Macedonian Journal of Medical Sciences*, 7(15), 2404–2412. https://doi.org/10.3889/oamjms.2019.741
	TCM Wiki. (2016, September 23). Oyster mushroom. https://tcmwiki.com/wiki/oyster-mushroom
Oyster shell	Other name: *Mu Li ke*
	Oyster shells contain mainly calcium carbonate. Other minerals include magnesium, copper, iron, nickel, and strontium. It also contains protein polysaccharides.
	It has cooling properties. It helps people with too much "Heat" in their body from Yang excess or Yin deficiency. It anchors and calms the spirit. It nourishes the Yin and quietens the overflowing of the Yang.
	It targets the liver, kidney, gallbladder, and bladder meridians. It is an assistant ingredient in Chinese polyherbal formulations.
	It is used to treat disorders caused by low calcium levels (osteoporosis, rickets, malnutrition, and hypoparathyroidism). It can strengthen bones and heal stomach ulcers.
	It can calm and tranquilize the mind. It is used to treat insomnia, anxiety, and restlessness. It has sedative properties.
	Side effects include constipation, stomach upset, and allergy reactions. It can decrease the absorption of some antibiotics and bisphosphonates.
	Me & Qi. (n.d.). Oyster shells. *Meandqi.com*. https://www.meandqi.com/herb-database/oyster-shells
	WebMD Editors. (2013). Natural Oyster shell calcium. *WebMD*. https://www.webmd.com/drugs/2/drug-16642/natural-oyster-shell-calcium-oral/details
Peach seed *Prunus persica*	Other names: *Tao Ren or Taoren, Semen persicae*
	In TCM, peach seeds are known to have bitter, sweet, and neutral properties. The seed is believed to invigorate the blood, remove stasis, and moisten the intestines.
	Amygdalin is the main compound found in peach seeds which helps in the treatment of hepatosplenomegaly.
	It is used to treat blood-related problems like amenorrhea and dysmenorrhea. It can also be used for constipation due to dry intestines or blood or Yin deficiency.
	Peach seeds contain hydrogen cyanide which in excess levels can cause headaches, blurred vision, and heart palpitations. These seeds should be avoided by pregnant women as it can promote the contraction of the uterus. It should also be avoided by patients with loose stools or diarrhea.
	Acupuncture Today. (n.d.). *Peach Seed (tao ren)*. Retrieved 27 C.E., from https://www.acupuncturetoday.com/herbcentral/peachseed.php

Ingredients	Mechanism of Action and Health Benefits
Pear/Chinese pear *Pyrus communi* *Pyrus pyrifolia*	Pears contain carotenoids, flavonoids, and anthocyanins. They are rich in antioxidants and fiber. It contains mainly vitamins (C and K) and potassium. It also has smaller amounts of calcium, iron, magnesium, riboflavin, vitamin B6, and folate. Pectin, a soluble fiber that is present, can nourish gut bacteria and improve gut health. The fiber can also improve healthy bowel function and reduce the risk of diverticulosis. It has antiinflammatory, antihypertensive, and detoxifying effects. It supports weight loss. It can reduce the risk of cancer, diabetes, and heart disease. Pears contain a higher content of fructose than glucose which makes them a high FODMAP (fermentable oligosaccharides, disaccharides, monosaccharides, and polyols) food. FODMAP food can increase gas and bloating, pain, and diarrhea in some people with IBS. Ware, M. (2019, November 1). What to know about pears. *MedicalNewsToday*. https://www.medical-newstoday.com/articles/285430 Wartenberg, L. (2019, July 12). 9 health and nutrition benefits of pears. *Healthline*. https://www.healthline.com/nutrition/benefits-of-pears
Pearl powder *Concha margaritifera usta*	Other names: *Zhen zhu, Zhen zhu mu, Nacre calcined* Pearl powder is made by boiling seawater or freshwater pearls to sterilize and then ground into fine powder. It is rich in minerals (mainly calcium carbonate, magnesium carbonate, some calcium phosphate, silica, trace elements), and amino acids. It also contains unique antiaging compounds, i.e., pearl signal proteins which are complex signaling proteins with regenerative properties (these include conchiolin, nacrein, mucoperlin, perlucin, and lustrin). It is regarded as a superfood. It has antioxidants (increases glutathione and superoxide dismutase levels), antiinflammatory, detoxifying, antiaging, and relaxing properties. It is a *Shen tonic*. It calms and soothes the nervous system, lowers stress levels, enhances relaxation and sleep. Pearl powder enters the heart meridian. It is a heart and liver tonic. It cools "toxic heat" in the liver. It improves circulation. It is a skin brightener and an antiwrinkling agent. It promotes smooth and clear skin and complexion. It is a mask ingredient and lightens age spots. It has moisturizing and antiaging properties. The signal proteins stimulate the regeneration of collagen. It improves bone density. The presence of nacre promotes collagen synthesis and wound healing. It promotes bright eyes with clear vision. Side effects include allergic reactions.
Peony *Radix Paeoniae alba* Chinese peony *Radix Paeoniae lactiflorae*	Other name: *Bai Shao* The main active compound present in peony is paeoniflorin which has antihypertensive action. It has antiinflammatory, antioxidation, and immunomodulatory effects. Peony has the effects of promoting blood circulation and nourishing blood, removing blood stasis and relieving pain. It is used for gout, osteoarthritis, fever, respiratory tract illnesses, and cough. It is also used by women for menstrual cramps, polycystic ovary syndrome, PMS, and for starting menstruation or causing an abortion. It is also used for viral hepatitis, liver cirrhosis, upset stomach, muscle cramps, and atherosclerosis. Peony is also used for spasms, whooping cough (pertussis), epilepsy, nerve pain (neuralgia), headache, and CFS. It can upset the stomach and cause rashes in sensitive people. It should not be used by people with bleeding disorders as peony can slow down blood clotting. RxList Staff. (2021, June 11). Peony. *RxList*. https://www.rxlist.com/peony/supplements.htm
Perilla leaf *Folium perillae*	Other name: *Zi su ye* The essential oil from perilla leaves contains mainly perillaldehyde and smaller amounts of limonene, linalool, β-caryophyllene, α-pinene, perillene, and elemicin. They also contain carotenoids, rosmarinic, ferulic, caffeic, and tormentic acids and luteolin, apigenin, and catechin. It is also rich in calcium. It has antioxidant, antiallergic, antiinflammatory, antidepressant, and anorexigen properties. The leaves can be used to treat wounds and cuts because of their antibacterial activity. Perilla leaves have tumor-preventing properties. The leaf powder and extract can be used for treating cold, cough, vomiting, abdominal pain, and constipation. It can also improve tyrosinase and melanin synthesis in skin. A decoction of perilla leaf can help in management of glomerulonephritis. Perilla ketone, a chemical related to ipomeanols, has toxic effects which are a potent agent for the induction of pulmonary edema. Thus, too many leaves should not be consumed at one time. Drugs.com. (n.d.). Perilla. https://www.drugs.com/npp/perilla.html

Ingredients	Mechanism of Action and Health Benefits
Phellodendron *Phellodendri cortex*	Other names: *Amur cork tree bark, Huang Bo, Huang Bai*

Phellodendri cortex is the dried bark of *Phellodendron chinense Schneid.* (Chuan Huang Bo) or *Phellodendron amurense Rupr.* (Guan Huang Bo). It contains several bioactive compounds including limonins (obaculactone and obacunone), alkaloids (berberine, magnoflorine, palmatine, and phellodendrine), and phytosterols (β-sitosterol and campesterol).

It covers the kidney, liver, and bladder meridians. It is cold in nature. It clears heat, purges fire, dries dampness, and eliminates toxicity.

It can treat UTI, vaginal discharge, and kidney stones.

It can also treat burns, skin sores, eczema, and abscesses.

It can also treat swollen and inflamed eyes. It can also help with diabetes.

Proven Herbal Remedies. (2021, July 2). Amur Cork Tree (Huang Bo). *Chinese Herbs Healing*. https://www.chineseherbshealing.com/proven-herbal-remedies/amur-cork-tree.html

TCM Wiki. (2016, September 23). Amur Corktree Bark. https://tcmwiki.com/wiki/amur-corktree-bark

Pinellia tuber
Pinellia ternata

Other names: *Ban Xia, Zhi Ban Xia*

Ban xia is the underground tuber of *Pinellia ternata.* The major chemical compounds present include triterpenes, sterols, fatty acids, cerebrosides, amino acids, total alkaloids, phenylpropanoids, and β-sitosterol.

In TCM, pinellia tuber is known to be pungent and warm. It is administered to the spleen, stomach, and lung Qi.

It is used for its antitussive, antiemetic, and anticancer actions.

It is used for morning sickness, birth control, influenza (flu), swine flu, and pain and swelling (inflammation). It also helps improve blood circulation in the body.

Ban xia contains chemicals called ephedrine alkaloids. These chemicals might cause serious side effects such as heart attack, stroke, or seizures.

Han, M. H., Yang, X. W., Zhang, M., & Zhong, G. Y. (2006). Phytochemical study of the rhizome of *Pinellia ternata* and quantification of phenylpropanoids in commercial Pinellia tuber by RP-LC. *Chromatographia*, *64*(11–12), 647–653. https://doi.org/10.1365/s10337-006-0103-8

RxList Editors. (2021, June 11). Pinellia Ternata. *RxList*. https://www.rxlist.com/pinellia_ternata/supplements.htm

Plantain seed
Plantago asiatica
Plantago depressa

Other name: *Che Qian Zi*

Refer under Indian "Psyllium husk."

Polyrhachis ant

Polyrhachis ant is a Chinese mountain black ant. It can strengthen the kidneys and the adrenal glands. It is an adaptogen similar to reishi, ginseng, and cordycep. It is a Qi tonic and is regarded as a superfood which is nutrient-dense with high proteins, minerals (high in zinc), and vitamins. Zinc is an essential element and cofactor in all the metabolic functions of the body.

It is an aphrodisiac in both males and females. It has antioxidant, immune-boosting, and detoxifying effects. It also supports digestive health and metabolism. It increases stamina, strength, endurance, vitality, and energy.

It also enhances mood and lowers depression and anger.

Health Wisdom™. (n.d.). Hei Ma Yi 黑蚂蚁, polyrhachis ants, northeast black ant, animal tonic. Retrieved September 8, 2021, from https://www.healthwisdom.shop/products/hei-ma-yi-polyrachis-ants-northeast-black-ant-animal-tonic

Ron Teeguarden Enterprises, Inc. (n.d.). Changbai Mountain Ant. *Dragon Herbs*. https://www.dragonherbs.com/changbai-mountain-ant

Polyporus
Polyporus umbrella

Other name: *Zhu Ling*

Polyporus is a large brown mushroom. In polyporus the main bioactive compounds are steroids and polysaccharides.

It has antiinflammatory, immune-boosting, and diuretic properties. It also has anticancer effects.

It can treat kidney disorders (including edema, UTI, and kidney stones) and vaginal discharge.

Acupuncture Today. (n.d.). Polyporus (zhu ling). *Acupuncturetoday.com*. https://www.acupuncturetoday.com/herbcentral/polyporus.php

Ingredients	Mechanism of Action and Health Benefits
Poria *Wolfiporia extensa*	Other names: *Poria cocos mushrooms, Fu ling, Tuckahoe* Poria is a mushroom that contains polysaccharides (known to enhance immune function) and triterpenoids (compounds with antioxidant effects). In TCM, it is used as a medicinal tonic to promote immune health. It has antidiabetic, hypolipidemic, antianxiety, and antidiarrheal properties. It is used in prevention of cancer, AD, and urination problems. It is also used for treating cough, fatigue, insomnia, kidney infection, and senile dementia. There are no known adverse side effects of poria mushrooms. They may cause allergic reactions such as vomiting or diarrhea. It should be avoided by pregnant and breastfeeding women. Wong, C., & Dashiell, E. (2021, January 19). The health benefits of Poria mushrooms. *Verywell Health*. https://www.verywellhealth.com/the-benefits-of-poria-88643
Pseudoginseng *Panax pseudoginseng*	Other names: *Tian Qi, San Qi* Pseudoginseng is referred to as San Qi which means "more precious than gold." The main active compounds present are panax notoginseng saponins (ginsenoside Rg1, ginsenoside Rb1, ginsenoside Re, and notoginsenoside R1). Notoginsenoside R1 helps reduce the risk of cardiovascular diseases. It has antihyperlipidemic, antihypertensive, antioxidant, and antiinflammatory properties. It can be used to stop or slow down bleeding. It is sometimes taken for nosebleeds (epistaxis), vomiting (hematemesis), coughing up blood (hematemesis), or passing blood in the urine (hematuria) or in the feces (melena). It can improve wound healing. Pseudoginseng is also used to relieve pain. It is also used for chest pain (angina), strokes, dizziness, and sore throat. San Qi can cause some side effects such as dry mouth, flushed skin, nervousness, sleep problems, nausea, and vomiting. It is also unsafe for pregnant and breastfeeding women. Pseudoginseng can act as an estrogen thus, it should be avoided by people with hormone-sensitive conditions such as breast cancer, uterine cancer, ovarian cancer, endometriosis, or uterine fibroids. NutritionReview.org. (2019, February 5). San Qi: The powerful Ginseng few people have heard of. *Nutrition Review*. https://nutritionreview.org/2019/02/san-qi-the-powerful-ginseng-few-people-have-heard-of/ RxList Editors. (2021, June 11). Panax Pseudoginseng. *RxList*. https://www.rxlist.com/panax_pseudoginseng/supplements.htm
Psoralea fruit *Psoralea corylifolia fructus*	Other names: *Malaytea Scurfpea Fruit, Bu Gu Zhi, Babchi, Psoralea fruit* Psoralea or Gu Zhi contains several bioactive compounds including coumarins (psoralen), phenols, flavonoids (psoromene and psorachalcones), sesquiterpenoids, and steroids. It is warm in nature. It covers the kidney, lung, and spleen meridians. It warms and invigorates the kidney and tonifies the Yang. It can strengthen bones, ligaments, and tendons. It is used in back pain and in osteoporosis. It has an antidiuretic effect and decreases urination. It can also treat diarrhea. It is also used to treat lung disorders associated with dyspnea (difficulty breathing). It is used in vitiligo, psoriasis, and alopecia. It can treat UTI and impotence. Side effects include possible phototoxicity from the furocoumarins. Shen-Nong Ltd. (n.d.). Herbal glossary: Fructus Psoraleae. *Shen-Nong*. http://www.shen-nong.com/eng/herbal/buguzhi.html TCM wiki. (2016, September 23). Bu Gu Zhi. https://tcmwiki.com/wiki/bu-gu-zhi
Pulsatilla *Pulsatilla chinensis* *Pulsatilla vulgaris*	Other names: *Chinese Anemone Root, Bai Tou Weng, Pasque flower, Meadow anemone, Windflower* There are more than 30 species of pulsatilla. The main active ingredient is anemonin. It is also widely used in homeopathy. It is cold in nature. It covers the large intestine and stomach meridians. It clears heat, dries dampness, and cools the blood. It has antiinflammatory, detoxifying, antispasmodic, and calming properties. It is used in bleeding disorders (dysentery, bleeding piles, and nosebleeds). It helps in anxiety, irritability, hyperactivity, nervous tension, stress, insomnia, and migraines. It can treat pain-related disorders in the digestive and reproductive systems. It can be used for skin disorders (including eczema).

Ingredients	Mechanism of Action and Health Benefits
	Side effects include allergic reactions, seizures, and gastric upset.
	Pulsatilla is used by homeopathic practitioners to treat toothaches, ear pain, digestive problems, and eye infections.
	Only dried pulsatilla must be used. Fresh pulsatilla contains ranunculin which is a toxic mucous membrane irritant.
	Acupuncture Today. (n.d.). Pulsatilla (bai tou weng). *Acupuncturetoday.com*. https://www.acupuncturetoday.com/herbcentral/pulsatilla.php
	WebMD Editors. (n.d.). Pulsatilla. *WebMD*. https://www.webmd.com/vitamins/ai/ingredientmono-633/pulsatilla
Purple Gromwell *Lithospermum erythrorhizon*	Other names: *Arnebia, Zi Cao*
	Purple gromwell contains hikonin, deoxyshikonin, caffeic acid, and naphthoquinone. It is cold in nature. It cools blood, clears heat, and expels fire toxins. It also clears damp-heat skin lesions.
	It supports skin health and is used to treat eczema, wounds, burns, and other skin conditions.
	It can also help in constipation and menstrual disorders (dysmenorrhea and amenorrhea).
	Overall, it is safe. It may cause allergic reactions.
	Hempen, D. (2009). Herbs that cool heat. *A materia medica for Chinese medicine*, 110–263. https://doi.org/10.1016/b978-0-443-10094-9.00007-8
	Sacred Lotus. (n.d.). Zi Cao (Groomwell Root or Arnebia or Lithospermum). https://www.sacredlotus.com/go/chinese-herbs/substance/zi-cao-groomwell-root-arnebia-lithospermum
Quince *Cydonia oblonga*	Other name: *Ma Gua*
	The *Cydonia oblonga* (quince)*, Pseudocydonia sinensis* (Chinese quince), and *Chaenomeles japonica* are related plants.
	Quince is warm in nature. It contains flavanols (kaempferol and quercetin). It is rich in fiber, vitamins (C, B6, and B1), and minerals (copper, potassium, and iron).
	It dispels wind and dampness. It also expels cold and warms the interior. It covers liver and spleen meridians.
	It has antimicrobial, antiinflammatory, antioxidant, hepatoprotective, and neuroprotective actions. It can lower blood glucose.
	It is used to treat rheumatoid arthritis, tendonitis, leg cramps or spasms, diarrhea, heatstroke, and swelling of legs.
	It can also increase libido.
	Hill, A. (2019, October 1). 8 emerging health benefits of quince (and how to eat it). *Healthline*. https://www.healthline.com/nutrition/what-is-quince-fruit
	Me and Qi. (2021). Flowering quince. *Meandqi.com*. https://www.meandqi.com/herb-database/flowering-quince
Radish seeds *Semen raphani sativi*	Other name: *Lai fu zi*
	Radish seeds are rich in minerals (magnesium, manganese, copper, and phosphorus) and vitamins (C and folate). It is also rich in antioxidants (flavonoids) and organic acids (linolenic acid, linoleic acid, sinapine, and erucic acid).
	Lai fu zi supports digestion and supports liver health.
	It reduces food stagnation, promotes digestion, and eliminates distention.
	It can also direct Qi downward and dissolve phlegm. It helps cough with copious sputum.
	Me & Qi. (n.d.). Radish seeds. *meandqi.com*. https://www.meandqi.com/herb-database/radish-seeds
Rangoon creeper *Combretum indicum*	Other names: *Quisqualis, Shi Jun Zi*
	Rangoon creeper or quisqualis is a climbing and creeping vine. It contains saponins, alkaloids, flavonoids, tannins, and steroids.
	It is warm in nature. It covers the stomach and spleen meridians.
	It has laxative, emetic, and anthelmintic properties.
	It treats indigestion and improves appetite.
	High doses may cause vomiting and dizziness.
	Acupuncture Today. (n.d.). Quisqualis (shi jun zi). *Acupuncturetoday.com*. https://www.acupuncturetoday.com/herbcentral/quisqualis.php
	Wijerathne, C.U.B., Park, H. S., Jeong, H. Y., Song, J. W., Moon, O. S., Seo, Y. W., et al. (2017). Quisqualis indica improves benign prostatic hyperplasia by regulating prostate cell proliferation and apoptosis. *Biological & Pharmaceutical Bulletin*, 40(12), 2125–2133. https://doi.org/10.1248/bpb.b17-00468

Ingredients	Mechanism of Action and Health Benefits
Red bean *Vigna angularis*	Other names: *Adzuki beans, Hong Dou, Chi Xiao Dou* Red beans or adzuki beans contain tocopherols, flavonoids, and phenolic compounds. It is rich in minerals, vitamins, and antioxidants. It covers the heart and small intestine meridians. It is neutral in nature. It expels the dampness and increases urination. It also improves blood circulation. It can replenish blood and Qi. It supports digestion and detoxification, lowers blood sugar and weight loss. It can enhance bone health and prevent osteoporosis. It has strengthening properties. It can treat edema and jaundice. Acupuncture Today. (n.d.). Adzuki beans. *Acupuncturetoday.com.* https://www.meandqi.com/herb-database/adzuki-beans Phoenix Medical. (n.d.). Red Bean (Hong Dou). https://www.phoenixmd.co.uk/red-bean
Red peony root *Radix paeoniae rubra*	Other name: *Chi shao* Red peony root contains mostly paeoniflorin as the bioactive ingredient. It is antiinflammatory and improves blood circulation. It clears the heat in the blood and cools it when there is fever with associated skin blotches and red-purple tongue. It also treats dysmenorrhea or menorrhagia. It invigorates blood, removes stagnation and swelling associated with acute inflammations, abdominal pain, and masses and abscess. It also clears ascending liver fire and treats the eyes problems with associated redness and swelling. It should not be used if there is a history of diarrhea, rupture of abscess, or use of anticoagulants. It should be used with caution if there is blood or cold deficiency. Tan, Y. Q., Chen, H. W., Li, J., & Wu, Q. J. (2020). Efficacy, chemical constituents, and pharmacological actions of *Radix paeoniae rubra* and *Radix paeoniae alba. Frontiers in Pharmacology, 11,* 1054. https://doi.org/10.3389/fphar.2020.01054
Red sage *Salvia miltiorrhiza*	Other names: *Salvia, Danshen or Dan Shen, Chinese red sage* Red sage is a rich source of chemical compounds such as tanshinone I, tanshinone II, miltirone, and salvianolic acid. It has antioxidant, antimicrobial, antivirus, anticancer, and antiinflammatory properties. It is a natural angiotensin-converting enzyme (ACE) inhibitor. It has blood-thinning properties and prevents platelets and blood from clotting. It can also cause blood vessels to widen, improving blood circulation. It also can increase osteoblast activity and early callus formation. Danshen can reduce the risk of cardiovascular problems including stroke, hypertension, angina pectoris, and other heart-related disorders. It can be used to treat menstrual disorders, chronic liver disease, and sleeping problems. It is also used for skin conditions including acne, psoriasis, and eczema, to relieve bruising, promote wound and fracture healing. Injecting red sage helps decrease cholesterol levels. Possible side effects include itching, upset stomach, and reduced appetite. It may also cause drowsiness, dizziness, and thrombocytopenia. RxList Editors. (2021, June 11). Danshen. *RxList.* https://www.rxlist.com/danshen/supplements.htm Wang, B. Q. (2010). Salvia miltiorrhiza: Chemical and pharmacological review of a medicinal plant. *Journal of Medicinal Plant Research, 425*(25), 2813–2820. https://www.researchgate.net/publication/228709331_Salvia_miltiorrhiza_Chemical_and_pharmacological_review_of_a_medicinal_plant
Reed rhizome *Rhizoma phragmitis*	Other name: *lú gēn* Reed rhizome contains bioactive compounds including tanin, terpenoids, glycosides, and flavonoids. It is also rich in vitamins A and C with some B vitamins. In TCM, reed rhizome is known to dispel heat in stomach, urinary tract, and lung. It has diuretic properties. It has anticancer, antihyperglycemic, and antioxidant properties. Lu gen can relieve fever, vomiting, dysuria, and constipation. It is applied on the skin for insect bites. It can also slow down acute reactions and detoxify the body. Reed rhizomes can replenish Qi and blood (tonic effect). The rhizome also improves kidney function. It should not be used by people who have weakness in stomach and spleen due to cold. Me & Qi. (n.d.). Common reed rhizomes. *Meandqi.com.* https://www.meandqi.com/herb-database/common-reed-rhizome

Ingredients	Mechanism of Action and Health Benefits
	Samir, D., Manel, A., & Abir, H. (2019). Phytochemical analysis and antioxidant property of rhizome extracts aqueous of *Phragmites australis* in alloxan diabetic rats. *Asian Journal of Pharmacy and Technology, 9*(4), 249. https://doi.org/10.5958/2231-5713.2019.00041.2
Reishi mushroom *Ganoderma lucidum*	Other name: *Lingzhi, Reishi* Read more under "Medicinal mushrooms" in Chinese natural ingredients. Reishi mushroom is a medicinal mushroom and is known as the divine mushroom of immortality. It contains several bioactive compounds including phenols, steroids, peptidoglycans, and triterpenes. It is an adaptogen. It has immune-boosting, antioxidant, antiviral, antibacterial, antiaging, antithrombotic, glucose-lowering hepatoprotective and anticancer properties. It has wide therapeutic indications. It can treat diabetes, allergies, urinary symptoms, and cancers. It may help improve attention and cognition in a child with developmental delay. It can be combined with other mushrooms and herbs.
Rice or geng mi *Oryza sativa*	Rice is rich in fiber such as hemicellulose and resistant starch. Resistant starch helps increase butyrate in the gut. Byurate promotes gut health by reducing inflammation, improving gut barrier function, and reducing the risk of colon cancer. It is rich with vitamins (niacin and thiamin) and minerals (manganese, selenium, and magnesium). Rice also contains some pantothenic acid, phosphorus, riboflavin, vitamin B6, copper, and folate. Brown rice is high in antioxidants such as lignans and ferulic acid. These antioxidants help lower risks of heart disease, menopausal symptoms, osteoporosis, and breast cancer. Ferulic acid also has antiinflammatory and antimicrobial effects. In TCM, geng mi is said to have sweet and cool properties. It influences the lungs, spleen, large intestine, and small intestine. Geng mi is used to treat diarrhea due to Yang deficiency and helps body fluid deficiency by generating fluids. Brown rice improves blood cholesterol levels and reduces the risk of heart disease, stroke, type 2 diabetes, and obesity. Regular consumption of large amounts of white rice may increase the risk of type 2 diabetes. Brown rice contains heavy metals including cadmium, chromium, lead, nickel, and arsenic. These heavy metals may accumulate overtime in the body leading to adverse health effects such as brain, kidney, liver, and lung disorders. Arnarson, A. (2020, May 15). What to know about rice. *MedicalNewsToday*. https://www.medicalnewstoday.com/articles/318699#nutrition Yin Yang House. (n.d.). Geng Mi. https://theory.yinyanghouse.com/theory/herbalmedicine/geng_mi_tcm_herbal_database.
Rice Paper Pith *Tetrapanax papyrifer*	Other name: *Tong Cao* Rice paper pith is derived from the dried hollow stem of *Tetrapanax papyrifer,* a shrub from the ginseng family. It contains sesquiterpenes (β-selinene and β-caryophyllene) and triterpenoid glycosides (papyriosides). It is slightly cold in nature and covers the lung and stomach meridians. It clears heat and acts as a diuretic. It also stimulates lactation in women. It can treat urinary problems like dysuria and frequency. It can interact with diuretic medications. AcupunctureToday. (n.d.). Rice paper pith (tong cao). https://www.acupuncturetoday.com/herbcentral/rice_paper_pith.php
Safflower *Carthamus tinctorius*	Other name: *Hong hua, Flos Carthami* Safflower has more than 100 phytochemicals present including flavonoids (quinochalcones, C-glycosides, O-glycosides, and kaempferol derivatives), alkaloids (N-feruloyl serotonin, N-feruloyl tryptamine, and serotonin derivatives), polyacetylenes, organic acids (linoleic acid, oleic acid, palmitic acid, and stearic acid), roseoside, uridine, and uracil. The alkaloids possess anticoagulant, hepatoprotective, neuroprotective, and antioxidant activities. It also has antihyperlipidemic, antimicrobial, antitumor, antiinflammatory, analgesic, antidiabetic, laxative, and antiperspirant properties. Safflower is used for the treatment of osteoporosis. The oil from safflower seeds can prevent heart diseases including atherosclerosis and stroke. It is also used for fever, tumors, coughs, breathing problems, chest pain, and traumatic injuries.

Ingredients	Mechanism of Action and Health Benefits

Safflower can also be used for absent or painful menstrual periods and to cause an abortion.

Safflower is safe for oral and topical use. It should be avoided in pregnancy, bleeding problems (hemorrhagic diseases, stomach or intestinal ulcers, or clotting disorders), and people who are allergic to the Asteraceae/Compositae family.

RxList Editors. (2021, June 11). Safflower. *RxList*. https://www.rxlist.com/safflower/supplements.htm

Zhang, L. L., Tian, K., Tang, Z. H., Chen, X. J., Bian, Z. X., Wang, Y. T., et al. (2016). Phytochemistry and pharmacology of *Carthamus tinctorius* L. *The American Journal of Chinese Medicine*, *44*(2), 197–226. https://doi.org/10.1142/s0192415x16500130

Scorpion
Centruroides gracilis

Other names: *Quan Xie or Quanxie, Buthus martensii*

Scorpions are toxic, venomous, and predatory arachnids which can thrive anywhere. There are many species. *Buthus martensii* is commonly used. They are caught, soaked in water, boiled, dried, and powdered for use in TCM. Usually the body and tail are used.

It covers the liver meridian. It dispels wind and toxins. It stops spasms. It has analgesic and anticancer actions. The analgesic potency is five times more in the scorpion tail than the body, making it very effective in pain management.

It is combined with other herbs and is used to treat seizures, spasms, stroke, and tetanus. It can also be used for headaches, joint pains, cancer, and tumors.

It should not be used in pregnancy.

Acupuncture Today. (n.d.). Scorpion (quan xie). https://www.acupuncturetoday.com/herbcentral/scorpion.php

Sea cucumber

Other names: *Hai shen, Gamat*

Sea cucumber is like slug and belongs to the echinoderms. There are many species. Bald, prickly, or white teat sea cucumbers are preferred. It is rich in fatty acids (arachidonic acid, palmitate, stearate, linoleic acid), chondroitin sulfate, collagen, amino acids, vitamins (B2 and niacin), and many bioactive compounds like squalene (which is part of endogenous steroids production), triterpenoids (which has antitumor effects) and coelomic fluid (which has antimicrobial properties).

It nourishes the Qi. It has antioxidant and antiinflammatory properties.

It also helps to rebuild cartilage and promotes wound healing. It can lower total cholesterol, triglycerides, and LDL-cholesterol and may reduce blood pressure.

It is used as a remedy in arthritis and heart problems. It can maintain blood, liver, and digestive health. It has been effective in oral thrush. The dried form is used as an aphrodisiac and health tonic. It has shown promising results in leukemia, liver, lung, colon, and breast cancers.

Allergic reactions may occur in those with shellfish allergy. It has blood-thinning properties, and caution has to be exercised when taken with anticoagulants. It should be avoided during pregnancy.

Brennan, D. (2020, September 18). Health benefits of sea cucumber. *WebMD*. https://www.webmd.com/diet/health-benefits-sea-cucumber#1

Seaweed

Seaweed is basically marine algae and is of mainly three types: red algae (Rhodophyta), brown algae (Phaeophyceae), and green algae (Chlorophyta).

It is high in protein and low in calories. Common edible varieties are red seaweed (nori) and brown seaweeds (kombu, wakame, and hijiki).

Seaweed contains iodine and tyrosine which are essential to make thyroid hormones. Brown seaweed contains fucoxanthin.

It is rich in antioxidants (flavonoids, carotenoids including fucoxanthin, vitamins A, C, and E). Others are vitamins (folate, B1, B2, B12, and K) and minerals (calcium, magnesium, sodium, zinc, manganese, and copper).

Its high fiber and sulfated polysaccharide contents promote gut health via more good gut bacteria and increased short-chain fatty acids.

It has antiobesity effects as it delays gastric emptying hence giving a sense of fullness. Also, it has near-zero calories.

It may support heart health by reducing blood pressure, cholesterol, and clotting tendency.

It can reduce blood glucose levels due to the presence of fucoxanthin and alginate and may prevent type 2 diabetes.

It is a safe food. Risk of iodine or heavy metal toxicity is low even with overconsumption of seaweed.

Mouristen, O. (2018, June 19). The science of seaweeds. *American Scientist*. https://www.american-scientist.org/article/the-science-of-seaweeds

O'Brien, S. (2018, May 28). 7 Surprising health benefits of eating seaweed. *Healthline*. https://www.healthline.com/nutrition/benefits-of-seaweed

Ingredients	Mechanism of Action and Health Benefits
Senna leaf *Cassia acutifolia* *Cassia angustifolia*	Other names: *Fan Xie Ye, Alexandrian senna* Refer to Cassia seed or *Cassiae semen* under *Indian Natural Ingredients.*
Siberian Ginseng *Acanthopanax senticosus* *Eleutherococcus senticosus*	Other names: *Acanthopanax Root, Wu Jia Pi* Siberian ginseng is from the root of *E. senticosus* and not from the Panax genus and its active compound is eleutherosides, hence it is not a ginseng. It is an adaptogen. It is less expensive compared to ginseng. It should not be used for more than 2 to 3 months at a time. Its health benefits are similar to ginseng. Refer under "Ginseng." RxList Editors. (2021, June 11). Siberian Ginseng. *RxList.* https://www.rxlist.com/siberian_ginseng/supplements.htm WebMD Editors. (2011). Siberian Ginseng capsule. *WebMD.* https://www.webmd.com/drugs/2/drug-735/siberian-ginseng-oral/details
Sichuan pepper *Zanthoxylum simulans* *Zanthoxylum bungeanum*	Other name: *Huājiāo* Sichuan pepper contains a variety of chemical compounds including quercitrin, kaempferol-3-rhamnoside, quercetin, sesamin, chlorogenic acid, hyperoside, trifolin, xanthyletin, and nitidine chloride. It contains minerals (potassium, iron, manganese, zinc, copper, and phosphorus) and vitamins A, B1, and B6, and carotenes. It has antiinflammatory, antioxidant, antimicrobial, antifungal, and antiphlogistic properties. In TCM, the pericarp can be used for gastralgia and dyspepsia. The leaves have carminative, stimulant, and sudorific effects. The roots are used for epigastric pains and bruises, eczema, and snakebites. Huājiāo can relieve toothache and boost gastrointestinal function. Sichuan pepper may cause some gastric irritation. It should be avoided in individuals with stomach ulcers, ulcerative colitis, and diverticulitis conditions. Rudrappa, U. (2019, April 5). Sichuan peppercorns (花椒) nutrition facts. *Nutrition And You.* https://www.nutrition-and-you.com/sichuan-peppercorns.html Zhang, Y., Luo, Z., Wang, D., He, F., & Li, D. (2014). Phytochemical profiles and antioxidant and antimicrobial activities of the leaves of *Zanthoxylum bungeanum*. *The Scientific World Journal*, *2014*, 1–13. https://doi.org/10.1155/2014/181072
Silkworm *Bombyx mori*	Other name: *Jiang Can* The dried silkworm feces or droppings is warm in nature. It covers the liver, lung, and stomach meridians. It eliminates dampness and expels wind. It has analgesic, tonic, astringent, antiinflammatory, and detoxifying properties. It is used to treat red eyes, headache, and sore throat. It is used in the treatment of itchy skin and eczema. It can also help in toothache and facial paralysis. Overall, it is safe. It should not be used in paralysis caused by blood deficiency. Me and Qi. (n.d.). Silkworm feces. *Meandqi.com.* https://www.meandqi.com/herb-database/silkworm-feces Proven Herbal Remedies. (2021, April 18). Bombyx Mori Feces (Can Sha). *Chinese Herbs Healing.* https://www.chineseherbshealing.com/proven-herbal-remedies/bombyx-mori-feces.html
Snakehead fish *Channa striata*	Other names: *Mudfish, Haruan fish* Snakehead fish is a medicinal freshwater fish popular in Asian countries. It is rich in fatty acids and essential amino acids which promote cell or tissue growth and wound healing. It is also rich in vitamin A. It has antimicrobial, antiinflammatory, antioxidant, and antinociceptive properties. It increases collagen fiber synthesis and reduces scars. It also contains arachidonic acid which is a precursor for prostaglandin and thromboxane synthesis that also help with wound healing and pain relief. It is consumed to improve postoperative wound-healing and muscle stamina. Snakehead fish contains polychlorinated biphenyls which in excess can lead to skin inflammation and liver damage. Rahman, M. A., Molla, M. H. R., Sarker, M. K., Chowdhury, S. H., & Shaikh, M. M. (2018). Snakehead fish (*Channa striata*) and its biochemical properties for therapeutics and health benefits. *SF Journal of Biotechnology and Biomedical Engineering*, *1*(1), 1–5. https://www.researchgate.net/publication/324731953_Snakehead_Fish_Channa_striata_and_Its_Biochemical_Properties_for_Therapeutics_and_Health_Benefits

Ingredients	Mechanism of Action and Health Benefits
Sodium sulfate *Natrii sulfas*	Sodium sulfate is a chemical with formula Na_2SO_4. It has antiseptic, antibiotic, and laxative properties. It is a bowel-cleansing agent used for large bowel examinations (for barium enema, x-ray, or colonoscopy). It is used to treat eye infections. It should not be used if there is an allergy to sulfate-based products. The International Pharmacopoeia. (2016). *Sodium sulfate, anhydrous (Natrii sulfas anhydricus)*. The International Pharmacopoeia (6th ed). https://www.who.int/medicines/publications/pharmaco-poeia/Sodium_sulfate_anhydrous.pdf?ua=1
Solomon seal *Polygonatum* spp. *Rhizoma Praeparata*	Other names: *Huang Jing, Yu Zhu, Siberian Solomon's Seal* "Yuzhu" includes the "Huang Jing" in ancient herbal text before the Qing Dynasty. Huang Jing is neutral in nature. It is a vital Qi building Yin tonic. It is slightly cooling and nourishes the Yin in the lung and stomach. It moistens the dryness in the lungs and strengthens the stomach. It can also be used directly to the skin for ulcers, bruises or boils, or hemorrhoids. Side effects are mild and include nausea, vomiting, and diarrhea. It may decrease blood sugar. 1st Chinese Herbs. (n.d.). Huang Jing. https://1stchineseherbs.com/herbs-a-z/h/huang-jing/ Acupuncture Today. (n.d.). Polygonatum (jing). *acupuncturetoday.com*. https://www.acupuncturetoday.com/herbcentral/polygonatum.php
Sophora japonica *Styphnolobium japonicum* *Flos Sophorae*	Other names: *Japanese pagoda tree flower, huai hua mi, huai hua wan* Sophora japonica has bitter and cool properties. It contains flavonoids, sophoradiol, triterpenoids, betulin, tannin, and sophoradiol. It influences the lung, liver, heart, and large intestine meridians. It clears heat and stops bleeding. It has hemostatic, astringent, and antiinflammatory properties. It is used to stop bleeding in hemorrhoids, anal fissure, rectal polyp, rectal prolapse, ulcerative colitis, dysentery, uterine bleeding, hemoptysis, and hematuria. It can also improve eyesight and relieve headaches. It should be avoided in fevers due to Yin deficiency and deficiency-cold in the spleen and stomach. Acupuncture Today Staff. (n.d.). Sophora flower (huai hua mi). *Acupuncture Today*. https://www.acupuncturetoday.com/herbcentral/sophoraflower.php Proven Herbal Remedies. (2021, August 4). Sophora Japonica (Huai Hua Mi). *Chinese Herbs Healing*. https://www.chineseherbshealing.com/proven-herbal-remedies/sophora-japonica.html
Sophora flavescens *Radix Sophorae Flavescentis* *Sophorae Flavescentis Radix*	Other name: *Ku Shen* *Sophora flavescens* has bitter and cool properties. It contains flavonoids (kushenol), matrine alkaloids, and saponin. It also acts as a phytoestrogen. It is associated with the liver, heart, large intestine, stomach, and urinary bladder meridians. It can dry dampness, clear heat, and purge fire. It can kill parasites and induce diuresis. It has antiinflammatory, antiviral, analgesic, and antitumor activities. It is used in the treatment of skin disorders such as eczema, scabies, fungal infection, chicken pox, and skin ulcers. It promotes wound healing. It also has skin-whitening effects. It is also used in ulcerative colitis. It is used in various cancers including liver, intestinal, lung, bone, and brain cancers. Side effects include stomach upset, heart rhythm abnormalities, breathing difficulties, palpitation, and abnormal gait. It should not be taken with hormone-sensitive cancer. Barrett, J. E. (2016). *Pharmacological mechanisms and the modulation of pain, Volume 75 (Advances in Pharmacology)* (1st ed.). London: Academic Press. Memorial Sloan Kettering Cancer Center Staff. (2014, February 12). *Sophora flavescens*. Memorial Sloan Kettering Cancer Center. https://www.mskcc.org/cancer-care/integrative-medicine/herbs/sophora-flavescens
Soy	Other names: *Soybeans, soya beans, soya, soy beans* Read more under "soybean sprouts." Soy is a legume and an edible bean. It is a complete protein. It is available in different colors. The *yellow* soybeans are commonly used to make unfermented soy products such as soy milk from which tofu and tofu skin are made. Fermented soy products include tempeh and tamari. The *green* soybeans (edamame) are often added into stir-fries or salads. The *black* soybeans are usually fermented for local traditional use.

Ingredients	Mechanism of Action and Health Benefits
	Soya is available in various forms: soy milk, flour, soy protein powder, and oil.

Soya is used extensively in Asian cuisine as a meat substitute.

It is high in protein, fibers (soluble and insoluble), omega-3 fatty acids, phytoestrogens, and antioxidants. It is cholesterol and lactose-free. It is gluten-free. 100% organic or nongenetically modified organism (non -GMO) soy products are preferred.

Metropulos, M. (2019, October 22). What to know about soy. *MedicalNewsToday*. https://www.medicalnewstoday.com/articles/320472#types-and-uses

Soybean sprouts

Other name: *Soya bean sprouts*

The active ingredients present in soybean sprouts include phenolic compounds, saponin, and isoflavone. They are rich in phytoestrogen, which reduces the risk of osteoporosis.

They have amino acids such as tryptophan, isoleucine, valine, histidine, and leucine. They are rich in vitamin K (55% of the DV), copper, manganese, phosphorus, and dietary fiber. They also contain vitamins (B9 and C) and minerals (iron, magnesium, and zinc).

They have antioxidant properties.

They help lower the risk of cancer and heart diseases. They can be used to treat anemia. During the sprouting process the antinutritional factors such as trypsin inhibitors, hemagglutinin, and lipoxygenase are reduced.

It helps in weight loss and constipation.

Soy reduces pigmentation. It lightens dark spots, sunspots, and dull complexion.

High amounts of soya can ruin the leptin sensitivity, provoke hunger pangs, and insulin resistance. This is also associated with infertility, breast cancer, and hormone imbalances. There are concerns about GMO soybeans.

Health Benefits Editors. (2018, July 5). Soybean sprouts fact, health benefits and nutritional value. *HealthBenefitstimes.com*. https://www.healthbenefitstimes.com/soybean-sprouts/

Stephania root

Stephania tetrandra

Other name: *Han Fang Ji*

Stephania contains several bioactive compounds including many alkaloids (including demethyl tetrandrine and tetrandrine), cepharanthine, and fangchinoline. It is cold in nature. It covers the bladder and lung meridians.

It dries dampness and clears heat.

It has diuretic, analgesic, and antiinflammatory properties. It increases urination.

It is cardioprotective. It can decrease blood pressure and can dilate coronary blood vessels. It also inhibits platelet aggregation.

It is used to treat rheumatoid arthritis, hypertension, and skin disorders (mainly eczema).

It also decreases edema.

No side effects have been recorded.

Me and Qi. (n.d.). Stephania roots. *Meandqi.com*. https://www.meandqi.com/herb-database/stephania-root

Proven Herbal Remedies. (2021, April 20). Stephania tetrandra (Han Fang Ji). Chinese Herbs Healing. https://www.chineseherbshealing.com/proven-herbal-remedies/stephania-tetrandra.html

Remali, J., & Aizat, W. M. (2021). A review on plant bioactive compounds and their modes of action against coronavirus infection. *Frontiers in Pharmacology*, 11, 589044. https://doi.org/10.3389/fphar.2020.589044

Szechuan lovage roots

Ligusticum chuanxiong

Ligusticum striatum

Other names: *Chuan Xiong (Ligusticum chuanxiong), Sichuan lovage rhizome, Chinese lovage root, Gao Ben (Ligusticum striatum)*

Ligusticum contains ligustrazine, alkaloids, phenolic acids, and phthalides. It is warm in nature. It covers the liver, gallbladder, and pericardium. It moves and invigorates blood. It relieves wind/cold.

It increases the blood flow through the whole body including coronary and cerebral blood vessels.

It has antioxidant, cardioprotective, and neuroprotective properties.

It can help in arthralgia and promote bone healing in fracture and bone loss conditions.

It can be used for menstrual problems (irregular menses and dysmenorrhea).

Side effects include allergic reactions, gastric upset, dry mouth, dizziness, and drowsiness.

Glenn, L. (2019, October 31). Szechuan Lovage. *American Botanical Council*. http://herbalgram.org/resources/herbclip/herbclip-news/2019/szechuan-lovage/

Me and Qi. (n.d.). Szechuan lovage roots. *meandqi.com*. https://www.meandqi.com/herb-database/szechuan-lovage-root

Proven Herbal Remedies. (2021, April 20). Lovage (Chuan Xiong). *Chinese Herbs Healing*. https://www.chineseherbshealing.com/proven-herbal-remedies/lovage.html

Ingredients	Mechanism of Action and Health Benefits
Szechuan Ox Knee *Radix cyathula officinalis*	Other name: *Chuan Niu Xi* *Cyathula* contains steroids (β-ecdysterone and cyasterone), oleanolic acid, β-sitosterol and triterpenoid saponins. It covers the kidney and liver meridians. It moves and invigorates blood. It removes blood stagnation. It drains dampness and increases urination. It tonifies the kidney and liver. It strengthens the bones, tendons, and ligaments. It is used in arthralgia, rheumatism, back ache, and knee pain. It helps in UTI and painful urination (dysuria). It is used to treat menstrual disorders (including dysmenorrhea and amenorrhea). It can also help with vertigo and headache. No side effects have been reported. 1st Chinese Herbs. (n.d.). Chuan Niu Xi. https://1stchineseherbs.com/c/chuan-niu-xi/ Me and Qi. (n.d.). Cyathula roots. *meandqi.com*. https://www.meandqi.com/herb-database/cyathula-root
Talcum	Other name: *Hua Shi* Talcum is hydrated magnesium silicate. It drains dampness and cold in nature. It covers the bladder and stomach meridians. It promotes urination. It is used to treat UTIs, oliguria, and eczema and other skin conditions. It can also be used to treat fevers. There may be an association of talc with stomach cancers. Me and Qi. (2021). Talc. *meandqi.com*. https://www.meandqi.com/herb-database/talc
Tangerine peel *Citrus reticulata*	Other name: *Chen Pi* Tangerine peel contains a super-flavonoid called tangeretin which is effective for hyperlipidemia. The peels are also rich in vitamins C and A. It has a bitter and pungent taste, and has a warm nature. It regulates spleen and lung Qi and disperses phlegm from lungs. It prevents stagnation caused by tonifying herbs. It also helps to drain dampness. It has antiinflammatory, antioxidant, and anticancer activities. Chen pi is known as "aged peel" and is believed to be able to stimulate digestion and hence improve appetite. It regulates the whole digestive system and activates liver detoxification. It can treat spleen and stomach issues. It relieves nausea, vomiting, belching, abdominal fullness, bloating, distention, and pain. It prevents indigestion, aids the digestion of fatty foods, and treats anorexia. Chen pi is also used to relieve skin inflammation, ringworm infections, aid in neuroprotection, and improve heart health. It can balance blood sugar. The peels are also used to treat colds, flu, coughs, stress, and menstrual disorders. There are no known side effects of using tangerine peels. Chen pi should not be used when there is a cough with Yin or Qi deficiency (this can be seen as dry cough or coughing blood). It should also be avoided when there is sticky yellow phlegm. Mao, S. N. (n.d.). Tangerine peel. *Dr. Mao*. https://askdrmao.com/natural-health-dictionary/tangerine-peel/index.html Me & Qi. (n.d.). Tangerine peel. *meandqi.com*. https://www.meandqi.com/herb-database/tangerine-peel
Teasels *Dipsacus* spp.	Other names: *Japanese or Chinese Teasel Roots, Xu Duan* Three common Dipsacus species are used—*D. asperoides* (Japanese or Chinese teasel), *D. sativus* (garden teasel), and *D. vulgaris* (wild teasel). Teasels contain several bioactive compounds including phenolic compounds (rutin, chlorogenic acid and caffeic acid), monoterpenes (iridoid and sylvestroside), and flavonoids (luteolin and apigenin). It is a bitter and pungent herb and is warm in nature. It covers the liver and kidney meridians. It removes blood stasis and enhances blood flow and circulation. It tonifies the liver and kidney. It also strengthens tendons, joints, and bones. It can treat back pain, joint stiffness, arthralgia, fractures, tendon injuries, and osteoporosis. It can stop bleeding in menorrhagia, endometriosis, and threatened miscarriage. Me & Qi. (n.d.). Japanese teasel roots (Xu Duan) in Chinese Medicine. *Meandqi.com*. https://www.meandqi.com/herb-database/japanese-teasel-root Vaher, M. (2018). Extraction and analysis of bioactive compounds from *Dipsacus fullonum* and *Galium verum* for Lyme Borreliosis Treatment. *Biomedical Journal of Scientific & Technical Research*, *11*(4), 1–3. https://doi.org/10.26717/bjstr.2018.11.002121

Ingredients	Mechanism of Action and Health Benefits
Thunder God vine *Tripterygium wilfordii Hook F.*	Other name: *Lei Gong Teng* Thunder god vine contains several bioactive compounds including terpenoids (tripdiolide, hypolide, and triptonoterpenol), alkaloids (wilforine, wilfordine, wilforidine, and euonine), and flavonoids. It is cold in nature. It covers the spleen and liver meridians. It clears heat, dispels wind, dampness, and toxicity. It has antiinflammatory, analgesic, antiinfective, and antirheumatic properties. It can treat arthralgia and arthritis of various causes such as psoriatic or rheumatoid. Side effects may include gut bleeding, liver and toxicity, low white cell count, and fertility issues. Chen, J. (2004, January 1). Lei Gong Teng (Radix Tripterygii Wilfordii): a blessing or a time bomb? *Acupuncture Today, 5*(1). https://www.acupuncturetoday.com/mpacms/at/article.php?id=28365 Me and Qi. (n.d.). Thunder god vines. *Meandqi.com*. https://www.meandqi.com/herb-database/thunder-god-vine National Center for Complementary and Integrative Medicine. (2021, January). *Thunder God Vine*. NCCIH. https://www.nccih.nih.gov/health/thunder-god-vine
True Indigo *Indigofera tinctoria*	Other names: *Avuri, Indigo naturalis or Qing Dai* Refer to "Avuri" under Indian Natural Ingredients
Turtle shell *Chinemys reevesii*	Other names: *Gui Ban, Gui Jia* Turtle shells are cold in nature. It covers kidney, heart, and liver meridians. It nourishes and tonifies the Yin. It can strengthen bones and help children with delayed bone growth. It can cool the blood and stop uterine bleeding. It is used in menorrhagia. It can also help with bleeding piles. Me and Qi. (n.d.). Tortoise plastrons. *meandqi.com*. https://www.meandqi.com/herb-database/tortoise-plastron
Walnut *Juglans regia*	Other names: *Hu Tao Ren, akhrot* There are about 20 species of walnut. The common ones are the English or Persian walnut *(Juglans regia)* and the black walnut *(Juglans nigra).* Black walnuts have more bioactive compounds and more health benefits. They also have 75% more protein than the English walnut. They are used mostly in TCM. Walnuts are rich in fiber, omega-3 fatty acids (lipoic acid), omega-6 fatty acids (linoleic acid), and antioxidants which help improve brain health and prevent heart disease and cancer. Other chemical compounds present include ellagic acid, ellagitannins, catechin, melatonin, and phytic acid. They also contain minerals (copper, phosphorus, and manganese) and vitamins including folic acid, vitamins B6, and E. In TCM, walnuts are associated with the lung, large intestine, and kidney Qi. They have sweet and warm properties. Walnuts are used to tonify the kidneys, nourish the blood, warm the lungs, and moisten the intestines. Typically, they are used to treat pain and weakness in the knees and back, aid in digestion, and relieve asthma. Black walnuts can nourish hair and treat dandruff. They have antihyperlipidemic and antiinflammatory properties. They can lower total cholesterol and LDL-cholesterol and raise HDL-cholesterol. They can help with weight loss. Walnut is generally safe. It can cause severe allergy or anaphylaxis. Phytic acid impairs the absorption of minerals such as iron and zinc. It is also high in oxalates. Excessive amounts of walnuts may cause diarrhea or risk of weight gain from the higher calories. Acupuncture Today. (n.d.). Walnut (hu tao ren). https://acupuncturetoday.com/herbcentral/walnut.php Arnarson, A. (2019, March 26). Walnuts 101: Nutrition facts and health benefits. *Healthline*. https://www.healthline.com/nutrition/foods/walnuts#benefits
Water caltrop *Trapa bicornis*	Other names: *Singhara, Li Xi, Li Tzu* Water caltrop contains antioxidants (including polyphenols and flavonoids). It is rich in minerals (potassium, copper, manganese, and iodine) and vitamin B6. It is cool in nature and is sweet. It covers the spleen, stomach, and kidney meridians. It clears heat. It tonifies the stomach and strengthens the spleen. It helps in various digestive disorders (diarrhea, gas and bloating, constipation, acid reflux, nausea, and jaundice). It can help in weight loss. It improves heart health, and lowers blood pressure and LDL cholesterol. It can regulate thyroid function. It promotes urination.

Ingredients	Mechanism of Action and Health Benefits

Arora, D. (2018, October 18). 7 health benefits of Singhara or water caltrops that you should know. *TheHealthSite*. https://www.thehealthsite.com/fitness/diet/health-benefits-of-singhara-or-water-caltrops-that-you-should-know-d1018-615944/

Chinese Medicine Living Admin. (2014, June 14). Chinese water chestnut. *Chinese Medicine Living*. https://www.chinesemedicineliving.com/chinese-medicine/chinese-water-chestnut/

White atractylodes rhizome

Atractylodes macrocephala

Other names: *Lion heart, Bai Zhu*

The active ingredient of white atractylodes rhizome is a volatile oil which contains actractylon, lactones, sesquiterpene, polysaccharides, and acetylenes. It is a Qi tonic.

Bai zhu is a spleen tonic and strengthens the digestive system. It also has diuretic properties and is a kidney tonic.

It is used to treat mental fatigue, dizziness, edema, diarrhea, and vomiting.

This rhizome is a safe herb and there are no known drug interactions. It should not be taken when there is dehydration.

White cnidium

Cnidium monnieri

Other name: *She Chuang Zi*

Cnidium contains terpenes, cnidiadin, bornyl isovalerate, oxol, parsley, berapten, and other active constituents which have antimicrobial and antiinflammatory effects.

It is used to treat impotency, erectile dysfunction, increase sex drive, and treat gynecological infections. It reduces itching in atopic dermatitis (eczema) and other skin conditions like tinea corporis. It is also used to treat hemorrhoids. It may also strengthen bones.

Side effects may include stomach upsets and bitter mouth.

Proven Herbal Remedies. (2021, April 20). Cnidium Monnieri (She Chuang Zi). *Chinese Herbs Healing*. https://www.chineseherbshealing.com/proven-herbal-remedies/cnidium-monnieri.html

White mulberry leaf

Morus alba

Other name: *Sang ye*

Mulberry includes many species including white mulberry *(Morus alba)*, red mulberry *(Morus rubra)*, and black mulberry *(Morus nigra)*.

White mulberry leaves are abundant in phytochemicals including phenolic acids, flavonoids, flavonols, benzofurans, coumarins, and anthocyanins. It is also rich in fiber, minerals (calcium, potassium, zinc, phosphorus, and magnesium), and vitamins (ascorbic acid and β-carotene).

It has antihyperglycemic, antioxidant, antiinflammatory, and antiglycation effects. The alkaloid, 1-deoxynojirimycin in the leaf prevents the absorption of carbohydrates in the intestine, hence lowering blood glucose.

Mulberry leaf has sweet, bitter, and cold properties in TCM. It is associated with the liver and lung Qi, functions to clear lung heat (fever, headache, sore throat, or cough) and clear fire in the liver (manifested as red, painful, and watery eyes).

It can lower blood glucose and insulin in type 2 diabetes. It is also used to stop bleeding, especially in patients who are vomiting blood. It is also used for muscle and joint pain. Other uses include for constipation, dizziness, asthma, and can prevent hair loss and premature graying. It may also reduce cholesterol and improve blood pressure.

It decreases appetite and helps in obesity.

This herb should not be used by those with weakness and cold in the lungs. It can interact with diabetic medications. Side effects include stomach upsets.

Chen, C., Mohamad Razali, U. H., Saikim, F. H., Mahyudin, A., & Mohd Noor, N. Q. I. (2021). *Morus alba* L. plant: bioactive compounds and potential as a functional food ingredient. *Foods, 10*(3), 689. https://doi.org/10.3390/foods10030689

Kubala, J. (2019, November 29). What is mulberry leaf? All you need to know. *Healthline*. https://www.healthline.com/nutrition/mulberry-leaf#benefits

White peony root

Paeoniae radix lactiflora

Other name: *Bai Shao*

White peony root is obtained from the tree *Paeonia lactiflora Pall*. Its main compound is paeoniflorin which helps increase the activity of aromatase, an enzyme that turns testosterone into estrogen.

It has antiinflammatory, analgesic, antianxiety, and antidepressant properties.

In TCM, bai shao is associated with liver and spleen Qi. It has bitter, sour, and slightly cold properties. It is thought to tonify the blood and relax the body.

It is used to treat fever, headaches, infertility, regulate the menstrual cycle, and also for night sweats.

This root should be avoided in liver disorders and by those taking anticoagulants.

Ingredients	Mechanism of Action and Health Benefits
	Eu Yan Sang. (n.d.). White Peony Root. *EuYanSang.com*. https://www.euyansang.com/en_US/white-peony-root/herb-WhitePeonyRoot.html
	Nunez, K. (2020, October 16). The potential benefits and side effects of the white peony root. *Healthline*. https://www.healthline.com/health/white-peony-root#benefits-of-white-peony-root-plant
Wolfberry/Goji berry *Lycium barbarum*	Other names: *Chinese Wolfberry, Gou Qi Zi* The fruit, root bark, and leaves of genus *Lycium* are used for medicine and culinary purposes. Lycium fruit is known as wolfberry or goji berry. The fruits of *L. barbarum* and *L. Chinense* are the most commonly used. The main bioactive compounds in wolfberry fruit (also called Lycii Fructus) are arabinogalactan proteins (AGPs), the carotenoid zeaxanthin, and 2-O-(β-D-glucopyranosyl) ascorbic acid. The AGPs have antiviral and antibacterial properties. It is rich in fiber, iron (11% of the DV), vitamin A (501% of the DV), and vitamin B (15% of the DV). It has antioxidant, antiinflammatory, antidiabetic, and immunomodulatory effects. In TCM, wolfberries are considered to be beneficial for strengthening the body, keeping fit, and prolonging life. It has sweet and calm properties. Wolfberry functions to nourish and tonify liver and kidney, and improve Qi. Wolfberry can reduce the risk of chronic conditions like cancer, heart diseases, and diabetes. It improves eye function and prevents disorders like macular degeneration. Wolfberries may interact with certain medications and trigger an allergic reaction in some people. Benzie, I. F. F., & Wachtel-Galor, S. (2011). *Chapter 14: Biomolecular and clinical aspects of Chinese wolfberry* (2nd ed.). Boca Raton: CRC Press. Link, R. (2020, September 8). What are Goji berries? This unique red fruit, explained. *Healthline*. https://www.healthline.com/nutrition/goji-berry#basics
Wolfberry root bark *Cortex lycii*	Other names: *Goji Tree Root Bark, Chinese Wolfberry Root Bark, Lycium Bark, Di Gu Pi* The Wolfberry root bark (also called *Lycii Radicis Cortex*) of the *L. barbarum* and *L. Chinense* are widely used. It contains several compounds including terpenoids, flavonoids, coumarins, alkaloids, lycium lignan D, and lycium phenylpropanoid A. It is cold in nature and is sweet. It covers the lung, liver, and kidney meridians. It cools the blood and clears lung heat. It is used to treat bleeding disorders including nosebleed, hemoptysis (blood in sputum), hematuria (blood in urine), hematemesis (blood in vomit), and menorrhagia (heavy menses). It can also treat cough with yellow phlegm. Me and Qi. (n.d.). Goji tree root bark. *Meandqi.com*. https://www.meandqi.com/herb-database/goji-tree-root-bark Yang, Y., An, Y., Wang, W., Du, N., Zhang, J., Feng, Z., et al. (2017). Nine compounds from the Root Bark of Lycium chinense and their anti-inflammatory activities. *Acta Pharmaceutica Sinica B*, 7(4), 491–495. https://doi.org/10.1016/j.apsb.2017.04.004
Wolfsbane *Aconitum carmichaeli*	Other name: *Fu Zi* Wolfsbane is a rich source of diterpene alkaloids and flavonoids. It also contains free fatty acids, polysaccharides, and different classes of alkaloids. It has analgesic, antiinflammatory, antihypertensive, and antianxiety properties. In TCM, it is associated with the spleen, kidney, and heart. Its nature is spicy, sweet, hot, and toxic. It is able to rescue Yang, tonify fire to raise Yang energy, and eliminate cold to stop pain. Wolfsbane is commonly used to reduce fever associated with colds, pneumonia, laryngitis, croup, and asthma. It is also used as a diuretic to induce sweating. It is made into a tincture and applied topically as a counter-irritant liniment for neuralgia, rheumatism, and sciatica. It can also be used for headaches, diarrhea, influenza or colds with congestion, and numbness. Fresh wolfsbane can be toxic as it contains aconitine. The symptoms of poisoning can be tongue numbness, limb numbness, tingling, dizziness, blurred vision, nausea, and vomiting. It should also be avoided by pregnant and breastfeeding women. Drugs.com. (2021). Aconite. https://www.drugs.com/npc/aconite.html Yao, H., & Ou, J. (2017, May 20). Understanding the Chinese Medical Herb Aconite (Fuzi). *AACMA*. https://www.aacmaonline.com/en/%E5%AD%A6%E6%9C%AF%E6%B4%BB%E5%8A%A8/understanding-the-chinese-medical-herb-aconite-fuzi/

Ingredients	Mechanism of Action and Health Benefits
Yam rhizome	Other names: *Wild Yam, Shan Yao*
Rhizoma dioscoreae	Shan yao is the rhizome of *Dioscorea opposita Thunb*. The chemical compounds present include phytosteroid sapogenins (diosgenin), saponin, choline, starch, and glycoprotein. The phytosteroids can affect hormone balance. The rhizome also contains amino acids, vitamins (B1, B2, and C), and minerals (calcium, phosphorus, and iron).
	It has antibiotic, antiinflammatory, antioxidant, and antiaging effects.
	Yam rhizome has a sweet taste and neutral properties in TCM. It is mainly associated with the spleen, kidney, and lung Qi. It can be used to replenish the Qi and tonify the spleen.
	Shan yao helps to boost and improve the digestive and respiratory functions. It can help relieve symptoms related to weak knees, sore lower back, frequent night urination, premature ejaculation, excessive vaginal discharge, and heavy menstrual bleeding. It can reduce thirst in diabetes.
	Yam should not be taken by itself when the user has accumulated dampness in the abdomen. It should not be used by pregnant or breastfeeding women without consulting a doctor.
	1st Chinese Herbs. (2021). Shan Yao. https://1stchineseherbs.com/s/shan-yao/
	Eu Yan Sang. (n.d.). Common Yam Rhizome. *EuYanSang.com*. http://euyansang.com/en_US/common-yam-rhizome/herb-CommonYamRhizome.html
Yerba de tajo herb	Other names: *False Daisy, Mo Han Lian*
Herba Ecliptae	Refer under "Bhringraj or False daisy."
Young tangerine peel	Other name: *Qing Pi*
Pericarpium citri reticulatae viride	Refer under "Tangerine peel."
Zao Jiao Ci	Other names: *Gleditsia spine, Chinese Honeylocust Spine*
Gleditsiae sinensis spina	Gleditsia spine is the dried thorn of *Gleditsia sinensis*. It contains more than 60 compounds including sterols (zizyberanalic acid and echinocystic acid), flavonoids (quercetin, luteolin, apigenin, and vitexin), triterpenoids (betulinic acid, stigmasterol, and alphitolic acid), phenols, and saponins (gleditsia saponin C).
	It is warm in nature. It covers the stomach, liver, and lung meridians. It expels phlegm. It also clears toxicity and invigorates blood.
	It has antiangiogenic properties.
	It is used topically on boils and abscesses.
	MedicineTraditions. (n.d.). Gleditsia Spina, Zao Jiao Ci 皂角刺. https://www.medicinetraditions.com/gleditsia-spina-zao-jiao-ci.html
	Zhang, J. P., Tian, X. H., Yang, Y. X., Liu, Q. X., Wang, Q., Chen, L. P., et al. (2016). Gleditsia species: An ethnomedical, phytochemical and pharmacological review. *Journal of Ethnopharmacology*, *178*, 155–171. https://doi.org/10.1016/j.jep.2015.11.044
Ze Xie	Other name: *Oriental water plantain rhizome*
Alisma *Plantain d'Eau*	It is a water plant and the roots are used to treat bladder and urinary tract diseases, high blood pressure, diabetes, and high cholesterol.
	Not much data is available.
	RxList Editors. (2021, June 11). Water plantain. *RxList*. https://www.rxlist.com/water_plantain/supplements.htm
	WebMD Editors. (n.d.). Asian water plantain. *WebMD*. https://www.webmd.com/vitamins/ai/ingredientmono-347/asian-water-plantain
Zedoary	Other names: *E Zhu, White Turmeric*
Curcuma zedoaria	Zedoary contains several bioactive compounds including polyphenols (curcumin), terpenoids (dihydrocurdione and curcumenol), and sesquiterpenes (zedoarofuran, gajutsulactones, curcumanolide, curcumenone, and zedoarolides). Its essential oils also contains 1,8-cineole, curzerenone, and germacrone.
	It has antiinflammatory, analgesic, and anticancer properties.
	Refer to "Turmeric."
	Lobo, R., Prabhu, K. S., Shirwaikar, A., & Shirwaikar, A. (2009). *Curcuma zedoaria* Rosc. (white turmeric): a review of its chemical, pharmacological and ethnomedicinal properties. *Journal of Pharmacy and Pharmacology*, *61*(1), 13–21. https://doi.org/10.1211/jpp/61.01.0003
	Proven Herbal Remedies. (2021, May 29). Turmeric Root (E Zhu). *Chinese Herbs Healing*. https://www.chineseherbshealing.com/proven-herbal-remedies/turmeric-root.html

Note: A TCM herb or ingredient is almost never used or eaten alone but always as part of a formula containing many herbs or ingredients that act synergistically.

Western/Others Natural Ingredients

Ingredients	Mechanism of Action and Health Benefits
Acetyl-L-carnitine	Carnitine is a natural amino acid derivative. It is made in the liver and kidney from lysine and methionine amino acids. Natural sources of carnitine include mainly meat and fish.
	There are many forms of carnitine. L-carnitine is biologically active. D-carnitine is the inactive form. Acetyl L-carnitine has neuroprotective properties. Propionyl-L-carnitine has more effect on the circulation. It can increase nitric oxide. L-carnitine L-tartrate is rapidly absorbed and is often used in postexercise fatigue.
	L-carnitine is essential for mitochondrial health. It transports fatty acids into the mitochondria. It is important for energy metabolism.
	L-carnitine is used for weight loss and is often regarded as a fat burner.
	It can also be used to improve brain function (in dementia, autism) even though acetyl-L-carnitine is preferred.
	Both forms can support heart health. It is used in heart failure, hypertension, and coronary artery disease. It can lower blood sugar and help in diabetes.
	It also increases stamina in exercise and sports performance.
	Side effects include gastric upset.
	Johnson, J. (2020, July 20). What to know about L-carnitine. *MedicalNewsToday*. https://www.medicalnewstoday.com/articles/l-carnitine
	Mawer, R. (2018, November 6). L-Carnitine: Benefits, side effects, sources and dosage. *Healthline*. https://www.healthline.com/nutrition/l-carnitine
African cherry *Prunus africana*	Other names: *African plum tree, Pyegeum africanum*
	The African cherry tree is a common forest canopy tree in the sub-Saharan countries.
	The bark of the African cherry tree contains atraric acid, atranorin, β-sitosterol ferulic acid, and other esters.
	Pygeum is an herbal extract taken from the bark of the African cherry tree.
	It has inflammatory properties. It supports prostate and kidney health. It may also treat fever including malaria.
	It is used to prevent and treat benign prostatic hyperplasia (BPH) and prostatic cancer.
	Side effects include gastric upsets, diarrhea, and constipation.
	Stewart, K. (2003). The African cherry (*Prunus africana*): Can lessons be learned from an overexploited medicinal tree? *Journal of Ethnopharmacology, 89*(1), 3–13. https://doi.org/10.1016/j.jep.2003.08.002
	Thompson, R. Q., Katz, D., & Sheehan, B. (2019). Chemical comparison of Prunus africana bark and pygeum products marketed for prostate health. *Journal of Pharmaceutical and Biomedical Analysis, 163*, 162–169. https://doi.org/10.1016/j.jpba.2018.10.004
African Mango *Irvingia gabonensis*	Other names: *Wild mango, Bush mango or Bika nut*
	African mango is used in Western Africa as a part of their diet. It is not the same as the common mango. It is rich in soluble fiber, minerals (calcium, magnesium, iron, and phosphorus), and vitamin C.
	It also has antioxidant properties.
	It helps with weight loss.
	Side effects include gas and bloating, constipation, and headache.
	McPherson, G. (2021, June 22). What is African mango and its extract? Weight Loss and More. *Healthline*. https://www.healthline.com/nutrition/african-mango
Agrimony *Agrimonia eupatoria*	Agrimony contains mostly tannins.
	It is used to treat diarrhea, stomach upsets, gallbladder problems, IBS, liver and kidney problems, and sore throat. It may lower blood glucose.
	It is an overall safe herb and not much data is available. Some gastric irritation or liver toxicity may occur with overuse. It can interact with diabetic medications.
	RxList Editors. (2021, June 11). Agrimony. *RxList*. https://www.rxlist.com/agrimony/supplements.htm
	WebMD Editors. (n.d.). Agrimony. *WebMD*. https://www.webmd.com/vitamins/ai/ingredient-mono-604/agrimony

Ingredients	Mechanism of Action and Health Benefits

Alfalfa
Medicago sativa

Alfalfa contains various bioactive components such as saponins, coumarins, flavonoids, phytosterols, phytoestrogens, and alkaloids. It also contains fiber, vitamins (A, B1, B6, C, E, and K), and minerals (calcium, potassium, iron, phosphorus, and zinc). The saponins present help in decreasing blood cholesterol levels. It is also an antioxidant. It has estrogenic activity.

It is used in treating diabetes, arthritis, UTIs, and menstrual problems. It can also stimulate breast milk production.

It may help prevent or clear kidney stones and metabolic health.

Alfalfa might be harmful to pregnant or breastfeeding women. It should also be avoided by those taking blood thinners, with an autoimmune disorder or a compromised immune system.

Cervoni, B., & Kroner, A. (2021, March 19). The health benefits of Alfalfa. *Verywell Health*. https://www.verywellhealth.com/health-benefits-of-alfalfa-4584280

Jones, T. (2016, September 3). Alfalfa. *Healthline*. https://www.healthline.com/nutrition/alfalfa#TOC_TITLE_HDR_4

Allspice
Pimenta dioica

Other names: *Jamaican pepper, Pimento, Myrtle pepper, Kurundu, Newspice*

It is a spice obtained from the dried unripe berry (fruit) of the *Pimenta dioica* shrub plant. Each berry is the size of a peppercorn. The dried berries are ground into a spice powder (which is used in meat marinades, soups, sauces, stews, curries, pickles, pies, puddings, and desserts). The allspice powder has a smell that resembles a mixture of ground cinnamon, cloves, nutmeg, and peppercorn. Essential oil (about 4%) is also extracted from the dried berries and it contains eugenol which has analgesic, antimicrobial, digestive aid, and insect-repellent properties. The dried leaves of allspice are used as bay leaves.

Allspice is rich in minerals (manganese, copper, iron, calcium, copper, potassium, and magnesium), vitamin C, and fiber.

It has antibacterial, antifungal, antiinflammatory antioxidant, immune-boosting, and antiaging effects.

It supports digestion and helps in nausea, vomiting, indigestion, dyspepsia, stomach cramps, colic, gas and bloating, flatulence, constipation, and diarrhea. It maintains oral and dental health and hygiene.

It maintains bone density (from manganese mainly) and can help in osteoporosis, arthritis, and gout.

It can help improve circulation (from iron and copper) and heart health (from potassium). It can also regulate blood glucose in diabetes and help with weight loss.

It can also reduce menstrual cramps.

Excessive use can cause gastric upsets, skin rash, and seizures. It should not be used in chronic IBD.

Lang, A. (2021, September 24). Allspice—a unique spice with surprising health benefits. *Healthline*. https://www.healthline.com/nutrition/allspice

Almond
Prunus dulcis

Other names: *Prunus amygdalus, Sweet almond, Badam*

Almond is the seed from the almond tree. There are sweet and bitter almond tree varieties. The sweet almond is safe and edible unlike the bitter almond. The active constituents in the sweet almond are globulins, albumin, and amino acids (arginine, histidine, lysine, phenylalanine, leucine, valine, tryptophan, methionine, and cystine). It is rich in dietary fiber, vitamin E, and minerals (manganese, magnesium, and calcium). It also contains trace amounts of copper, phosphorus, and vitamin B2. Vitamin E contains tocopherol, an antioxidant.

Although it is high in unsaturated fats, it can lower total cholesterol, decrease low-density lipoproteins levels (LDL or bad cholesterol), and raise HDL cholesterol (good cholesterol).

It can lower blood sugar. It also reduces the risk of breast cancer. It helps in weight loss. It has mild laxative action and can help in constipation.

The almonds can be eaten raw, blanched, or roasted. Almond milk is a dairy-free plant milk. Almond flour or almond meal is finely ground blanched almonds and is gluten-free. Almond butter is blended dry roasted almonds and is a substitute for peanut allergy. Almond oil is cold-pressed from the almonds.

Almond oil is beneficial for treatment of head lice, and various skin diseases like eczema and acne.

Sweet almonds contain trace amounts of amygdalin, a toxic cyanogenic glycoside which gets broken into hydrocyanic acid (prussic acid). Bitter almonds are lethal due to higher amygdalin.

Rao, H. J., & Lakshmi. (2012). Therapeutic applications of almonds (*Prunus amygdalus* L.): a review. *Journal of Clinical and Diagnostic Research*, 6(1), 130–135. https://www.jcdr.net/articles/PDF/1836/38%20-%203719.(A).pdf

Times of India Editors. (2020, September 11). Surprising side effects of eating too many almonds. *The Times of India*. https://timesofindia.indiatimes.com/life-style/health-fitness/photo-stories/5-surprising-side-effects-of-eating-too-many-almonds/photostory/60747918.cms

Ingredients	Mechanism of Action and Health Benefits
Alpha-lipoic acid	Other name: Lipoic acid
	Alpha-lipoic is present in natural or in synthetic forms. It is made in the mitochondria of the cells and is also present in small amounts in red meat, organ meat, and some plants (spinach, watercress, brussel sprouts, broccoli, beet, yam, and rice bran). It is also available as a dietary supplement.
	It is a vitamin B-like antioxidant. It can also boost levels of glutathione. It also has antiinflammatory actions.
	It can lower blood glucose by decreasing insulin resistance and inhibiting the enzyme AMP-activated protein kinase (AMPK) so that hunger is reduced. It can also reduce the risk of diabetic retinopathy and neuropathy.
	It helps with weight loss. It can improve skin health making it smooth and wrinkle-free.
	It can help in many chronic diseases including heart disease, cancer, AD dementia (improves memory), neuropathy (improves nerve function in diabetic neuropathy and carpal tunnel syndrome), rheumatoid arthritis, and others.
	Overall, it is safe. Side effects include rash, nausea, and itching.
	Raman, R. (2019, September 26). Alpha-lipoic acid: weight loss, other benefits and side effects. *Healthline*. https://www.healthline.com/nutrition/alpha-lipoic-acid
American pawpaw *Asimina triloba*	The bark, roots, twigs, and seeds of American paw paw contain acetogenins. They have antitumor, pesticidal, antimalarial, anthelmintic, antiviral, and antimicrobial effects. Its essential oil contains sesquiterpenes. The fruit contains phenolic acids and flavonoids that have antioxidant properties.
	It is rich in vitamins A, B, and C. Vitamin A present is beneficial for eyesight and vitamin B for the nerves and muscles. Vitamin C helps in improving the immune system.
	It has antiinflammatory, antidiabetic, antimicrobial, and antiulcer properties.
	It is also used in the treatment of malaria, asthma, bronchitis, skin conditions (eczema and acne), piles, and impotence.
	Drugs.com. (2021, March 22). *Pawpaw*. https://www.drugs.com/npp/pawpaw.html
	Health Benefits Times. (2017, December 25). Paw Paw facts and health benefits. *HealthBenefitstimes.com*. https://www.healthbenefitstimes.com/paw-paw/
Apple cider vinegar *Malus pumila Mill*	It contains natural probiotics that can improve the immune system and gut health. It also has vitamins (B, C), antioxidants, and small amounts of the minerals (sodium, phosphorus, potassium, calcium, iron, and magnesium). It can restore and maintain pH balance.
	It has antiinflammatory, antistress, and antioxidant properties.
	It helps in weight loss, lowers blood sugar and cholesterol levels, and improves blood pressure. It is also used for skin conditions like eczema, psoriasis, and dandruff. It is also used in psoriatic arthritis, infections, and sore throats. It may also help with acid reflux, yeast infections, and ulcerative colitis.
	MedicineNet. (2021, June 11). *Apple cider vinegar supplement: Uses, benefits, side effects, dose, precautions & warnings*. https://www.medicinenet.com/apple_cider_vinegar/supplements-vitamins.htm
	Migala, J., & Grieger, L. R. (2020, February 10). Apple cider vinegar: Benefits, side effects, uses, dosage, and more. *EverydayHealth.com*. https://www.everydayhealth.com/diet-nutrition/diet/apple-cider-vinegar-nutrition-facts-health-benefits-risks-more/
Apple (Green & Red) *Malus domestica*	Apples contain several bioactive compounds including phenols (caffeic acid, cinnamic acid, and ferulic acid), flavonoids (quercetin, quercetin glycosides, and anthocyanins), triterpenoids, and phytosterol. It is also rich in soluble and insoluble fibers and vitamin C.
	It has antiinflammatory, antioxidant, and immune-boosting properties.
	It can reduce the risk of cardiovascular diseases (such as stroke, heart disease, and atherosclerosis) by reducing cholesterol, triglycerides, blood sugar, and blood pressure. It also helps in healthy weight loss.
	It supports digestion, improves regularity, and prevents constipation.
	It can help reduce the risk of AD.
	It may also help prevent certain cancers including colorectal, breast, esophageal, and oral cavity cancers.
	It is a versatile fruit and used in many ways. It is usually eaten as a fresh whole fruit to boost immune and gut health, as apple juice for gallstones, as stewed apple for diarrhea, as apple milk for depression, as apple puree for baby's weaning food, as apple paste for head lice, and as apple soup for eczema.

Ingredients	Mechanism of Action and Health Benefits
	Overall, it is safe. Overconsumption can cause bloating and constipation.

Barrie, L., & Kennedy, K. (2020, October 2). 7 outstanding health benefits of apples. *EverydayHealth.com*. https://www.everydayhealth.com/diet-nutrition/impressive-health-benefits-of-apples/

Patocka, J., Bhardwaj, K., Klimova, B., Nepovimova, E., Wu, Q., Landi, M., et al. (2020). Malus domestica: A review on nutritional features, chemical composition, traditional and medicinal value. *Plants*, *9*(11), 1408–1427. https://doi.org/10.3390/plants9111408

Aquaporins

Aquaporins (AQPs) are water channel proteins found in the cell membranes of the outer layer of the skin epidermis i.e., stratum corneum layer. They are transmembrane proteins. It acts as a natural protective skin moisture barrier. It transports water and glycerol. It maintains skin hydration. There are many types of aquaporins. Aquaglyceroporin AQP3 is the most abundant type and is commonly found in the keratinocytes of the stratum corneum cells. AQP5 is involved in sweat secretion.

It can also be synthetically made from plant extracts or human recombinant technology. Artificial water channels or artificial aquaporins are used in many skin care products and also in wound healing. They can be incorporated into liposome systems to facilitate delivery of the AQPs.

Boury-Jamot, M., Sougrat, R., Tailhardat, M., Varlet, B. L., Bonté, F., Dumas, M., et al. (2006). Expression and function of aquaporins in human skin: Is aquaporin-3 just a glycerol transporter? *Biochimica et Biophysica Acta (BBA)—Biomembranes, 1758*(8), 1034–1042. https://doi.org/10.1016/j.bbamem.2006.06.013

Arctic root
Rhodiola rosea

Other name: *Rhodiola*

Rhodiola is an herbal root that grows in cold mountains. It is an adaptogen and contains more than 140 bioactive compounds of which rosavin and salidroside are the most potent.

It is helpful in stress and stress-related symptoms including anxiety, depression, and insomnia. It also reduces chronic and mental fatigue and increases cognitive performance. It can also improve exercise performance and endurance.

It can also lower blood sugar and diabetes.

There are no significant side effects reported.

Walle, G. V. D. (2018, March 3). 7 science-backed health benefits of Rhodiola rosea. *Healthline*. https://www.healthline.com/nutrition/rhodiola-rosea

Arnica
Arnica montana

Other name: *Mountain Arnica*

Arnica contains bioactive compounds including flavonoids (quercetin, kaempferol, and patuletin glucoside), sterols, and polyphenols (chlorogenic acid).

It has antiinflammatory and analgesic properties.

Homeopathic form is used to treat arthralgia, arthritis, bruises, hair loss, and other painful conditions.

The nonhomeopathic form if consumed can be life threatening. Topical use can cause skin dryness.

Ciuperca, O. T., Țebrencu, C. E., Iacob, E., Cretu, R. M., Chiriac, M., & Ionescu, E. (2016). Phytochemical screening and chromatographic fingerprint studies on ethanolic extract of *Arnica montana* L. *Analele Științifice Ale Universității, 62*(2), 53–60.

Davidson, K. (2020, July 20). Arnica homeopathic medicine: Overview, uses, and benefits. *Healthline*. https://www.healthline.com/nutrition/arnica-homeopathic

WebMD Editors. (n.d.). Arnica. *WebMD*. https://www.webmd.com/vitamins/ai/ingredientmono-721/arnica

Artemisia
- **Mugwort**
Artemisia vulgaris
- **Wormwood**
Artemisia absinthium
- **Sagebrush**
Artemisia tridentata

Artemisia contains more than 200 species including wormwood, mugwort, and sagebrush.

Wormwood

Wormwood contains strong bitter compounds, i.e., absinthin and anabsinthin, which stimulate bile flow and digestive juices. Absinthin is an appetite stimulant and is an ingredient in the spirit, absinthe. The essential oils in wormwood include thujone (α- and β-thujone), chamazulene (an antioxidant), and artemisinin (a terpene with antiinflammatory and antimalarial effects). Thujone blocks GABA, hence stimulates the brain and can cause seizures.

Wormwood is a potent antifungal, antibacterial, and antiparasitic herb and can treat candida infection, bacterial vaginosis, and malaria.

It is also a remedy for stomach, gallbladder, and liver disorders. It can treat intestinal worms. It can also be used as an insect repellent.

It can relieve pain in osteoarthritis and reduce inflammation in Crohn's disease.

Side effects include allergic reactions, digestive upsets, risk of seizures, and kidney failure. It can interact with anticoagulants.

Ingredients	Mechanism of Action and Health Benefits

Mugwort

Mugwort contains more than 24 bioactive compounds including terpenes (camphor, sabinene, chrysanthenone, and β-thujone), flavonoids (luteolin, rutin, and morin), and phenols.

It is used as a tonic and can boost energy.

It increases bile and gastric juice production. It helps in digestive disorders including diarrhea, constipation, vomiting, stomach cramps, and worm infestations. It can also be used as an insect repellent.

It calms the nerves and can help in insomnia, epilepsy, depression, and anxiety.

It is an emmenagogue. It stimulates the uterus and regulates the menstrual cycle.

It has mild psychoactive and hallucinogenic effects. Allergic reactions (including sneezing and skin rash) can occur as adverse reactions.

Sagebrush

It is rarely used by herbalists.

Morris, R. (2016, December 19). Mugwort: A weed with potential. *Healthline*. https://www.healthline.com/health/mugwort-weed-with-potential

Pandey, B. P., Thapa, R., & Upreti, A. (2017). Chemical composition, antioxidant and antibacterial activities of essential oil and methanol extract of *Artemisia vulgaris* and *Gaultheria fragrantissima* collected from Nepal. *Asian Pacific Journal of Tropical Medicine*, 10(10), 952–959. https://doi.org/10.1016/j.apjtm.2017.09.005

Stuart, A. G. (n.d.). *Wormwood*. The University of Texas, Herbal Safety. https://www.utep.edu/herbal-safety/herbal-facts/herbal%20facts%20sheet/wormwood.html

The Editors of Encyclopaedia Britannica. (2009, February 5). Artemisia. *Encyclopedia Britannica*. https://www.britannica.com/plant/artemisia-plant

Wartenberg, L. (2020, January 16). What is wormwood, and how is it used? *Healthline*. https://www.healthline.com/nutrition/what-is-wormwood

WebMD Editors. (n.d.). Mugwort. *WebMD*. https://www.webmd.com/vitamins/ai/ingredientmono-123/mugwort

Artichoke

Cynara cardunculus var. scolymus

Cynara scolymus

Other names: *Globe artichoke, French artichoke, Green artichoke*

Artichoke is rich in fiber, vitamins (folate, C, and K), minerals (iron, magnesium, potassium, and phosphorus), and antioxidants (luteolin which prevents cholesterol formation, cynarin and silymarin which are hepatoprotective). It contains inulin which is a prebiotic that promotes healthy gut bacteria. It is a cholagogue. The cynarin stimulates bile production and increases peristalsis. It also has a diuretic effect.

Artichoke extract can slow the activity of α-glucosidase which is an enzyme that breaks down starch into glucose.

It promotes digestive health and reduces flatulence. It can stimulate bile production and help with liver and gallbladder metabolism. It can treat gallstones.

It can reduce LDL cholesterol, lower blood pressure and blood glucose. It reduces fat deposits in nonalcoholic fatty liver disease and improves IBS symptoms. It helps with obesity.

Side effects include upset stomach, gas, diarrhea, and allergic reactions.

Brown, M. J. (2019, January 16). Top 8 health benefits of Artichokes and Artichoke extract. *Healthline*. https://www.healthline.com/nutrition/artichoke-benefits#TOC_TITLE_HDR_6

Aspartic acid

Aspartic acid is a natural amino acid that is present in the D and L forms. The D-aspartic acid has an effect on the hormones.

It increases the testosterone levels by increasing the FSH and LH.

It may improve sperm count and motility.

It can improve muscle stamina and strength. It is often used to boost sports performance. It can help with muscle fatigue.

Overall, it is safe.

Tinsley, G. (2018, January 3). D-Aspartic acid: Does it boost testosterone? *Healthline*. https://www.healthline.com/nutrition/d-aspartic-acid-and-testosterone#TOC_TITLE_HDR_2

WebMD Editors. (2011). Aspartic acid. *WebMD*. https://www.webmd.com/vitamins/ai/ingredient-mono-12/aspartic-acid

Ingredients	Mechanism of Action and Health Benefits
Avocado *Persea americana*	Avocado is a nutrient-dense superfood. There are many varieties. The most common type is Hass avocado which has a green alligator type of skin. It contains bioactive compounds such as flavonoids (luteolin, β-carotene, and citraurin), phenolic acids (gallic acid, vanillic acid, and ferulic acid), terpenoids (perseanol and indicol), and tannins. It is also rich in lutein and zeaxanthin. It also has healthy monounsaturated fats (oleic acid) and polyunsaturated omega-3 and some omega-6 fatty acids), vitamins (folate, K, C, E, B5, and B6), and minerals (potassium, copper, magnesium, and manganese). It contains more insoluble fiber (75%) than soluble fiber (25%). It does not contain any cholesterol. Avocados are rich in plant sterols which act as selective estrogen receptor modulators. Hence, it has hormonal balancing effects. It blocks the absorption of estrogen. There is reduced excess estrogen, increased progesterone in women, and increased testosterone in men. The high potassium content supports heart health. It lowers LDL cholesterol and triglycerides and increases HDL cholesterol. It can also increase insulin sensitivity. The presence of the antioxidants supports eye health and can prevent cataract and macular degeneration. It can help in weight loss. It may also prevent prostate cancer. Side effects may include latex allergy. Bhuyan, D. P., Alsherbiny, M. A., Perera, S., Low, M., Basu, A., Devi, O. A., et al. (2019). The Odyssey of bioactive compounds in avocado (*Persea americana*) and their health benefits. *Antioxidants*, *8*(10), 426–479. https://doi.org/10.3390/antiox8100426 Gunnars, K. (2018, June 29). 12 proven health benefits of avocado. *Healthline*. https://www.healthline.com/nutrition/12-proven-benefits-of-avocado
Azelaic acid	Azelaic acid is a natural dicarboxylic acid. It is made by the yeast on the skin. It is also produced from various grains such as wheat, barley, and rye. It is also synthesized in the lab. It maintains skin health. It has antioxidant, antiinflammatory, antibacterial, skin-lightening, keratolytic, and exfoliating actions. It inhibits the enzyme tyrosinase and hence can lighten the melanin pigment. It also inhibits 5-alpha reductase and promotes hair growth. It can treat acne, rosacea, hyperpigmentation, melasma, clogged pores, and alopecia. It can smoothen rough or uneven skin. It is very safe, gentle, and effective. Side effects include mild irritation and tingling. Rarely, allergic reactions may occur. It is safe to use in pregnancy. Watson, K. (2018, December 19). Treating acne with azelaic acid. *Healthline*. https://www.healthline.com/health/azelaic-acid-acne
Baking soda *Sodium bicarbonate*	Sodium bicarbonate is derived from soda ash. It is alkaline, has antacid properties, neutralizes stomach acid quickly and relieves mild stomach pain, indigestion, and bloating and gas after a meal. It can treat heartburn and acid reflux. It has antiseptic and antibacterial properties. It also is used as a mouthwash and to treat mouth ulcers. By increasing saliva pH, there is reduced bacterial growth and oral hygiene is improved. It can be used as a teeth whitener. It neutralizes the acidity of urine and may ease the discomfort in UTIs. It can also reduce the uric acid levels in the body and hence useful in gout. Overuse and long-term use can result in hypokalemia and hypochloremia. Raman, R. (2020, July 13). 22 benefits and uses for baking soda. *Healthline*. https://www.healthline.com/nutrition/baking-soda-benefits-uses
Banana Musa	Bananas contain fiber (mainly pectin), minerals (including manganese, copper, potassium, and magnesium), and vitamins (B6, C, and β-carotene). It contains dopamine (a neurotransmitter) and tryptophan. It has antioxidant, antiobesity, laxative, and anticancer activities. Pectin helps in lowering blood sugar levels, improves digestion, and reduces the risk of leukemia and stomach ulcers. It can also help with constipation and diarrhea. It improves heart health by managing blood pressure levels. It can also help improve kidney function. The tryptophan boosts mind health, improves memory, and regulates the mood. It can also boost energy. It may help in weight loss by reducing appetite. The banana peel and leaves can help with itchy skin, psoriasis, warts, and insect bites.

Ingredients	Mechanism of Action and Health Benefits
	Overall, it is safe. Rare allergic reactions can occur. It should not be taken with beta-blockers due to the high potassium content in both.

Bjarnadottir, A. (2018, October 18). 11 evidence-based health benefits of bananas. *Healthline*. https://www.healthline.com/nutrition/11-proven-benefits-of-bananas

Hagy, C. (2017, November 15). 11 banana health benefits you might not know about. *Everyday-Health.com*. https://www.everydayhealth.com/diet-nutrition/11-banana-health-benefits-you-might-not-know-about/

Bee products
The main bee products include *bee pollen, beeswax, honeycomb, honey, royal jelly*, and *propolis*. All are edible and also used topically. Honey is the most common product. Bee venom is also a bee product used as a medicine. Apitherapy is using bee products for therapeutic use.

Bee pollen
Key benefit

Bee pollen: Good source of proteins, vitamins, and minerals.

Beeswax: Used in cosmetics for skin health.

Honeycomb:

Honey: Natural and nutrient-rich sweetener.

Royal jelly: Excellent superfood and nutraceutical for the elderly.

Propolis: Natural antibiotic.

Bee venom: Medicine to desensitize those with bee allergy. It is also used as a Botox substitute.

<u>Bee pollen</u> is nutritional food for the bee. Worker or field honeybees get covered with pollen and collect nectar and from different plant anthers. The bees return to the beehive with pollen and nectar which then becomes enriched food for the colony of bees. It is a fermented mixture of flower pollen, enzymes, bees' secretion or saliva, honey, nectar, and beeswax which are packed and deposited in the honeycomb cells.

Bee pollen appears as dark brown, black, or orangish balls/granules or pellets. It is a nutrient-rich superfood. These balls of pollen are extracted from the honeycomb cells to produce bee bread.

Bee pollen contains several vitamins (mainly Bs), minerals (calcium, magnesium, iron, copper, and selenium), proteins (28%) including several amino acids, essential fatty acids (phospholipids and triglycerides), and simple sugars.

It has antimicrobial, antiviral, antifungal, antiinflammatory, immune-boosting, hepatoprotective, and anticancer actions. It also has antiallergy effects.

It is used in children who have loss of appetite, malnutrition, mental delay, and physical and mental fatigue. It can also help in dyslexia.

It can also be used for burns and wounds.

Komosinska-Vassev, K., Olczyk, P., Kaźmierczak, J., Mencner, L., & Olczyk, K. (2015). Bee Pollen: chemical composition and therapeutic application. *Evidence-Based Complementary and Alternative Medicine*, *2015*, 1–6. https://doi.org/10.1155/2015/297425

Beeswax
Beeswax is made from the honeycomb of honeybees. Beeswax can be natural or synthetic.

The yellow beeswax is obtained directly from the honeycomb. The white or bleached beeswax is derived from the yellow beeswax. Beeswax absolute is yellow beeswax which has been treated with alcohol. The above types are widely used as stiffening agents in the cosmetic, food, and beverage industries.

Beeswax pastilles or pellets are smaller broken pieces from the original beeswax blocks and are more convenient to use.

Beeswax is rich in vitamin A. It has antiinflammatory, antiviral, antibacterial, and analgesic properties. It can be consumed or used topically.

It acts as a protective barrier, humectant and protects the skin. It also exfoliates the dead skin and slough. It helps in wound healing and can decrease inflamed swellings.

It can help with gastric ulcers. It can also lower cholesterol.

Overall, it is safe.

RxList Editors. (2021, June 11). Beeswax. *RxList*. https://www.rxlist.com/beeswax/supplements.htm

WebMD Editors. (2014). Beeswax. *WebMD*. https://www.webmd.com/vitamins/ai/ingredient-mono-305/beeswax

Honeycomb is a hexagonal mass of cells made from beeswax secretions of worker honeybees in their nest. It contains larvae, honey, and bee pollen. The honeycomb is removed to harvest and extract the honey.

Ingredients	Mechanism of Action and Health Benefits
Honeycomb	Cohen-Garcia, X. (2017, September 1). Why are honeycomb cells hexagonal? *Science Friday*. https://www.sciencefriday.com/educational-resources/why-do-bees-build-hexagonal-honeycomb-cells/
Honey	*Honey* is extracted from the honeycomb which is built by the honeybees. Honey is made from nectar which is collected by worker bees. It is eaten by all adult bees except the queen bee (who eats royal jelly).
	The main active compounds in honey are flavonoids including pinocembrin, pinobanksin, chrysin, galagin, acacetin, and kaempferol. Honey contains enzymes (invertase and catalase) and amino acids of which the most abundant is proline. It also contains trace amounts of B vitamins (B2, B3, B9, B5, and B6) and vitamin C. The minerals calcium, iron, zinc, potassium, phosphorus, magnesium, selenium, chromium, and manganese are also present.
	It has antioxidant, antiinflammatory, and antibacterial effects. It also has antidepressant, anticonvulsant, and antianxiety benefits.
	It is used in the treatment of wounds, particularly burns. It is also commonly used orally to treat coughs. Antioxidants in honey help prevent or reduce the risk of cardiovascular diseases.
	It might also help relieve GI tract conditions such as diarrhea associated with gastroenteritis. It can also be used for oral rehydration therapy.
	Loveridge, J. (n.d.). *Chemical composition of honey*. chm.bris.ac.uk. http://www.chm.bris.ac.uk/webprojects2001/loveridge/index-page3.html
	Mayo Clinic Staff. (2020, November 14). *Honey*. Mayo Clinic. https://www.mayoclinic.org/drugs-supplements-honey/art-20363819
Royal jelly	*Royal jelly* (also called bee milk) is a thick gelatinous milky fluid and a superfood secreted from the glands of worker honeybees (nurse bees) to feed only the queen bee and her larvae. It contains flavonoids (catechin, pinocembrin, kaempferol, apigenin, rutin, and luteolin) and polyphenols.
	It is also rich in B vitamins, trace minerals, specific major royal jelly proteins, and unique fatty acids.
	It has antiaging, antioxidant, and immune-boosting properties. It promotes erythropoiesis and muscle performance.
	It is neuroprotective. It can boost memory, cognition, and mental activities.
	It is also a digestive stimulant.
	It supports reproductive health and is used for premenstrual and menopausal symptoms. It can also help in obesity and fertility.
	It promotes wound healing.
	It can cause insomnia with excessive consumption.
	Hill, A. (2018, October 3). 12 potential health benefits of royal jelly. *Healthline*. https://www.healthline.com/nutrition/royal-jelly
	Pasupuleti, V. R., Sammugam, L., Ramesh, N., & Gan, S. H. (2017). Honey, propolis, and royal jelly: A comprehensive review of their biological actions and health benefits. *Oxidative Medicine and Cellular Longevity, 2017*, 1–21. https://doi.org/10.1155/2017/1259510
	Science Direct. (2017). Royal jelly—An overview.| *ScienceDirect*. https://www.sciencedirect.com/topics/agricultural-and-biological-sciences/royal-jelly
Propolis	*Propolis* is produced by bees from the sap of needle-leaved evergreens. It is combined with beeswax and its own fluids. It is greenish-brown and sticky and is used to build the hives.
	It is rich in flavonoid polyphenols. It has antimicrobial and antiinflammatory properties. The antifungal effect is due to the presence of pinocembrin, a flavonoid.
	Topical propolis is used to treat cold sores and genital herpes. It is also used to treat breast cancer.
	Goldman, R. (2018, September 29). The benefits and uses of propolis. *Healthline*. https://www.healthline.com/health/propolis-an-ancient-healer
	In general, all bee products, especially honey should not be given to babies under the age of 1 year as it can cause GI conditions (infant botulism) in rare cases. Acute allergic reactions, anaphylaxis, or contact dermatitis can also occur especially in those who have pollen allergy.
	Marko, S. (2018). Honey and other bee products. *Celebrate World Bee Day*. https://www.worldbeeday.org/en/did-you-know/92-honey-and-other-bee-products.html

Ingredients	Mechanism of Action and Health Benefits
Beetroot *Beta vulgaris*	Other names: *Sugar beet, Red garden beet, Blood turnip, Spinach beet, Chukkander*

Beetroot contains glycosides (betanin), glutamine, vulgaxanthin, and inorganic nitrate. It is a good source of fiber, vitamins (folate and C), and minerals (iron, manganese, and potassium).

Beetroot also contains bioactive pigments called betalains. These are mainly betacyanin pigments which include betanin (red-violet in color) and betaxanthin pigments (yellow-orange).

Betacyanin helps the liver clear toxins from the body. The alkaline nature of beetroot also helps balance the acidity in the system. It is helpful in PCOS. It can regulate blood sugar.

It has antioxidant, antiinflammatory, and anticancer properties.

The nitrates present boost heart health by improving blood pressure levels and blood flow. It also reduces the risk of heart diseases and stroke.

Glutamine, an amino acid present supports the healthy gut bacteria and improves gut health. The high fiber content supports bowel function.

It can increase stamina, improve oxygen use, and enhance physical activity.

It can improve immune function and skin health.

Overall, it is safe. Overconsumption of beetroot causes beeturia which gives urine a red or pink color (it is harmless). The beet greens and roots are rich in oxalates which can contribute to kidney stones and can interfere with nutrient absorption. Beetroot should not be taken in case of IBS as it contains fructans which can cause stomach upset. |

Bjarnadottir, A. (2019, March 8). Beetroot 101: Nutrition facts and health benefits. *Healthline*. https://www.healthline.com/nutrition/foods/beetroot

Lewin, J. (2021, February 8). Top 5 health benefits of beetroot. *BBC Good Food*. https://www.bbcgoodfood.com/howto/guide/ingredient-focus-beetroot

Bilberry *Vaccinium myrtillus*	Bilberry is similar to blueberry but is smaller and darker. It contains anthocyanosides which may protect the retina from free radical damage. It may also aid the body to produce rhodopsin, a compound responsible for good night vision. It contains minerals (manganese) and vitamins (C and K).

It has antioxidant, neuroprotective, and antiinflammatory properties.

It can reduce eye fatigue and dryness and improve vision in people with glaucoma.

It can lower blood sugar by stimulating insulin secretion.

It can support heart health by lowering blood pressure, blood sugar, and LDL cholesterol.

It can improve memory and learning.

Overall, it is safe. It can cause diarrhea. It can interact with blood-thinning and diabetic medications. |

National Center for Complementary and Integrative. (2020, August). *Bilberry*. NCCIH. https://www.nccih.nih.gov/health/bilberry

Petre, A. (2019, August 13). 9 Emerging Health Benefits of Bilberries. *Healthline*. https://www.healthline.com/nutrition/bilberry-benefits

Birch *Betula* spp.	There are many species of birch. Common medicinal birches include white birch *(B. alba)* and black birch *(B. lenta or sweet birch)* mostly, and also yellow birch *(B. alleghaniensis or golden birch)* and silver birch *(B. pendula)*. The inner bark, twigs, and leaves have medicinal properties.

It is rich in phenols (flavonoids and tannins), betulin, betulinic acid (which are triterpenes mostly in the bark), salicylin (which has aspirin-like activity and mostly in the young twig bark), and saponins. It is high in vitamin C.

It has detoxifying, blood-purifying, antiseptic, antiinflammatory, astringent, and diuretic properties. It also can lower blood glucose and lipids.

It can treat rheumatism, arthritis, bone fracture, kidney stones and urinary tract infection.

It enhances skin and hair health. It can treat dandruff and hair loss. Birch water is the sap obtained from birch trees. It is rich in minerals (manganese and magnesium) and antioxidants and has a mild sweet taste. It can improve skin, hair, and bone health.

Side effects include birch pollen allergy and risk of manganese toxicity. |

WebMd. (n.d.). BIRCH: Overview, uses, side effects, precautions, interactions, dosing and reviews. *WebMD*. https://www.webmd.com/vitamins/ai/ingredientmono-352/birch

Ingredients	Mechanism of Action and Health Benefits
Bitterwood *Picrasma excelsa*	Other names: *Jamaican quassia, Quassia* Bitterwood contains alkaloids (canthin-6-one and others), terpenoids (quassin and its derivatives), coumarins, β-sitosterol, β-sitostenone, and thiamine. It is a bitter tonic. It has antimicrobial, antitumor, and insecticidal actions. It is used in the treatment of fevers, diabetes, head lice, intestinal worms, seborrheic dermatitis, indigestion, and constipation. In high doses, it can cause gastric irritation and vomiting. It can interact with drugs like diuretics, antacids, and digoxin. WebMD Editors. (n.d.). Quassia. *WebMD*. https://www.webmd.com/vitamins/ai/ingredientmono-290/quassia
Blackberry *Rubus fruticosus*	Blackberry fruit contains anthocyanins, polyphenols, tannins, and flavonoids. It is rich in vitamins (C, K, E, and A), minerals (calcium, manganese, and potassium), and fiber. It is best eaten fresh. It has antioxidant, anticancer, and neuroprotective properties. Blackberry leaves contain more chlorogenic acid (polyphenol antioxidant) than the berries. The tannins in the leaves have astringent properties. Blackberry aids digestive health and can relieve acid reflux and constipation. It can lower insulin resistance and triglycerides. It helps in obesity and diabetes. Decoction from the leaves can treat anemia, acute diarrhea, oral thrush, regulate the menses, and also be used as mouthwash. Overall, it is safe. Rarely, it causes allergies. Honeycutt, L. (2019, December 27). What are the benefits of blackberry leaves? *livestrong.com*. https://www.livestrong.com/article/257328-what-are-the-benefits-of-blackberry-leaves/ Kandola, A. (2018, June 7). What are the benefits of blackberries? *MedicalNewsToday*. https://www.medicalnewstoday.com/articles/322052 WebMD Editorial Contributors. (2020, September 1). Health benefits of blackberries. *WebMD*. https://www.webmd.com/diet/health-benefits-blackberries#2
Black cohosh *Cimicifuga racemosa* *Actaea racemosa*	Other names: *Black snakeroot, Bug bane* Black cohosh is different from blue cohosh (blue cohosh ripens the uterus to facilitate labor and delivery). Black cohosh contains triterpene glycosides, alkaloids, and phenolic acids (caffeic acid and ferulic acid). It acts as a phytoestrogen and balances hormones. It is a "women's herb." It is used for fertility and menopausal symptoms (reduces hot flashes and body aches). It is also used in PMS, PCOS, irregular periods, menstrual cramps, menorrhagia, and fibroids. It can improve sleep, mental health, and weight gain in menopausal women. It can reduce bone loss and improve fracturing in early osteoporosis. Side effects are mild and include skin rash, digestive upset, breast enlargement or pain, and occasional vaginal spotting. Rare hepatotoxicity and anemia has been reported. Lin, Y. (2021, July 27). *What black cohosh can (and can't) do for menopause symptoms*. Cleveland Clinic. https://health.clevelandclinic.org/what-is-black-cohosh/ Nikolić, D., Lankin, D. C., Cisowska, T., Chen, S. N., Pauli, G. F., & van Breemen, R. B. (2015). Nitrogen-containing constituents of black cohosh: Chemistry, structure elucidation, and biological activities. *The Formation, Structure and Activity of Phytochemicals*, 45, 31–75. https://doi.org/10.1007/978-3-319-20397-3_2 Shoemaker, S. (2020, May 27). Black cohosh: Benefits, dosage, side effects, and more. *Healthline*. https://www.healthline.com/health/food-nutrition/black-cohosh
Blackcurrant *Ribes nigrum*	All parts of the blackcurrant plant can be used. It can be consumed as dried fruit, tablets, capsules, oil, or powder. It contains antioxidants (such as phenolic compounds and anthocyanins). The seed oil contains gamma linoleic acid (omega-6 fatty acid). It is rich in vitamins (C, A, E, B1, B5, and B6) and minerals (potassium). It has antiinflammatory, antimicrobial, immune-boosting, anticancer, and neuroprotective effects. It is used to treat sore throat, cough, and flus. It supports heart health. It can lower blood pressure, cholesterol, and blood sugar. It prevents atherosclerosis plaque buildup and improves blood flow. It prevents anemia. The oil can be applied for psoriasis and eczema. It can improve vision and eye fatigue.

Ingredients	Mechanism of Action and Health Benefits
	It can also be used in arthritis.
	Overall, it is safe. Side effects may include mild diarrhea and gas and bloating. It interacts with blood-thinning medications.

Health Benefits Times. (2017, July 6). Health benefits of black currants. *HealthBenefitstimes.com*. https://www.healthbenefitstimes.com/black-currants/

Morris, R. (2017, September 14). 6 health benefits of black currant. *Healthline*. https://www.healthline.com/health/health-benefits-black-currant

Ingredients	Mechanism of Action and Health Benefits
Black haw *Viburnum prunifolium*	Black haw contains several compounds including tannins, salicin, scopoletin, and volatile oils. It is high in oxalate and salicylate.
	It is uterine antispasmodic. It is also a diuretic and can relieve fluid retention.
	It is used to treat heavy (menorrhagia) and painful (dysmenorrhea) periods. It can prevent miscarriages, uterine prolapse, and uterine atony after childbirth.
	Side effects with overuse include nausea, seizures, and bradycardia.

Health Benefits Times. (2018, February 8). Facts about Blackhaw Viburnum. *HealthBenefitstimes.com*. https://www.healthbenefitstimes.com/blackhaw-viburnum/

RxList Editors. (2021, June 11). Black Haw. *RxList*. https://www.rxlist.com/black_haw/supplements.htm#UsesAndEffectiveness

Ingredients	Mechanism of Action and Health Benefits
Bladderwrack *Fucus vesiculosus*	Bladderwrack is a brown seaweed rich in antioxidants (fucoxanthin, alginic acid, fucoidans, and phlorotannins) proteins, vitamins (C and A), minerals (iodine, calcium, potassium, magnesium, zinc, and sodium), and fiber. It is high in mucilage. It demonstrates antiestrogenic and progestogenic effects and prolongs the menstrual cycle length. This can improve the irregular menstrual cycles in premenopausal women.
	It also has antiinflammatory and diuretic actions.
	The iodine content in bladderwrack supports thyroid health. It can be used to treat hypothyroidism.
	It also supports skin health. It boosts collagen synthesis, promotes healing and antiaging.
	It can also be used for obesity, UTIs, digestive problems (acid reflux, gastritis and constipation) and arthritis.
	Read more under "Seaweed."

Davidson, K. (2020, July 8). Bladderwrack: Benefits, uses, and side effects. *Healthline*. https://www.healthline.com/nutrition/bladderwrack-benefits

TraceGains, Inc. (2015, June 5). Bladderwrack. *Kaiser Permanente*. https://wa.kaiserpermanente.org/kbase/topic.jhtml?docId=hn-3653002

WebMD Editors. (n.d.). Bladderwrack. *WebMD*. https://www.webmd.com/vitamins/ai/ingredient-mono-726/bladderwrack

Ingredients	Mechanism of Action and Health Benefits
Blue cohosh *Caulophyllum* *thalictroides*	Other names: *Caulophylle, Blue ginseng, Papoose root, Squaw root, Blueberry root*
	Blue cohosh is unrelated to black cohosh.
	Blue cohosh or Squaw root is used to treat symptoms of menstruation, menopause, and induce labor.
	It is a strong emmenagogue. It can also initiate menstruation, suppress heavy menstrual flow, and relieve menstrual cramps and pain.
	The flower is an effective parturifacient and facilitates childbirth. For a week or two before the expected date of delivery, pregnant squaw women would drink tea infused with powdered Blue Cohosh roots. The tea was believed to induce a rapid and painless labor. Blue cohosh ripens and stimulates the uterus to initiate labor pains and facilitate delivery.
	It also helps in endometriosis and pelvic inflammatory disease.
	It should not be used when a pregnancy is confirmed.
	It has antispasmodic properties. It is also used as a laxative.
	It can treat colic, cramps, epilepsy, and sore throats.
	The roasted seeds of blue cohosh can be consumed as coffee substitute.

WebMD. (n.d.). BLUE COHOSH: Overview, uses, side effects, precautions, interactions, dosing and reviews. https://www.webmd.com/vitamins/ai/ingredientmono-987/blue-cohosh

Ingredients	Mechanism of Action and Health Benefits
Borage *Borago officinalis*	Borage contains GLA which has antiinflammatory actions. It increases the prostaglandin PGE1 levels, (PGE1) which increases cyclic AMP (cAMP) and inhibits tumor necrosis factor formation.
	It has antiarthritic activity. It is also used in skin disorders (eczema, acne, and rosacea), premenstrual symptoms, menopause, and cardiovascular diseases. It may also help to increase breast milk production.
	Side effects include mainly dyspeptic symptoms (burp, bloating, nausea, indigestion) and worsening of seizures.

RxList Editors. (2021, June 11). Borage. *RxList*. https://www.rxlist.com/borage/supplements.htm

Ingredients	Mechanism of Action and Health Benefits
Broccoli *Brassica oleracea*	Broccoli contains several bioactive compounds including carotenoids (lutein and zeaxanthin), phenols (caffeic acid), isothiocyanates, and glucosinolates. It is a rich source of minerals (potassium, iron, calcium, magnesium, and selenium), vitamins (A, K, E, C, and folic acid), and antioxidants (sulforaphane and indole-3-carbinol). Refer to "Broccoli sprouts." Ware, M. (2020, January 9). The health benefits of broccoli. *MedicalNewsToday*. https://www.medicalnewstoday.com/articles/266765
Broccoli sprout	Broccoli sprout is a cruciferous vegetable. It is rich in sulforaphane which is a sulfur-rich compound. Its precursor is glucoraphanin. Broccoli sprouts contain 10 to 100 times more glucoraphanin than mature broccoli. It contains myrosinase enzymes which activate the glucoraphanin to sulforaphane. It is rich in antioxidants including phenolic compounds (chlorogenic acid, p-coumaric acid, and ferulic acid) and flavonoids (robinin and luteolin). Sulforaphane has anticancer, blood-sugar-lowering, and immune-boosting properties. It also supports heart and digestive health. It can be used to treat constipation and autoimmune diseases. It can also detoxify environmental toxins and chemicals. It can also be used in autism to improve some social and verbal skills. Overall, it is safe. Overconsumption may lead to digestive upset including gas and bloating. Coyle, D. (2019, February 26). Sulforaphane: Benefits, side effects, and food sources. *Healthline*. https://www.healthline.com/nutrition/sulforaphane Paśko, P., Tyszka-Czochara, M., Galanty, A., Gdula-Argasińska, J., Żmudzki, P., Bartoń, H., et al. (2018). Comparative study of predominant phytochemical compounds and proapoptotic potential of broccoli sprouts and florets. *Plant Foods for Human Nutrition*, 73(2), 95–100. https://doi.org/10.1007/s11130-018-0665-2
Boneset *Eupatorium* *perfoliatum*	Other names: *Crosswort, Thoroughwort, Teasel, Eupatoire, Eupatorio, Feverwort, Indian Sage, Sweating Plant,* The roots and leaves contain various phytoactive compounds including triterpenes, tannins, alkaloids and flavonoids, (kaempferol, quercetin, and caffeic acid). It also contains allantoin, minerals (calcium, phosphorus, and potassium) and vitamins (C and A). The dried leaf and flowers are used to make tea. Boneset has been used for fever, flu, cough and common cold. It is also used to treat fracture and osteoporosis. WebMD. (2020). BONESET: Overview, Uses, Side Effects, Precautions, Interactions, Dosing and Reviews. WebMD. https://www.webmd.com/vitamins/ai/ingredientmono-594/boneset
Buchu *Agathosma betulina*	The active constituents in buchu include limonene, menthone, psi-diosphenol, and pulegone. Limonene promotes weight loss and anticancer activity. It is used for treating UTIs such as in the urethra (urethritis) and kidneys (pyelonephritis) or STDs. It is also used in treating inflamed prostate (prostatitis), BPH, high blood pressure, fever, cough, common cold, upset stomach, stomach ulcers, IBS, gout, and STDs. It can be hepatotoxic. WebMD Editors. (n.d.). BUCHU. *WebMD*. https://www.webmd.com/vitamins/ai/ingredientmono-180/buchu
Burdock *Arctium lappa*	Burdock contains several antioxidants including flavonoids (luteolin and quercetin), phenolic acids, and lignans. It is also rich in inulin (a prebiotic) that supports gut health and digestion. It facilitates estrogen metabolism in the liver and hence it can reduce the size of uterine fibroids. It has antiinflammatory, antiseptic, antimicrobial, skin-toning, and diuretic effects. It can also purify the blood and eliminate toxins. It is used to treat osteoarthritis, skin disorders (acne, eczema, psoriasis, and wrinkles), and pancreatic cancer. Overall, it is safe. Side effects include allergic reactions, gas and bloating, and dehydration. It can interact with blood thinners and diabetic medications. Brennan, D. (2020, November 12). Health benefits of burdock root. *WebMD*. https://www.webmd.com/diet/health-benefits-burdock-root#1 Gotter, A. (2021, January 12). *What Is Burdock Root?* Healthline. https://www.healthline.com/health/burdock-root#recipes

Ingredients	Mechanism of Action and Health Benefits
Burning bush *Dictamnus albus*	Burning bush leaves, bark, and roots are used. It is rich in polyphenols, phenolic acids (gallic acid, salicylic acid, ferulic acid, and sinapic acid), coumarins (auraptene, xanthotoxin, and umbelliferone), flavonoids (luteolin), and alkaloids. It has antibacterial, antifungal, antihelminthic, carminative, and contraceptive properties. It is hepatoprotective and is a liver tonic. It can treat jaundice. It supports digestive health including stomach ache and cramps. It can also treat epilepsy. It is also used for eczema, psoriasis, scabies, wound healing, and hair loss. It is also used for arthritis. Side effects include stomach upset with overconsumption and increased sunburn risk (photodermatitis). Health Benefits Times. (2018, February 16). Know about the burning bush. *HealthBenefitstimes.com.* https://www.healthbenefitstimes.com/burning-bush/ WebMD Editors. (n.d.). Burning bush. *WebMD.* https://www.webmd.com/vitamins/ai/ingredient-mono-599/burning-bush Zhao, Y., Wu, Y., & Wang, M. (2015). Bioactive substances of plant origin. In P. Cheung, B. Mehta (Eds.), *Handbook of food chemistry.* Berlin, Heidelberg: Springer. https://doi.org/10.1007/978-3-642-36605-5_13
Butcher's broom *Ruscus aculeatus*	Other name: *Kneeholly, Sweetbroom* Butcher's broom contains flavonoids and saponins. It has antiinflammatory properties (from the ruscogenin presence) and venotonic actions. It also has laxative and diuretic functions. It is used in chronic venous insufficiency disorders like hemorrhoids, varicose veins, and gallstones. Overall, it is safe. Occasional gastric upsets may occur. Raman, M. R. S. (2018, October 26). *Butcher's broom: a shrub with surprising benefits?* Healthline. https://www.healthline.com/nutrition/butchers-broom#benefits
Butterbur *Petasites*	Other name: *Coltsfoots* Butterbur contains bioactive compounds such as terpenes (linalool and fukinanolide), sequestrepenes (eremophilene), and alkaloids. The leaves and roots are used to make butterbur extracts. It has antispasmodic and antiinflammatory properties. It is used to prevent and relieve migraines and headaches. It can help in cough, bronchitis, asthma, and allergic rhinitis (hay fever). It is also used in stomach upset. It can also reduce symptoms in UTIs. Side effects include stomach upset, gas, headache, and allergic reactions. Butterbur products which are pyrrolizidine alkaloid (PA)-free are used. Burgess, L. (2017, October 11). What are the health benefits of butterbur? *MedicalNewsToday.* https://www.medicalnewstoday.com/articles/319667 Mihajilov-Krstev, T., Jovanović, B., Zlatković, B., Matejić, J., Vitorović, J., Cvetković, V., et al. (2020). Phytochemistry, toxicology and therapeutic value of *Petasites hybridus* subsp. ochroleucus (common butterbur) from the Balkans. *Plants, 9*(6), 700. https://doi.org/10.3390/plants9060700 WebMD Editors. (n.d.). Butterbur. *WebMD.* https://www.webmd.com/vitamins/ai/ingredientmono-649/butterbur
Cajeput oil *Melaleuca cajuputi*	Other names: *White wood, White tree, Kayu Putih, Cajuput, White samet, Melaleuca leucadendron* Cajeput oil is distilled from the fresh leaves and twigs of the cajeput tree *(Melaleuca leucadendron)* usually and *(Melaleuca quinquenervia)*. It is similar to the tea tree oil which is from *Melaleuca alternifolia* (same family) but is different. It contains a higher concentration of 1.8-cineole compared to tea tree oil. Other bioactive compounds include linalool, terpineol, terpinolene, myrcene, pinenes, and caryophyllene. It has antiinflammatory, analgesic, antioxidant, antibacterial, decongestant, expectorant, and insecticide properties. It is mostly for external use. It is more effective in respiratory infections compared to tea tree oil. It can loosen phlegm in cough, cold, sore throat, sinusitis, and chest infections. It can be applied for toothache, headache, and rheumatism. It can be applied to eczema, acne, boils, scabies, wounds, fungal infection, and dandruff. It is used in skin care products and cosmetic products. It is often added to other herbs.

Ingredients	Mechanism of Action and Health Benefits
	Overall, it is safe. It should not be taken in asthma.
	Health Benefits Times. (2017, August 10). Health benefits of cajeput essential oil. *HealthBenefitstimes.com*. https://www.healthbenefitstimes.com/5142-2/
	RxList Editors. (2021, June 11). Cajeput oil. *RxList*. https://www.rxlist.com/cajeput_oil/supplements.htm
Calendula *Calendula officinalis*	Other name: *Pot marigold*
	Calendula contains polyphenols, flavonoids, triterpenes, and carotenoids. It is widely available as creams or ointments in cosmetics.
	It has antiinflammatory, antioxidant, wound healing, antifungal, and antimicrobial effects.
	It moisturizes the skin and is used to treat eczema, diaper rash, and also fungal nails.
	It is used as a mouthwash for inflamed gums. It can lower blood lipids and glucose.
	Overall, it is safe. It may cause drowsiness and can interact with sedatives or antihypertensive medications. Rare mild local skin irritation may occur.
	Health Benefits Times. (2019, June 3). Calendula facts and health benefits. *HealthBenefitstimes.com*. https://www.healthbenefitstimes.com/health-benefits-of-calendula/
	Lang, A. (2020, April 8). 7 potential benefits of calendula tea and extract. *Healthline*. https://www.healthline.com/nutrition/calendula-tea
	RxList Editors. (2021, June 11). Calendula. *RxList*. https://www.rxlist.com/calendula/supplements.htm
California poppy *Eschscholzia californica*	California poppy stems, leaves, and flowers are used. It contains isoquinoline alkaloids (including californidine, sanguinarine, protopine, allocryptopine, escholzine, and chelidonine), flavone glycosides (including rutin, quercetin, and isorhamnetin), carotenoids, and essential oil.
	It has sedative, nervine, anxiolytic, analgesic, febrifuge, antispasmodic, and antihistamine properties. It is also an uterine stimulant.
	The alkaloids i.e., protopine and allocryptopine stimulate and increase the neurotransmitter GABA receptors to calm the nervous system. It also has mood-stabilizing (thymoleptic) and sleep-promoting effects.
	It is used to treat insomnia, nervous agitation, stress, and mild to moderate anxiety. It is helpful in tension, headaches, ADD/ADHD, IBS, spasmodic cough, and bedwetting in children.
	Unlike opium poppy, California poppy is nonaddictive and is not a narcotic. It is a safe and effective alternative.
	Side effects may include excessive sleepiness.
	Health Benefits Times. (2018, March 2). Facts about California Poppy. *HealthBenefitstimes.com*. https://www.healthbenefitstimes.com/california-poppy/
Carrot *Daucus carota*	Carrots contain several bioactive compounds including several carotenoids (lutein, β-carotene, α-carotene, and lycopene), anthocyanins, and polyacetylenes. They also contain vitamins A, B6, and K and potassium.
	It is rich in soluble (mainly pectin) and insoluble (hemicellulose, cellulose, and lignin) fibers. The soluble fibers help in lowering blood sugar and LDL cholesterol while insoluble fibers help in smooth bowel movement and reduce the risk of constipation.
	It has antioxidant, anticancer, antiinflammatory, and immunomodulatory properties.
	It can reduce the risk of heart diseases and stroke.
	The carotenoids and vitamin A present can improve eyesight, reduce the risk of night blindness, and age-related macular degeneration.
	It can prevent the risk of certain cancers (including prostate, stomach, colon, and leukemia).
	It can help in weight loss by increasing fullness. It also promotes healthy skin and nails.
	Overall, it is safe. Too much carotene can cause skin to become yellow or orange.
	Bjarnadottir, A. (2019, May 3). Carrots 101: Nutrition facts and health benefits. *Healthline*. https://www.healthline.com/nutrition/foods/carrots#plant-compounds
	Sengupta, S. (2019, June 19). 8 amazing health benefits of carrots: From weight-loss to healthy eyesight. *NDTV Food*. https://food.ndtv.com/food-drinks/8-amazing-health-benefits-of-carrots-from-weight-loss-to-healthy-eyesight-1767963

Ingredients	Mechanism of Action and Health Benefits
Cashew Nut *Anacardium occidentale*	Other names: *Cashew, Gajus, Jagus* Cashew nuts contain several bioactive compounds including lutein, β-carotene, stearic acid, proanthocyanidins, polyphenols, antioxidants, linoleic acid, and tocopherols. It contains monounsaturated (i.e., oleic acid which is an omega-3 fatty acid) and polyunsaturated good fats and insoluble fiber. It is rich in various vitamins (including vitamin E, C, thiamine, and folate), minerals (magnesium, copper, manganese, potassium, and phosphorus), and protein. Although it contains stearic acid which is a saturated fatty acid, it does not affect heart health. It can be used as a dairy-free substitute. Cashews help in weight loss and reduce the risk of obesity. It supports heart health and can regulate cholesterol, sugar, and blood pressure. The protein, magnesium, copper, and calcium content help to strengthen and preserve bones. It can reduce the risk of gallstones. Adverse reactions include acute allergic reactions. Raw cashews contain urushiol, a toxin. It is also high in oxalate which can lead to kidney stones. Trox, J., Vadivel, V., Vetter, W., Stuetz, W., Scherbaum, V., Gola, U., et al. (2010). Bioactive compounds in cashew nut (*Anacardium occidentale* L.) kernels: Effect of different shelling methods. *Journal of Agricultural and Food Chemistry*, 58(9), 5341–5346. https://doi.org/10.1021/jf904580k Ware, M. (2018, June 18). Health benefits of cashews. *MedicalNewsToday*. https://www.medicalnewstoday.com/articles/309369 WebMD Editorial Contributors. (2020, September 2). Health benefits of cashews. *WebMD*. https://www.webmd.com/diet/health-benefits-cashews#1
Catnip *Nepeta cataria*	Catnip is rich in antioxidants such as flavonoids, phenolic acids (caffeic acid, rosmarinic acid, and coumaric acid), and volatile oils (including thymol, nepetalactone, and pinene). It also possesses antiinflammatory, antidiabetic, and antimicrobial activities. It is commonly used for treating nervousness, anxiety, and insomnia. It is also used for treatment of coughs and asthma. It may be used to treat GI conditions, including indigestion, cramping, gas and bloating, and diarrhea. It also has insect-repellent properties. Overall, it is safe. It can cause vomiting, headache, and increased menstrual flow. It can interact with sedatives. WebMD Editors. (2020, December 3). Catnip tea: Are there health benefits? *WebMD*. https://www.webmd.com/diet/catnip-tea-health-benefits#1
Cayenne pepper *Capsicum annuum*	Other name: *Capsicum* spp. Cayenne pepper contains several antioxidants (vitamins C and E, β-carotene, lutein, choline, zeaxanthin, and cryptoxanthin) which support the immune system and remove toxins. It also contains capsaicin, a phytochemical that binds to neuroreceptors and causes a calcium influx. This causes the levels of antioxidant enzymes in the body to increase hence facilitating toxin excretion from the body. It can boost metabolism as well as suppresses appetite. Topical capsaicin (cream, patch, and spray) has analgesic, rubefacient, and circulatory stimulating effects. It can provide pain relief by decreasing the amount of a neuropeptide known as substance P that goes to the brain to signal pain. Less substance P produced means less pain. Capsaicin desensitizes the trigeminal nerve so that less calcitonin gene-related peptide is produced. Cayenne pepper can also improve hormone imbalance and blood circulation. It can relieve nasal and sinus congestion (stuffy nose), colds, and postnasal drip. The capsaicin may constrict the dilated and congested blood vessels in the nose and throat. Intranasal capsaicin can relieve migraine or cluster headaches. Too much cayenne can cause gastric irritation, burning sensation, cough, and flushing. Raman, R. (2017, March 18). 8 impressive health benefits of cayenne pepper. *Healthline*. https://www.healthline.com/nutrition/8-benefits-of-cayenne-pepper Ware, M. (2020, January 3). The health benefits of cayenne pepper. *MedicalNewsToday*. https://www.medicalnewstoday.com/articles/267248

Ingredients	Mechanism of Action and Health Benefits

CBD oil
(Medical Cannabis)

Other name: *Marijuana, Cannabidiol, Cannabis*

Marijuana is a nonopiate narcotic psychoactive drug. It is from the *Cannabis sativa* plant. Cannabidiol, or CBD, and THC are two of many different phytocannabinoids present in marijuana. CBD is non-psychoactive. THC is psychoactive.

There are 3 types of CBD oil extracts.

Full-spectrum CBD oil contains all complete hemp components and THC (up to 0.3%)

Broad-spectrum CBD oil contains all hemp components (including essential fatty acids, flavonoids, terpenes, cannabinol, and cannabigerol). There is no tetrahydrocannabinol (THC) or only trace amount.

Isolate CBD oil contains only pure cannabidiol extract with neglible or less than 0.3 % THC.

Any of the above CBD oil extract type is blended with a carrier oil (such as olive oil, coconut oil).

Standard CBD oil is obtained from carbon dioxide extraction. CBD tincture is via alcohol extraction. The next generation CBD uses a new delivery system for higher cell absorption.

A CBD or cannabis product can be in:

- *Edible/oral forms* ie as oil, tincture, capsule, sublingual, gummy forms or in food products (candy, chocolate, cake, ice cream, baked goods, beverages, butter, oil etc).

(The balanced cannabis edible contains near equal amounts of CBD and THC. The CBD-dominant edible contains no or trace THC).

- *Topical forms* ie as cream, ointment, gel, lotion, salve, balm.
- *Others:* Mist spray, vaping liquid.

Medical marijuana or CBD has been used to treat intractable epilepsy. CBD also has many potential uses such as an antiinflammatory, pain relief in nicotine and drug withdrawal symptoms, multiple sclerosis, motor neuron disease, schizophrenia, cancer, anxiety disorders, and AD.

There are very few side effects with CBD which include dry mouth, nausea, and red eyes.

Kubala, J. (2018, February 26). 7 benefits and uses of CBD oil (plus side effects). *Healthline.* https://www.healthline.com/nutrition/cbd-oil-benefits

Celery
Apium graveolens

Celery contains the following bioactive compounds: apigenin, and luteolin along with selinene, limonene, kaempferol, and p coumaric acid which have powerful antioxidant properties. It also contains fiber, vitamins (A, C, K, and folate), and minerals (potassium, magnesium, calcium, iron, and sodium). It has an alkalizing effect.

Apigenin has antiinflammatory, antibacterial, antiviral, antiseptic, detoxifying, and antioxidant effects. Apiuman, a pectin-based polysaccharide that is present, supports digestive health. It can prevent stomach ulcers, constipation, and improve other stomach disorders.

The stem, leaves, or seeds can reduce high blood pressure and high cholesterol levels. It is also used commonly to treat bronchitis, asthma, vomiting, fever, psoriasis, and other skin disorders.

It may also be helpful in the treatment of urinary tract obstruction, UTIs, gout, rheumatic disorders, and jaundice in liver disease.

Celery can increase the male pheromone (androsterone) in sweat which is an aphrodisiac. It may improve male fertility.

It may have neuroprotective effects.

Rarely, allergic reactions or drowsiness may occur. It should not be taken with sedatives.

Overconsumption can interfere with iodine uptake by thyroid gland. It is high in oxalate. Celery seed supplements can cause uterine stimulation, so it should be avoided by pregnant women.

Brazier, Y. (2019, December 4). Health benefits and risks of celery. MedicalNewsToday. https://www.medicalnewstoday.com/articles/270678

Timmons, J. (2019, June 10). 5 healthy benefits of adding celery to your diet. Healthline. https://www.healthline.com/health/food-nutrition/health-benefits-of-celery

Ceramide

The skin consists of natural fats i.e., cholesterol, fatty acids, and ceramide. These fats act as a natural protective skin moisture barrier against the environmental elements. It has antiaging effects and keeps the skin smooth, soft, and supple.

Ceramide is a natural fatty acid i.e., a form of sphingolipid. It is produced from the sebaceous glands. There are nine types of ceramides, and the differences are based on the carbon chain.

Ceramide can be made synthetically, and it is added to moisturizers and various skin care products.

Local allergic reactions may occur.

Spada, F., Barnes, T. M., & Greive, K. A. (2018). Skin hydration is significantly increased by a cream formulated to mimic the skin's own natural moisturizing systems. *Clinical, Cosmetic and Investigational Dermatology, 11,* 491–497. https://doi.org/10.2147/ccid.s177697

Ingredients	Mechanism of Action and Health Benefits
Cetyl Myristoleate (CMO)	Cetyl Myristoleate (CMO) is a natural fatty acid complex which exists in the oleate form. It is a fatty acid ester i.e., a cetylated fatty acid (CFA).
	CFAs are natural fats (from beef tallow, whale blubber) or synthetic fats (two common ones are cetyl myristoleate and cetyl myristate).
	CFA has antiinflammatory and antiarthritic actions. It can help to lubricate joints and improve soft tissue and joint flexibility.
	CMO, especially from beef-tallow extract, is used to treat arthritis, osteoarthritis, and fibromyalgia.
	It is available as nutraceuticals or in topical forms.
	Cetylated Fatty Acids (CFAs): Overview, uses, side effects, precautions, interactions, dosing and reviews. (n.d.). WebMD. https://www.webmd.com/vitamins/ai/ingredientmono-400/cetylated-fatty-acids-cfas
	Lee, S. C., Jin, H. S., Joo, Y., Kim, Y. C., & Moon, J. Y. (2017). The minimal effective dose of cis-9-cetylmyristoleate (CMO) in persons presenting with knee joint pain. *Medicine, 96*(9), e6149. https://doi.org/10.1097/md.0000000000006149
Charcoal or *Activated charcoal*	Activated charcoal is made by heating common charcoal at very high temperatures to create more pores so that it can trap toxins or chemicals.
	It is a universal antidote and is given by mouth to treat most poisonings or drug overdoses (if given within 1 hour of the poison ingestion). It also relieves abdominal gas and bloating and indigestion. It can reduce the cholestasis (bile flow stasis) during pregnancy. It may lower cholesterol or reduce alcohol hangover symptoms. It can also reduce high phosphate levels and toxins in kidney failure.
	It is applied to wounds as part of dressings to trap odors and toxins from wounds.
	It can impair digestion and absorption of nutrients, medications and supplements, rendering the latter to be less effective. Side effects include nausea, vomiting, black stools, and constipation. It should not be used in intestinal obstruction.
	Petre, A. (2017, June 29). What is activated charcoal good for? Benefits and uses. *Healthline*. https://www.healthline.com/nutrition/activated-charcoal
	WebMD Editors. (n.d.). Activated charcoal. *WebMD*. https://www.webmd.com/vitamins/ai/ingredient-mono-269/activated-charcoal
Chamomile *Matricaria chamomilla* *Chamaemelum nobile*	Three popular varieties of chamomile are the German Chamomile *(Matricaria recutita)*, Roman or English Chamomile *(Chamaemelum nobile)*, and the Egyptian chamomile.
	The chamomile flowers contain polyphenol flavonoids compounds, (apigenin, quercetin, patuletin, and luteolin). Other constituents include coumarin (herniarin and umbelliferone), glycoside, farnesol, nerolidol, and germacranolide. It has antiestrogenic effects. Chamomile also has antimicrobial and antiinflammatory properties and can be used for wound healing. It contains bisabolol (colorless oil in the flowers).
	It is also a mild sedative. It promotes relaxation, sleep, and reduces anxiety.
	It is mainly used for digestive problems (infant colic, heartburn, nausea, vomiting). It can reduce menstrual pain and regulate blood sugar.
	It relieves the inflammation and itchiness of eczema.
	It helps to soothe and calm the irritated bladder.
	There are herb–drug interactions. Apigenin in the chamomile can interact with nonsteroidal antiinflammatory drugs (NSAIDs) including aspirin and anticoagulant agents. Hence, they should not be consumed together. Chamomile should also not be taken if there is a history of pollen allergy or cancer of breast, uterus, or ovaries.
	Villines, Z. (2020, January 6). What are the benefits of chamomile tea? *MedicalNewsToday*. https://www.medicalnewstoday.com/articles/320031#benefits-of-chamomile-tea
Chasteberry *Vitex agnus-castus* *Vitex trifolia*	Other names: *Chaste tree, Monk's pepper, Man Jingzi (Vitex trifolia)*
	Vitex is a large genus. *Vitex agnus-castus* is the most common species for medicinal use. Its fruit is called chasteberry or monk's pepper. It contains several bioactive compounds including flavonoids, iridoid glycosides, diterpenes, and essential fatty acids.
	It has antiinflammatory, antispasmodic, antifungal, antibacterial, diuretic, sedative, and insect-repellent properties. Despite its name, it has some aphrodisiac actions and can balance libido.
	Chasteberry is regarded as a women's herb or hormonal tonic. It balances the female hormones. It can improve symptoms related to the female reproductive system. It can treat infertility, decreases prolactin levels, PMS (headache, mood changes, constipation, breast engorgement, and cravings), menstrual (it relieves pain and regulates menstrual flow), and menopausal (hot flushes, night sweat, and sleep) problems.

Ingredients	Mechanism of Action and Health Benefits
	Vitex trifolia is more effective for skin disorders, rheumatism, and dizziness.
	Overall, it is safe. Side effects include stomach upset, skin rash, and headache. It can interact with oral contraceptives and hormone replacement therapy.
	Kamari, F. L., Ousaaid, D., Taroq, A., Aouam, I., Lyoussi, B., Abdellaoui, A., et al. (2021). Bioactive ingredients of different extracts of *Vitex agnus-castus* L. Fruits from Morocco and their antioxidant potential. *Jordan Journal of Biological Sciences*, *14*(2), 267–270. http://jjbs.hu.edu.jo/files/vol14/n2/Paper%20Number%2010.pdf
	Petre, A. (2019, August 9). Vitex agnus-castus: Which benefits of chasteberry are backed by science? *Healthline*. https://www.healthline.com/nutrition/vitex
Chickweed *Stellaria media*	Chickweed is rich in alkaloids, flavonoids, saponins, tannins, phenols, and terpenoids. The young shoots are eaten as salad greens.
	It has antioxidant, antiinflammatory, antimicrobial, and calming and soothing properties.
	It is often used externally for skin disorders (such as eczema, wounds, and psoriasis) and conjunctivitis.
	It can be use internally as demulcent and expectorant in respiratory problems such as asthma.
	It is also used as salve or poultice for joint pain.
	Side effects mainly include allergic reactions.
	Drugs.com. (n.d.). Chickweed. https://www.drugs.com/npc/chickweed.html
	Oladeji, O. S., & Oyebamiji, A. K. (2020). *Stellaria media* (L.) Vill.—a plant with immense therapeutic potentials: phytochemistry and pharmacology. *Heliyon*, *6*(6), e04150. https://doi.org/10.1016/j.heliyon.2020.e04150
	WebMD Editors. (2011). Chickweed. *WebMD*. https://www.webmd.com/vitamins/ai/ingredient-mono-622/chickweed
Chitosan	Chitosan is derived from chitin. Chitin is the hard fibrous compound in the exoskeleton of crustaceans (prawns, crabs, and lobsters) and also from the cell wall of certain fungi.
	Chitosan can lower cholesterol and is used as a dietary supplement in obesity. When chitosan is consumed, it becomes gel-like in the gut and prevents fats being absorbed.
	It is also used in wound dressings.
	Side effects include shellfish allergy and gastric upsets. The absorption of fat-soluble vitamins may also be reduced.
	Knudsen, M. (2021, September 7). Shells for weight loss? Here's the science behind chitosan supplements. *Healthline*. https://www.healthline.com/nutrition/chitosan-supplements
Chocolate *Cocoa butter*	Chocolate is derived from the pods of the cacao tree *(Theobroma cacao)*. The cacao pods contain cacao beans. The beans are fermented and dried. The dried cacao beans are then roasted, cracked, and winnowed to separate the cocoa nibs (cocoa bean kernels) from the cocoa bean shells.
	The cocoa nibs are then ground and conched into a thick paste called cocoa mass or cocoa liquor (which consists of 47% to 56% cocoa butter and the dark bitter cocoa solids). The cocoa mass/liquor is then tempered, and it is the base ingredient to make chocolate, to which milk, sugar, and vanilla are added.
	The cocoa mass can further be dried and ground to make pure unsweetened cacao or cocoa powder, from which most of the cocoa butter is removed.
	Cocoa butter contains antioxidants, fatty acids (to moisturize baby's skin), and cocoa mass polyphenol, which inhibits the production of IgE.
	Chocolate contains several bioactive compounds including resveratrol, flavanols (epicatechins and catechin), polyphenols, and phenolic acids. Dark chocolate also has less fat and sugar. Hence, unsweetened dark chocolate with 100% cocoa is a healthy choice.
	It is rich in minerals (magnesium, copper, iron, manganese, potassium, selenium, and zinc) and soluble fiber. It contains monounsaturated (i.e., oleic acid which is an omega-3 fatty acid) and polyunsaturated fats. Some saturated fats (such as palmitic acid and stearic acid) are also present.
	It helps reduce the risk of heart diseases. It can lower LDL cholesterol and blood pressure. Epicatechins can increase nitric oxide production which helps with vasodilation. Cerebral blood flow is increased, and this can improve cognitive function and reduce the risk of stroke.
	Theobromine and caffeine are stimulants present in chocolate which can help in ADHD.
	Chocolate can also promote fetus growth and development in early pregnancy.
	Dark chocolate has higher cocoa solid content (30% to 80%) with little or no added sugar or milk. It has more antioxidants.

Ingredients	Mechanism of Action and Health Benefits
	Milk chocolate has cocoa solids (7% to 12%), milk solids (up to 12%), milk fats (4%), and some cocoa butter, cocoa liquor, and vanilla.
	White chocolate has no cocoa solids. It contains milk solids, sugar, vanilla, and some cocoa butter.
	High sugar and fat content can lead to hypertension, acne, and diabetes. In some people chocolate can trigger migraines. Lead and cadmium are heavy metals that can be high in some cocoa powder. There may also be some risk of bone loss in menopause.
	Gunnars, K. (2021, July 27). 7 proven health benefits of dark chocolate. *Healthline*. https://www.healthline.com/nutrition/7-health-benefits-dark-chocolate
	Nordqvist, J. (2018, July 17). Health benefits and risks of chocolate. *MedicalNewsToday*. https://www.medicalnewstoday.com/articles/270272
	Scapagnini, G., Davinelli, S., di Renzo, L., de Lorenzo, A., Olarte, H., Micali, G., et al. (2014). Cocoa bioactive compounds: significance and potential for the maintenance of skin health. *Nutrients*, 6(8), 3202–3213. https://doi.org/10.3390/nu6083202
Chondroitin sulfate	Chondroitin sulfate is a natural component of the extracellular matrix in cartilages, bones, ligaments, tendons, and skin. It is mainly obtained from bovine, porcine, or shark cartilage.
	It has antiinflammatory and antioxidant effects.
	It has a slow onset of action, and the effects of joint pain relief are felt after several months.
	Side effects are similar as in glucosamine.
	Drugs.com. (n.d.). Chondroitin. https://www.drugs.com/npp/chondroitin.html#
Chromium	Chromium is an essential trace element in the body. It acts as a cofactor in insulin action and also facilitates fat and carbohydrate metabolism.
	It occurs in 2 forms ie trivalent and hexavalent chromium. The hexavalent form is a toxic mineral. Trivalent chromium is safe. Natural sources of chromium include meat, whole grains and broccoli. The nutritional supplement (trivalent form) is usually available as chromium picolinate.
	Chromium toxicity can arise from prolonged high dose ingestion or from industrial pollution.
	Chromium is a part of chromodulin which regulates blood sugar via insulin.
	It may be used to treat diabetes type 2.
	It helps in weight loss by reducing hunger pangs and cravings.
	It can interact with non-steroidal anti-inflammatory drugs (NSAIDs), psychiatric medications and beta-blockers.
	Side effects include gastric irritation, headaches, sleeplessness and changes in mood. Liver, kidney and possible DNA damage can occur with prolonged use.
	Tinsley, G. (2018, March 23). Chromium Picolinate: What Are the Benefits? Healthline. https://www.healthline.com/nutrition/chromium-picolinate#supplements
Cilantro	Cilantro, like coriander, is derived from the same plant *Coriandrum sativum*. There is often confusion between the two names (Coriander refers to the stalk and leaves of *Coriandrum sativum*. The coriander seeds are the dried seeds of this plant).
	Although they are from the same plant, the nutritional content and taste are different. Fresh cilantro is widely used as garnish in Oriental and South American cooking.
	Cilantro leaves have more vitamins (A, K, and C) compared to coriander. However, it has lower minerals (iron, manganese, calcium, magnesium, zinc, and selenium) compared to coriander. The water content is higher in fresh cilantro.
	It has antiinflammatory and antioxidant effects.
	It can lower blood sugar and reduce the risk of heart disease.
	Raman, R. (2018, February 22). Cilantro vs coriander: What's the difference? *Healthline*. https://www.healthline.com/nutrition/cilantro-vs-coriander
Cleavers *Galium aparine*	The bioactive constituents in cleavers include iridoids (asperulosidic acid, monotropein, and asperuloside), flavonoids (kaempferol glycosides and quercetin), steroids, and alkaloids. It can be used both internally and externally.
	It has diuretic, antispasmodic, antiinflammatory, blood- and lymphatic-purifying, and detoxifying actions.
	It can be used to treat skin conditions including psoriasis, eczema, acne, and wounds.
	It can treat UTIs, reduce edema, and can dissolve kidney stones.
	It can treat the premenstrual symptoms of water retention.
	Health Benefits Times. (2018, September 13). Health benefits of cleavers. *HealthBenefitstimes.com*. https://www.healthbenefitstimes.com/cleavers/

Ingredients	Mechanism of Action and Health Benefits

Ilina, T., Skowrońska, W., Kashpur, N., Granica, S., Bazylko, A., Kovalyova, A., et al. (2020). Immuno-modulatory activity and phytochemical profile of infusions from cleavers herb. *Molecules*, 25(16), 3721–3735. https://doi.org/10.3390/molecules25163721

Cod liver oil

Cod liver oil is derived from the livers of the cod fish. The fish eats phytoplanktons which absorb microalgae. Microalgae has high omega-3 fatty acids content, i.e., docosahexaenoic acid (DHA) and eicosapentaenoic acid (EPA). It is rich in vitamins A and D.

It has antiinflammatory and immune-boosting properties.

It maintains strong and healthy bones. It can reduce joint pain in arthritis and rickets.

It can support eye health.

It can reduce the risk of heart diseases. It increases HDL cholesterol, lowers triglycerides, lowers blood pressure, and reduces arterial plaque formation.

It prevents frequent coughs and colds.

It also promotes fetal brain development. During pregnancy, it can reduce the risk of type 1 diabetes.

It may lower anxiety and depression.

Side effects may include acid reflux, nosebleeds, and gas and bloating.

Raman, R. (2017, June 20). 9 science-backed benefits of cod liver oil. *Healthline*. https://www.healthline.com/nutrition/9-benefits-of-cod-liver-oil

WebMD Editors. (n.d.). Cod liver oil. *WebMD*. https://www.webmd.com/vitamins/ai/ingredient-mono-1040/cod-liver-oil

Coenzyme Q

Other name: *Ubiquinol*

Coenzyme Q10 (ubiquinone or ubidecarenone) is present naturally in all the cells but is highest in the heart, kidneys, liver, and pancreas. It is necessary for biochemical reactions in the cells to provide energy. It has antioxidant activity. Ubiquinone is converted to ubiquinol (reduced form). Ubiquinol is the bioavailable and active form of CoQ10 in the plasma. It decreases with age and chronic diseases.

It has been found to aid in maintaining healthy LDL levels in the body and increase cardiac output, which is a measure of the heart's strength.

It maintains heart health after age 40 years and is used to treat heart failure, hypertension, and angina. It can also prevent migraine headaches, PD, and inflammatory arthritis. The onset of action is 4 to 12 weeks.

Side effects are rare and include digestive upset, appetite loss, insomnia, dizziness, headache, itchy rash, and fatigue. There can be drug interactions with anticoagulants and insulin.

National Center for Complementary and Integrative Medicine. (2019, January). *Coenzyme Q10*. NCCIH. https://www.nccih.nih.gov/health/coenzyme-q10

Coffee

Coffee is derived from coffee beans which are from the *Coffea* plant. The main bioactive compounds in coffee are alkaloids (caffeine and xanthines) and other antioxidants (chlorogenic acid, diterpenes, and trigonelline).

Coffee silverskin or coffee chaff is the epidermis of the coffee bean that comes off during the high heat roasting. It is used in skin care products and cosmetics.

Caffeine improves mood, alertness, mental performance, and metabolism. It triggers the release of adrenaline and blocks the effects of adenosine so as to increase physical energy.

Coffee is known to stimulate bowel movements and relieves constipation. It has a laxative effect as it releases the gastrin hormone from the stomach. The xanthine component causes bronchodilation, helps to clear mucus from the airways, and hence relieves coughs.

Drinking coffee in moderation (1 to 3 cups per day) can maintain heart health and reduce risk of coronary heart disease, stroke, diabetes, and kidney disease especially in women. There may also be lower risk of PD, AD, and colon cancers. It may also maintain liver functions and prevent DNA breakages.

Excessive consumption can cause palpitations, high blood pressure, agitation, tremors, headache, insomnia, loose stools, or worsening of GERD. Caffeine remains in the system for an average of 5 h (range of 1.5 to 9 hours).

The Johns Hopkins University Staff. (2021). 9 reasons why (the right amount of) coffee is good for you. *Johns Hopkins Medicine*. https://www.hopkinsmedicine.org/health/wellness-and-prevention/9-reasons-why-the-right-amount-of-coffee-is-good-for-you

Ingredients	Mechanism of Action and Health Benefits
Comfrey leaf *Symphytum officinale*	Other name: *Knitbone* The leaves and roots of comfrey plant are used. The active constituents in comfrey include allantoin and mucilaginous substances. Allantoin can promote epithelial formation in wound healing and constrict blood vessels. Rosmarinic acid and other hydroxycinnamic acid derivatives (including caffeic acid and chlorogenic acid) and gamma linoleic acid (omega-6 fatty acid) are also present. Comfrey leaf speeds up tissue healing and bone repair. Topical formulations with comfrey root are used to treat poorly healing wounds, eczema, bedsores, sore nipples, eye inflammation, bruises, bites, sprains, swellings, pulled muscles and tendons, tenosynovitis, and muscle and joint disorders including osteoarthritis, periosteum problems, bone fractures, promotion of callus formation, and neuralgia after fractures and hematoma. It also promotes hair growth. Internal use as a tea is used for menorrhagia, gastritis, peptic ulcers, diarrhea, bronchitis, and rheumatism. It contains PAs which are potentially toxic. Hence, topical ointments or creams are PA-free or have low PA. Excessive oral consumption can be carcinogenic to the liver. Berst, T. (2019, March 28). Comfrey leaf. *Herbal Health Review*. https://herbalhealthreview.com/comfrey-leaf/ RxList Editors. (2021, June 11). Comfrey. *RxList*. https://www.rxlist.com/comfrey/supplements.htm TraceGains, Inc. (2015, May 23). Comfrey. *Kaiser Permanente*. https://wa.kaiserpermanente.org/kbase/topic.jhtml?docId=hn-2073000
Common ivy Hedera helix	Other name: *English ivy* Common ivy is an ornamental evergreen plant. It is different from poison ivy. The main bioactive compounds are triterpenoid saponins and flavonoids. It has antiinflammatory, antioxidant, antiarthritic, and antimicrobial activities. It is used to treat respiratory conditions such as bronchitis, asthma, and chronic obstructive lung disease. The saponins help to dilate the airway, liquify the mucus, and reduce the cough. It can also remove and reduce biological (molds) and chemical toxins (formaldehyde, toluene, benzene, and xylene) from the air, which contribute to the sick building syndrome. It is also used to treat arthritis. Side effects include hypersensitivity reaction and stomach upset. Goldman, R. (2016, November 3). Everything you want to know about English ivies. *Healthline*. https://www.healthline.com/health/5-fast-facts-english-ivy
Common rue *Ruta graveolens L*	Common rue contains flavonoids (quercetin and rutin), furoquinoline alkaloids (arborinine and arborine), acridone alkaloids, other alkaloids (graveoline and rutacridone), and furocoumarins (psoralen, rutamarin, and bergapten). It has antispasmodic, antiinflammatory, antifungal, emmenagogue, antifertility, and abortifacient actions. It is a potassium channel blocker. It is used to treat neuromuscular disorders, multiple sclerosis, eye strain, arthritis, epilepsy, and cardiac disorders. Rue essential oil is extracted from the fresh common rue plant by steam distillation. It is a homeopathic remedy used for wound healing, skin conditions, and hemorrhoids. Side effects may include stomach upset, dizziness, and risk of photosensitivity if combined with certain prescription medication. Drugs.com. (2021, July 5). Rue. https://www.drugs.com/npp/rue.html WebMD Editors. (2010). Rue. *WebMD*. https://www.webmd.com/vitamins/ai/ingredientmono-885/rue Health Benefits Times. (2019, September 16). Rue health benefits. *HealthBenefitstimes.com*. https://www.healthbenefitstimes.com/rue/
Cornflower *Centaurea cynaus*	The active ingredients in cornflower are flavonoids, sesquiterpene lactones, and coumarins found in the petals, leaves, and seeds. It is a bitter tonic and can support digestion, protect the liver and gallbladder, and relieve constipation. It is also used to treat fever and UTIs. Topically, it is used as an eyewash in conjunctivitis or to restore tired eyes, as a vaginal wash in yeast infections, and also applied on small wounds to stop bleeding. It may also relieve chest congestion. RxList Editors. (2021, June 11). Cornflower: Health benefits, side effects, uses, dose & precautions. *RxList*. https://www.rxlist.com/cornflower/supplements.htm

Ingredients	Mechanism of Action and Health Benefits
Corn silk *Zea mays*	Other name: *Stigma maydis, Corn hair* Corn silk refers to the natural fiber which is the long silky thread that is present in the corncob. It has medicinal uses although it is often thrown away before eating. It contains several bioactive compounds including flavone glycosides, terpenoids, carotenoids, and tannins. It is also used in TCM. It has diuretic and antiinflammatory properties. It is helpful in UTIs and prostate problems. It may lower blood pressure and blood sugar. Overall, it is safe. Side effects include allergic reactions and low potassium. Hill, A. (2019, June 12). What is corn silk, and does it have benefits? *Healthline.* https://www.health-line.com/nutrition/corn-silk#benefits Nawaz, H., Muzaffar, S., Aslam, M., & Ahmad, S. (2018). Phytochemical composition: Antioxidant potential and biological activities of corn. *Corn—Production and human health in changing climate.* Published. https://doi.org/10.5772/intechopen.79648 WebMD Editorial Contributors. (2020, December 21). Corn Silk Tea: Are There Health Benefits? *WebMD.* https://www.webmd.com/diet/health-benefits-corn-silk-tea
Cottonwood *Populus balsamifera or P. trichocarpa*	Other names: *Balm of Gilead* It is a tree that belongs to the willow family. There are many species. The cottonwood leaf buds contain resins which are rich in tannins, flavones and salicylates. They have anti-pyretic, anti-inflammatory, antimicrobial and antifungal and anti-arthritic properties. Cottonwood bud oil is made from the resin. It is applied topically to promote wound healing, treat cold sores and arthritis, and muscle sprains. The buds steeped in honey has expectorant properties and can help sore throat and cough with phlegm. Overall, it is safe. Local allergic reactions are rare. Forêt, R. (n.d.). Cottonwood Benefits. HerbalRemediesAdvice.Org. https://www.herbalremediesad-vice.org/cottonwood-benefits.html#:%7E:text=The%20Iroquois%20used%20cottonwood%20to,as%20a%20salve%20for%20wounds
Couch grass *Elymus repens*	Other names: *Common couch, Quick grass, Quack grass, Dog grass, Agropyron repens* Common couch is an invasive weed. The roots and leaves are used for medicinal purposes. The main bioactive compounds include triticin, Inositol (polysaccharides), mucilage, volatile oils, and silica. It has antiinflammatory, diuretic, expectorant, and demulcent effects. It is used to treat UTIs (in bladder, ureter, kidneys, or prostrate), kidney stones, and water retention. It can be used to treat cough, sore throat, bronchitis, and chest infections. It can soothe the gut mucosal lining, block absorption of toxins and bacteria, lower cholesterol, and prevent fatty liver. It can also improve hair loss. Side effects include diarrhea. Health Benefits Times. (2017, September 14). Health benefits of Couch Grass. *HealthBenefitstimes.com.* https://www.healthbenefitstimes.com/couch-grass/ RxList Editors. (2021, June 11). Couch Grass. *RxList.* https://www.rxlist.com/couch_grass/supplements.htm#UsesAndEffectiveness
Cowslip *Primula veris*	Cowslip has both culinary and medicinal uses. It contains triterpenoid saponins which have powerful expectorant properties. It can liquify and loosen mucus. It is effective in sore throat, sinusitis, bronchitis, cough, asthma, and cold. It is also used in insomnia. Side effects include stomach upset, vomiting, and diarrhea. Health Benefits Times. (2017, September 14). Health benefits of cowslip. *HealthBenefitstimes.com.* https://www.healthbenefitstimes.com/cowslip/
Cranberry *Vaccinium oxycoccos*	Other names: *Vaccinium macrocarpon* (large cranberry), *Vaccinium oxycoccos* (small cranberry) Cranberry contains antioxidant polyphenols including flavonoids (proanthocyanidins, anthocyanins, quercetin and myricetin flavonols, catechin, and flavanols), hydroxycinnamic, and other phenolic acids and triterpenoids. Cyanidin and peonidin give it a rich red color. It is rich in vitamins C and E (antioxidants), K1, and B6 and minerals (copper and manganese). The proanthocyanidins prevent bacteria from adhering to the urinary tract lining. This may prevent UTI. It can improve digestive health. Drinking the cranberry juice daily may also reduce *H. pylori* infections and stomach ulcers.

Ingredients	Mechanism of Action and Health Benefits
	It can improve heart health as it can lower blood pressure, blood cholesterol, and homocysteine levels. Excessive consumption may cause stomach upset, diarrhea, and risk of kidney oxalate stones.

Arnarson, A. (2019, February 15). Cranberries 101: Nutrition Facts and Health Benefits. *Healthline*. https://www.healthline.com/nutrition/foods/cranberries

Ware, M. (2019, November 1). What to know about cranberries. *MedicalNewsToday*. https://www.medicalnewstoday.com/articles/269142

Cucumber
Cucumis sativus
Chinese cucumber or *guālóu*
Trichosanthes kirilowii

The chemical compounds present in Chinese cucumbers are fatty acids, glucosides (arvenins III and opercurins A), triterpenes (bluemenol A), sterols (alpha-spinasterol and stigmasterol), and flavones.

Chinese cucumbers have antibiotic, antidiabetic, and anticancer effects (especially antineoplastic effects against hepatic cancer cells).

The fruit is commonly used to boost immunity and to treat coughs, especially those with thick phlegm that is difficult to cough up. It helps relieve sensations of pressure and stifling in the chest, and treat abscesses of the breasts and lungs. It may provide protection against stomach ulcers.

The seeds of guālóu can help decrease pain and swelling (inflammation). The roots can be taken orally or injected for HIV/AIDS, cough, and cancer.

Guālóu can have mild side effects such as diarrhea and upset stomach. Unprocessed roots can cause severe side effects, including allergic reactions, seizures, fever, fluid buildup in the lungs and brain, bleeding in the brain, heart damage, and even death.

Mao, S. N. (n.d.). Chinese cucumber. *Ask Dr. Mao*. https://askdrmao.com/natural-health-dictionary/chinese-cucumber/index.html

WebMD Editors. (n.d.). Chinese cucumber. *WebMD*. https://www.webmd.com/vitamins/ai/ingredient-mono-112/chinese-cucumber

Xu, Y., Chen, G., Lu, X., Li, Z. Q., Su, S. S., Zhou, C., et al. (2012). Chemical constituents from *Trichosanthes kirilowii* Maxim. *Biochemical Systematics and Ecology*, *43*, 114–116. https://doi.org/10.1016/j.bse.2012.03.002

Damiana
Turnera diffusa

Damiana contains several bioactive compounds including flavonoids (apigenin and gonzalitosin I), phenolic glycosides (arbutin), and terpenes (1,8-cineole).

It is an aphrodisiac and a sexual stimulant. It is used by both males and females. In females, it increases sexual desire, clitoral sensation, and orgasm.

It is also an appetite suppressant.

Overall, it is safe. Overconsumption may cause seizures, low sugar, and symptoms mimicking strychnine poisoning or rabies.

Kumar, S., Madaan, R., & Sharma, A. (2008). Pharmacological evaluation of the bioactive principle of *Turnera aphrodisiaca*. *Indian Journal of Pharmaceutical Sciences*, *70*(6), 740–744. https://doi.org/10.4103/0250-474x.49095

WebMD Editors. (n.d.). Damiana. *WebMD*. https://www.webmd.com/vitamins/ai/ingredientmono-703/damiana

Wong, C., & Butner, L. (2021, January 19). The health benefits of Damiana. *Verywell Health*. https://www.verywellhealth.com/damiana-what-should-i-know-about-it-89557

Dandelion
Taraxacum officinale

Dandelion contains active constituents that include sesquiterpene lactones, taraxasterol, taraxerol, and chlorogenic acid. These have antiinflammatory, antioxidative, antirheumatic, and choleretic properties. It is rich in fiber, vitamins (A, C, E, and K), and minerals (iron, calcium, magnesium, phosphorus, zinc, and potassium). It also contains small amounts of folate and other B vitamins.

It has antidiabetic, hepatoprotective, anticancer, and antiobesity properties. It may help reduce blood pressure and lower cholesterol levels. It may relieve constipation. The sesquiterpene lactones glycosides in the dandelion stimulate bile excretion from a sluggish liver and helps in the detoxification process and fat metabolism. It is commonly used to treat loss of appetite and poor digestion.

It has diuretic action and can flush out bladder irritants.

It has low toxicity and is safe when consumed with other foods. It can cause contact dermatitis for those with sensitive skin. It may interact negatively with certain medications, particularly diuretics and antibiotics.

Hill, A. (2018, July 18). 13 potential health benefits of dandelion. *Healthline*. https://www.healthline.com/nutrition/dandelion-benefits

Wirngo, F. E., Lambert, M. N., & Jeppesen, P. B. (2016). The physiological effects of dandelion (*Taraxacum officinale*) in type 2 diabetes. *The Review of Diabetic Studies*, *13*(2–3), 113–131. https://doi.org/10.1900/rds.2016.13.113

Ingredients	Mechanism of Action and Health Benefits

Date

Phoenix dactylifera L.

Other names: *Date palm, Brown date*

Refer to Jujube (Chinese date or red date, under Chinese remedy)

Brown dates are sweeter than red dates.

Devil's claw

Harpagophytum procumbens

Devil's claw contains various iridoid glycosides, of which harpagoside is the main bioactive constituent. It has antioxidant and antiinflammatory properties.

It is used to treat osteoarthritis, back pain, rheumatoid disorders, and gout.

It may also help with weight loss as it can suppress the ghrelin, the hunger hormone.

Side effects include stomach upsets, diarrhea, and allergic reactions.

It can interact with the NSAIDs, proton pump inhibitors (PPIs), statin drugs, and blood thinners.

Meixner, M. (2018, August 27). Devil's claw: Benefits, side effects and dosage. *Healthline.* https://www.healthline.com/nutrition/devils-claw#what-it-is

Ectoine

Ectoine is a compatible solute, osmolyte, and stress protectant which is biosynthesized in the cytoplasm of most free-living microorganisms, including Gram-negative and Gram-positive bacteria, to adapt and survive fluctuations in environmental pH, temperature, and salinity.

It is also produced commercially by fermentation in a bioreactor by cultivating *Halomonas elongata*, a nonGMO bacteria.

Ectoine is an active ingredient in skin care products and sun blocks. It stabilizes cellular matrices and protects the skin from dryness, heat, and UV light.

It is used to treat inflammation of skin and mucous membranes as in allergic eye disease, eczema, allergic rhinitis, and psoriasis.

Overall, it is very safe.

Richter, A. A., Mais, C. N., Czech, L., Geyer, K., Hoeppner, A., Smits, S. H. J., et al. (2019). Biosynthesis of the stress-protectant and chemical chaperon ectoine: biochemistry of the transaminase EctB. *Frontiers in Microbiology, 10*, 2811. https://doi.org/10.3389/fmicb.2019.02811

Salapatek, A. M., Werkhäuser, N., Ismail, B., Mösges, R., Raskopf, E., & Bilstein, A. (2021). Effects of ectoine containing nasal spray and eye drops on symptoms of seasonal allergic rhinoconjunctivitis. *Clinical and Translational Allergy, 11*(1), e12006. https://doi.org/10.1002/clt2.12006

Eggplant

Solanum melongena

Other names: *Aubergine, Oriental Charm, qié zi, Pingtung Long, makhuca*

Eggplant is a nightshade plant which is a fruit. It comes in various shapes and color shades (purple, green, and white). The common ones are globe or *American* eggplant (dark purple and large), *Italian* eggplant (dark purple and smaller than American eggplant), *Japanese or Chinese* eggplant (thin, long, and bright purple), *Indian* eggplant (dull purple and round), *Thai* eggplant (green-white, smaller, and more bitter or small, purple-white), rosa bianca (purple and white stripes), and white eggplant.

It is rich in antioxidants such as polyphenols (including chlorogenic acid) and flavonoids (including anthocyanins such as nasunin, lutein, and zeaxanthin).

It also contains vitamins (B6 and C) and potassium. It is high in fiber and low in calories.

It promotes heart health. It can lower blood cholesterol and help in weight loss. It may also reduce neuroinflammation and improve cognitive performance.

It also supports eye health.

Rarely there is eggplant allergy with hypersensitivity reaction. It also contains a small amount of solanine, a toxic alkaloid. The presence of oxalate in eggplant may predispose to kidney stones.

Ware, M. (2019, November 8). Eggplant health benefits and tasty tips. *MedicalNewsToday.* https://www.medicalnewstoday.com/articles/279359

Eggs

Eggs are wholesome, complete, and perfect foods. They are rich in protein, vitamins (A, B2, B5, B12, K, and folate), minerals (iodine, selenium, and phosphorus), and choline. It also contains antioxidants (including zeaxanthin and lutein) that improve eye health, help prevent cataracts and macular degeneration. It is also low in calories. It also contains vitamin D which aids in bone health and lowers the risk of rickets and osteoporosis.

It helps increase HDL cholesterol levels and reduce heart problems (stroke and heart disease). The iodine and selenium present in the egg yolk help in regulating thyroid hormones. It can help in hypothyroidism.

Eggs are filling. It increases satiety, increases the GLP-1 and PYY and can help in weight loss.

Topical application can improve hair growth and reduce hair fall.

Overall, it is safe. Overconsumption may lead to high cholesterol and heart-related risks.

Gunnars, K. (2018, June 28). Top 10 health benefits of eating eggs. *Healthline.* https://www.healthline.com/nutrition/10-proven-health-benefits-of-eggs

Lewin, J. (2019, November 6). The health benefits of eggs. *BBC Good Food.* https://www.bbcgoodfood.com/howto/guide/ingredient-focus-eggs

Ingredients	Mechanism of Action and Health Benefits
Elderberry *Sambucus* *Sambucus canadensis*	There are many varieties of elderberry. *Sambucus nigra* (Black or European elderberry) is the most common type. Many parts of the plants are used for both medicinal and culinary purposes. It is rich in flavonols, phenolic acid, and anthocyanins which have strong antiinflammatory and antioxidant properties. It is also high in vitamins C and A. These compounds can boost and strengthen the immune system. It also contains fiber and other minerals including iron, calcium, and potassium. It also contains alpha-glucosidase (α-glucosidase) which has glucose-lowering properties. It is used to treat colds and flu and helps to reduce the severity and duration of the influenza illness. It is also used for bronchitis and sinusitis. It is also used to treat *H. pylori* gastritis. It can support heart health, lowers blood pressure, cholesterol, blood sugar, and uric acid. It also has diuretic properties. Side effects include gastroenteritis, dizziness, and weakness if the uncooked parts of the plant are consumed as it contains cyanide and lectin. Barrell, A. (2018, October 9). Health benefits of elderberry. *MedicalNewsToday*. https://www.medical-newstoday.com/articles/323288 Mandl, E. (2021, March 12). Elderberry: Benefits and dangers. *Healthline*. https://www.healthline.com/nutrition/elderberry#health-benefits
Elemi	The oil extracted from gum of the Elemi tree contains 10% to 25% essential oils which have limonene, elemicin, elemol, terpinolene, terpineol, carvone, dipentene, phellandrene, and others. The essential oil is used in aromatherapy or via steam inhalation or as an expectorant to reduce mucus in the respiratory tract or sinuses, to moisturize and rejuvenate the skin, and to repair fractures. Overall, it is safe. Gamble, L. (2019, February 23). Elemi essential oil—The complete uses and benefits guide. *Mom Prepares*. https://momprepares.com/essential-oils/elemi/ WebMD Editors. (2013). Elemi. *WebMD*. https://www.webmd.com/vitamins/ai/ingredientmono-430/elemi
Emu oil	Emu oil is derived from the fat of the emu bird. It contains mostly monounsaturated (such as oleic acid) and polyunsaturated (including linoleic acid and linolenic acid) fatty acids. It is absorbed by the skin and penetrates deeply. It has pain-relieving and antioxidant effects. It is used topically for various skin conditions such as eczema, dry skin, and chronic skin conditions. It is also used as a moisturizer. It also promotes wound healing and is also used for bruises, cuts, and burns. It also reduces acne scars and age spots. It also improves hair, seborrheic dermatitis, and nail growth. Ingestion of Emu oil by mouth is controversial. There are no significant side effects. Pointer, K. (2019, August 13). Everything you need to know about emu oil. *Healthline*. https://www.healthline.com/health/emu-oil#TOC_TITLE_HDR_1 WebMD Editors. (n.d.). Emu oil. *WebMD*. https://www.webmd.com/vitamins/ai/ingredientmono-825/emu-oil
Epsom salt	Epsom salt is also called magnesium sulfate. Magnesium is an important mineral in the body after sodium, potassium, and calcium. It is important for cell health and it is beneficial for melatonin. It reduces stress and promotes nerve function. Magnesium is also used to treat constipation. It is used to relieve sore and aching muscles. It can also improve symptoms in arthritis and fibromyalgia. It is often added to a bath. Epsom salt has antiinflammatory and muscle-relaxing properties. It contains magnesium and hence stimulates bowel muscle contractions. It should not be used long term as a laxative and magnesium overdose can cause flushing, nausea, weakness, headache, and coma. Elliott, B. (2018, December 13). Epsom salt: Benefits, uses, and side effects. *Healthline*. https://www.healthline.com/nutrition/epsom-salt-benefits-uses

Ingredients	Mechanism of Action and Health Benefits
Eucalyptus oil	Eucalyptus essential oil is widely used in Chinese, Ayurvedic, and European medicine. There are more than 400 species of Eucalyptus. *Eucalyptus globulus* (Blue gum) is the main source of this essential oil.
	The leaves are steam distilled to extract the essential oil which contains eucalyptol. It also has flavonoids (antioxidants) and tannins which have antiinflammatory properties.
	It has antimicrobial properties against various bacteria such as *Haemophilus influenzae* and streptococcus.
	It is used mostly in respiratory disorders and it can relieve cold, flu, sinusitis, sore throat, bronchitis, and asthma. It is used in aromatherapy.
	It can also be applied topically as Vicks VapoRub. It reduces lung congestion and loosens the phlegm.
	It is also used as a mouthwash or chewing gum to promote teeth and gum health.
	It has analgesic properties and can relieve muscle and joint pain in arthritis, strains, and sprains. It is also used in wound healing and fungal infections.
	It is also an effective insect repellent and insecticide.
	Side effects include local skin irritation (if used undiluted) and allergic reactions. It should not be taken orally or used near the eye. It can interact with diabetes and asthma medications.
	Nordqvist, J. (2018, January 5). The health benefits of eucalyptus. *MedicalNewsToday*. https://www.medicalnewstoday.com/articles/266580#eucalyptus_health_benefits
	WebMD Editors. (n.d.). Eucalyptus. *WebMD*. https://www.webmd.com/vitamins/ai/Ingredient-mono-700/eucalyptus
European or purple cyclamen *Cyclamen purpurascens*	Cyclamen roots contain triterpene saponins including cyclamen.
	It is used to treat rhinitis and sinusitis. When given as a nose spray it reduces mucus. It helps with anxiety.
	It is also used to treat skin rash. It may also help menstrual pain, can induce menstrual cycle, and expel the placenta after birth. It also helps digestive problems.
	The juice from the root when applied externally over the lower abdomen has laxative properties and also can increase the flow of urine.
	Oral consumption is generally not advised. Side effects include GIT upset, breathing difficulties, and spasms. Not much information is available on drug interactions.
	Sturluson, T. (2019, August 18). Cyclamen herb uses, health benefits and side effects. *The Herbal Resource*. https://www.herbal-supplement-resource.com/cyclamen-herbal-medicine.html
	WebMD Editors. (n.d.). Cyclamen. *WebMD*. https://www.webmd.com/vitamins/ai/ingredient-mono-420/cyclamen
Evening primrose *Oenothera*	The seeds of the evening primrose flower are used to produce evening primrose oil. It is rich in GLA. GLA is an omega-6 fatty acid with antiinflammatory, antioxidant, and pain-relieving effects. The GLA can also help reduce neuropathy symptoms such as numbness, hot and cold sensitivity, tingling, and weakness.
	It has antidiabetic, hypotensive, and hypolipidemic properties.
	Evening primrose can improve the skin moisture, roughness, firmness, and elasticity. It is used to treat acne and eczema.
	The oil can also help relieve PMS symptoms like digestive issues, backache, fatigue, tenderness, irritability, and depression. It can also relieve hot flashes in menopausal women.
	Evening primrose oil is considered safe for use. Minor side effects include stomach pain, digestive problems, and headaches. It should not be taken alongside blood thinners or antiplatelet medications as it can increase bleeding risk in people taking them. It should also be avoided by cancer patients and pregnant women.
	McDermott, A. (2019, March 7). 10 benefits of evening primrose oil and how to use it. *Healthline*. https://www.healthline.com/health/evening-primrose-oil
Eyebright *Euphrasia officinalis*	Eyebright is rich in polyphenolic flavonoids (including quercetin and luteolin) which gives it antiallergy and antihistamine properties. It also contains compounds such as tannins, glycosides (aucubin), and terpenoids (iridoids). It has antiinflammatory properties.
	It is used to treat eye allergy, eye irritation, eye fatigue, eye strain, and eye infections.
	Side effects include allergic reactions, headache, and insomnia. It may lower blood sugar.
	McCulloch, M. (2019, April 11). Do eyebright drops and supplements benefit health? *Healthline*. https://www.healthline.com/nutrition/eyebright#plant-compounds
	TraceGains, Inc. (2015, May 23). Eyebright. *Kaiser Permanente*. https://wa.kaiserpermanente.org/kbase/topic.jhtml?docId=hn-2087000

Ingredients	Mechanism of Action and Health Benefits
Feverfew *Tanacetum parthenium*	Feverfew leaves contain several bioactive compounds including volatile oils and flavonoids. Parthenolide, a sesquiterpene lactone and tanetin, a flavonoid can reduce migraine headaches via multiple mechanisms. It has analgesic and antiinflammatory properties. It is used to treat frequent migraine headaches and is given as prophylaxis for 3 to 4 months. It can also be used to treat an acute migraine headache. It can reduce fever. It may also help in tinnitus, dizziness, vomiting, and arthritis. It can also induce onset of menstrual periods, treat dysmenorrhea, and enhance uterine contractions so as to shorten labor time during childbirth. Side effects include allergic reactions, gastric upsets, and gas and bloating. Raman, R. (2019, January 25). What is feverfew, and does it work for migraines? *Healthline*. https://www.healthline.com/nutrition/feverfew WebMD Editors. (n.d.). Feverfew. *WebMD*. https://www.webmd.com/vitamins/ai/ingredientmono-933/feverfew
Fig and Fig Oil *Ficus carica*	Figs are rich in many vitamins (K, B6, C, A, and β-carotene) and minerals (calcium, copper, iron, and magnesium). Dried figs contain a higher sugar content compared to fresh figs. Fig oil is derived from the seed via the cold press method. It has antioxidant, antiinflammatory, and anticancer properties. The high fiber content in figs helps to promote digestion, reduce constipation, IBS, and colitis. It also acts as a prebiotic. It may also improve heart health. It can lower blood pressure, LDL cholesterol, and blood sugar. It also reduces the risk of macular degeneration of the eye. Fig oil is a moisturizer and can help with skin barrier repair. Topical use of fig oil can also help dry and itchy skin in allergic dermatitis. The fig tree latex is also effective for skin warts. Dried fig leaves can be brewed as tea or can be used as a wrap for cooking. Adverse effects can include fig allergy. There is interaction with blood thinners in view of its vitamin K content. Akers, A. S. (2021, July 23). What is a macro diet, and how does it work? *MedicalNewsToday*. https://www.medicalnewstoday.com/articles/macro-diet#summary Shoemaker, S. (2020, June 3). All you need to know about figs. *Healthline*. https://www.healthline.com/nutrition/figs-benefits
Flaxseed *Linum usitatissimum*	Flaxseeds are available whole or milled. Whole flaxseeds function as insoluble fiber (cellulose and lignin). Milled flaxseeds function as both mucilage gum containing soluble (20% to 40%) and insoluble (60% to 80%) fibers. It is rich in omega-3 fatty acids (especially ALA), polyunsaturated and monounsaturated fats and lignans. It has antioxidant and estrogen properties. It can reduce the risk of breast cancer in post-menopausal women and prostate cancer. It is also high in plant proteins. The omega-3 fatty acids can lower blood pressure and are heart-healthy. The presence of soluble fiber helps to regulate blood sugar and reduce blood cholesterol. The insoluble fiber results in regular bowel movements and softer stools. It is helpful for chronic constipation, IBS, and diverticulosis. It can reduce hunger pangs and may help in weight loss. There is a risk of thyroid dysfunction due to the presence of thiocyanates (produced by the interaction of cyanogenic glycosides and sulfur in the body). The presence of phytates in flaxseed reduces the absorption of iron and zinc. The presence of fiber may also cause gas and bloating. There is risk of blood-thinning effects and should not be used alongside blood thinners. Due to the presence of phytoestrogens caution must be exercised during pregnancy and breastfeeding. Tan, V., (2017, April 26). Top 10 health benefits of flax seeds. *Healthline*. https://www.healthline.com/nutrition/benefits-of-flaxseeds#TOC_TITLE_HDR_1

Ingredients	Mechanism of Action and Health Benefits
Fleabane	Other names: *Canada fleabane, Canadian horseweed, horseweed, butterweed, fleabane daisy, bitter weed, fireweed, butter weed*

There are many fleabane species in the Erigeron genus. Some of these include Eastern daisy fleabane, *Erigeron annuus, Erigeron canadensis or Conyza canadensis.*

Although all parts of the plant are used, the leaves and flowers have the most active phytoconstituents. The leaves can be eaten as a part of salad or cooked.

Fleabane contains tannins and flavonoids. It is rich in potassium and calcium.

It is a common weed. It has astringent, diuretic, hemostatic, and antimicrobial actions.

It has caffeic acid (polyphenol) which helps with diabetes and obesity. It can also stop bleeding in piles. It can be used for dysentery and diarrhea.

It can treat rheumatism, bronchitis, sore throat, UTI, and menorrhagia. It can be applied as a liniment or poultice over sore joints.

RxList. (2021, June 11). Canadian fleabane: Health benefits, side effects, uses, dose & precautions. https://www.rxlist.com/canadian_fleabane/supplements.htm

Floating pennywort	Other name: *Marsh penny*
Hydrocotyle ranunculoides	Refer to "Gotu kola or Indian pennywort."

Gelatin	Other name: *Gelatine*

Gelatin is usually an animal protein product obtained from the cow (sometimes pig) carcass which contains bones, tendons, skin and ligaments. Donkey hide gelatin is used in TCM. Vegan-derived gelatin is obtained from seaweed and it is called agar agar. Gelatin is a translucent, tasteless powder and is used as a gelling agent in foods, beverages, and medications. Bone broth is made from the whole animal and hence it is more wholesome and nutritious (with more vitamins, minerals, and protein in addition to gelatin). Gelatin contains collagen.

It can help in osteoarthritis, osteoporosis, and aging skin. It can promote hair growth. Consuming gelatin can help build collagen which is a component in skin, cartilage, and bones.

Side effects include stomach heaviness, bloating and gas, rarely allergic reactions and mad cow disease transmission risk.

WebMD. (n.d.). GELATIN: Overview, uses, side effects, precautions, interactions, dosing and reviews. https://www.webmd.com/vitamins/ai/ingredientmono-1051/gelatin

Geranium	Other names and also includes: *Cranesbill/Cranesbill geranium flower, Alumroot, Hardy geranium/ Hardy cranesbill geranium (Geranium maculatum) Rose geranium*

Geranium is an ornamental plant often found on balconies. There are many varieties of geranium. Basically, they are scented and unscented. The scented varieties (examples include Rose geranium, *Pelargonium Graveolens* and Robert geranium i.e., *Geranium robertianum*) have more medicinal value. Geranium flowers are edible and can be used for garnishing.

Cranesbill is rich in essential oils. It also contains tannins and gallic acid.

It has astringent properties and is used as a mouthwash to relieve painful mouth sores. It can also stop bleeding piles, dysentery, and bleeding wounds. Wild geranium also has astringent and hemostatic properties.

The essential oils from the rose geranium have antiinflammatory, antiseptic, antibacterial, antioxidant, and antiaging effects. It is also added to food products as a flavoring agent. The fresh rose geranium flowers are also edible and can be added to desserts or salads.

It promotes skin health and is used to treat acne, eczema, and skin rash. It is an ingredient in cosmetics, perfumes, and skin and body products.

The crushed leaves poultices can help with wound healing and breast engorgement after birth.

The essential oil also has calming and sedating effects. It can be used to enhance deep sleep, relieve stress, anxiety, and depression via massage therapy or aromatherapy. It is often blended with other essential oils.

It has antispasmodic and astringent activities and can be used in diarrhea. It may help gallstones.

It can also lower blood glucose. It can relieve sore throat.

Overall, it is safe. Local allergic reactions or eye irritation may occur from the sap.

Staughton, J. (2021, July 16). 9 amazing benefits of geranium. *Organic Facts*. https://www.organic-facts.net/health-benefits/herbs-and-spices/geranium.html

Ingredients	Mechanism of Action and Health Benefits
Glucomannan	Glucomannan is a soluble fiber and a complex sugar. It is derived from konjac roots mostly and other plants such as orchid, lily, redwood, and white pine.
	It is very hygroscopic and absorbs water quickly. It is used in the food industry as a thickening agent.
	It can lower blood glucose and cholesterol. It is used to treat diabetes, obesity, and constipation. It decreases ghrelin levels (the hunger hormone), makes the stomach feel full, decreases absorption of glucose, lipids, and proteins, sequestrates bile acids, and improves the gut flora.
	It can also improve skin health and may help in hyperthyroidism.
	Overall, it is safe. It must be taken with plenty of water.
	WebMD. (n.d.-a). GLUCOMANNAN: Overview, uses, side effects, precautions, interactions, dosing and reviews. https://www.webmd.com/vitamins/ai/ingredientmono-205/glucomannan
Glucosamine	It is an amino-acid sugar and is part of normal cartilage. As a dietary supplement, glucosamine is extracted from the shells of shellfish (crabs, prawns, or lobsters) or animal bones. It slows down the degeneration of joint cartilage.
	Adverse reactions of glucosamine include GI symptoms (nausea, constipation or diarrhea, bloating, and heartburn) mainly and, rarely, hair loss, irregular heartbeat, and eye or leg swelling.
	It may also be used in the treatment of a variety of chronic inflammatory diseases such as interstitial cystitis, IBD, multiple sclerosis, glaucoma, and temporomandibular joint.
	Glucosamine may affect blood sugar or insulin levels.
	Hill, A. (2018, September 26). Does glucosamine work? Benefits, dosage and side effects. *Healthline.* https://www.healthline.com/nutrition/lucosamine#effectiveness
Glutathione	Glutathione is a tripeptide containing three amino acids i.e., glutamate, glycine, and cysteine. It is a powerful antioxidant which scavenges free radicals. It is a thiol compound (also called mercaptans) which contains organosulfur moleculesi.e., carbon, hydrogen, and sulfur are present which give the pungent odor. It exists in the oxidized form (GSSG) and reduced form (GSH).
	Glutathione is essential for cell detoxification of toxic chemicals and xenobiotics [via the enzyme glutathione-S-transferase (GST)], antioxidant functions, biosynthesis pathways [via γ-glutamylcysteine synthetase (GSH1) and glutathione synthase], and redox homeostasis (via GSSG and GSH recycling).
	Plant foods that are glutathione-rich include avocado, asparagus, spinach, okra, onions, garlic, cruciferous vegetables, and watermelon.
	Glutathione boosters include lipoic acid, l-cysteine, and methylsulfonylmethane.
	Glutathione—an overview|ScienceDirect Topics. (n.d.). https://www.sciencedirect.com/topics/agricultural-and-biological-sciences/glutathione
Goldenrod *Solidago* spp.	Other names: *Solidago virgaurea, European goldenrod, Canadian goldenrod or Solidago canadensis*
	Goldenrod has many species and the names are often used interchangeably. The dried flowers and leaves of goldenrod are used. It contains phenolic compounds (hyperoside, quercitrin, and leiocarposide), terpenes, and flavonoids.
	It has antiinflammatory, analgesic, antispasmodic, antimicrobial, antifungal, and diuretic properties.
	It is used to treat UTI, kidney stones, arthritis, gout, rheumatism, hemorrhoids, and skin conditions (eczema). It also aids in wound healing.
	Side effects include heartburn. It can interact with diuretics.
	Toiu, A., Vlase, L., Vodnar, D. C., Gheldiu, A. M., & Oniga, I. (2019). *Solidago graminifolia* L. Salisb. (Asteraceae) as a valuable source of bioactive polyphenols: HPLC profile, in vitro antioxidant and antimicrobial potential. *Molecules, 24*(14), 2666. https://doi.org/10.3390/molecules24142666
	WebMD Editors. (2011). *Goldenrod.* WebMD. https://www.webmd.com/vitamins/ai/ingredient-mono-84/goldenrod

Ingredients	Mechanism of Action and Health Benefits
Goldenseal *Hydrastis canadensis*	Goldenseal is rich in alkaloid compounds such as berberine, hydrastine, and canadine. These alkaloids have antiinflammatory and antibacterial properties. Berberine has antiviral effects that can help in the treatment of chlamydia and herpes.

Goldenseal is rich in alkaloid compounds such as berberine, hydrastine, and canadine. These alkaloids have antiinflammatory and antibacterial properties. Berberine has antiviral effects that can help in the treatment of chlamydia and herpes.

It has antidiabetic and hypolipidemic properties.

It is used to treat colds, hay fever, digestive problems, sore gums, and skin problems (acne and psoriasis). It is commonly used to prevent or treat upper respiratory tract infections and the common cold. It may also be used to treat lack of appetite, heavy or painful periods, sinus infections, and indigestion.

It may also be used as a detox agent to get rid of toxins and harmful substances in the body and reduce the risk of tooth infections.

Goldenseal is also used in several over-the-counter remedies including ear drops, feminine hygiene products, eyewash formulations, cold and flu remedies, allergy relief products, laxatives, and digestive aids.

It is advisable to consume goldenseal in small doses for a short period of time. Side effects are rare but may include nausea, vomiting, and reduced liver function.

Petre, A. (2020, June 18). *Goldenseal: Benefits, dosage, side effects, and more*. Healthline. https://www.healthline.com/health/goldenseal-cure-for-everything#benefits-uses

Grapeseed oil and Grapeseed extract (GSE)

Grapeseed oil is extracted (via cold press or chemical press) from leftover grape seeds after grapes are pressed to make wine. It contains linoleic acid, oleic acid (omega-6 PUFAs), and vitamin E. It also contains proanthocyanidin, a powerful antioxidant. It has antiinflammatory and antimicrobial effects.

It has skin-moisturizing and skin-lightening effects. It can improve acne and lessen scars. It promotes healthy hair growth.

It can decrease insulin resistance and risk of heart disease.

Grapeseed extract (GSE) is obtained from the ground-up seeds of red wine grapes. It contains proanthocyanidins and resveratrol. It can help in chronic venous insufficiency, macular degeneration, diabetic eye disease, atherosclerosis, wound healing, and antiaging.

Side effects of GSE include sore throat, nausea, and headaches. It can interact with blood thinners or NSAIDs.

Adcox, M. (2017, July 12). The health and beauty benefits of grapeseed oil. *MedicalNewsToday*. https://www.medicalnewstoday.com/articles/318395

Griffin, M. (2009, May 12). Grape Seed Extract. *WebMD*. https://www.webmd.com/diet/grape-seed-extract

Watson, K. (2019, October 3). Grapeseed oil for skin: Benefits and uses. *Healthline*. https://www.healthline.com/health/grapeseed-oil-for-skin

Green-lipped mussel

Green-lipped mussel is a shellfish. Oral form is available as capsules, freeze-dried or ground form.

Oil is also available. Usually New Zealand green-lipped mussels are said to be the best quality.

Mussels are rich in minerals (zinc, iron, and selenium), B-vitamins. Its antiinflammatory properties are due to contains and chondroitin sulfate and omega-3 fatty acids.

It can be used for arthritis (osteoarthritis and rheumatoid arthritis). It can also help with delayed onset exercise-induced muscle soreness.

It can help with children with ADHD.

Side effects include allergic reactions and intolerance.

Walle, G. V. D. (2021, February 1). Green-lipped mussel supplements: All you need to know. *Healthline*. https://www.healthline.com/nutrition/green-lipped-mussel

WebMD Editors. (n.d.). New Zealand green-lipped mussel. *WebMD*. https://www.webmd.com/vitamins/ai/ingredientmono-830/new-zealand-green-lipped-mussel

Griffonia simplicifolia

Other name: *Bandeiraea simplicifolia*

It is a plant shrub that grows in West and Central Africa.

The seeds contain 5 HTP (5-hydroxytryptophan) which is converted to serotonin (5-hydroxytryptamine), a neurotransmitter in the brain. It is used to treat anxiety, depression, insomnia, mood disorders, attention deficit disorder, fibromyalgia, and obesity.

Side effects include mild GI upsets and CNS effects (irritability and agitation). It can interact with MAOI and SSRI drugs.

Science Direct. (1997). Griffonia simplicifolia—an overview. *ScienceDirect*. https://www.sciencedirect.com/topics/agricultural-and-biological-sciences/griffonia-simplicifolia

Ingredients	Mechanism of Action and Health Benefits
Guaifenesin	Guaifenesin is derived from the guaiac tree. It is now synthesized in the lab.
	It has mucolytic and expectorant properties. It is used to relieve the cough from nasal and chest congestion as in common colds, acute respiratory infections, sinusitis, acute or chronic bronchitis, asthma.
	It is a generally safe and effective expectorant after age 2 years. Side effects may include diarrhea, rash, stomach upset, headache, and dizziness.
	Mayo Clinic Staff. (2021, February 1). *Guaifenesin (Oral Route)*. Mayo Clinic. https://www.mayoclinic.org/drugs-supplements/guaifenesin-oral-route/side-effects/drg-20068720?p=1
Guarana	Other name: *Paullinia cupana*
	Guarana is a plant which grows in the Amazon region. The black guarana seeds contain caffeine more than coffee beans.
	The guarana seeds are harvested, roasted, and ground into powder. It is brewed to make caffeinated beverages and tonics.
	It improves physical energy and mental alertness. It is used in obesity and in sports.
	Side effects include gastric upsets, irritability, and insomnia.
	WebMD. (n.d.-b). GUARANA: Overview, uses, side effects, precautions, interactions, dosing and reviews. https://www.webmd.com/vitamins/ai/ingredientmono-935/guarana
Guelder rose bark *Viburnum opulus*	Other name: *Cramp bark*
	Guelder rose or cramp bark contains esculetin and viopudial which are antispasmodic. It can relax blood vessels and muscles and help reduce blood pressure and pain. It is high in citrate and antioxidants (carotenoids, flavonoids, and others).
	It also has antiinflammatory, emmenagogic, nervine, hypotensive, astringent, and sedative effects.
	It is used to treat cramps, colics, or pain due to menstrual cramps/PMS, endometriosis, constipation, IBS, muscle cramps, and kidney stones. The presence of high citrate also helps to prevent kidney stones.
	It may also help with anxiety and insomnia.
	It is prepared as a decoction (water extract), tincture (alcoholic extract), or a lotion.
	No side effects are reported with the bark supplements. The raw berries may cause stomach upsets. It should not be taken during pregnancy.
	Shoemaker, S. (2019, October 3). *What is cramp bark, and what is it used for?* Healthline. https://www.healthline.com/nutrition/cramp-bark-guelder-rose
Helichrysum italicum	This essential oil has antimicrobial and antiinflammatory properties. The active ingredient is arzanol.
	It maintains, nourishes, and rejuvenates healthy skin. It promotes wound healing.
	It can help in cough, colds, and flu.
	It can also be used in digestive ailments.
	Overall, it is safe.
	Hersh, E. (2019, May 9). *Everything you need to know about Helichrysum essential oil*. Healthline. https://www.healthline.com/health/helichrysum-essential-oil#claims
Hesperidin	It is a bioflavonoid derived from citrus fruits. It has antiinflammatory and antioxidant properties. It can also lower blood pressure.
	It is used for varicose veins, hemorrhoids, venous stasis from poor circulation, lymphedema, and hypertension.
	Side effects include nausea and increased risk of bleeding as it can slow blood clotting.
	Wong, C., & Kroner, A. (2021, March 20). *The potential benefits of hesperidin*. Verywell Health. https://www.verywellhealth.com/what-you-need-to-know-about-hesperidin-89462
Hibiscus *Hibiscus rosa-sinensis*	The hibiscus flowers contain flavonoids, anthocyanins, organic acids, (citric, malic, tartaric acids, and allo-HCA lactone), and polysaccharides. Many minerals such as iron, calcium, magnesium, phosphorus, and potassium are present.
	It has antioxidant, antiinflammatory, diuretic, antidiabetic, and mild laxative effects (it can stimulate bowel movements).
	It can help to lower blood pressure, glucose, and cholesterol. It is a natural ACE inhibitor. It is cardiotonic and used to treat hypertension, dyslipidemia, and heart failure. Hibiscus tea has been found to increase uric acid excretion and hence prevent kidney stone formation.
	Overall, it is safe. Excessive consumption may have a laxative effect.
	Hudson, T. (2011). Hibiscus, Hawthorn, and the Heart: Modern research supports the use of traditional plants. *Natural Medicine Journal3*, 3(7). https://www.naturalmedicinejournal.com/journal/2011-07-hibiscus-hawthorn-and-heart

Ingredients	Mechanism of Action and Health Benefits

Hordenine

Hordenine is a natural or synthetic product. It is present in various plants including barley (*Hordeum vulgare*), cacti, algae, seaweed, and bitter orange (*Citrus aurantium*).

It has stimulant actions and it has a similar structure to ephedrine.

Hordenine is present in diet pills and is used for obesity.

It also can increase physical and athletic performance.

Side effects include tachycardia and hypertension. It can interact with MAO-I and other stimulants medications (caffeine, amphetamine, methylphenidate, and more).

WebMD. (n.d.-c). HORDENINE: Overview, uses, side effects, precautions, interactions, dosing and reviews. *WebMD*. https://www.webmd.com/vitamins/ai/ingredientmono-1528/hordenine

Horehound Leaf
Marrubium vulgare

Other name: *White horehound*

Horehound contains many active compounds including several triterpenoids of which marrubiin is the main constituent. It also contains steroids, tannins, flavonoids, saponins, and volatile oils.

It has antispasmodic, gastroprotective, antidiabetic, antiinflammatory, and antimicrobial properties.

It is a mucolytic and expectorant especially in wet coughs and relieves bronchospasm. It is used to treat nasal and chest congestion, sinus infections, allergies, and postnasal drip.

It also supports digestive health and is used for gas and bloating, indigestion, constipation, diarrhea, and jaundice.

It can also kill parasites. It promotes wound healing and can be applied topically. It can also lower blood sugar and is used to treat diabetes.

White horehounds are generally safe. Vomiting may occur from overconsumption. No drug interactions are known.

WebMD Editors. (2014). White horehound. *WebMD*. https://www.webmd.com/vitamins/ai/ingredient-mono-886/white-horehound

Horse chestnut
Aesculus hippocastanum

It contains triterpene saponins (aescin 3% to 6%), tannins, flavonoids (including kaempferol and quercetin), sterols, quinines, fatty acids (linolenic acid, palmitic acid, and stearic acid), coumarins (esculetin, fraxin), and scopolin glucoside. The aescin active ingredient acts on capillary membranes to improve vascular permeability.

Raw horse chestnuts are not edible. It contains esculin poison which is fatal if consumed raw.

It also has antiinflammatory, antioxidant, and anticancer properties.

It is used to treat the symptoms of leg edema, leg pain and ulcers from varicose veins, chronic venous infection or poor circulation.

It can also reduce the swelling and pain in hemorrhoids.

It may also help with sperm quality when there is associated varicocele and male infertility.

It may also help certain cancers like leukemia, multiple myeloma, and liver cancer.

Side effects include digestive upset, headache, dizziness, and allergic reaction.

It can interact with diabetic medication, blood thinners, lithium, and NSAIDs.

Kharlamenko, A. (2019, April 2). 7 health benefits of horse chestnut extract. *Healthline*. https://www.healthline.com/nutrition/horse-chestnut-benefits#TOC_TITLE_HDR_8

Horsetail
Equisetum arvense

Horsetail contains several antioxidants (mostly phenolic compounds). It is rich in silica, selenium, cysteine, and calcium which are important for hair, nail, skin, and bone health. It also contains nicotine and also thiaminase enzymes.

It has antiinflammatory, antioxidant, antidiabetic, and antimicrobial (against various bacteria and fungi including *S. aureus, E. coli, Aspergillus niger*, and *Candida albicans*) activities.

It can also lower blood glucose levels.

Silica helps with bone remodeling, and bone and blood vessel healing. It can stimulate bone osteoblasts and inhibit osteoclasts. It improves bone density and cartilage by facilitating collagen synthesis. It is used to treat osteoporosis and fractures. It also promotes wound healing.

It is also a natural diuretic. It is also used to treat kidney stones, UTIs, and urinary incontinence.

It is overall a safe herb. It should not be taken by those who want to quit smoking. It can reduce thiamine levels. It has interactions with prescription drugs.

Lang, A. (2020, May 28). Horsetail: Benefits, uses, and side effects. *Healthline*. https://www.healthline.com/nutrition/horsetail#uses-dosage

Ingredients	Mechanism of Action and Health Benefits
Hops *Humulus lupulus*	Hops is a flowering plant. It is mostly used in the food and beverage industry. In beer fermentation, it is added as a flavor, bitter, and stability agent. It has sleep-promoting and sedative properties. It is used to treat insomnia, anxiety, nervous tension, and ADHD. It has a mild estrogen effect and may help menopausal symptoms or hot flashes. It can increase appetite, promote urination, and treat indigestion. It is also used in lotions and skin creams. Overall, it is safe. It should not be used with antidepressants or in estrogen-sensitive cancers. It can interact with birth control pills, PPIs, sedatives, and steroids. RxList Editors. (2021, June 11). Hops. *RxList.* https://www.rxlist.com/hops/supplements.htm
Hyaluronic acid	Hyaluronic acid (HA) is a natural polysaccharide sugar-amino acid molecule i.e., glycosaminoglycan. It is present in the connective tissue of the synovial fluid in joints, skin, and eyes. It lubricates and protects the joints. HA is present in the dermis of the skin and acts as a natural humectant and keeps the skin firm, full, hydrated, and elastic. Foods that can boost HA production in the body include bone broth, magnesium-rich foods (like almonds, kale, and sweet potato as magnesium is required in HA synthesis), soy products (tofu, tempeh, and edamame contain phytoestrogens which can increase HA levels), and oranges (it contains naringenin which inhibits HA breakdown so that HA levels remain normal). HA decreases with age. Synthetic HA is available as intra-articular injections where it is injected into joints with osteoarthritis) to reduce stiffness and pain. HA is widely available for topical use in skin care products as a skin humectant or hydrator (in creams, serum, or moisturizer). Dermal fillers are available as injectable HA gels to address sagging cheeks, sunken eyes, and deep wrinkles. It also promotes wound healing. There are different molecular weights of HA. Low molecular weight nano-HA around 130 kDa are preferred for topical skin use as it can penetrate more deeply into the skin. HA-based eye drops can prevent dry eyes. HA is also injected into the eyes during cataract surgery. Oral HA supplements are also taken for skin health, acid reflux, and UTIs. Overall, HAs are safe. Rarely, allergic reactions occur. WebMD. (n.d.-d). Hyaluronic acid: Overview, uses, side effects, precautions, interactions, dosing and reviews. https://www.webmd.com/vitamins/ai/ingredientmono-1062/hyaluronic-acid Wilson, D. (2019, March 8). Why science says hyaluronic acid is the holy grail to wrinkle-free, youthful hydration. *Healthline.* https://www.healthline.com/health/beauty-skin-care/hyaluronic-acid#benefits
Hydrangea *Hydrangea paniculata*	Hydrangea has more than 70 species of which *H. paniculata, H. macrophylla*, and *H. arborescens* are used for medicinal purposes. The flowers contain amygdalin which can give euphoria. It contains coumarin and skimmin, which have antiinflammatory properties. Other compounds include saponin, volatile oil, and flavonoid antioxidants (kaempferol and quercetin). It is also rich in minerals (magnesium, calcium, iron, potassium, sulfur, and phosphorus). It is bladder protective. The underground root and rhizome of hydrangea plant is used for various medical purposes. It is used to treat kidney stones and UTIs in the bladder, and enlarged prostate. It also has a diuretic effect. The breakdown of amygdalin can produce cyanide. Overconsumption can cause severe bloody diarrhea, dizziness, chest tightness, or allergic reactions. Not much data is available on adverse effects. It can interact with lithium. Health Benefits Times. (2017, October 6). Hydrangea facts and health benefits. *HealthBenefitstimes. com.* https://www.healthbenefitstimes.com/hydrangea/ Lang, A. (2021, February 25). Hydrangea root: Supplements, uses, and benefits. *Healthline.* https://www.healthline.com/nutrition/hydrangea-root#what-it-is
Hydrogen Peroxide (H_2O_2)	Hydrogen peroxide has mild antiseptic and disinfectant action. It is a powerful oxidizing agent. It has multiple applications for home use. H_2O_2 has antibacterial and antiyeast properties. It is often used to clean minor wounds, burns, medical equipment and surfaces. It can also be used for oral hygiene. However, it is not generally recommended for wound care nowadays as it can delay healing.

Ingredients	Mechanism of Action and Health Benefits
	Three percent H_2P_2 is generally safe. Side effects include burning sensation, skin irritation, difficulty breathing, and it can splash in the eyes.
	Stanborough, R. J. (2019, November 13). 22 healthy uses for hydrogen peroxide (and a few you should avoid). *Healthline*. https://www.healthline.com/health/hydrogen-peroxide-uses#health
Hydroxy Acids	Hydroxy acids are of two types: alpha hydroxy acid (AHA) and beta hydroxy acid (BHA). They are present in skin care products and have antiinflammatory, antioxidant, antibacterial, exfoliating, skin-lightening, antiaging, and moisturizing effects (varying effects with different hydroxy acids). They are used as quick "lunch time" beauty chemical peels to keep the skin smooth, soft, and shiny.
	AHA is widely used. It is more water-soluble and works well for dry skin. There are many types of AHAs. Lactic acid (from lactose milk sugar) and glycolic acid (from sugar cane) are the common AHAs. Others are malic acid (from apples), tartaric acid (from grapes), citric acid (from citrus fruits), mandelic acid (from almonds), kojic acid (from rice fermentation), and ferulic acid (from wheat bran, rice, oats. and citrus).
	BHA is more oil-soluble and penetrating and works well for more oily skin. It helps better in acne. Salicylic acid is a BHA.
	AHA and BHA ingredients can be combined or used alternately in skin care daily routine.
	Cherney, K. (2019, March 8). AHA vs. BHA: What's the difference? *Healthline*. https://www.healthline.com/health/aha-vs-bha
	Cherney, K. (2019, January 29). Ferulic acid: The antioxidant-boosting skin care ingredient. *Healthline*. https://www.healthline.com/health/ferulic-acid
Irish moss *Chondrus crispus*	Other names: *Sea moss, Red seaweed*
	Irish moss or sea moss is an algae seaweed. The red variety is the most common. Carrageenan (or carragelose) is a sulfated polysaccharide gelling agent that is extracted from the red seaweed and is used widely in foods and cosmetics.
	It is rich in minerals and vitamins including iodine. It is low in calories. It has immune-boosting properties.
	It can support thyroid health and gut health and facilitate weight loss.
	It can help PD.
	Refer under "Seaweed."
	Panoff, L. (2021, February 12). Sea moss: Benefits, nutrition, and how to prepare it. *Healthline*. https://www.healthline.com/nutrition/seamoss
	WebMD Editorial Contributors. (2020, September 24). Health benefits of sea moss. *WebMD*. https://www.webmd.com/diet/health-benefits-sea-moss#1
Joe Pye weed *Eutrochium purpureum*	Other names: *Kidney root, Gravel root*
	Joe pye weed contains euparin, euparone, and benzofurans.
	It has diuretic and tonic properties.
	It can dissolve stones in the kidney and gallbladder. It can also help with painful urination and increase the flow of urine in UTIs.
	It is also used for rheumatism, gout, and arthritis.
	It may contain PAs which are hepatotoxic.
	Medicinal Herb Info Staff. (n.d.). Joe-Pye Weed. *Medicinal Herb Info*. http://medicinalherbinfo.org/000Herbs2016/1herbs/joe-pye-weed/
	WebMD. (2012). Gravel Root. https://www.webmd.com/vitamins/ai/ingredientmono-672/gravel-root
Juniper *Juniperus communis*	Juniper belongs to the Cypress family and there are many species. Some species are poisonous.
	Juniper berries (seed cones) are used for culinary and medicinal uses. It is added as a flavor and bitter agent in gin, other beverages, and foods. It contains several active compounds including sesquiterpenes (α-cadinol, germacrene D, spathulenol, and α-humulene), terpenes (β-myrcene and α-pinene), flavonoids, and phenols. The essential oil from juniper berries contains monoterpenes (camphor, limonene, and β-pinene). It is rich in vitamin C. Essential oil can also be extracted from the leaves or needles, but they are different in composition from the berries essential oil although they have similar healing or therapeutic properties.
	Juniper berries have antiinflammatory, antioxidant, antidiabetic, antibacterial, and antifungal properties. It also has diuretic, carminative, detoxifying, and antiarthritic effects. Juniper essential oil has calming properties and is used in aromatherapy. The oil is also added to cosmetic products.
	It helps in digestive disorders including stomach ache, acid reflux, and loss of appetite.

Ingredients	Mechanism of Action and Health Benefits
	It helps in wound healing.
	It is used for arthritis. It can also be used for UTIs and kidney stones.
	It supports heart health. It can lower triglycerides and LDL cholesterol and increase HDL cholesterol.
	Overall, it is safe. Side effects include allergic reactions. Long-term use may cause seizures and nephrotoxicity.

Bais, S., Gill, N. S., Rana, N., & Shandil, S. (2014). A phytopharmacological review on a medicinal plant: *Juniperus communis*. *International Scholarly Research Notices*, *2014*, 1–6. https://doi.org/10.1155/2014/634723

Kubala, J. (2019, August 30). 5 emerging benefits of juniper berries. *Healthline*. https://www.health-line.com/nutrition/juniper-berries

RxList Editors. (2021, June 11). Juniper. *RxList*. https://www.rxlist.com/juniper/supplements.htm

Hyssop
Hyssopus officinalis

Unlike many medicinal plants, in hyssop the above-ground parts of the plant are used instead of its roots. It has a bitter taste and is used in food flavoring. The hyssop oil is used in makeup and body-care products due to its fragrance.

The bioactive ingredients constituents of hyssop include flavonoids, volatile oils (pinocamphone), and tannins.

It has antiinflammatory, antioxidant, and antimicrobial properties.

It is also used in the treatment of asthma, coughs, colds, and sore throat.

It is used for the treatment of digestive ailments including stomach ulcers, indigestion, and gas.

The essential oil of hyssop can be used topically for mild skin irritations such as frostbite, burns, bruises, and small cuts. It can also be used for other skin diseases like psoriasis, and eczema.

The oil is also used in aromatherapy for boosting the mood. It may also be used for menstrual cramps.

Symptoms of possible hyssop allergy are swelling, dryness and peeling, sneezing and runny nose, red rash and itchy skin.

Cherney, K. (2019, August 9). What you need to know about hyssop essential oil. *Healthline*. https://www.healthline.com/health/hyssop-oil#precautions

Dellwo, A., & Bull, M. (2020, December 7). The health benefits of hyssop. *Verywell Health*. https://www.verywellhealth.com/hyssop-benefits-4588178

Kava root
Piper methysticum

Kava belongs to the nightshade family. It is used as a social and ceremonial drink in the South Pacific Islands. It has a relaxing and euphoric effect.

The main active ingredients in the root are kavalactones which promote relaxation, calmness, lowers stress, anxiety, and pain sensations. It is also neuroprotective. It can also promote sleep.

Overall, it is safe. Unlike prescription drugs, it does not cause withdrawal symptoms or dependency. Some cases of liver toxicity have been reported. It should not be taken with alcohol, antidepressants, and benzodiazepines.

Kandola, A. (2018, December 17). Kava kava: Benefits and safety concerns. *MedicalNewsToday*. https://www.medicalnewstoday.com/articles/324015#summary

Walle, G. V. D. (2018, February 10). Kava Kava: Benefits, side effects and dosage. *Healthline*. https://www.healthline.com/nutrition/kava-kava#TOC_TITLE_HDR_3

Kelp

Kelp is a large brown algae seaweed of the Laminariaceae family. There are several varieties of kelp. Common ones include *kombu* (*Saccharina japonica*), *wakame*, Laminaria, giant kelp, and bull kelp.

Kelp contains flavonoids and carotenoids. It is rich in vitamins (K and A), and minerals (including iodine, iron, calcium, and magnesium). The high iodine content helps in the production of thyroid hormone.

Kelp also contains vanadium, which mimics insulin hence can lower blood sugar in diabetes.

Sodium alginate, a natural gelling agent, is extracted from kelp and is used as an emulsifier in the food industry. It also acts as an insoluble fiber and fat blocker to stop the absorption of fat in the gut.

Glutamate (an amino acid) is high in kelp and this imparts the umami taste.

Kelp also contains fucoidan (a polysaccharide) which has antioxidant, antiinflammatory, anticlotting, and anticancer effects.

Fucoxanthin is a carotenoid pigment in brown seaweed or kelp which helps with weight loss.

It can induce labor and also enhance termination of pregnancy. It can also treat anemia.

Xanthigen is a nutraceutical product containing brown seaweed kelp (which is fucoxanthin-rich) and pomegranate seed oil (which is punicic acid-rich). It is used for weight loss.

Ingredients	Mechanism of Action and Health Benefits

Laminaria sticks (a type of brown seaweed kelp) are inserted into the cervix to ripen the cervix and induce labor for birth or earlier to induce abortions. The sticks cause the release of prostaglandins to dilate the cervix.

See further under "Seaweed."

Deep Ocean Facts. (2017, August 31). 10 types of kelp—Characteristics—Benefits. *DeepOceanFacts.com*. https://deepoceanfacts.com/types-of-kelp

Forge, T. L. (2019, March 8). How kelp can actually help you lose weight and balance your hormones. *Healthline*. https://www.healthline.com/health/food-nutrition/ways-to-eat-kelp-or-seaweed#health-benefits-of-kelp

WebMD Editorial Contributors. (2020, September 17). Health benefits of kelp. *WebMD*. https://www.webmd.com/diet/health-benefits-kelp#1

Lady's mantle
Alchemilla mollis or
Alchemilla vulgaris or
Alchemilla xanthochlora

Lady's mantle contains flavonoids (rutin, kaempferol, and quercetin), phenolic acids (caffeic and gallic acids), tannins (ellagitannins including alchemillin and pedunculagin), and essential oils.

It is largely a women's herb.

It has antiinflammatory, antioxidant, astringent, antifungal, and nootropic properties.

It acts as a uterine tonic. It can treat infertility, menstrual (it relieves pain and regulates menstrual flow), and menopausal (hot flushes and night sweat) problems. It improves the luteal phase and thickens the endometrium so that implantation is better should pregnancy occur. Lady's mantle can also stop spotting between periods as well as reduce blood flow.

It can promote sleep. It is also used to treat cough, colds, and sore throat.

Overall, it is safe. Overconsumption can cause hepatotoxicity.

Lady's Mantle. (2020, August 24). Drugs.com. https://www.drugs.com/npp/lady-s-mantle.html

Baeva V. M. (2019). Prospects for the use of the herb lady's mantle in geriatrics. *Advances in gerontology = Uspekhi gerontologii, 32*(1–2), 180–184.

Lavender
Lavandula angustifolia

There are many species of lavender. It can be used for cooking, bathing, scenting the air, and for medicinal needs. *L. angustifolia* has relaxant and sedative properties. *L. latifolia* has expectorant and stimulant properties. It contains linalool, linalyl acetate (these have sedative properties), cis-beta-ocimene, trans-beta-ocimene, and terpinen-4-ol.

It helps with digestive issues (nausea, vomiting, gas and bloating, and indigestion). It is used for culinary purposes and the leaves or flowers are often added to baked goods, desserts, or dressings. The English lavender is more used for cooking than the French lavender.

It has antibacterial, antifungal, antiseptic, and antiinflammatory properties. It also reduces itchiness. It can hasten wound healing and reduce scarring, treat minor burns including sunburns, insect bites, skin irritation, fungal infections, and hair loss.

Inhaling lavender aromatherapy oil can treat insomnia, restlessness, anxiety, depression, and headaches. The scent is calming and relaxing and can reduce stress levels, hence it can also lower blood pressure.

The essential oil is toxic if swallowed. Excessive topical use may lead to prepubertal gynecomastia. There are drug–herb interactions with other CNS depressants (barbiturates and benzodiazepines) causing more drowsiness and with antihypertensives (sartans and ACE inhibitors) causing low blood pressure.

Buckle, J. (2014). Chapter 3—Basic plant taxonomy, basic essential oil chemistry, extraction, biosynthesis, and analysis. In *Clinical Aromatherapy: Essential Oils in Healthcare* (3rd ed., pp. 37–72). Edinburgh: Churchill Livingstone. https://doi.org/10.1016/B978-0-7020-5440-2.00003-6

Nordqvist, J. (2019, March 4). What are the health benefits and risks of lavender? *MedicalNewsToday*. https://www.medicalnewstoday.com/articles/265922

Ingredients	Mechanism of Action and Health Benefits
Lemon balm *Melissa officinalis*	Lemon balm belongs to the mint family. The active constituents are rosmarinic acid, flavonoids (apigenin, kaempferol, quercetin, and luteolin), phenols (caffeic acid and chlorogenic acid), tannins, terpenes (ursolic and oleanolic acids), and eugenol. The aroma is from citronellal, neral, and geranial.

It has a calming and sedative effect. It has antiviral properties. It is rich in antioxidants.

It is used for anxiety, stress relief, and insomnia. It is antispasmodic and is used to treat indigestion (dyspepsia, acid reflux, nausea, bloating, and colic). It can relieve premenstrual symptoms and menstrual pain. It can treat early herpes infections.

It is available as tea, tincture, capsules, or as cream. Overall, it is safe if used short term. Rare side effects include palpitations, rash, nausea, and headaches. It should not be used in pregnant women or young children. There is drug interaction with thyroid medications or sedatives.

Fletcher, J. (2020, March 3). Lemon balm: Uses and health benefits. *MedicalNewsToday*. https://www.medicalnewstoday.com/articles/lemon-balm-uses#_noHeaderPrefixedContent

Lily of the valley
Convallaria majalis

Lily of the valley contains many types of steroidal glycosides (cardenolide, convalloside, convallatoxin, bufadienolide, and others), triterpenoids (withanolide), and aglycon. The dried flower tip, stem, and root are used.

It is a cardiotonic herb. It can treat heart disorders including heart failure and irregular heartbeat.

It is also used to treat UTI, kidney stones, and edema.

It helps in epilepsy and depression.

Side effects include gastric upset, headache, decreased responsiveness, visual disturbances, and abnormal heart rhythms.

Liang, X., Nielsen, N. J., & Christensen, J. H. (2020). Selective pressurized liquid extraction of plant secondary metabolites: *Convallaria majalis* L. as a case. *Analytica Chimica Acta: X, 4*, 100040. https://doi.org/10.1016/j.acax.2020.100040

RxList Editors. (2021, June 11). Lily-of-the-valley. *RxList*. https://www.rxlist.com/lily-of-the-valley/supplements.htm

WebMD Editors. (2015). Lily-of-the-valley. *WebMD*. https://www.webmd.com/vitamins/ai/ingredient-mono-289/lily-of-the-valley

Lime
Citrus aurantiifolia
Lemon
Citrus limon

Lime and lemon are citrus fruits. There are many species. There are minor differences between lime and lemon but the health benefits are similar. Lemon is sweeter. Lime is more bitter. It has both culinary and medicinal uses.

The active compounds in the essential oil are d-limonene, γ-terpinene, linalool, linalyl acetate, α-terpineol, terpinolene, β-pinene, borneol, citral, neral acetate, and geranyl acetate.

They have antioxidant, antiinflammatory, antidepressant, and antifungal, and anticarcinogenic properties.

It is rich in antioxidants (especially vitamin C which is higher in lemon). Vitamins (B1 and B6) and minerals (iron, calcium, and potassium) are also present.

It contains citrate which binds with calcium in the urine and hence prevents kidney stone formation.

It boosts immunity, decreases heart disease risk, increases iron absorption, and promotes healthy skin.

It is a safe herb. The high acidity may worsen acid reflux (GERD) or erode the enamel of teeth.

Raman, R. (2019, March 21). Limes: A Citrus Fruit with Powerful Benefits. *Healthline*. https://www.healthline.com/nutrition/limes

West, H. (2019, January 7). 6 Evidence-Based Health Benefits of Lemons. *Healthline*. https://www.healthline.com/nutrition/6-lemon-health-benefits

Linden tea
Tilia cordata

Linden contains quercetin, kaempferol, rutin, volatile oils, mucilage, tannins, and other flavonoids. Others phytoconstituents include chlorogenic and caffeic acids, amino acids (alanine, cysteine, cystine, and phenylalanine).

The flavonoids and p-coumaric acid give the diaphoretic properties and induce sweating in fevers and also its antispasmodic effects. Linden also has diuretic, expectorant, antitussive, and sedative properties.

It is used in the treatment of influenza, cough, migraine, anxiety and stress, spasms from various causes, liver and gallbladder disorders, diarrhea, and hypertension associated with arteriosclerosis.

It is safe to consume in moderation. Side effects include drowsiness, risk of botulism (from *Clostridium botulinum* spores) dehydration, and risk of cardiotoxicity with excessive consumption.

Drugs.com. (2021, April 1). Linden. https://www.drugs.com/npp/linden.html

Ingredients	Mechanism of Action and Health Benefits
Lobelia *Lobelia inflata*	Other names: *Indian tobacco, puke weed* Lobelia is a flowering plant. It contains many alkaloids including lobeline, lobinaline caffeine, nicotine, and morphine. Others include apigenin, isolobelanine, lobelanidine, quercetin, coumarins, glucosides, and other flavonoids. Lobelin, the most important constituent, has antiinflammatory effects. It helps to improve breathing, relax the airways, thin and clear mucus in asthma, bronchitis, and pneumonia. Lobinaline has antioxidant effects and may help in PD and depression. Due to the presence of nicotine, it may be helpful in smokers who want to quit. It also improves the release and uptake of dopamine in the brain and may help with the focus and hyperactivity in ADHD. Excessive amounts can cause nausea, vomiting, profuse sweating, and even death. Streit, L. (2020, May 8). *What is Lobelia, and how is it used?* Healthline. https://www.healthline.com/nutrition/lobelia#benefits
Maca *Lepidium meyenii*	Other names: *Peruvian Viagra* Maca is a root vegetable known as "Peruvian Viagra." The root contains flavonoids, alkaloids, macamides, and macaridine. It balances the hormones. It is rich in iron, iodine, calcium, and potassium. It has antioxidant properties and can also boost the body's endogenous antioxidants i.e., glutathione and superoxide dismutase. It can improve male sexual health. It helps to increase male libodo, erectile function, and increase sperm count. It can also increase physical energy, endurance, and sports performance. It can lower anxiety, depression, improve mood, and reduce menopausal symptoms in postmenopausal women. It is also neuroprotective and can improve memory and learning. Overall, it is safe. It may interact with thyroid hormone. Kandola, A. (2020, January 30). What are the benefits of maca root? *MedicalNewsToday*. https://www.medicalnewstoday.com/articles/322511#ten-benefits Khatri, M. (2020, August 17). All About Maca Root. *WebMD*. https://www.webmd.com/diet/ss/slideshow-diet-maca root
Magnesium	Magnesium is the fourth most prominent mineral in the body. The serum magnesium level (like potassium) does not reflect the total body magnesium content. It represents only less than 1% of the total body concentration. In the body, 60% of the magnesium is stored in the bones, 25% in the muscles, and less than 1% in the blood. The ideal ratio of magnesium to calcium should be 1:1 but in the modern diet, it is 1:5. Food sources of magnesium include whole grains, nuts, sea food, berries, and legumes. Magnesium is an important mineral for all cellular and biochemical functions. It is a cofactor for more than 300 enzyme reactions in the body. Magnesium is required for muscle contraction. Too much calcium can interfere with this. It helps blood pressure and blood glucose regulation, muscle contraction, brain and nerve function, and energy production. It is important for heart health and maintains stable electrophysiological action and hemodynamics. It can help in heart failure, insomnia, stress, migraine headaches, anxiety, depression, constipation, and diabetes. It decreases the overactive bladder muscle spasms and promotes bladder emptying. Most people are deficient in magnesium. There are many magnesium salts available. Magnesium citrate, magnesium glycinate, magnesium threonate, and magnesium amino acid chelate are easily absorbed and have high bioavailability. Others with lesser bioavailability include magnesium oxide, magnesium hydroxide, and magnesium carbonate. The bioavailability of magnesium may be different from the percentage of elemental magnesium present in the magnesium salt. Magnesium toxicity is rare and supplementation must be cautious in kidney failure. Ware, M. R. (2020, January 6). Why do we need magnesium? *MedicalNewsToday*. https://www.medicalnewstoday.com/articles/286839#benefits

Ingredients	Mechanism of Action and Health Benefits
Mallow *Malva sylvestris*	Other names: *Common mallow, Blue mallow, Wood mallow, Tree mallow, High mallow, Cheese flower, Cheeses* Mallow is a flowering plant and there are many species. It contains flavonoids, phenols, terpenoids, fatty acids (omega-3 and omega-6), vitamins (C, E, β-carotene), and abundant mucilage. Although common mallow and marshmallow have similar medicinal uses, common mallow is inferior in its actions and efficacy. Mallow has antimicrobial, antiinflammatory, antioxidant, expectorant, laxative, demulcent, diuretic, wound-healing, and salve actions. The leaves and flowers are mainly used. The fruit and seeds have more mucilage content than the leaves (but less than marshmallow). The leaves are used to make poultices to heal wounds, rashes, insect bites, and other skin problems. Common mallow is effective in respiratory (for sore throat and dry cough) and oral/digestive problems (dry mouth, constipation). Health Benefits Times. (2019, February 11). Common Mallow facts and health benefits. *HealthBenefitstimes.com*. https://www.healthbenefitstimes.com/common-mallow/
Manuka Honey	Manuka is produced in New Zealand and Australia. The bees pollinate the tea tree bush (*Leptospermum scoparium* bush). This manuka tea tree is different from the tea tree oil of the Melaleuca alternifolia tree. The nectar of the manuka flowers contain leptosperin and have a higher concentration of dihydroxyacetone (DHA) which gets converted into methylglyoxal (MGO). Manuka honey has antiseptic, antibacterial, antiinflammatory, and osmotic (humectant) properties. It acts as a natural antibiotic. The antibacterial properties are due to the presence of H_2P_2, MGO, and DHA. It has an acidic pH 3.2–4.5. The antibacterial potency is measured by the Unique Manuka Factor (UMF) rating, which is based on the concentration of the three compounds (MGO, DHA, and leptosperin). The UMF rating or scores are 0 to 4 = undetectable, 5 to 9 = low level, 10 to 15 = useful levels, .16 = superior. A high UMF is a better quality honey. It is used to treat sore throat, cough, and bronchitis. It helps in wound infection and wound healing. It is also used in eczema and acne. It can also help improve the gut flora and gut health. Side effects include high blood sugar and allergic reactions. Connor, E. (2020, August 18). Everything you should know about manuka honey. *Healthline*. https://www.healthline.com/health/manuka-honey#risks-and-warnings
Marjoram *Origanum majorana*	Other name: Sweet marjoram Marjoram has culinary and medicinal uses. The active ingredients include carvacrol, rosmarinic acid, coumarinic acid, sinapic acid, vanillic acid, caffeic acid, ferulic acid, and syringic acid. It also contains potassium, β-carotene, lutein, folate, and vitamins A and K. It has antioxidant, antiinflammatory, and antimicrobial activities. It has antitussive effects. Marjoram essential oil can be used for steam inhalation to treat colds, flu, asthma, and sinus-related headaches. It also has carminative effects and can treat stomach ulcers and cramps. It regulates the menstrual cycle. It can promote menstrual blood flow, balance the hormones, and reduce menopause symptoms. It can also treat PCOS. It can also be added to baths to reduce stress. It can also be applied topically to treat fungal skin infections. Overall, it is safe. It can cause eye irritation or allergic reactions. It can interact with anticholinergic drugs or blood thinners and diabetic medications. Preiato, D. (2019, September 5). What is marjoram? Benefits, side effects, and uses. *Healthline*. https://www.healthline.com/nutrition/marjoram
Marshmallow root *Althaea officinalis*	The marshmallow root contains more mucilage than the common mallow. Today's candy marshmallows in confectioneries are synthetic (made from sugar, corn syrup, animal gelatine, vanillin, and starch and rarely egg white) and do not contain the natural marshmallow roots (the original marshmallow contained the natural mucilage). It has antioxidant, antiinflammatory, and antibacterial activities. It also has pain-relieving properties. It is helpful in treating dry coughs, colds, bronchitis, or respiratory tract diseases with mucus formation. It also improves chronic dry mouth (xerostomia).

Ingredients	Mechanism of Action and Health Benefits
	It is also used to treat many digestive ailments such as heartburn, gastric ulcers, intestinal colic, inflammation in digestive tract, and constipation.

It also relieves skin irritation due to conditions like eczema and furunculosis. It also improves skin health and wound healing.

The root may also act as a diuretic and can also improve overall urinary health. It has demulcent action and soothes the irritation in the mucus membrane of the urinary tract. The flowers can lower LDL cholesterol levels, and treat platelet aggregation.

Marshmallow roots are generally safe. Overconsumption can cause dizziness, skin irritation, and stomach upsets. It should be avoided by diabetes patients.

Berry, J. (2019, April 2). What are the benefits of marshmallow root? *MedicalNewsToday*. https://www.medicalnewstoday.com/articles/324860#summary

Cronkleton, E. (2019, March 29). Everything you need to know about marshmallow root. *Healthline*. https://www.healthline.com/health/food-nutrition/marshmallow-root

Mastic gum
Pistacia lentiscus

Other names: *Teardrops of Chios, Arabic gum, Yemen gum*

Mastic tree is a shrub. The leaves and the bark contain tannins and terpenes (linalool), which have antiseptic and antiinflammatory functions. Mastic trees produce a natural resin in the shape of tears. Mastic gum is used mostly in cosmetics, oral hygiene products, and also added to food. It is also used as a varnish. It does not produce edible nuts like the pistachio tree (*Pistacia vera*).

It is often chewed as a chewing gum for breath freshener. It maintains oral hygiene, prevents dental plaque, bad breath, and maintains healthy gums and teeth. It can help in periodontitis.

It also helps in gastric ulcers, acid reflux, indigestion, and it may also be effective against *H. pylori*.

It can also be used in wound healing.

Overall, it is safe. Rarely, allergy may occur. It is related to pistachio trees and there can be reactivity between mastic gum and pistachio nuts.

Meadowsweet
Filipendula ulmaria

Other names: *Mead wort, queen of the meadow, pride of the meadow, meadsweet, ulmaira, bridewort*

Meadowsweet grows in the damp meadows. It contains salicylic acid (salicylates) which have antipyretic and analgesic properties (from which aspirin is derived). It helps with colds and flus to bring down the fever and reduce body or muscle aches. Other active constituents include tannins, flavone glycosides, and essential oils. The tannins help to decrease phlegm.

It can also help in arthritis or gout, heartburn, headache, and migraine.

It has some diuretic effect and can be used in bladder infections.

Excessive or prolonged consumption of meadowsweet causes salicylate poisoning with gastric upsets, melena (blood in stools), skin rash, difficulty breathing, tinnitus, and kidney impairment. If there is history of aspirin allergy or sensitivity, meadowsweet should not be used.

Streit, M. L. S. (2021, March 3). Meadowsweet herb: Benefits, uses, tea, and more. *Healthline*. https://www.healthline.com/nutrition/meadowsweet-herb

Milk thistle
Silybum marianum

Milk thistle is an excellent liver cleansing herb. The bioactive compound in milk thistle is silymarin which contains silicristin, silydianin, and silibinin. It also contains isosilybin, silydianin, and silybin.

It has antiinflammatory, antioxidant, and neuroprotective properties.

It supports liver health and can prevent fatty change in nonalcoholic liver disease. It can also be used to treat hepatitis.

It also improves bone health and increases mineralization.

It increases breast milk production.

It can promote healthy skin and treat acne and eczema.

It can reduce insulin resistance and blood sugar.

Overall, it is safe. Side effects can include stomach upset and bloating. It can interact with oral contraceptives. It should be avoided if there is a history of estrogen-sensitive tumors.

West, H. (2018, January 19). 7 science-based benefits of milk thistle. *Healthline*. https://www.healthline.com/nutrition/milk-thistle-benefits

Ingredients	Mechanism of Action and Health Benefits
Mint or **Bo he** *Mentha Family* • **Peppermint** *Mentha piperita* • **Spearmint** (*Mentha spicata*) • **Wild or field mint** *Mentha arvensis* • **Apple mint** *Mentha suaveolens* • **Pineapple mint** *Mentha suaveolens— variegata variety* • **Pennyroyal** *Mentha pulegium* • **Watermint** *Mentha aquatica*	Mint family has about 20 species. These six types of mints—peppermint, spearmint, wild mint, apple mint, pineapple mint, pennyroyal, and watermint—are commonly grown in home gardens. The essential oil is extracted from the leaves. The dilute form of the extract is used as a flavor in foods and beverages. It is also available as a capsule supplement. The oil has antispasmodic, mild antimicrobial, neuroprotective, and antianalgesic properties. They have antiinflammatory and antioxidant properties due to the presence of rosmarinic acid. Menthol is the main bioactive essential volatile oil found in the leaves and flowers which gives the cool sensation. Other essential oils include menthone, and limonene, cineol, and other volatile oils. Pulegone is another constituent which has pesticide effects. Other active ingredients include terpenoids (such as d (-)-carvone and limonene). There are subtle changes among the mint varieties but most of their health benefits and uses remain the same. It helps in nausea, indigestion, gas and bloating, abdominal cramps, IBS, flatulence, diarrhea, and dissolution of gallstones. It also helps in cough and colds. It is a decongestant and expectorant. It can also reduce stress and anxiety, muscle and nerve pain. It is effective against staphylococcus and candida. It can also promote hair growth, and decrease skin itching. It can treat and heal chronic wounds. It is used in oral hygiene and is effective against dental caries. It is also used in many products such as toothpaste and mouthwash. Side effects include gastric upset, acid reflux, and allergic reactions. If consumed excessively it can cause skin irritation. It can interact with antacids, antihypertensive and antidiabetic drugs. **Peppermint** Peppermint is a hybrid of spearmint and watermint. It has antibacterial and antispasmodic activities and can be used to treat urine infection. It helps to calm the bladder. **Spearmint** It supports hormonal imbalance in women, increasing the estrogen and decreasing testosterone. **Apple mint** Apple mint and pineapple mint are similar. Pineapple mint is a variegated cultivar of the apple mint. **European Pennyroyal** It can be consumed as essential oil and can abort pregnancy. It is also used for pest control. **Wild mint** It can also be used as a pesticide. Brazier, Y. (2017, June 27). Health benefits and risks of peppermint. *MedicalNewsToday*. https://www.medicalnewstoday.com/articles/265214 Groves, M. (2018, October 24). 11 surprising benefits of spearmint tea and essential oil. *Healthline*. https://www.healthline.com/nutrition/spearmint#TOC_TITLE_HDR_4 Max. (2020, December 18). 6 types of mints you can grow in the garden. *Trees.com*. https://www.trees.com/herb-plants/mint Nordqvist, J. (2018, January 11). Spearmint: Health benefits and more. *MedicalNewsToday*. https://www.medicalnewstoday.com/articles/266128#possible-health-benefits-of-spearmint Pearson, K. (2017, December 13). 8 health benefits of mint. *Healthline*. https://www.healthline.com/nutrition/mint-benefits#TOC_TITLE_HDR_3 Seladi-Schulman, J. (2019, April 25). About peppermint oil uses and benefits. *Healthline*. https://www.healthline.com/health/benefits-of-peppermint-oil#pain
Mistletoe *Viscum album*	Other name: *European mistletoe* Mistletoe contains several bioactive ingredients including thionins (viscotoxins), triterpene, flavonoids, and phenylpropanoids. It is widely used in Europe to treat different types of cancers as an alternative therapy. It has antiinflammatory, immunomodulating, and reported anticancer properties. It can treat headache, epilepsy, menopausal symptoms, hypertension, and rheumatism. Side effects include fever, chills, headache, and acute allergic reactions. Kubala, J. (2021, August 25). Does mistletoe help treat cancer? An evidence-based look. *Healthline*. https://www.healthline.com/nutrition/mistletoe-and-cancer

Ingredients	Mechanism of Action and Health Benefits

Nazaruk, J., & Orlikowski, P. (2015). Phytochemical profile and therapeutic potential of Viscum album L. *Natural Product Research*, 30(4), 373–385. https://doi.org/10.1080/14786419.2015.1022776

Rx List Editors. (2021, June 11). European mistletoe. *RxList*. https://www.rxlist.com/european_mistletoe/supplements.htm

Molasses

Molasses is a thick syrup that is a by-product of the sugar-making process. It contains antioxidants, several minerals (including magnesium, manganese, copper, potassium, selenium, iron, and calcium) and also vitamin B6. It is amber to red in color and is sweet and acidic. Blackstrap molasses, also a by-product but from triple processing, is very dark, bitter, salty with lower GI and higher nutritional value compared to regular molasses.

The potassium content promotes heart health and lowers blood pressure.

It may also lower blood sugar levels in diabetes.

Molasses may relieve constipation due to its high magnesium content. It can also improve bone health.

Overall, it is safe. Overconsumption may cause digestive disorders like loose stools or diarrhea. It should be avoided by those with IBS or other digestive discomforts.

McDonell, K. (2020, March 16). Everything you need to know about molasses. *MedicalNewsToday*. https://www.medicalnewstoday.com/articles/318719

Motherwort
Leonurus cardiaca
Leonurus japonicus

Other names: *Chinese Motherwort, Yi Mu Cao*

Motherwort contains sterols, flavonoids, tannins, and triterpenes.

It has antioxidant properties. It is also a nerve tonic.

It supports heart health and acts as a diuretic. It lowers blood pressure and heart rate. It can treat irregular heartbeat and palpitations associated with anxiety and hyperthyroidism.

It has estrogen-like properties and can reduce menopausal symptoms. It can treat postpartum bleeding. It can also regulate the menstrual cycle. It can reduce period cramps by lessening uterine muscle spasms.

Side effects include uterine bleeding, diarrhea, and stomach pain. It can interact with blood thinners.

McGrane, K. (2019, October 16). What is motherwort? Benefits, side effects, and dosage. *Healthline*. https://www.healthline.com/nutrition/motherwort

TraceGains, Inc. (2015, May 24). Motherwort. *Kaiser Permanente*. https://wa.kaiserpermanente.org/kbase/topic.jhtml?docId=hn-2132004

WebMD Editors. (2014). Motherwort. *WebMD*. https://www.webmd.com/vitamins/ai/ingredient-mono-126/motherwort

Mullein Leaf
Verbascum thapsus

Mullein leaf and flowers contain mucilage, which is soothing to the irritated mucous membranes. It also has saponins which are natural detergents that have expectorant and antiinflammatory effects. The flavonoids, phenylethanoid glycosides, and iridoids present also have antiinflammatory properties. It has antiviral (against influenza A and herpes) and antibacterial (against Klebsiella, *E. coli*) effects.

It is an excellent respiratory tonic which relieves airway spasm, chest tightness, cough and irritation in asthma, bronchitis, COPD, and lung congestion. The oil can be used to treat earaches.

It is also a diuretic and can be used in urinary tract inflammation.

It is generally safe. Some allergic rash may occur on contact with the leaves.

Brennan, D. (2020, November 10). Health benefits of mullein tea. *WebMD*. https://www.webmd.com/diet/health-benefits-mullein-tea#1

Ghoshal, M. (2020, March 13). Mulling over mullein leaf. *Healthline*. https://www.healthline.com/health/mullein-leaf

Myo-inositol

Inositol is a B-like vitamin (vitamin B8) found in plant foods (seeds, nuts, whole grains, beans, and fresh fruit). It occurs in many isomer forms and myo-inositol (MI) is one of the commonest isomers. It is also made in the body or is available as a supplement.

MI can increase insulin sensitivity, decrease hyperandrogenism, and improve the menstrual cycle. It is used to treat metabolic syndrome and polycystic ovary syndrome (PCOS). It helps to lower serum insulin, testosterone, cholesterol, and inflammatory markers.

There are mixed views for its use in diabetic neuropathy, AD, anxiety, panic disorder, and depression.

Mild side effects include nausea, stomach upsets, gas, fatigue, dizziness, and headaches.

Ingredients	Mechanism of Action and Health Benefits
Naringenin	It is a natural flavonoid found in citrus fruits (grapefruit, orange, lemon, and bergamot) and tomato. It is also available as a nutritional supplement. It has antioxidant, antiinflammatory, immunomodulating, and anticancer actions. It can increase insulin sensitivity. It can help in obesity, metabolic syndromes, and lower the risk of cardiovascular diseases. It can also be used in certain types of cancers and hepatitis C. Salehi, B., Fokou, P., Sharifi-Rad, M., Zucca, P., Pezzani, R., Martins, N., et al. (2019). The therapeutic potential of naringenin: A review of clinical trials. *Pharmaceuticals, 12*(1), 11. https://doi.org/10.3390/ph12010011
Natural moisturizing factor	Natural moisturizing factor (NMF) is present and formed in the stratum corneum layer of the epidermis from filaggrin proteolysis. It acts as a natural protective skin moisture barrier. It consists of water-attracting molecules (hydrophilic molecules). These include free amino acids or their derivatives including urea, urocanic acid, lactic acid, pyrrolidone carboxylic acid (PCA), HA, and other inorganic salts. NMF decreases with aging, baths, sun exposure or other environmental elements, and in many skin disorders. NMF are natural hydrators and humectants and they are often added to cosmetic products so that the skin will not become dry, dull, and lusterless. Robinson, M., Visscher, M., Laruffa, A., & Wickett, R. (2010). Abstracts: natural moisturizing factors in the stratum corneum I. Effects of lipid extraction and soaking. *International Journal of Cosmetic Science, 32*(5), 394. https://doi.org/10.1111/j.1468-2494.2010.00591_2.x
Nobiletin	Nobiletin is found in the peel of Citrus fruits including Citrus nobilis (mandarin orange) Citrus aurantium (seville orange) and kumquat. It is a flavonoid. It has anti-oxidant, anti-inflammatory, anti-cancer and anti-angiogenic actions. It is neuroprotective and is a novel therapy for Alzheimer's disease (AD) and Parkinson's disease. It can reduce the amyloid-β (Aβ) plaques and improve the cognitive deficits in AD. It can also reduce bone loss, lower blood glucose and cholesterol. Overall, it is safe. Drugs.com. (2022, July). Nobiletin. https://www.drugs.com/npp/nobiletin.html# Nakajima, A., & Ohizumi, Y. (2019). Potential Benefits of Nobiletin, A Citrus Flavonoid, against Alzheimer's Disease and Parkinson's Disease. International journal of molecular sciences, 20(14), 3380. https://doi.org/10.3390/ijms20143380
Oats *Avena sativa*	Oats are nearly gluten-free whole cereal grains. • *Oat groat* is the hulled whole oat kernel. It contains the outer oat bran, endosperm, and innermost germ (or embryo). The oat groat is most nutritious. • *Oat bran* is the oat groat without the endosperm and germ. It contains beta-glucan, a soluble fiber in the oat bran. • *Rolled oats* are steamed oat groats and then steel-rolled into thick oat flakes (also called regular or old-fashioned oats). • *Instant or quick oats* are rolled oats which are more processed. They are precooked, dried, and rolled into thin oat flakes. • *Steel cut oats* are oat groats which have coarsely chopped by steel blades and not rolled. • *Oatmeal* is stone-ground or stone-milled oat groats (as in Scottish oatmeal). • *Oat flour* is finely ground rolled oats. • *Oat milk* is a plant casein-free and nearly gluten-free milk. • *Oat malt* and *oatmeal stout* are fermented oat liquors. • *Oat grass* has some medicinal use. *Oat straw* is used as animal bedding. Oats are abundant in minerals (including manganese, phosphorus, magnesium, iron, and copper), vitamins (B1, B5, and folate), antioxidants (avenanthramides, polyphenols, and ferulic acid), and fiber (beta-glucan). Avenalin is the main protein content. Avenin is a minor protein which is similar to gliadin in wheat. There is also some gluten in oats. Oats have antiinflammatory, antioxidant, and antiitching effects. It promotes the growth of healthy gut bacteria. The beta-glucans and avenanthramides support heart health. It reduces blood sugar and cholesterol levels. It can also lower blood pressure levels and improve blood flow. The fiber helps in weight loss by increasing fullness. It can relieve constipation.

Ingredients	Mechanism of Action and Health Benefits

Oat extracts are also used in a variety of skin care products and are useful in the treatment of itchy and dry skin and eczema. Oats contain prebiotic fiber which helps nourish the skin microbiome.

Oats are generally considered safe. Allergic reactions can occur.

Migala, J., & Kennedy, K. (2019, July 1). What is oatmeal? Benefits, risks, recipes, more. Everyday Health. *EverydayHealth.com*. https://www.everydayhealth.com/diet-nutrition/diet/oatmeal-benefits-risks-recipes-more/

Palsdottir, H. (2016, July 19). 9 health benefits of eating oats and oatmeal. *Healthline*. https://www.healthline.com/nutrition/9-benefits-oats-oatmeal

Olive
Olea europaea

Olives have both medicinal and culinary uses. The bioactive compounds include phenolic compounds (including oleuropein, oleocanthal, hydroxytyrosol, and tyrosol), flavonoids (quercetin), and triterpenoids (oleanolic acid). It is also rich in oleic acid, a monounsaturated fatty acid.

It has antioxidant, antiinflammatory, and antihypertensive properties.

Olives also contain vitamin E and minerals (including iron, copper, calcium, and sodium).

It can lower the risk of heart disease and stroke by maintaining the blood cholesterol and pressure. It may also prevent chronic disorders and cancers (including breast cancer).

Olive oil is produced by extracting the oil from the fruit. The oil can help reduce the risk of osteoporosis and bone fractures.

Olives and olive oil can also reduce the risk of AD and other brain-related disorders due to the presence of oleocanthal.

Overall, olive fruits are safe. Rarely, allergic reactions may occur in the mouth or throat. Olives are high in heavy metals such as tin, lithium, sulfur, and boron with potential risk of cancer and chronic diseases.

Bjarnadottir, A. (2019, May 21). Olives 101: Nutrition facts and health benefits. *Healthline*. https://www.healthline.com/nutrition/foods/olives

Brennan, D. (2020, November 20). Health benefits of olives. *WebMD*. https://www.webmd.com/diet/health-benefits-olives#

Olive Leaf Extract

Olive leaves are rich in polyphenols, especially oleuropein and oleacein.

The olive leaf extract has antiinflammatory, antioxidant, antimicrobial, gastroprotective, neuroprotective, and anticancer actions. It maintains healthy gut flora.

It can support heart health and weight loss and may prevent AD and dementia.

It can lower blood pressure and cholesterol and improve heart health. It can lower the serum insulin and blood glucose in diabetes.

Overall, it is safe.

Cronkleton, E. (2018, August 16). Olive leaf extract: Dosage, benefits, side effects, and more. *Healthline*. https://www.healthline.com/health/olive-leaf-extract#side-effects

Omega-3 fish oil

Omega-3 fatty acids are polyunsaturated fats and essential fatty acids. The three common types of omega-3 fatty acids are ALA, EPA, and DHA.

ALA is mostly found in plant foods. EPA and DHA are mostly found in animal foods, mostly fatty fish and sometimes from krill, a small shrimp-like crustacean. DHA is found in large amounts in the retina of the fish eye. DHA is found in large amounts in the retina.

Fish oil is obtained by extracting oil from oily fish such as tuna, sardines or herring. It is yellow or gold color. Krill oil is from the krill and it is red in color. Fish or krill oil contains omega-3 fatty acids (EPA and DHA). It is also rich in vitamin A and D.

It has antiinflammatory, antidiabetic, and antihyperlipidemic properties.

It improves heart health and also reduces cholesterol levels, triglycerides, arterial plaques, blood pressure, and fatal arrhythmias.

Omega-3 fatty acids improve brain function and can reduce symptoms of bipolar disorder and schizophrenia. It can improve depression and mental decline.

It helps prevent eye diseases and improve vision.

The omega-3 content also promotes bone health and helps prevent bone diseases.

Fish oil supplements can reduce rheumatoid arthritis symptoms such as joint stiffness and pain. It also improves infant's early life development and growth. It can also reduce the risk of childhood asthma and allergies and symptoms of ADHD.

It also helps reduce weight and waist circumference. It can also improve liver function and liver fat.

Overall, it is safe. Side effects may include stomach upset, nausea, loose stools, and fishy breath.

Ingredients	Mechanism of Action and Health Benefits

Bruce, D. F. (2009, January 26). Omega-3 fish oil supplements: Benefits, side effects, and uses. *WebMD*. https://www.webmd.com/hypertension-high-blood-pressure/guide/omega-3-fish-oil-supplements-for-high-blood-pressure

Robertson, R. (2018, December 18). 13 benefits of taking fish oil. *Healthline*. https://www.healthline.com/nutrition/13-benefits-of-fish-oil

Oregano
Origanum vulgare

Oregano contains several bioactive compounds such as phenols (mainly carvacrol and thymol), terpenoids, and terpenes. It has antioxidant, antiinflammatory, antimicrobial, and antilithogenic activities.

It is effective against several bacteria including *E. coli, S. aureus*, and *Pseudomonas* infection.

It also supports digestive health in diarrhea, gas and bloating, and IBS. It can lower blood sugar and cholesterol and help in weight loss. It can also kill intestinal parasites.

It also has anticancer effects for liver, lung, and breast cancers.

It can also prevent kidney stone formation.

Side effects include stomach upsets if over consumed. It can cause eye or skin irritation or allergy.

Whelan, C. (2018, September 17). Oregano oil side effects. *Healthline*. https://www.healthline.com/health/oregano-oil-side-effects

Ozone

Ozone is O_3. It has sterilizing and disinfecting properties. It can be administered into the body in many ways via the ears, bladder, rectum, intravenously, intramuscularly, intravaginally, and subcutaneously. Ozonated water can be applied as a spray or a compress to the wound or during dental treatment. It should never be inhaled. It has widespread clinical use.

It has antiinfective, antimicrobial, antiinflammatory, analgesic, antioxidant, immune-boosting, detoxifying, and anticancer activities. It boosts the antioxidant pathway in the body. Hence, reducing inflammation.

It improves skin health. It helps with chronic wounds, diabetic foot ulcer healing, and vaginal discharge (especially in recurrent candida vulvovaginitis).

It can also treat brain injury, arthritis, ischemic heart disease, and macular degeneration.

It is used to sterilize medical equipment.

Overall, it is safe. Side effects include nausea, headache, eye irritation, loss of vision, coughing, and air embolism.

Zhang, Q. Q., Zhang, L., Liu, Y., Wang, Y., Chen, R., Huang, Z. Y., et al. (2019). Effect of ozonated water on normal vaginal microecology and Lactobacillus. *Chinese Medical Journal, 132*(9), 1125–1127. https://doi.org/10.1097/cm9.0000000000000216

Paracress
Acmella oleracea

Other name: *Toothache plant*

Paracress contains spilanthol, tannins, carotenoids, steroids, sesquiterpenes (α- and β-bisabolene), phytosterols (stigmasterol, β-sitosterol, α- and β-amyrins), essential oils (limonene and β-caryophyllene), and flavonoid glucoside (cadinenes).

It has antiinflammatory, analgesic, and diuretic properties. The spilanthol has local anesthetic effects.

It helps to relieve toothache and can treat inflamed gums, mouth ulcers, stomatitis, throat pain, and gastric ulcers. It can also induce more salivation when there is a dry mouth.

Side effects include allergic reactions.

Nunez, K. (2020, September 23). What you need to know about the medicinal benefits of the toothache plant. *Healthline*. https://www.healthline.com/health/toothache-plant

Lalthanpuii, P. B., Lalawmpuii, R., Lalremsanga, H. T., & Lalchhandama, K. (2018, June). Pharmacognostic study of the medicinal plant *Acmella oleracea*: Analysis of its chemical components and properties. *Biodiversity Conservation: Strategies and Applications*, 303–313.

Passion flower
Passiflora incarnata

Refer to "*Passion fruit Under Indian Natural Ingredients.*"

There are several species of passion flower. *P. incarnata* has more medicinal value than *Passiflora edulis*.

Peacock flower
Caesalpinia nuga

Other names: *Caesalpinia nuga, Pride of Barbados or Barbados Pride, Paradise flower, Peacock tree, Bird of paradise flower, Paradise flower, Poinciana, Bunga Merak*

There are many varieties of Caesalpinia. It is native to the West Indies and South America.

It has antiinflammatory properties.

Various parts of the plants i.e., leaves, roots, and bark are boiled together to make tea. This is used to treat fever, kidney, and GI problems such as diarrhea. It can also be used as a gargle to treat sore throat and mouth ulcers.

The flower decoction has expectorant properties and is used in chronic cough with phlegm.

The seeds are toxic and poisonous. Although the seeds are toxic, the young green seeds are widely used in Indonesia and Thailand.

M, S. (2018, March 29). Poinciana facts and medicinal uses. *HealthBenefitstimes.com*. https://www.healthbenefitstimes.com/poinciana/

Ingredients	Mechanism of Action and Health Benefits
Peanut *Arachis hypogaea*	Other name: *Groundnut* Peanuts are legumes. It contains 25% proteins but lacks cysteine and methionine amino acids (which are abundant in animal protein). They are rich in polyphenols including p-coumaric acid, resveratrol, and isoflavones. The presence of phytosterols lowers the absorption of cholesterol from the intestine. It contains monounsaturated (i.e., oleic acid which is an omega-3 fatty acid) and polyunsaturated fats and insoluble fiber. It also contains various vitamins (including biotin, niacin, vitamin E, thiamine, and folate) and minerals (magnesium, copper, manganese, and phosphorus). The presence of phytate can reduce the absorption of iron and zinc. It has antioxidant (from the p-coumaric acid and resveratrol) and vasodilator (from the arginine) properties. Peanuts help in weight loss and reduce the risk of obesity. It supports heart health and can regulate cholesterol, sugar, and blood pressure. The protein, magnesium, copper, and calcium content help to strengthen and preserve bones. Adverse reactions include acute allergic effects or anaphylaxis and liver failure from aflatoxin poisoning from the mold *Aspergillus flavus.* Arnarson, A. (2019, May 7). Peanuts 101: Nutrition facts and health benefits. *Healthline.* https://www.healthline.com/nutrition/foods/peanuts Burgess, L. (2019, April 18). What are the nutritional benefits of peanuts? *MedicalNewsToday.* https://www.medicalnewstoday.com/articles/325003
Peanut butter	This is a nut butter and is made from ground peanuts. Pure peanut butter, unlike commercial ones, has excellent nutritional value without added sugar or trans fats. Refer to "Peanuts." Gunnars, K. (2021, June 30). Is peanut butter good or bad for your health? *Healthline.* https://www.healthline.com/nutrition/is-peanut-butter-bad-for-you WebMD Editorial Contributors. (2020, September 30). Peanut butter: Is it good for you? *WebMD.* https://www.webmd.com/diet/peanut-butter-good-for-you#1
Petrolatum & **Paraffin**	Other names for Petrolatum: *Petroleum jelly, Soft paraffin, White petrolatum, Multi-hydrocarbon.* Petroleum jelly consists of a mixture of hydrocarbons and it is semi-solid. It is extracted from petroleum (crude oil). Vaseline is a brand name. It consists of petroleum jelly with added minerals, microcrystalline wax (microwax), and fragrances (lavender oil baby powder). Microcrystalline wax is produced by de-oiling the petrolatum. Vaseline is a common home remedy for dry skin especially in the elderly, diaper rash from urine incontinence, chapped lips, nasal crusting, and epistaxis. It is used in skin and hair care (as hair pomade) products. Waxelene is a nonpetroleum jelly alternative product which consists of nonGMO organic soy oil, organic rosemary oil, raw unbleached beeswax, and vitamin E oil. Paraffin oil (also called liquid paraffin oil or mineral oil) is distilled from crude oil. It is an emollient and lubricant. Liquid paraffin acts as a laxative. Paraffin wax can be petroleum paraffin wax or synthetic paraffin wax. Paraffin wax bath is used to treat painful joints, muscle sprain, and muscle spasms. It increases blood flow and decreases stiffness. It is also used in salons for nail and skin care. It is used as an embedding medium to make histology slides. Side effects include heat rash and chemical allergy. Paraffin oil and paraffin wax also have wide cosmetic, medical, and industrial application (for candles, crayons, polishes [floor, wood, leather] etc.). Microcrystalline wax is more tough and flexible compared to paraffin wax and has more industrial application. Gillespie, C. (2019, March 8). The benefits of paraffin wax and how to use it at home. *Healthline.* https://www.healthline.com/health/paraffin-wax ScienceDirect. (2019). Paraffin Oil—an overview. *ScienceDirect.* https://www.sciencedirect.com/topics/engineering/paraffin-oil Phosphatidylserine (PS) is a part of the cell membrane. It is mainly made in the body. It is also available from foods. The supplements are derived from animal source (cow brain) and plant source (cabbage or soya). The animal source is more effective.

Ingredients	Mechanism of Action and Health Benefits
Phosphatidylserine	PS is essential for brain function including memory, attention, focus, cognition, and mood. It can be used in dementia, ADHD, and autism.

It can also help reduce stress, insomnia, and anxiety in young adults.

Side effects include gastric upset and insomnia. There is a risk of mad cow disease if from a bovine source.

Graff-Radford, J. (2019, April 20). *Phosphatidylserine supplements: Can they improve memory?* Mayo Clinic. https://www.mayoclinic.org/diseases-conditions/alzheimers-disease/expert-answers/phosphatidylserine/faq-20057764

WebMD Editors. (n.d.). Phosphatidylserine. *WebMD*. https://www.webmd.com/vitamins/ai/ingredient-mono-992/phosphatidylserine

Pine bark
Pinus spp.

Other names: *Pinus pinaster (maritime or cluster pines)*

There are more than 100 species of pine or conifer trees. The *Pine* family consists of *Pinus* (Pine), *Picea* (Spruce), *Abies* (Fir), and *Larix* (Larch) *and Tsuga* (Hemlock) *genera*.

Various parts have medicinal value including needles, bark, cones, nuts, and resin. *Pinus pinaster* is most commonly found in Mediterranean countries. *Pinus eldarica* is also called *Afghan pine*.

Pine bark contains several bioactive constituents including phenolic compounds (procyanidins, caffeic acid, ferulic acid, catechins, and taxifolin), terpenes (α-pinene, myrtenal, and δ-3-carene), and sesquiterpene (β-caryophyllene). It is also rich in vitamins and minerals. Pine bark is commonly called pycnogenol.

The pine bark is ground, washed and then soaked in hot water and strained. The liquid extract is then freeze-dried. Then, it is ground into powder which is available as tablets or capsules.

It has antioxidant, antiinflammatory, antimicrobial, antiaging, and neuroprotective properties.

It can support heart health, relieve coughs and colds, and help in cancers.

It can help with ADHD, cognition, and other neurodegenerative disorders.

It can lower blood sugar and blood pressure and also help with metabolic syndrome.

Overall, it is safe. It should be avoided during pregnancy due to the presence of taxine (a toxic alkaloid). Some pine tree needles and barks are poisonous like yew and ponderosa pines.

Iravani, S., & Zolfaghari, B. (2014). Phytochemical analysis of *Pinus eldarica* bark. *Research in Pharmaceutical Sciences, 9*(4), 243–250.

Snyder, C. (2021, February 11). Pine bark extract: Uses, benefits, and side effects. *Healthline.* https://www.healthline.com/nutrition/pine-bark-extract

Pineapple
Ananas comosus

Pineapple is a low calorie fruit. It is rich in vitamin C, β-carotene, manganese, and calcium. It contains a digestive protease enzyme called bromelain which is used as a meat tenderizer. It is also rich in antioxidants such as phenolic acids and flavonoids. It has a high water and high fiber content. It has antiinflammatory, antioxidant, and anticancer effects.

The digestive enzyme is used to treat pancreatic insufficiency. The high fiber and water content is effective at relieving constipation. It may reduce GI cancers.

It is used to treat bronchitis and sinusitis. The bromelain also helps to loosen the mucus and improve symptoms of asthma and also decrease the symptoms in UTI. In some, it can paradoxically cause more bladder irritation.

It can lower the risk of diabetes, heart disease, obesity, and osteoporosis.

Side effects include pineapple allergy with itching or sore lips. It can worsen acid reflux.

Raman, R. (2018, May 26). 8 impressive health benefits of pineapple. *Healthline.* https://www.healthline.com/nutrition/benefits-of-pineapple

Ware, M. (2018, July 26). Everything you need to know about pineapple. *MedicalNewsToday.* https://www.medicalnewstoday.com/articles/276903#risks

Plantain weed/leaf
Plantago major

Other name: *Great plantain*

The major bioactive compounds in plantain weed include flavonoids (luteolin and apigenin), iridoid glycosides (aucubin), alkaloids, terpenoids, phenolic acid derivatives, and fatty acids.

It has antiinflammatory, antiseptic, astringent, diuretic, and detoxifying effects. It also contains epidermal growth factors which promote wound healing.

It can reduce mucus production in bronchitis, sinusitis, cough, cold, and flu.

It can help in constipation, hemorrhoids, mouth and gastric ulcers, and bleeding gums.

It can also be applied to wounds on eczema, diaper rash, cuts, bruises, insect bites, and psoriasis.

It may help reduce heavy bleeding in menorrhagia and also help in bladder infection.

Overall, it is a safe herb.

Ingredients	Mechanism of Action and Health Benefits
	Adom, M. B., Taher, M., Mutalabisin, M. F., Amri, M. S., Abdul Kudos, M. B., Wan Sulaiman, M. W. A., et al. (2017). Chemical constituents and medical benefits of *Plantago major*. *Biomedicine & Pharmacotherapy*, *96*, 348–360. https://doi.org/10.1016/j.biopha.2017.09.152
	Health Benefits Times. (2017, October 31). Health benefits of Plantain herb. *HealthBenefitstimes.com*. https://www.healthbenefitstimes.com/plantain-herb/
	WebMD Editors. (2013). Great Plantain. *WebMD*. https://www.thelancet.com/journals/lancet/article/PIIS0140-6736(12)61312-9/fulltext
Potato *Solanum tuberosum*	Potato is a plant from the nightshade family. The phytoconstituents in the skin include polyphenols (chlorogenic acid, catechin), carotenoids (lutein), kukoamines, and glycoalkaloids (solanine and chaconine). It is high in water, potassium, and vitamin C. It contains several other vitamins and minerals including vitamin B6, folate, choline, calcium, phosphorus, and iron. It also contains dietary fiber. It is a very filling food.
	It can help improve heart health by reducing high blood pressure and high blood sugar levels.
	It can help prevent skin damage from pollution, sun, and smoke. It can also improve skin rashes, acne, and overall skin health.
	Choline can help with improving mood, muscle movement, learning, and memory.
	The fiber present promotes digestion and helps prevent constipation.
	Generally it is safe. Potato allergy and allergy to glycoalkaloids can rarely occur. Long-term exposure to acrylamides (when frying potatoes) can increase the risk of certain cancers (such as mouth, kidneys, breast, ovaries, and esophagus). Excess consumption of potatoes can lead to weight gain and diabetes.
	Arnarson, A. (2019, March 7). Potatoes 101: Nutrition facts and health effects. *Healthline*. https://www.healthline.com/nutrition/foods/potatoes
	Ware, M. (2017, October 13). How can potatoes benefit my health? *MedicalNewsToday*. https://www.medicalnewstoday.com/articles/280579
Pokeweed *Phytolacca americana*	Other names: *American pokeweed, P. decandra, Indian pokeweed, dragonberries, American Nightshade, American Spinach, inkberry, chui xu shang*
	Pokeweed is a toxic and poisonous plant. It is used by native Indians and is generally not recommended.
	The pokeweed young leaves if cooked properly and the roots have antiinflammatory, purgative, and emetic properties.
	The root poultices are used to treat sprains, swellings, bruises, and arthritic joints.
	The leaf poultices can treat acne, eczema, and psoriasis. It acts as salve.
	It is used as homeopathic tinctures for tonsillitis and weight loss.
	Pokeweed contains phytolaccine, a toxic gastric irritant. Other side effects include hypotension, thirst, and urine incontinence.
	WebMD. (n.d.). POKEWEED: Overview, uses, side effects, precautions, interactions, dosing and reviews. https://www.webmd.com/vitamins/ai/ingredientmono-220/pokeweed
Pomegranate *Punica granatum*	Other names: *Shi liu, Dadima*
	Pomegranate is rich in antioxidants especially punicalagin (present in juice) and punicic acid (fatty acid in the seeds). It is rich in vitamins (C, A, E, and folic acid) and fiber.
	It has antiinflammatory, antioxidant, antiviral, antitumor, and immune-boosting properties. It has three times more antioxidants compared to red wine or green tea.
	It supports heart health, prevents atherosclerosis, and lowers blood pressure, cholesterol, and glucose.
	It also supports digestive health. It can prevent yeast and bacterial infections.
	The astringent and antioxidant properties prevent kidney stone formation. It also lowers the urine acidity.
	It boosts female fertility by improving blood circulation, thickening the endometrial lining, and enhances fetal growth. It can help in erectile dysfunction.
	It can improve memory and help in AD.
	It can prevent arthritis and strengthen the bones. It can also improve exercise strength and stamina.
	It may also reduce the risk of prostate and breast cancers.
	Apart from possible allergies, it is otherwise a safe and healthy super fruit. It can interact with antihypertensive, blood thinners, and diabetic medications.
	Leech, J. (2018, August 15). 12 health benefits of pomegranate. *Healthline*. https://www.healthline.com/nutrition/12-proven-benefits-of-pomegranate#TOC_TITLE_HDR_7

Ingredients	Mechanism of Action and Health Benefits
Prickly pear cactus *Opuntia*	Other name: *Nopal cactus* Prickly pear cactus is rich in antioxidants, fiber, and carotenoids. Flowers, leaves, and fruits are edible. It is also rich in vitamin C and flavonoids (kaempferol and quercetin). It has antiviral, antioxidant, and neuroprotective properties. It is rich in pectin and can lower blood glucose, cholesterol, and lipids. It is used to treat prostate enlargement. It can prevent hangovers before consuming alcohol. It is generally safe. Side effects can include gas and bloating, nausea, diarrhea, and headache. Gotter, A. (2017, May 25). Nopal cactus: Benefits and uses. *Healthline*. https://www.healthline.com/health/nopal#recipes Zeratsky, K. (2020, December 15). *Does prickly pear cactus have health benefits?* Mayo Clinic. https://www.mayoclinic.org/healthy-lifestyle/consumer-health/expert-answers/prickly-pear-cactus/faq-20057771
Prebiotics	*Prebiotics* are natural sugars (xylitol, rhamnose, fructo-oligosaccharides, and glucomannan) and indigestible food fibers. They are found in many fruits and vegetables. Prebiotic-containing foods include inulin (found in chicory root), onions, garlic, wheat bran, oats, barley, asparagus, bananas, and flaxseed. Prebiotics are added to cosmetics products including serums or moisturizers to maintain a healthy skin microbiome balance. Prebiotics are essentially foods consumed by probiotics. They feed on the good gut bacteria.
Probiotics	*Probiotics* are the good bacteria in and on the body that keep our bodies balanced and healthy inside and out. They are living bacteria that are ingested to give several health benefits. Probiotic foods include yogurt, kimchi, tempeh, kefir, and sauerkraut. Lactobacillus and Bifidobacteria are common strains of the beneficial bacteria. Others include Saccharomyces, Bacillus, Streptococcus, Escherichia and Enterococcus. It regulates the gut flora and gut microbiome. It supports digestive health and can treat or prevent diarrhea, constipation, IBS, and weight loss. It can also help reduce autism symptoms. It helps with immune system, allergies and helps reduce inflammation. It may help with cold and flu prevention. It can also prevent UTIs. Taking probiotics with at least 10 billion colony-forming units' dose during a cold/flu may reduce the symptoms. It should be taken at bedtime or on an empty stomach in the morning.
Postbiotics	*Postbiotics* are bioactive functional "waste products" which are produced by the probiotic bacteria when they eat and ferment prebiotic fiber and sugars. These products include mainly short-chain fatty acids (i.e., butyrate), bacterial lysates, enzymes, polysaccharides, and others. Short-chain fatty acids are low in leaky gut syndrome, IBD, and IBS. Taking butyrate supplements can be beneficial in these conditions. Postbiotics may also help with immunity and prevent colds and flu. *Synbiotics* refers to a combination of prebiotics and probiotics. Overall prebiotics, probiotics, and postbiotics are safe. Rarely, there is gas and bloating. Gunnars, K. (2020, December 9). Probiotics 101: A simple beginner's guide. *Healthline*. https://www.healthline.com/nutrition/probiotics-101 Nordqvist, J. (2020, June 25). Benefits of probiotics. *MedicalNewsToday*. https://www.medicalnewstoday.com/articles/264721 Wegh, C. A. M., Geerlings, S. Y., Knol, J., Roeselers, G., & Belzer, C. (2019). Postbiotics and their potential applications in early life nutrition and beyond. *International Journal of Molecular Sciences, 20*(19), 4673. https://doi.org/10.3390/ijms20194673
Prune *Prunus domestica*	Other name: *Dried European plum* Prunes are dried plums. There are two main types: the European plum (smaller and darker) and Japanese plum (larger and yellow-red). It is rich in antioxidants (mainly caffeoylquinic acids i.e., chlorogenic acid and neochlorogenic acid). It also contains minerals (especially potassium, iron, manganese, and boron) and vitamins (A, B6, C, and K). It is also rich in soluble and insoluble fibers, cholorogenic acid and sorbitol. These increase bowel movements and can prevent haemorrhoids. The soluble fiber also improves digestion and absorption of nutrients. It prevents bone and muscle loss and supports bone health. It supports heart health and prevents atherosclerosis. It also lowers the LDL cholesterol. Potassium helps with heart rhythms, maintains cardiac muscle contractions and blood pressure.

Ingredients	Mechanism of Action and Health Benefits
	Prunes can prevent anemia. It can reduce the risk of colon cancer. It can also lower appetite and help in weight loss.
	It can lower the bladder pH and make the environment more hostile for bacteria in UTI. It can also control the urge to urinate in an overactive bladder.
	Overconsumption of prunes may cause diarrhea and gas and bloating.
	Brennan, D. (2020, October 17). Prunes: Are there health benefits? *WebMD*. https://www.webmd.com/diet/prunes-health-benefits#2
	Fanous, S. (2019, March 7). The top health benefits of prunes and prune juice. *Healthline*. https://www.healthline.com/health/food-nutrition/top-benefits-of-prunes-prune-juice#iron
Pumpkin Seed *Cucurbita*	Pumpkin seeds contain several bioactive compounds including lutein, phenolic acids, and flavonoles. It contains monounsaturated (i.e., oleic acid which is an omega-3 fatty acid) and polyunsaturated (i.e., linoleic acid) good fats and insoluble fiber. Some saturated fat (i.e., palmitic acid) is also present. It is rich in various vitamins (including vitamins E, K, and carotenoid), minerals (zinc, copper, iron, manganese, phosphorus, and magnesium), and protein.
	It has antioxidant and antiinflammatory properties.
	It can reduce the risk of several cancers including prostate, lung, breast, stomach, and colon.
	It improves prostate and bladder health. It can relieve symptoms of enlarged prostate and ease urination. It can help with overactive bladder and UTIs.
	Pumpkin seeds help in weight loss and reduce the risk of obesity. It supports heart health and can regulate cholesterol, blood sugar, and blood pressure.
	The protein, magnesium, copper, and calcium content help to strengthen and preserve bones.
	It can help with insomnia.
	It can also improve sperm quality and help in infertility.
	The presence of phytate can reduce the absorption of iron and zinc. Allergic reactions are rare.
	Brown, M. J. (2018, September 24). Top 11 science-based health benefits of pumpkin seeds. *Healthline*. https://www.healthline.com/nutrition/11-benefits-of-pumpkin-seeds
	Kulczyński, B., Sidor, A., & Gramza-Micha≈Çowska, A. (2020). Antioxidant potential of phytochemicals in pumpkin varieties belonging to *Cucurbita moschata* and *Cucurbita pepo* species. *CyTA—Journal of Food, 18*(1), 472–484. https://doi.org/10.1080/19476337.2020.1778092
	WebMD Editorial Contributors. (2020, November 18). Health benefits of pumpkin seeds. *WebMD*. https://www.webmd.com/diet/health-benefits-pumpkin-seeds#1
Purple coneflower *Echinacea purpurea*	There are several species of purple coneflower but only three are used as medicinal herbs i.e., *Echinacea angustifolia*, *Echinacea purpurea*, and *Echinacea pallida*. The flowers, leaves, and roots are used.
	It contains several bioactive compounds such as phenolic acids (cichoric acid), alkamides, caffeic acid, flavonoid, polyacetylenes, and rosmarinic acid.
	It has antiinflammatory, antioxidant, antimicrobial, and immune-boosting properties.
	It is used for treating colds and flu. It can lower blood sugar and help reduce anxiety.
	It can improve eczema and acne. It can soothe and repair skin.
	Side effects include allergic reactions and nausea. It should not be taken in autoimmune disorders.
	Raman, R. (2018, October 25). Echinacea: Benefits, uses, side effects and dosage. *Healthline*. https://www.healthline.com/nutrition/echinacea
Purslane *Portulaca oleracea*	Other names: *Pigweed, Little hogweed, Fatweed*
	Purslane is a weed but also an edible superfood vegetable. It is a vegan omega-3 superfood with high omega-3 fatty acids i.e., ALA, GLA, and EPA. It contains several minerals (iron, magnesium, manganese, calcium, and potassium) and vitamins (A and B). It is low in calories. It can be eaten raw or cooked.
	It has antiinflammatory, antioxidant, laxative, and diuretic properties.
	It supports heart health. It can lower cholesterol and triglycerides. It is used as a heart tonic. It can also lower blood glucose.
	As an essential fatty acid, it is important for cell growth and development. It has immune-boosting properties.
	It can also be used for osteoporosis.
	Palsdottir, H. (2017, June 16). Purslane—A tasty "weed" that is loaded with nutrients. *Healthline*. https://www.healthline.com/nutrition/purslane

Ingredients	Mechanism of Action and Health Benefits
	Uddin, M. K., Juraimi, A. S., Hossain, M. S., Nahar, M. A. U., Ali, M. E., & Rahman, M. M. (2014). Purslane weed (*Portulaca oleracea*): a prospective plant source of nutrition, omega-3 fatty acid, and antioxidant attributes. *The Scientific World Journal, 2014*, 1–6. https://doi. org/10.1155/2014/951019
Raspberry leaf *Rubus idaeus*	Other name: *Red raspberry leaf*
	Red raspberry leaves contain several bioactive compounds including antioxidants and polyphenols (such as flavonoids, tannins, and ellagic acids). The antispasmodic effects are due to the presence of fragarine.
	It is rich in vitamins (B and C) and several minerals (including magnesium, potassium, phosphorus, zinc, and iron).
	It is referred to as a "woman's herb." It can reduce premenstrual symptoms and menstrual cramps. It may reduce morning sickness during pregnancy, strengthen the uterus, induce and shorten labor during pregnancy, and also prevent postpartum bleeding after childbirth.
	Tea from the leaves and the fruit are effective to expel calcium oxalate kidney stones.
	Raspberry ketones (rheosmin or frambinone) are natural compounds that are found in the red raspberry fruit that give its aroma. It is also present in rhubarb, pine tree bark, and other fruits (kiwi, peach, and apple) and it can help with weight loss.
	Overconsumption of the leaves may cause diuresis and increased bowel movements.
	Goodson, A. (2018, July 30). Red raspberry leaf tea: Pregnancy, benefits and side effects. *Healthline.* https://www.healthline.com/nutrition/red-raspberry-leaf-tea#benefits
Red Clover *Trifolium pratense* White Clover *Trifolium repens*	Other names: *Clover, Trefoil, Dutch clover or White clover (Trifolium repens)*
	There are more than 300 species of clover. Commonly cultivated clovers are white clover *(Trifolium repens)* and red clover *(Trifolium pratense)*. They are grown for grazing by livestock (as animal fodder).
	Sweet clover is not a true clover. They are also grown for livestock and are also usually eaten by wildlife and birds. There are two common types: yellow sweet clover *(Melilotus officinalis)* and white sweet clover *(Melilotus alba)*.
	Based on the number of leaflets, clovers are classified as three-leaf clover (commonest), four-leaf clover, and the five-leaf clover. Trifolium refers to the three-leaf clover.
	Red clover contains isoflavones, flavonoids, coumarins, and tyramine. The isoflavones (like biochanin A, formononetin, and daidzein) demonstrate phytoestrogenic activity.
	It has antioxidant and antiinflammatory properties.
	It strengthens the bones and improves bone health. It is used in the treatment of osteoporosis and arthritis.
	The high isoflavone content helps in lowering menopause symptoms such as night sweats and hot flashes. It can also improve depression, anxiety, and vaginal dryness in menopausal women.
	It also promotes hair growth and improves skin health. It also improves heart health and lowers LDL cholesterol.
	It can also help in weight loss, cough, asthma, and cancer.
	Red clover is generally considered safe. Potential side effects include nausea, headache, prolonged menstruation, vaginal spotting, and skin irritation. It should be avoided by those with hormone-sensitive conditions like ovarian and breast cancer or endometriosis and those taking blood thinners and oral contraceptives.
	Davidson, K. (2020, August 20). Red clover: Benefits, uses, and side effects. *Healthline.* https://www. healthline.com/nutrition/red-clover#benefits
	A. Romm, S. S. Weed, P. Gardiner, B. Bhattacharya, & C. A. Lennox (Eds.) (2009). Chapter 19— Menopausal Health. In *Botanical Medicine for Women's Health* (1st ed., pp. 455–520). Edinburgh: Churchill Livingstone. https://doi.org/10.1016/B978-0-443-07277-2.00021-0
Resveratrol	Resveratrol is a polyphenol. The main sources of resveratrol are red wine, skin and seeds of grapes and berries, and also peanuts.
	It has antioxidant, antiinflammatory, anticancer, estrogenic, detoxifying, and neuroprotective properties. It can increase longevity.
	It supports heart health. It can lower blood sugar, blood pressure, and LDL cholesterol. It increases insulin sensitivity and activates AMPK protein. It promotes vasodilation via the nitric oxide pathway.
	It can also help in arthralgia and arthritis.

Ingredients	Mechanism of Action and Health Benefits
	Overall, it is safe.
	Jennings, K. (2017, March 3). 7 health benefits of resveratrol supplements. *Healthline*. https://www.healthline.com/nutrition/resveratrol#TOC_TITLE_HDR_3
	Watson, S. (2009, October 20). Resveratrol supplements. *WebMD*. https://www.webmd.com/heart-disease/resveratrol-supplements
Rhubarb *Rheum rhabarbarum* *Rheum palmatum*	Other name: *Da Huang, Chinese rhubarb (Rheum palmatum)* Rhubarb contains various bioactive compounds including stilbenes, anthraquinones, and flavonoids. It is also rich in antioxidants (anthocyanins and proanthocyanidins). It is also an excellent source of vitamin K which is essential for bones and blood clotting. It also contains other vitamins (A, C, and folate) and minerals (calcium, potassium, magnesium, and manganese). It has antiinflammatory, anticancer, and antimicrobial properties. In TCM, rhubarb is believed to eliminate dampness and drain the excess heat. It can also cool the blood and stop bleeding. Rhubarb root is also commonly used as a purgative agent due to its laxative properties. It is used to treat liver, spleen, and stomach dysfunctions as well as blood purification. It is also known to prevent cardiovascular disorders and help reduce cholesterol levels. Rhubarb (mainly leaves) is high in calcium oxalate. Too much consumption of calcium oxalate can lead to hyperoxaluria, which is the buildup of oxalate crystals in different organs. This can also promote kidney stones. Brennan, D. (2020, September 24). Health benefits of Rhubarb. *WebMD*. https://www.webmd.com/diet/health-benefits-rhubarb#2 Kołodziejczyk-Czepas, J., & Liudvytska, O. (2020). *Rheum rhaponticum* and *Rheum rhabarbarum*: a review of phytochemistry, biological activities and therapeutic potential. *Phytochemistry Reviews*, *20*(3), 589–607. https://doi.org/10.1007/s11101-020-09715-3 Me and Qi. (n.d.). Rhubarb. *meandqi.com*. https://www.meandqi.com/herb-database/rhubarb
Rooibos *Aspalathus linearis*	Other name: *Red bush tea* There are two types of rooibos tea i.e., red and green. The common red rooibos tea is fermented or oxidized and tastes sweet like hibiscus tea. The green rooibos is nonoxidized and tastes earthy like yerba mate. Rooibos contains flavonoids (quercetin and chrysoeriol), polyphenol glucoside (aspalathin), and tannins. The chrysoeriol has bronchodilator effects. Rooibos also has natural ACE inhibitor properties to relax blood vessels. It has antioxidant, antiinflammatory, antispasmodic, and immune-boosting effects. It aids in digestion and can prevent bloating and cramps. It helps reduce diarrhea. It can support heart health. It lowers the LDL cholesterol and blood pressure, improves circulation, and decreases atherosclerotic plaque buildup. It can also reduce insulin resistance and blood sugar. Overall, it is safe. Very rare cases of raised liver enzymes and estrogen have been reported. Brown, M. J. (2018, November 13). 5 health benefits of rooibos tea (plus side effects). *Healthline*. https://www.healthline.com/nutrition/rooibos-tea-benefits WebMD Editorial Contributors. (2020, September 30). Are there health benefits to drinking rooibos tea? *WebMD*. https://www.webmd.com/diet/health-benefits-rooibos-tea#1
Rose hip/Rosehip *Rosa canina L.*	Other names: *Dog rose* Rose hip is at the base of the petals which is red-orange in color. It has both culinary and medicinal uses. It is rich in antioxidants such as quercetin, catechin, ellagic acid, tiliroside and carotenoids (beta-carotene and lycopene). It also contains polyunsaturated fats. *Rosehip oil* is cold-pressed oil extracted from the seeds or pseudo-fruit (usually from *Rosa canina, Rosa rubiginosa* or *Rosa moschata*). It has high essential fatty acids, polyphenols, vitamin A (carotenoids including lycopene) and Vitamin E (tocopherols) mainly and also vitamins C, K, B1, B2 and B3. It has analgesic, anti-inflammatory, antiseptic, anti-aging and anti-arthritic properties. It helps in skin rejuvenation and skin cell regeneration. It maintains skin health and can reduce wrinkles, acne, eczema, scars, stretch marks and skin hyperpigmentation. It also helps with wound healing. It stimulates hair growth.

Ingredients	Mechanism of Action and Health Benefits
	It can prevent kidney stone formation. It increases urinary citrate.
	It may also lower cholesterol, blood pressure and promote fat loss.
	It can relieve joint inflammation in osteoarthritis and other rheumatoid disorders.
	Rosehip is also functional food. It can also be consumed as rosehip jam, jelly or juice.
	Side effects may include stomach upset.
	Davidson, K. (2019, December 4). *What Are Rose Hips, and Do They Have Benefits?* Healthline. https://www.healthline.com/nutrition/rose-hips#side-effects
Rosemary *Rosmarinus officinalis*	Rosemary is an herb in the mint family. It has culinary and medicinal uses. It contains triterpenes (ursolic acid), phenolic diterpenes (carnosic acid, rosmanol, and carnosol), and flavonoids. It is rich in vitamins (B and C) and minerals (including iron and calcium).
	It has antioxidant, antiinflammatory, analgesic, neuroprotective, antiarthritic, antispasmodic, and immune-boosting activities. It can reduce cortisol hormone. It can act synergistically with certain antibiotics.
	Rosemary helps to boost digestion and metabolism. It may improve the release of bile. It is used to treat indigestion, constipation, and food poisoning.
	It can also improve memory, focus, performance, concentration, mood, energy, and speed. It can prevent aging and may help in AD, stroke, and macular degeneration. It can reduce stress, mental fatigue, and anxiety.
	It may also help in rheumatoid arthritis and osteoporosis.
	It can kill *Propionibacterium acnes (P. acnes)* bacteria found under skin in acne. It can also be used for eczema. It can clear dandruff and promote hair growth.
	It is also an insect repellent against Aedes aegypti mosquitoes and head lice.
	Side effects include nausea, vomiting, pulmonary edema, and coma due to overconsumption. It can interact with ACE inhibitor antihypertensives, diuretics, and blood thinners.
	McCulloch, M. (2018, November 15). 14 benefits and uses of rosemary essential oil. *Healthline*. https://www.healthline.com/nutrition/rosemary-oil-benefits
	Nordqvist, J. (2017, December 13). Everything you need to know about rosemary. *MedicalNews Today*. https://www.medicalnewstoday.com/articles/266370#benefits
Rutabaga	Other names: *Swede, Swedish turnip*
	It is a root vegetable that is a hybrid between a turnip and a cabbage. It belongs to the cruciferous family. It is rich in antioxidants (vitamins A, i.e., carotenoids, C, and E). It contains minerals (magnesium, calcium, and potassium). The presence of glucosinolates are heart-protective and may also prevent cancers. It is also high in fiber.
	Excessive consumption can cause bloating.
	Davidson, K. (2019, July 10). 7 powerful health benefits of rutabagas. *Healthline*. https://www.healthline.com/nutrition/rutabagas
Sacha inchi *Plukenetia volubilis*	Other names: *Mountain peanut, Inca nut*
	The seeds of the sacha inchi plant are pressed to extract oil or roasted and ground into fine powder. The leaves are dried to make tea. It is a vegan omega-3 superfood. It contains several bioactive compounds including phenolic compounds and flavonoids.
	It is rich in protein, fiber, minerals (potassium, magnesium, phosphorus, zinc, and calcium) and vitamins (E and carotenoids). It is high in unsaturated fats.
	It has antiinflammatory and antioxidant properties.
	It lowers LDL and cholesterol and increases HDL cholesterol.
	It supports gut health and can help with IBS, piles, and diverticulitis. It also enhances weight loss.
	Gonzales, G. F., & Gonzales, C. (2014). A randomized, double-blind placebo-controlled study on acceptability, safety and efficacy of oral administration of sacha inchi oil (*Plukenetia volubilis* L.) in adult human subjects. *Food and Chemical Toxicology*, 65, 168–176. https://doi.org/10.1016/j.fct.2013.12.039
	Link, R. (2021, June 11). What is sacha inchi? Uses, benefits, side effects, and forms. *Healthline*. https://www.healthline.com/nutrition/what-is-sacha-inchi#benefits

Ingredients	Mechanism of Action and Health Benefits
Sage *Salvia officinalis*	Sage has culinary and medicinal uses. It contains flavonoids (such as apigenin, luteolin, and quercetin), phenolic acids (rosmarinic acid, caffeic acid, ferulic acid, chlorogenic acid, and ellagic acid), and glycoside (rutin). It is rich in vitamins (especially K and A, C, and E) and minerals (magnesium and copper). It has antioxidant, antiinflammatory, antimicrobial, antiaging, neuroprotective, and estrogen-like properties. The essential oil has uropathogenic actions. It can treat indigestion (including nausea, gas and bloating). Sage mouthwash can kill streptococcus bacteria and candida yeast. It can prevent or treat dental caries, infected gums, mouth ulcers, and throat infection. It can improve memory, mood, and alertness. It can help AD, dementia, and stroke. It can lower blood sugar levels by improving insulin sensitivity. It can also reduce LDL cholesterol levels. It may reduce menopausal symptoms. It may prevent GI and breast and kidney tumors. Side effects include vomiting, agitation, tethytheria, dizziness, tremors, convulsion, and kidney failure. Raman, R. (2018, December 14). 12 health benefits and uses of sage. *Healthline*. https://www.healthline.com/nutrition/sage#TOC_TITLE_HDR_2
Salt *Sodium Chloride*	Other name: Saline Salt consists of 60% chloride and 40% sodium. Some salts may contain trace amounts of iron, potassium, calcium, and zinc. Iodine is also added to salt. Iodide salt can help improve thyroid function. Salt promotes electron balance and helps in keeping the body hydrated. It can also improve cystic fibrosis symptoms, used as a nasal spray for coughs, colds, and flus, to prevent hypotension. Overall, salt is safe. Excess salt can cause water retention, bloating, stroke, heart attack, stomach cancer, and osteoporosis. Higuera, V., & Kennedy, K. (2019, July 7). All about salt: Health benefits, risks, types, and how to cut back. *EverydayHealth.com*. https://www.everydayhealth.com/diet-nutrition/diet/salt-health-benefits-risks-types-how-cut-back-more/
Salvia *Salvia divinorum*	Salvia belongs to the mint family. The main bioactive compound is salvinorin A, a terpenoid. It activates k-neuroreceptors. It has antioxidant properties. It is neuroprotective and can increase blood flow to the brain. It can improve memory, reaction time, cognition, and child's developmental milestones. Side effects include nausea, hallucination, and dizziness if it is inhaled or chewed as psychedelic drug. It can also lead to drug dependency. Brito-da-Costa, A. M., & Carvalho, A. M. (2021, March 3). Salvia divinorum. *encyclopedia.ub*. https://encyclopedia.pub/8665#:%7E:text=divinorum%20was%20brought%20to%20the,divinorum%20in%201982. Holland, K. (2018, September 18). What is Salvia Divinorum? *Healthline*. https://www.healthline.com/health/what-is-salvia RxList Editors. (2021, June 11). Salvia Divinorum. *RxList*. https://www.rxlist.com/salvia_divinorum/supplements.htm
S-adenosylmethionine *SAMe*	S-adenosylmethionie is a part of the cell membrane. It regulates hormones and maintains cell structure integrity. It is mainly made in the body. It is available as a dietary supplement (in oral, intravenous, and intramuscular forms). It is used to treat depression, osteoarthritis, and liver disease. It can also help in dementia including AD, CFS, anxiety, and PD. In osteoarthritis, it can reduce knee pain. It can stimulate some cartilage to be produced. It may also help in other musculoskeletal problems including backache, tendonitis, and bursitis. In liver disease, it can improve the bile flow from the liver (cholestasis). Side effects include gastric upset, irritability, sleeplessness, and anxiety. It should not be taken if there is an immune deficiency or in bipolar disorder. It can interact with antidepressants or antipsychotics, St. John's Wort or L-Dopa and causes serotonin syndrome. Mayo Clinic Staff. (2020, November 18). *SAMe*. Mayo Clinic. https://www.mayoclinic.org/drugs-supplements-same/art-20364924 WebMD Editors. (n.d.). *SAMe*. WebMD.https://www.webmd.com/vitamins/ai/ingredientmono-786/same

Ingredients	Mechanism of Action and Health Benefits
Saw Palmetto *Serenoa repens*	Saw palmetto contains phytosterols (mainly β-sitosterol), antioxidants (epicatechin and methyl gallate), and fatty acids (including linoleic acid, oleic acid, stearic acid, and palmitic acid). It has antiinflammatory properties. It helps block the activity of 5-alpha reductase (5α-R) which helps reduce hair loss and improves hair growth. It improves urinary tract symptoms associated with benign prostate hyperplasia (BPH). It is also used for difficulty urinating and urinary incontinence. It may help lower the risk of prostate cancer. It can also help maintain testosterone levels. Overall, it is safe. Side effects may include dizziness, headache, nausea, and constipation. Link, R. (2019, March 20). 5 Promising benefits and uses of saw palmetto. *Healthline*. https://www.healthline.com/nutrition/saw-palmetto-benefits Maya-Luevano, R. (2017). Nutrition and functional foods for healthy aging. In J. A. Clor & M. P. Ferreira (Eds.), *Chapter 25—North American natural health products and sexual function in aging adults* (1st ed., pp. 293–303). London: Academic Press. https://doi.org/10.1016/B978-0-12-805376-8.00025-3
Selenium	It is a micronutrient trace mineral that is essential for cell metabolism. It is present in organic form (as selenocysteine, seleno-L-methionine [SLM], and Se-methylselenocysteine [MSC]) and inorganic form (as selenates, selenades and selenites). There are also many other forms. Only seleno-L-methionine (SLM) form is used as a nutritional supplement. Natural dietary sources of selenium include Brazil nuts, seafood (tuna and sardine), organ meats, dairy products, broccoli, barley, and whole grains. Selenium metabolism is a complex process. It has immunomodulatory, antioxidant, anti-inflammatory and anti-cancer (chemopreventive) properties. It can repair DNA. Some data indicate that selenium may have tumor-promoting effects although most studies show that selenium deficiency in blood is associated with higher cancer incidence and also more viral infections. Intravenous high dose inorganic selenium is used as adjunctive treatment with chemotherapy to treat cancers, improve tumour biomarkers and reduce chemotherapy-induced side effects such as peripheral neuropathy by paclitaxel. Selenium also maintains thyroid health and cognitive fuctions. Side effects include gastric upsets, hypersensitivity reactions and garlic odour. WebMD Editorial Contributors. (2020, November 11). Healthy Foods High in Selenium. WebMD. https://www.webmd.com/diet/foods-high-in-selenium#1 Rataan, A. O., Geary, S. M., Zakharia, Y., Rustum, Y. M., & Salem, A. K. (2022). Potential Role of Selenium in the Treatment of Cancer and Viral Infections. *International Journal of Molecular Sciences*, 23(4), 2215. https://doi.org/10.3390/ijms23042215
Sheep sorrel *Rumex acetosella*	Other names: *Red sorrel, Garden sorrel, Common sorrel* Sheep sorrel contains tannins (it dries mucus secretion), anthraquinones (antioxidants), and oxalates. It is mostly used for respiratory ailments. It is different from the Indian sorrel which is used more for digestive disorders. Sheep sorrel has antiinflammatory and anticancer properties. It also has diuretic, laxative, and blood-thinning effects. It is often combined with several other Western herbs for the treatment of sinusitis and bronchitis. Overall, it is safe. Occasional side effects include oxalate kidney stones, diarrhea, and allergic rash with overconsumption. Memorial Sloan Kettering Cancer Center. (2019, November 15). *Sheep Sorrel*. https://www.mskcc.org/cancer-care/integrative-medicine/herbs/sheep-sorrel RxList Editors. (2021, June 11). Sorrel. *RxList*. https://www.rxlist.com/sorrel/supplements.htm
Shepherd's purse leaf *Capsella bursa – pastoris*	Shepherd's purse leaf belongs to the mustard family. It contains flavonoids and phenolic acids. It has antiinflammatory and antioxidant properties. It can reduce clotting. It is used in heavy menstrual bleeding and postpartum bleeding. It also helps in nosebleeds, lowers blood pressure, and promotes wound healing. Side effects include drowsiness, weakness, and shortness of breath with high doses. There may be drug interactions with sedatives, blood thinners, and thyroid medications. Shoemaker, S. (2020, June 26). Shepherd's purse: Benefits, dosage, side effects, and more. *Healthline*. https://www.healthline.com/health/shepherds-purse

Ingredients	Mechanism of Action and Health Benefits

Slippery elm
Ulmus rubra

The inner bark of slippery elm contains mucilage which gives soothing and demulcent effects on the throat, gut, and skin.

It is antitussive and can relieve the coughs in sore throat, bronchitis, and asthma.

It also stimulates the nerve endings in the gut to increase more mucus secretion which may protect and heal the gut in ulcers and excess acidity. It can help inflammatory bowel disorders like Crohn's disease or ulcerative colitis and IBS. It also contains soluble polysaccharides which act like a fiber laxative. The presence of antioxidants also can heal colitis.

It can also be soothing in urinary tract irritation from cystitis.

It can be used as a poultice or salve for burns, wounds, boils, and skin ulcers or inflammation.

It is generally safe. There is risk of hepatotoxicity due to the presence of PAs. The presence of mucilage may affect the absorption of other medications hence affecting its efficacy.

Griffin, R. M. (2013, October 21). Slippery elm: Uses and risks. *WebMD*. https://www.webmd.com/vitamins-and-supplements/slippery-elm-uses-and-risks

Silver, N. (2018, August 20). Can you use slippery elm to treat acid reflux? *Healthline*. https://www.healthline.com/health/digestive-health/slippery-elm-for-acid-reflux

Snowdrop
Galanthus woronowii

Other names: Kemularia, Fair Maid of February

There are many *Galanthus* species. The common ones are *G. woronowii, G. nivalis* and *G. elwesii*. It is a small early spring plant with white flowers.

The main phytoactive compounds in the bulbs are the alkaloids (galanthamine and lycorine) which have acetylcholinesterase activity. There are many other alkaloids (isoquinoline-like compounds) which have antibacterial, antiviral, anti-inflammatory, antioxidant and anticancer actions. Lectin may have anti-HIV effects.

Snowdrop was widely used as folk medicine. The plant bulb and leaves were rubbed on the forehead to relieve headache, migraine and to improve memory and focus. Galantamine is a competitive, reversible, acetylcholinesterase inhibitor. It increases brain acetylcholine, a neurotransmitter.

It is also used to treat traumatic brain injuries. Galantamine is now widely used as a memory supplement in Alzheimer disease and mild dementia.

It is an emmenagogue and increases menstrual flow.

Overall, it is safe. It can induce miscarriage and should not be used during pregnancy.

Royal College of Physicians. (2017, February 24). White here, white now: The medicinal power of the dainty snowdrop. https://www.rcplondon.ac.uk/news/white-here-white-now-medicinal-power-dainty-snowdrop

Kong, C. K., Low, L. E., Siew, W. S., Yap, W. H., Khaw, K. Y., Ming, L. C., Mocan, A., Goh, B. H., & Goh, P. H. (2021). Biological Activities of Snowdrop (Galanthus spp., Family Amaryllidaceae). Frontiers in Pharmacology, 11. https://doi.org/10.3389/fphar.2020.552453

Stinging nettle
Urtica dioica

Other names: *Nettle, Common nettle, Nettle leaf, Bichu.*

Cooked and steamed stinging nettle is edible. Fresh leaves should not be eaten. It contains polyphenols (including quercetin, acetylcholine, coumarins, and caffeic acid), tannins, and lectin. The nettle hairs contain serotonin and acetylcholine.

It has antiinflammatory, antioxidant, and antiallergic properties. It prevents the conversion of testosterone into dihydrotestosterone (antiandrogenic activity).

It is rich in minerals (calcium and iron), vitamins (A, D, K, and C), and chlorophyll. It is used as a general health tonic and can help in anemia. It can regulate hormone balance, ovulation, and menstrual cycles. It helps with menorrhagia and PCOS. It is a fertility tonic and can prepare the uterus for pregnancy.

It is a natural diuretic and can treat incontinence, enlarged prostate, kidney stones, and UTI.

It can lower blood sugar and blood pressure.

It can reduce postoperative bleeding.

It promotes wound healing when applied topically. It is a great hair tonic and is used in hair loss.

Oral or topical forms of nettle can also reduce pain in arthritis. It can help in hay fever by decreasing histamine release.

Side effects include allergic reactions, stomach upsets, and diarrhea from the fresh leaves. There is drug interaction with diuretic, blood thinners, and diabetes medications.

Raman, R. (2018, November 21). 6 evidence-based benefits of stinging nettle. *Healthline*. https://www.healthline.com/nutrition/stinging-nettle#TOC_TITLE_HDR_3

Ingredients	Mechanism of Action and Health Benefits
St John's wort *Hypericum perforatum*	St John's wort contains several bioactive compounds including hyperforin, hypericin, pseudohypericin, and hyperforin. It stimulates the GABA receptors and regulates serotonin. These active ingredients can be denatured by light. It is used in the treatment of anxiety, depression, CFS, fibromyalgia, and insomnia. It can also be used for PMS, menopausal symptoms, and ADHD. It can also help indigestion. It is effective in treating burns, wounds, bruises, and sores. It should not be taken with **Monoamine oxidase inhibitors** (MAOIs) inhibitors because of serotonin syndrome risk. It may also cause restlessness, vivid dreams, and stomach irritation and hence difficulty sleeping. It can interact with benzodiazepine, digoxin, oral contraceptives, and PPIs. It should be used with caution in major depression as it may trigger mania. Pietrangelo, A. (2018, June 7). St. John's Wort: The benefits and the dangers. *Healthline*. https://www.healthline.com/health-news/is-st-johns-wort-safe-080615#The-benefits-of-St.-Johns-wort RxList Editors. (2021, June 11). St. John's Wort. *RxList*. https://www.rxlist.com/st_johns_wort/supplements.htm
Sumac *Rhus coriaria*	Other name: *Syrian sumac* Sumac has many species. It is a plant herb which has culinary and medicinal uses. The red fruits are dried and used as a seasoning. It is rich in antioxidants including flavonoids, tannins, and anthocyanins. It also contains monounsaturated fats i.e., oleic acid and linoleic acid. It has antidiabetic actions. Rare allergic reactions may occur. It must be differentiated from poison. Hill, A. (2020, November 5). Sumac: Benefits, uses, and forms. *Healthline*. https://www.healthline.com/nutrition/sumac-benefits-uses-and-forms
Sunflower oil *Helianthus annuus*	Sunflower oil is made by pressing *Helianthus annuus* plant seeds. It contains unsaturated fatty acids (such as linoleic acid and oleic acid) and saturated fatty acids (stearic acid). It is rich in vitamins E and K. It has antiinflammatory and antibacterial properties. The high content of unsaturated fatty acids helps in lowering the LDL cholesterol and triglyceride levels. This reduces the risk of heart disease. Sunflower oil also improves brain function and reduces the progress of AD. It is used to moisturize the skin in eczema. Overconsumption can lead to obesity, heart-related disorders. Heating of sunflower oil releases aldehydes that can increase the risk of cancer. Brennan, D. (2020, October 30). Sunflower oil: Is it good for you? *WebMD*. https://www.webmd.com/diet/sunflower-oil-good-for-you#1-3 Streit, L. (2020, March 3). Is sunflower oil healthy? *Healthline*. https://www.healthline.com/nutrition/is-sunflower-oil-healthy
Sunflower seed *Helianthus annuus*	Sunflower seeds are the fruits of the sunflower plant (*Helianthus annuus*). The phytochemical constituents present in sunflower seed include phenolic acids, flavonoids, and tocopherols. It is rich in fiber, vitamins (E, B1, and B6), and minerals (iron, copper, selenium, manganese, potassium, and zinc). The selenium and zinc present have immunomodulatory and antimicrobial effects. It has antiinflammatory, antioxidant, and wound-healing properties. Consumption of sunflower seeds can reduce the risk of developing high blood pressure, high cholesterol, or cardiovascular diseases. It is used for treating bronchial, laryngeal, and pulmonary infections. It is also useful for treatment of coughs and colds and whooping cough. Sunflower seeds should be taken in moderation due to its high calorie and sodium content. It also contains cadmium which is a heavy metal that can harm the kidneys from long-term exposure. Eating a large number of sunflower seeds can also cause fecal impaction in both children and adults. Acute allergy reactions are relatively uncommon. Guo, S., Ge, Y., & Na Jom, K. (2017). A review of phytochemistry, metabolite changes, and medicinal uses of the common sunflower seed and sprouts (*Helianthus annuus* L.). *Chemistry Central Journal*, *11*(95). https://doi.org/10.1186/s13065-017-0328-7 McCulloch, M. (2018, November 22). Are sunflower seeds good for you? Nutrition, benefits and more. *Healthline*. https://www.healthline.com/nutrition/sunflower-seeds

Ingredients	Mechanism of Action and Health Benefits
Sour cherry *Prunus cerasus*	Other name: *Tart cherry*

There are two common varieties of tart cherries, i.e., Montmorency and Morello varieties.

Tart cherries contain quercetin, anthocyanins, and tryptophan. They are rich in several vitamins (such as A, C, and K) and minerals (manganese, copper, and potassium). It has more anthocyanins compared to black cherries. They are usually used for cooking or making fresh juice.

It has antioxidant and antiinflammatory properties.

It contains natural melatonin and also increases the bioavailability of tryptophan which is a substrate for melatonin synthesis. Melatonin is a natural sleep hormone in the body. Tart cherry juice helps insomnia and improves sleep quality and duration by increasing melatonin in the body.

It also can reduce muscle soreness and muscle strength loss. It may also reduce arthritis and gout symptoms such as joint pain and swelling.

It can improve brain function and reduce symptoms of mild-to-moderate dementia, AD, and PD.

Overall, it is safe. It contains a high content of sorbitol which can cause diarrhea and stomach pain. Quercetin can interact with blood thinner medications.

Petre, A. (2017, June 10). 10 health benefits of Tart cherry juice. *Healthline*. https://www.healthline.com/nutrition/10-tart-cherry-juice-benefits

Sweet Cherry *Prunus serontina*

Other names: *Black cherry, Wild black cherry*

There are many varieties of sweet cherries (from dark to light colors), the common ones being Bing, Maraschino, Black Chelan, Lapin, Tulare, Lambert, and Rainier varieties. They are usually eaten fresh.

Sweet cherries contain active compounds including flavonoids (anthocyanin), carotenoids (β-carotene), polyphenols, terpenes, and tocopherols. It is also rich in iron and melatonin. Sweet cherries have higher protein, calories (sugar), and sodium and lesser anthocyanins, iron, and acidity compared to tart cherries.

It has antiinflammatory, antioxidant, antiaging, and anticancer properties.

It is beneficial for heart health. It helps lower cholesterol levels and reduce the risk of stroke and heart disease.

It can also help arthritis. It can decrease the uric acid levels in gout. It can prevent dental plaque and cavities.

It is effective against insomnia, migraine, and depression. It also improves skin health and improves hair growth. It can also be used to treat anemia.

It is effective for dry spasmodic cough and throat irritation and can open the airways.

The seeds and leaves are rich in hydrogen cyanide which in excess can cause poisoning, respiratory failure, and even death.

Health Benefits Times. (2018, September 5). Health benefits of black cherry. *HealthBenefitstimes.com*. https://www.healthbenefitstimes.com/black-cherry/

Sweet broom *Scoparia dulcis*

Other names: *Kallurukki ("stone melter"), Sweet broom (Scoparia dulcis), Common sweet broom (Cytisus racemosus), Common broom or Scotch broom (Cytisus scoparius).*

There are two main species in Broom plants, i.e., *Cytisus* spp. and *Genista* spp. The common sweet broom is *Cytisus racemosus* syn *Genista racemosa*. *Cytisus scoparius* is common broom or Scotch broom. They are invasive weeds and are largely ornamental plants. It contains scoparin (a diuretic) and sparteine (an antiarrhythmic).

Scoparia dulcis, also commonly known as sweet broom, is a weed and has more traditional medicine uses. It contains terpenes (scoparic acids A–C, scopadulciol, and scopadulin), flavones, and steroids.

It has analgesic, antipyretic, antiinflammatory, antimicrobial, hypoglycemic, and antihyperlipidemic actions.

It can treat kidney stones, urinary disorders, stomach ailments, hypertension, diabetes, bronchitis, and hemorrhoids.

Adverse reactions include sympathetic effects.

Drugs.com. (2021, March 22). *Sweet broomweed*. https://www.drugs.com/npp/sweet-broomweed.html

Heath, S. (2021, July 3). Broom plants: Care & growing guide. *The Spruce*. https://www.thespruce.com/growing-broom-plants-5089367

Prasad, S. (2020, September 26). 16 uses of sweetbroom in folk medicine. *Things Guyana*. https://www.thingsguyana.com/16-uses-of-sweetbroom-in-folk-medicine/

Ingredients	Mechanism of Action and Health Benefits
Tea Tree oil *Melaleuca* *alternifolia*	Tea tree oil contains a number of active compounds including terpinols (terpinen-4-ol) and terpenoids (1.8-cineole). It has antifungal, antiinflammatory, antiseptic, and antibiotic properties. It can be used for acne, contact dermatitis, psoriasis, dandruff, and head lice. It can soothe and repair the skin in eczema. It is also used for nail fungal infections. It can be used to treat bacterial infections (*staphylococcus*). The oil can also be used to make mouthwash for reducing dental plaque and bad breath. It may be used as an insect repellent. Overall, it is safe. Oral consumption should be avoided as it might be toxic. It may cause allergic reactions. Khan, N. (2017, April 21). 14 everyday uses for tea tree oil. *Healthline*. https://www.healthline.com/nutrition/tea-tree-oil#The-Bottom-Line Mayo Clinic Staff. (2020, November 14). *Tea tree oil*. Mayo Clinic. https://www.mayoclinic.org/drugs-supplements-tea-tree-oil/art-20364246
Thyme *Thymus vulgaris*	Thyme is used for both culinary and medicinal purposes. There are many varieties. *Thymus vulgaris* is commonly used for cooking. It contains several active ingredients including volatile oils (mainly thymol and carvacrol), flavonoids (thymonin, apigenin, luteolin, and naringenin), terpenes (camphene and caryophyllene), and tannins. Thymol is a natural phenol found in the oil of thyme. It is rich in minerals (iron, copper, potassium, and manganese) and vitamins (C and A). It has antiinflammatory (effect on inflammatory cytokines), diuretic, antioxidant, antimicrobial, antifungal, insecticidal, anticancer, antispasmodic, and immune-boosting effects. It is also carminative. It is used for cough, sore throat, and bronchitis. It can eliminate airborne bacteria and molds. It supports digestive health. It decreases intestinal cramps, gas and bloating. It can help increase appetite and produces more protective gastric mucus. It can lower blood pressure and cholesterol and can maintain blood flow. It also promotes regular urination. It can be mood uplifting. It can also be used to repel insects including mosquitoes. It can help with wound healing and acne. Overall, it is safe. Side effects include digestive upset, dizziness, and headache. Fanous, S. (2018, September 17). 9 health benefits of thyme. *Healthline*. https://www.healthline.com/health/health-benefits-of-thyme
Tiger Nuts Cyperus esculentus	Other names: Yellow nutsedge, Zulu nuts, Chufa, Earth almonds It is related to the nutgrass family. These are small edible tubers and not nuts. They are brown, black or yellow and are nutrient-dense. It is rich in resistant starch, insoluble fiber, monounsaturated fats, minerals (chromium, iron, zinc, copper, magnesium, manganese and sodium), vitamins (E and C), and amino acids (especially arginine). It is regarded as a superfood. It can be sprouted or roasted or dried. It can lower blood glucose and lipids. It helps in diabetes and improves circulation. They are rich in insoluble fiber, resistant starch and enzymes and help in constipation, indigestion, gas and bloating. It contains anti-nutrients (eg phytates and oxalates) which can inhibit absorption of essential minerals Petre, M. A. S. (2022, January 6). 6 Emerging Health Benefits of Tiger Nuts. Healthline. https://www.healthline.com/nutrition/tiger-nuts
Valerian *Valeriana officinalis*	Other names: *Indian valerian (Tagar, Tagara, Valeriana jatamansi, Sugandhbala)* There are many species of valerian. *V. officinalis* is usually used for medicinal purposes. Valerian contains several bioactive compounds including flavonoids (such as hesperidin and linarin), terpenoids (Volvalerine A and valerenic acid), and isovaleric acid. It stimulates the GABA receptors, raises the GABA level, and regulates serotonin. It has sedative, muscle-relaxant, antispasmodic, and mild antidepressant properties. It is used in the treatment of acute stress, anxiety, insomnia, migraine, ADHD, and obsessive-compulsive disorder. The sleep onset is faster and there is better quality deep sleep. It is not habit-forming and there are no hangover effects. It can also be used for PMS and menopausal symptoms. It is usually combined with lemon balm.

Ingredients	Mechanism of Action and Health Benefits
	Overall, it is safe. Side effects include dizziness, restlessness, itching, and stomach upset. It should not be taken with tranquilizers, pain, or diarrhea medications.

Spritzler, F. (2017, April 16). How valerian root helps you relax and sleep better. *Healthline*. https://www.healthline.com/nutrition/valerian-root#TOC_TITLE_HDR_3

Wexler, A. (2017, June 25). Does valerian root treat anxiety and insomnia? *MedicalNewsToday*. https://www.medicalnewstoday.com/articles/318088

Verbena
Verbena officinalis

Other names: *Common Vervain, Blue Vervain, European Vervain, Common Verbena, Herb of Grace, Pigeonweed.*

There are many species of Verbena which are trailing or vertical plants. Lemon verbena (*Aloysia citriodora/ Lippia citriodora*) is one of the species.

The leaves and flower tops contain various bioactive phenolic compounds (verbascoside) and terpenoids which have antioxidant (limonene, luteolin, geranial and neral) and anti-inflammatory actions. It has antipyretic, antispasmodic, diuretic and astringent effects. It increases GABA neurotransmitter levels in the brain.

It is consumed as a tea. The essential oil is also used in fragrances, foods (beverages, alcohol and herbal teas) and also in aromatherapy.

It acts as a nasal decongestant in rhinosinusitis and colds, sore throat and asthma.

It is used as a mouth wash or gargle in mild gingivitis (gum inflammation) and sore throat. It helps in digestive problems such as constipation, diarrhoea, intestinal colic, gas and indigestion.

It can promote sleep and helps in insomnia, anxiety, depression and seizures.

It helps with wound healing, burns, itchy skin conditions.

It promotes lactation in breast feeding mothers. It is a uterus stimulant and helps in irregular and painful menstruation and perimenopausal symptoms.

Overall, it is safe. Rarely, skin rash occurs. Caution should be exercised in hypertension and kidney disorders. It should not be used in pregnancy.

WebMD. (2020b). Verbena - Uses, Side Effects, and More. https://www.webmd.com/vitamins/ai/ingredientmono-88/verbena

RxList. (2021, November 6). Lemon Verbena. RxList. https://www.rxlist.com/body_vitamin_e_benefits_for_your/article.htm

Watermelon
Citrullus lanatus

Watermelon is low in calories and rich in vitamins A and C. It also has a high water content. It also contains several minerals (such as potassium and magnesium) along with trace contents of vitamins B1, B5, and B6. It also contains plant compounds such as carotenoids (including lycopene, α-carotene, and β-carotene), terpenoids (cucurbitacin E), and citrulline, an amino acid.

It has antioxidant, antiinflammatory, and anticancer properties.

The high water content in watermelon helps in weight loss by making one feel full.

It helps reduce the risk of heart disease or stroke by lowering blood pressure and cholesterol levels. Lycopene can reduce thickness and stiffness of artery walls. It can also help maintain eye health and reduce the risk of age-related macular degeneration.

It can also improve brain health and delay progression of AD and other chronic disorders.

The rich vitamins A and C content may help in skin protection and hair growth.

Citrulline can increase nitric oxide production which helps with vasodilatation. This can improve exercise performance, endurance, and may reduce muscle soreness.

Overall, it is safe. Overconsumption may cause digestive disorders (including gas and bloating, diarrhea, and flatulence), diabetes, overhydration, and cardiovascular problems (like weak pulse rate and irregular heartbeat).

Jennings, K. (2018, August 9). Top 9 health benefits of eating watermelon. *Healthline*. https://www.healthline.com/nutrition/watermelon-health-benefits

Rana, S. (2018, April 26). 5 side effects of eating too much watermelon. *NDTV Food*. https://food.ndtv.com/health/5-side-effects-of-eating-too-much-watermelon-1843398

Ingredients	Mechanism of Action and Health Benefits
Wheatgrass *Triticum aestivum*	Wheatgrass is considered a superfood. The active ingredients are mugineic acid, phenolic acids, tannin, and saponins. It contains several minerals (including calcium, iron, and magnesium) and vitamins (A, C, E, K, and B).

It has antioxidant, antiinflammatory, antimicrobial, and neuroprotective properties. It also has detoxifying effects.

The high content of enzymes in wheatgrass helps in digestion and relieves IBS, constipation, gas and bloating, and stomach discomfort.

It promotes heart health and reduces LDL cholesterol, blood sugar, and blood pressure.

It also improves immune function. It may possibly reduce infections and disease risk.

It can improve cognitive and mental functions. It also helps relieve anxiety, prevent memory loss, treat AD, and improve hand-eye coordination.

It helps in weight loss by reducing cravings. It can also improve bone function and arthritis symptoms such as pain, swelling, and stiffness.

It may reduce the risk of certain cancers (such as oral, colon, and leukemia).

Overall, it is safe. Side effects include rashes, nausea, constipation, headache, fever, and stomach upset. It should be avoided by people with celiac disease and gluten sensitivity.

Cronkleton, E. (2017, October 12). Wheatgrass benefits: 11 reasons to enjoy. *Healthline*. https://www.healthline.com/health/food-nutrition/wheatgrass-benefits

Villines, Z. (2019, October 17). What are the benefits of wheatgrass? *MedicalNewsToday*. https://www.medicalnewstoday.com/articles/320210

Whey

Whey is a protein in milk that is separated during cheese production. It contains essential amino acids, high proteins, and low lactose content.

It has antiinflammatory, antioxidant, and anticancer effects.

It can also help in weight loss.

It contains leucine, an amino acid that can prevent age-related muscle loss and improve muscle strength.

It can reduce blood pressure and blood sugar levels. It can also reduce blood cholesterol.

It may improve irritable bowel disease symptoms. It can also be used in the treatment of asthma.

Overconsumption can cause digestive problems including bloating, nausea, cramping, diarrhea, and flatulence. High doses of whey can cause acne. It should also be avoided by those with lactose intolerance.

Arnarson, A., (2017, June 12). 10 evidence-based health benefits of whey protein. *Healthline*. https://www.healthline.com/nutrition/10-health-benefits-of-whey-protein#TOC_TITLE_HDR_1

Nordqvist, J. (2017, November 27). What are the benefits and risks of whey protein? *MedicalNewsToday*. https://www.medicalnewstoday.com/articles/263371#dangers

White oak bark
Quercus alba

Other name: *Oak bark*

The bark, leaves, and acorns of oak trees contain tannin which is toxic.

However, the very young leaf shoots and roasted or boiled acorns are edible.

The inner white oak bark is dried and ground for topical or oral use. The tannins in the bark have astringent, antiinflammatory, and antibacterial properties.

Topically, it can be used to treat piles and bleeding or swollen gums. It can also calm and soothe itchy skin rash.

As a tea, it can treat indigestion and diarrhea. It is an appetite stimulant.

It can also help with sore throat, cough, and colds.

Oral use should be limited for 3 days and topical use for 2 to 3 weeks. Side effects include gastric upsets, liver and kidney toxicity. It should not be taken with iron supplements.

White lupin
Lupinus albinus

Other names: *Field lupine, White lupine, Termis seeds, Lupini beans or Lupin beans*

Lupin is a legume or pulse crop which is cultivated. The lupin beans are a rich source of protein (especially arginine), minerals (copper, manganese, iron), and vitamins (vitamin C, folate). It is rich in phenolic antioxidants.

It is used to prevent and treat digestive problems such as constipation, IBS, and helps in weight loss. It has prebiotics from the high fiber content.

It can lower blood pressure.

It supports skin and hair health and strengthens bones. It also helps in wound healing.

Lupin seeds can be cooked as a savory dish or eaten as a snack. The lupin flour is made from ground lupin seeds. Lupin oil is derived from the seeds. The roasted seeds are used as a caffeine-free coffee substitute.

S. (2017, September 20). Lupin bean facts and health benefits. *HealthBenefitstimes.com*. https://www.healthbenefitstimes.com/lupin/

Ingredients	Mechanism of Action and Health Benefits
Willow Bark *Salix* spp.	Other name: *White willow (Salix alba), Black willow (Salix nigra)* Willow bark is obtained from the willow tree. There are different varieties of willow trees including white willow *(Salix alba)*, black willow *(Salix nigra)*, and many others. Willow bark contains salicin (a β-glucoside) as the main bioactive compound. Others include flavonoids (flavanols and procyanidins), phenolic glycosides, and shikimic acid. It has analgesic, antipyretic, antiinflammatory, and exfoliating effects. It is used to relieve pain in various arthritis including osteoarthritis, rheumatoid arthritis, and gout. It is used for joint and muscle pain. It can be used in fevers. It can also be used for headaches and period cramps. Side effects include gastric upset and rare risk of Reye syndrome if used in young children. Goldman, R. (2017, February 14). Willow Bark: Nature's Aspirin. *Healthline.* https://www.healthline.com/health/willow-bark-natures-aspirin Piątczak, E., Dybowska, M., Płuciennik, E., Kośla, K., Kolniak-Ostek, J., & Kalinowska-Lis, U. (2020). Identification and accumulation of phenolic compounds in the leaves and bark of *Salix alba* (L.) and their biological potential. *Biomolecules, 10*(10), 1391–1408. https://doi.org/10.3390/biom10101391 Tyśkiewicz, K., Konkol, M., Kowalski, R., Rój, E., Warmiński, K., Krzyňaniak, M., et al. (2019). Characterization of bioactive compounds in the biomass of black locust, poplar and willow. *Trees, 33*(5), 1235–1263. https://doi.org/10.1007/s00468-019-01837-2 WebMD Editors. (n.d.). Willow Bark. *WebMD.* https://www.webmd.com/vitamins/ai/ingredient-mono-955/willow-bark
Witch hazel *Hamamelis virginiana*	Other name: *Common witch hazel* Witch hazel contains resin, flavonoids (including procyanidins), phenolic acids (gallic acid), and tannins. It has antiinflammatory, hemostatic, astringent, and antiviral properties. It can treat hemorrhoids and also reduces the itching, irritation, and bleeding. It is used in eczema, acne, psoriasis, seborrheic dermatitis, and dandruff. Accidental overconsumption may cause stomach irritation. Link, R. (2018, July 16). 8 benefits and uses of witch hazel. *Healthline.* https://www.healthline.com/nutrition/witch-hazel-benefits-uses#TOC_TITLE_HDR_2
Wooly lamb's ear *Stachys byzantina*	Other names: *Lamb's ear, Donkey's ears, Jesus Flannel, Lamb's wool, Big ears, Silver carpet.* Lamb's ear grows as a wild groundcover plant. The phytoactive compounds include tannins and alkaloids (stachydrene, betonicine, and trigonelline) It has antiseptic, anti-inflammatory, anti-bacterial and hemostatic properties. It improves coagulation in bleeding wounds. The crushed leaves can be applied on wounds as a poultice or bandage. The dried leaves can be used to make tea and consumed during coughs, sore throat and also for internal bleeding. The Complete Medicinal Herbal: A Practical Guide to the Healing Properties of Herbs by Penelope Ody Medicinal Herb Info. (1993). Lamb's Ear. http://medicinalherbinfo.org/000Herbs2016/1herbs/lambs-ear/
Yarrow leaf *Achillea millefolium*	Yarrow contains flavonoids (such as hyperoside, luteolin, myricetin, and kaempferol), alkaloids, tannins, phenols, and steroids. It is also rich in potassium. It has antiinflammatory, antioxidant, and neuroprotective properties. It can relieve cough, cold, and sore throat. It can treat digestive problems including IBS, gas and bloating, and stomach ulcers. It can promote wound healing and treat eczema. It can also help in menorrhagia. It may support brain health in PD, AD, and multiple sclerosis. It may also be used to treat anxiety and depression. Overall, it is safe. It may cause an allergic reaction. It should not be used in bleeding disorders. It can interact with sedatives. Georgieva, L., Gadjalova, A., Mihaylova, D., & Pavlov, A. (2015). *Achillea millefolium* L.—Phytochemical profile and in vitro antioxidant activity. *International Food Research Journal, 22*(4), 1347–1352. https://www.researchgate.net/publication/282889888_Achillea_millefolium_L_-_Phytochemical_profile_and_in_vitro_antioxidant_activity WebMD Editors. (n.d.). Yarrow. *WebMD.* https://www.webmd.com/vitamins/ai/ingredientmono-151/yarrow

Ingredients	Mechanism of Action and Health Benefits
Yerba mate *Ilex paraguariensis*	Yerba mate is an herbal tea. The yerba mate plant is native to South America and contains polyphenols and xanthines (including caffeine stimulants). It is made by drying leaves and twigs of the *Ilex paraguariensis* (yerba mate) plant over fire and steeping it in hot water. Traditionally, Yerba mate is consumed from a container called a gourd and shared with others as a sign of friendship and bonding. It is an earthy, herbaceous, bittersweet, healthy, and stimulating drink. It contains 35 mg of caffeine per 8 oz. serving and also vitamin C, magnesium, manganese, and potassium. It has been found to suppress hunger pangs, which aids with weight loss. Overall, it is safe. Overconsumption may increase the risk of oral, throat, and lung cancer. Mayo Clinic Staff. (2021, March 6). *Yerba mate: Is it safe to drink?* Mayo Clinic. https://www.mayo-clinic.org/healthy-lifestyle/nutrition-and-healthy-eating/expert-answers/yerba-mate/faq-20058343?reDate=05082021 Petre, A. (2018, December 17). 8 health benefits of yerba mate (backed by science). *Healthline.* https://www.healthline.com/nutrition/8-benefits-of-yerba-mate
Yogurt	Other names: *Curd, Thayir, Dahi* Yogurt contains several important minerals (calcium, phosphorus, magnesium, and potassium) and vitamins (B12 and riboflavin). It is also rich in proteins which helps in weight loss and appetite control. It has antiinflammatory properties. The probiotics present in yogurt promote digestive health and lessen the symptoms of IBS such as constipation, bloating, and diarrhea. It can strengthen bones and teeth and prevent osteoporosis. It can also help in reducing painful menstrual cramps. It can also improve the immune system and reduce the risk of illnesses. It can be used as a beauty aid in improving hair growth and skin. It promotes heart health and reduces high blood pressure, blood sugar, and LDL cholesterol. Yogurt should be avoided by people with lactose intolerance. Most yogurts contain high amounts of added sugar which from overconsumption can cause obesity and diabetes. Elliott, B. (2017, January 20). 7 impressive health benefits of yogurt. *Healthline.* https://www.healthline.com/nutrition/7-benefits-of-yogurt Ware, M. (2018, January 11). Everything you need to know about yogurt. *MedicalNewsToday.* https://www.medicalnewstoday.com/articles/295714#nutrition
Yohimbine *Pausinystalia yohimbe*	Other names: *Yohimbe, Corynanthe Yohimbe, Corynanthe* Yohimbine is a compound isolated from the bark of the tree, *Pausinystalia yohimbe,* which grows in Africa. It is an alpha-2 adrenergic receptor blocker. It also can break down fats and can help with weight loss. It can also treat erectile dysfunction and male impotency. It can improve mood and increase athletic performance. Side effects include sympathetic stimulation causing tachycardia, hypertension, and anxiety. It can interact with blood pressure medications. WebMD. (n.d.-e). YOHIMBE: Overview, uses, side effects, precautions, interactions, dosing and reviews. https://www.webmd.com/vitamins/ai/ingredientmono-759/yohimbe

Index

Page number followed by "*b*" indicates boxes, and "*t*" indicates tables.